Taylor's Clinical Nursing Skills

A Nursing Process Approach

Fifth Edition

Pamela Lynn, EdD, MSN, RN
Assistant Professor
Gwynedd Mercy University
Frances M. Maguire School of Nursing and Health Professions
Gwynedd Valley, Pennsylvania

 Wolters Kluwer

Philadelphia • Baltimore • New York • London
Buenos Aires • Hong Kong • Sydney • Tokyo

Vice President and Publisher: Julie K. Stegman
Digital Product Manager: Betsy Gentzler
Director of Product Development: Jennifer K. Forestieri
Senior Development Editor: Michael Kerns
Editorial Coordinators: Emily Buccieri and Lindsay Ries
Marketing Manager: Brittany Clements
Editorial Assistant: Leo Gray
Design Coordinator: Holly Reid McLaughlin
Art Director, Illustration: Jennifer Clements
Production Project Manager: Bridgett Dougherty
Manufacturing Coordinator: Karin Duffield
Prepress Vendor: Aptara, Inc.

5th Edition

Library of Congress Cataloging-in-Publication Data

Names: Lynn, Pamela (Pamela Barbara), 1961- , author.
Title: Taylor's clinical nursing skills : a nursing process approach / Pamela
   Lynn.
Other titles: Clinical nursing skills
Description: Fifth edition. | Philadelphia, PA : Wolters Kluwer Health,
   [2019] | Includes bibliographical references and index.
Identifiers: LCCN 2018027966 | ISBN 9781496384881
Subjects: | MESH: Nursing Process | Nursing Care–methods
Classification: LCC RT51 | NLM WY 100.1 | DDC 610.73–dc23 LC record available at https://lccn.loc.gov/
2018027966 https://lccn.loc.gov/2018027966

CCS0818

In remembrance of Carol Lillis and Priscilla Koeplin who offered unlimited and genuine support, encouragement, and guidance from the beginning of this adventure. I could not have asked for better mentors or friends.

Contributor to This Edition

Patricia Brown-O'Hara, PhD, RN
Assistant Professor
Gwynedd Mercy University
Frances M. Maguire School of Nursing and Health Professions
Gwynedd Valley, Pennsylvania
Chapter 9: Activity

For a list of the contributors to the Student and
Instructor Resources accompanying this book,
please visit thePoint®.

Reviewers

Elizabeth Hammond-Ritschard, MSN
Associate Clinical Professor
Drexel University
Philadelphia, Pennsylvania

Susan M. Randol, MSN, RN, CNE
Master Instructor/Semester Coordinator
University of Louisiana
Lafayette, Louisiana

Faith Richardson, DNP, MSN (FNP), MA, BSc, BA
Assistant Professor of Nursing
Trinity Western University
Langley, British Columbia

Judy Sabel, MSN
Nursing Instructor
Waukesha County Technical College
Pewaukee, Wisconsin

Sally Saites, MSN/Ed, RN
Lecturer
California State University San Marcos
San Marcos, California

Alnisa Shabazz, MS, RN
Assistant Professor
Bronx Community College
Bronx, New York

Nicole Smith, MS, BSN
Instructor, Clinical Simulation Laboratory Coordinator
University of Maryland School of Nursing
Rockville, Maryland

Diane Spoljoric, PhD, RNC, FNP
Associate Professor of Nursing
Purdue University Northwest
Westville, Indiana

Ruth Swart, EdD, MHS, BSc, BN, RN
Instructor
University of Calgary
Calgary, Alberta

Lori Theodore, EdD, MSN
Professor of Nursing
Seminole State College of Florida
Altamonte Springs, Florida

Alice Tobin, MSN, BSN, AAS/RN
Professor of Nursing
Suffolk County Community College
Brentwood, New York

Susan Tucker, DNP, MSN, RN, CNE
Program Director
Gadsden State Community College
Gadsden, Alabama

Kimberly Valich, MSN
Professor of Nursing
University of St. Francis
Lowell, Indiana

Amy Wall, MSN, BSN
Instructor
Wharton County Junior College
Sugar Land, Texas

Sherylyn Watson, PhD, MSN, RN, CNE
Assistant Dean
Sacred Heart University
Fairfield, Connecticut

Anne Wilkinson, MSN, RN
Instructor, Divisional Program Chair
Gateway Technical College
Kenosha, Wisconsin

Liza Willis, MSN
Associate Professor
St. Charles Community College
Cottleville, Missouri

Kelly Winters, MSN
Director Workforce Development
College of Southern Maryland
La Plata, Maryland

Jean Yockey, PhD
Assistant Professor
University of South Dakota
Vermillion, South Dakota

For a list of the reviewers of the Test Generator accompanying this book, please visit thePoint®.

Taylor's Clinical Nursing Skills: A Nursing Process Approach aims to help nursing students or graduate nurses incorporate cognitive, technical, interpersonal, and ethical/legal skills into safe and effective person-centered care. This book is written to meet the needs of novice to advanced nurses. Many of the skills shown in this book may not be encountered by the student while in school, but may be encountered once the graduate nurse has entered the workforce.

Because it emphasizes the basic principles of patient care, we believe this book can easily be used with any Fundamentals text. However, this Skills book was specifically designed to accompany *Fundamentals of Nursing: The Art and Science of Person-Centered Nursing Care,* Ninth Edition, by Taylor, Lynn, and Bartlett, to provide a seamless learning experience. Some of the Skills and Guidelines for Nursing Care from the Taylor *Fundamentals* book may also be found in this book, but its content has been embellished here to:

- Highlight the nursing process
- Emphasize unexpected situations that the nurse may encounter, along with related interventions for how to respond to these unexpected situations
- Draw attention to critical actions within skills
- Illustrate specific actions within a skill through the use of nearly 1,000 four-color photographs and illustrations
- Highlight available best practice guidelines and/or research-based evidence to support the skills
- Reference appropriate case study or studies included at the end of the book, emphasizing which case studies utilize and enhance the content of each chapter.

In addition, this book contains numerous higher-level skills that are not addressed in the Taylor *Fundamentals* book.

Learning Experience

This text and the entire Taylor Suite have been created with the student's experience in mind. Care has been taken to appeal to all learning styles. The student-friendly writing style ensures that students will comprehend and retain information. The extensive art program enhances understanding of important actions. Free video clips 🎬 clearly demonstrate and reinforce important skill steps; as students watch and listen to the videos, comprehension increases. In addition, each element of the Taylor Suite, which is described later in the preface, coordinates to provide a consistent and cohesive learning experience.

Organization

Taylor's Clinical Nursing Skills is organized into three units. Ideally, the text will be followed sequentially, but every effort has been made to respect the differing needs of diverse curricula and students. Thus, each chapter stands on its own merit and may be read independently of others.

Unit I: Actions Basic to Nursing Care

This unit introduces the foundational skills used by nurses: maintaining asepsis, measuring vital signs, assessing health, promoting safety, administering medication, and caring for surgical patients.

In Chapter 3, Health Assessment, revised physical assessment content reflects the practice needs of beginning and general nurses. Assessment procedures performed by advanced practice professionals are clearly identified. Assessments identified as advanced procedures and skills are available on thePoint°.

Unit II: Promoting Healthy Physiologic Responses

This unit focuses on the physiologic needs of patients: hygiene; skin integrity and wound care; activity; comfort and pain management; nutrition; urinary elimination; bowel elimination; oxygenation; fluid, electrolyte, and acid–base balance; neurologic care; cardiovascular care; and specimen collection.

Unit III: Integrated Case Studies

Although nursing skills textbooks generally present content in a linear fashion for ease of understanding, in reality, many nursing skills are performed in combination for patients with complicated health needs. The integrated case studies in this unit are designed to challenge the reader to think critically and outside the norm, consider the multiple needs of patients, and prioritize care appropriately—ultimately preparing the student and graduate nurse for complex situations that may arise in everyday practice.

Teaching/Learning Package

To facilitate mastery of this text's content, a comprehensive teaching/learning package has been developed to assist faculty and students.

Resources for Instructors

Tools to assist you with teaching your course are available upon adoption of this text on thePoint at http://thepoint.lww.com/Lynn5e.

- The **Test Generator** has over 500 NCLEX®-Style questions to help you put together exclusive new tests from a bank with questions spanning the book's topics, which will assist you in assessing your students' understanding of the material.
- **PowerPoint Presentations,** provided for each book chapter, enhance teaching by providing key visuals and reinforcing content. These provide an easy way for you to integrate the textbook with your students' learning experience, either via slide shows or handouts.
- **Skills Lab Teaching Plans** walk you through each chapter, objective by objective, and provide a lecture outline and teaching guidelines. In addition to one teaching plan for each chapter, there is one bonus teaching plan to assist with lab simulations.
- A **Master Checklist for Skills Competency** is provided to help you track your students' progress on all the skills in this book.
- A **QSEN Competency Map** shows where in the text to find the Knowledge, Skills, and Attitudes (KSAs) that students will need to develop so they can ensure quality and safety in patient care.
- A sample **Syllabus** is provided to help you organize your course.
- **Strategies for Effective Teaching** to help you prepare your course materials and effectively meet your students' needs.
- **Journal Articles** offer access to current research available in Wolters Kluwer journals.
- **WebCT/Blackboard-Ready Materials** can be accessed on thePoint, plus access to all Student Resources, including Watch & Learn video clips, Practice & Learn activities, and Concepts in Action Animations.
- The **Image Bank** provides free access to illustrations and photos from the textbook for use in PowerPoint presentations and handouts.

Resources for Students

Valuable learning tools for students are available on thePoint at http://thepoint.lww.com/Lynn4e, including:

- **NCLEX®-Style Review Questions** correspond with each book chapter for review of important concepts and to help practice for the NCLEX examination. Nearly 400 questions are included.
- **Watch & Learn** video clips 📹, **Practice & Learn** activities 🔬, and **Concepts in Action Animations** demonstrate important concepts related to skills.
- **Journal Articles** offer access to current research available in Wolters Kluwer journals.

- A **Spanish–English Audio Glossary** provides helpful terms and phrases for communicating with patients who speak Spanish.
- **Dosage Calculation Quizzes** provide opportunities for students to practice math skills and calculate drug dosages.

Taylor Suite Resources

From traditional texts to video and interactive products, the Taylor Fundamentals/Skills suite is tailored to fit every learning style. This integrated suite of products offers students a seamless learning experience not found elsewhere. To learn more about any solution with the Taylor suite, please contact your local Wolters Kluwer representative.

- *Fundamentals of Nursing: The Art and Science of Person-Centered Nursing Care*, **9th Edition,** by Carol Taylor, Pamela Lynn, and Jennifer Bartlett. This Fundamentals text promotes nursing as an evolving art and science, directed to human health and well-being. It challenges students to cultivate the Quality and Safety Education for Nurses (QSEN) and blended competencies they will need to serve patients and the public well. The aim is to prepare nurses who combine the highest level of scientific knowledge and technologic skill with responsible, caring practice. The text challenges students to identify and master the cognitive and technical skills as well as the interpersonal and ethical/legal skills they will need to effectively nurse the patients in their care. The text includes engaging features to promote critical thinking and clinical decision-making and comprehension.
- *Taylor's Video Guide to Clinical Nursing Skills,* **4th Edition.** With more than 12 hours of video footage and over 170 video clips, this updated series follows nursing students and their instructors as they perform a range of essential nursing procedures. Institutions and students can purchase them for convenient streaming access.
- *Skill Checklists for Taylor's Clinical Nursing Skills,* **5th Edition.** This collection of checklists with convenient perforated pages is designed to accompany the Skills textbook and promote proper technique while increasing students' confidence.

Lippincott
CoursePoint+

A Comprehensive, Digital, Integrated Course Solution

Lippincott CoursePoint+ for Taylor's Clinical Nursing Skills offers an integrated learning solution for nursing skills, including a complete, enhanced skills eBook and integrated video series illustrating the most important skills. Practice & Learn Interactive Case Studies and Skill Checklists give students opportunities for application, practice, and competency demonstration.

Lippincott CoursePoint+ is designed for the way students learn, providing content in context, exactly where and when students need it. Features include:

- **Leading content in context:** Digital content is embedded in our powerful tools, engaging students and encouraging interaction and learning on a deeper level.

  - The complete interactive eBook, *Taylor's Clinical Nursing Skills: A Nursing Process Approach,* **5th Edition,** aims to help nursing students and graduate nurses incorporate cognitive, technical, interpersonal, and ethical/legal skills into safe and effective patient care. With nearly 1,000 photographs, it provides students a step-by-step photo atlas of each skill, all within the context of the full nursing process.

  - The eBook features annual content updates based on the latest evidence-based practices and provides students with anytime, anywhere access on multiple devices.

  - Multimedia resources, including animations and interactive case studies, walk students through knowledge application and address multiple learning styles.

  - Full online access to *Stedman's Medical Dictionary for the Health Professions and Nursing* ensures students work with the best medical dictionary available.

- **Powerful tools to maximize performance:** Course-specific tools provide experiential learning for every student:

  - *Taylor's Video Guide to Clinical Nursing Skills,* **4th Edition,** follows nursing students and their instructors as they perform a range of essential nursing procedures. Step-by-step skill demonstration to match the skills textbook is accompanied by model communication skills. By watching the videos and completing related activities, students will enhance their understanding and prepare for skills lab, clinicals, and nursing practice.

  - *vSim for Nursing | Fundamentals, a new virtual simulation platform* (*available via* thePoint®). Codeveloped by Laerdal Medical and Wolters Kluwer, *vSim for Nursing | Fundamentals* helps students develop clinical competence and decision-making skills as they interact with virtual patients in a safe, realistic environment. *vSim for Nursing* records and assesses student decisions throughout the simulation, then provides a personalized feedback log highlighting areas needing improvement.

Pamela Lynn, EdD, MSN, RN

FOCUS ON PATIENT CARE!

Each chapter in Units I and II begins with a description of three real-world case scenarios that put the skills into context. These scenarios provide a framework for the chapter content to be covered.

GET READY TO LEARN!

Before reading the chapter content, read the **Learning Objectives**. These roadmaps help you understand what is important and why. Create your own learning outline or use them for self-testing.

Review the **Key Terms** lists to become familiar with new vocabulary presented throughout the narrative. Look for them in bold type throughout the chapter.

2

Vital Signs

Focusing on Patient Care

This chapter will explain some of the skills related to vital signs necessary to care for the following patients:

Tyrone Jeffries, age 5, is in the emergency department with a temperature of 101.3°F (38.9°C).

Toby White, age 26, has a history of asthma and is now breathing 32 times per minute.

Carl Glatz, age 58, has recently started taking medications to control his hypertension (high blood pressure).

Refer to Focusing on Patient Care: Developing Clinical Reasoning at the end of the chapter to apply what you learn.

Learning Objectives

After completing the chapter, you will be able to accomplish the following:

1. Assess body temperature via the oral, tympanic, temporal, axillary, and rectal routes.
2. Regulate an infant's temperature using an overhead radiant warmer.
3. Regulate temperature using a hypothermia blanket.
4. Assess peripheral pulses by palpation.
5. Assess an apical pulse by auscultation.
6. Assess peripheral pulses using Doppler ultrasound.
7. Assess respiration.
8. Assess blood pressure by auscultation or using an automatic electronic blood pressure monitor.
9. Assess systolic blood pressure using Doppler ultrasound.

Key Terms

apnea: absence of breathing
bell: (of stethoscope) hollowed, upright, curved portion used to auscultate low-pitched sounds, such as murmurs
blood pressure: force of blood against arterial walls
bradypnea: abnormally slow rate of breathing
diaphragm: (of stethoscope) large, flat disk on the stethoscope used to auscultate high-pitched sounds, such as respiratory sounds
diastolic pressure: least amount of pressure exerted on arterial walls, which occurs when the heart is at rest between ventricular contractions

38

DEVELOP CRITICAL THINKING AND CLINICAL REASONING!

Fundamentals Review. Because of the breadth and depth of nursing knowledge that must be absorbed, nursing students and graduate nurses can easily become overwhelmed. Thus, this book is designed to eliminate excessive content and redundancy and to better focus the reader's attention. To this end, each chapter in Units I and II includes several boxes, tables, or figures that summarize important concepts that should be understood before performing a skill. For a more in-depth study of these concepts, readers are encouraged to refer to their Fundamentals textbook.

Fundamentals Review 2-1

AGE-RELATED VARIATIONS IN NORMAL VITAL SIGNS

Age	Temperature °C °F	Pulse beats/min	Respirations breaths/min	Blood Pressure mm Hg
Infants (temporal)	37.1–38.1 98.7–100.5	80–150	25–55	85/37
Toddler (temporal)	37.1–38.1 98.7–100.5	70–120	20–40	89/46
Child (tympanic)	36.8–37.8 98.2–100	60–100	15–25	95/57
Adolescent (oral)	35.8–37.5 96.4–99.5	55–95	12–18	102/61
Adult (oral)	35.8–37.5 96.4–99.5	60–100	12–20	120/80

Source: Adapted from Hogan-Quigley, B., Palm, M. L., & Bickley, L. S. (2017). *Bates' nursing guide to physical examination and history taking* (2nd ed.). Philadelphia, PA: Wolters Kluwer; Kyle, T., & Carman, S. (2017). *Essentials of pediatric nursing* (3rd ed.). Philadelphia, PA: Wolters Kluwer.

Enhance Your Understanding, located at the end of each chapter, gives readers an opportunity to further their understanding and apply what they have learned. It includes three sections:

Focusing on Patient Care: Developing Clinical Reasoning asks readers to consider questions that reflect back to the opening scenarios for added cohesion throughout the chapters. Readers are challenged to apply the skills and use the new knowledge they have gained to "think through" learning exercises designed to show how critical thinking and clinical reasoning can result in a clinical judgment, leading to a possible change in outcomes and an impact on patient care.

Suggested Answers for Focusing on Patient Care: Developing Clinical Reasoning represent possible nursing care solutions to the problems. The answers can be found after the bibliography section at the end of the chapter.

Integrated Case Study Connection refers readers to the appropriate case study or studies discussion in Unit III, emphasizing which case studies utilize and enhance the content of that chapter.

Enhance Your Understanding

Focusing on Patient Care: Developing Clinical Reasoning

Consider the case scenarios at the beginning of the chapter as you answer the following questions to enhance your understanding and apply what you have learned.

QUESTIONS

1. Tyrone Jeffries, the 5 year old with a fever of 101.3°F (38.5°C), is suspected of having a middle-ear infection. You need to obtain another set of vital signs for him. As you approach with the electronic thermometer, Tyrone begins to scream, saying, "Go away. I don't want it!" How would you respond?

2. Toby White, who is 26 years old with a history of asthma, has a respiratory rate of 32 breaths per minute. What other assessments would be most important to make?

3. Carl Glatz, the 58-year-old man receiving medications for hypertension, asks you about how he should monitor his blood pressure at home. What information would you suggest?

You can find suggested answers after the Bibliography at the end of this chapter.

Integrated Case Study Connection

The case studies in the back of the book focus on integrating concepts. Refer to the following case studies to enhance your understanding of the concepts and skills in this chapter.

- Basic Case Studies: Abigail Cantonelli, page 1099; James White, page 1102; Naomi Bell, page 1103; Joe LeRoy, page 1108.
- Intermediate Case Studies: Olivia Greenbaum, page 1113; Victoria Holly, page 1115; Lucille Howard, page 1123; Janice Romero, page 1124; Gwen Galloway, page 1125.
- Advanced Case Studies: Cole McKean, page 1128.

Taylor Suite Resources

Explore these additional resources to enhance learning for this chapter:

- NCLEX-Style Questions and other resources on thePoint®, http://thePoint.lww.com/Lynn5e
- Skill Checklists for *Taylor's Clinical Nursing Skills*, 5e
- *Taylor's Video Guide to Clinical Nursing Skills:* Vital Signs
- *Fundamentals of Nursing:* Chapter 25, Vital Signs
- *Lippincott DocuCare* Fundamentals cases

Delegation Considerations assist students and graduate nurses in developing the critical decision-making skills necessary to transfer responsibility for the performance of an activity to another person and to ensure safe and effective nursing care. Delegation decision-making information is provided in each skill and Appendix A, using delegation guidelines based on American Nurses Association (ANA) and National Council of State Boards of Nursing (NCSBN) principles and recommendations.

DELEGATION CONSIDERATIONS	Measurement of body temperature may be delegated to nursing assistive personnel (NAP) or to unlicensed assistive personnel (UAP), as well as to licensed practical/vocational nurses (LPN/LVNs). The decision to delegate must be based on careful analysis of the patient's needs and circumstances, as well as the qualifications of the person to whom the task is being delegated. Refer to the Delegation Guidelines in Appendix A.

Skill 2-1 ▶ Assessing Body Temperature *(continued)*

Infant and Child Considerations

- Pull the pinna back and down when measuring tympanic temperature on a child younger than 3 years of age. For children older than 3 years of age, there is no need to manipulate the pinna (Kyle & Carman, 2017).
- Small children have a limited attention span and difficulty keeping their lips closed long enough to obtain an accurate oral temperature reading. Based on an assessment of the child's ability to cooperate, it may be more appropriate to use the temporal or tympanic site.
- Chemical dot thermometers (liquid crystal skin contact thermometers) are sometimes used as alternatives in pediatric settings. These single-use, disposable, flexible thermometers have specific chemical mixtures in circles on the thermometer that change color to measure temperature increments of two tenths of a degree. Place the thermometer in the mouth with the dot side (sensor) down, into the posterior sublingual pocket. Keep this type of thermometer in the mouth for 1 minute, in the axilla 3 minutes, and in the rectum 3 minutes. Read the color change 10 to 15 seconds after removing the thermometer. Read away from any heat source. Wearable, continuous-use chemical dot thermometers are available. These are placed under the axilla and must remain in place at least 2 to 3 minutes before taking the first reading; continuously thereafter. Replace thermometer and assess the underlying skin every 48 hours (Higgins, 2008; Perry et al., 2014).
- The Society of Pediatric Nurses (SPN) recognizes that temporal artery thermometry is accurate for infants less than 90 days old without fever, as well as for all patients more than 90 days of age with or without fever, ill, or well. The SPN recommends that the temporal artery method should not be used in infants 90 days or younger who are ill, have a fever, or have an ill diagnosis (Asher & Northington, 2008, p. 235). The rectal method should be used for these infants unless contraindicated by diagnosis, in which case the axillary method should be used. In addition, in children 6 months of age or older, the tympanic or oral methods may be used with correct positioning of the ear (tympanic) and if the patient can cooperate (oral) (Asher & Northington, 2008).

Home Care Considerations

- Teach patients who use electronic or digital thermometers to clean the probe after use to prevent transmission of microorganisms among family members. Clean according to manufacturer's directions.
- Teach patients using nonmercury glass thermometers to clean the thermometer after use in lukewarm soapy water and rinse in cool water. Store it in an appropriate place to prevent breakage and injury from the glass.
- Pacifier thermometers, which use the supralingual area, are available to screen for fever. Leave this thermometer in place for 3 to 6 minutes, based on the manufacturer's recommendations (Mayo Clinic, 2015b; Braun, 2006).

Evidence for Practice highlights available best practice guidelines and/or research-based evidence to support the skills.

→

EVIDENCE FOR PRACTICE ▶

FEVER AND ANTIPYRESIS
Temperature increase and fever are common clinical symptoms. Most fevers, unless extremely high (above 40°C/104°F), are not harmful (Grossman & Porth, 2014). Fever is an important part of a person's defense mechanisms against infection. Findings about antipyretic treatment have further challenged the need for routine or aggressive fever suppression. Unfortunately, many nurses continue to be fever phobic, while their attitudes toward fever and antipyresis considerably affect antipyretic practice (Kiekkas et al, 2014). What are nurses' attitudes toward fever and antipyresis? Is nursing practice based on traditional beliefs that fever is harmful? Do nurses over-treat fever?

Related Research
Kiekkas, P., Konstantinou, E., Psychogiou, K. S., Tsampoula, I., Stefanopoulos, N., & Bakalis, N. (2014). Nursing personnel's attitudes towards fever and antipyresis of adult patients: cross-sectional survey. *Journal of Clinical Nursing, 23*(19/20), 2949–2957.
   This prospective, cross-sectional, multicenter study evaluated nurses' attitudes toward fever and antipyresis or knowledge about fever and antipyresis in adults via questionnaire. The questionnaire included knowledge-evaluating items about fever and antipyresis, as well as attitude-evaluating items toward fever and antipyresis. Multiple linear regression analysis was

MASTER NURSING PROCESS!

The **nursing process** framework is used to integrate related nursing responsibilities for each of the five steps: Assessment, Nursing Diagnoses,* Outcome Identification and Planning, Implementation, and Evaluation, as well as Documentation.

Documentation Guidelines direct students and graduate nurses in accurate documentation of the skill and their findings. **Sample Documentation** demonstrates proper documentation.

*Material related to nursing diagnoses is from T. Heather Herdman/ Shigemi Kamitsuru (Eds.), NANDA International, Inc. *Nursing Diagnoses: Definitions and Classification 2018–2020,* Eleventh Edition © 2017 NANDA International, ISBN 978-1-62623-929-6. Used by arrangement with the Thieme Group, Stuttgart/ New York. To make safe and effective judgments using NANDA-I nursing diagnoses, it is essential that nurses refer to the definitions and defining characteristics of the diagnoses listed in the Appendix found on thePoint®.

Skill 2-4 ▶ Assessing a Peripheral Pulse by Palpation (continued)

EQUIPMENT
- Watch with second hand or digital readout
- Electronic record, or a pen, paper or flow sheet
- Nonsterile gloves, if appropriate; additional PPE, as indicated

ASSESSMENT
Choose a site to assess the pulse. For an adult patient, adolescent, and older child, the most common site for obtaining a peripheral pulse is the radial pulse. Apical pulse measurement is the preferred method of pulse assessment for infants and children less than 2 years of age (Jarvis, 2016). (Refer to Skill 2-5.) Assess for factors that could affect pulse characteristics, such as the patient's age, amount of exercise, fluid balance, and medications. Note baseline or previous pulse measurements.

NURSING DIAGNOSIS
Determine the related factors for the nursing diagnoses based on the patient's current status. Appropriate nursing diagnoses may include:
- Decreased cardiac output
- Ineffective peripheral tissue perfusion
- Risk for ineffective peripheral tissue perfusion

OUTCOME IDENTIFICATION AND PLANNING
The expected outcomes to achieve when measuring a pulse rate are that the patient's pulse is assessed accurately without injury and that the patient experiences minimal discomfort. Other outcomes may be appropriate, depending on the patient's nursing diagnosis.

IMPLEMENTATION

ACTION	RATIONALE
1. Check medical order or nursing care plan for frequency of pulse assessment. More frequent pulse measurement may be appropriate based on nursing judgment.	Assessment and measurement of vital signs at appropriate intervals provide important data about the patient's health status.
2. Perform hand hygiene and put on PPE, if indicated.	Hand hygiene and PPE prevent the spread of microorganisms. PPE is required based on transmission precautions.
3. Identify the patient.	Identifying the patient ensures the right patient receives the intervention and helps prevent errors.
4. Close the curtains around the bed and close the door to the room, if possible. Discuss the procedure with the patient and assess the patient's ability to assist with the procedure.	This ensures the patient's privacy. Explanation relieves anxiety and facilitates cooperation.
5. Put on gloves, if indicated.	Gloves are not usually worn to obtain a pulse measurement unless contact with blood or body fluids is anticipated. Gloves prevent contact with blood and body fluids.
6. Select the appropriate peripheral site based on assessment data.	Ensures safety and accuracy of measurement.
7. Move the patient's clothing to expose only the site chosen.	The site must be exposed for pulse assessment. Exposing only the site keeps the patient warm and maintains his or her dignity.
8. Place your first, second, and third fingers over the artery (Figure 1). Place your fingers over the artery so that the	The sensitive fingertips can feel the pulsation of the artery.

ACTION	RATIONALE
9. Using a watch with a second hand, count the number of pulsations felt for 30 seconds (Figure 2). Multiply this number by 2 to calculate the rate for 1 minute. If the rate, rhythm, or amplitude of the pulse is abnormal in any way, palpate and count the pulse for 1 minute.	Ensures accuracy of measurement and assessment.

FIGURE 1. Palpating the radial pulse.

FIGURE 2. Counting the pulse.

ACTION	RATIONALE
10. Note the rhythm and amplitude of the pulse.	Provides additional assessment data regarding the patient's cardiovascular status.
11. When measurement is completed, remove gloves, if worn. Cover the patient and help him or her to a position of comfort.	Proper removal of gloves reduces the risk for infection transmission and contamination of other items. Ensures patient comfort.
12. Remove additional PPE, if used. Perform hand hygiene.	Proper removal of PPE reduces the risk for infection transmission and contamination of other items. Hand hygiene prevents the spread of microorganisms.

EVALUATION
The expected outcomes have been met when the patient's pulse is assessed accurately without injury and the patient experiences minimal discomfort.

DOCUMENTATION
Guidelines
Record pulse rate, amplitude, and rhythm in the electronic record or flow sheet. Identify site of assessment. Report abnormal findings to the primary care provider.

Sample Documentation

 Practice documenting pulse and other vital signs in Lippincott DocuCare.

2/6/120 1000 Pulses 84, regular, 2+ and equal bilaterally in radial, popliteal, and dorsalis pedis sites.

—*M. Evans, RN*

UNEXPECTED SITUATIONS AND ASSOCIATED INTERVENTIONS
- *The pulse is irregular:* Monitor the pulse for a full minute. If the pulse is difficult to assess, validate pulse measurement by taking the apical pulse for 1 minute. If this is a change for the patient, notify the primary care provider.
- *The pulse is palpated easily, but then disappears:* Apply only moderate pressure to the pulse. Applying too much pressure may obliterate the pulse.
- *You cannot palpate a pulse:* Use a portable Doppler ultrasound to assess the pulse. If this is a change in assessment or if you cannot find the pulse using a Doppler ultrasound, notify the primary care provider. If you can find the pulse using a Doppler ultrasound, place a small X over the spot where the pulse is located. This can make palpating the pulse easier because the exact location of the pulse is known.

(continued)

DEVELOP THE NECESSARY SKILLS!

Step-by-Step Skills. Each chapter presents numerous related step-by-step skills. The skills are presented in a concise, straightforward, and simplified two-column format to facilitate competent performance of nursing skills.

Scientific Rationales accompany each nursing action to promote a deeper understanding of the basic principles supporting nursing care.

Nursing Alerts draw attention to crucial information.

Photo Atlas Approach. When learning a new skill, it is often overwhelming to only *read* how to perform a skill. With nearly 1,000 photographs, this book offers a pictorial guide to performing each skill. The skill will not only be learned but also remembered through the use of text with pictures.

 Hand Hygiene icons alert you to this crucial step that is the best way to prevent the spread of microorganisms. Important information related to this icon is included inside the back cover.

 Patient Identification icons alert you to this critical step ensuring the right patient receives the intervention, to help prevent errors. Important information related to this icon is included inside the back cover.

Skill 2-5 — Assessing the Apical Pulse by Auscultation *(continued)*

ACTION	RATIONALE
3. Identify the patient.	Identifying the patient ensures the right patient receives the intervention and helps prevent errors.
4. Close curtains around the bed and close the door to the room, if possible. Discuss the procedure with the patient and assess the patient's ability to assist with the procedure.	This ensures the patient's privacy. Explanation relieves anxiety and facilitates cooperation.
5. Put on gloves, if indicated.	Gloves are not usually worn to obtain a pulse measurement unless contact with blood or body fluids is anticipated. Gloves prevent contact with blood and body fluids.
6. Use an alcohol swab to clean the diaphragm of the stethoscope. Use another swab to clean the earpieces, if necessary.	Cleaning with alcohol deters transmission of microorganisms.
7. Assist the patient to a sitting or reclining position and expose the chest area.	This position facilitates identification of the site for stethoscope placement.
8. Move the patient's clothing to expose only the apical site.	The site must be exposed for pulse assessment. Exposing only the apical site keeps the patient warm and maintains his or her dignity.
9. Hold the stethoscope diaphragm against the palm of your hand for a few seconds.	Warming the diaphragm promotes patient comfort.
10. Palpate the space between the fifth and sixth ribs (fifth intercostal space), and move to the left midclavicular line. Place the stethoscope diaphragm over the apex of the heart (Figures 1 and 2).	Position the stethoscope over the apex of the heart, where the heartbeat is best heard.

Apex area
Place diaphragm here

Midsternum   Midclavicular line

FIGURE 1. Locating the apical pulse: apex area.

A

B

FIGURE 2. The apical pulse is usually found at (**A**) the fifth intercostal space just inside the midclavicular line and can be heard (**B**) over the apex of the heart.

OUTCOME IDENTIFICATION AND PLANNING	The expected outcomes to achieve when performing temperature assessment are that the patient's temperature is assessed accurately without injury and the patient experiences minimal discomfort. Other outcomes may be appropriate, depending on the patient's nursing diagnosis.

IMPLEMENTATION

ACTION	RATIONALE
1. Check the medical order or nursing care plan for frequency of measurement and route. More frequent temperature measurement may be appropriate based on nursing judgment.	Assessment and measurement of vital signs at appropriate intervals provide important data about the patient's health status.
2. Perform hand hygiene and put on PPE, if indicated.	Hand hygiene and PPE prevent the spread of microorganisms. PPE is required based on transmission precautions.
3. Identify the patient.	Identifying the patient ensures that the right patient receives the intervention and helps prevent errors.
4. Close the curtains around the bed and close the door to the room, if possible. Discuss the procedure with the patient and assess the patient's ability to assist with the procedure.	This ensures the patient's privacy. Explanation relieves anxiety and facilitates cooperation. Dialogue encourages patient participation and allows for individualized nursing care.
5. Assemble equipment on the overbed table within reach.	Organization facilitates performance of task.
6. Ensure that the electronic or digital thermometer is in working condition.	Improperly functioning thermometer may not give an accurate reading.
7. Put on gloves, if indicated.	Gloves prevent contact with blood and body fluids. Gloves are usually not required for an oral, axillary, or tympanic temperature measurement, unless contact with blood or body fluids is anticipated. Gloves should be worn for rectal temperature measurement.
8. Select the appropriate site based on assessment data.	This ensures safety and accuracy of measurement.
9. Follow the steps as outlined below for the appropriate type of thermometer.	

Skill Variations provide clear, start-to-finish instructions for variations in equipment or technique.

Skill 2-7 | Assessing Blood Pressure by Auscultation *(continued)*

Home Care Considerations

• Automated blood pressure devices in public locations are generally inaccurate and inconsistent. In addition, the cuffs on these devices are inadequate for people with large arms (Pickering et al., 2005).
• Explain to the patient that it is important to use a cuff size appropriate for limb circumference. Inform the patient that cuff sizes range from a pediatric cuff to a large thigh cuff and that a poorly fitting cuff can result in an inaccurate measurement.
• Inform the patient about digital blood pressure monitoring equipment. Although more costly than manual cuffs, most provide an easy-to-read recording of systolic and diastolic measurements.
• Explain that three readings, at least 1 minute apart, should be taken while in a sitting position, both in the morning and at night. Measurement should occur after resting quietly in a chair for 3 to 5 minutes, with the upper arm at heart level. The readings should be recorded to show to the health care provider.
• Explain that home monitoring devices should be checked for accuracy every 1 to 2 years. Readings should be compared with auscultated measurement by a health care provider to ensure accuracy.

Skill Variation | Assessing Blood Pressure Using an Automatic Electronic Blood Pressure Monitor

Automatic, electronic equipment may be used to monitor blood pressure any time frequent assessments are necessary (Figure A). These monitors determine blood pressure by analyzing the sounds of blood flow or measuring oscillations (fluctuations) in blood flow. The machine can be set to take and record blood pressure readings at preset intervals. Irregular heart rates, excessive patient movement, and environmental noise can interfere with the readings. Because electronic equipment is more sensitive to outside interference, these readings are susceptible to error. The cuff is applied in the same manner as the auscultatory method, with the microphone or pressure sensor positioned directly over the artery. When using an automatic blood pressure device for serial readings, check the cuffed limb frequently. Incomplete deflation of the cuff between measurements can lead to inadequate arterial perfusion and venous drainage, compromising the circulation in the limb (Bern et al., 2007; Pickering et al., 2004).

FIGURE A. Electronic blood pressure device. *(Photo by B. Proud.)*

1. Check the medical order or nursing care plan for frequency of blood pressure measurement. More frequent measurement may be appropriate based on nursing judgment.

 2. Perform hand hygiene and put on PPE, if indicated.

 3. Identify the patient.

4. Close the curtains around the bed and close the door to the room, if possible.
5. Discuss the procedure with the patient and assess the patient's ability to assist with the procedure.
6. Validate that the patient has relaxed for several minutes.
7. Select the appropriate limb for application of cuff.
8. Have the patient assume a comfortable lying or sitting position with the limb exposed.
9. Center the bladder of the cuff over the artery, lining up the artery mark on the cuff with the limb artery.
10. Wrap the cuff around the limb smoothly and snugly, and fasten it. Do not allow any clothing to interfere with the proper placement of the cuff.
11. Turn on the machine. If the machine has different settings for infants, children, and adults, select the appropriate setting. Push the start button. Instruct the patient to hold the limb still.
12. Wait until the machine beeps and the blood pressure reading appears. Remove the cuff from the patient's limb and clean and store the equipment.
13. Remove PPE, if used. Perform hand hygiene.
14. Record the findings on electronic record or flow sheet. Report abnormal findings to the appropriate person. Identify arm used and site of assessment if other than brachial.

Special Considerations, including **Infant, Child, Older Adult,** and **Home Care Considerations** (e.g., modifications and home care), appear throughout to explain the varying needs of patients across the lifespan and in various settings.

SPECIAL CONSIDERATIONS

General Considerations

• If respiratory rate is irregular, count respirations for 1 minute.

Infant and Child Considerations

• For infants, count respirations for 1 full minute due to a normally irregular rhythm.
• Assess respirations in infants and children when the child is resting or sitting quietly, because respiratory rate often changes when infants or young children cry, feed, or become more active. The most accurate respiratory rate is obtained when the infant or child is at rest (Jensen, 2015).
• Infants' respirations are primarily diaphragmatic; count abdominal movements to measure respiratory rate (Jensen, 2015). After 1 year of age, count thoracic movements (Kyle & Carman, 2017).

Unexpected Situations are provided after the explanation of normal outcomes. Each situation is followed by an explanation of how best to react, with rationales. This feature serves as a starting point for group discussion.

UNEXPECTED SITUATIONS AND ASSOCIATED INTERVENTIONS

• *Temperature reading is higher or lower than expected based on your assessment:* Reassess temperature with a different thermometer. The thermometer may not be calibrated correctly. If using a tympanic thermometer, you will get lower readings if the probe is not inserted far enough into the ear.
• *During rectal temperature assessment, the patient reports feeling light-headed or passes out:* Remove the thermometer immediately. Quickly assess the patient's blood pressure and heart rate. Notify the health care provider. Do not attempt to take another rectal temperature on this patient.

Many skills have free accompanying video clips, indicated by the **Watch & Learn** icon , or free accompanying activities, indicated by the **Practice & Learn** icon . All of these are available on thePoint® website at http://thepoint.lww.com/Lynn5e.

CONTENTS

Chapter 8   **Skin Integrity and Wound Care   415**

Chapter 9   **Activity   503**

Chapter 10   **Comfort and Pain Management   596**

Chapter 15 Fluid, Electrolyte, and Acid–Base Balance 884

Chapter 16 Cardiovascular Care 953

Chapter 17 Neurologic Care 1000

Chapter 18 Laboratory Specimen Collection 1031

Integrated Case Studies

UNIT III

ACKNOWLEDGMENTS

This updated edition is the work of many talented people. I would like to acknowledge the hard work of all who have contributed to the completion of this project. Thanks to Carol Taylor and Jennifer Bartlett for offering generous support and encouragement.

The work of this revision was skillfully coordinated by my dedicated team in the Nursing Education division of Wolters Kluwer. I am grateful to each of you for your patience, support, unending encouragement, and total commitment. My thanks to Michael Kerns, Senior Developmental Editor, for his insight and tireless work on this edition. My thanks to Betsy Gentzler, Digital Product Manager, for her hard work and guidance throughout the project; and to Emily Buccieri and Lindsay Ries, Editorial Coordinators; Bridgett Dougherty, Production Project Manager; Holly Reid McLaughlin, Design Coordinator; and Jennifer Clements, Art Director, Illustration.

A special thanks to my colleagues at Gwynedd Mercy University who offer unending support and professional guidance.

Finally, I would like to gratefully acknowledge my husband and daughters, for their love, understanding, and encouragement. Their support was essential during the long hours of research and writing.

Pamela Lynn

Actions Basic
to Nursing Care

Asepsis and Infection Control

Focusing on Patient Care

This chapter will help you develop some of the skills related to asepsis and infection control necessary to care for the following patients:

Joe Wilson, age 64, is scheduled to undergo a cardiac catheterization later this morning.

Sheri Lawrence, age 28, has been ordered to have an indwelling urinary catheter inserted.

Edgar Barowski, age 78, is suspected of having tuberculosis and requires infection control precautions.

Refer to Focusing on Patient Care: Developing Clinical Reasoning at the end of the chapter to apply what you learn.

Learning Objectives

After completing the chapter, you will be able to accomplish the following:

1. Perform hand hygiene using an alcohol-based handrub.
2. Perform hand hygiene using soap and water (handwashing).
3. Put on and remove personal protective equipment safely.
4. Prepare a sterile field.
5. Add sterile items to a sterile field.
6. Put on sterile gloves and remove soiled gloves.

Key Terms

health care–associated infection (HAI): infection not present on admission to a health care setting; acquired during the course of treatment for other conditions

medical asepsis: clean technique; involves procedures and practices that reduce the number and transfer of pathogens

pathogen: disease-producing microorganism

personal protective equipment (PPE): equipment and supplies necessary to minimize or prevent exposure to infectious material, including gloves, gowns, masks, and protective eye gear

standard precautions: precautions used in the care of all hospitalized patients regardless of their diagnosis or possible infection status; these precautions apply to blood, all body fluids, secretions and excretions (except sweat), nonintact skin, and mucous membranes

surgical asepsis: sterile technique; involves practices used to render and keep objects and areas free from microorganisms

transmission-based precautions: precautions used in addition to *Standard Precautions* for patients in hospitals who are suspected of being infected with pathogens that can be transmitted by airborne, droplet, or contact routes; these precautions encompass all the diseases or conditions previously listed in the disease-specific or category-specific classifications

Nurses and other health care workers play a key role in reducing the spread of disease, minimizing complications, and reducing adverse outcomes for their patients. Prevention of **health care–associated infections (HAIs)** is a major challenge for health care providers. In the United States, over a million HAIs occur every year, accounting for tens of thousands of deaths and billions of dollars in health care costs (AHRQ, 2015). Limiting the spread of microorganisms is accomplished by breaking the chain of infection. The practice of asepsis includes all activities to prevent infection or break the chain of infection. **Medical asepsis**, or clean technique, involves procedures and practices that reduce the number and transfer of **pathogens** (disease-producing microorganisms). Procedures incorporating medical asepsis include, for example, performing hand hygiene and wearing gloves. Refer to Fundamentals Review 1-1. **Surgical asepsis**, or sterile technique, includes practices used to render and keep objects and areas free from microorganisms. Procedures incorporating surgical asepsis include, for example, inserting an indwelling urinary catheter or inserting an intravenous catheter. Refer to Fundamentals Review 1-2.

Hand hygiene is the most effective way to help prevent the spread of infectious agents. The Joint Commission has included a recommendation to use hand hygiene as part of the 2018 Patient Safety Goal to "prevent infection" (The Joint Commission, 2018b). In addition, as part of their "Hand Hygiene Project," The Joint Commission Center for Transforming Healthcare (2014) has identified the need for hand hygiene upon entering and exiting a patient care area and before and after patient care. The World Health Organization (WHO, 2009) has identified the "My 5 Moments for Hand Hygiene" approach to define the key moments when health care workers should perform hand hygiene. These include:

- Moment 1: Before touching a patient
- Moment 2: Before a clean or aseptic procedure
- Moment 3: After body fluid exposure risk
- Moment 4: After touching a patient
- Moment 5: After touching patient surroundings

If the health care worker's hands are not visibly soiled, alcohol-based handrubs are recommended because they save time, are more accessible and easy to use, and reduce bacterial count on the hands (CDC, 2002). Refer to Fundamentals Review 1-3 for general guidelines regarding hand hygiene for health care workers.

Fundamentals Review 1-4 and 1-5 outline a summary of CDC-recommended practices for *Standard* and *Transmission-Based Precautions*, an important part of protecting patients and health care providers and preventing the spread of infection.

This chapter focuses on nursing skills to assist in preventing the spread of infection. These skills include performing hand hygiene, using personal protective equipment (PPE), preparing a sterile field, adding sterile items to a sterile field, and putting on and removing sterile gloves.

Fundamentals Review 1-1

BASIC PRINCIPLES OF MEDICAL ASEPSIS IN PATIENT CARE

- Practice good hand hygiene techniques.
- Carry soiled items, including linens, equipment, and other used articles, away from the body to prevent them from touching the clothing.
- Do not place soiled bed linen or any other items on the floor, which is grossly contaminated. It increases contamination of both surfaces.
- Avoid allowing patients to cough, sneeze, or breathe directly on others. Provide patients with disposable tissues, and instruct them, as indicated, to cover their mouth and nose to prevent spread by airborne droplets.
- Move equipment away from you when brushing, dusting, or scrubbing articles. This helps prevent

contaminated particles from settling on your hair, face, and uniform.
- Avoid raising dust. Use a specially treated or a dampened cloth. Do not shake linens. Dust and lint particles constitute a vehicle by which organisms can be transported from one area to another.
- Clean the least soiled areas first and then move to the more soiled ones. This helps prevent having the cleaner areas soiled by the dirtier areas.
- Dispose of soiled or used items directly into appropriate containers. Wrap items that are moist from body discharge or drainage in waterproof containers, such as plastic bags, before discarding into the refuse

Fundamentals Review 1-1 continued

BASIC PRINCIPLES OF MEDICAL ASEPSIS IN PATIENT CARE

holder so that handlers will not come in contact with them.
- Pour liquids that are to be discarded, such as bath water, mouth rinse, and the like, directly into the drain to avoid splattering in the sink and onto you.
- Sterilize items that are suspected of containing pathogens. After sterilization, they can be managed as clean items if appropriate.

- Use personal grooming habits that help prevent spreading microorganisms. Shampoo your hair regularly; keep your fingernails short and free of broken cuticles and ragged edges; do not wear artificial nails; and do not wear rings with grooves and stones that might harbor microorganisms.
- Follow guidelines conscientiously for infection control or barrier techniques as prescribed by your facility.

Fundamentals Review 1-2

BASIC PRINCIPLES OF SURGICAL ASEPSIS IN PATIENT CARE

- Only a sterile object can touch another sterile object. Unsterile touching sterile means contamination has occurred.
- Open sterile packages so that the first edge of the wrapper is directed away from you to avoid the possibility of a sterile surface touching unsterile clothing. The outside of the sterile package is considered contaminated.
- Avoid spilling any solution on a cloth or paper used as a field for a sterile setup. The moisture penetrates the sterile cloth or paper and carries organisms by capillary action to contaminate the field. A wet field is considered contaminated if the surface immediately below it is not sterile.
- Hold sterile objects above waist level. This will ensure keeping the object within sight and preventing accidental contamination.
- Avoid talking, coughing, sneezing, or reaching over a sterile field or object. This helps to prevent

contamination by droplets from the nose and the mouth or by particles dropping from your arm.
- Never walk away from or turn your back on a sterile field. This prevents possible contamination while the field is out of your view.
- All items brought into contact with broken skin, used to penetrate the skin to inject substances into the body, or used to enter normally sterile body cavities should be sterile. These items include dressings used to cover wounds and incisions, needles for injection, and tubes (catheters) used to drain urine from the bladder.
- Use dry, sterile forceps when necessary. Forceps soaked in disinfectant are not considered sterile.
- Consider the outer 1-in edge of a sterile field to be contaminated.
- Consider an object contaminated if you have any doubt about its sterility.

Fundamentals Review 1-3

HAND HYGIENE FOR HEALTH CARE WORKERS

HAND HYGIENE IS REQUIRED

- Before and after contact with each patient
- Before putting on gloves
- Before performing any invasive procedure, such as placement of a peripheral vascular catheter
- After accidental contact with body fluids or excretions, mucous membranes, nonintact skin, and wound dressings, even if hands are not visibly soiled
- When moving from a contaminated body site to a clean body site during patient care
- After contact with inanimate objects near the patient
- After removal of gloves

ADDITIONAL GUIDELINES

- The use of gloves does not eliminate the need for hand hygiene.
- The use of hand hygiene does not eliminate the need for gloves.
- Natural fingernails should be kept less than 1/4 in long.
- Artificial fingernails or extenders should not be worn when having direct contact with patients at high risk.
- Gloves should be worn when contact with blood, infectious material, mucous membranes, and nonintact skin could occur.
- Hand lotions or creams are recommended to moisturize and protect skin related to the occurrence of irritant dermatitis associated with hand hygiene.

Source: Modified with permission from Centers for Disease Control and Prevention. (2002). Guidelines for hand hygiene in health-care settings. *Morbidity and Mortality Weekly Report, 51*(RR-16), 1–45.

Fundamentals Review 1-4

STANDARD PRECAUTIONS

Standard Precautions are to be used for all patients receiving care in hospitals without regard to their diagnosis or presumed infection status. *Standard Precautions* apply to blood; all body fluids, secretions, and excretions except sweat, whether or not blood is present or visible; nonintact skin; and mucous membranes. *Standard Precautions* reduce the risk of transmission of microorganisms that cause infections in hospitals.

STANDARD PRECAUTIONS (TIER 1)

- Follow hand hygiene techniques.
- Wear clean nonsterile gloves when touching blood, body fluids, excretions, secretions, contaminated items, mucous membranes, and nonintact skin. Change gloves between tasks on the same patient, as necessary, and remove gloves promptly after use.
- Wear personal protective equipment such as mask, eye protection, face shield, or fluid-repellent gown during procedures and care activities that are likely to generate splashes or sprays of blood or body fluids. Use gown to protect skin and prevent soiling of clothing.
- Avoid recapping used needles. If you must recap, never use two hands. Use a needle-recapping device or the one-handed scoop technique. Place needles, sharps, and scalpels in appropriate puncture-resistant containers after use.
- Wear gloves to handle used patient care equipment that is soiled with blood or identified body fluids, secretions, and excretions to prevent transfer of microorganisms. Clean and reprocess items appropriately if used for another patient.

- Follow respiratory hygiene/cough etiquette. These strategies are targeted at patients and accompanying family members and friends with undiagnosed transmissible respiratory infections. These strategies apply to any person entering a health care facility with signs of illness, including cough, congestion, rhinorrhea, or increased production of respiratory secretions. Educate patients and visitors to health care facilities to cover the mouth/nose with a tissue when coughing; to dispose of used tissues promptly; to use surgical masks on the coughing person when tolerated and appropriate; to use hand hygiene after contact with respiratory secretions; and to use spatial separation, ideally >3 ft, between people with respiratory infections in common waiting areas when possible. Health care personnel are advised to observe *Droplet Precautions* (i.e., wear a mask) and perform hand hygiene when examining and caring for patients with signs and symptoms of a respiratory infection. Health care personnel who have a respiratory infection are advised to avoid direct patient contact, especially with high-risk patients. If this is not possible, then a mask should be worn while providing patient care.
- Use safe injection practices: Use basic principles of aseptic technique for the preparation and administration of parenteral medications, including the use of a sterile, single-use, disposable needle and syringe for each injection given and prevention of contamination of injection equipment and medication. Whenever possible, use of single-dose vials is preferred over multiple-dose vials, especially when medications will be administered to multiple patients.
- Wear a face mask if placing a catheter or injecting material into the spinal or epidural space.

Fundamentals Review 1-5

TRANSMISSION-BASED PRECAUTIONS

Transmission-Based Precautions are used in addition to *Standard Precautions* for patients with suspected infection with pathogens that can be transmitted by airborne, droplet, or contact routes. Any of the three types can be used in combination with the others. Equipment required for patient care, such as a thermometer, sphygmomanometer, and stethoscope, should be disposable, kept in the patient's room, and not used for other patients. The 2007 CDC guidelines include a directive to put on personal protective equipment (PPE) when entering the room of a patient with transmission-based precautions, and to remove the PPE only when leaving the room. These categories recognize that a disease may have multiple routes of transmission (Taylor et al., 2019).

AIRBORNE PRECAUTIONS (TIER 2)

- Use *Airborne Precautions* for patients who have infections that spread through the air such as tuberculosis, varicella (chicken pox), rubeola (measles), and possibly severe acute respiratory syndrome (SARS).
- Place patient in a private room that has monitored negative air pressure in relation to surrounding areas, 6 to 12 air changes per hour, and appropriate discharge of air outside or monitored filtration if air is recirculated. Keep door closed and patient in room.

Fundamentals Review 1-5 continued

TRANSMISSION-BASED PRECAUTIONS

- Use respiratory protection when entering room of patient with known or suspected tuberculosis. If patient has known or suspected rubeola or varicella, respiratory protection should be worn unless the person entering the room is immune to these diseases.
- Transport patient out of room only when necessary and place a surgical mask on the patient if possible.
- Consult CDC Guidelines for additional prevention strategies for tuberculosis.

DROPLET PRECAUTIONS

- Use *Droplet Precautions* for patients with an infection that is spread by large-particle droplets, such as rubella, mumps, diphtheria, and the adenovirus infection in infants and young children.
- Use a private room, if available. Door may remain open.
- Wear PPE upon entry into the room for all interactions that may involve contact with the patient and potentially contaminated areas in the patient's environment.
- Transport patient out of the room only when necessary and place a surgical mask on the patient if possible.
- Keep visitors 3 ft away from the infected person.

CONTACT PRECAUTIONS

- *Contact Precautions* are intended to prevent transmission of infectious agents that are spread by direct or indirect contact with the patient or the patient's environment.
- Use *Contact Precautions* for patients who are infected or colonized by a multidrug-resistant organism (MDRO).
- Observe *Contact Precautions* in the presence of excessive wound drainage, fecal incontinence, or other discharges from the body that suggest an increased potential for extensive environmental contamination and risk of transmission.
- Place patient in a private room if available.
- Wear PPE whenever you enter the room for all interactions that may involve contact with the patient and potentially contaminated areas in the patient's environment. Change gloves after having contact with infective material. Remove PPE before leaving the patient environment, and wash hands with an antimicrobial or waterless antiseptic agent.
- Limit movement of the patient out of the room.
- Avoid sharing patient care equipment.

Source: Adapted from Centers for Disease Control and Prevention (CDC). (2007d). *Guideline for isolation precautions: Preventing transmission of infectious agents in healthcare settings.* Retrieved https://www.cdc.gov/infectioncontrol/pdf/guidelines/isolation-guidelines.pdf.

 Skill 1-1 ▶ **Performing Hand Hygiene Using an Alcohol-Based Handrub**

Alcohol-based handrubs can be used in the health care setting. Alcohol-based handrubs have an alcohol concentration between 60% and 95% and are available as foam, gel, or lotions. When using these products, check the product labeling for correct amount of product needed. Alcohol-based handrubs (CDC, 2002):

- may be used if hands are not visibly soiled or have not come in contact with blood or body fluids.
- may be used before inserting urinary catheters, peripheral vascular catheters, or invasive devices that do not require surgical placement; before donning sterile gloves prior to an invasive procedure (e.g., inserting a central intravascular catheter); and if moving from a contaminated body site to a clean body site during patient care.
- should be used before and after each patient contact, after contact with surfaces in the patient's environment, and after removing gloves.
- significantly reduce the number of microorganisms on skin.
- are fast-acting and cause less skin irritation than other skin cleansers.

Skill 1-2 provides guidelines for situations requiring handwashing, as opposed to hand hygiene with an alcohol-based rub (CDC, 2002).

(continued)

Skill 1-1 ▶ Performing Hand Hygiene Using an Alcohol-Based Handrub *(continued)*

DELEGATION CONSIDERATIONS	The application and use of hand hygiene are appropriate for all health care providers.
EQUIPMENT	• Alcohol-based handrub • Oil-free lotion (optional)
ASSESSMENT	• Assess hands for any visible soiling or contact with blood or body fluids. Alcohol-based handrubs can be used if hands are not visibly soiled, or have not come in contact with blood or body fluids. Wash hands with soap and water before eating and after using the restroom. In addition, if hands are visibly soiled, proceed with washing the hands with soap and water. If hands have been in contact with blood or body fluids, even if there is no visible soiling, proceed with washing the hands with soap and water. Handwashing is required if exposure to certain organisms, such as those causing anthrax, norovirus or *Clostridium difficile*, is known or suspected. Alcohol-based handrubs have poor activity against these organisms.
NURSING DIAGNOSIS	Determine the related factors for the nursing diagnosis based on the patient's current status. An appropriate nursing diagnosis may include Risk for infection.
OUTCOME IDENTIFICATION AND PLANNING	The expected outcome to achieve when performing hand decontamination with alcohol-based rubs is that transient microorganisms will be eliminated from the hands. Other outcomes may be appropriate, depending on the specific nursing diagnosis identified for the patient.

IMPLEMENTATION

ACTION	RATIONALE
1. Remove jewelry prior to patient contact, if possible, and secure in a safe place. (A plain wedding band may remain in place.)	Microorganisms may accumulate in settings of jewelry, so it should not be worn during patient care. If jewelry was worn during patient care, it should be left on during handwashing.
2. Check the product labeling for correct amount of product needed.	Amount of product required to be effective varies from manufacturer to manufacturer, but is usually 1 to 3 mL.
3. Apply the product to the palm of one hand (Figure 1). Ensure use of the correct amount of product (Figure 2).	Adequate amount of product is required to cover hand surfaces thoroughly.

FIGURE 1. Applying the correct amount of product to the palm of one hand.

FIGURE 2. Ensuring use of the correct amount of product.

ACTION

4. Rub hands together, covering all surfaces of hands and fingers, and between fingers. Also clean the fingertips and the area beneath the fingernails.

5. Rub hands together until they are dry (at least 15 seconds) (Figure 3).

6. Use oil-free lotion on hands, if use of lotion is desired.

RATIONALE

All surfaces must be treated to prevent disease transmission.

Drying ensures antiseptic effect.

Oil-free lotion helps to keep the skin soft and prevents chapping. It is best applied after patient care is complete, and from a small, personal container, according to facility policy. Avoid use of oil-based lotions because they can cause deterioration of gloves.

FIGURE 3. Rubbing hands together until dry.

EVALUATION	The expected outcome has been met when transient microorganisms are eliminated from the hands.
DOCUMENTATION	The performance of hand hygiene using an alcohol-based handrub is not generally documented.

SPECIAL CONSIDERATIONS

General Considerations

- Hand hygiene performance by patients may be an important intervention to reduce acquisition and transmission of health care–associated pathogens (Sunkesula et al., 2015, p. 986).
- Health care providers should educate patients on the importance of hand hygiene. Informed patients have the ability to be better engaged as members of the health care team and are better able to advocate for themselves (Busby, Kennedy, Davis, Thompson, & Jones, 2015; Sunkesula et al., 2015).

Home Care Considerations

- Proper hand hygiene, including the use of alcohol-based handrubs, is useful to reduce the risk of spread of viral infections among family members (Tamimi, Maxwell, Edmonds, & Gerba, 2015). Patients and their families should be taught and encouraged to use hand hygiene techniques.

(continued)

Skill 1-1 ▶ Performing Hand Hygiene Using an Alcohol-Based Handrub *(continued)*

EVIDENCE FOR PRACTICE ▶

IMPROVING THE USE OF HAND HYGIENE MEASURES

Prevention of health care–associated infections is a major challenge for health care providers. Hand hygiene is regarded as an effective preventive measure. What types of interventions can be used to increase adherence to hand hygiene guidelines by health care workers?

Johnson, L., Grueber, S., Schlotzhauer, C., et al. (2014). A multifactorial action plan improves hand hygiene adherence and significantly reduces central line–associated bloodstream infections. *American Journal of Infection Control, 42*(11), 1146–1151.

This collaborative quality-improvement project utilized multiple interventions in a hospital over the course of 6 years. This multimodal plan included interventions related to staff education, staff accountability, hand sanitizer product selection and accessibility, and changes in organizational culture. Adherence to hand hygiene and central line–associated bloodstream infection rates were monitored as outcome measures. Hand hygiene adherence rates among all hospital units and among all health care worker categories increased from 58% to 98% over the 6-year timeframe. Central line–associated bloodstream infection rates decreased over the 6 years from 4.08 infections per 1,000 device-days to 0.42 infections per 1,000 device-days. The authors concluded that interventions by health care institutions to address adherence to hand hygiene should involve a multidisciplinary team and multimodal approach.

Relevance for Nursing Practice

There are numerous interventions that can be used to increase adherence to hand hygiene guidelines. Nurses are in a position to advocate for and introduce ideas to increase compliance related to hand hygiene adherence, resulting in improved patient care.

Refer to Skill 1-2 for additional research related to hand hygiene.

Refer to thePoint® for additional research on related nursing topics.

Skill 1-2 ▶ Performing Hand Hygiene Using Soap and Water (Handwashing)

Handwashing, as opposed to hand hygiene with an alcohol-based rub, is required (CDC, 2002):

- when hands are visibly soiled.
- when hands are contaminated with blood or other body fluids.
- before eating and after using the restroom.
- if exposure to certain organisms, such as those causing anthrax, norovirus, or *C. difficile*, is known or suspected. (Other agents, such as alcohol-based handrubs, have poor activity against these organisms.)

Using handwashing products that contain an antimicrobial (agent that kills microorganisms) or antibacterial ingredient is recommended in any setting where the risk for infection is high. When present in certain concentrations, these agents can kill bacteria or suppress their growth (Taylor, Lynn & Bartlett, 2019).

DELEGATION CONSIDERATIONS	The application and use of hand hygiene are appropriate for all health care providers.
EQUIPMENT	• Antimicrobial or nonantimicrobial soap (if in bar form, soap must be placed on a soap rack) • Paper towels • Oil-free lotion (optional)
ASSESSMENT	Assess for any of the above requirements for handwashing. If no requirements are fulfilled, the caregiver has the option of decontaminating hands with soap and water or using an alcohol-based handrub.
NURSING DIAGNOSIS	Determine the related factors for the nursing diagnosis based on the patient's current status. An appropriate nursing diagnosis may include Risk for infection.
OUTCOME IDENTIFICATION AND PLANNING	The expected outcome to achieve when performing handwashing is that the hands will be free of visible soiling and transient microorganisms will be eliminated. Other outcomes may be appropriate, depending on the specific nursing diagnosis identified for the patient.

IMPLEMENTATION

ACTION	RATIONALE
1. Gather the necessary supplies. Stand in front of the sink. Do not allow your clothing to touch the sink during the washing procedure (Figure 1).	The sink is considered contaminated. Clothing may carry organisms from place to place.
2. Remove jewelry, if possible, and secure in a safe place. A plain wedding band may remain in place.	Removal of jewelry facilitates proper cleansing. Microorganisms may accumulate in settings of jewelry. If jewelry was worn during care, it should be left on during handwashing.
3. Turn on water and adjust force (Figure 2). Regulate the temperature until the water is warm.	Water splashed from the contaminated sink will contaminate clothing. Warm water is more comfortable and is less likely to open pores and remove oils from the skin. Organisms can lodge in roughened and broken areas of chapped skin.

FIGURE 1. Standing in front of sink.

FIGURE 2. Turning on the water at the sink.

(*continued*)

Skill 1-2 ▶ Performing Hand Hygiene Using Soap and Water (Handwashing) *(continued)*

ACTION	RATIONALE
4. Wet the hands and wrist area. Keep hands lower than elbows to allow water to flow toward fingertips (Figure 3).	Water should flow from the cleaner area toward the more contaminated area. Hands are more contaminated than forearms.
5. Use about 1 teaspoon liquid soap from dispenser or rinse bar of soap and lather thoroughly (Figure 4). Cover all areas of hands with the soap product. If using bar soap, rinse soap bar again and return to soap rack without touching the rack.	Rinsing the soap before and after use removes the lather, which may contain microorganisms.

FIGURE 3. Wetting hands to the wrist.

FIGURE 4. Lathering hands with soap and rubbing with firm circular motion.

6. With firm rubbing and circular motions, wash the palms and backs of the hands, each finger, the areas between the fingers (Figure 5), and the knuckles, wrists, and forearms. **Wash at least 1 in above area of contamination.** If hands are not visibly soiled, wash to 1 in above the wrists (Figure 6).	Friction caused by firm rubbing and circular motions helps to loosen dirt and organisms that can lodge between the fingers, in skin crevices of knuckles, on the palms and backs of the hands, and on the wrists and forearms. Cleaning less contaminated areas (forearms and wrists) after hands are clean prevents spreading microorganisms from the hands to the forearms and wrists.

FIGURE 5. Washing areas between fingers.

FIGURE 6. Washing to 1 inch above the wrist.

7. Continue this friction motion for at least 20 seconds.	Effective handwashing requires at least a 20-second scrub with plain soap or disinfectant and warm water. Length of handwashing is determined by degree of contamination. Hands that are visibly soiled need a longer scrub.

ACTION	**RATIONALE**
8. Use fingernails of the opposite hand or a clean orangewood stick to clean under fingernails (Figure 7).	Area under nails has a high microorganism count, and organisms may remain under the nails, where they can grow and be spread to other people.
9. Rinse thoroughly with water flowing toward fingertips (Figure 8).	Running water rinses microorganisms and dirt into the sink.

FIGURE 7. Using fingernails to clean under nails of opposite hand.

FIGURE 8. Rinsing hands under running water with water flowing toward fingertips.

ACTION	**RATIONALE**
10. Pat hands dry with a paper towel, beginning with the fingers and moving upward toward forearms, and discard it immediately. Use another clean towel to turn off the faucet. Discard towel immediately without touching other clean hand.	Patting the skin dry prevents chapping. Dry hands first because they are considered the cleanest and least contaminated area. Turning the faucet off with a clean paper towel protects the clean hands from contact with a soiled surface.
11. Use oil-free lotion on hands, if desired.	Oil-free lotion helps to keep the skin soft and prevents chapping. It is best to apply after patient care is complete and from a small, personal container. Oil-based lotions should be avoided because they can cause deterioration of gloves.

EVALUATION   The expected outcome has been met when the hands are free of visible soiling and transient microorganisms are eliminated.

DOCUMENTATION   The performance of handwashing is not generally documented.

SPECIAL CONSIDERATIONS

General Considerations

- In September, 2016, the U.S. Food & Drug Administration issued a final rule establishing that over-the-counter consumer antiseptic wash products containing certain active ingredients can no longer be marketed. This decision was the result of a lack of evidence that the ingredients are both safe for long-term daily use and more effective than plain soap and water in preventing illness and the spread of certain infections. This rule does not affect consumer hand "sanitizers" or wipes, or antibacterial products used in health care settings (U.S. FDA, 2016).
- Hand hygiene performance by patients may be an important intervention to reduce acquisition and transmission of health care–associated pathogens (Sunkesula et al., 2015, p. 986).
- Health care providers should educate patients on the importance of hand hygiene. Informed patients have the ability to be better engaged as members of the health care team and are better able to advocate for themselves (Busby et al., 2015; Sunkesula et al., 2015).

(continued)

Skill 1-2 ▶ Performing Hand Hygiene Using Soap and Water (Handwashing) *(continued)*

Home Care Considerations

- Proper hand hygiene, including the use of alcohol-based handrubs, is useful to reduce the risk of spread of viral infections among family members (Tamimi et al., 2015). Patients and their families should be taught and encouraged to use hand hygiene techniques.

EVIDENCE FOR PRACTICE ▶

IMPROVING THE USE OF HAND HYGIENE MEASURES

Health care providers are the focus of many hand hygiene initiatives in health care facilities. Hand hygiene by patients may also be an important means to prevent acquisition and dissemination of health care–associated pathogens (Ardizzone, Smolowitz, Kline, Thom, & Larson, 2013).

Related Research

O'Donnell, M., Harris, T., Horn, T., et al. (2015). Sustained increase in resident meal time hand hygiene through an interdisciplinary intervention engaging long-term care facility residents and staff. *American Journal of Infection Control, 43*(2), 162–164.

The objectives of this quality-improvement initiative were to evaluate the frequency of resident hand hygiene prior to meals in a long-term care facility, identify factors that limit hand hygiene, and examine the impact of an interdisciplinary intervention to improve meal time hand hygiene practices. A sink and alcohol-based handrub dispensers were available at the entrance of each resident room and towelettes were provided with meals. However, residents shared common cafeteria and recreation areas and often required assistance with hand hygiene due to multiple underlying conditions, including dementia and decreased manual dexterity. Over the course of 1 month, the meal time hand hygiene performance by residents was observed from the time the meal was announced through the beginning of the meal. The use of soap and water, alcohol-based rub, or towelettes was recorded as hand hygiene. After the 1-month observation period, residents were surveyed regarding knowledge of hand hygiene and perceived barriers to performance of hand hygiene in general, as well as to barriers before meals. An education intervention based on the results of the observations and survey was implemented over the course of the next 6 months. The intervention included education on the importance of hand hygiene, reminders by staff to perform hand hygiene, a hand hygiene station at the dining room entrance with antimicrobial towelettes and an automated dispenser of alcohol-based gel, and resident participation in education and distribution of towelettes. Additional observations of meal-time resident hand hygiene were performed 1 day/wk during the 6-month intervention period. Comparison of the percentages of hand hygiene performance before versus during the intervention was completed. The educational intervention resulted in a significant increase in the percentage of hand hygiene opportunities during which hand hygiene was performed prior to meals; hand hygiene was performed 4 times out of 240 opportunities (2%) before versus 1,025 times out of 1,206 opportunities (85%) ($p < 0.0001$). The authors concluded residents were aware of the importance of hand hygiene, but performance before meals was uncommon due to multiple barriers. It was also concluded that an interdisciplinary intervention addressing these identified barriers was effective in improving premeal hand hygiene. The authors identified the importance of ease of accessibility and visibility of hand hygiene materials, as well as ease of use, and active involvement of health care personnel.

Relevance for Nursing Practice

Effective hand hygiene is a critical means to help prevent the spread of microorganisms and infectious agents. Simple interventions, such as removing barriers and providing assistance, can make significant contributions to effective hand hygiene implementation. Nurses should consider undertaking studies related to improving hand hygiene compliance to ensure safe patient care. Such studies would also add to the body of knowledge to support evidence-based nursing practice.

Refer to Skill 1-1 for additional research related to hand hygiene.

Refer to thePoint® for additional research on related nursing topics.

EVIDENCE FOR PRACTICE ▶

IMPROVING THE USE OF HAND HYGIENE MEASURES

Effective hand hygiene practices are a critical method to reduce the prevalence of health care–associated infections (HAIs). However, this procedure is still not performed consistently in health care settings, and many infections are transmitted by health care personnel (The Joint Commission Center for Transforming Healthcare, 2014). Patients play a role in effective use of hand hygiene, but often encounter barriers to adequate hand hygiene for themselves (Korniewicz & El-Masri, 2010; Burnett et al., 2008, as cited in Fox et al., 2015, p. 217).

Related Research

Fox, C., Wavra, T., Ash Drake, D., et al. (2015). Use of a patient hand hygiene protocol to reduce hospital-acquired infections and improve nurses' hand washing. *American Journal of Critical Care, 24*(3), 216–224.

This quality-improvement project investigated the use of a hand hygiene protocol designed to reduce HAI rates and improve nurses' handwashing compliance in one adult cardiovascular intensive care unit at a community hospital. A pre-experimental design was used to compare 12-month rates of central catheter–associated bloodstream infection, catheter-associated urinary tract infection, and nurses' handwashing compliance measured before and during use of the hand hygiene protocol. Patient hand hygiene, using chlorhexidine gluconate wipes, was provided three times a day. Nurses' performance of hand hygiene before entering and after leaving intensive care unit patients' rooms was monitored to identify compliance. Reductions in 12-month infection rates were reported for both central catheter–associated bloodstream infections and catheter-associated urinary tract infections. Twelve-month nurse hand hygiene compliance also improved. The authors concluded that the use of this type of hand hygiene protocol was effective in reducing health care–associated infections and providing a means for quality improvement.

Relevance for Nursing Practice

Nurses are in an important position to investigate strategies to prevent HAIs and to implement quality-improvement efforts. Such studies would add to the body of knowledge supporting evidence-based nursing practice and result in improved patient care and outcomes.

Refer to Skill 1-1 for additional research related to hand hygiene.

Refer to thePoint® for additional research on related nursing topics.

Skill 1-3 ▶ Using Personal Protective Equipment

Personal protective equipment (PPE) refers to specialized clothing or equipment worn by an employee for protection against infectious materials. PPE is used in health care settings to improve personnel safety in the health care environment (CDC, 2014b). This equipment includes clean (nonsterile) and sterile gloves, impervious gowns/aprons, surgical and high-efficiency particulate air (HEPA) masks, N95 disposable masks, face shields, and protective eyewear/goggles.

Understanding the potential contamination hazards related to the patient's diagnosis and condition and the institutional policies governing PPE is very important. The type of PPE used will vary based on the type of exposure anticipated and category of precautions: **standard precautions** and **transmission-based precautions**, including contact, droplet, or airborne precautions. It is the nurse's responsibility to enforce the proper wearing of PPE during patient care for members of the health care team. Refer to Fundamentals Review 1-4 and 1-5 for a summary of CDC-recommended practices for standard and transmission-based precautions. Box 1-1 provides Guidelines for Effective Use of PPE.

(continued)

Skill 1-3 ▶ Using Personal Protective Equipment *(continued)*

Box 1-1   Guidelines for Effective Use of PPE

- Put on PPE before contact with the patient, preferably before entering the patient's room. When using transmission-based precautions, put on PPE before entering the patient's room.
- Choose appropriate PPE based on the type of exposure anticipated and type of transmission-based precautions.
- When wearing gloves, work from "clean" areas to "dirty" areas.
- Touch as few surfaces and items with your PPE as possible.
- Avoid touching or adjusting other PPE.

- Keep gloved hands away from your face.
- If gloves become torn or heavily soiled, remove and replace. Perform hand hygiene before putting on the new gloves.
- Personal glasses are not a substitute for goggles.
- As diseases/infections/conditions emerge or their prevalence increases, guidelines need to evolve. The CDC issued revised guidelines related to Ebola virus disease (EVD), which are available at http://www.cdc.gov/vhf/ebola/healthcare-us/ppe/guidance.html.

Source: Adapted from Centers for Disease Control and Prevention (CDC). (2007e). (Updated 2012). Personal protective equipment for healthcare personnel. Excerpted from guideline for isolation precautions: Preventing transmission of infectious agents in healthcare settings. Retrieved www.cdc.gov/hicpac/pdf/isolation/Isolation2007.pdf.

DELEGATION CONSIDERATIONS	The application and use of PPE are appropriate for all health care providers.
EQUIPMENT	• Gloves • Mask (surgical or particulate respirator) • Impervious gown • Protective eyewear (does not include eyeglasses) *Note: Equipment for PPE may vary depending on facility policy.*
ASSESSMENT	Assess the situation to determine the necessity for PPE. In addition, check the patient's chart for information about a suspected or diagnosed infection or communicable disease. Determine the possibility of exposure to blood and body fluids and identify the necessary equipment to prevent exposure; refer to the infection control manual provided by your facility.
NURSING DIAGNOSIS	Determine the related factors for the nursing diagnoses based on the patient's current status. Appropriate nursing diagnoses may include: • Risk for infection • Ineffective protection • Diarrhea
OUTCOME IDENTIFICATION AND PLANNING	The expected outcome to achieve when using PPE is prevention of microorganism transmission. Other outcomes that may be appropriate include the following: patient and staff remain free of exposure to potentially infectious microorganisms; and patient verbalizes information about the rationale for use of PPE.

IMPLEMENTATION

ACTION	RATIONALE
1. Check medical record and nursing care plan for type of precautions and review precautions in infection control manual.	Mode of transmission of organism determines type of precautions required.
2. Plan nursing activities before entering patient's room.	Organization facilitates performance of task and adherence to precautions.
3. Provide instruction about precautions to patient, family members, and visitors.	Explanation encourages cooperation of patient and family, and reduces apprehension about precaution procedures.

ACTION	**RATIONALE**

4. Perform hand hygiene.

Hand hygiene prevents the spread of microorganisms.

5. Put on gown, mask, protective eyewear, and gloves based on the type of exposure anticipated and category of isolation precautions.

Use of PPE interrupts chain of infection and protects patient and nurse. Gown should protect entire uniform. Gloves protect hands and wrists from microorganisms. Masks protect nurse or patient from droplet nuclei and large-particle aerosols. Eyewear protects mucous membranes in the eye from splashes.

a. Put on the gown, with the opening in the back. Tie gown securely at neck and waist (Figure 1).

Gown should fully cover the torso from the neck to knees, arms to the end of wrists, and wrap around the back.

b. Put on the mask or respirator over your nose, mouth, and chin (Figure 2). Secure ties or elastic bands at the middle of the head and neck. If respirator is used, perform a fit check. Inhale; the respirator should collapse. Exhale; air should not leak out.

Masks protect nurse or patient from droplet nuclei and large-particle aerosols. A mask must fit securely to provide protection.

c. Put on goggles (Figure 3). Place over eyes and adjust to fit. Alternately, a face shield could be used to take the place of the mask and goggles (Figure 4).

Eyewear protects mucous membranes in the eye from splashes. Must fit securely to provide protection.

FIGURE 1. Tying gown at neck and waist.

FIGURE 2. Applying mask over nose, mouth, and chin.

FIGURE 3. Putting on goggles.

FIGURE 4. Putting on face shield.

(continued)

Skill 1-3 ▶ Using Personal Protective Equipment *(continued)*

ACTION	RATIONALE

d. Put on clean disposable gloves. Extend gloves to cover the cuffs of the gown (Figure 5).

Gloves protect hands and wrists from microorganisms.

FIGURE 5. Putting on gloves, ensuring gloves cover gown cuffs.

6. Identify the patient. Explain the procedure to the patient. Continue with patient care as appropriate.

Patient identification validates the correct patient and correct procedure. Discussion and explanation help allay anxiety and prepare the patient for what to expect.

Remove PPE

7. Remove PPE: Except for respirator, remove PPE at the doorway or in an anteroom. **Remove respirator after leaving the patient's room and closing the door.**

Proper removal prevents contact with and the spread of microorganisms. Removing respirator outside the patient's room prevents contact with airborne microorganisms.

a. If impervious gown has been tied in front of the body at the waistline, untie waist strings before removing gloves.

Outside front of equipment is considered contaminated. The inside, outside back, ties on head and back are considered clean, which are areas of PPE that are not likely to have been in contact with infectious organisms. Front of gown, including waist strings, are contaminated. If tied in front of body, the ties must be untied before removing gloves.

b. Grasp the outside of one glove with the opposite gloved hand and peel off, turning the glove inside out as you pull it off (Figure 6). Hold the removed glove in the remaining gloved hand.

Outside of gloves are contaminated.

c. Slide fingers of ungloved hand under the remaining glove at the wrist, **taking care not to touch the outer surface of the glove** (Figure 7).

Ungloved hand is clean and should not touch contaminated areas.

FIGURE 6. Grasping the outside of one glove and peeling off.

FIGURE 7. Sliding fingers of ungloved hand under the remaining glove at the wrist.

ACTION

d. Peel off the glove over the first glove, containing the one glove inside the other (Figure 8). Discard in appropriate container.

e. To remove the goggles or face shield: Handle by the head-band or earpieces (Figure 9). Lift away from the face. Place in designated receptacle for reprocessing or in an appropriate waste container.

f. To remove gown: Unfasten ties, if at the neck and back. Allow the gown to fall away from shoulders. **Touching only the inside of the gown**, pull away from the torso. Keeping hands on the inner surface of the gown, pull gown from arms. Turn gown inside out. Fold or roll into a bundle and discard.

g. To remove mask or respirator: Grasp the neck ties or elastic, then top ties or elastic and remove. **Take care to avoid touching front of mask or respirator** (Figure 10). Discard in waste container. If using a respirator, save for future use in the designated area.

RATIONALE

Proper disposal prevents transmission of microorganisms.

Outside of goggles or face shield is contaminated; **do not touch.** Handling by headband or earpieces and lifting away from face prevents transmission of microorganisms. Proper disposal prevents transmission of microorganisms.

Gown front and sleeves are contaminated. Touching only the inside of the gown and pulling it away from the torso prevents transmission of microorganisms. Proper disposal prevents transmission of microorganisms.

Front of mask or respirator is contaminated; **do not touch.** Not touching the front of the mask and disposing the mask properly prevent transmission of microorganisms.

FIGURE 8. Pulling glove off the hand and over the other glove.

FIGURE 9. Removing goggles by grasping earpieces.

8. Perform hand hygiene immediately after removing all PPE.

FIGURE 10. Removing mask or respirator, grasping the neck ties or elastic, taking care to avoid touching the front.

Hand hygiene prevents spread of microorganisms.

(continued)

Skill 1-3 ▶ Using Personal Protective Equipment *(continued)*

EVALUATION

The expected outcomes have been met when the transmission of microorganisms is prevented; the patient and staff remain free from exposure to potentially infectious microorganisms; and the patient verbalizes an understanding about the rationale for use of PPE.

DOCUMENTATION

It is not usually necessary to document the use of specific articles of PPE or each application of PPE. However, document the implementation and continuation of specific transmission-based precautions as part of the patient's care.

UNEXPECTED SITUATIONS AND ASSOCIATED INTERVENTIONS

- *You did not realize the need for protective equipment at beginning of task:* Stop task and obtain appropriate protective wear.
- *You are accidentally exposed to blood and body fluids:* Stop task and immediately follow facility protocol for exposure, including reporting the exposure.

EVIDENCE FOR PRACTICE ▶

PPE AND PREVENTION OF TRANSFER OF MICROORGANISMS

Prevention of health care–associated infections is a major challenge for health care providers. The removal of PPE after patient care may result in transfer of microorganisms to the skin and clothing of health care workers, contributing to the transfer of microorganisms and increased risk of infection. How can this risk of transfer be reduced?

Related Research

Tomas, M. E., Kundrapu, S., Thota, P., et al. (2015). Contamination of health care personnel during removal of personal protective equipment. *JAMA Internal Medicine, 175*(12), 1904–1910.

The focus of this study was to determine the frequency and sites of contamination of the skin and clothing of personnel during PPE removal. The study also evaluated the effect of educational interventions on the frequency of contamination. Participants conducted simulations of contaminated PPE removal using fluorescent lotion to identify the frequency and sites of contamination after removal of contaminated gloves or gown and establish a baseline for comparison. Contamination of skin or clothing with the fluorescent lotion occurred in 60% of the simulations, with contamination occurring more frequently during removal of contaminated gloves than gowns. Education and supervised practice in removal of contaminated PPE with immediate visual feedback related to skin and clothing contamination was provided. After the education and supervised practice intervention, a reduction in skin and clothing contamination during glove and gown removal was identified (60% before the intervention vs. 18.9% after, $p < 0.001$). This reduction was sustained after 1 and 3 months (12% at both time points, $p < 0.001$ compared with before the intervention). The authors concluded that contamination of the skin and clothing of health care personnel occurs frequently during removal of contaminated gloves or gowns. Educational interventions can significantly reduce the risk of contamination during removal of PPE.

Relevance for Nursing Practice

Nurses should constantly strive to improve practice and be alert for interventions to help achieve better practice. As responsible practitioners, nurses and other health care personnel should continually review infection control standards and guidelines for best practice. It is important to examine and reflect on individual practice to ensure appropriate use of infection control measures, including use of PPE, to provide safe and responsible nursing care.

Refer to thePoint® for additional research on related nursing topics.

Skill 1-4 ▶ Preparing a Sterile Field Using a Packaged Sterile Drape

A sterile field is created to provide a surgically aseptic workspace. It should be considered a restricted area. A sterile drape may be used to establish a sterile field or to extend the sterile working area. The sterile drape should be waterproof on one side, with that side placed down on the work surface. After establishing the sterile field, add other sterile items, as needed, including solutions. Sterile items and sterile-gloved hands are the only objects allowed in the sterile field. Refer to Fundamentals Review 1-2 to review basic principles of surgical asepsis.

DELEGATION CONSIDERATIONS	Procedures requiring the use of a sterile field and other sterile items are not delegated to nursing assistive personnel (NAP) or unlicensed assistive personnel (UAP). Depending on the state's nurse practice act and the organization's policies and procedures, these procedures may be delegated to licensed practical/vocational nurses (LPN/LVNs). The decision to delegate must be based on careful analysis of the patient's needs and circumstances, as well as the qualifications of the person to whom the task is being delegated. Refer to the Delegation Guidelines in Appendix A.
EQUIPMENT	• Sterile-wrapped drape • Additional sterile supplies, such as dressings, containers, or solutions, as needed • PPE, as indicated
ASSESSMENT	Assess the situation to determine the necessity for creating a sterile field. Assess the area in which the sterile field is to be prepared. Move any unnecessary equipment out of the immediate vicinity.
NURSING DIAGNOSIS	Determine the related factors for the nursing diagnoses based on the patient's current status. Appropriate nursing diagnoses may include: • Risk for infection • Ineffective protection
OUTCOME IDENTIFICATION AND PLANNING	The expected outcome to achieve when preparing a sterile field is that the sterile field is created without contamination and the patient remains free of exposure to pathogens.

IMPLEMENTATION

ACTION	RATIONALE
1. Perform hand hygiene and put on PPE, if indicated.	Hand hygiene and PPE prevent the spread of microorganisms. PPE is required based on transmission precautions.
2. Identify the patient. Explain the procedure to the patient.	Patient identification validates the correct patient and correct procedure. Discussion and explanation help allay anxiety and prepare the patient for what to expect.
3. Check that the packaged sterile drape is dry and unopened. Also note expiration date, making sure that the date is still valid.	Moisture contaminates a sterile package. Expiration date indicates period that package remains sterile.
4. Select a work area that is waist level or higher.	Work area is within sight. Bacteria tend to settle, so there is less contamination above the waist.
5. Open the outer covering of the drape. Remove sterile drape, lifting it carefully by its corners. Hold away from body and above the waist and work surface.	Outer 1 in (2.5 cm) of drape is considered contaminated. Any item touching this area is also considered contaminated.

(continued)

Skill 1-4 ▶ Preparing a Sterile Field Using a Packaged Sterile Drape *(continued)*

ACTION

6. Continue to hold only by the corners. Allow the drape to unfold, away from your body and any other surface (Figure 1).

7. Position the drape on the work surface with the moisture-proof side down (Figure 2). This would be the shiny or blue side. Avoid touching any other surface or object with the drape. If any portion of the drape hangs off the work surface, that part of the drape is considered contaminated.

RATIONALE

Touching the outer side of the wrapper maintains the sterile field. Contact with any surface would contaminate the field.

Moisture-proof side prevents contamination of the field if it becomes wet. The moisture penetrates the sterile cloth or paper and carries organisms by capillary action to contaminate the field. A wet field is considered contaminated if the surface immediately below it is not sterile.

FIGURE 1. Holding drape by corners and allowing it to unfold away from body and surfaces.

FIGURE 2. Positioning drape on work surface with the moisture-proof side down.

8. Place additional sterile items on field as needed. Refer to Skill 1-6. Continue with the procedure as indicated.

9. When procedure is completed, remove PPE, if used. Perform hand hygiene.

Sterility of the field is maintained.

Proper removal of PPE reduces the risk for infection transmission and contamination of other items. Hand hygiene prevents the spread of microorganisms.

EVALUATION

The expected outcome has been met when the sterile field is prepared without contamination and the patient has remained free of exposure to pathogens.

DOCUMENTATION

It is not usually necessary to document the preparation of a sterile field. However, document the use of sterile technique for any procedure performed using sterile technique.

UNEXPECTED SITUATIONS AND ASSOCIATED INTERVENTIONS

- *A part of the sterile field becomes contaminated:* When any portion of the sterile field becomes contaminated, discard the sterile field and any items on the field, and start over.
- *The nurse realizes a supply is missing after setting up the sterile field:* Call for help. Do not leave the sterile field unattended. If the nurse is not able to directly see the sterile field at all times, it is considered contaminated.
- *The patient touches the sterile field:* If the patient touches the sterile field, discard the supplies and prepare a new sterile field. If the patient is confused, have someone assist by holding the patient's hands and/or provide reassurance and explanation of the procedure.

EVIDENCE FOR PRACTICE ▶

SIMULATION-BASED TRAINING AND STERILE TECHNIQUE

Use of strict sterile technique is critical to prevent contamination and possible infection. Nurses routinely provide care interventions that require the use of sterile technique, as well as playing a key role in assisting and monitoring implementation of sterile technique as part of patient care interventions by other health care practitioners. Do nurses have adequate knowledge of the steps in sterile technique?

Related Research

Gerolemou, L., Fidellaga, A., Rose, K., et al. (2014). Simulation-based training for nurses in sterile techniques during central vein catheterization. *American Journal of Critical Care, 23*(1), 40–48.

This study evaluated the effectiveness of simulation-based training of critical care nurses related to use of sterile techniques during central vein catheterization and the effect of such training on catheter-related bloodstream infection rates. Forty-six critical care nurses participated in the study. Forty-six critical care nurses participated in the study. Using simulation, the nurses' baseline skills related to the steps in sterile technique preparation during central venous catheter insertion according to facility practice, up to the point of needle insertion, were observed and recorded via video. Observers used an assessment tool based on CDC's recommendations to evaluate and score the nurses' performance in nonsterile preparation, handwashing, sterile field/supply preparation, sterile gowning, sterile gloving, and sterile draping. Participants then received individualized debriefing on her or his baseline performance, including a review of the video-recorded demonstration by the nurse. Debriefing included feedback, comments on individual steps when appropriate, and hands-on training and repetitive practice in sterile technique based on the nurse's performance. After the debriefing and subsequent training, each nurse underwent reassessment of her or his sterile technique skills. Data were also reviewed related to the rate of catheter-related bloodstream infections in the medical, surgical, neurologic critical care unit for the 12 months before and 12 months after the simulation-based study intervention. Performance scores at baseline were poor; median total score on the evaluation instrument was 7 out of a maximum score of 24. After simulation-based training, the nurses' median total score significantly increased to 23 ($p < 0.01$). After completion of the simulation-based training, the mean infection rate in the unit was reduced by 85% from 2.61 to 0.4 infections per 1,000 catheter-days ($p = 0.02$). The authors concluded that simulation-based training of critical care nurses in sterile technique is an important component in strategies to reduce the occurrence of catheter-related bloodstream infections and to promote patient safety.

Relevance to Nursing Practice

This study highlights the importance of awareness of best practice and the development of adequate skill in implementation of sterile technique in providing patient care interventions. Similar interventions might be implemented to improve the use of sterile technique related to other patient care practices and interventions. Nurses are in an important position to investigate strategies to prevent health care–associated infections and to implement quality-improvement efforts.

Refer to thePoint° for additional research on related nursing topics.

Skill 1-5 ▶ Preparing a Sterile Field Using a Commercially Prepared Sterile Kit or Tray

A sterile field is created to provide a surgically aseptic workspace. Consider it a restricted area. Commercially prepared sterile kits and trays are wrapped in a sterile wrapper that, once opened, becomes the sterile field. Sterile items and sterile-gloved hands are the only objects allowed in the sterile field. If the area is breached, the entire sterile field is considered contaminated. Refer to Fundamentals Review 1-2 to review basic principles of surgical asepsis.

DELEGATION CONSIDERATIONS

Procedures requiring the use of a sterile field and other sterile items are not delegated to nursing assistive personnel (NAP) or unlicensed assistive personnel (UAP). Depending on the state's nurse practice act and the organization's policies and procedures, these procedures may be delegated to licensed practical/vocational nurses (LPN/LVNs). The decision to delegate must be based on careful analysis of the patient's needs and circumstances, as well as the qualifications of the person to whom the task is being delegated. Refer to the Delegation Guidelines in Appendix A.

EQUIPMENT

- Commercially prepared sterile package
- Additional sterile supplies, such as dressings, containers, or solutions, as needed
- PPE, as indicated

ASSESSMENT

Assess the situation to determine the necessity for creating a sterile field. Assess the area in which the sterile field is to be prepared. Move any unnecessary equipment out of the immediate vicinity.

NURSING DIAGNOSIS

Determine the related factors for the nursing diagnoses based on the patient's current status. Appropriate nursing diagnoses may include:

- Risk for infection
- Ineffective protection

OUTCOME IDENTIFICATION AND PLANNING

The expected outcome to achieve when opening a commercially packaged sterile kit or tray is that a sterile field is created without contamination, the contents of the package remain sterile, and the patient remains free of exposure to pathogens.

IMPLEMENTATION

ACTION	RATIONALE

1. Perform hand hygiene and put on PPE, if indicated.

Hand hygiene and PPE prevent the spread of microorganisms. PPE is required based on transmission precautions.

2. Identify the patient. Explain the procedure to the patient.

Patient identification validates the correct patient and correct procedure. Discussion and explanation help allay anxiety and prepare the patient for what to expect.

3. Check that the packaged kit or tray is dry and unopened. Also note expiration date, making sure that the date is still valid.

Moisture contaminates a sterile package. Expiration date indicates period that package remains sterile.

4. Select a work area that is waist level or higher.

Work area is within sight. Bacteria tend to settle, so there is less contamination above the waist.

ACTION	RATIONALE

ACTION

5. Open the outside cover of the package and remove the kit or tray (Figure 1). Place in the center of the work surface, with the topmost flap positioned on the far side of the package. Discard outside cover.

6. Reach around the package and grasp the outer surface of the end of the topmost flap, holding no more than 1 in from the border of the flap. Pull open away from the body, keeping the arm outstretched and away from the inside of the wrapper (Figure 2). Allow the wrapper to lie flat on the work surface.

RATIONALE

This allows sufficient room for sterile field.

This maintains sterility of inside of wrapper, which is to become the sterile field. Outer surface of the wrapper is considered unsterile. Outer 1-in border of the wrapper is considered contaminated.

FIGURE 1. Opening outside cover of package.

FIGURE 2. Pulling top flap open, away from body.

7. Reach around the package and grasp the outer surface of the first side flap, holding no more than 1 in from the border of the flap. Pull open to the side of the package, keeping the arm outstretched and away from the inside of the wrapper (Figure 3). Allow the wrapper to lie flat on the work surface.

8. Reach around the package and grasp the outer surface of the remaining side flap, holding no more than 1 in from the border of the flap. Pull open to the side of the package, keeping the arm outstretched and away from the inside of the wrapper (Figure 4). Allow the wrapper to lie flat on the work surface.

This maintains sterility of inside of wrapper, which is to become the sterile field. Outer surface of the wrapper is considered unsterile. Outer 1-in border of the wrapper is considered contaminated.

This maintains sterility of inside of wrapper, which is to become the sterile field. Outer surface of the wrapper is considered unsterile. Outer 1-in border of the wrapper is considered contaminated.

FIGURE 3. Pulling open the first side flap.

FIGURE 4. Pulling open the remaining side flap.

(continued)

Skill 1-5 ▶ Preparing a Sterile Field Using a Commercially Prepared Sterile Kit or Tray *(continued)*

ACTION

9. Stand away from the package and work surface. Grasp the outer surface of the remaining flap closest to the body, holding not more than 1 in from the border of the flap. Pull the flap back toward the body, keeping arm outstretched and away from the inside of the wrapper (Figure 5). Keep this hand in place. Use other hand to grasp the wrapper on the underside (the side that is down to the work surface). Position the wrapper so that when flat, edges are on the work surface, and do not hang down over sides of work surface (Figure 6). Allow the wrapper to lie flat on the work surface.

FIGURE 5. Pulling open flap closest to body.

10. The outer wrapper of the package has become a sterile field with the packaged supplies in the center (Figure 7). Do not touch or reach over the sterile field. Place additional sterile items on field as needed. Refer to Skill 1-6. Continue with the procedure as indicated.

11. When procedure is completed, remove PPE, if used. Perform hand hygiene.

RATIONALE

This maintains sterility of the inside of the wrapper, which is to become the sterile field. Outer surface of the wrapper is considered unsterile. Outer 1-in border of the wrapper is considered contaminated.

FIGURE 6. Positioning wrapper on work surface.

Sterility of the field and contents are maintained.

FIGURE 7. Outside wrapper of package is now sterile field.

Proper removal of PPE reduces the risk for infection transmission and contamination of other items. Hand hygiene prevents the spread of microorganisms.

EVALUATION	The expected outcome has been met when the sterile field is prepared without contamination, the contents of the package remain sterile, and the patient remains free of exposure to pathogens.
DOCUMENTATION	It is not usually necessary to document the preparation of a sterile field. However, do document the use of sterile technique for any procedure performed using sterile technique.
UNEXPECTED SITUATIONS AND ASSOCIATED INTERVENTIONS	• *A part of the sterile field becomes contaminated:* When any portion of the sterile field becomes contaminated, discard the sterile field and any items on the field and start over. • *You realize a supply is missing after setting up the sterile field:* Call for help. Do not leave the sterile field unattended. If you are unable to directly see the sterile field at all times, it is considered contaminated. • *The patient touches the sterile field:* If the patient touches the sterile field, discard the supplies and prepare a new sterile field. If the patient is confused, have someone assist by holding the patient's hands and/or provide reassurance and explanation of the procedure.

EVIDENCE FOR PRACTICE ▶	**SIMULATION-BASED TRAINING AND STERILE TECHNIQUE** Use of strict sterile technique is critical to prevent contamination and possible infection. Nurses routinely provide care interventions that require the use of sterile technique. Nurses also play a key role in assisting and monitoring implementation of sterile technique as part of patient care interventions by other health care practitioners. Do nurses have adequate knowledge of the steps in sterile technique? **Related Research** Gerolemou, L., Fidellaga, A., Rose, K., et al. (2014). Simulation-based training for nurses in sterile techniques during central vein catheterization. *American Journal of Critical Care, 23*(1), 40–48. Refer to details in Skill 1-4, Evidence for Practice, and to thePoint˚ for additional research on related nursing topics.

Skill 1-6 ▶ Adding Sterile Items to a Sterile Field

	A sterile field is created to provide a surgically aseptic workspace. It should be considered a restricted area. After establishing the sterile field, add other sterile items, including solutions, as needed. Items can be wrapped and sterilized within the facility, or they can be commercially prepared. Take care to ensure that nothing unsterile touches the field or other items in the field, including hands or clothes. Refer to Fundamentals Review 1-2 to review basic principles of surgical asepsis.
DELEGATION CONSIDERATIONS	Procedures requiring the use of a sterile field and other sterile items are not delegated to nursing assistive personnel (NAP) or unlicensed assistive personnel (UAP). Depending on the state's nurse practice act and the organization's policies and procedures, these procedures may be delegated to licensed practical/vocational nurses (LPN/LVNs). The decision to delegate must be based on careful analysis of the patient's needs and circumstances, as well as the qualifications of the person to whom the task is being delegated. Refer to the Delegation Guidelines in Appendix A.
EQUIPMENT	• Sterile field • Sterile gauze, forceps, dressings, containers, solutions, or other sterile supplies, as needed • PPE, as indicated

(continued)

Skill 1-6 ▶ Adding Sterile Items to a Sterile Field *(continued)*

ASSESSMENT	Assess the situation to determine the necessity for creating a sterile field. Assess the area in which the sterile field is to be prepared. Move any unnecessary equipment out of the immediate vicinity. Identify additional supplies needed for the procedure.
NURSING DIAGNOSIS	Determine the related factors for the nursing diagnoses based on the patient's current status. Appropriate nursing diagnoses may include: • Risk for infection • Ineffective protection
OUTCOME IDENTIFICATION AND PLANNING	The expected outcomes to achieve when adding items to a sterile field are that the sterile field is created without contamination; the sterile supplies are not contaminated; and the patient remains free of exposure to pathogens.

IMPLEMENTATION

ACTION	RATIONALE
1. Perform hand hygiene and put on PPE, if indicated.	Hand hygiene and PPE prevent the spread of microorganisms. PPE is required based on transmission precautions.
2. Identify the patient. Explain the procedure to the patient.	Patient identification validates the correct patient and correct procedure. Discussion and explanation help allay anxiety and prepare the patient for what to expect.
3. Check that the sterile, packaged drape and supplies are dry and unopened. Also note expiration date, making sure that the date is still valid.	Moisture contaminates a sterile package. Expiration date indicates period that package remains sterile.
4. Select a work area that is waist level or higher.	Work area is within sight. Bacteria tend to settle, so there is less contamination above the waist.
5. Prepare sterile field as described in Skill 1-4 or Skill 1-5.	Proper technique maintains sterility.
6. Add sterile item:	
To Add a Facility-Wrapped and Sterilized Item	
a. Hold facility-wrapped item in the dominant hand, with top flap opening away from the body. With other hand, reach around the package and unfold top flap and both sides.	Only sterile surface and item are exposed before dropping onto sterile field.
b. Keep a secure hold on the item through the wrapper with the dominant hand. Grasp the remaining flap of the wrapper closest to the body, taking care not to touch the inner surface of the wrapper or the item. Pull the flap back toward the wrist, so the wrapper covers the hand and wrist.	Only sterile surface and item are exposed before dropping onto sterile field.
c. Grasp all the corners of the wrapper together with the nondominant hand and pull back toward wrist, covering hand and wrist. Hold in place.	Only sterile surface and item are exposed before dropping onto sterile field.
d. Hold the item 6 in above the surface of the sterile field and drop onto the field. Be careful to avoid touching the surface or other items or dropping any item onto the 1-in border.	This prevents contamination of the field and inadvertent dropping of the sterile item too close to the edge or off the field. Any items landing on the 1-in border are considered contaminated.

ACTION	**RATIONALE**

To Add a Commercially Wrapped and Sterilized Item

a. Hold package in one hand. Pull back top cover with other hand. Alternately, carefully peel the edges apart using both hands (Figure 1).

Contents remain uncontaminated by hands.

b. After top cover or edges are partially separated, hold the item 6 in above the surface of the sterile field. Continue opening the package and drop the item onto the field (Figure 2). **Be careful to avoid touching the surface or other items or dropping an item onto the 1-in border.**

This prevents contamination of the field and inadvertent dropping of the sterile item too close to the edge or off the field. Any items landing on the 1-in border are considered contaminated.

c. Discard wrapper.

A neat work area promotes proper technique and avoids inadvertent contamination of the field.

FIGURE 1. Carefully peeling edges apart.

FIGURE 2. Dropping sterile item onto sterile field.

To Add a Sterile Solution

a. Obtain appropriate solution and check expiration date.

Once opened, label any bottles with date and time. Solution remains sterile for 24 hours once opened.

b. Open solution container according to directions and **place cap on table away from the field with edges up** (Figure 3).

Sterility of inside cap is maintained.

c. Hold bottle outside the edge of the sterile field with the label side facing the palm of your hand and prepare to pour from a height of 4 to 6 in (10 to 15 cm). **Never touch the tip of the bottle to the sterile container or field.**

Label remains dry, and solution may be poured without reaching across sterile field. Minimal splashing occurs from that height. Accidentally touching the tip of the bottle to a container or dressing contaminates them both.

d. Pour required amount of solution steadily into sterile container previously added to the sterile field and positioned at side of sterile field or onto dressings (Figure 4). **Avoid splashing any liquid.**

A steady stream minimizes the risk of splashing; moisture contaminates sterile field.

e. Touch only the outside of the lid when recapping. Label solution with date and time of opening.

Solution remains uncontaminated and available for future use.

FIGURE 3. Opening bottle of sterile solution and placing cap on table with edges up.

FIGURE 4. Pouring solution into sterile container.

(*continued*)

Skill 1-6 ▶ Adding Sterile Items to a Sterile Field *(continued)*

ACTION	RATIONALE

7. Continue with procedure as indicated.

 8. When procedure is completed, remove PPE, if used. Perform hand hygiene.

Proper removal of PPE reduces the risk for infection transmission and contamination of other items. Hand hygiene prevents the spread of microorganisms.

EVALUATION

The expected outcome to achieve when adding items to a sterile field have been met when the sterile field is created without contamination; the sterile supplies are not contaminated; and the patient remains free of exposure to pathogens.

DOCUMENTATION

It is not usually necessary to document the addition of sterile items to a sterile field. However, document the use of performing sterile technique for any procedure.

UNEXPECTED SITUATIONS AND ASSOCIATED INTERVENTIONS

- *The item being added falls close to or on the edge of the field:* Consider the outer 1-in edge of a sterile field to be contaminated. Any item within the outer 1-in is considered contaminated.
- *A part of the sterile field becomes contaminated:* When any portion of the sterile field becomes contaminated, discard the sterile field and any items on the field and start over.
- *The nurse realizes a supply is missing after setting up the sterile field:* Call for help. Do not leave the sterile field unattended. If you are unable to visualize the sterile field at all times, it is considered contaminated.
- *The patient touches the sterile field:* If the patient touches the sterile field, discard the supplies and prepare a new sterile field. If the patient is confused, have someone assist by holding the patient's hands and/or reinforcing what is happening.

EVIDENCE FOR PRACTICE ▶

SIMULATION-BASED TRAINING AND STERILE TECHNIQUE
Use of strict sterile technique is critical to prevent contamination and possible infection. Nurses routinely provide care interventions that require the use of sterile technique. They also play a key role in assisting and monitoring implementation of sterile technique as part of patient care interventions by other health care practitioners. Do nurses have adequate knowledge of the steps in sterile technique?

Related Research
Gerolemou, L., Fidellaga, A., Rose, K., et al. (2014). Simulation-based training for nurses in sterile techniques during central vein catheterization. *American Journal of Critical Care,* *23*(1), 40–48.

Refer to details in Skill 1-4, Evidence for Practice, and to thePoint° for additional research on related nursing topics.

Skill 1-7 ▶ Putting on Sterile Gloves and Removing Soiled Gloves

When applying and wearing sterile gloves, keep hands above waist level and away from nonsterile surfaces. Replace gloves if they develop an opening or tear; the integrity of the material becomes compromised; or the gloves come in contact with any nonsterile surface or nonsterile item. Refer to Fundamentals Review 1-2 for additional guidelines related to working with sterile gloves. It is a good idea to bring an extra pair of gloves with you when gathering supplies, according to facility policy. That way, if the first pair is contaminated in some way and needs to be replaced, you will not have to leave the procedure to get a new pair.

DELEGATION CONSIDERATIONS	Procedures requiring the use of sterile gloves and other sterile items are not delegated to nursing assistive personnel (NAP) or unlicensed assistive personnel (UAP). Depending on the state's nurse practice act and the organization's policies and procedures, these procedures may be delegated to licensed practical/vocational nurses (LPN/LVNs). The decision to delegate must be based on careful analysis of the patient's needs and circumstances, as well as the qualifications of the person to whom the task is being delegated. Refer to the Delegation Guidelines in Appendix A.
EQUIPMENT	• Sterile gloves of the appropriate size • PPE, as indicated
ASSESSMENT	Assess the situation to determine the necessity for sterile gloves. In addition, check the patient's medical record for information about a possible latex allergy. Also, question the patient about any history of allergy, including latex allergy, or sensitivity and signs and symptoms that have occurred. If the patient has a latex allergy, anticipate the need for latex-free gloves.
NURSING DIAGNOSIS	Determine the related factors for the nursing diagnoses based on the patient's current status. Appropriate nursing diagnoses may include: • Risk for infection • Ineffective protection • Risk for latex allergy reaction
OUTCOME IDENTIFICATION AND PLANNING	The expected outcome to achieve when putting on and removing sterile gloves is that the gloves are applied and removed without contamination. Other outcomes that may be appropriate include: the patient remains free of exposure to infectious microorganisms; and the patient does not exhibit signs and symptoms of a latex allergy response.

IMPLEMENTATION

ACTION	RATIONALE
1. Perform hand hygiene and put on PPE, if indicated.	Hand hygiene and PPE prevent the spread of microorganisms. PPE is required based on transmission precautions.
2. Identify the patient. Explain the procedure to the patient.	Patient identification validates the correct patient and correct procedure. Discussion and explanation help allay anxiety and prepare the patient for what to expect.
3. Check that the sterile glove package is dry and unopened. Also note expiration date, making sure that the date is still valid.	Moisture contaminates a sterile package. Expiration date indicates the period that the package remains sterile.

(continued)

Skill 1-7 ▶ Putting on Sterile Gloves and Removing Soiled Gloves *(continued)*

ACTION	RATIONALE
4. Place sterile glove package on clean, dry surface at or above your waist.	Moisture could contaminate the sterile gloves. Any sterile object held below the waist is considered contaminated.
5. Open the outside wrapper by carefully peeling the top layer back (Figure 1). Remove inner package, handling only the outside of it.	This maintains sterility of gloves in inner packet.
6. Place the inner package on the work surface with the side labeled "cuff end" closest to the body.	Allows for ease of glove application.
7. Carefully open the inner package. Fold open the top flap, then the bottom and sides (Figure 2). **Do not touch the inner surface of the package or the gloves.**	The inner surface of the package is considered sterile. The outer 1-in border of the inner package is considered contaminated. The sterile gloves are exposed with the cuff end closest to the nurse.

FIGURE 1. Pulling top layer of outside wrapper back.

FIGURE 2. Folding back side flaps.

8. With the thumb and forefinger of the nondominant hand, grasp the folded cuff of the glove for the dominant hand, touching only the exposed inside of the glove (Figure 3).	Unsterile hand touches only inside of glove. Outside remains sterile.
9. Keeping the hands above the waistline, lift and hold the glove up and off the inner package with fingers down (Figure 4). **Do not let it touch any unsterile object.**	Glove is contaminated if it touches any unsterile objects.

FIGURE 3. Grasping cuff of glove for dominant hand.

FIGURE 4. Lifting glove from package.

ACTION

10. Carefully insert dominant hand palm up into glove (Figure 5) and pull glove on. Leave the cuff folded until the opposite hand is gloved.

11. Hold the thumb of the gloved hand outward. Place the fingers of the gloved hand inside the cuff of the remaining glove (Figure 6). Lift it from the wrapper, taking care not to touch anything with the gloves or hands.

RATIONALE

Attempting to turn upward with unsterile hand may result in contamination of sterile glove.

Thumb is less likely to become contaminated if held outward. Sterile surface touching sterile surface prevents contamination.

FIGURE 5. Inserting dominant hand into glove.

FIGURE 6. Sliding fingers under cuff of glove for nondominant hand.

12. Carefully insert nondominant hand into glove. Pull the glove on, taking care that the skin does not touch any of the outer surfaces of the gloves.

13. **Slide the fingers of one hand under the cuff of the other and fully extend the cuff down the arm, touching only the sterile outside of the glove (Figure 7). Repeat for the remaining hand.**

14. **Adjust gloves on both hands, if necessary, touching only sterile areas with other sterile areas (Figure 8).**

15. Continue with procedure as indicated.

Sterile surface touching sterile surface prevents contamination.

Sterile surface touching sterile surface prevents contamination.

Sterile surface touching sterile surface prevents contamination.

FIGURE 7. Sliding fingers of one hand under cuff of other hand and extending cuff down the arm.

FIGURE 8. Adjusting gloves as necessary.

(*continued*)

Skill 1-7 ▶ Putting on Sterile Gloves and Removing Soiled Gloves (continued)

ACTION	**RATIONALE**

Removing Soiled Gloves

16. Use dominant hand to grasp the opposite glove **near cuff end on the outside exposed area.** Remove it by pulling it off, inverting it as it is pulled, keeping the contaminated area on the inside (Figure 9). Hold the removed glove in the remaining gloved hand.

Contaminated area does not come in contact with hands or wrists.

FIGURE 9. Inverting glove as it is removed.

17. Slide fingers of ungloved hand between the remaining glove and the wrist (Figure 10). **Take care to avoid touching the outside surface of the glove.** Remove it by pulling it off, inverting it as it is pulled, keeping the contaminated area on the inside, and securing the first glove inside the second (Figure 11).

Contaminated area does not come in contact with hands or wrists.

 18. Discard gloves in appropriate container. Remove additional PPE, if used. Perform hand hygiene.

Proper removal and disposal of PPE reduces the risk for infection transmission and contamination of other items. Hand hygiene prevents the spread of microorganisms.

FIGURE 10. Sliding fingers of ungloved hand inside remaining glove.

FIGURE 11. Inverting glove as it is removed, securing first glove inside it.

EVALUATION	The expected outcome has been met when gloves are applied and removed without contamination. Other expected outcomes are met when the patient remains free of exposure to pathogens, and does not exhibit signs and symptoms of a latex allergy response.
DOCUMENTATION	It is not usually necessary to document the application and removal of sterile gloves. However, document the use of sterile technique for any procedure performed using sterile technique.
UNEXPECTED SITUATIONS AND ASSOCIATED INTERVENTIONS	• *Contamination occurs during application of the sterile gloves:* Discard gloves and open new package of sterile gloves. • *A hole or tear is noticed in one of the gloves:* Discard gloves and open a new package of sterile gloves. • *A hole or tear is noticed in one of the gloves during the procedure:* Stop procedure. Remove damaged gloves. Wash hands or perform hand hygiene (depending on whether soiled or not) and put on new sterile gloves. • *The patient touches the nurse's hands or the sterile field:* If the patient touches your hands and nothing else, you may remove the contaminated gloves and put on new, sterile gloves. It is a good idea to bring two pairs of sterile gloves into the room, depending on facility policy. If the patient touches the sterile field, discard the supplies and prepare a new sterile field. If the patient is confused, have someone assist you by holding the patient's hands or reinforcing what is happening. • *Patient has a latex allergy:* Obtain latex-free sterile gloves.

EVIDENCE FOR PRACTICE ▶

PPE AND PREVENTION OF TRANSFER OF MICROORGANISMS

Prevention of health care–associated infections is a major challenge for health care providers. The removal of PPE after patient care may result in transfer of microorganisms to the skin and clothing of health care workers, contributing to the transfer of microorganisms and increased risk of infection. How can this risk of transfer be reduced?

Related Research

Tomas, M. E., Kundrapu, S., Thota, P., et al. (2015). Contamination of health care personnel during removal of personal protective equipment. *JAMA Internal Medicine, 175*(12), 1904–1910.

Refer to details in Skill 1-3, Evidence for Practice, and to thePoint® for additional research on related nursing topics.

EVIDENCE FOR PRACTICE ▶

SIMULATION-BASED TRAINING AND STERILE TECHNIQUE

Use of strict sterile technique is critical to prevent contamination and possible infection. Nurses routinely provide care interventions that require the use of sterile technique. They also play a key role in assisting and monitoring implementation of sterile technique as part of patient care interventions by other health care practitioners. Do nurses have adequate knowledge of the steps in sterile technique?

Related Research

Gerolemou, L., Fidellaga, A., Rose, K., et al. (2014). Simulation-based training for nurses in sterile techniques during central vein catheterization. *American Journal of Critical Care, 23*(1), 40–48.

Refer to details in Skill 1-4, Evidence for Practice, and to thePoint® for additional research on related nursing topics.

Enhance Your Understanding

Focusing on Patient Care: Developing Clinical Reasoning

Consider the case scenarios at the beginning of the chapter as you answer the following questions to enhance your understanding and apply what you have learned.

QUESTIONS

1. While preparing the sterile table in the cardiac catheterization lab for Mr. Wilson, you realize that a sterile bowl is missing. How can you obtain a sterile bowl?

2. While you are putting on sterile gloves in preparation for an indwelling urinary catheter insertion, your patient, Sheri Lawrence, moves her leg. You do not think that Sheri's leg touched the glove, but you are not positive. What should you do?

3. Edgar Barowski's son is visiting and asks you why the masks that are outside Edgar's room are different from the ones that people wear in the operating room. What should you tell Edgar's son?

You can find suggested answers after the Bibliography at the end of this chapter.

Integrated Case Study Connection

The case studies in the back of the book focus on integrating concepts. Refer to the following case studies to enhance your understanding of the concepts and skills in this chapter.

- Basic Case Studies: Tiffany Jones, page 1100; John Willis, page 1104.
- Intermediate Case Studies: Tula Stillwater, page 1117; Gwen Galloway, page 1125; George Patel, page 1126.

Taylor Suite Resources

Explore these additional resources to enhance learning for this chapter:

- NCLEX-Style Questions and other resources on thePoint*, http://thePoint.lww.com/Lynn5e
- *Skill Checklists for Taylor's Clinical Nursing Skills*, 5e
- *Taylor's Video Guide to Clinical Nursing Skills*: Asepsis
- *Fundamentals of Nursing*: Chapter 24, Asepsis and Infection Control

Bibliography

Agency for Healthcare Research and Quality (AHRQ). (2015). *AHRQ's healthcare-associated infections program.* Retrieved http://www.ahrq.gov/professionals/quality-patient-safety/hais/index.html

Akpaka, C. C. (2014). Best practices for hand hygiene compliance by health care providers in the inpatient setting. *American Journal of Infectious Diseases, 10*(2), 84–87.

Allegranzi, B., Memish, Z. A., Donaldson, L., Pittet, D.; World Health Organization Global Patient Safety Challenge Task Force on Religious and Cultural Aspects of Hand Hygiene; World Alliance for Patient Safety. (2009). Religion and culture: Potential undercurrents influencing hand hygiene promotion in health care. *American Journal of Infection Control, 37*(1), 28–34.

Ardizzone, L. L., Smolowitz, J., Kline, N., Thom, B., & Larson, E. L. (2013). Patient hand hygiene practices in surgical patients. *American Journal of Infection Control, 41*(6), 487–491.

Association for Professionals in Infection Control and Epidemiology (APIC). (2010). *Guide to the elimination of methicillin-resistant Staphylococcus aureus (MRSA) transmission in hospital settings* (2nd ed.). Washington, DC: Author. Retrieved http://www.apic.org/Resource_/EliminationGuideForm/631fcd91-8773-4067-9f85-ab2a5b157eab/File/MRSA-elimination-guide-2010.pdf

Association for Professionals in Infection Control and Epidemiology (APIC). (2015). *Guide to hand hygiene programs for infection prevention.* Retrieved http://apic.org/Professional-Practice/Implementation-guides#HandHygiene

Association of periOperative Registered Nurses (AORN). (2015). *Perioperative standards and recommended practices.* Denver, CO: AORN, Inc.

Busby, S. R., Kennedy, B., Davis, S. C., Thompson, H. A., & Jones, J. W. (2015). Assessing patient awareness of proper hand hygiene. *Nursing, 45*(5), 27–30.

Buser, G. L., Fisher, B. T., Shea, J. A., & Coffin, S. E. (2013). Parent willingness to remind health care workers to perform hand hygiene. *American Journal of Infection Control, 41*(6), 492–496.

Centers for Disease Control and Prevention. (2002). Guidelines for hand hygiene in health-care settings. *Morbidity and Mortality Weekly Report, 51*(RR-16), 1–45. Retrieved http://www.cdc.gov/mmwr/PDF/rr/rr5116.pdf

Centers for Disease Control and Prevention (CDC). (2007a). *Part III.B.3. Airborne precautions. 2007 Guideline for isolation precautions: Preventing transmission of infectious agents in healthcare settings. [Excerpt].* Retrieved http://www.cdc.gov/hicpac/pdf/isolation/Isolation2007.pdf

Centers for Disease Control and Prevention (CDC). (2007b). *Part III.B.1. Contact precautions. 2007 Guideline for isolation precautions: Preventing transmission of infectious agents in healthcare settings. [Excerpt].* Retrieved http://www.cdc.gov/hicpac/pdf/isolation/Isolation2007.pdf

Centers for Disease Control and Prevention (CDC). (2007c). *Part III.B.2. Droplet precautions. 2007 Guideline for isolation precautions: Preventing transmission of infectious agents in healthcare settings. [Excerpt].* Retrieved http://www.cdc.gov/hicpac/pdf/isolation/Isolation2007.pdf

Centers for Disease Control and Prevention (CDC). (2007d). *Part III.A.1. New elements of standard precautions. 2007 Guideline for isolation precautions: Preventing transmission of infectious agents in healthcare settings. [Excerpt].* Retrieved http://www.cdc.gov/hicpac/pdf/isolation/Isolation2007.pdf

Centers for Disease Control and Prevention (CDC). (2007e). *Part II.E. Personal protective equipment (PPE) for healthcare personnel. 2007 Guideline for isolation precautions: Preventing transmission of infectious agents in healthcare settings. [Excerpt].* Retrieved http://www.cdc.gov/hicpac/pdf/isolation/Isolation2007.pdf

Centers for Disease Control and Prevention (CDC). (2014a). Sequence for putting on and removing personal protective equipment (PPE). [Poster]. Retrieved from http://www.cdc.gov/hai/pdfs/ppe/PPE-Sequence.pdf

Centers for Disease Control and Prevention (CDC). (2014b). *Guidance for the selection and use of personal protective equipment (PPE) in healthcare settings.* Retrieved http://www.cdc.gov/HAI/pdfs/ppe/PPEslides6-29-04.pdf

Centers for Disease Control and Prevention (CDC). (2015a). *Hand hygiene in healthcare settings.* Retrieved http://www.cdc.gov/handhygiene

Centers for Disease Control and Prevention (CDC). (2015b). *Guidance on personal protective equipment (PPE) to be used by healthcare workers during management of patients with confirmed Ebola or persons under investigation (PUIs) for Ebola who are clinically unstable or have bleeding, vomiting, or diarrhea in U.S. hospitals, including procedures for donning and doffing PPE.* Retrieved http://www.cdc.gov/vhf/ebola/healthcare-us/ppe/guidance.html

Chassin, M. R., Mayer, C., & Nether, K. (2015). Improving hand hygiene at eight hospitals in the United States by targeting specific causes of noncompliance. *The Joint Commission Journal on Quality and Patient Safety, 41*(1), 1–12. Retrieved http://www.centerfortransforminghealthcare.org/assets/4/6/JQPS_Jan2015_Chassin.pdf

D'Alesandro, M. A. (2015). Avoiding common breaks in sterile technique. *OR Nurse, 9*(5), 12–13.

Doenges, M. E., Moorhouse, M. F., & Murr, A. (2016). *Nursing diagnoses manual. Planning, individualizing, and documenting client care* (5th ed.). Philadelphia, PA: F.A. Davis Company.

Eaves, K., Thornton, J., & Chapman, A. L. (2013). Patient retention of training in self-administration of intravenous antibiotic therapy in an outpatient parenteral antibiotic therapy service. *Journal of Clinical Nursing, 23*(9–10), 1318–1322.

Fox, C., Wavra, T., Ash Drake, D., et al. (2015). Use of a patient hand hygiene protocol to reduce hospital-acquired infections and improve nurses' hand washing. *American Journal of Critical Care, 24*(3), 216–224.

Gerolemou, L., Fidellaga, A., Rose, K., et al. (2014). Simulation-based training for nurses in sterile techniques during central vein catheterization. *American Journal of Critical Care, 23*(1), 40–48.

Ghezeljeh, T. N., Abbasnejad, Z., Rafii, F., & Haghani, H. (2015). Effect of a multimodal training program and traditional lecture method on nurses' hand hygiene knowledge, belief, and practice: A brief report. *American Journal of Infection Control, 43*(7), 762–764.

Grossman, S., & Porth, C. M. (2014). *Porth's pathophysiology: Concepts of altered health states* (9th ed.). Philadelphia, PA: Wolters Kluwer Health.

Healthy People 2020. (n.d.). *Healthcare-associated infections.* Retrieved http://www.healthypeople.gov/2020/topics-objectives/topic/healthcare-associated-infections?topicid=17

Hinkle, J. L., & Cheever, K. H. (2014). *Brunner & Suddarth's textbook of medical-surgical nursing* (13th ed.). Philadelphia, PA: Wolters Kluwer Health.

Institute for Healthcare Improvement (IHI). (2006). *How-to guide: Improving hand hygiene.* Retrieved http://www.ihi.org/resources/Pages/Tools/HowtoGuideImprovingHandHygiene.aspx

Jabbar, U., Leischner, J., Kasper, D., et al. (2010). Effectiveness of alcohol-based hand rubs for removal of Clostridium difficile spores from hands. *Infection Control & Hospital Epidemiology, 31*(6), 565–570.

Johnson, L., Grueber, S., Schlotzhauer, C., et al. (2014). A multifactorial action plan improves hand hygiene adherence and significantly reduces central line-associated bloodstream infections. *American Journal of Infection Control, 42*(11), 1146–1151.

The Joint Commission. (2018a). *National patient safety goals. Hospital: 2018 National patient safety goals.* Retrieved http://www.jointcommission.org/standards_information.aspx

The Joint Commission. (2018b). National patient safety goals. Hospital: 2018 National patient safety goals. NPSG.07.01.01. Retrieved https://www.jointcommission.org/assets/1/6/2018_HAP_NPSG_goals_final.pdf

The Joint Commission Center for Transforming Healthcare. (2014). *Facts about the hand hygiene project.* Retrieved http://www.centerfortransforminghealthcare.org/assets/4/6/CTH_HH_Fact_Sheet.pdf

NANDA International, Inc.: Nursing Diagnoses - Definitions and Classification 2018–2020 © 2017 NANDA International, ISBN 978-1-62623-929-6. Used by arrangement with the Thieme Group, Stuttgart/New York.

O'Donnell, M., Harris, T., Horn, T., et al. (2015). Sustained increase in resident meal time hand hygiene through an interdisciplinary intervention engaging long-term care facility residents and staff. *American Journal of Infection Control, 43*(2), 162–164.

Office of Disease Prevention and Health Promotion. (n.d.). *Health care-associated infections (HAIs): National action plan to prevent health care-associated infections: Road map to elimination.* Retrieved http://health.gov/hcq/prevent-hai.asp

Spruce, L. (2013). Back to basics: Hand hygiene and surgical hand antisepsis. *AORN Journal, 98*(5),449–457.

Sunkesula, V. C., Knighton, S., Zabarsky, T. F., Kundrapu, S., Higgins, P. A., & Donskey, C. J. (2015). Four moments for patient hand hygiene: A patient-centered, provider-facilitated model to improve patient hand hygiene. *Infection Control & Hospital Epidemiology, 36*(8), 986–989.

Tamimi, A. H., Maxwell, S., Edmonds, S. L., & Gerba, C. P. (2015). Impact of the use of an alcohol-based hand sanitizer in the home on reduction in probability of infection by respiratory and enteric viruses. *Epidemiology & Infection, 143*(15), 3335–3341.

Taylor, C., Lynn, P., & Bartlett, J. (2019). *Fundamentals of nursing: The art and science of person-centered care* (9th ed.). Philadelphia, PA: Wolters Kluwer.

Tomas, M. E., Kundrapu, S., Thota, P., et al. (2015). Contamination of health care personnel during removal of personal protective equipment. *JAMA Internal Medicine, 175*(12), 1904–1910.

U.S. Food & Drug Administration (FDA). (2016). *FDA issues final rule on safety and effectiveness of antibacterial soaps.* Retrieved http://www.fda.gov/NewsEvents/Newsroom/PressAnnouncements/ucm517478.htm

Walker, B. W. (2007). New guidelines for fighting multidrug-resistant organisms. *Nursing, 37*(5), 20.

World Health Organization. (2009). *Save lives: Clean your hands.* Retrieved http://www.who.int/gpsc/5may/en

Wyeth, J. (2013). Hand hygiene and the use of personal protective equipment. *British Journal of Nursing, 22*(16), 920–925.

SUGGESTED ANSWERS FOR FOCUSING ON PATIENT CARE: DEVELOPING CLINICAL REASONING

1. You should call for or ask another staff member to obtain the bowl. Never walk away from or turn your back on a sterile field. This prevents possible contamination while the field is out of your view.

2. You should change gloves. Only a sterile object can touch another sterile object. Nonsterile touching sterile means contamination has occurred. Consider an object contaminated if you have any doubt about its sterility.

3. You should explain the rationale for transmission-based precautions, including specific information about airborne precautions. Airborne precautions are used for patients who have infections that spread through the air, such as tuberculosis, varicella (chicken pox), rubeola (measles), and possibly SARS. Place patient in a private room that has monitored negative air pressure in relation to surrounding areas, 6 to 12 air changes per hour, and appropriate discharge of air outside or monitored filtration if air is recirculated. Keep door closed and patient in room.

Vital Signs

2

Focusing on Patient Care

This chapter will explain some of the skills related to vital signs necessary to care for the following patients:

Tyrone Jeffries, age 5, is in the emergency department with a temperature of 101.3°F (38.9°C).

Toby White, age 26, has a history of asthma and is now breathing 32 times per minute.

Carl Glatz, age 58, has recently started taking medications to control his hypertension (high blood pressure).

Refer to Focusing on Patient Care: Developing Clinical Reasoning at the end of the chapter to apply what you learn.

Learning Objectives

After completing the chapter, you will be able to accomplish the following:

1. Assess body temperature via the oral, tympanic, temporal, axillary, and rectal routes.
2. Regulate an infant's temperature using an overhead radiant warmer.
3. Regulate temperature using a hypothermia blanket.
4. Assess peripheral pulses by palpation.
5. Assess an apical pulse by auscultation.
6. Assess peripheral pulses using Doppler ultrasound.
7. Assess respiration.
8. Assess blood pressure by auscultation or using an automatic electronic blood pressure monitor.
9. Assess systolic blood pressure using Doppler ultrasound.

Key Terms

apnea: absence of breathing

bell: (of stethoscope) hollowed, upright, curved portion used to auscultate low-pitched sounds, such as murmurs

blood pressure: force of blood against arterial walls

bradypnea: abnormally slow rate of breathing

diaphragm: (of stethoscope) large, flat disk on the stethoscope used to auscultate high-pitched sounds, such as respiratory sounds

diastolic pressure: least amount of pressure exerted on arterial walls, which occurs when the heart is at rest between ventricular contractions

expiration: act of breathing out; synonym is exhalation

febrile: a condition in which the body temperature is elevated

hypertension: blood pressure elevated above the upper limit of normal

hypotension: blood pressure below the lower limit of normal

hypothermia: body temperature below the lower limit of normal

inspiration: act of breathing in; synonym is inhalation

Korotkoff sounds: series of sounds that correspond to changes in blood flow through an artery as pressure is released

orthopnea: a condition in which people with dyspnea can often breath more easily in an upright position

orthostatic hypotension: temporary fall in blood pressure associated with assuming an upright position; synonym for postural hypotension

pulse (peripheral): a throbbing sensation that can be palpated (felt) over a peripheral artery, such as the radial artery or the carotid artery

pulse pressure: the difference between the systolic and diastolic blood pressures

respiration: act of breathing and using oxygen in body cells

systolic pressure: highest point of pressure on arterial walls when the ventricles contract

tachypnea: abnormally rapid rate of breathing

temperature: the difference between the amount of heat produced by the body and the amount of heat lost to the environment measured in degrees

vital signs: indicators of physiologic functioning; body temperature, pulse, respiratory rates, and blood pressure

Vital signs are indicators of physiologic functioning and include a person's temperature, pulse, respiration, and blood pressure, abbreviated as T, P, R, and BP. The health status of a person is reflected in these indicators of body function. A change in vital signs may indicate a change in health. Pain assessment is often included along with measurement of vital signs and is discussed in Chapter 10. Pulse oximetry, the noninvasive measurement of arterial oxyhemoglobin saturation of arterial blood, is also often included with the measurement of vital signs and is discussed in Chapter 14.

Vital signs are assessed and compared with accepted normal values and the patient's usual patterns in a wide variety of instances. Examples of appropriate times to measure vital signs include, but are not limited to, screenings at health fairs and clinics, in the home, upon admission to a health care setting, when medications are given that may affect one of the vital signs, before and after invasive diagnostic and surgical procedures, and in emergency situations. Nurses take vital signs as often as the condition of a patient requires such assessment, prioritizing and adapting assessment of vital signs to address the patient's unique situation. Frequency of assessment should be based on the patient's medical diagnosis, comorbidities, types of treatments received, and the patient's level of acuity (Burchill, Anderson, & O'Connor, 2015).

Although vital sign measurement may be delegated to other health care personnel when the condition of the patient is stable, it is the nurse's responsibility to ensure the accuracy of the data, interpret vital sign findings, and report abnormal findings. Principles of delegation should be followed (see Appendix A). If a patient has abnormal or unusual physical signs or symptoms (e.g., chest pain or dizziness) or has unexpected changes in vital signs, the nurse should validate the findings and further assess the patient. Techniques for measuring each of the vital signs are presented in this chapter. Fundamentals Review 2-1 outlines age-related variations in normal vital signs. Fundamentals Review 2-2 provides guidelines for obtaining vital signs for infants and children.

Fundamentals Review 2-1

AGE-RELATED VARIATIONS IN NORMAL VITAL SIGNS

Age	Temperature °C °F	Pulse beats/min	Respirations breaths/min	Blood Pressure mm Hg
Infants (temporal)	37.1–38.1 98.7–100.5	80–150	25–55	85/37
Toddler (temporal)	37.1–38.1 98.7–100.5	70–120	20–40	89/46
Child (tympanic)	36.8–37.8 98.2–100	60–100	15–25	95/57
Adolescent (oral)	35.8–37.5 96.4–99.5	55–95	12–18	102/61
Adult (oral)	35.8–37.5 96.4–99.5	60–100	12–20	120/80

Source: Adapted from Hogan-Quigley, B., Palm, M. L., & Bickley, L. S. (2017). *Bates' nursing guide to physical examination and history taking* (2nd ed.). Philadelphia, PA: Wolters Kluwer; Kyle, T., & Carman, S. (2017). *Essentials of pediatric nursing* (3rd ed.). Philadelphia, PA: Wolters Kluwer.

Fundamentals Review 2-2

TECHNIQUES FOR OBTAINING VITAL SIGNS OF INFANTS AND CHILDREN

- Due to the "fear factor" of blood pressure measurement, save the blood pressure measurement for last. Children and infants often begin to cry during blood pressure assessment, and this may affect the respiration and pulse rate assessment.
- Perform as many tasks as possible while the child is sitting on the parent's lap or in a chair next to the parent.
- Let the child see and touch the equipment before you begin to use it.

- Make measuring vital signs a game. For instance, if you are using a tympanic thermometer that makes a chirping sound, tell the child you are looking for "birdies" in the ear. While auscultating the pulse, tell the child you are listening for another type of animal.
- If the child has a doll or stuffed animal, pretend to take the doll's vital signs first.

Skill 2-1   ▶   Assessing Body Temperature

Body **temperature** is the difference between the amount of heat produced by the body and the amount of heat lost to the environment, measured in degrees. Heat is generated by metabolic processes in the core tissues of the body, transferred to the skin surface by the circulating blood, and then dissipated to the environment. Core body temperature (intracranial, intrathoracic, and intra-abdominal) is higher than surface body temperature. Normal body temperature is 35.9° to 38°C (96.7° to 100.5°F), depending on the route used for measurement (Jensen, 2015). There are individual variations of these temperatures as well as variations related to age, biological sex, physical activity, state of health, and environmental temperatures. Body temperature also varies during the day, with temperatures being lowest in the early morning and highest in the late afternoon (Grossman & Porth, 2014).

Health facility policies and procedures often specify the site to be used for assessing patients' temperatures. However, the nurse is expected to choose an appropriate site, and the correct equipment, based on the patient's condition, facility policy, and medical orders. Factors affecting the site selection include the patient's age, state of consciousness, amount of pain, and other care or treatments (e.g., oxygen administration) being provided.

Several types of equipment and different procedures might be used to measure body temperature. Different types of thermometers are illustrated in Figure 1. To obtain an accurate measurement, choose an appropriate site, the correct equipment, and the appropriate tool based on the patient's condition. If a temperature reading is obtained from a site other than the oral route, document the site used along with the measurement. If no site is listed with the documentation, it is generally assumed to be the oral route.

Although bulb-type glass thermometers containing liquids other than mercury are available, they should never be used to measure the temperature of a person who is unconscious or irrational, or of infants and young children, because the glass could break.

FIGURE 1. Types of thermometers. **A.** Electronic thermometer. **B.** Tympanic membrane thermometer. **C.** Disposable thermometer for measuring oral temperature; the dots change color to indicate temperature. **D.** Temporal artery thermometer. (Part **C** Timby, B. K. [2005]. *Fundamental nursing skills and concepts* [8th ed.]. Philadelphia, PA: Lippincott Williams & Wilkins.)

DELEGATION CONSIDERATIONS

Measurement of body temperature may be delegated to nursing assistive personnel (NAP) or to unlicensed assistive personnel (UAP), as well as to licensed practical/vocational nurses (LPN/ LVNs). The decision to delegate must be based on careful analysis of the patient's needs and circumstances, as well as the qualifications of the person to whom the task is being delegated. Refer to the Delegation Guidelines in Appendix A.

EQUIPMENT

- Digital or electronic thermometer, appropriate for site to be used
- Disposable probe covers
- Water-soluble lubricant for rectal temperature measurement
- Nonsterile gloves, if appropriate
- Additional personal protective equipment (PPE), as indicated
- Toilet tissue, if needed
- Electronic record, or a pen, paper or flow sheet

(continued)

Skill 2-1 ▶ Assessing Body Temperature *(continued)*

ASSESSMENT

Note baseline or previous temperature measurements. Assess the patient to ensure that his or her cognitive functioning is intact. When selecting the oral site, the patient must be able to close his or her mouth around the probe. Therefore, this site is not suitable for use in children less than 5 years old, in some children with developmental delay, in patients who are unable to follow directions, nor in patients who are confused or comatose (El-Radhi, 2013; Sund-Levander & Grodzinsky, 2013). If a patient has had either hot or cold food or fluids or has been smoking or chewing gum, the general recommendation is to wait 15 to 30 minutes to allow the oral tissues to return to normal temperature. Mouth breathing can influence the results (El-Radhi, 2013; Sund-Levander & Grodzinsky). Oral temperatures should not be taken in people with diseases of the oral cavity, in those who have had surgery of the nose or mouth, or when there is a risk of seizures (Sund-Levander & Grodzinsky). In addition, oral temperatures should not be assessed in patients receiving oxygen by mask, because the time it takes to assess a reading is likely to result in a serious drop in the patient's blood oxygen level. Oral temperature readings range from 36.5° to 37.5°C (97.7° to 99.5°F) (Jensen, 2015). The probe must remain in the sublingual pocket for the full period of measurement (El-Radhi, 2013; Davie & Amoore, 2010).

If a patient has an earache, do not use the affected ear to take a tympanic temperature. The movement of the tragus may cause severe discomfort. Assess the patient for significant ear drainage or a scarred tympanic membrane. These conditions can provide inaccurate results and could cause problems for the patient. However, an ear infection or the presence of earwax in the canal will not significantly affect a tympanic thermometer reading. If the patient has been sleeping with the head turned to one side, take a tympanic temperature in the other ear. Heat may be increased on the side that was against the pillow, especially if it is a plastic-covered pillow. Otherwise, either ear can be used. Tympanic temperature readings range from 36.8° to 37.8°C (98.2° to 100°F) (Jensen, 2015).

When taking a temporal artery temperature, assess for head coverings. Anything covering the area, such as a hat, hair, wigs, or bandages, would insulate the area, resulting in falsely high readings. If a patient is lying on his or her side, measure only the side of the head exposed to the environment. Do not measure temporal artery temperature over scar tissue, open lesions, or abrasions. Move the thermometer across the forehead slowly and remain in contact with the skin to ensure accurate results. Temporal artery temperature readings are more accurate than axillary temperature measurements (McConnell et al., 2013). Temporal artery temperature readings range from 37.1° to 38.1°C (98.7° to 100.5°F) (Jensen, 2015).

The axillary site may be used when both oral and rectal sites are contraindicated or when these sites are inaccessible, but should not be used where accurate temperature measurement is required (El-Radhi, 2013). Axillary readings are affected by ambient temperature, local blood flow, appropriate placement of the probe, and closure of the axillary cavity (Sund-Levander & Grodzinsky, 2013). Place the probe in the center of the axilla; hold the patient's arm by the patient's side until the measurement is complete. Axillary temperature readings range from 35.9° to 36.9°C (96.7° to 98.5°F) (Jensen, 2015).

The rectal site should not be used in newborns, children with diarrhea, nor in patients who have undergone rectal surgery or have a disease of the rectum. Because the insertion of the thermometer into the rectum can slow the heart rate by stimulating the vagus nerve, assessing a rectal temperature for patients with heart disease or after cardiac surgery may not be allowed in some institutions. In addition, assessing a rectal temperature is contraindicated in patients who are neutropenic (have low white blood cell counts, such as in leukemia) and in patients who have certain neurologic disorders (e.g., spinal cord injuries). Do not insert a rectal thermometer into a patient who has a low platelet count. The rectum is very vascular, and a thermometer could cause rectal bleeding. Rectal temperature readings range from 37.1° to 38.1°C (98.7° to 100.5°F) (Jensen, 2015).

NURSING DIAGNOSIS

Determine related factors for the nursing diagnoses based on the patient's current status. Appropriate nursing diagnoses may include:

- Hyperthermia
- Hypothermia
- Ineffective thermoregulation

OUTCOME IDENTIFICATION AND PLANNING	The expected outcomes to achieve when performing temperature assessment are that the patient's temperature is assessed accurately without injury and the patient experiences minimal discomfort. Other outcomes may be appropriate, depending on the patient's nursing diagnosis.

IMPLEMENTATION

ACTION	RATIONALE
1. Check the medical order or nursing care plan for frequency of measurement and route. More frequent temperature measurement may be appropriate based on nursing judgment.	Assessment and measurement of vital signs at appropriate intervals provide important data about the patient's health status.
2. Perform hand hygiene and put on PPE, if indicated.	Hand hygiene and PPE prevent the spread of microorganisms. PPE is required based on transmission precautions.
3. Identify the patient.	Identifying the patient ensures that the right patient receives the intervention and helps prevent errors.
4. Close the curtains around the bed and close the door to the room, if possible. Discuss the procedure with the patient and assess the patient's ability to assist with the procedure.	This ensures the patient's privacy. Explanation relieves anxiety and facilitates cooperation. Dialogue encourages patient participation and allows for individualized nursing care.
5. Assemble equipment on the overbed table within reach.	Organization facilitates performance of task.
6. Ensure that the electronic or digital thermometer is in working condition.	Improperly functioning thermometer may not give an accurate reading.
7. Put on gloves, if indicated.	Gloves prevent contact with blood and body fluids. Gloves are usually not required for an oral, axillary, or tympanic temperature measurement, unless contact with blood or body fluids is anticipated. Gloves should be worn for rectal temperature measurement.
8. Select the appropriate site based on assessment data.	This ensures safety and accuracy of measurement.
9. Follow the steps as outlined below for the appropriate type of thermometer.	
10. When measurement is completed, remove gloves, if worn. Remove additional PPE, if used. Perform hand hygiene.	Proper removal of PPE reduces the risk for infection transmission and contamination of other items. Hand hygiene prevents the spread of microorganisms.

Measuring an Oral Temperature

11. Remove the electronic unit from the charging unit, and remove the probe from within the recording unit.	Electronic unit must be taken into the patient's room to assess the patient's temperature. On some models, the machine is turned on when the probe is removed.

(continued)

Skill 2-1 ▶ Assessing Body Temperature *(continued)*

ACTION

12. Cover thermometer probe with disposable probe cover and slide it on until it snaps into place (Figure 2).

13. **Place the probe beneath the patient's tongue in the posterior sublingual pocket (Figure 3). Ask the patient to close his or her lips around the probe.**

FIGURE 2. Putting probe cover on the thermometer.

14. Continue to hold the probe until you hear a beep (Figure 4). Note the temperature reading.

15. Remove the probe from the patient's mouth. Dispose of the probe cover by holding the probe over an appropriate receptacle and pressing the probe-release button (Figure 5).

16. Return the thermometer probe to the storage place within the unit. Return the electronic unit to the charging unit, if appropriate.

FIGURE 4. Holding probe in the patient's mouth.

RATIONALE

Using a cover prevents contamination of the thermometer probe.

When the probe rests deep in the posterior sublingual pocket, it is in contact with blood vessels lying close to the surface.

FIGURE 3. Inserting thermometer under the tongue in the posterior sublingual pocket.

If left unsupported, the weight of the probe tends to pull it away from the correct location. The signal indicates that the measurement is completed. The electronic thermometer provides a digital display of the measured temperature.

Disposing of the probe cover ensures that it will not be reused accidentally on another patient. Proper disposal prevents spread of microorganisms.

The thermometer needs to be recharged for future use. If necessary, the thermometer should stay on the charger so that it is ready to use at all times.

FIGURE 5. Pushing button to dispose of cover.

ACTION

Measuring a Tympanic Membrane Temperature

17. If necessary, push the "ON" button and wait for the "ready" signal on the unit.

18. Attach the disposable cover onto the tympanic probe (Figure 6).

19. **Insert the probe snugly into the external ear using gentle but firm pressure, angling the thermometer toward the patient's jaw line (Figure 7). Pull the pinna up and back to straighten the ear canal in an adult.**

RATIONALE

For proper function, the thermometer must be turned on and warmed up.

Use of a disposable cover deters the spread of microorganisms.

If the probe is not inserted correctly, the patient's temperature may be noted as lower than normal.

FIGURE 6. Turning unit on and awaiting the ready signal.

FIGURE 7. Thermometer in patient's ear canal with pinna pulled up and back.

20. Activate the unit by pushing the trigger button. The reading is immediate (usually within 2 seconds). Note the reading.

21. Discard the probe cover in an appropriate receptacle by pushing the probe-release button or use the rim of cover to remove it from the probe (Figure 8). Replace the thermometer in its charger, if necessary.

The digital thermometer must be activated to record the temperature.

Discarding the probe cover ensures that it will not be reused accidentally on another patient. Proper disposal prevents the spread of microorganisms. If necessary, the thermometer should stay on the charger so that it is ready to use at all times.

FIGURE 8. Disposing of probe cover.

(continued)

Skill 2-1 ▶ Assessing Body Temperature *(continued)*

ACTION

RATIONALE

Measuring Temporal Artery Temperature

22. Brush the patient's hair aside if it is covering the temporal artery area.

Anything covering the area—such as a hat, hair, wigs, or bandages—would insulate the area, resulting in falsely high readings. Measure only the side of the head exposed to the environment.

23. Apply a probe cover.

Using a cover prevents contamination of the thermometer probe.

24. Hold the thermometer like a remote control device, with your thumb on the red "ON" button. Place the probe flush on the center of the forehead, with the body of the instrument sideways (not straight up and down) so that it is not in the patient's face (Figure 9).

Allows for easy use of the device and reading of the display. Holding the instrument straight up and down could be intimidating for the patient, particularly young patients and/or those with alterations in mental status.

25. Depress the "ON" button. Keep the button depressed throughout the measurement.

26. Slowly slide the probe straight across the forehead, midline, to the hairline (Figure 10). The thermometer will click; fast clicking indicates a rise to a higher temperature, slow clicking indicates that the instrument is still scanning, but not finding any higher temperature.

Midline on the forehead, the temporal artery is less than 2 mm below the skin; whereas at the side of the face, the temporal artery is much deeper. Measuring there would result in falsely low readings.

FIGURE 9. Placing the thermometer probe on the center of the forehead.

FIGURE 10. Sliding the probe across the forehead to the hairline.

27. If required, based on specific thermometer in use, brush hair aside if it is covering the ear, exposing the area of the neck under the ear lobe. Lift the probe from the forehead and touch on the neck just behind the ear lobe, in the depression just below the mastoid (Figure 11).

Sweat causes evaporative cooling of the skin on the forehead, possibly leading to a falsely low reading. During diaphoresis, the area on the head behind the ear lobe exhibits high blood flow necessary for the arterial measurement; it is a double check for the thermometer (Exergen, 2007; update 2014).

FIGURE 11. Touching the probe behind the ear.

ACTION

28. Release the button and read the thermometer measurement.

29. Hold the thermometer over a waste receptacle. Gently push the probe cover with your thumb against the proximal edge to dispose of the probe cover.

30. The instrument will automatically turn off in 30 seconds, or press and release the power button.

Measuring Axillary Temperature

31. Move the patient's clothing to expose only the axilla (Figure 12).

32. Remove the probe from the recording unit of the electronic thermometer. Place a disposable probe cover on by sliding it on and snapping it securely.

33. **Place the end of the probe in the center of the axilla (Figure 13). Have the patient bring the arm down and close to the body.**

FIGURE 12. Exposing axilla to assess temperature.

34. Hold the probe in place until you hear a beep, and then carefully remove the probe. Note the temperature reading.

35. Cover the patient and help him or her to a position of comfort.

36. Dispose of the probe cover by holding the probe over an appropriate waste receptacle and pushing the release button.

37. Place the bed in the lowest position and elevate rails, as needed. Leave the patient clean and comfortable.

38. Return the electronic thermometer to the charging unit.

Measuring Rectal Temperature

39. Adjust the bed to a comfortable working height, usually elbow height of the caregiver (VHACEOSH, 2016). Put on nonsterile gloves.

40. Assist the patient to a side-lying position. Pull back the covers sufficiently to expose only the buttocks.

RATIONALE

Discarding the probe cover ensures that it will not be reused accidentally on another patient.

Turns thermometer off.

The axilla must be exposed for placement of the thermometer. Exposing only the axilla keeps the patient warm and maintains his or her dignity.

Using a cover prevents contamination of the thermometer probe.

The deepest area of the axilla provides the most accurate measurement; surrounding the bulb with skin surface provides a more reliable measurement.

FIGURE 13. Placing thermometer in the center of the axilla.

Axillary thermometers must be held in place to obtain an accurate temperature.

Ensures patient comfort.

Discarding the probe cover ensures that it will not be reused accidentally on another patient.

Low bed position and elevated side rails provide for patient safety.

Thermometer needs to be recharged for future use.

Having the bed at the proper height prevents back and muscle strain. Gloves prevent contact with contaminants and body fluids.

The side-lying position allows the nurse to see the buttocks. Exposing only the buttocks keeps the patient warm and maintains his or her dignity.

(continued)

Skill 2-1 ▶ Assessing Body Temperature *(continued)*

ACTION	**RATIONALE**

41. Remove the rectal probe from within the recording unit of the electronic thermometer. Cover the probe with a disposable probe cover and slide it until it snaps in place (Figure 14).

Using a cover prevents contamination of the thermometer.

42. **Lubricate about 1 in of the probe with a water-soluble lubricant (Figure 15).**

Lubrication reduces friction and facilitates insertion, minimizing the risk of irritation or injury to the rectal mucous membranes.

FIGURE 14. Removing appropriate probe and attaching disposable probe cover.

FIGURE 15. Lubricating thermometer tip.

43. Reassure the patient. Separate the buttocks until the anal sphincter is clearly visible.

If not placed directly into the anal opening, the thermometer probe may injure adjacent tissue or cause discomfort.

44. **Insert the thermometer probe into the anus about 1.5 in in an adult or no more than 1 in in a child (Figure 16).**

Depth of insertion must be adjusted based on the patient's age. Rectal temperatures are not normally taken in an infant, but may be indicated. Refer to the Special Considerations section at the end of the skill.

FIGURE 16. Inserting thermometer into the anus.

45. Hold the probe in place until you hear a beep, then carefully remove the probe. Note the temperature reading on the display.

If left unsupported, movement of the probe in the rectum could cause injury and/or discomfort. The signal indicates that the measurement is completed. The electronic thermometer provides a digital display of the measured temperature.

ACTION	**RATIONALE**
46. Dispose of the probe cover by holding the probe over an appropriate waste receptacle and pressing the release button.	Proper probe cover disposal reduces risk of microorganism transmission.
47. Using toilet tissue, wipe the anus of any feces or excess lubricant. Dispose of the toilet tissue. Remove gloves and discard them.	Wiping promotes cleanliness. Disposing of the toilet tissue avoids transmission of microorganisms.
48. Cover the patient and help him or her to a position of comfort.	Ensures patient comfort.
49. Place the bed in the lowest position; elevate rails as needed.	These actions provide for the patient's safety.
50. Perform hand hygiene.	Hand hygiene prevents the spread of microorganisms.
51. Return the thermometer to the charging unit.	The thermometer needs to be recharged for future use.

EVALUATION

The expected outcomes have been met when the patient's temperature has been assessed accurately without injury and the patient has experienced minimal discomfort.

DOCUMENTATION

Guidelines

Record temperature in electronic record or flow sheet. Report abnormal findings to the appropriate person. Identify the site of assessment used if other than oral.

Sample Documentation

DocuCare Practice documenting body temperature and other vital signs in *Lippincott DocuCare*.

10/20/20 Tympanic temperature assessed. Temperature 102.5°F. Patient states she has "a pounding" headache; denies chills, malaise. Physician notified. Received order to give 650 mg PO acetaminophen now. Incentive spirometer × 10 q 2 hours.
—*M. Evans, RN*

UNEXPECTED SITUATIONS AND ASSOCIATED INTERVENTIONS

- *Temperature reading is higher or lower than expected based on your assessment:* Reassess temperature with a different thermometer. The thermometer may not be calibrated correctly. If using a tympanic thermometer, you will get lower readings if the probe is not inserted far enough into the ear.
- *During rectal temperature assessment, the patient reports feeling light-headed or passes out:* Remove the thermometer immediately. Quickly assess the patient's **blood pressure** and heart rate. Notify the health care provider. Do not attempt to take another rectal temperature on this patient.

SPECIAL CONSIDERATIONS

General Considerations

- If the patient smoked, chewed gum, or consumed hot or cold food or fluids recently, wait 30 minutes before taking an oral temperature to allow the oral tissues to return to baseline temperature.
- Nasal oxygen is not thought to affect oral temperature readings. Do not assess oral temperatures in patients receiving oxygen by mask. Removal of the mask for the time period required for assessment could result in a serious drop in the patient's blood oxygen level.
- When using a tympanic thermometer, make sure to insert the probe into the ear canal sufficiently tightly to seal the opening to ensure an accurate reading.
- A dirty probe lens and cone on the temporal artery thermometer can cause a falsely low reading. If the lens is not shiny in appearance, clean the lens and cone with an alcohol preparation or swab moistened in alcohol.
- If the patient's axilla has been washed recently, wait 15 to 30 minutes before taking an axillary temperature to allow the skin to return to baseline temperature.

(continued)

Skill 2-1 ▶ Assessing Body Temperature *(continued)*

Infant and Child Considerations

- Pull the pinna back and down when measuring tympanic temperature on a child younger than 3 years of age. For children older than 3 years of age, there is no need to manipulate the pinna (Kyle & Carman, 2017).
- Small children have a limited attention span and difficulty keeping their lips closed long enough to obtain an accurate oral temperature reading. Based on an assessment of the child's ability to cooperate, it may be more appropriate to use the temporal or tympanic site.
- Chemical dot thermometers (liquid crystal skin contact thermometers) are sometimes used as alternatives in pediatric settings. These single-use, disposable, flexible thermometers have specific chemical mixtures in circles on the thermometer that change color to measure temperature increments of two tenths of a degree. Place the thermometer in the mouth with the dot side (sensor) down, into the posterior sublingual pocket. Keep this type of thermometer in the mouth for 1 minute, in the axilla 3 minutes, and in the rectum 3 minutes. Read the color change 10 to 15 seconds after removing the thermometer. Read away from any heat source. Wearable, continuous-use chemical dot thermometers are available. These are placed under the axilla and must remain in place at least 2 to 3 minutes before taking the first reading; continuously thereafter. Replace thermometer and assess the underlying skin every 48 hours (Higgins, 2008; Perry et al., 2014).
- The Society of Pediatric Nurses (SPN) recognizes that temporal artery thermometry is accurate for infants less than 90 days old without fever, as well as for all patients more than 90 days of age with or without fever, ill, or well. The SPN recommends that the temporal artery method should not be used in infants 90 days or younger who are ill, have a fever, or have an ill diagnosis (Asher & Northington, 2008, p. 235). The rectal method should be used for these infants unless contraindicated by diagnosis, in which case the axillary method should be used. In addition, in children 6 months of age or older, the tympanic or oral methods may be used with correct positioning of the ear (tympanic) and if the patient can cooperate (oral) (Asher & Northington, 2008).

Home Care Considerations

- Teach patients who use electronic or digital thermometers to clean the probe after use to prevent transmission of microorganisms among family members. Clean according to manufacturer's directions.
- Teach patients using nonmercury glass thermometers to clean the thermometer after use in lukewarm soapy water and rinse in cool water. Store it in an appropriate place to prevent breakage and injury from the glass.
- Pacifier thermometers, which use the supralingual area, are available to screen for fever. Leave this thermometer in place for 3 to 6 minutes, based on the manufacturer's recommendations (Mayo Clinic, 2015b; Braun, 2006).

EVIDENCE FOR PRACTICE ▶

FEVER AND ANTIPYRESIS

Temperature increase and fever are common clinical symptoms. Most fevers, unless extremely high (above 40°C/104°F), are not harmful (Grossman & Porth, 2014). Fever is an important part of a person's defense mechanisms against infection. Findings about antipyretic treatment have further challenged the need for routine or aggressive fever suppression. Unfortunately, many nurses continue to be fever phobic, while their attitudes toward fever and antipyresis considerably affect antipyretic practice (Kiekkas et al, 2014). What are nurses' attitudes toward fever and antipyresis? Is nursing practice based on traditional beliefs that fever is harmful? Do nurses over-treat fever?

Related Research

Kiekkas, P., Konstantinou, E., Psychogiou, K. S., Tsampoula, I., Stefanopoulos, N., & Bakalis, N. (2014). Nursing personnel's attitudes towards fever and antipyresis of adult patients: cross-sectional survey. *Journal of Clinical Nursing, 23*(19/20), 2949–2957.

This prospective, cross-sectional, multicenter study evaluated nurses' attitudes toward fever and antipyresis or knowledge about fever and antipyresis in adults via questionnaire. The questionnaire included knowledge-evaluating items about fever and antipyresis, as well as attitude-evaluating items toward fever and antipyresis. Multiple linear regression analysis was used to identify the predictors of attitudes toward fever and antipyresis. The attitudes of the 458 participants were relatively positive toward fever and antipyresis, indicating intention to treat to achieve fever suppression, despite lack of evidence to support such intervention. Nurses' fever/antipyresis knowledge was relatively low, indicating a general lack of knowledge. However, high fever/antipyresis knowledge scores were an independent predictor of both more positive attitudes toward fever and less positive attitude toward antipyresis. The authors concluded that nurses with high fever/antipyresis knowledge keep abreast of current evidence and are more likely to adapt their attitudes toward fever and antipyresis according to research evidence. The authors suggest the need for continuing education to overcome nurses' traditional misconceptions about the need for suppressing any fever and to develop a more progressive attitude toward fever treatment.

Relevance to Nursing Practice

Nurses must engage in lifelong education to engage in evidence-based practice. There is a need for continuing education of nursing professionals in relation to fever and antipyresis that includes knowledge, clinical skills, attitudes, and barriers to change in practice. Advancing nurses' knowledge will contribute to the elimination of "fever phobia" and promote implementation of evidence-based nursing care (Kiekkas et al., 2014).

Refer to thePoint° for additional research on related nursing topics.

Skill 2-2 ▶ Regulating Temperature Using an Overhead Radiant Warmer

Neonates, infants who are exposed to stressors or chilling (e.g., from undergoing numerous procedures), and infants who have an underlying condition that interferes with thermoregulation (e.g., prematurity) are highly susceptible to heat loss. Therefore, radiant warmers are used for infants who have trouble maintaining body temperature. In addition, use of a radiant warmer minimizes the oxygen and calories that the infant would expend to maintain body temperature, thereby minimizing the effects of body temperature changes on metabolic activity.

An overhead radiant warmer uses infrared light to warm the infant. The infant's skin is warmed, causing an increase in blood flow, which heats both the underlying blood and tissue surfaces. The warmed blood and tissue transfer this heat to the rest of the body (Dondelinger, 2010). The warmer is adjusted to maintain an anterior abdominal skin temperature of 36.5°C (97.7°F), but at least 36°C (96.8°F), using servo-control (automatic thermostat) (Bell, 2015; Dondelinger, 2010).

DELEGATION CONSIDERATIONS

Measurement of body temperature for an infant in a radiant warmer is not delegated to nursing assistive personnel (NAP) nor to unlicensed assistive personnel (UAP). Depending on the state's nurse practice act and the organization's policies and procedures, the measurement of body temperature for an infant in a radiant warmer may be delegated to a licensed practical/vocational nurse (LPN/LVN). The decision to delegate must be based on careful analysis of the patient's needs and circumstances, as well as the qualifications of the person to whom the task is being delegated. Refer to the Delegation Guidelines in Appendix A.

(continued)

Skill 2-2 ▶ Regulating Temperature Using an Overhead Radiant Warmer *(continued)*

EQUIPMENT
- Overhead warmer
- Temperature probe
- Aluminum foil probe cover
- Axillary or rectal thermometer, based on facility policy
- PPE, as indicated

ASSESSMENT

Assess the patient's temperature using the route specified in facility policy, and assess the patient's fluid intake and output.

NURSING DIAGNOSIS

Determine the related factors for the nursing diagnoses based on the patient's current status. Appropriate nursing diagnoses may include:
- Hyperthermia
- Hypothermia
- Ineffective thermoregulation

OUTCOME IDENTIFICATION AND PLANNING

The expected outcomes to achieve when using an overhead warmer are that the infant's temperature is maintained within normal limits without injury.

IMPLEMENTATION

ACTION	RATIONALE
1. Check the medical order or nursing care plan for the use of a radiant warmer.	Provides for patient safety and appropriate care.
2. Perform hand hygiene and put on PPE, if indicated.	Hand hygiene and PPE prevent the spread of microorganisms. PPE is required based on transmission precautions.
3. Identify the patient.	Identifying the patient ensures the right patient receives the intervention and helps prevent errors.
4. Close curtains around the bed and close the door to the room, if possible. Discuss the procedure with the patient's family.	This ensures the patient's privacy. Explanation reduces the family's apprehension and encourages family cooperation.
5. Plug in the warmer. Turn the warmer to the manual setting. Allow the blankets to warm before placing the infant under the warmer.	By allowing the blankets to warm before placing the infant under the warmer, you are preventing heat loss through conduction. By placing the warmer on the manual setting, you are keeping the warmer at a set temperature no matter how warm the blankets become.
6. Switch the warmer setting to automatic. Set the warmer to the desired abdominal skin temperature, usually 36.5°C (97.7°F).	The automatic setting ensures that the warmer will regulate the amount of radiant heat, depending on the temperature of the infant's skin. The temperature should be adjusted so that the infant does not become too warm or too cold.

ACTION

7. Place the infant under the warmer. Attach the probe to the infant's abdominal skin at mid-epigastrium, halfway between the xiphoid and the umbilicus. Cover with a foil-backed shield (Figure 1). If the infant is prone, attach the probe to the skin over either flank (not between the scapulae) (Bell, 2015).

8. When the abdominal skin temperature reaches the desired set point, check the patient's temperature using the route specified in facility policy to be sure it is within the normal range (Figure 2).

FIGURE 1. Probe in place with foil cover. (*Photo by Joe Mitchell.*)

9. Adjust the warmer's set point slightly, as needed, if the patient's temperature is abnormal. Do not change the set point if the temperature is normal.

10. Remove additional PPE, if used. Perform hand hygiene.

11. Check the position of the probe frequently to ensure the probe maintains contact with the patient's skin. Continue to monitor temperature measurement and other vital signs.

RATIONALE

The foil-backed shield prevents direct warming of the probe, allowing the probe to read only the infant's temperature.

By monitoring the infant's temperature, you are watching for signs of hyperthermia or **hypothermia**.

FIGURE 2. Taking infant's axillary temperature. (*Photo by Joe Mitchell.*)

By monitoring the infant's temperature, you are watching for signs of hyperthermia or hypothermia. This prevents the infant from becoming too warm or too cool.

Proper removal of PPE reduces the risk for infection transmission and contamination of other items. Hand hygiene deters the spread of microorganisms.

Poor contact will cause overheating. Entrapment of the probe under the arm or between the infant and mattress will cause under-heating (Bell, 2015). Monitoring of vital signs assesses patient status.

EVALUATION

The expected outcomes have been met when the infant is placed under the radiant warmer, the infant's temperature is well controlled, and the infant experiences no injury.

DOCUMENTATION

Guidelines

Document initial assessment of the infant, including body temperature; the placement of the infant under the radiant warmer; and the settings of the radiant warmer. Document incubator air temperatures, as well as subsequent skin and axillary or rectal temperatures, and other vital sign measurements.

Sample Documentation

<u>10/13/20</u> 1110 Infant placed under radiant warmer. Warmer on automatic setting 36.7°C (98°F), baby's skin temperature 36.8°C (98.2°F), rectal temperature 37°C (98.6°F), warmer air temperature 36.7°C (98°F).

—*M. Evans, RN*

(continued)

Skill 2-2 ▶ Regulating Temperature Using an Overhead Radiant Warmer *(continued)*

UNEXPECTED SITUATIONS AND ASSOCIATED INTERVENTIONS

- *The infant becomes **febrile** under the radiant warmer:* Do not turn the warmer off and leave the infant naked. This could cause cold stress and even death. Leave the warmer on automatic and lower the set temperature. Notify the primary care provider.
- *The warmer's temperature is fluctuating constantly or is inaccurate:* Change the probe cover. If this does not improve the temperature variations, change the probe as well.

SPECIAL CONSIDERATIONS

Infant and Child Considerations

- Radiant warmers result in increased insensible water loss. This water loss needs to be taken into account when daily fluid requirements are calculated.

Skill 2-3 ▶ Regulating Temperature Using a Hypothermia Blanket

A hypothermia blanket, or cooling pad, is a blanket-sized aquathermia pad that conducts a cooled solution, usually distilled water, through coils in a plastic blanket or pad (Figure 1). Placing a patient on a hypothermia blanket or pad helps to lower body temperature. The nurse monitors the patient's body temperature and can reset the blanket setting accordingly. The blanket also can be preset to maintain a specific body temperature; the device continually monitors the patient's body temperature using a temperature probe (which is inserted rectally or in the esophagus, or placed on the skin) and adjusts the temperature of the circulating liquid accordingly.

FIGURE 1. Hypothermia blanket.

DELEGATION CONSIDERATIONS

The application of a hypothermia pad is not delegated to nursing assistive personnel (NAP) or to unlicensed assistive personnel (UAP). The measurement of a patient's body temperature while a hypothermia pad is in use may be delegated to nursing assistive personnel (NAP) or unlicensed assistive personnel (UAP). Depending on the state's nurse practice act and the organization's policies and procedures, the application of a hypothermia pad may be delegated to a licensed practical/vocational nurse (LPN/LVN). The decision to delegate must be based on careful analysis of the patient's needs and circumstances, as well as the qualifications of the person to whom the task is being delegated. Refer to the Delegation Guidelines in Appendix A.

EQUIPMENT	• Disposable hypothermia blanket or pad • Electronic control panel • Distilled water to fill the device, if necessary • Thermometer, if needed to monitor the patient's temperature • Sphygmomanometer • Stethoscope • Temperature probe, if needed • Thin blanket or sheet • Towels • Clean gloves • Additional PPE, as indicated
ASSESSMENT	Assess the patient's condition, including current body temperature, to determine the need for the hypothermia blanket. Consider alternative measures to help lower the patient's body temperature before implementing the blanket. Also verify the medical order for the application of a hypothermia blanket. Assess the patient's vital signs, neurologic status, peripheral circulation, and skin integrity. Assess the equipment to be used, including the condition of cords, plugs, and cooling elements. Look for fluid leaks. Once the equipment is turned on, make sure there is a consistent distribution of cooling.
NURSING DIAGNOSIS	Determine the related factors for the nursing diagnoses based on the patient's current status. Appropriate nursing diagnoses may include: • Risk for injury • Risk for impaired skin integrity • Hyperthermia
OUTCOME IDENTIFICATION AND PLANNING	The expected outcome to achieve when using a hypothermia blanket is that the patient maintains the desired body temperature. Other outcomes that may be appropriate include: the patient does not experience shivering; the patient's vital signs are within normal limits; and the patient does not experience alterations in skin integrity, neurologic status, peripheral circulation, or fluid and electrolyte status and edema.

IMPLEMENTATION

ACTION	RATIONALE
1. Review the medical order for the application of the hypothermia blanket. Obtain consent for the therapy per facility policy.	Reviewing the order validates the correct patient and correct procedure.
2. Perform hand hygiene and put on PPE, if indicated.	Hand hygiene and PPE prevent the spread of microorganisms. PPE is required based on transmission precautions.
3. Identify the patient. Determine if the patient has had any previous adverse reaction to hypothermia therapy.	Identifying the patient ensures the right patient receives the intervention and helps prevent errors. Individual differences exist in tolerating specific therapies.
4. Assemble equipment on the overbed table within reach.	Organization facilitates performance of task.
5. Close curtains around the bed and close the door to the room, if possible. Explain what you are going to do and why you are going to do it to the patient.	This ensures the patient's privacy. Explanation relieves anxiety and facilitates cooperation.

(continued)

Skill 2-3 ▶ Regulating Temperature Using a Hypothermia Blanket *(continued)*

ACTION	**RATIONALE**
6. Check that the water in the electronic unit is at the appropriate level. Fill the unit two thirds full with distilled water, or to the fill mark, if necessary. Check the temperature setting on the unit to ensure it is within the safe range.	Sufficient water in the unit is necessary to ensure proper function of the unit. Tap water leaves mineral deposits in the unit. Checking the temperature setting helps to prevent skin or tissue damage.
7. Assess the patient's vital signs, neurologic status, peripheral circulation, and skin integrity.	Assessment supplies baseline data for comparison during therapy and identifies conditions that may contraindicate the application.
8. Adjust bed to comfortable working height, usually elbow height of the caregiver (VHACEOSH, 2016).	Having the bed at the proper height prevents back and muscle strain.
9. Make sure the patient's gown has cloth ties, not snaps or pins.	Cloth ties minimize the risk of cold injury.
10. Apply lanolin or a mixture of lanolin and cold cream to the patient's skin where it will be in contact with the blanket.	These agents help protect the skin from cold.
11. Turn on the blanket and make sure the cooling light is on. **Verify that the temperature limits are set within the desired safety range (Figure 2).**	Turning on the blanket prepares it for use. Keeping temperature within the safety range prevents excessive cooling.
12. Cover the hypothermia blanket with a thin sheet or bath blanket.	A sheet or blanket protects the patient's skin from direct contact with the cooling surface, reducing the risk for injury.
13. Position the blanket under the patient so that the top edge of the pad is aligned with the patient's neck (Figure 3).	The blanket's rigid surface may be uncomfortable. The cold may lead to tissue breakdown.

FIGURE 2. Checking the settings on the hypothermia blanket control unit and turning it on.

FIGURE 3. Aligning hypothermia blanket on bed.

ACTION	**RATIONALE**
14. Put on gloves. Lubricate the rectal probe and insert it into the patient's rectum unless contraindicated. Or tuck the skin probe deep into the patient's axilla and tape it in place. For patients who are comatose or anesthetized, use an esophageal probe. Remove gloves. Perform hand hygiene. Attach the probe to the control panel for the blanket.	The probe allows continuous monitoring of the patient's core body temperature. Rectal insertion may be contraindicated in patients with a low white blood cell or platelet count.
15. Wrap the patient's hands and feet in gauze if ordered, or if the patient desires. For male patients, elevate the scrotum off the hypothermia blanket with towels.	These actions minimize chilling, promote comfort, and protect sensitive tissues from direct contact with cold.
16. Place the patient in a comfortable position. Lower the bed. Dispose of any other supplies appropriately.	Repositioning promotes patient comfort and safety.
17. Recheck the thermometer and settings on the control panel.	Rechecking verifies that the blanket temperature is maintained at a safe level.

ACTION	RATIONALE
18. Remove any additional PPE, if used. Perform hand hygiene.	Proper removal of PPE reduces the risk for infection transmission and contamination of other items. Hand hygiene prevents the spread of microorganisms.
19. **Turn and position the patient regularly (every 30 minutes to 1 hour). Keep linens free from condensation. Reapply cream, as needed. Observe the patient's skin for change in color, changes in lips and nail beds, edema, pain, and sensory impairment.**	Turning and repositioning prevent alterations in skin integrity and provide for assessment of potential skin injuries.
20. **Monitor vital signs and perform a neurologic assessment, per facility policy, usually every 15 minutes, until the body temperature is stable. In addition, monitor the** patient's skin integrity, peripheral circulation and fluid and electrolyte status, as per facility policy.	Continuous monitoring provides evaluation of the patient's response to the therapy and permits early identification and intervention if adverse effects occur.
21. Avoid cooling to the point of shivering (Morton & Fontaine, 2018). Observe for signs of shivering, including verbalized sensations, facial muscle twitching, hyperventilation, or twitching of extremities.	Shivering increases heat production, and is often controlled with medications.
22. Assess the patient's level of comfort.	Hypothermia therapy can cause discomfort. Prompt assessment and action can prevent injuries.
23. Turn off the blanket according to facility policy, usually when the patient's body temperature reaches 1 degree above the desired temperature. **Continue to monitor the patient's temperature until it stabilizes.**	Body temperature can continue to fall after this therapy.

EVALUATION

The expected outcome has been met when the patient maintains the desired body temperature and other vital signs within acceptable parameters. In addition, the patient remains free from shivering; does not experience alterations in skin integrity, neurologic status, peripheral circulation, fluid and electrolyte status, or edema.

DOCUMENTATION

Guidelines

Document assessments, such as vital signs, neurologic, peripheral circulation, and skin integrity status prior to use of the hypothermia blanket. Record verification of medical order and that the procedure was explained to the patient. Document the control settings, time of application and removal, and the route of the temperature monitoring. Include the application of lanolin cream to the skin as well as the frequency of position changes. Document the patient's response to the therapy, especially noting a decrease in temperature and level of discomfort. Record the use of medication to reduce shivering or other discomforts, if implemented. Include any pertinent patient and family teaching.

Sample Documentation

11/10/20 1800 Patient's temperature 106°F (41°C), pulse 122, respirations 24, BP 118/72. Dr. Fenter notified. Order received for application of hypothermia blanket. Procedure explained to patient. Lanolin applied to skin, bath sheet applied between blanket and patient, axillary probe applied, hypothermia blanket setting 99°F (37.2°C) per order. Vital signs, neurologic, neurovascular, and skin assessment every 30 minutes; see electronic flow sheets. Patient without evidence of shivering.
—J. Lee, RN

11/10/20 1930 Patient reports chills and shivering. Temperature 100°F (37.8°C), pulse 104, respirations 20, BP 114/68. Dr. Fenter notified. Hypothermia blanket discontinued per order.
—J. Lee, RN

(continued)

Skill 2-3 ▶ Regulating Temperature Using a Hypothermia Blanket *(continued)*

UNEXPECTED SITUATIONS AND ASSOCIATED INTERVENTIONS

- *The patient states he is cold and has chills. You observe shivering of his extremities:* Obtain vital signs. Assess for other symptoms. Increase the blanket temperature to a more comfortable range. If shivering persists or is excessive, discontinue the therapy. Notify the primary care provider of the findings and document the event in the patient's record.
- *When performing a skin assessment during therapy, you note increased pallor on pressure points and sluggish capillary refill. The patient reports alterations in sensation on these points:* Discontinue therapy, obtain vital signs, assess for other symptoms, notify the primary care provider, and document the event in the patient's record.

SPECIAL CONSIDERATIONS

Older Adult Considerations

- Older adults are more at risk for skin and tissue damage because of their thin skin, loss of cold sensation, decreased subcutaneous tissue, and changes in the body's ability to regulate temperature. Check these patients more frequently during therapy.

Skill 2-4 ▶ Assessing a Peripheral Pulse by Palpation

The peripheral **pulse** is a throbbing sensation that can be palpated (felt) over a peripheral artery, such as the radial artery or the carotid artery. Peripheral pulses result from a wave of blood being pumped into the arterial circulation by the contraction of the left ventricle. Each time the left ventricle contracts to eject blood into an already full aorta, the arterial walls in the cardiovascular system expand to compensate for the increase in pressure of the blood. The peripheral pulses may be felt wherever an artery passes over a solid structure, such as bone or cartilage. Characteristics of the peripheral pulse include rate, rhythm, and amplitude (quality; strong or weak). These characteristics are indicators of the effectiveness of the heart as a pump, the volume of blood ejected with each heartbeat (stroke volume), and the adequacy of peripheral blood flow.

Pulse rates are measured in beats per minute. The normal pulse rate for adolescents and adults ranges from 60 to 100 beats per minute. Pulse amplitude (quality) describes the quality of the pulse in terms of its fullness—strong or weak. It is assessed by the feel of the blood flow through the vessel. Pulse rhythm is the pattern of the pulsations and the pauses between them. Pulse rhythm is normally regular; the pulsations and the pauses between occur at regular intervals. An irregular pulse rhythm occurs when the pulsations and pauses between beats occur at unequal intervals.

Assess the pulse by palpating peripheral arteries, by auscultating the apical pulse with a stethoscope, or by using a portable Doppler ultrasound (see the accompanying Skill Variation). To assess the pulse accurately, you need to know which site to choose and what method is most appropriate for the patient.

The most commonly used sites to palpate peripheral pulses and a scale used to describe pulse amplitude are illustrated in Box 2-1. Place your fingers over the artery so that the ends of your fingers are flat against the patient's skin when palpating peripheral pulses. Do not press with the tip of the fingers only (refer to Figure 1, Step 8).

Box 2-1 Pulse Sites and Pulse Amplitude

Pulse Sites

Arteries commonly used for assessing the pulse include the temporal, carotid, brachial, radial, femoral, popliteal, posterior tibial, and dorsalis pedis.

Pulse Amplitude

- 0: Absent, unable to palpate
- +1: Diminished, weaker than expected
- +2: Brisk, expected (normal)
- +3: Bounding

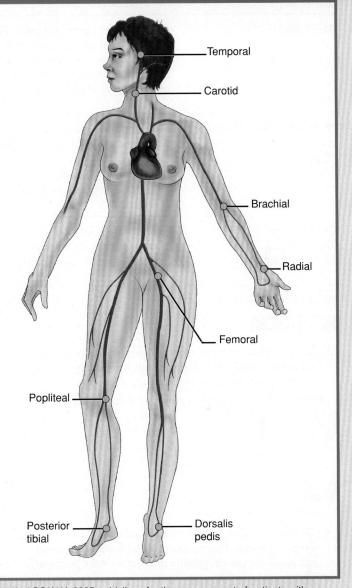

Source: Adapted from Hirsch, A.T., Haskal, Z. J., Hertzer, N. R., et al. (2006). ACC/AHA 2005 guidelines for the management of patients with peripheral arterial disease (lower extremity, renal, mesenteric, and abdominal aortic): Executive summary, a collaborative report from the American Association for Vascular Surgery/Society for Vascular Surgery, Society for Cardiovascular Angiography and Interventions, Society for Vascular Medicine and Biology, Society of Interventional Radiology, and the ACC/AHA Task Force on Practice Guidelines (Writing Committee to Develop Guidelines for the Management of Patients with Peripheral Arterial Disease). *Circulation, 113*(11), e463–e654.

DELEGATION CONSIDERATIONS

The measurement of the radial and brachial peripheral pulses may be delegated to nursing assistive personnel (NAP) or to unlicensed assistive personnel (UAP). The measurement of peripheral pulses may be delegated to licensed practical/vocational nurses (LPN/LVNs). The decision to delegate must be based on careful analysis of the patient's needs and circumstances, as well as the qualifications of the person to whom the task is being delegated. Refer to the Delegation Guidelines in Appendix A.

(continued)

Skill 2-4 ▶ Assessing a Peripheral Pulse by Palpation *(continued)*

EQUIPMENT	• Watch with second hand or digital readout • Electronic record, or a pen, paper or flow sheet • Nonsterile gloves, if appropriate; additional PPE, as indicated
ASSESSMENT	Choose a site to assess the pulse. For an adult patient, adolescent, and older child, the most common site for obtaining a peripheral pulse is the radial pulse. Apical pulse measurement is the preferred method of pulse assessment for infants and children less than 2 years of age (Jarvis, 2016). (Refer to Skill 2-5.) Assess for factors that could affect pulse characteristics, such as the patient's age, amount of exercise, fluid balance, and medications. Note baseline or previous pulse measurements.
NURSING DIAGNOSIS	Determine the related factors for the nursing diagnoses based on the patient's current status. Appropriate nursing diagnoses may include: • Decreased cardiac output • Ineffective peripheral tissue perfusion • Risk for ineffective peripheral tissue perfusion
OUTCOME IDENTIFICATION AND PLANNING	The expected outcomes to achieve when measuring a pulse rate are that the patient's pulse is assessed accurately without injury and that the patient experiences minimal discomfort. Other outcomes may be appropriate, depending on the patient's nursing diagnosis.

IMPLEMENTATION

ACTION	**RATIONALE**
1. Check medical order or nursing care plan for frequency of pulse assessment. More frequent pulse measurement may be appropriate based on nursing judgment.	Assessment and measurement of vital signs at appropriate intervals provide important data about the patient's health status.
2. Perform hand hygiene and put on PPE, if indicated.	Hand hygiene and PPE prevent the spread of microorganisms. PPE is required based on transmission precautions.
3. Identify the patient.	Identifying the patient ensures the right patient receives the intervention and helps prevent errors.
4. Close the curtains around the bed and close the door to the room, if possible. Discuss the procedure with the patient and assess the patient's ability to assist with the procedure.	This ensures the patient's privacy. Explanation relieves anxiety and facilitates cooperation.
5. Put on gloves, if indicated.	Gloves are not usually worn to obtain a pulse measurement unless contact with blood or body fluids is anticipated. Gloves prevent contact with blood and body fluids.
6. Select the appropriate peripheral site based on assessment data.	Ensures safety and accuracy of measurement.
7. Move the patient's clothing to expose only the site chosen.	The site must be exposed for pulse assessment. Exposing only the site keeps the patient warm and maintains his or her dignity.
8. Place your first, second, and third fingers over the artery (Figure 1). Place your fingers over the artery so that the ends of your fingers are flat against the patient's skin when palpating peripheral pulses. Do not press with the tip of the fingers only. **Lightly compress the artery so pulsations can be felt and counted.**	The sensitive fingertips can feel the pulsation of the artery.

ACTION	**RATIONALE**
9. Using a watch with a second hand, count the number of pulsations felt for 30 seconds (Figure 2). Multiply this number by 2 to calculate the rate for 1 minute. **If the rate, rhythm, or amplitude of the pulse is abnormal in any way, palpate and count the pulse for 1 minute.**	Ensures accuracy of measurement and assessment.

FIGURE 1. Palpating the radial pulse.

FIGURE 2. Counting the pulse.

ACTION	**RATIONALE**
10. Note the rhythm and amplitude of the pulse.	Provides additional assessment data regarding the patient's cardiovascular status.
11. When measurement is completed, remove gloves, if worn. Cover the patient and help him or her to a position of comfort.	Proper removal of gloves reduces the risk for infection transmission and contamination of other items. Ensures patient comfort.
12. Remove additional PPE, if used. Perform hand hygiene.	Proper removal of PPE reduces the risk for infection transmission and contamination of other items. Hand hygiene prevents the spread of microorganisms.

EVALUATION The expected outcomes have been met when the patient's pulse is assessed accurately without injury and the patient experiences minimal discomfort.

DOCUMENTATION

Guidelines Record pulse rate, amplitude, and rhythm in the electronic record or flow sheet. Identify site of assessment. Report abnormal findings to the primary care provider.

Sample Documentation

DocuCare Practice documenting pulse and other vital signs in *Lippincott DocuCare.*

> 2/6/120 1000 Pulses 84, regular, 2+ and equal bilaterally in radial, popliteal, and dorsalis pedis sites.
>
> —*M. Evans, RN*

UNEXPECTED SITUATIONS AND ASSOCIATED INTERVENTIONS

- *The pulse is irregular*: Monitor the pulse for a full minute. If the pulse is difficult to assess, validate pulse measurement by taking the apical pulse for 1 minute. If this is a change for the patient, notify the primary care provider.
- *The pulse is palpated easily, but then disappears*: Apply only moderate pressure to the pulse. Applying too much pressure may obliterate the pulse.
- *You cannot palpate a pulse*: Use a portable Doppler ultrasound to assess the pulse. If this is a change in assessment or if you cannot find the pulse using a Doppler ultrasound, notify the primary care provider. If you can find the pulse using a Doppler ultrasound, place a small X over the spot where the pulse is located. This can make palpating the pulse easier because the exact location of the pulse is known.

(continued)

Skill 2-4 Assessing a Peripheral Pulse by Palpation *(continued)*

SPECIAL CONSIDERATIONS

General Considerations
- The normal heart rate varies by age.
- The carotid pulse should be palpated only in the lower third of the neck to avoid stimulation of the carotid sinus (Jensen, 2015, p. 94). When palpating a carotid pulse, lightly press only one side of the neck at a time. Never attempt to palpate both carotid arteries at the same time. Bilateral palpation could result in reduced cerebral blood flow and cause the patient to lose consciousness (Jensen, 2015).
- If a peripheral pulse is difficult to assess accurately because it is irregular, feeble, or extremely rapid, assess the apical rate.

Infant and Child Considerations
- In infants and toddlers, palpate or auscultate an apical rate (see Skill 2-5) (Jarvis, 2016).
- In children older than 2 years, use the radial site for pulse assessment and count for 1 minute (Jarvis, 2016; Perry et al., 2014). Do not measure the radial pulse in children younger than 2 years of age, because it is difficult to palpate accurately in this age group (Perry et al.). In older children, measure the radial pulse for a full minute.
- Measure the apical rate if the child has a cardiac problem or congenital heart defect (see Skill 2-5).

Home Care Considerations
- Teach the patient and family members how to take the patient's pulse, if appropriate.
- Inform the patient and family about digital pulse monitoring devices.
- Teach family members how to locate and monitor peripheral pulse sites, if appropriate.

Skill Variation Assessing Peripheral Pulse Using a Portable Doppler Ultrasound

1. Check medical order or nursing care plan for frequency of pulse assessment. More frequent pulse measurement may be appropriate based on nursing judgment. Determine the need to use a Doppler ultrasound device for pulse assessment.

2. Perform hand hygiene and put on PPE, if indicated.

3. Identify the patient.

4. Assemble equipment on the overbed table within reach.
5. Close curtains around the bed and close the door to the room, if possible.
6. Explain the procedure to the patient.
7. Put on gloves, if indicated. Gloves are not usually worn to obtain a pulse measurement unless contact with blood or body fluids is anticipated.
8. Select the appropriate peripheral site based on assessment data.
9. Move the patient's clothing to expose only the site chosen.
10. Remove Doppler from charger and turn it on. Make sure that volume is set at low.
11. Apply conducting gel to the site where you expect to auscultate the pulse.
12. Hold the Doppler base in your nondominant hand. With your dominant hand, touch the probe lightly to the skin with the probe tip in the gel. Adjust the volume, as needed. Hold the probe perpendicular to the skin. Slowly move the Doppler tip around until the pulse is heard (Figure A).
13. **Using a watch with a second hand, count the heartbeat for 1 minute. Note the rhythm of the pulse.**

FIGURE A. Moving the Doppler tip until pulse is heard.

14. Remove the Doppler tip and turn the Doppler off. Wipe excess gel off of the patient's skin with a tissue.
15. Place a small X over the spot where the pulse is located with an indelible pen, depending on facility policy. Marking the site allows for easier future assessment. It can also make palpating the pulse easier because the exact location of the pulse is known.
16. Cover the patient and help him or her to a position of comfort.
17. Wipe any gel remaining on the Doppler probe off with a tissue. Clean the Doppler probe per facility policy or manufacturer's recommendations.

18. Remove PPE, if used. Perform hand hygiene.

19. Return the Doppler ultrasound device to the charge base.
20. Record pulse rate, rhythm, and site, and that it was obtained with a Doppler ultrasound device.

Skill 2-5 ▶ Assessing the Apical Pulse by Auscultation

An apical pulse is auscultated (listened to) over the apex of the heart, as the heart beats. Heart sounds, which are produced by closure of the valves of the heart, are characterized as "lub-dub." The apical pulse is the result of closure of the mitral and tricuspid valves ("lub") and the aortic and pulmonic valves ("dub"). The combination of the two sounds is counted as one beat. Pulse rates are measured in beats per minute. The normal pulse rate for adolescents and adults ranges from 60 to 100 beats per minute. Pulse rhythm is also assessed. Pulse rhythm is the pattern of the beats and the pauses between them. Pulse rhythm is normally regular; the beats and the pauses between occur at regular intervals. An irregular pulse rhythm occurs when the beats and pauses between beats occur at unequal intervals.

An apical pulse is assessed when giving medications that alter heart rate and rhythm. In addition, if a peripheral pulse is difficult to assess accurately because it is irregular, feeble, or extremely rapid, assess the apical rate. In adults, the apical rate is counted for 1 full minute by listening with a stethoscope over the apex of the heart. Apical pulse measurement is also the preferred method of pulse assessment in children less than 2 years of age (Jarvis, 2016; Perry et al., 2014).

DELEGATION CONSIDERATIONS	The assessment of an apical pulse is not delegated to nursing assistive personnel (NAP) or to unlicensed assistive personnel (UAP). The measurement of an apical pulse may be delegated to a licensed practical/vocational nurse (LPN/LVN). The decision to delegate must be based on careful analysis of the patient's needs and circumstances, as well as the qualifications of the person to whom the task is being delegated. Refer to the Delegation Guidelines in Appendix A.
EQUIPMENT	• Watch with second hand or digital readout • Stethoscope • Alcohol swab • Electronic record, or a pen, paper or flow sheet • Nonsterile gloves, if appropriate; additional PPE, as indicated
ASSESSMENT	Assess for factors that could affect apical pulse rate and rhythm, such as the patient's age, amount of exercise, fluid balance, and medications. Note baseline or previous apical pulse measurements.
NURSING DIAGNOSIS	Determine the related factors for the nursing diagnoses based on the patient's current status. Appropriate nursing diagnoses may include: • Decreased cardiac output • Deficient fluid volume • Risk for decreased cardiac tissue perfusion
OUTCOME IDENTIFICATION AND PLANNING	The expected outcomes to achieve when measuring an apical pulse rate are that the patient's pulse is assessed accurately without injury and the patient experiences minimal discomfort. Other outcomes may be appropriate, depending on the patient's nursing diagnosis.

IMPLEMENTATION

ACTION	RATIONALE
1. Check medical order or nursing care plan for frequency of pulse assessment. More frequent pulse measurement may be appropriate based on nursing judgment. Identify the need to obtain an apical pulse measurement.	Provides for patient safety and appropriate care.
2. Perform hand hygiene and put on PPE, if indicated.	Hand hygiene and PPE prevent the spread of microorganisms. PPE is required based on transmission precautions.

(continued)

Skill 2-5 ▶ Assessing the Apical Pulse by Auscultation *(continued)*

ACTION	RATIONALE
3. Identify the patient.	Identifying the patient ensures the right patient receives the intervention and helps prevent errors.
4. Close curtains around the bed and close the door to the room, if possible. Discuss the procedure with the patient and assess the patient's ability to assist with the procedure.	This ensures the patient's privacy. Explanation relieves anxiety and facilitates cooperation.
5. Put on gloves, if indicated.	Gloves are not usually worn to obtain a pulse measurement unless contact with blood or body fluids is anticipated. Gloves prevent contact with blood and body fluids.
6. Use an alcohol swab to clean the **diaphragm** of the stethoscope. Use another swab to clean the earpieces, if necessary.	Cleaning with alcohol deters transmission of microorganisms.
7. Assist the patient to a sitting or reclining position and expose the chest area.	This position facilitates identification of the site for stethoscope placement.
8. Move the patient's clothing to expose only the apical site.	The site must be exposed for pulse assessment. Exposing only the apical site keeps the patient warm and maintains his or her dignity.
9. Hold the stethoscope diaphragm against the palm of your hand for a few seconds.	Warming the diaphragm promotes patient comfort.
10. **Palpate the space between the fifth and sixth ribs (fifth intercostal space), and move to the left midclavicular line.** Place the stethoscope diaphragm over the apex of the heart (Figures 1 and 2).	Position the stethoscope over the apex of the heart, where the heartbeat is best heard.

FIGURE 1. Locating the apical pulse: apex area.

Apex area

Place diaphragm here

Midsternum   Midclavicular line

A

B

FIGURE 2. The apical pulse is usually found at (**A**) the fifth intercostal space just inside the midclavicular line and can be heard (**B**) over the apex of the heart.

ACTION	RATIONALE
11. Listen for heart sounds ("lub-dub"). Each "lub-dub" counts as one beat.	These sounds occur as the heart valves close.
12. Using a watch with a second hand, count the heartbeat for 1 minute.	Counting for a full minute increases the accuracy of assessment.
13. Note the rhythm of the beats.	Provides additional assessment data regarding the patient's cardiovascular status.
14. When measurement is completed, cover the patient and help him or her to a position of comfort.	Ensures patient comfort.
15. Clean the diaphragm of the stethoscope with an alcohol swab.	Cleaning with alcohol deters transmission of microorganisms.
16. Remove gloves and additional PPE, if used. Perform hand hygiene.	Proper removal of PPE reduces the risk for infection transmission and contamination of other items. Hand hygiene prevents the spread of microorganisms.

EVALUATION

The expected outcomes have been met when the patient's apical pulse is assessed accurately without injury and the patient experiences minimal discomfort.

DOCUMENTATION

Guidelines

Record pulse rate and rhythm in electronic record or flow sheet. Report abnormal findings to the appropriate person. Identify site of assessment.

Sample Documentation

Lippincott **DocuCare** Practice documenting the apical pulse and other vital signs in *Lippincott DocuCare.*

> 2/6/20 1000 Apical pulse 82 and regular. Digoxin 0.125 mg administered orally per order. Patient verbalized understanding of actions and untoward effects of medication.
> —B. Clapp, RN

UNEXPECTED SITUATIONS AND ASSOCIATED INTERVENTIONS

- If the apical rate is irregular, assess the patient for other symptoms, such as lightheadedness, dizziness, shortness of breath, or palpitations. Notify appropriate health care provider of findings.

SPECIAL CONSIDERATIONS

Infant and Child Considerations

- Assess the apical pulse just above and outside the left nipple of the infant at the third or fourth intercostal space. As the child ages, the location for assessment moves to a more medial and slightly lower area until 7 years of age. In children age 7 years or older, assess the apical pulse at the fourth or fifth intercostal space at the midclavicular line (Jensen, 2015).
- The apical pulse is most reliable for infants and small children. Count the rate for 1 full minute in infants and children because of possible rhythm irregularities (Perry et al., 2014).
- Allow the young child to examine or handle the stethoscope to become familiar with the equipment.
- Apical rate of infants is easily palpated with the fingertips.

(continued)

Skill 2-5 ▶ Assessing the Apical Pulse by Auscultation *(continued)*

Skill Variation ▶ Assessing the Apical–Radial Pulse Deficit

Measurement of the apical–radial pulse deficit may be utilized to assess the effectiveness of the contractions of the heart, specifically the left ventricle. Counting of the pulse at the apex of the heart and at the radial artery simultaneously is used to assess the apical–radial pulse deficit. A difference between the apical and radial pulse rates is called the pulse deficit and indicates that all of the heartbeats are not reaching the peripheral arteries or are too weak to be palpated (Taylor et al., 2019). Two nurses are required to perform this skill; one listens with a stethoscope over the apex of the heart for the apical heart rate and the other counts the pulse rate at the radial artery.

1. Perform hand hygiene and put on PPE, if indicated.

2. Identify the patient.

3. Close curtains around the bed and close the door to the room, if possible.
4. Explain the procedure to the patient.
5. Put on gloves, if indicated. Gloves are not usually worn to obtain a pulse measurement unless contact with blood or body fluids is anticipated.
6. Expose the patient's chest wall so that the stethoscope can be placed directly on the skin of the chest wall.
7. One watch with a sweep second hand is placed so that both nurses can read it simultaneously.
8. The nurses determine where they can best hear and feel the pulse and decide on a time to start counting, such as when the second hand on the watch is at a specified place (e.g., the number 12).
9. Both nurses count for 1 full minute and record their counts. The difference between the apical and radial pulse rates is the pulse deficit.

10. Remove PPE and gloves, if used. Perform hand hygiene.

Skill 2-6 ▶ Assessing Respiration

Under normal conditions, healthy adults breathe about 12 to 20 times per minute (**respirations per minute**). Infants and children breathe more rapidly. Fundamentals Review 2-1 outlines respiratory rate ranges for different age groups. The depth of respirations varies normally from shallow to deep. The rhythm of respirations is normally regular, with each inhalation/exhalation and the pauses between occurring at regular intervals. An irregular respiratory rhythm occurs when the inhalation/exhalation cycle and the pauses between occur at unequal intervals. Table 2-1 outlines various respiratory patterns.

Assess respiratory rate, depth, and rhythm by inspection (observing and listening) or by listening with the stethoscope. Determine the rate by counting the number of breaths per minute. If respirations are very shallow and difficult to detect, observe the sternal notch, where respiration is more apparent. With an infant or young child, assess respirations before taking the temperature so that the child is not crying, which would alter the respiratory status.

Move immediately from the pulse assessment to counting the respiratory rate to avoid letting the patient know you are counting respirations. Patients should be unaware of the respiratory assessment because, if they are conscious of the procedure, they might alter their breathing patterns or rate.

DELEGATION CONSIDERATIONS	The measurement of respirations may be delegated to nursing assistive personnel (NAP) or to unlicensed assistive personnel (UAP), as well as to licensed practical/vocational nurses (LPN/LVNs). The decision to delegate must be based on careful analysis of the patient's needs and circumstances, as well as the qualifications of the person to whom the task is being delegated. Refer to the Delegation Guidelines in Appendix A.

Table 2-1 Patterns of Respiration

	DESCRIPTION	PATTERN	ASSOCIATED FEATURES
Normal	12–20 breaths/min; Regular		Normal pattern
Tachypnea	>24 breaths/min; Shallow		Fever, anxiety, exercise, respiratory disorders
Bradypnea	<10 breaths/min; Regular		Depression of the respiratory center by medications, brain damage
Hyperventilation	Increased rate and depth		Extreme exercise, fear, diabetic ketoacidosis (Kussmaul's respirations), overdose of aspirin
Hypoventilation	Decreased rate and depth; irregular		Overdose of narcotics or anesthetics
Cheyne–Stokes respirations	Alternating periods of deep, rapid breathing followed by periods of **apnea**; regular		Drug overdose, heart failure, increased intracranial pressure, renal failure
Biot's respirations	Varying depth and rate of breathing, followed by periods of apnea; irregular		Meningitis, severe brain damage

EQUIPMENT	• Watch with second hand or digital readout • Electronic record, or a pen, paper or flow sheet • PPE, as indicated
ASSESSMENT	Assess the patient for factors that could affect respirations, such as exercise, medications, smoking, chronic illness or conditions, neurologic injury, pain, and anxiety. Note baseline or previous respiratory measurements. Assess patient for any signs of respiratory distress, which include retractions, nasal flaring, grunting, **orthopnea**, or **tachypnea**.
NURSING DIAGNOSIS	Determine the related factors for the nursing diagnoses based on the patient's current status. Appropriate nursing diagnoses may include: • Ineffective breathing pattern • Impaired gas exchange • Ineffective airway clearance
OUTCOME IDENTIFICATION AND PLANNING	The expected outcomes to achieve when assessing respirations are that the patient's respirations are assessed accurately without injury and the patient experiences minimal discomfort. Other outcomes may be appropriate depending on the patient's nursing diagnosis.

(continued)

Skill 2-6 ▶ Assessing Respiration *(continued)*

IMPLEMENTATION

ACTION	RATIONALE
1. While your fingers are still in place for the pulse measurement, after counting the pulse rate, observe the patient's respirations (Figure 1).	The patient may alter the rate of respirations if he or she is aware they are being counted.

FIGURE 1. Assessing respirations.

ACTION	RATIONALE
2. Note the rise and fall of the patient's chest.	A complete cycle of an **inspiration** and an **expiration** composes one respiration.
3. Using a watch with a second hand, count the number of respirations for 30 seconds. Multiply this number by 2 to calculate the respiratory rate per minute.	Sufficient time is necessary to observe the rate, depth, and other characteristics.
4. If respirations are abnormal in any way, count the respirations for at least 1 full minute.	Increased time allows the detection of unequal timing between respirations.
5. Note the depth and rhythm of the respirations.	Provides additional assessment data regarding the patient's respiratory status.
6. When measurement is completed, remove gloves, if worn. Cover the patient and help him or her to a position of comfort.	Proper removal of gloves reduces the risk for infection transmission and contamination of other items. Ensures patient comfort.
7. Remove additional PPE, if used. Perform hand hygiene.	Proper removal of PPE reduces the risk for infection transmission and contamination of other items. Hand hygiene deters the spread of microorganisms.

EVALUATION

The expected outcome has been met when the patient's respirations are assessed accurately without injury and the patient experiences minimal discomfort.

DOCUMENTATION

Guidelines

Document respiratory rate, depth, and rhythm on electronic record or flow sheet. Report any abnormal findings to the appropriate person.

Sample Documentation

DocuCare Practice documenting respiration and other vital signs in *Lippincott DocuCare.*

> <u>10/23/20</u> 0830 Patient breathing at a rate of 16 respirations per minute. Respirations regular and unlabored.
>
> —M. Evans, RN

| UNEXPECTED SITUATIONS AND ASSOCIATED INTERVENTIONS | • *The patient is breathing with such shallow respirations that you cannot count the rate:* Sometimes it is easier to count respirations by auscultating the lung sounds. Auscultate lung sounds and count respirations for 30 seconds. Multiply by 2 to calculate the respiratory rate per minute. If the respiratory rate is irregular, count for a full minute. Notify the primary health care provider of the respiratory rate and the shallowness and irregularity of the respirations. |

SPECIAL CONSIDERATIONS	
General Considerations	• If respiratory rate is irregular, count respirations for 1 minute.
Infant and Child Considerations	• For infants, count respirations for 1 full minute due to a normally irregular rhythm. • Assess respirations in infants and children when the child is resting or sitting quietly, because respiratory rate often changes when infants or young children cry, feed, or become more active. The most accurate respiratory rate is obtained when the infant or child is at rest (Jensen, 2015). • Infants' respirations are primarily diaphragmatic; count abdominal movements to measure respiratory rate (Jensen, 2015). After 1 year of age, count thoracic movements (Kyle & Carman, 2017).

  Skill 2-7 ▶ **Assessing Blood Pressure by Auscultation**

Blood pressure refers to the force of the blood against arterial walls. **Systolic pressure** is the highest point of pressure on arterial walls when the ventricles contract and push blood through the arteries at the beginning of systole. When the heart rests between beats during diastole, the pressure drops. The lowest pressure present on arterial walls during diastole is the **diastolic pressure** (Taylor et al., 2019). Blood pressure, measured in millimeters of mercury (mm Hg), is recorded as a fraction. The numerator is the systolic pressure; the denominator is the diastolic pressure. The difference between the two is called the **pulse pressure**. For example, if the blood pressure is 120/80 mm Hg, 120 is the systolic pressure and 80 is the diastolic pressure. The pulse pressure, in this case, is 40. Table 2-2 outlines categories of blood pressure levels for adults.

To get an accurate assessment of blood pressure, you must know what equipment to use, which site to choose, and how to identify the sounds you hear. Take routine measurements after the patient has rested for a minimum of 5 minutes. In addition, make sure the patient does not have any caffeine or nicotine 30 minutes before measuring blood pressure. The American Heart Association recommends that blood pressure readings be measured on two or more subsequent occasions before determining if the blood pressure is outside acceptable parameters (AHA, 2015).

Table 2-2	Categories for Blood Pressure Levels in Adults (Ages 18 and Older)		
	BLOOD PRESSURE LEVEL (MM HG)		
CATEGORY	*Systolic*		*Diastolic*
Normal[a]	<120	AND	Less than 80
Prehypertension	120–139	OR	80–89
High blood pressure			
Stage 1	140–159	OR	90–99
Stage 2	≥160	OR	100 or higher

[a]In regard to risk of heart disease, optimal is defined as less than 120/80 mm Hg.
Source: National Heart, Lung, and Blood Institute (NHLBI). (2015a). National Institutes of Health (NIH). Description of high blood pressure. Retrieved http://www.nhlbi.nih.gov/health/health-topics/topics/hbp.

(*continued*)

Skill 2-7 ▶ Assessing Blood Pressure by Auscultation *(continued)*

The series of sounds for which to listen when assessing blood pressure are called **Korotkoff sounds**. Table 2-3 describes and illustrates these sounds. Blood pressure can be assessed with different types of devices. Commonly, it is assessed by using a stethoscope and sphygmomanometer, obtaining a measurement by auscultation. Blood pressure can also be estimated with a Doppler ultrasound device, by palpation, and with electronic or automated devices. Auscultation is the preferred method of obtaining blood pressure readings in adults and children older than 1 year (Cincinnati Children's Hospital Medical Center, 2009; Ogedegbe & Pickering, 2010; Pickering et al., 2005). It is very important to use the correct technique and properly functioning equipment when assessing blood pressure to avoid errors in measurement. Use of a cuff of the correct size for the patient, correct limb placement, recommended deflation rate, and correct interpretation of the sounds heard are also necessary to ensure accurate blood pressure measurement (Hinkle & Cheever, 2018; Pickering et al., 2005). Table 2-4 outlines common errors in blood pressure measurement.

Table 2-3 | Korotkoff Sounds

PHASE	DESCRIPTION	ILLUSTRATION
Phase I	Characterized by the first appearance of faint, but clear tapping sounds that gradually increase in intensity; the first tapping sound is the systolic pressure.	 **FIGURE A.** Blood flow interrupted by inflated cuff.
Phase II	Characterized by muffled or swishing sounds; these sounds may temporarily disappear, especially in hypertensive people; the disappearance of the sound during the latter part of phase I and during phase II is called the *auscultatory gap* and may cover a range of as much as 40 mm Hg; failing to recognize this gap may cause serious errors of underestimating systolic pressure or overestimating diastolic pressure.	 **FIGURE B.** As the pressure in the cuff is released, blood starts flowing again and Korotkoff sounds are audible.
Phase III	Characterized by distinct, loud sounds as the blood flows relatively freely through an increasingly open artery.	
Phase IV	Characterized by a distinct, abrupt, muffling sound with a soft, blowing quality; in adults, the onset of this phase is considered to be the first diastolic pressure.	
Phase V	The last sound heard before a period of continuous silence; the pressure at which the last sound is heard is the second diastolic pressure.	 **FIGURE C.** Cuff is completely deflated after Phase V, restoring complete blood flow.

At times, it is necessary to assess a patient for **orthostatic hypotension** (postural hypotension). Orthostatic hypotension is a low blood pressure; it is defined as a decrease in systolic blood pressure of 20 mm Hg or a decrease in diastolic blood pressure of 10 mm Hg within 3 minutes of standing when compared with blood pressure from the sitting or supine position (Angelousi et al., 2014). Box 2-2 outlines the procedure for blood pressure measurement to assess for orthostatic hypotension.

Various sites can be used to assess blood pressure. The brachial artery and the popliteal artery are used most commonly. This skill discusses using the brachial artery site to obtain a blood pressure measurement. The skill begins with the procedure for estimating systolic pressure. Estimation of systolic pressure prevents inaccurate readings in the presence of an auscultatory gap (a pause in the auscultated sounds). To identify the first Korotkoff sound accurately, the cuff must be inflated to a pressure above the point at which the pulse can no longer be felt.

Table 2-4 — Blood Pressure Assessment Errors and Contributing Causes

ERROR	CONTRIBUTING CAUSES
Falsely low assessments	• Hearing deficit • Noise in the environment • Viewing the meniscus from above eye level • Applying too wide a cuff • Inserting ear tips of stethoscope incorrectly • Using cracked or kinked tubing • Releasing the valve rapidly • Misplacing the bell beyond the direct area of the artery • Failing to pump the cuff 20–30 mm Hg above the disappearance of the pulse
Falsely high assessments	• Using a manometer not calibrated at the zero mark • Assessing the blood pressure immediately after exercise • Viewing the meniscus from below eye level • Applying a cuff that is too narrow • Releasing the valve too slowly • Reinflating the bladder during auscultation

Box 2-2 — Blood Pressure Measurement to Assess for Orthostatic Hypotension

Assess for signs and symptoms of hypotension, such as dizziness, lightheadedness, pallor, diaphoresis, or syncope throughout the procedure. If the patient is attached to a cardiac monitor, assess for arrhythmias. Immediately return the patient to a supine position if symptoms appear during the procedure. Do not have the patient stand if symptoms of hypotension occur when the patient is sitting. Use the following guidelines to assess for orthostatic hypotension:

• Lower the head of the bed. Place the bed in a low position.
• Ask the patient to lie in a supine position for 3 to 10 minutes. At the end of this time, take initial blood pressure and pulse measurements.

• Assist the patient to a sitting position on the side of the bed with the legs dangling. After 1 to 3 minutes, take the blood pressure and pulse measurements.
• Assist the patient to stand, unless standing is contraindicated. Wait 2 to 3 minutes, then take blood pressure and pulse measurements.
• Record the measurements for each position, noting the position with the readings. A decrease in systolic blood pressure of ≥20 mm Hg or a decrease in diastolic blood pressure of ≥10 mm Hg within 3 minutes of standing when compared with blood pressure from the sitting or supine position is significant for orthostatic hypotension (Angelousi et al., 2014).

Source: Adapted from Angelousi, A., Gererd, N., Benetos, A., et al. (2014). Association between orthostatic hypotension and cardiovascular risk, cerebrovascular risk, cognitive decline and falls as well as overall mortality: A systematic review and meta-analysis. *Journal of Hypertension, 32*(8), 1562–1571; Lanier, J. B., Mote, M. B., & Clay, E. C. (2011). Evaluation and management of orthostatic hypotension. *American Family Physician, 84*(5), 527–536; and Pickering, T. G., Hall, J. E., Appel, L. J., et al. (2005). American Heart Association Scientific Statement. Recommendations for blood pressure measurement in humans and experimental animals. Part 1: Blood pressure measurement in humans: A statement for professionals from the subcommittee of professional and public education of the American Heart Association Council on High Blood Pressure Research. *Circulation, 111*(5), 697–716. Retrieved http://circ.ahajournals.org/content/111/5/697.abstract.

(continued)

Skill 2-7 ▶ Assessing Blood Pressure by Auscultation *(continued)*

DELEGATION CONSIDERATIONS	The measurement of brachial artery blood pressure may be delegated to nursing assistive personnel (NAP) or unlicensed assistive personnel (UAP), as well as to licensed practical/vocational nurses (LPN/LVNs). The decision to delegate must be based on careful analysis of the patient's needs and circumstances, as well as the qualifications of the person to whom the task is being delegated. Refer to the Delegation Guidelines in Appendix A.

EQUIPMENT

- Stethoscope
- Sphygmomanometer
- Blood pressure cuff of appropriate size
- Electronic record, or a pen, paper or flow sheet
- Alcohol swab
- PPE, as indicated

ASSESSMENT

Assess the brachial pulse, or the pulse appropriate for the site being used. Assess for an intravenous infusion or breast or axilla surgery on the side of the body corresponding to the arm used. Assess for the presence of a cast, arteriovenous shunt, or injured or diseased limb. If any of these conditions are present, do not use the affected arm to monitor blood pressure. Assess the size of the limb so that the appropriate-sized blood pressure cuff can be used. The correct cuff should have a bladder length that is 80% of the arm circumference and a width that is at least 40% of the arm circumference: a length to width ratio of 2:1. Refer to Table 2-5 for recommended cuff sizes based on arm circumference. Assess for factors that could affect blood pressure reading, such as the patient's age, exercise, position, weight, fluid balance, smoking, and medications. Note baseline or previous blood pressure measurements. Assess the patient for pain. If the patient reports pain, give pain medication as ordered before assessing blood pressure. If the blood pressure is taken while the patient is in pain, make a notation concerning the pain if the blood pressure is elevated.

Table 2-5 Recommended Blood Pressure Cuff Sizes

CUFF SIZE	CUFF MEASUREMENTS (CM)	ARM CIRCUMFERENCE[a] (CM)
Newborn–premature infants	4 × 8	22–26
Infants	6 × 12	27–34
Older children	9 × 18	35–44
Small adult size	12 × 22	45–52
Adult size	16 × 30	
Large adult size	16 × 36	
Adult thigh size	16 × 42	

[a]Select a blood pressure cuff that has a bladder width that is at least 40% of the arm circumference midway between the olecranon and the acromion.
Source: Data from Pickering, T. G., Hall, J. E., Appel, L. J., et al. (2005). American Heart Association Scientific Statement. Recommendations for blood pressure measurement in humans and experimental animals. Part 1: Blood pressure measurement in humans: A statement for professionals from the subcommittee of professional and public education of the American Heart Association Council on High Blood Pressure Research. *Circulation, 111*(5), 697–716. Retrieved http://circ.ahajournals.org/content/111/5/697.abstract.

NURSING DIAGNOSIS

Determine the related factors for the nursing diagnoses based on the patient's current status. Appropriate nursing diagnoses may include:

- Decreased cardiac output
- Risk for falls
- Risk for unstable blood pressure

OUTCOME IDENTIFICATION AND PLANNING

The expected outcome to achieve when measuring blood pressure is that the patient's blood pressure is measured accurately without injury. Other outcomes may be appropriate depending on the patient's nursing diagnosis.

IMPLEMENTATION

| ACTION |

1. Check the medical order or nursing care plan for frequency of blood pressure measurement. More frequent measurement may be appropriate based on nursing judgment.

2. Perform hand hygiene and put on PPE, if indicated.

3. Identify the patient.

4. Close the curtains around the bed and close the door to the room, if possible. Discuss the procedure with the patient and assess patient's ability to assist with the procedure. Validate that the patient has relaxed for several minutes.

5. Put on gloves, if indicated.

6. Select the appropriate arm for application of the cuff.

7. Have the patient assume a comfortable lying or sitting position with the forearm supported at the level of the heart and the palm of the hand upward (Figure 1). If the measurement is taken in the supine position, support the arm with a pillow. In the sitting position, support the arm yourself or by using the bedside table. If the patient is sitting, have the patient sit back in the chair so that the chair supports his or her back. In addition, make sure the patient keeps the legs uncrossed.

8. Expose the brachial artery by removing garments or move a sleeve if it is not too tight, above the area where the cuff will be placed.

| RATIONALE |

Provides for patient safety.

Hand hygiene and PPE prevent the spread of microorganisms. PPE is required based on transmission precautions.

Identifying the patient ensures the right patient receives the intervention and helps prevent errors.

This ensures the patient's privacy. Explanation relieves anxiety and facilitates cooperation. Activity immediately before measurement can result in inaccurate results.

Gloves prevent contact with blood and body fluids. Gloves are usually not required for measurement of blood pressure, unless contact with blood or body fluids is anticipated.

Measurement of blood pressure may temporarily impede circulation to the extremity.

The position of the arm can have a major influence when the blood pressure is measured; if the upper arm is below the level of the right atrium, the readings will be too high. If the arm is above the level of the heart, the readings will be too low (Pickering et al., 2005). If the back is not supported, the diastolic pressure may be elevated falsely; if the legs are crossed, the systolic pressure may be elevated falsely (Pickering et al., 2005). This position places the brachial artery on the inner aspect of the elbow so that the **bell** or diaphragm of the stethoscope can rest on it easily. This sitting position ensures accuracy.

FIGURE 1. Proper positioning for blood pressure assessment using brachial artery. (*Photo by B. Proud.*)

Clothing over the artery interferes with the ability to hear sounds and can cause inaccurate blood pressure readings. A tight sleeve would cause congestion of blood and possibly inaccurate readings.

Skill 2-7 ▶ Assessing Blood Pressure by Auscultation *(continued)*

ACTION	RATIONALE
9. Palpate the location of the brachial artery. **Center the bladder of the cuff over the brachial artery, about midway on the arm, so that the lower edge of the cuff is about 2.5 to 5 cm (1 to 2 in) above the inner aspect of the elbow. Line up the artery marking on the cuff with the patient's brachial artery. The tubing should extend from the edge of the cuff nearer the patient's elbow (Figure 2).**	Pressure in the cuff applied directly to the artery provides the most accurate readings. If the cuff gets in the way of the stethoscope, readings are likely to be inaccurate. A cuff placed upside down with the tubing toward the patient's head may give a false reading.
10. Wrap the cuff around the arm smoothly and snugly, and fasten it. Do not allow any clothing to interfere with the proper placement of the cuff.	A smooth cuff and snug wrapping produce equal pressure and help promote an accurate measurement. A cuff wrapped too loosely results in an inaccurate reading.
11. Check that the needle on the aneroid gauge is within the zero mark (Figure 3). If using a mercury manometer, check to see that the manometer is in the vertical position and that the mercury is within the zero level with the gauge at eye level.	If the needle is not in the zero area, the blood pressure reading may not be accurate. Tilting a mercury manometer, inaccurate calibration, or improper height for reading the gauge can lead to errors in determining the pressure measurements.

FIGURE 2. Placing the blood pressure cuff. (*Photo by B. Proud.*)

FIGURE 3. Ensuring gauge starts at zero. (*Photo by B. Proud.*)

Estimating Systolic Pressure

12. Palpate the pulse at the brachial or radial artery by pressing gently with the fingertips (Figure 4).	Palpation allows for measurement of the approximate systolic reading.

FIGURE 4. Palpating the brachial pulse. (*Photo by B. Proud.*)

13. Tighten the screw valve on the air pump.	The bladder within the cuff will not inflate with the valve open.

ACTION

14. **Inflate the cuff while continuing to palpate the artery. Note the point on the gauge where the pulse disappears.**

15. Deflate the cuff and wait 1 minute.

Obtaining Blood Pressure Measurement

16. Assume a position that is no more than 3 ft away from the gauge.

17. Place the stethoscope earpieces in your ears. Direct the earpieces forward into the canal and not against the ear itself.

18. Place the bell or diaphragm of the stethoscope firmly but with as little pressure as possible over the brachial artery (Figure 5). Do not allow the stethoscope to touch clothing or the cuff.

19. Pump the pressure 30 mm Hg above the point at which the systolic pressure was palpated and estimated. Open the valve on the manometer and allow air to escape slowly (allowing the gauge to drop 2 to 3 mm per second).

20. **Note the point on the gauge at which the first faint, but clear, sound appears that slowly increases in intensity. Note this number as the systolic pressure (Figure 6). Read the pressure to the closest 2 mm Hg.**

RATIONALE

The point where the pulse disappears provides an estimate of the systolic pressure. To identify the first Korotkoff sound accurately, the cuff must be inflated to a pressure above the point at which the pulse can no longer be felt.

Allowing a brief pause before continuing permits the blood to refill and circulate through the arm.

A distance of more than about 3 ft can interfere with accurate reading of the numbers on the gauge.

Proper placement blocks extraneous noise and allows sound to travel more clearly.

Having the bell or diaphragm directly over the artery allows more accurate readings. Heavy pressure on the brachial artery distorts the shape of the artery and the sound. Placing the bell or diaphragm away from clothing and the cuff prevents noise, which would distract from the sounds made by blood flowing through the artery.

Increasing the pressure above the point where the pulse disappeared ensures a period before hearing the first sound that corresponds with the systolic pressure. It prevents misinterpreting phase II sounds as phase I sounds.

Systolic pressure is the point at which the blood in the artery is first able to force its way through the vessel at a similar pressure exerted by the air bladder in the cuff. The first sound is phase I of Korotkoff sounds.

FIGURE 5. Proper placement of diaphragm of stethoscope. (*Photo by B. Proud.*)

FIGURE 6. Measuring systolic blood pressure. (*Photo by B. Proud.*)

21. Do not reinflate the cuff once the air is being released to recheck the systolic pressure reading.

Reinflating the cuff while obtaining the blood pressure is uncomfortable for the patient and can cause an inaccurate reading. Reinflating the cuff causes congestion of blood in the lower arm, which lessens the loudness of Korotkoff sounds.

Skill 2-7 ▶ Assessing Blood Pressure by Auscultation (continued)

ACTION	RATIONALE
22. Note the point at which the sound completely disappears. Note this number as the diastolic pressure (Figure 7). Read the pressure to the closest 2 mm Hg.	The point at which the sound disappears corresponds to the beginning of phase V Korotkoff sounds and is generally considered the diastolic pressure reading (Pickering et al., 2005).

FIGURE 7. Measuring diastolic blood pressure. (*Photo by B. Proud.*)

ACTION	RATIONALE
23. Allow the remaining air to escape quickly. Repeat any suspicious reading, but wait at least 1 minute. Deflate the cuff completely between attempts to check the blood pressure.	False readings are likely to occur if there is congestion of blood in the limb while obtaining repeated readings.
24. When measurement is completed, remove the cuff. Remove gloves, if worn. Cover the patient and help him or her to a position of comfort.	Removing gloves properly reduces the risk for infection transmission and contamination of other items. Ensures patient comfort.
25. Clean the bell or diaphragm of the stethoscope with the alcohol wipe. Clean and store the sphygmomanometer, according to facility policy.	Appropriate cleaning deters the spread of microorganisms. Equipment should be left ready for use.
26. Remove additional PPE, if used. Perform hand hygiene.	Proper removal of PPE reduces the risk for infection transmission and contamination of other items. Hand hygiene deters the spread of microorganisms.

EVALUATION

The expected outcome has been met when the blood pressure is measured accurately without injury and with minimal patient discomfort.

DOCUMENTATION

Guidelines

Record the findings on electronic record or flow sheet. Report abnormal findings to the primary health care provider. Identify arm used and site of assessment if other than brachial.

Sample Documentation

DocuCare Practice documenting blood pressure and other vital signs in *Lippincott DocuCare*.

> 10/18/20 0945 Blood pressure taken in right arm 180/88. Dr. Brown notified. Ordered captopril 25 mg PO b.i.d. Blood pressure to be repeated 30 minutes after administering medication.
>
> —*M. Evans, RN*

SPECIAL CONSIDERATIONS

General Considerations

- It is recommended that blood pressure measurements should be checked in both arms at the first examination (Pickering et al., 2005). Most people have differences in blood pressure readings between arms. When there is a consistent interarm difference, use the arm with the higher pressure (Pickering et al., 2005).
- If you have difficulty hearing the blood pressure sounds, raise the patient's arm, with cuff in place, over his or her head for 30 seconds before rechecking the blood pressure. Inflate the cuff while the arm is elevated, and then gently lower the arm while continuing to support it. Position the stethoscope and deflate the cuff at the usual rate while listening for Korotkoff sounds. Raising the arm over the head reduces vascular volume in the limb and improves blood flow to enhance the Korotkoff sounds (Pickering et al., 2005).
- Blood pressure can be assessed using an automatic electronic blood pressure monitor or Doppler ultrasound (see the accompanying Skill Variation).
- Many versions of automatic electronic blood pressure monitors are not recommended for patients with irregular heart rates, tremors, or the inability to hold the extremity still. The presence of these conditions may cause the monitor to incorrectly overinflate the cuff, causing pain for the patient. Check the manufacturer's guidelines when considering use with these patients.
- Diastolic pressure measured while the patient is sitting is approximately 5 mm Hg higher than when measured while the patient is supine; systolic pressure measured while the patient is supine is approximately 8 mm Hg higher than when measured in the patient who is sitting (Pickering et al., 2005).
- Measuring blood pressure in the forearm by auscultating the radial artery for the Korotkoff sounds is becoming more common. Forearm measurements tend to be higher than the upper arm measurements (Halm, 2014). The accuracy of readings with forearm monitors is affected by the position of the wrist relative to the heart. This can be avoided if the wrist is always at heart level when the reading is taken (Pickering et al., 2005). This site for measurement has been suggested as an alternative for obtaining blood pressure readings in people who are obese. It is often difficult to obtain the appropriately sized cuff for the upper arm, given arm circumference and conical-shaped upper arms common in obesity. The conical shape of the upper arm makes it difficult to fit the cuff to the arm, increasing the likelihood of inaccurate blood pressure measurement (Halm, 2014). Thus, measurement in the forearm can be a possible solution to this problem.
- When the patient's brachial artery is inaccessible and/or the use of the upper arm is contraindicated, you can assess the blood pressure using the popliteal artery in the leg. The systolic pressure is normally 10 to 40 mm Hg higher at this site than the arm, although the diastolic pressure is the same (Jensen, 2015).

Infant and Child Considerations

In infants and small children, the lower extremities are commonly used for blood pressure monitoring. The more common sites are the popliteal, dorsalis pedis, and posterior tibial. Blood pressures obtained in the lower extremities are generally higher than if taken in the upper extremities. In children over 1 year of age, the systolic pressure in the thigh tends to be 10 to 40 mm Hg higher than in the arm; the diastolic pressure remains the same (Kyle & Carman, 2017).

- Infants and children presenting with cardiac complaints may have blood pressures assessed in all four extremities. Large differences among blood pressure readings can indicate heart defects.
- The fifth Korotkoff sound corresponds to diastolic blood pressure in children. In some children, the Korotkoff sounds continue to 0 mm Hg. In this situation, document the reading as systolic pressure over "P" for pulse (Kyle & Carman, 2017).

Skill 2-7 ▶ Assessing Blood Pressure by Auscultation *(continued)*

Home Care Considerations

- Automated blood pressure devices in public locations are generally inaccurate and inconsistent. In addition, the cuffs on these devices are inadequate for people with large arms (Pickering et al., 2005).
- Explain to the patient that it is important to use a cuff size appropriate for limb circumference. Inform the patient that cuff sizes range from a pediatric cuff to a large thigh cuff and that a poorly fitting cuff can result in an inaccurate measurement.
- Inform the patient about digital blood pressure monitoring equipment. Although more costly than manual cuffs, most provide an easy-to-read recording of systolic and diastolic measurements.
- Explain that three readings, at least 1 minute apart, should be taken while in a sitting position, both in the morning and at night. Measurement should occur after resting quietly in a chair for 3 to 5 minutes, with the upper arm at heart level. The readings should be recorded to show to the health care provider.
- Explain that home monitoring devices should be checked for accuracy every 1 to 2 years. Readings should be compared with auscultated measurement by a health care provider to ensure accuracy.

Skill Variation ▶ Assessing Blood Pressure Using an Automatic Electronic Blood Pressure Monitor

Automatic, electronic equipment may be used to monitor blood pressure any time frequent assessments are necessary (Figure A). These monitors determine blood pressure by analyzing the sounds of blood flow or measuring oscillations (fluctuations) in blood flow. The machine can be set to take and record blood pressure readings at preset intervals. Irregular heart rates, excessive patient movement, and environmental noise can interfere with the readings. Because electronic equipment is more sensitive to outside interference, these readings are susceptible to error. The cuff is applied in the same manner as the auscultatory method, with the microphone or pressure sensor positioned directly over the artery. When using an automatic blood pressure device for serial readings, check the cuffed limb frequently. Incomplete deflation of the cuff between measurements can lead to inadequate arterial perfusion and venous drainage, compromising the circulation in the limb (Bern et al., 2007; Pickering et al., 2004).

FIGURE A. Electronic blood pressure device. (*Photo by B. Proud.*)

1. Check the medical order or nursing care plan for frequency of blood pressure measurement. More frequent measurement may be appropriate based on nursing judgment.

2. Perform hand hygiene and put on PPE, if indicated.

3. Identify the patient.

4. Close the curtains around the bed and close the door to the room, if possible.
5. Discuss the procedure with the patient and assess the patient's ability to assist with the procedure.
6. Validate that the patient has relaxed for several minutes.
7. Select the appropriate limb for application of cuff.
8. Have the patient assume a comfortable lying or sitting position with the limb exposed.
9. **Center the bladder of the cuff over the artery, lining up the artery mark on the cuff with the limb artery.**
10. Wrap the cuff around the limb smoothly and snugly, and fasten it. Do not allow any clothing to interfere with the proper placement of the cuff.
11. Turn on the machine. **If the machine has different settings for infants, children, and adults, select the appropriate setting.** Push the start button. Instruct the patient to hold the limb still.
12. Wait until the machine beeps and the blood pressure reading appears. Remove the cuff from the patient's limb and clean and store the equipment.
13. Remove PPE, if used. Perform hand hygiene.
14. Record the findings on electronic record or flow sheet. Report abnormal findings to the appropriate person. Identify arm used and site of assessment if other than brachial.

Skill Variation ▶ Assessing Systolic Blood Pressure Using Doppler Ultrasound

Blood pressure can be measured with a Doppler ultrasound device, which amplifies sound. It is especially useful if the sounds are indistinct or inaudible with a regular stethoscope. This method provides only an estimate of systolic blood pressure.

1. Check the medical order or nursing care plan for frequency of blood pressure measurement. More frequent measurement may be appropriate based on nursing judgment.

2. Perform hand hygiene and put on PPE, if indicated.

3. Identify the patient.

4. Explain the procedure to the patient.
5. Close the curtains around the bed and close the door to the room, if possible.
6. Select the appropriate limb for application of cuff.
7. Have the patient assume a comfortable lying or sitting position with the appropriate limb exposed.
8. Center the bladder of the cuff over the artery, lining up the artery marker on the cuff with the artery.
9. Wrap the cuff around the limb smoothly and snugly, and fasten it. Do not allow any clothing to interfere with the proper placement of the cuff.
10. Check that the needle on the aneroid gauge is within the zero mark. If using a mercury manometer, check to see that the manometer is in the vertical position and that the mercury is within the zero level with the gauge at eye level.
11. Place a small amount of conducting gel to the site where you expect to auscultate the pulse.
12. Hold the Doppler device in your nondominant hand. Using your dominant hand, touch the probe lightly to the skin with the probe tip in the gel. Adjust the volume, as needed. Hold the probe perpendicular to the skin. Slowly move the Doppler tip around until you hear the pulse.
13. Once the pulse is found using the Doppler device, close the valve to the sphygmomanometer. Tighten the screw valve on the air pump.

14. Inflate the cuff while continuing to use the Doppler device on the artery. Note the point on the gauge where the pulse disappears (Figure B).

FIGURE B. Inflating cuff while listening to artery pulsations. (*Photo by B. Proud.*)

15. Open the valve on the manometer and allow air to escape quickly. Repeat the measurement if a suspicious reading is obtained, but wait at least 1 minute between readings to allow normal circulation to return in the limb. Deflate the cuff completely between attempts to check the blood pressure.
16. Remove the Doppler tip and turn off the Doppler device. Wipe excess gel off the patient's skin with tissue. Remove the cuff.
17. Wipe any gel remaining on the Doppler probe off with a tissue. Clean the Doppler device according to facility policy or manufacturer's recommendations.
18. Return the Doppler device to the charge base.
19. Remove PPE, if used. Perform hand hygiene.

20. Record the findings on electronic record or flow sheet. Report abnormal findings to the appropriate person. Identify arm used and site of assessment if other than brachial.

Skill 2-7 ▶ Assessing Blood Pressure by Auscultation *(continued)*

EVIDENCE FOR PRACTICE ▶

HOME BLOOD PRESSURE MONITORING

Patients and/or their family members often need to check their own temperature, pulse, and/or blood pressure at home. Home blood pressure monitoring (HBPM) is being increasingly recommended and has been shown to improve blood pressure control (Crabtree & Stuart-Shor, 2014; Pickering et al., 2005). Research has shown that readings at home are often lower than those taken in a health care provider setting, contribute to better adherence treatment, and provide multiple readings taken over prolonged periods, giving a better picture of the patient's status and response to treatment (Lamble, 2014; Shimbo et al., 2015).

Related Research

Crabtree, M. M., & Stuart-Shor, E. (2014). Implementing home blood pressure monitoring into usual care. *Journal for Nurse Practitioners, 10*(8), 607–610.

This study investigated the incorporation of a culturally tailored HBPM program into primary care in a Federally Qualified Community Health Center in the Northeast region of the United States. Patients with **hypertension** or at risk for hypertension were supplied with a validated HBPM device. Registered nurses provided patient education in HBPM and self-management strategies using culturally/linguistically tailored visual handouts. Patients were asked to measure and record their blood pressure daily three or four times per week, and bring the information to follow-up appointments. Information was collected related to the number of clinical sessions attended, baseline (pre) and 12-month (post) measures of mean blood pressure, proportion of patients at blood pressure goal, change in systolic and diastolic blood pressure, and pre/post percentage improvement in blood pressure. Patients reported assessment of self-care skills and satisfaction with HBPM via surveys. The nurses also provided outreach for continued motivation and adherence. The proportion of patients at goal blood pressure improved from pre (30%) to post (90%). Significant reductions were noted pre/post for systolic and diastolic blood pressure. The majority (84%) of patients reported HBPM improved their understanding and management of their blood pressure and they would continue to use the HBPM. The authors concluded that it is possible to implement HBPM in an underserved, high-risk population and that control of blood pressure can be improved by this type of intervention.

Relevance to Nursing Practice

Patient education is an important part of nursing care. Nurses can play an important role in assisting patients with hypertension to learn to measure their blood pressure accurately and in improving management of care for patients with hypertension.

Refer to thePoint® for additional research on related nursing topics.

Enhance Your Understanding

Focusing on Patient Care: Developing Clinical Reasoning

Consider the case scenarios at the beginning of the chapter as you answer the following questions to enhance your understanding and apply what you have learned.

QUESTIONS

1. Tyrone Jeffries, the 5 year old with a fever of 101.3°F (38.5°C), is suspected of having a middle-ear infection. You need to obtain another set of vital signs for him. As you approach with the electronic thermometer, Tyrone begins to scream, saying, "Go away. I don't want it!" How would you respond?

2. Toby White, who is 26 years old with a history of asthma, has a respiratory rate of 32 breaths per minute. What other assessments would be most important to make?

3. Carl Glatz, the 58-year-old man receiving medications for hypertension, asks you about how he should monitor his blood pressure at home. What information would you suggest?

You can find suggested answers after the Bibliography at the end of this chapter.

Integrated Case Study Connection

The case studies in the back of the book focus on integrating concepts. Refer to the following case studies to enhance your understanding of the concepts and skills in this chapter.

- Basic Case Studies: Abigail Cantonelli, page 1099; James White, page 1102; Naomi Bell, page 1103; Joe LeRoy, page 1108.
- Intermediate Case Studies: Olivia Greenbaum, page 1113; Victoria Holly, page 1115; Lucille Howard, page 1123; Janice Romero, page 1124; Gwen Galloway, page 1125.
- Advanced Case Studies: Cole McKean, page 1128.

Taylor Suite Resources

Explore these additional resources to enhance learning for this chapter:

- NCLEX-Style Questions and other resources on thePoint°, http://thePoint.lww.com/Lynn5e
- *Skill Checklists for Taylor's Clinical Nursing Skills*, 5e
- *Taylor's Video Guide to Clinical Nursing Skills:* Vital Signs
- *Fundamentals of Nursing:* Chapter 25, Vital Signs
- *Lippincott DocuCare* Fundamentals cases

Bibliography

Allegaert, K., Casteels, K., van Gorp, I., & Bogaert, G. (2014). Tympanic, infrared skin, and temporal artery scan thermometers compared with rectal measurement in children: A real-life assessment. *Current Therapeutic Research, 76,* 34–38.

American Heart Association. (2017). Understanding blood pressure readings. Retrieved http://www.heart.org/HEARTORG/Conditions/HighBloodPressure/KnowYourNumbers/Understanding-Blood-Pressure-Readings_UCM_301764_Article.jsp#.WrZcg4jwaUl

Angelousi, A., Gererd, N., Benetos, A., et al. (2014). Association between orthostatic hypotension and cardiovascular risk, cerebrovascular risk, cognitive decline and falls as well as overall mortality: A systematic review and meta-analysis. *Journal of Hypertension, 32*(8), 1562–1571.

Ansell, H., Meyer, A., & Thompson, S. (2014). Why don't nurses consistently take patient respiratory rates? *British Journal of Nursing, 23*(8), 414–418.

Asher, C., & Northington, L. (2008). Society of Pediatric Nurses. Position statement for measurement of temperature/fever in children. *Journal of Pediatric Nursing, 23*(3), 234–326.

Bell, E. (2015). University of Iowa Children's Hospital. Iowa neonatology handbook: Temperature. Servocontrol: Incubator and radiant warmer. Retrieved http://www.uichildrens.org/childrens-content.aspx?id=234214

Bern, L., Brandt, M., Mbeiu, N., et al. (2007). Differences in blood pressure values obtained with automated and manual methods in medical inpatients. *Medsurg Nursing, 16*(6), 356–361.

Brady, T. M., Redwine, K. M., & Flynn, J. T. (2013). Screening blood pressure measurement in children: Are we saving lives? *Pediatric Nephrology, 29*(6), 947–950.

Braun, C. (2006). Accuracy of pacifier thermometers in young children. *Pediatric Nursing, 32*(5), 413–418.

Burchill, C., Anderson, B., & O'Connor, P. (2015). Exploration of nurse practices and attitudes related to postoperative vital signs. *Medsurg Nursing, 24*(4), 249–255.

Cincinnati Children's Hospital Medical Center. (2009). Best evidence statement. Blood pressure measurement in children. Retrieved file:///C:/Users/John%20and%20Pam/Downloads/NephroBPMeasureFINALBESt023.1-9-2009a.pdf

Cohen, B. J., & Taylor, J. J. (2013). *Memmler's structure and function of the human body* (10th ed.). Philadelphia, PA: Wolters Kluwer.

Collins, S. A., Cato, K., Albers, D., et al. (2013). Nursing documentation and patients' mortality. *American Journal of Critical Care, 22*(4). 306–313.

Coogan, N., Marra, A., & Lomonaco, E. (2015). Assessing accurate BP measurement: Size and technique matter! *Nursing, 45*(4), 16–18.

Crabtree, M. M., & Stuart-Shor, E. (2014). Implementing home blood pressure monitoring into usual care. *Journal for Nurse Practitioners, 10*(8), 607–610.

Davie, A., & Amoore, J. (2010). Best practice in the measurement of body temperature. *Nursing Standard, 24*(42), 42–49.

Dondelinger, R. M. (2010). The fundamentals of… Infant warmers. *Biomedical Instrumentation & Technology, 44*(6), 485–487.

Elliott, M., & Coventry, A. (2012). Critical care: the eight vital signs of patient monitoring. *British Journal of Nursing, 21*(10), 621–625.

El-Radhi, A. S. (2013). Temperature measurement: The right thermometer and site. *British Journal of Nursing, 22*(4), 208–211.

El-Radhi, A. S. (2014). Determining fever in children: The search for an ideal thermometer. *British Journal of Nursing, 23*(2), 91–94.

Eliopoulos, C. (2014). *Gerontological Nursing* (8th ed.). Philadelphia, PA: Wolters Kluwer.

Exergen. (2007, update 2014). *Temporal scanner reference manual.* Watertown, MA: Author. Retrieved http://www.exergen.com/medical/PDFs/tat2000c-manual.pdf

Flynn, J. T., Daniels, S. R., Hayman, L. L., et al. (2014). AHA scientific statement. Update: Ambulatory blood pressure monitoring in children and adolescents. *Hypertension, 63*(5), 1116–1135.

Furlong, D., Carroll, D. L., Finn, C., Gay, D., Gryglik, C., & Donahue, V. (2015). Comparison of temporal to pulmonary artery temperature in febrile patients. *Dimensions of Critical Care Nursing, 34*(1), 47–52.

Grossman, S., & Porth, C. M. (2014). *Porth's pathophysiology: Concepts of altered health states* (9th ed.). Philadelphia, PA: Wolters Kluwer.

Halm, M. A. (2014). Arm circumference, shape, and length: How interplaying variables affect blood pressure measurement in obese persons. *American Journal of Critical Care, 23*(2), 166–170.

Hamilton, P. A., Marcos, L. S., & Secic, M. (2013). Performance of infrared ear and forehead thermometers: A comparative study in 205 febrile and afebrile children. *Journal of Clinical Nursing, 22*(17–18), 2509–2518.

Haugan, B., Langerud, A. K., Kalvøy, H., Frøslie, K. F., Riise, E., & Kapstad, H. (2012). Can we trust the new generation of infrared tympanic thermometers in clinical practice? *Journal of Clinical Nursing, 22*(5/6), 698–709.

Henley, N., Quatrara, B., & Conaway, M. (2015). A pilot study: Comparison of arm versus ankle noninvasive blood pressure measurement at 2 different levels of backrest elevation. *Dimensions of Critical Care Nursing, 34*(4), 232–235.

Higgins, D. (2008). Patient assessment Part 2: Measuring oral temperature. *Nursing Times, 104*(8), 24–25.

Hinkle, J. L., & Cheever, K. H. (2018). *Brunner & Suddarth's textbook of medical-surgical nursing* (14th ed.). Philadelphia, PA: Wolters Kluwer.

Hirsch, A. T., Haskal, Z. J., Hertzer, N. R., et al. (2006). ACC/AHA 2005 guidelines for the management of patients with peripheral arterial disease (lower extremity, renal, mesenteric, and abdominal aortic): A collaborative report from the American Association for Vascular Surgery/Society for Vascular Surgery, Society for Cardiovascular Angiography and Interventions, Society for Vascular Medicine and Biology, Society of Interventional Radiology, and the ACC/AHA Task Force on Practice Guidelines (Writing Committee to Develop Guidelines for the Management of Patients with Peripheral Arterial Disease). *Circulation, 113*(11), e463–e654.

Hogan-Quigley, B., Palm, M. L., & Bickley, L. S. (2017). *Bates' nursing guide to physical examination and history taking* (2nd ed.). Philadelphia, PA: Wolters Kluwer.

Holland, M., & Lewis, P. S. (2014). An audit and suggested guidelines for in-patient blood pressure measurement. *Journal of Hypertension, 32*(11), 2166–2170.

Hurwitz, B., Brown, J., & Altmiller, G. (2015). Improving pediatric temperature measurement in the ED. *American Journal of Nursing, 115*(9), 48–55.

Jarvis, C. (2016). *Physical examination & health assessment* (7th ed.). St. Louis, MO: Elsevier.

Jensen, S. (2015.) *Nursing health assessment: A best practice approach* (2nd ed.). Philadelphia, PA: Wolters Kluwer.

Kiekkas, P., Konstantinou, E., Psychogiou, K. S., Tsampoula, I., Stefanopoulos, N., & Bakalis, N. (2014). Nursing personnel's attitudes towards fever and antipyresis of adult patients: cross-sectional survey. *Journal of Clinical Nursing, 23*(19/20), 2949–2957.

Kyle, T., & Carman, S. (2017). *Essentials of pediatric nursing* (3rd ed.). Philadelphia, PA: Wolters Kluwer.

Lamble, J. (2014). Home blood pressure monitoring in hypertension. *British Journal of Cardiac Nursing, 9*(1), 13–17.

Leblanc, M. E., Cloutier, L., & Poirier, P. (2015). Sensitivity, specificity, and predictive values of a forearm blood pressure measurement method in severe obesity. *Blood Pressure Monitoring, 20*(2), 79–82.

Makic, M. B., Martin, S. A., Burns, S., Phhilbrick, D., & Rauen, C. (2013). Putting evidence into nursing practice: Four traditional practices not supported by evidence. *Critical Care Nurse, 33*(2), 28–43.

Mayo Clinic. (2015a). High blood pressure (hypertension). Get the most out of home blood pressure monitoring. Retrieved http://www.mayoclinic.com/health/high-blood-pressure/HI00016

Mayo Clinic. (2015b). Thermometers: Understand the options. Retrieved http://www.mayoclinic.org/diseases-conditions/fever/in-depth/thermometers/art-20046737

McConnell, E., Senseney, D., George, S. S., & Whipple, D. (2013). Reliability of temporal artery thermometers. *Medsurg Nursing, 22*(6), 387–392.

Mills, P., Gray, D., & Krassioukov, A. (2014). Five things to know about orthostatic hypotension and aging. *Journal of the American Geriatrics Society, 62*(9), 1822–1823.

Morton, P. G., & Fontaine, D. K. (2018). *Critical care nursing. A holistic approach* (11th ed.). Philadelphia, PA: Wolters Kluwer.

NANDA International, Inc.: Nursing Diagnoses - Definitions and Classification 2018–2020 © 2017 NANDA International, ISBN 978-1-62623-929-6. Used by arrangement with the Thieme Group, Stuttgart/New York.

National Heart, Lung, and Blood Institute (NHLBI). (2010). National Institutes of Health. (NIH). What is hypotension? Retrieved http://www.nhlbi.nih.gov/health/health-topics/topics/hyp

National Heart, Lung, and Blood Institute (NHLBI). (2015a). National Institutes of Health. (NIH). Description of high blood pressure. Retrieved http://www.nhlbi.nih.gov/health/health-topics/topics/hbp

National Heart, Lung, and Blood Institute (NHLBI). (2015b). National Institutes of Health. (NIH). Risk factors for high blood pressure. Retrieved http://www.nhlbi.nih.gov/health/health-topics/topics/hbp/atrisk

Ogedegbe, G., & Pickering, T. (2010). Principles and techniques of blood pressure measurement. *Cardiology Clinics, 28*(4), 571–586.

Ogunlesi, T. A. (2009). *Radiant warmers versus incubators for regulating body temperature in newborn infants: RHL commentary. The WHO Reproductive Health Library.* Geneva: World Health Organization. Retrieved http://apps.who.int/rhl/newborn/cd000435_ogunlesita_com/en/index.html#

Parkes, R. (2011). Rate of respiration: The forgotten vital sign. *Emergency Nurse, 19*(2), 12–17.

Perry, S. E., Hockenberry, M. J., Lowdermilk, D. L., & Wilson, D. (2014). *Maternal child nursing care* (5th ed.). St. Louis, MO: Elsevier.

Philip, K., Richardson, R., & Cohen, J. (2013). Staff perceptions of respiratory rate measurement in a general hospital. *British Journal of Nursing, 22*(10), 570–574.

Pickering, T. G., Hall, J. E., Appel, L. J., et al. (2005). American Heart Association Scientific Statement. Recommendations for blood pressure measurement in humans and experimental animals. Part 1: Blood pressure measurement in humans: A statement for professionals from the subcommittee of professional and public education of the American Heart Association Council on High Blood Pressure Research. *Circulation, 111*(5), 697–716. Retrieved http://circ.ahajournals.org/content/111/5/697.abstract

Reddy, A. K., Jogendra, M. R. D., & Rosendorff, C. (2014). Blood pressure measurement in the geriatric population. *Blood Pressure Monitoring, 19*(2), 59–63.

Schimanski, K., Jull, A., Mitchell, N., & McLay, J. (2014). Comparison study of upper arm and forearm non-invasive blood pressures in adult emergency department patients. *International Journal of Nursing Studies, 51*(12), 1575–1584.

Shimbo, D., Abdalla, M., Falzon, L., Townsend, R. R., & Muntner, P. (2015). Role of ambulatory and home blood pressure monitoring in clinical practice. A narrative review. *Annals of Internal Medicine, 163*(9), 691–700.

Singler, K., Bertsch, T., Juergen Heppner, H., et al. (2013). Diagnostic accuracy of three different methods of temperature measurement in acutely ill geriatric patients. *Age and Ageing, 42*(6), 740–746.

Smith, J., Alcock, G., & Usher, K. (2013). Temperature measurement in the preterm and term neonate: A review of the literature. *Neonatal Network, 32*(1), 16–25.

Storm-Versloot, M. N., Verweij, L., Lucas, C., et al. (2014). Clinical relevance of routinely measured vital signs in hospitalized patients: A systematic review. *Journal of Nursing Scholarship, 46*(1), 39–49.

Sund-Levander, M., & Grodzinsky, E. (2013). Assessment of body temperature measurement options. *British Journal of Nursing, 22*(15), 880–888.

Taylor, C., Lynn, P., & Bartlett, J. (2019). *Fundamentals of nursing: The art and science of person-centered care* (9th ed.). Philadelphia, PA: Wolters Kluwer.

Tysinger, E. L. (2015). How vital are vital signs? A systematic review of vital sign compliance and accuracy in nursing. *Journal of Science & Medicine,* 68–75. Retrieved http://www.wakehealth.edu/uploadedFiles/User_Content/SchoolOfMedicine/_MD_Program/WFJSM/Documents/2015_May/wfjsm2015v1i1p68.pdf

U.S. Environmental Protection Facility (EPA). (2015). Mercury. Thermometers. Retrieved http://epa.gov/hg/thermometer-main.html

Van Kuiken, D., & Huth, M. M. (2013). What is 'normal'? Evaluating vital signs. *Pediatric Nursing, 39*(5), 216–224.

VHA Center for Engineering & Occupational Safety and Health (CEOSH). (2016). *Safe patient handling and mobility guidebook.* St. Louis, MO: Author. Retrieved http://www.tampavaref.org/safe-patient-handling.htm

SUGGESTED ANSWERS FOR FOCUSING ON PATIENT CARE: DEVELOPING CLINICAL REASONING

1. First, assess the problem, talking with Tyrone and his mother, using age-appropriate communication with Tyrone. Because potentially he is thought to have an ear infection, he may be having pain in one or both ears. Assess his status and ability to cooperate and consider another route for temperature measurement. Temporal artery or axillary measurement may be indicated, based on your assessment and facility policy.

2. In addition to the respiratory rate, note the depth and rhythm of the respirations. Auscultate lung sounds. Measure the patient's oxygen saturation level with pulse oximetry. Ask the patient about recent activity and the presence of factors that may have caused an acute asthma attack, and for factors that could affect respirations, such as exercise, medications, smoking, chronic illness or conditions, neurologic injury, pain, and anxiety. Note baseline or previous respiratory measurements. Assess patient for any signs of respiratory distress, which include retractions, nasal flaring, grunting, and orthopnea (breathing more easily in an upright position).

3. Home monitoring of blood pressure for patients with hypertension is strongly recommended. Advise Mr. Glatz that automated blood pressure devices in public areas are generally inaccurate and inconsistent. Use a cuff size appropriate for limb circumference. Inform him that cuff sizes range from a pediatric cuff to a large thigh cuff and that a poorly fitting cuff can result in an inaccurate measurement. Discuss digital blood pressure monitoring equipment. Although more costly than manual cuffs, most provide an easy-to-read recording of systolic and diastolic measurements.

Health Assessment

3

Focusing on Patient Care

This chapter will help you develop some of the physical assessment skills related to health assessment necessary to care for the following patients:

William Lincoln, age 54, comes to the clinic for a routine checkup.

Lois Felker, age 30, has a history of type 1 diabetes. She is a patient in the hospital.

Bobby Williams, age 14, has been brought to the emergency department by his parents and is suspected of having appendicitis.

Refer to Focusing on Patient Care: Developing Clinical Reasoning at the end of the chapter to apply what you learn.

Learning Objectives

After completing the chapter, you will be able to accomplish the following:

1. Describe and perform the components of a general survey.
2. Weigh a patient using a bed scale.
3. Use appropriate equipment while performing a head-to-toe physical assessment.
4. Position the patient correctly to perform a head-to-toe physical assessment.
5. Verbalize the appropriate rationales for performing the specific head-to-toe assessment techniques.
6. Assess the skin, hair, and nails.
7. Assess the head and neck.
8. Assess the thorax, lungs, and breasts.
9. Assess the cardiovascular system.
10. Assess the abdomen.
11. Assess female genitalia.
12. Assess male genitalia.
13. Assess the neurologic, musculoskeletal, and peripheral vascular systems.

Key Terms

activities of daily living (ADLs): daily self-care activities within person's place of residence and/or in outdoor environments

adventitious breath sounds: sounds that are not normally heard in the lungs on auscultation

ascites: accumulation of serous fluid in the peritoneal cavity

auscultation: act of listening with a stethoscope to sounds produced within the body

body mass index (BMI): a ratio of weight (in kilograms) to height (in meters), used as an indicator of total body fat stores in the general population, and to estimate relative risk for diseases such as cardiovascular disease, high blood pressure, and type 2 diabetes

bruits: abnormal "swooshing" sounds heard on auscultation, indicating turbulent blood flow

cyanosis: bluish or grayish skin discoloration in response to inadequate oxygenation

ecchymosis: a collection of blood in the subcutaneous tissues, causing purplish discoloration

edema: excess fluid in the tissues, characterized by swelling

erythema: redness of the skin

general survey: overall impression of a person by the health care provider; includes physical appearance, body structure, mobility, and behavior

health history: a collection of subjective data that provides information about the patient's health status

inspection: process of performing purposeful observations in a systematic manner

instrumental activities of daily living (IADLs): daily self-care activities needed for independent living; for example, housekeeping, meal preparation, management of finances, and transportation

jaundice: yellow color of the skin resulting from liver and gallbladder diseases, some types of anemia, and hemolysis

pallor: paleness of the skin

palpation: an assessment technique that uses the sense of touch

percussion: the act of striking one object against another to produce sound

physical assessment: a collection of objective data that provides information about changes in the patient's body systems

precordium: the area on the anterior chest over the heart and lower thorax, encompassing the aortic, pulmonic, tricuspid, and mitral (apical) areas, and Erb's point

turgor: fullness or elasticity of the skin

Health assessment involves gathering information about the overall level of physical, psychological, sociocultural, developmental, functional, and spiritual health of a patient. The nurse gathers, evaluates, and synthesizes information (data). Based on these findings, the nurse plans appropriate nursing interventions and evaluates patient care outcomes to deliver the best possible care for each patient. A health assessment includes a health history and a physical assessment.

A **health history** is a collection of subjective data that provides information about the patient's health status. Components of the health history include biographical data; the reason the patient is seeking health care; present health concerns or history of those health concerns; health history; family history; functional health; psychosocial and lifestyle factors; and a review of systems. The nurse should adapt questions to the individual patient, omitting questions that do not apply and adding questions that seem pertinent, based on the setting, situation, the individual patient, and ongoing information as the health assessment proceeds. Be sure to use language the patient can understand; avoid using medical terms and jargon. Nurses use therapeutic communication skills, including interviewing techniques, during the health history to gather data to identify actual and potential health problems as well as sources of patient strength. In addition, during the health history, the nurse begins to establish an effective nurse–patient relationship. Fundamentals Review 3-1 summarizes major components of a health history. Examples of health history questions related to each body system (review of systems) are included in the discussion of each region of the physical examination discussed in this chapter.

In general, a physical assessment is performed after taking the health history. **Physical assessment** is a collection of objective data that provides information about changes in the patient's body systems. These data are obtained through direct observation or elicited through examination techniques, such as **inspection, palpation, percussion,** and **auscultation** (Fundamentals Review 3-2). The use of percussion and deep palpation are advanced physical assessment skills, usually performed by advanced practice profession-als, health care providers with advanced education. *Percussion and deep palpation will not be discussed as part of physical assessment in this chapter. Refer to information on* thePoint® *or a health assessment text for details of these advanced assessment skills.* To perform a physical examination, the nurse requires knowledge of anatomy and physiology, the equipment used for assessing body systems, and proper patient positioning and draping.

Nurses should be familiar with the general health beliefs of various cultural and ethnic groups to improve the effectiveness of health care services and provide care within a cul-tural context (Purnell, 2013). Nurses should know risk factors for alterations in health that are based on racial inheritance and ethnic backgrounds. They should also be aware of the normal variations that occur within races, and should understand how religion and spirituality may impact health. In addition, laboratory and diagnostic tests provide crucial information about a patient's health. These results become a part of the total health assessment.

For a comprehensive assessment, the nurse integrates individual assessments following a systematic head-to-toe format. *However, not all assessments included in a comprehensive physical assessment are covered in this chapter.* Advanced practice professionals (health care providers with advanced education) typically perform some of the assessments included in a comprehensive or focused exam, such as an internal eye examination, a vaginal examina-tion, or a rectal examination. *Refer to information on* thePoint® *or a health assessment text for details of these advanced assessment skills.*

It is often not necessary to perform a comprehensive assessment during each patient encounter. Assessment focused on the circumstances and the needs of a particular patient can help to prioritize care. A short, focused general assessment can be used to establish a baseline to prioritize nursing care. The nurse can then gather more data about the patient at a later time. This basic assessment based on the patient's diagnosis, individual circumstances, and potential complications helps to quickly identify changes in the patent's clinical status (Henley Haugh, 2015). Nursing knowledge, expertise, judgment, and clinical experience guide the nurse in decisions about which assessments are a priority for an individual patient. This prioritized initial assessment may also identify specific findings to follow up on later. Fundamentals Review 3-3 provides an example of a brief, general physical assessment to gather pertinent data to provide a basis for prioritizing nursing care. Nurses should use clinical judg-ment to adapt this generic assessment to the individual circumstances of an individual patient and to monitor for changes that might require further intervention (Henley Haugh, 2015).

Fundamentals Review 3-1

COMPONENTS OF A HEALTH HISTORY

BIOGRAPHIC DATA

Biographic information is often collected during admis-sion to a health care facility and documented on a specific form; it helps to identify the patient. Depending on the health care setting, some biographic data may be collected by people other than the nurse.

Biographic data include the patient's name, address, billing, and insurance information. Additional biographi-cal information includes biological sex, age and birth date, marital status, occupation, race, ethnic origin, religious preference, presence of an advance directive/living will, and the patient's primary health care provider.

The source of the information is also recorded. Dif-ferences in language and culture may have an effect on the quality and safety of health care. Language has been

identified as the biggest barrier to health care and appears to increase the risks to patient safety (Purnell, 2013). It is important to note the patient's preferred language for discussing health care, as well as any sensory or commu-nication needs.

REASON FOR SEEKING HEALTH CARE

The reason for seeking care is a statement in the patient's own words that describes the patient's reason for seeking care. This can help to focus the rest of the assessment. Ask an open-ended question, such as, "Tell me why you are here today." **Record whatever it is the person says; his or her description in exact words. Avoid paraphrasing or interpreting.**

(continued)

COMPONENTS OF A HEALTH HISTORY

HISTORY OF PRESENT HEALTH CONCERN

When taking the patient's history of present health concern, be sure to explore the symptoms thoroughly. Encourage the patient to describe and explain any symptoms. The description should include information regarding the onset of the problem; location; duration; intensity; quality/description; relieving/exacerbating factors; associated factors; past occurrences; any treatments; and how the problem has affected the patient.

PAST MEDICAL HISTORY

A patient's past health history may provide insight to causes of current symptoms. It also alerts the nurse to certain risk factors. A past health history includes childhood and adult illnesses, chronic health problems and treatment, and previous surgeries or hospitalizations. This history should also include accidents or injuries, obstetric history, allergies, and the date of most recent immunizations. Vaccine recommendations are updated each year by the Centers for Disease Control and Prevention (CDC). Current guidelines for different age groups can be found on the CDC's website at www.cdc.gov (CDC, n.d. b). Ask the patient about health maintenance screenings, such as routine mammograms and colorectal tests, including dates and results, as well as the use of safety measures. Ask the patient about prescribed and over-the-counter medications, including vitamins, supplements, and any home or herbal remedies. Include the name, dose, route, frequency, and purpose for each medication.

FAMILY HISTORY

A person's family history will provide information about diseases and conditions for which a patient may be at increased risk. Certain disorders have genetic links. Information regarding contact with family members with communicable diseases or environmental hazards can provide clues to the patient's current health or risk factors for health issues. This information can also identify important topics for health teaching and counseling.

FUNCTIONAL HEALTH ASSESSMENT

A functional health assessment focuses on the effects of health or illness on a patient's quality of life, including the strengths of the patient and areas that need to improve. Assess the patient's ability to perform **activities of daily living (ADLs)**. Eating, bathing, dressing, and toileting are examples of ADLs. Assess the patient's ability to perform **instrumental activities of daily living (IADLs)**. Housekeeping, meal preparation, management of finances, and transportation are examples of IADLs. Functional health may be further assessed using a formal tool, such as the Katz Index of Independence in Activities of Daily Living, which is used with older adults (Figure 1).

ACTIVITIES POINTS (1 OR 0)	**INDEPENDENCE:** (1 POINT) **NO** supervision, direction, or personal assistance	**DEPENDENCE:** (0 POINTS) **WITH** supervision, direction, personal assistance, or total care
BATHING POINTS:_____	**(1 POINT)** Bathes self completely or needs help in bathing only a single part of the body such as the back, genital area, or disabled extremity.	**(0 POINTS)** Needs help with bathing more than one part of the body, getting in or out of the tub or shower. Requires total bathing.
DRESSING POINTS:_____	**(1 POINT)** Gets clothes from closets and drawers and puts on clothes and outer garments complete with fasteners. May have help tying shoes.	**(0 POINTS)** Needs help with dressing self or needs to be completely dressed.
TOILETING POINTS:_____	**(1 POINT)** Goes to toilet, gets on and off, arranges clothes, cleans genital area without help.	**(0 POINTS)** Needs help transferring to the toilet, cleaning self, or uses bedpan or commode.
TRANSFERRING POINTS:_____	**(1 POINT)** Moves in and out of bed or chair unassisted. Mechanical transferring aides are acceptable.	**(0 POINTS)** Needs help in moving from bed to chair or requires a complete transfer.
CONTINENCE POINTS:_____	**(1 POINT)** Exercises complete self-control over urination and defecation.	**(0 POINTS)** Is partially or totally incontinent of bowel or bladder.
FEEDING POINTS:_____	**(1 POINT)** Gets food from plate into mouth without help. Preparation of food may be done by another person.	**(0 POINTS)** Needs partial or total help with feeding or requires parenteral feeding.
TOTAL POINTS = _____ 6 = High (*patient independent*) 0 = Low (*patient very dependent*)		

FIGURE 1. Katz Index of Independence in Activities of Daily Living. (Slightly adapted from Katz, S., Down, T. D., Cash, H. R., & Grotz, R. C. [1970]. Progress in the development of the index of ADL. *The Gerontologist, 10*[1], 20–30. Copyright © The Gerontological Society of America. Reproduced [Adapted] by permission of the publisher.)

Fundamentals Review 3-1   continued

COMPONENTS OF A HEALTH HISTORY

PSYCHOSOCIAL AND LIFESTYLE FACTORS

A patient's lifestyle contributes to his or her overall health and well-being. Ask about the patient's social support and network of available assistance. Ask about confidants, skillful supporters, and people who can help the patient cope with any health alteration, illness, or other change. Ask about the patient's level of activity and exercise; sleep and rest; and nutrition. Obtain information related to the patient's interpersonal relationships and resources; values, beliefs, and spiritual resources; self-esteem and self-concept; and coping and stress management. Question the patient regarding personal habits, including use of alcohol, illicit drugs, and/or tobacco; environmental and occupational hazards; intimate partner and family violence; sexual history and orientation; and mental health.

Regular screenings in primary care and other health care settings enable earlier identification of mental health and substance use disorders, leading to earlier treatment and care. Screenings should be provided to people of all ages, even the young and older adults (Substance Abuse and Mental Health Services Administration [SAMHSA] and the Health Resources and Services Administration [HRSA], SAMHSA-HRSA Center for Integrated Health Solutions [CIHS], 2012). There are many assessment tools available to assist with screening for mental health disorders. Specific tools are available to screen for depression or suicide, for example, and to be used with specific populations, such as adolescents or older adults. The Patient Health Questionnaire-9 (PHQ-9), the most common screening tool to identify depression, is one example of a mental health assessment tool (Figure 2).

Over the last 2 weeks, how often have you been bothered by any of the following problems? (Use "✓" to indicate your answer)	Not At All	Several Days	More Than Half the Days	Nearly Every Day
1. Little interest or pleasure in doing things	0	1	2	3
2. Feeling down, depressed, or hopeless	0	1	2	3
3. Trouble falling or staying asleep, or sleeping too much	0	1	2	3
4. Feeling tired or having little energy	0	1	2	3
5. Poor appetite or overeating	0	1	2	3
6. Feeling bad about yourself—or that you are a failure or have let yourself or your family down	0	1	2	3
7. Trouble concentrating on things, such as reading the newspaper or watching television	0	1	2	3
8. Moving or speaking so slowly that other people could have noticed. Or the opposite—being so fidgety or restless that you have been moving around a lot more than usual	0	1	2	3
9. Thoughts that you would be better off dead or of hurting yourself in some way	0	1	2	3

FOR OFFICE CODING 0 + _____ + _____ + _____

= Total Score: _____

If you checked off any problems, how difficult have these problems made it for you to do your work, take care of things at home, or get along with other people?

Not difficult at all ☐	Somewhat difficult ☐	Very difficult ☐	Extremely difficult ☐

How to Score PHQ-9

Major Depressive Syndrome is suggested if:

• Of the 9 items, 5 or more are checked as at least "More than half the days"
• Either item #1 or #2 is positive, that is, at least "More than half the days"

Other Depressive Syndrome is suggested if:

• Of the 9 items, 2, 3, or 4 are check as at least "More than half the days"
• Either item #1 or #2 is positive, that is, at least "More than half the days"

FIGURE 2. From Patient Health Questionnaire (PHQ) Screeners. Developed by Dr. Robert L. Spitzer, Dr. Janet B. W. Williams, Dr. Kurt Kroenke, and colleagues, with an educational grant from Pfizer Inc. No permission required to reproduce, translate, display, or distribute. Retrieved http://www.phqscreeners.com.

Fundamentals Review 3-2

ASSESSMENT TECHNIQUES

Inspection is the process of performing deliberate, purposeful observations in a systematic manner. The nurse closely observes visually, but also uses hearing and smell to gather data throughout the assessment. The nurse assesses details of the patient's appearance, behavior, and movement. Inspection begins with the initial patient contact and continues through the entire assessment. Adequate natural or artificial lighting is essential for distinguishing the color, texture, and moisture of body surfaces. The nurse inspects each area of the body for size, color, shape, position, movement, and symmetry, noting normal findings and any deviations from normal.

Palpation uses the sense of touch. The hands and fingers are sensitive tools that can assess skin temperature, turgor, texture, and moisture, as well as vibrations within the body (e.g., the heart) and shape or structures within the body (e.g., the bones). Specific parts of the hand are more effective at assessing different qualities. The dorsum (back) surfaces of the hand and fingers are used for gross measure of temperature. The palmar (front) surfaces of the fingers and fingerpads are used to assess firmness, contour, shape, tenderness, and consistency. The fingerpads are best at fine discrimination. Use fingerpads to locate pulses, lymph nodes, and other small lumps, and to assess skin texture and edema. Vibration is palpated best with the ulnar, or outside, surface of the hand. For light palpation, apply light pressure with the dominant hand, using a circular motion to feel the surface structure; press down no more than 1 cm (0.5 in). *Advanced health care providers usually perform deep palpation. Refer to information on* thePoint® *or a health assessment text for details of this advanced assessment skill.*

Percussion is the act of striking one object against another to produce sound. The fingertips are used to tap the body over body tissues to produce vibrations and sound waves. The characteristics of the sounds produced are used to assess the location, shape, size, and density of tissues. Abnormal sounds suggest alteration of tissues, such as an emphysematous lung, or the presence of a mass, such as an abdominal tumor. A quiet environment allows sounds to be heard. *Advanced health care providers usually perform percussion. Refer to information on* thePoint® *or a health assessment text for details of this advanced assessment skill.*

Auscultation is the act of listening with a stethoscope to sounds produced within the body. This technique is used to listen for blood pressure, and heart, lung, and bowel sounds. Four characteristics of sound are assessed by auscultation: (1) pitch (ranging from high to low); (2) loudness (ranging from soft to loud); (3) quality (e.g., gurgling or swishing); and (4) duration (short, medium, or long). When auscultating, use the proper part of the stethoscope (diaphragm or bell) for specific sounds. Use the *bell* of the stethoscope to detect low-pitched sounds (such as some heart murmurs). Hold the bell lightly against the body part being auscultated. Use the *diaphragm* of the stethoscope to detect high-pitched sounds (such as normal heart sounds, breath sounds, and bowel sounds). Hold the diaphragm firmly against the body part being auscultated.

Fundamentals Review 3-3

BRIEF GENERAL PHYSICAL ASSESSMENT

Assessment	Components
Safety	Assess: bed position, call bell location, appropriate emergency equipment, assistive devices, fall risk/hazards
Vital signs	Assess: temperature, pulse, respirations, blood pressure, oxygen saturation, pain assessment
Mental status	Assess: level of consciousness; orientation to person, place, and time; speech
Psychosocial	Assess: behavior and affect
Head, eyes, ears, nose, throat, neck	Assess: eyes, pupils, mouth, carotid arteries, swallowing, facial color, moisture, lesions, wounds, glasses, hearing aid, ability to hear conversation, ability to see
Chest	Assess: chest color, moisture, lesions, wounds, quality of respirations, heart sounds, lung sounds, cough, sputum
Abdomen	Assess: abdomen color, moisture, lesions, wounds, bowel sounds, tenderness, distention, pain/discomfort, ability to eat, urine elimination pattern and urine characteristics, bowel elimination pattern and stool characteristics
Upper and lower extremities	Assess: skin, color, pulses, temperature, tenderness, edema, capillary refill, strength, sensation, range of motion, lesions, wounds
Activity	Assess: movement and ambulation, ability to move in bed, ability to get out of bed, ability to walk and distance, gait
Therapeutic devices	Assess: peripheral and central venous access devices, supplemental oxygen setting, pacemaker, cardiac monitor, urinary catheters, gastric tubes, chest tubes, dressings, braces, slings

Nurses should use clinical judgment to adapt this generic assessment to the individual circumstances of an individual patient and to monitor for changes that might require further intervention (Henley Haugh, 2015).

Source: Adapted from Henley Haugh, K. (2015). Head-to-toe: Organizing your baseline patient physical assessment. *Nursing, 45*(12), 58–61. Used with permission; Anderson, B., Nix, E., Norman, B., & McPike, H. D. (2014). An evidence based approach to undergraduate physical assessment practicum course development. *Nurse Education in Practice, 14*(3), 242–246.

Skill 3-1 ▶ Performing a General Survey

The **general survey** is the first component of the physical assessment, beginning with the first moment of patient contact and continuing throughout the nurse–patient relationship. The general survey contributes to an overall impression of the patient. It includes observing the patient's overall appearance and behavior; taking vital signs; measuring height, weight, and waist circumference; and calculating the **body mass index (BMI)**. BMI and waist circumference are indicators of risk for developing obesity-associated diseases or conditions, such as cardiovascular disease, high blood pressure, and type 2 diabetes (National Heart, Lung, and Blood Institute, n.d.).

DELEGATION CONSIDERATIONS

Measurement of the patient's weight and height, and vital signs may be delegated to nursing assistive personnel (NAP) or unlicensed assistive personnel (UAP). Depending on the state's nurse practice act and the organization's policies and procedures, the licensed practical/vocational nurses (LPN/LVNs) may perform some or all of the parts of the general survey. The decision to delegate must be based on careful analysis of the patient's needs and circumstances, as well as the qualifications of the person to whom the task is being delegated. Refer to the Delegation Guidelines in Appendix A.

(continued)

Skill 3-1 ▶ Performing a General Survey *(continued)*

EQUIPMENT	• Adequate lighting • Tape measure • A scale with height attachment; chair scale; or bed scale • PPE, as indicated
ASSESSMENT	Develop an overall impression of the patient, focusing on appearance and behavior, vital signs, height, and weight. Ask the patient about any changes in weight, pain or discomfort, sleeping patterns, and any difficulty sleeping.
NURSING DIAGNOSIS	Determine the related factors for the nursing diagnosis based on the patient's current status. Appropriate nursing diagnoses may include: • (Bathing; Dressing; Feeding; Toileting) self-care deficit • Anxiety • Ineffective coping
OUTCOME IDENTIFICATION AND PLANNING	The expected outcome to achieve in performing a general survey is that the assessment is completed without the patient experiencing anxiety or discomfort, an overall impression of the patient is formulated, the findings are documented, and the appropriate referral is made to other health care professionals, as needed, for further evaluation. Other specific outcomes will depend on the identified nursing diagnosis.

IMPLEMENTATION

ACTION	**RATIONALE**
1. Perform hand hygiene and put on PPE, if indicated.	Hand hygiene and PPE prevent the spread of microorganisms. PPE is required based on transmission precautions.
2. Identify the patient.	Identifying the patient ensures the right patient receives the intervention and helps prevent errors.
3. Close curtains around the bed and the door to the room, if possible. Explain the purpose of the health examination and what you are going to do. Answer any questions.	This ensures the patient's privacy. Explanation relieves anxiety and facilitates cooperation.
4. Assess the patient's overall appearance and behavior. Observe if the patient appears to be his or her stated age. Note the patient's mental status. Is the person alert and oriented, responsive to questions, and responding appropriately? Are the facial features symmetric? Note any signs of acute distress, such as shortness of breath, pain, or anxiousness.	Appearance provides information about various aspects of the patient's health. Changes in cognitive processes, asymmetry, and signs of distress can be indicators of health abnormalities.
5. Assess the patient's body structure. Does the person's height appear within normal range for stated age and genetic heritage? Does the person's weight appear within normal range for height and body build? Note if body fat is evenly distributed. Do body parts appear equal bilaterally and relatively proportionate? Is the patient's posture erect and appropriate for age?	Height that is excessively short or tall, asymmetry, one-sided atrophy or hypertrophy, abnormal posture, and abnormal body proportion can be indicators of health problems.

ACTION	RATIONALE
6. Assess the patient's mobility. Is the patient's gait smooth, even, well balanced, and coordinated? Is joint mobility smooth and coordinated with a general full range of motion (ROM)? Are involuntary movements evident?	Abnormalities in gait and ROM can indicate health concerns.
7. Assess the patient's behavior. Are facial expressions appropriate for the situation? Does the patient maintain eye contact, based on cultural norms? Does the person appear comfortable and relaxed with you? Is the patient's speech clear and understandable? Observe the person's hygiene and grooming. Is the clothing appropriate for climate, fit well, appear clean, and appropriate for the person's culture and age group? Does the person appear clean and well groomed, appropriate for age and culture?	Facial expressions, speech, eye contact, and other behaviors provide clues to mood and mental health. Deficits in hygiene and grooming may indicate alterations in health.
8. Assess for pain. (Refer to Chapter 10.)	Pain can indicate alterations in physical and psychological health.
9. Have the patient remove shoes and heavy outer clothing. Weigh the patient using a scale (Figure 1). Compare the measurement with previous weight measurements and recommended range for height.	Weight loss or gain may indicate health problems.
10. With shoes off, and standing erect, measure the patient's height using a wall-mounted measuring device or measuring pole (Figure 2).	Ratio of height and weight is a general assessment of overall health, hydration, and nutrition.

FIGURE 1. Weighing patient using scale. (*Photo by B. Proud.*)

FIGURE 2. Measuring patient's height. (*Photo by B. Proud.*)

(*continued*)

Skill 3-1 ▶ Performing a General Survey *(continued)*

ACTION	RATIONALE
11. Use the patient's weight and height measurements to calculate the patient's BMI. $$\text{Body mass index} = \frac{\text{weight in kilograms}}{\text{height in meters}^2}$$	BMI, an indicator of total body fat stores in the general population, provides a more accurate weight calculation than weight measurement alone. In addition, it provides an estimation of risk for diseases, such as heart disease, diabetes, and hypertension (National Heart, Lung, and Blood Institute, n.d.).
12. Using the tape measure, measure the patient's waist circumference. Place the tape measure snugly around the patient's waist at the level of the umbilicus.	Waist circumference is a good indicator of abdominal fat. It is thought to be an important and reliable indicator of risk for obesity-associated diseases or conditions (National Heart, Lung, and Blood Institute, n.d.).
13. Measure the patient's temperature, pulse, respirations, blood pressure, and oxygen saturation. (Refer to Chapter 2, and Chapter 14, for specific techniques.)	Vital signs and oxygen saturation are measured to establish a baseline for the database and to detect actual or potential health problems.
14. Remove PPE, if used. Clean equipment, based on facility policy. Perform hand hygiene. Continue with assessments of specific body systems as appropriate or indicated. Initiate appropriate referral to other health care providers for further evaluation as indicated.	Proper removal of PPE reduces the risk for infection transmission and contamination of other items. Cleaning of equipment prevents transmission of microorganisms. Hand hygiene prevents the spread of microorganisms. Additional assessments should be completed, as indicated, to evaluate the patient's health status. Intervention by other health care providers may be indicated to evaluate and treat the patient's health status.

EVALUATION

The expected outcomes have been met when the assessment is completed without the patient experiencing anxiety or discomfort, an overall impression of the patient is formulated, the findings are documented, and the appropriate referral is made to other health care professionals, as needed, for further evaluation.

DOCUMENTATION

Guidelines

Document findings related to assessment of the patient's physical appearance, body structure, mobility, and behavior. Document the patient's height, weight, BMI, and waist circumference. Document the presence or absence of pain, as well as an initial pain assessment if present. Record the patient's temperature (T), pulse (P), respiration (R), and blood pressure (BP) measurements, as well as the oxygen saturation measurement. Note any referrals.

Sample Documentation

DocuCare Practice documenting assessment techniques and findings in *Lippincott DocuCare.*

> 1/26/20 1015 Patient admitted to room 432. Patient is a 23-year-old Asian female graduate student at a local university, living in an apartment with three other female students. Appears well nourished, disheveled, clothing appropriate for age and season, and tired. Oriented, cooperative, with no signs of acute distress; patient denies pain at present. T 98.9°F, P 78, R 16, BP 114/58 mm Hg (left arm), sitting O$_2$ sat 96% on room air. Height 144 cm (5 ft). Weight 55 kg (121 lb). BMI 26.5. Waist circumference 32 in. Information provided regarding use of call bell, lights, and phone, and location of bathroom. Patient verbalizes an understanding of information.
>
> —R. Robinson, RN

UNEXPECTED SITUATIONS AND ASSOCIATED INTERVENTIONS

- *Patient is unable to tolerate standing for height or weight measurement:* Obtain a chair scale or bed scale to measure weight (see Skill 3-2). Obtain a measuring stick to measure height. Alternately, use tape to mark the patient's length in the bed with the patient supine, the head in the midline position, and the legs extended flat on the bed. Measure the resulting length.

SPECIAL CONSIDERATIONS

General Considerations

- BMI may not be accurate for people, such as athletes, with a large muscle mass; people with **edema** or dehydration; older adults and others who have lost muscle mass (Dudek, 2014; NIH, 2012).
- According to the guidelines published by the National Heart, Lung, and Blood Institute, an adult with a BMI below 18.5 is underweight; a BMI of 25 to 29.9 indicates that a person is overweight; a BMI of 30 or greater indicates obesity; and a BMI of 40 or greater indicates extreme obesity (NIH, 2012).
- Disease risk increases with a waist measurement of more than 40 in in men and 35 in in women (NIH, 2012).

Infant and Child Considerations

- Measure height in children up to 2 years of age in the recumbent position with legs fully extended.
- Weigh infants without clothing.
- Weigh children in their underwear.
- Overweight and obesity are defined differently for children and teens than for adults. Children are still growing, and boys and girls mature at different rates (NIH, 2012).
- BMIs for children and teens compare their heights and weights against growth charts that take age and sex into account. This is called BMI-for-age percentile. A child or teen's BMI-for-age percentile shows how his or her BMI compares with other boys and girls of the same age (NIH, 2012).
- Information about BMI-for-age and growth charts for children can be found at the Centers for Disease Control and Prevention (CDC)'s BMI-for-age calculator (CDC, n.d. a).

Skill 3-2 ▶ Using a Portable Bed Scale

Obtaining a patient's weight is an important component of assessment. In addition to providing baseline information of the patient's overall status, weight is a valuable indicator of nutritional status and fluid balance. Changes in a patient's weight can provide clues to underlying problems, such as nutritional deficiencies or fluid excess or deficiency, or it can indicate the development of new problems, such as fluid overload.

Typically, the nurse will measure weight by having the patient stand on an upright scale. However, doing so requires that the patient is mobile and can maintain his or her balance. Chair scales are available for patients who are unable to stand. For patients who are confined to the bed, have limited mobility, or cannot maintain a balanced upright or standing position for a short period of time, a bed scale can be used. With a bed scale, the nurse places the patient in a sling and raises the patient above the bed. To ensure safety, a second nurse should be on hand to assist with weighing the patient. Many facilities provide beds with built-in scales. The following procedure explains how to weigh the patient with a portable bed scale.

DELEGATION CONSIDERATIONS

Measurement of body weight may be delegated to nursing assistive personnel (NAP) or unlicensed assistive personnel (UAP), as well as to licensed practical/vocational nurses (LPN/LVNs). The decision to delegate must be based on careful analysis of the patient's needs and circumstances, as well as the qualifications of the person to whom the task is being delegated. Refer to the Delegation Guidelines in Appendix A.

(continued)

Skill 3-2 ▶ Using a Portable Bed Scale (continued)

EQUIPMENT	• Bed scale with sling • Cover for sling • Sheet or bath blanket • PPE, as indicated

---

ASSESSMENT

Assess the patient's ability to stand for a weight measurement. If the patient cannot stand, assess the patient's ability to sit in a chair or to lie still for a weight measurement. Assess the patient for pain. If necessary, give medication for pain or sedation before placing the patient on a bed scale. Assess for the presence of any material, such as tubes, drains, or IV tubing, which could become entangled in the scale or pulled during the weighing procedure.

NURSING DIAGNOSIS

Determine the related factors for the nursing diagnoses based on the patient's current status. Appropriate nursing diagnoses may include:

• Impaired physical mobility
• Imbalanced nutrition: less than body requirements
• Overweight

OUTCOME IDENTIFICATION AND PLANNING

The expected outcomes to achieve when weighing a patient using a portable bed scale are that the patient's weight is measured accurately without injury, and the patient experiences minimal discomfort.

IMPLEMENTATION

ACTION	RATIONALE
1. Check the medical order or nursing care plan for frequency of weight measurement. More frequent measurement of the patient's weight may be appropriate based on nursing judgment. Obtain the assistance of a second caregiver, based on the patient's mobility and ability to cooperate with the procedure.	This provides for patient safety and appropriate care.
2. Perform hand hygiene and put on PPE, if indicated.	Hand hygiene and PPE prevent the spread of microorganisms. PPE is required based on transmission precautions.
3. Identify the patient.	Identifying the patient ensures that the right patient receives the intervention and helps prevent errors.
4. Close the curtains around the bed and close the door to the room if possible. Discuss the procedure with the patient and assess the patient's ability to assist with the procedure.	This ensures the patient's privacy. Explanation relieves anxiety and facilitates cooperation.
5. Place a cover over the sling of the bed scale.	Using a cover deters the spread of microorganisms.
6. Attach the sling to the bed scale. Lay the sheet or bath blanket in the sling. Turn on the scale. Balance the scale so that weight reads 0.0.	Scale will add the sling, blanket, and cover into the weight unless it is zeroed with the sling, blanket, and cover.
7. Adjust the bed to a comfortable working position, usually elbow height of the caregiver (VHACEOSH, 2016). Position one caregiver on each side of the bed, if two caregivers are present. Raise side rail on the opposite side of the bed from where the scale is located, if not already in place. Cover the patient with the sheet or bath blanket. Remove other covers and any pillows.	Having the bed at the proper height prevents back and muscle strain. Having one caregiver on each side of the bed provides for patient safety and appropriate care. Side rail assists patient with movement. Blanket maintains patient's dignity and provides warmth.

ACTION	**RATIONALE**
8. Turn the patient onto his or her side facing the side rail, keeping his or her body covered with the sheet or blanket. Remove the sling from the scale. Place the cover on the sling. Roll cover and sling lengthwise. Place rolled sling under the patient, making sure the patient is centered in the sling.	Rolling the patient onto his or her side facilitates placing the patient onto the sling. Blanket maintains patient's dignity and provides warmth.
9. Roll the patient back over the sling and onto the other side. Pull the sling through, as if placing sheet under patient, unrolling the sling as it is pulled through.	This facilitates placing the patient onto the sling.
10. Roll the scale over the bed so that the arms of the scale are directly over the patient. **Spread the base of the scale.** Lower the arms of the scale and place the arm hooks into the holes on the sling.	By spreading the base, you are giving the scale a wider base, thus preventing the scale from toppling over with the patient. Hooking sling to scale provides secure attachment to the scale and prevents injury.
11. Once the scale arms are hooked onto the sling, gradually elevate the sling so that the patient is lifted up off the bed (Figure 1). **Assess all tubes and drains, making sure that none have tension placed on them as the scale is lifted. Once the sling is no longer touching the bed, ensure that nothing else is hanging onto the sling (e.g., ventilator or IV tubing). If any tubing is connected to the patient, raise it up so that it is not adding any weight to the patient.**	The scale must be hanging free to obtain an accurate weight. Any tubing that is hanging off the scale will add weight to the patient.

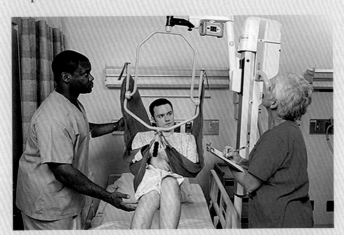

FIGURE 1. Using a bed scale.

12. Note the weight reading on the scale. Slowly and gently, lower the patient back onto the bed. Disconnect the scale arms from the sling. Close the base of the scale and pull it away from the bed.	Lowering the patient slowly does not alarm the patient. Closing the base of the scale facilitates moving the scale.
13. Raise the side rail. Turn the patient to the side rail. Roll the sling up against the patient's backside.	Raising the side rail is a safety measure.
14. Raise the other side rail. Roll the patient back over the sling and up facing the other side rail. Remove the sling from the bed. Remove gloves, if used. Raise the remaining side rail.	The patient needs to be removed from the sling before it can be removed from the bed.
15. Cover the patient and help him or her to a position of comfort. Place the bed in the lowest position.	Ensures patient comfort and safety.
16. Remove the disposable cover from the sling and discard in the appropriate receptacle.	Using a cover deters the spread of microorganisms.

(continued)

Skill 3-2 ▶ Using a Portable Bed Scale *(continued)*

ACTION	**RATIONALE**
17. Remove additional PPE, if used. Clean equipment based on facility policy. Perform hand hygiene.	Proper removal of PPE reduces the risk for infection transmission and contamination of other items. Cleaning equipment prevents transmission of microorganisms. Hand hygiene deters the spread of microorganisms.
18. Replace the scale and sling in the appropriate spot. Plug the scale into the electrical outlet.	Scale should be ready for use at any time.

EVALUATION

The expected outcome has been met when the patient is weighed accurately without injury.

DOCUMENTATION

Guidelines

Document weight, unit of measurement, and scale used.

Sample Documentation

> 10/15/20 0230 Patient reports pain in legs 5/10. Premedicated with oxycodone 5 mg and acetaminophen 325 mg 2 tabs PO before obtaining weight per order. Patient weighed using bed scale, 75.2 kg.
>
> —M. Evans, RN

UNEXPECTED SITUATIONS AND ASSOCIATED INTERVENTIONS

- *As the patient is being lifted, the scale begins to tip over:* Stop lifting the patient. Slowly lower the patient back to the bed. Ensure that the base of the scale is spread wide enough before attempting to weigh the patient.
- *Weight differs from the previous day's weight by more than 1 kg:* Weigh the patient using the same scale at the same time each day. Check scale calibration. Make sure that the patient is wearing the same clothing. Make sure that no tubes or containers are hanging on the scale. If the patient is incontinent, make sure undergarments are clean and dry.
- *Patient becomes agitated as the sling is raised into the air:* Stop lifting the patient and reassure him or her. If the patient continues to be agitated, lower him or her back to the bed. Reevaluate necessity of obtaining weight at that exact time. If appropriate, obtain an order for sedation before attempting to obtain another weight measurement.

 # Skill 3-3 ▶ Assessing the Skin, Hair, and Nails

The integumentary system includes the skin, hair, nails, sweat glands, and sebaceous glands. Assessment of the skin, hair, and nails provides information about the nutritional and hydration status and overall health of the patient. In addition, this assessment can provide information associated with certain systemic diseases, infection, immobility, excessive sun exposure, and allergic reactions. Assessment often begins with an overall inspection of the skin's condition and skin assessment is integrated throughout the entire health assessment. Assessment of specific regions is usually integrated into specific body system assessments. Skin assessment is presented separately in this text for learning purposes.

DELEGATION CONSIDERATIONS

The assessment of the patient's skin, hair, and nails should not be delegated to nursing assistive personnel (NAP) or unlicensed assistive personnel (UAP). However, the NAP or UAP may notice some items while providing care. The nurse must then validate, analyze, document, communicate, and act on these findings, as appropriate. Depending on the state's nurse practice act and the organization's policies and procedures, the licensed practical/vocational nurses (LPN/LVNs) may perform some or all of the parts of assessment of the patient's skin, hair, and nails. The decision to delegate must be based on careful analysis of the patient's needs and circumstances, as well as the qualifications of the person to whom the task is being delegated. Refer to the Delegation Guidelines in Appendix A.

EQUIPMENT	• Gloves • Additional PPE, as indicated • Bath blanket or other drape • Measuring tape or ruler • Adequate light source

ASSESSMENT

Complete a health history, focusing on the integumentary system. Identify risk factors for altered health by asking about the following:

- History of rashes, lesions, change in color, or itching
- History of bruising or bleeding in the skin
- History of allergies to medications, plants, foods, or other substances
- History of bathing routines and products
- Exposure to the sun and sunburn history
- Presence of lesions (wounds, bruises, abrasions, or burns)
- Presence of body piercings and/or tattoos
- Change in the color, size, or shape of a mole
- Exposure to chemicals that may be harmful to the skin, hair, or nails
- Degree of mobility
- Types of food eaten and liquids consumed each day
- Cultural practices related to skin

NURSING DIAGNOSIS

Determine the related factors for the nursing diagnoses based on the patient's current health status. Appropriate nursing diagnoses may include:

- Impaired skin integrity
- Disturbed body image

OUTCOME IDENTIFICATION AND PLANNING

The expected outcome to achieve in performing assessment of the skin, hair, and nails is that the assessment is completed without the patient experiencing anxiety or discomfort, the findings are documented, and the appropriate referral is made to the other health care professionals, as needed, for further evaluation. Other specific outcomes will be expected depending on the identified nursing diagnosis.

IMPLEMENTATION

ACTION	RATIONALE
1. Perform hand hygiene and put on PPE, if indicated.	Hand hygiene and PPE prevent the spread of microorganisms. PPE is required based on transmission precautions.
2. Identify the patient.	Identifying the patient ensures the right patient receives the intervention and helps prevent errors.
3. Close curtains around the bed and the door to room, if possible. Explain the purpose of the integumentary examination and what you are going to do. Answer any questions.	This ensures the patient's privacy. Explanation relieves anxiety and facilitates cooperation.
4. Ask the patient to remove all clothing and put on an examination gown (if appropriate). The patient remains in the sitting position for most of the examination, but will need to stand or lie on the side when the posterior part of the body is examined, exposing only the body part being examined.	Exposing only the body part being examined provides privacy for the patient. During the initial part of the examination, assess the skin areas that are exposed (e.g., face, arms, and hands). As the different assessments are completed, incorporate skin examination within these systems.

(continued)

Skill 3-3 ▶ Assessing the Skin, Hair, and Nails *(continued)*

ACTION	RATIONALE

5. Use the bath blanket or drape to cover any exposed area other than the one being assessed. Inspect the overall skin coloration (Figure 1).

Use of a bath blanket or drape provides for comfort and warmth. Overall coloration is a good indication of health status. Skin color varies among races and people; individual skin color should be relatively consistent across the body. Abnormal findings include **cyanosis, pallor, jaundice,** and **erythema.**

6. Inspect skin for vascularity, bleeding, or **ecchymosis.**

These signs may relate to injury or cardiovascular, hematologic, or liver dysfunction.

7. Inspect the skin for lesions. Note bruises, scratches, cuts, insect bites, and wounds. (Refer to General Wound Assessment [Fundamentals Review 8-1] in Chapter 8.) If present, note size, shape, color, exudates, and distribution/ pattern, and presence of drainage or odor. Assess the location and condition of body piercings and/or tattoos.

Lesions can be normal variations, such as a macule or freckle, or an abnormal lesion, such as a melanoma.

8. Palpate skin using the backs of your hands to assess temperature. Wear gloves when palpating any potentially open area of the skin (Figure 2).

The back of the hand is more sensitive to temperature. Increase in skin temperature may indicate elevated body temperature.

FIGURE 1. Inspecting overall skin coloration. (*Photo by B. Proud.*)

FIGURE 2. Assessing skin temperature. (*Photo by B. Proud.*)

9. Palpate for texture and moisture.

In a dehydrated patient, skin is dry, loose, and wrinkled. Elevated body temperature may result in increased perspiration.

10. Assess skin **turgor** by gently pinching the skin under the clavicle (Figure 3).

Provides information about the patient's hydration status as well as skin mobility and elasticity. Decreased elasticity may be present in dehydrated patients.

FIGURE 3. Assessing skin turgor. (*Photo by B. Proud.*)

11. Palpate for edema, which is characterized by swelling, with taut and shiny skin over the edematous area.

Edema may be the result of overhydration, heart failure, kidney dysfunction, or peripheral vascular disease.

ACTION	RATIONALE
12. If lesions are present, put on gloves and palpate the lesion.	Palpation of lesions may result in drainage, which provides clues to the type or cause of the lesion. Gloves prevent contact with blood and body fluids.
13. Inspect the nail condition, including the shape, texture, and color as well as the nail angle; note if any clubbing is present.	Nail condition provides information about underlying illness and oxygenation status. Nails are normally convex and the cuticle is pink and intact. The angle of nail attachment is 160 degrees. Clubbing is present when the nail angle base exceeds 180 degrees.
14. Palpate nails for texture and capillary refill.	Normally, nails are firm and smooth and capillary refill should be brisk, less than 3 seconds.
15. Inspect the hair and scalp for color, texture, and distribution (Figure 4). Wear gloves for palpation if lesions or infestation is suspected or if hygiene is poor.	Hair condition provides information about nutritional and oxygenation status. Hair should be evenly distributed over the scalp. There are variations in hair color. Scalp should feel mobile and nontender.

FIGURE 4. Inspecting the scalp and hair. (*Photo by B. Proud.*)

16. Remove gloves and any additional PPE, if used. Perform hand hygiene. Continue with assessments of specific body systems, as appropriate or indicated. Initiate appropriate referral to other health care providers for further evaluation, as indicated.	Proper removal of PPE reduces the risk for infection transmission and contamination of other items. Hand hygiene prevents the spread of microorganisms. Additional assessments should be completed, as indicated, to evaluate the patient's health status. Intervention by other health care providers may be indicated to evaluate and treat the patient's health status.

EVALUATION

The expected outcomes have been met when the patient participates in the integumentary assessment, the assessment has been completed without the patient experiencing anxiety or discomfort, the findings are documented, and the appropriate referrals are made to the other health care professionals, as needed for further evaluation.

DOCUMENTATION

Guidelines

Describe specific findings, including coloration, texture, moisture, temperature, turgor, capillary refill, and edema. Note hair distribution and texture. Describe the condition of nails, including any abnormal findings. If lesions are present, document specifics, describing type, size, shape (use tape measure if necessary), elevation, coloring, location, drainage, distribution, and patterns.

Sample Documentation

> <u>5/2/20</u> 1030 Skin assessment performed. Patient reports history of atopic dermatitis. Uniform skin coloring (tan) with pink undertones. Skin on all areas, but the hands, is soft and warm. Skin returns to position when pinched. Multiple lesions, consistent with dermatitis, observed on the hands. Lesions are red, scaly, and dry. Brown hair, shiny and evenly distributed. Nails are firm and the cuticle is pink and intact and without ridging or pitting.
>
> —*B. Gentzler, RN*

(continued)

Skill 3-3 ▶ Assessing the Skin, Hair, and Nails (continued)

UNEXPECTED OUTCOMES AND ASSOCIATED INTERVENTIONS

- *While assessing the skin of a patient with dark skin tone, you are unsure if the change in coloration in a particular area of the body is normal or abnormal:* It is especially important when assessing people with dark skin tones to conduct the assessment with natural light rather than artificial lighting. When an abnormal condition is present, first examining an area of the skin that is not affected by the dermatologic disorder provides a comparison for identifying abnormal color conditions. Skin temperature becomes important to detect erythema in people with dark skin tones; areas of erythema will feel warm compared with surrounding skin. Pallor in patients with dark skin tones is seen as an ashen gray or yellow tinge. Also, lesions that look red or brown on light skin may present as black or purple on dark skin.

SPECIAL CONSIDERATIONS

Older Adult Considerations

In the older adult patient expect to find overall thinning of the skin, reduced sweating and oil, and reduced skin turgor.

Cultural Considerations

- Pallor in people with dark skin tones appears as absence of the "glow" of brown or black skin, or may appear as ashen gray or yellow tinged. Lighter skin appears more yellowish brown; darker skin looks ashen. Assess cyanosis in people with darker skin tones by examining the oral mucosa, the lips, nail beds, and the conjunctiva. Assess jaundice by observing the sclera of the eyes, the palms of the hands, and soles of the feet for a yellowish discoloration.
- Mongolian spot is a common variation of hyperpigmentation in newborns of African, African American, Turkish, Asian, American Indian, and Hispanic heritage. It is a blue black to purple macular area of hyperpigmentation that is usually located at the sacrum or buttocks, but sometimes occurs on the abdomen, thighs, shoulders, or arms. Mongolian spot gradually fades during the first year of life. It is important not to confuse these areas of hyperpigmentation with bruises (Jarvis, 2016).
- Asian patients may exhibit normal variations in physical features, such as a decrease in body hair and coarse head hair.

 # Skill 3-4 ▶ Assessing the Head and Neck

Examination of the head and neck region includes the assessment of multiple structures and body systems. The eyes, ears, nose, mouth, and throat are located within the facial structures. Anterior neck structures include the trachea, esophagus, and the thyroid gland, as well as the arteries, veins, and lymph nodes. Posterior neck areas involve the upper portion of the spine.

DELEGATION CONSIDERATIONS

Assessment of the patient's head and neck should not be delegated to nursing assistive personnel (NAP) or unlicensed assistive personnel (UAP). However, the NAP or UAP may notice some items while providing care. The nurse must then validate, analyze, document, communicate, and act on these findings, as appropriate. Depending on the state's nurse practice act and the organization's policies and procedures, the licensed practical/vocational nurses (LPN/LVNs) may perform some or all of the parts of assessment of the patient's head and neck. The decision to delegate must be based on careful analysis of the patient's needs and circumstances, as well as the qualifications of the person to whom the task is being delegated. Refer to the Delegation Guidelines in Appendix A.

EQUIPMENT

- Stethoscope
- Gloves
- Additional PPE, as indicated
- Bath blanket or other drape
- Lighting, including a penlight
- Tongue blades
- Visual acuity chart

| **ASSESSMENT** | Complete a health history, focusing on the head and neck. Identify risk factors for altered health by asking about the following: |

- Changes with aging in vision or hearing
- History of use of corrective lenses or hearing aids
- History of allergies
- History of disturbances in vision or hearing
- History of chronic illnesses, such as hypertension, diabetes mellitus, or thyroid disease
- Exposure to harmful substances or loud noises
- History of smoking, chewing tobacco, or cocaine use
- History of eye or ear infections
- Presence of body piercings and/or tattoos
- Oral and dental care practices

NURSING DIAGNOSIS

Determine the related factors for the nursing diagnoses based on the patient's current health status. Appropriate nursing diagnoses may include:

- Impaired swallowing
- Impaired dentition
- Impaired oral mucous membrane integrity

OUTCOME IDENTIFICATION AND PLANNING

The expected outcome to achieve in performing an examination of the structures in the head and neck region is that the assessment is completed without the patient experiencing anxiety or discomfort, the findings are documented, and the appropriate referral is made to the other health care professionals, as needed, for further evaluation. Other specific outcomes will be expected depending on the identified nursing diagnosis.

IMPLEMENTATION

ACTION	RATIONALE
1. Perform hand hygiene and put on PPE, if indicated.	Hand hygiene and PPE prevent the spread of microorganisms. PPE is required based on transmission precautions.
2. Identify the patient.	Identifying the patient ensures the right patient receives the intervention and helps prevent errors.
3. Close the curtains around the bed and close the door to the room, if possible. Explain the purpose of the head and neck examination and what you are going to do. Answer any questions.	This ensures the patient's privacy. Explanation relieves anxiety and facilitates cooperation.
4. Inspect the head for size and shape. Inspect the face for color, symmetry, lesions, and distribution of facial hair. Note facial expression. Palpate the skull.	In general, the shape of the head is normocephalic and symmetric. Abnormal findings include a lack of symmetry or unusual size or contour of the head, which may be a result of trauma or disease. Facial expression is appropriate. Skull should be mobile and nontender.
5. Inspect the external eye structures (eyelids, eyelashes, eyeball, and eyebrows), cornea, conjunctiva, and sclera. Note color, edema, symmetry, and alignment.	Inspection detects abnormalities, such as ptosis, styes, conjunctivitis, or scleral color. Some abnormalities are associated with systemic disorders.

(continued)

Skill 3-4 ▶ Assessing the Head and Neck   *(continued)*

ACTION

6. Examine the pupils for equality of size and shape (Figure 1). Examine the pupillary reaction to light:

   a. Darken the room.

   b. Ask the patient to look straight ahead.

   c. Bring the penlight from the side of the patient's face and briefly shine the light on the pupil (Figure 2).

   d. Observe the pupil's reaction; it normally constricts rapidly (direct response). Note pupil size.

   e. Repeat the procedure and observe the other eye; it too normally will constrict (consensual reflex).

   f. Repeat the procedure with the other eye.

RATIONALE

Testing pupillary response to light and accommodation assesses cranial nerve III, the oculomotor nerve. The pupils are normally black, equal in size, round, and smooth. The normal and consensual pupillary response is constriction.

● • • ● ● ● ● ●
1   2   3   4   5   6   7

FIGURE 1. Pupillary gauge measures pupils in millimeters (mm).

FIGURE 2. Assessing pupillary reaction to light.

7. Test for pupillary accommodation:

   a. Hold the forefinger, a pencil, or other straight object about 10 to 15 cm (4 to 6 in) from the bridge of the patient's nose.

   b. Ask the patient to first look at the object, then at a distant object, and then back to the object being held. The pupil normally constricts when looking at a near object and dilates when looking at a distant object (Figure 3).

Testing pupillary response to light and accommodation assesses cranial nerve III, the oculomotor nerve. The normal pupillary response is constriction when focusing on a near object.

FIGURE 3. Assessing pupillary accommodation.

ACTION

RATIONALE

8. Assess extraocular movements.

   a. Ask the patient to hold the head still and follow the movement of your forefinger or a penlight with the eyes as you move the patient's eyes through the six cardinal positions of gaze.

   b. Keeping your finger or penlight about 1 ft from the patient's face, move it slowly through the cardinal positions: up and down, right and left, diagonally up and down to the left (Figure 4A), diagonally up and down to the right (Figure 4B).

This evaluates the function of each of the six extraocular eye muscles (EOM) and tests cranial nerves III, IV, and VI (oculomotor, trochlear, and abducens nerves). Normally, both eyes move together, are coordinated, and are parallel.

FIGURE 4. Assessing extraocular movements.

9. Test convergence:

   a. Hold your finger about 6 to 8 in from the bridge of the patient's nose.

   b. Move your finger toward the patient's nose (Figure 5). The patient's eyes should normally converge (assume a cross-eyed appearance).

10. Test the patient's visual acuity with a Snellen chart. Have the patient stand 20 ft from the chart and ask the patient to read the smallest line of letters possible, first with both eyes and then with one eye at a time (with the opposite eye covered). Note whether the patient's vision is being tested with or without corrective lenses (Figure 6).

The patient's eyes should normally converge; converging eyes normally follow the object to within 5 cm of the nose (assume a cross-eyed appearance).

Evaluates the patient's distance vision and function of cranial nerve II (optic nerve). Additional tools are used to test for color perception.

FIGURE 5. Assessing convergence.

FIGURE 6. Testing visual acuity with a Snellen chart.

(continued)

Skill 3-4 ▶ Assessing the Head and Neck   *(continued)*

ACTION	RATIONALE
11. Inspect the external ear bilaterally for shape, size, and lesions. Palpate the ear and mastoid process. Inspect the visible portion of the ear canal. Note cerumen (wax), edema, discharge, or foreign bodies.	Inspection may reveal abnormalities, such as uneven color, size, drainage, or lesions; inflammation (edema) or infection; nodules, lesions, or tenderness. Cerumen may normally be dark orange, brown, yellow, gray, or black and soft, moist, dry, or hard.
12. Use a whispered voice to test hearing. Stand about 1 to 2 ft away from the patient out of the patient's line of vision. Ask the patient to cover the ear not being tested. Determine whether the patient can hear a whispered sentence or group of numbers from a distance of 1 to 2 ft. Perform test on each ear.	Provides a gross assessment of cranial nerve VIII (acoustic nerve). The patient should repeat what has been said.
13. Put on gloves. Inspect and palpate the external nose (Figure 7).	Gloves prevent contact with blood and body fluids. These actions assess for the color, shape, consistency, and tenderness of the nose.
14. Palpate over the frontal and maxillary sinuses (Figure 8).	Sinus palpation is used to elicit tenderness, which may indicate sinus congestion or infection. Normally, the sinuses are not painful when palpated.

FIGURE 7. Palpating the nose. *(Photo by B. Proud.)*

FIGURE 8. Palpating the sinuses. *(Photo by B. Proud.)*

15. Occlude one nostril externally with a finger while patient breathes through the other; repeat for the other side.	This technique checks the patency of the nasal passages.
16. Inspect each anterior nares and turbinates by tipping the patient's head back slightly and shining a light into the nares. Examine the mucous membranes for color and the presence of lesions, exudate, or growths.	This technique can detect edema, inflammation, and excessive drainage. The nasal mucosa is moist and darker red than the oral mucosa.
17. Inspect the lips, oral mucosa, hard and soft palates, gingivae, teeth, and salivary gland openings. Ask the patient to open the mouth wide and use a tongue blade and penlight to visualize structures.	Evaluates the condition of the oral structures and hydration level of the patient. The lips should be pink, moist, and smooth. The gums should be pink and smooth. The teeth should be regular and free of cavities or have dental restoration. The tonsils, if present, are small, pink, and symmetric in size.

ACTION

18. Inspect the tongue. Ask the patient to stick out the tongue. Place a tongue blade at the side of the tongue while patient pushes it to the left and right with the tongue. Inspect the uvula by asking the patient to say "ahh" while sticking out the tongue (Figure 9). Palpate the tongue for muscle tone and tenderness. Remove gloves.

RATIONALE

Sticking out the tongue evaluates the function of cranial nerve XII (hypoglossal nerve). Saying "ahh" checks for movement of the uvula and soft palate.

The tongue and mucous membranes are normally pink, moist, and free of swelling or lesions. The uvula is normally centered and freely movable. Tongue should feel soft with positive muscle tone and be nontender.

FIGURE 9. Inspecting the mouth using a tongue blade and penlight. (*Photo by B. Proud.*)

19. Inspect and palpate the lymph nodes (Figure 10) for enlargement, tenderness, and mobility, using the fingerpads in a slow, circular motion (Figure 11).

Palpation can determine size, shape, mobility, consistency, and/or tenderness of enlarged lymph nodes.

Preauricular
Parotid
Posterior auricular
Occipital
Tonsillar
Posterior cervical
Submaxillary
Submental
Anterior or deep cervical chain
Supraclavicular

FIGURE 10. Location of lymph nodes in neck.

FIGURE 11. Palpating lymph nodes. (*Photo by B. Proud.*)

(*continued*)

Skill 3-4 ▶ Assessing the Head and Neck *(continued)*

ACTION	**RATIONALE**
20. Inspect and palpate (Figure 12A) the left and then the right carotid arteries. **Palpate only one carotid artery at a time.** Note the strength of the pulse and grade it as with peripheral pulses. Use the bell of the stethoscope to auscultate the carotid arteries (Figure 12B).	Palpation of this area evaluates circulation through the arteries. Palpating both arteries at once can reduce blood flow to the brain, potentially causing dizziness or loss of consciousness. Auscultation can detect a **bruit**.

A **B**

FIGURE 12. Palpating (**A**) and auscultating (**B**) the carotid arteries. (*Photos by B. Proud.*)

21. Inspect and palpate the trachea (Figure 13).	Inspection and palpation of the trachea evaluate its midline position.
22. Assess the thyroid gland with the patient's neck slightly hyperextended. Observe the lower portion of the neck overlying the thyroid gland (Figure 14). Assess for symmetry and visible masses. Ask the patient to swallow. Observe the area while the patient swallows. Offer a glass of water, if necessary, to make it easier for the patient to swallow.	Abnormal findings include asymmetry, enlargement, lumps, and bulging. These findings may indicate the presence of enlargement of the thyroid (a goiter), inflammation of the thyroid (thyroiditis), or cancer of the thyroid.

FIGURE 13. Palpating to determine position of trachea. (*Photo by B. Proud.*)

Thyroid cartilage

Cricoid cartilage

Thyroid gland

FIGURE 14. Assessing the thyroid gland. (From Hogan-Quigley, et al. [2012]. Bates' nursing guide to physical examination and history taking. 1st Edition, P. 200; Wolters Kluwer Health | Lippincott Williams & Wilkins; Philadelphia, PA.)

ACTION	**RATIONALE**
23. Inspect the ability of the patient to move the neck. Ask the patient to touch chin to chest and to each shoulder, each ear to the corresponding shoulder, and then tip the head back as far as possible.	These actions assess neck ROM, which is normally smooth and controlled.
24. Remove any additional PPE, if used. Perform hand hygiene. Continue with assessments of specific body systems, as appropriate or indicated. Initiate appropriate referral to other health care providers for further evaluation, as indicated.	Proper removal of PPE reduces the risk for infection transmission and contamination of other items. Hand hygiene prevents the spread of microorganisms. Additional assessments should be completed, as indicated, to evaluate the patient's health status. Intervention by other health care providers may be indicated to evaluate and treat the patient's health status.

EVALUATION

The expected outcomes have been met when the patient participates in head and neck assessment, the assessment is completed without the patient experiencing anxiety or discomfort, the findings are documented, and the appropriate referrals are made to the other health care professionals, as needed, for further evaluation.

DOCUMENTATION

Guidelines

Describe specific findings. For the head and face, document symmetry, coloration, and presence of lesions or edema. Note visual acuity, pupillary reaction, and condition of the external eye. Document results of tests for accommodation, convergence, and extraocular muscles. Describe condition of the ear, noting any lesions or discharge. Document results of any hearing tests. Note condition of the nose and sinuses. Describe condition of lips, gums, tongue, and buccal mucosa. Document quality of carotid pulse. Note position of trachea and any enlargement of the thyroid. Describe quality of any lymph nodes palpable. Note ROM of the neck. Document presence of pain or discomfort.

Sample Documentation

6/10/20 1545 Head and neck examination completed. Patient denies history of any sensory changes or sensory difficulties, but states, "I have some sores in my mouth." Overall skin coloring consistent, with pink undertones. Head symmetric and normal in size. Eyes are symmetric. No lesions or redness noted. Pupils equal and reactive to light; positive accommodation and convergence. Visual acuity 20/20 in both eyes. Eyes move smoothly through six fields of gaze. External ears and canal free of discharge, lesions, or tenderness. Whisper test negative for hearing loss. Nose and sinuses nontender. Minimal clear discharge present in the nostrils; nostrils patent. Lips free of lesions. Multiple white lesions approximately 1 cm in diameter noted on buccal mucosa and tongue. Uvula rise normal. No palpable lymph nodes. Carotid pulse strong bilaterally. Trachea midline. Thyroid not enlarged.

—B. Gentzler, RN

UNEXPECTED SITUATIONS AND ASSOCIATED INTERVENTIONS

- *While you are testing a patient's visual acuity, the patient states that he can't see anything without his glasses:* Stop the test. Instruct the patient to put on his glasses, and then resume testing.
- *While performing an examination of the regional lymph nodes in the neck area, you palpate a lymph node that feels hard and fixed:* Ask the patient if he has felt this node before and, if so, for how long it has been present and if it is painful. Refer the patient to a primary health care provider for follow-up care.

(continued)

Skill 3-4 ▶ Assessing the Head and Neck (continued)

SPECIAL CONSIDERATIONS

General Considerations

- A patient who wears corrective lenses should have them on when visual acuity is being tested.
- A Snellen picture chart or Snellen E-chart can be used to test vision in children and in patients who are unable to read English. The E-chart uses the capital letter E in varying sizes pointing in different directions. The patient points his or her fingers in the direction the legs of the E are pointing.
- Near vision is tested with a handheld vision screen with varying sizes of print. A Jaeger card can be used for this measurement. The patient holds the card 14 in from the eyes. Ask the patient to read the smallest line of letters possible, with one eye at a time (with the opposite eye covered), and corrective lenses in place, if used. The results are recorded as a fraction and written as 14 over the smallest line read by the patient. A normal result is 14/14.

Infant and Child Considerations

- When examining the neck of an infant or child, the preferred approach to assess ROM of the neck is to assess one movement at a time, rather than a full rotation of the neck, to avoid dizziness on movement.
- When examining the head of an infant, inspect and gently palpate the fontanels and sutures.
- Keep in mind that an infant's nose is usually slightly flattened.
- For a child under age 8 years, do not assess the frontal sinuses; they are usually too small to assess.
- Be aware that lymph nodes may be palpable in children under age 12 years, which is considered a normal variation.
- Note the number of teeth in a child; a child may have up to 20 temporary teeth.

Older Adult Considerations

- Look for a thin, grayish ring in the cornea (arcus senilis). This may be a normal finding in an older adult.
- When evaluating the older adult patient, expect to find normal age-related changes, such as a decrease in vision, hearing, smell, and taste.
- If the patient wears dentures, ask him or her to remove them for inspection of the gums and roof of the mouth.

Cultural Considerations

- Exophthalmos, protrusion of the eyeball, can be a normal finding in an African American patient.

EVIDENCE FOR PRACTICE ▶

INTERPROFESSIONAL ORAL ASSESSMENT AND SCREENING

Assessment of the mouth can provide information about the status of the patient's oral cavity, as well as dental problems, oral hygiene status, salivary conditions, hydration, localized infection, and possible nutritional concerns. Timely assessment of the oral cavity provides the opportunity for referral to appropriate health care providers, such as dietetics and speech pathology, as well as implementation of appropriate oral hygiene interventions. The identification of high-risk patients in relation to mouth care requirements and/or malnutrition is an area that is often overlooked (Hill, Tuck, Ranner, Davies, & Bolieiro-Amaral, 2014). What effect can a systematic interprofessional process for oral screening have?

Related Research

Hill, K. E., Tuck, A., Ranner, S., Davies, N., & Bolieiro-Amaral, K. (2014). The use of a nursing oral and nutritional assessment tool to improve patient outcomes – one centre's experience. *Renal Society of Australasia Journal, 10*(1), 6–10.

This participatory action research study was undertaken as a clinical practice improvement, with the idea that resistance to change in practice could be overcome (Hill et al., 2014). A nursing oral and nutritional assessment tool was created and implemented by the research team, comprised of staff nurses, speech pathologists, and dieticians. All patients admitted or transferred to the acute renal/medical step-down patient care unit were assessed using the developed tool. Based on screening results, nutrition and oral care pathways were implemented. After initial screening, oral assessment was performed daily and an oral and nutritional assessment was performed weekly. Patient records were audited 2 and 5 months after the introduction of the assessment tool. Seventy-four percent (74%) of the nursing staff agree the assessment tool assisted them in the care of patients; 82% of staff felt supported by dietetics in assessing patient's dietary needs; and 79% of staff reported being confident to plan oral care needs independently. Anecdotal experience from the speech pathologist provided support that the mouth care of patients had significantly improved and that the nursing staff had begun to proactively describe care plans and seek support when providing mouth care for patients with dysphagia. The authors concluded that implementation of a standardized assessment tool can improve the provision of patient care.

Relevance to Nursing Practice

Increased awareness of the relationship between inadequate nutrition and poor oral health, and awareness of the consequences of poor oral hygiene and the importance of oral assessment enables nurses to place oral care as a priority in patient care. Progressive oral assessment can provide information related to deterioration or improvement in oral health, as well as provide the ability to initiate interventions related to nutritional support.

Refer to thePoint® for additional research on related nursing topics.

EVIDENCE FOR PRACTICE ▶

SCREENING FOR HEARING AND VISUAL IMPAIRMENT

Hearing and visual impairment are common age-associated changes in older adults. Despite being considered part of the normal aging process, age-related sensory impairment can have significant impact on the functional status of older adults. Communication, interpretation, mobility support, and environmental alterations are often required to address these sensory changes. Many assessment tools used to screen for sensory impairments are self-report tools and cannot be used as observational tools for care staff (Roets-Merken, Zuidema, Vernooij-Dassen, & Kempen, 2014). Is there a reliable objective means for nurses and other caregivers to assess for behavioral cues related to sensory impairments to identify older adults in need of communication and functional support?

Related Research

Roets-Merken, L. M., Zuidema, S. U., Vernooij-Dassen, M. J., & Kempen, G. I. (2014). Screening for hearing, visual and dual sensory impairment in older adults using behavioral cures: A validation study. *International Journal of Nursing Studies, 51*(11), 1434–1440.

The aim of this comparative study was to assess the reliability, validity, and feasibility of a previously developed screening tool used to observe behavior related to sensory impairment (Lyng & Svingen, 2006, as cited in Roets-Merken et al., 2014). The Severe Dual Sensory Loss in Old Age (SDSL) screening tool is a nurse-rated checklist on hearing- and visual-related behavior. The instrument items focus on participation and daily activities identified as being behavioral consequences and adaptations to age-related decline of the auditory and visual system and its neurologic processes. Fifty-six older adults receiving aged care, and 12 nurses and care assistants, participated in the study. Nurses and care assistants received a written version of the tool and instructions. For each participating older adult, the tool was administered by two different staff members independently of each other. After completing the SDSL screening, audiometry was tested in each older adult by a speech-language specialist, and visual acuity, visual field, and contrast sensitivity were tested by a low-vision specialist. The SDSL screening tool was compared with the criterion standards for hearing and visual impairment and was found to be a valid and reliable tool. The SDSL enables nurses and care assistants to identify hearing and visual impairment in older adults.

Relevance to Nursing Practice

Sensory impairment can have negative effects on communication and functional abilities of older adults. Nurses and care assistants play a key role in recognizing sensory impairment in older adults and implementing interventions to support older adults. Nurses and other care givers could benefit from an easy-to-use screening tool to identify hearing and/or visual impairment, leading to improved care for older adults.

Refer to thePoint® for additional research on related nursing topics.

Skill 3-5 ▶ Assessing the Thorax, Lungs, and Breasts

The thorax is composed of the lungs, rib cage, cartilage, and intercostal muscles. A thorough examination of the respiratory system is essential because the primary purpose of this system is to supply oxygen to, and remove carbon dioxide from, the body. Recognizing and identifying normal and abnormal breath sounds, a crucial component of lung assessment, takes practice (Tables 3-1 and 3-2). Assessment of the breasts and axillae is also included in this assessment.

Table 3-1 Normal Breath Sounds

TYPE, DESCRIPTION, AND LOCATION	RATIO OF INSPIRATION TO EXPIRATION
Bronchial or Tubular	
Blowing, hollow sounds; auscultated over the larynx and trachea	Sound on expiration is longer, lower, and higher-pitched than inspiration
Bronchovesicular	
Medium-pitched, medium intensity, blowing sounds; auscultated over the first and second intercostal spaces anteriorly and the scapula posteriorly	Inspiration and expiration sounds have similar pitch and duration
Vesicular	
Soft, low-pitched, whispering sounds; heard over most of the lung fields	Sound on inspiration is longer, louder, and higher-pitched than expiration

Table 3-2 Adventitious Breath Sounds

TYPE AND CHARACTERISTICS	ILLUSTRATION
Wheeze (Sibilant) • Musical or squeaking • High-pitched, continuous sounds • Auscultated during inspiration and expiration • Air passing through narrowed airways	
Rhonchi (Sonorous Wheeze) • Sonorous or coarse; snoring quality • Low-pitched, continuous sounds • Auscultated during inspiration and expiration • Coughing may somewhat clear the sound • Air passing through or around secretions	
Crackles • Bubbling, crackling, popping • Low- to high-pitched, discontinuous sounds • Auscultated during inspiration and expiration • Opening of deflated small airways and alveoli; air passing through fluid in the airways	
Stridor • Harsh, loud, high-pitched • Auscultated on inspiration • Narrowing of upper airway (larynx or trachea); presence of foreign body in airway	
Friction Rub • Rubbing or grating • Loudest over lower lateral anterior surface • Auscultated during inspiration and expiration • Inflamed pleura rubbing against chest wall	

DELEGATION CONSIDERATIONS	Assessment of the patient's thorax, breasts, axillae, and lungs should not be delegated to nursing assistive personnel (NAP) or unlicensed assistive personnel (UAP). However, the NAP or UAP may notice some items while providing care. The nurse must then validate, analyze, document, communicate, and act on these findings, as appropriate. Depending on the state's nurse practice act and the organization's policies and procedures, the licensed practical/vocational nurses (LPN/LVNs) may perform some or all of the parts of assessment of the patient's thorax, breasts, axillae, and lungs. The decision to delegate must be based on careful analysis of the patient's needs and circumstances, as well as the qualifications of the person to whom the task is being delegated. Refer to the Delegation Guidelines in Appendix A.

EQUIPMENT

- Bath blanket or other drape
- Examination gown
- Light source
- Stethoscope
- PPE, as indicated

ASSESSMENT

Complete a health history, focusing on the thorax and lungs. Identify risk factors for altered health by asking about the following:

- History of trauma to the ribs or history of lung surgery
- Number of pillows used when sleeping
- History of persistent cough with or without producing sputum
- History of allergies
- Environmental exposure to chemicals, asbestos, or smoke
- History of smoking (including pack-years)
- History of lung disease in family members or self
- History of frequent or chronic respiratory infections
- Breast discomfort, masses, or lumps, nipple discharge
- History of breast disease, biopsy, or surgeries
- Menstrual and pregnancy history, breastfeeding

NURSING DIAGNOSIS

Determine the related factors for the nursing diagnoses based on the patient's current health status. Appropriate nursing diagnoses may include:

- Ineffective airway clearance
- Impaired gas exchange
- Ineffective health management

OUTCOME IDENTIFICATION AND PLANNING

The expected outcome to achieve in performing an examination of the thorax, lungs, breasts, and axillae is that the assessment is completed without the patient experiencing anxiety or discomfort, the findings are documented, and the appropriate referral is made to the other health care professionals, as needed, for further evaluation. Other specific outcomes will be expected, depending on the identified nursing diagnosis.

IMPLEMENTATION

ACTION	RATIONALE
1. Perform hand hygiene and put on PPE, if indicated.	Hand hygiene and PPE prevent the spread of microorganisms. PPE is required based on transmission precautions.
2. Identify the patient.	Identifying the patient ensures the right patient receives the intervention and helps prevent errors.

(continued)

Skill 3-5 ▶ Assessing the Thorax, Lungs, and Breasts *(continued)*

ACTION	RATIONALE
3. Close the curtains around the bed and close the door to the room, if possible. Explain the purpose of the thorax, lung, breast, and axillae examination and what you are going to do. Answer any questions.	This ensures the patient's privacy. Explanation relieves anxiety and facilitates cooperation.
4. Help the patient undress, if needed, and provide a patient gown. Assist the patient to a sitting position and expose the posterior thorax.	Having the patient wear a gown facilitates examination of the thorax while maintaining the patient's privacy.
5. Use the bath blanket to cover any exposed area other than the one being assessed.	Use of a bath blanket provides for comfort and warmth.
6. Inspect the posterior thorax. Examine the skin (Figure 1), bones, and muscles of the spine, shoulder blades, and back as well as symmetry of expansion and accessory muscle use during respirations.	Examination provides information about lung expansion and accessory muscle use during respiration. Inspection of skin reveals color, presence of lesions, rashes, or masses.
7. Assess the anteroposterior (AP) and lateral diameters of the thorax.	This assessment helps to detect deformities, such as a barrel chest. Normally, the AP is less than the transverse diameter (1:2 ratio).
8. Palpate over the spine and posterior thorax. Use the dorsal surface of the hand to palpate for temperature. Use the palmar surface of the hand to palpate in a sequential pattern for tenderness, muscle development, and masses (Figure 2).	Palpation may reveal abnormal findings, such as excessively dry or moist skin, muscle asymmetry, masses, tenderness, or vibrations.

FIGURE 1. Inspecting the skin for abnormalities and variations. Any lesion or mole noted during inspection of the patient's back should be documented in the patient's medical record for follow-up evaluation. (*Photo by B. Proud.*)

FIGURE 2. Palpating the posterior thorax.

9. Assess thoracic expansion by standing behind the patient and placing both thumbs on either side of the patient's spine at the level of T9 or T10 (Figure 3A). Ask the patient to take a deep breath and note movement of your hands (Figure 3B).	Movement should be symmetric bilaterally.

ACTION	RATIONALE

FIGURE 3. Palpating posterior thoracic excursion. **A.** The examiner's hands are placed symmetrically on the patient's back. **B.** As the patient inhales, the examiner's hands should move apart symmetrically. (*Photos by B. Proud.*)

10. As the patient breathes slowly and deeply through the mouth, auscultate the lungs across and down the posterior thorax to the bases of lungs in a sequential pattern, comparing sides (Figure 4).

11. Inspect the anterior thorax. With the patient sitting, rearrange the gown so the anterior chest is exposed. Inspect the skin, bones, and muscles, as well as symmetry of lung expansion and accessory muscle use.

12. Palpate the anterior thorax across and down the anterior thorax to the bases of lungs in a sequential pattern (Figure 5). Use the palmar surface of the hand to palpate for temperature, tenderness, muscle development, and masses.

Lung auscultation assesses for normal breath sounds and for **adventitious breath sounds**. Abnormal breath sounds indicate respiratory compromise or diseases, such as asthma or bronchitis.

Examination of the anterior thorax provides information about lung expansion and accessory muscle use during respiration. Inspection of skin reveals color, presence of lesions, rashes, or masses.

Palpation may reveal abnormal findings, such as excessively dry or moist skin, muscle asymmetry, masses, tenderness, or vibrations.

FIGURE 4. Auscultating the posterior thorax.

FIGURE 5. Palpating the anterior thorax.

(*continued*)

Skill 3-5 ▶ Assessing the Thorax, Lungs, and Breasts (continued)

ACTION	RATIONALE

13. As the patient breathes slowly and deeply through the mouth, auscultate the lungs across and down the anterior thorax to the bases of lungs in a sequential pattern, comparing sides (Figure 6).

Lung auscultation assesses for normal breath and abnormal (adventitious) breath sounds. Abnormal breath sounds indicate respiratory compromise or diseases, such as asthma or bronchitis.

FIGURE 6. Auscultating the anterior thorax. (From Hogan-Quigley, et al. [2012]. Bates' nursing guide to physical examination and history taking. 1st Edition, P. 318; Wolters Kluwer Health | Lippincott Williams & Wilkins; Philadelphia, PA.)

14. If assessment of the breasts is required, inspect the breasts. Ask the patient to rest hands on both sides of the body, then on the hips and finally above the head. With the patient holding each position, inspect the breasts for size, shape, symmetry, color, texture, and skin lesions. Inspect the areola and nipples for size and shape and the nipples for discharge, crusting, and inversion.

This technique evaluates the general condition of the breasts and helps to identify any abnormalities.

15. Palpate the axillae with the patient's arms resting against the side of the body. If any nodes are palpable, assess their location, size, shape, consistency, tenderness, and mobility.

Palpating the axillae helps to detect nodular enlargement, tenderness, and other abnormalities.

16. Assist the patient into a supine position. Place a small pillow or towel under the patient's back and ask the patient to place a hand on the side being examined under the head, if possible.

Positioning facilitates the exam.

17. Wear gloves if there is any discharge from the nipples or if a lesion is present. Palpate each quadrant of each breast in a systematic method, using either the circular, wedge, or vertical strip technique (see Box 3-1). Palpate the nipple and areola and gently compress the nipple between the thumb and forefinger to assess for discharge.

Gloves prevent contact with blood and body fluids. Palpating the breasts evaluates the consistency and elasticity of breast tissue and nipples and for presence of lumps, masses, or discharge.

18. Assist the patient into a comfortable position and in replacing the gown. Remove gloves and any additional PPE, if used. Perform hand hygiene. Continue with assessments of specific body systems, as appropriate or indicated. Initiate appropriate referral to other health care providers for further evaluation, as indicated.

Replacing the gown ensures patient comfort. Proper removal of PPE reduces the risk for infection transmission and contamination of other items. Hand hygiene prevents the spread of microorganisms. Additional assessments should be completed, as indicated, to evaluate the patient's health status. Intervention by other health care providers may be indicated to evaluate and treat the patient's health status.

Box 3-1 Methods for Palpating the Breasts

Wedge Method

- Work in a clockwise direction and palpate from the periphery toward the areola.
- Use the pads of the first three fingers to gently compress the breast tissue against the chest wall.

Circular Method

- Start at the tail of Spence and move in increasing smaller circles, moving in toward areola.
- Use the pads of the first three fingers to gently compress the breast tissue against the chest wall.

Vertical Strip Method

- Start at the outer edge of the breast and palpate up and down the breast.
- Use the pads of the first three fingers to gently compress the breast tissue against the chest wall.

EVALUATION

The expected outcomes have been met when the patient participates in the assessment of the thorax, lungs, breasts, and axillae; the patient verbalizes understanding of these assessment techniques as appropriate; the assessment is completed without the patient experiencing anxiety or discomfort; the findings are documented; and the appropriate referrals are made to the other health care professionals, as needed, for further evaluation.

DOCUMENTATION

Guidelines

Describe specific findings. Include specific findings for all assessment techniques performed. Note the location of elicited abnormalities. For breast assessment, clock position (using the positioning of the hands of an analog clock) is often used to describe the location of findings.

Sample Documentation

DocuCare Practice documenting assessment techniques and findings in *Lippincott DocuCare*.

6/10/20 2025 Patient states that she "has had a dry cough for the past week and feels weak." Skin pale. RR 30. Breathing effort moderately labored; right-sided intercostal retraction noted. Barrel-shaped chest. Vibrations palpated on right anterior and posterior chest. Rhonchi (sonorous wheezes) auscultated in RUL, RML, and RLL of lung fields. Breasts symmetric, skin smooth with even tone. Breasts and axillae without lumps, masses, dimpling, or discharge.

—B. Gentzler, RN

UNEXPECTED SITUATIONS AND ASSOCIATED INTERVENTIONS

- *When assessing a patient's lungs, you hear short, high-pitched popping sounds on inspiration:* Ask the patient to cough and auscultate again. If the sounds remain, suspect fine crackles and ask the patient if he or she is experiencing any difficulty in breathing or shortness of breath. Crackles may indicate disease, such as pneumonia or heart failure. Document the findings. Continue to assess the patient and notify the primary care provider, as indicated.

(continued)

Skill 3-5 ▶ Assessing the Thorax, Lungs, and Breasts (continued)

SPECIAL CONSIDERATIONS

General Considerations
- Warm equipment, such as a stethoscope, before using it to prevent chilling the patient.
- Warm hands before palpating thorax and breasts to prevent chilling the patient and causing any discomfort.
- Attempt to reduce the noise level in the room while auscultating for breath sounds to ensure accuracy in listening. Also, the presence of chest hair may mimic the sound of crackles and bumping the stethoscope against clothing may distort the sound.

Infant and Child Considerations
- Auscultate a child's lungs before performing other assessment techniques that may cause crying.
- Expect to hear breath sounds that are harsher or more bronchial than those of an adult.

Older Adult Considerations
- In the older adult patient, expect to find a reduction in respiratory effort due to age-related changes. A common finding in the older adult is kyphoscoliosis, a skeletal deformity affecting the spinal column, which causes the AP diameter to increase and the thorax to shorten.

Skill 3-6 ▶ Assessing the Cardiovascular System

The cardiovascular system transports oxygen, nutrients, and other substances to the body tissues and removes metabolic waste products to the kidneys and lungs. Careful assessment of this vital system is essential. In this skill, assessment data associated with the heart will be presented. The peripheral vascular system assessment is included in Skill 3-10, because peripheral vascular, neurologic, and musculoskeletal systems are usually combined when performing a head-to-toe assessment. While assessing the heart, careful auscultation is important. Identifying heart sounds takes practice. Table 3-3 provides a review of normal heart sounds in relation to the cardiac cycle and information about abnormal heart sounds.

DELEGATION CONSIDERATIONS

Assessment of the patient's cardiovascular system should not be delegated to nursing assistive personnel (NAP) or unlicensed assistive personnel (UAP). However, the NAP or UAP may notice some items while providing care. The nurse must then validate, analyze, document, communicate, and act on these findings, as appropriate. Depending on the state's nurse practice act and the organization's policies and procedures, the licensed practical/vocational nurses (LPN/LVNs) may perform some or all of the parts of assessment of the patient's cardiovascular system. The decision to delegate must be based on careful analysis of the patient's needs and circumstances, as well as the qualifications of the person to whom the task is being delegated. Refer to the Delegation Guidelines in Appendix A.

EQUIPMENT

- Bath blanket or other drape
- Examination gown
- Stethoscope
- Centimeter ruler
- PPE, as indicated

ASSESSMENT

Complete a health history, focusing on the heart. Identify risk factors for altered health by asking about the following:

- History of chest pain, tightness, palpitations, dizziness, or fatigue
- Swelling in the ankles and feet
- Number of pillows used to sleep
- Type and amount of medications taken daily

Table 3-3 | Heart Sounds

Normal Heart Sounds

During auscultation, the first heart sound, S_1, is heard as the "lub" of "lub-dub." This sound occurs when the mitral and tricuspid valves close, and it corresponds to the onset of ventricular contraction. The sound, low-pitched and dull, is heard best at the apical area. The second heart sound, S_2, occurs at the termination of systole and corresponds to the onset of ventricular diastole. The "dub" of "lub-dub," it represents the closure of the aortic and pulmonic valves. The sound of S_2 is higher-pitched and shorter than S_1. The two sounds occur within 1 second or less, depending on the heart rate. Normal findings include S_1 that is louder at the tricuspid and apical areas, with S_2 louder at the aortic and pulmonic areas.

A Electrocardiogram

B Heart sounds

Heart sounds in relation to the cardiac cycle and an electrocardiogram.

Abnormal Heart Sounds

Abnormal findings include extra heart sounds at any of the cardiac landmarks and abnormal rate or rhythm. A wide variety of conditions may alter the normal heart rate or rhythm, including serious infections, anemia, diseases of the heart muscle or conducting system, dehydration or overhydration, endocrine disorders, respiratory disorders, and head trauma. Extra heart sounds may be S_3, S_4, or murmurs.

- S_3, known as the third heart sound, follows S_2 and is often represented by a "lub-dub-dee" pattern ("dee" being S_3). This sound is best heard with the stethoscope bell at the mitral area, with the patient lying on the left side. S_3 is considered normal in children and young adults and abnormal in middle-aged and older adults.
- S_4 is the fourth heart sound, occurring right before S1, and is often represented by a "dee-lub-dub" pattern ("dee" being S_4). S_4 is considered normal in older adults but abnormal in children and adults.
- Heart murmurs are extra heart sounds caused by some disruption of blood flow through the heart. The characteristics of a murmur and grading depend on the adequacy of valve function, rate of blood flow, and size of the valve opening. Usually, nurses are more concerned with recognizing changes in murmurs rather than in diagnosing and labeling them (Jensen, 2015, p. 475). Refer to information on the**Point** or a health assessment text for grading details and additional information related to assessment of heart sounds.

- History of heart defect, rheumatic fever, or chest or heart surgery
- Family history of hypertension (high blood pressure), myocardial infarction (heart attack), coronary artery disease, high blood cholesterol levels, or diabetes mellitus
- History of smoking (including pack-years)
- Alcohol use
- Type and amount of exercise
- Usual foods eaten each day

NURSING DIAGNOSIS

Determine the related factors for the nursing diagnoses based on the patient's current health status. Appropriate nursing diagnoses may include:

- Decreased cardiac output
- Impaired gas exchange
- Risk for decreased cardiac tissue perfusion

OUTCOME IDENTIFICATION AND PLANNING

The expected outcome to achieve in performing an examination of the cardiovascular structures is that the assessment is completed without causing the patient to experience anxiety or discomfort, the findings are documented, and the appropriate referral is made to other health care professionals, as needed, for further evaluation. Other specific outcomes will be formulated, depending on the identified nursing diagnosis.

(continued)

Skill 3-6 ▶ Assessing the Cardiovascular System *(continued)*

IMPLEMENTATION

ACTION	RATIONALE
1. Perform hand hygiene and put on PPE, if indicated.	Hand hygiene and PPE prevent the spread of microorganisms. PPE is required based on transmission precautions.
2. Identify the patient.	Identifying the patient ensures the right patient receives the intervention and helps prevent errors.
3. Close the curtains around the bed and close the door to the room, if possible. Explain the purpose of the cardiovascular examination and what you are going to do. Answer any questions.	This ensures the patient's privacy. Explanation relieves anxiety and facilitates cooperation.
4. Help the patient undress, if needed, and provide a patient gown. Assist the patient to a supine position with the head elevated about 30 to 45 degrees, if possible, and expose the anterior chest. Use the bath blanket to cover any exposed area other than the one being assessed.	Having the patient wear a gown facilitates examination of the cardiovascular system. Use of a bath blanket provides for comfort and warmth.
5. If not performed previously with the assessment of the head and neck, inspect and palpate the left and then the right carotid arteries. **Palpate only one carotid artery at a time.** Note the strength of the pulse and grade it as with peripheral pulses.	Palpation of this area evaluates circulation through the arteries. Palpating both arteries at once can reduce blood flow to the brain, potentially causing dizziness or loss of consciousness.
6. Inspect the neck for distention of the jugular veins.	Jugular venous distention (fullness) is associated with heart failure and fluid volume overload.
7. Inspect the **precordium** for contour, pulsations, and heaves (Figure 1). Observe for the apical impulse at the fourth to fifth intercostal space (ICS) at the left midclavicular line.	Precordium inspection helps detect pulsations. There are normally no pulsations, except for the apical impulse.
8. Using the palmar surface, with the four fingers held together, gently palpate the precordium for pulsations. Remember that hands should be warm. Palpation proceeds in a systematic manner, with assessment of specific cardiac landmarks—the aortic, pulmonic, tricuspid, and mitral areas and Erb's point (Refer to Figure 1). Palpate the apical impulse in the mitral area (Figure 2). Note size, duration, force, and location in relationship to the midclavicular line.	Normal findings include no pulsation palpable over the aortic and pulmonic areas, with a palpable apical impulse. Abnormal findings include precordial thrills, which are fine, palpable, rushing vibrations over the right or left second ICS, and any lifts or heaves, which involve a rise along the border of the sternum with each heartbeat.

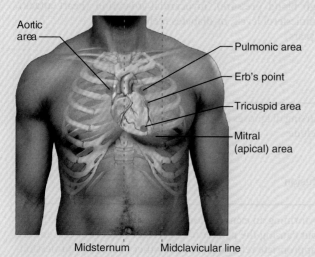

Aortic area — Pulmonic area — Erb's point — Tricuspid area — Mitral (apical) area — Midsternum — Midclavicular line

FIGURE 1. Precordium cardiac landmarks.

FIGURE 2. Palpating the apical impulse in the mitral area.

ACTION	**RATIONALE**

9. Auscultate heart sounds. Ask the patient to breathe normally. Use the diaphragm of the stethoscope first to listen to high-pitched sounds. Then use the bell to listen to low-pitched sounds. Focus on the overall rate and rhythm of the heart and the normal heart sounds (Table 3-3). Begin at the aortic area, move to the pulmonic area, then to Erb's point, then the tricuspid area, and finally listen at the mitral area (Figures 1 and 3).

Auscultation evaluates heart rate and rhythm and assesses for normal sounds (the lub, S_1; the dub, S_2) and abnormal heart sounds. The normal heart sounds (S_1 and S_2) are generated by the closing of the valves (the aortic, pulmonic, tricuspid, mitral). Extra heart sounds are often heard when the patient has anemia or heart disease. A wide variety of conditions may alter the normal heart rate or rhythm, including serious infections, diseases of the heart muscle or conducting system, dehydration or overhydration, endocrine disorders, respiratory disorders, and head trauma. Extra heart sounds may be S_3, S_4, or murmurs.

FIGURE 3. Auscultating the mitral area. (*Photo by B. Proud.*)

10. Assist the patient in replacing the gown. Remove PPE, if used. Perform hand hygiene. Continue with assessments of specific body systems as appropriate or indicated. Initiate appropriate referral to other health care providers for further evaluation, as indicated.

Replacing the gown ensures patient comfort. Proper removal of PPE reduces the risk for infection transmission and contamination of other items. Hand hygiene prevents the spread of microorganisms. Additional assessments should be completed as indicated to evaluate the patient's health status. Intervention by other health care providers may be indicated to evaluate and treat the patient's health status.

EVALUATION

The expected outcomes have been met when the patient participates in the assessment of the cardiovascular system, the patient verbalizes understanding of these assessment techniques as appropriate, the assessment is completed without the patient experiencing anxiety or discomfort, the findings are documented, and the appropriate referrals are made to the other health care professionals, as needed, for further evaluation.

DOCUMENTATION

Guidelines

Document assessment techniques performed, along with specific findings. Note assessment data related to color and temperature of the skin. Record inspection findings related to the carotid arteries, jugular veins, and anterior chest wall area. Document findings related to palpation of anterior chest wall for presence of pulsations, thrills, lifts, and heaves. Note auscultation findings, including rate, rhythm, pitch, and location of sounds. Record the normal heart sounds (S_1 and S_2) as well as the presence of any extra (abnormal) sounds.

Sample Documentation

DocuCare Practice documenting assessment techniques and findings in *Lippincott DocuCare.*

5/10/20 1015 Patient denies chest pain but states, "I have palpitations occurring about once a week." Skin pale, cool to touch, brisk capillary refill. Inspection and palpation of chest: no lifts, pulsations, or heaves were noted. Auscultation: S_1 loudest at the apex; S_2 loudest at the base; no extra sounds auscultated. Carotid pulse 88, regular rhythm, +2, equal bilaterally.

—S. Moses, RN

(continued)

Skill 3-6 ▶ Assessing the Cardiovascular System   *(continued)*

SPECIAL CONSIDERATIONS

General Considerations
- Warm equipment, such as a stethoscope, before using it to prevent chilling the patient.

Infant and Child Considerations
- The presence of abnormal heart sound S_3 is considered normal in children and young adults.
- The presence of abnormal heart sound S_4 is considered abnormal in children.

Older Adult Considerations
- The presence of abnormal heart sound S_3 is considered abnormal in middle-aged and older adults.
- The presence of abnormal heart sound S_4 is considered normal in older adults.

Skill 3-7 ▶ Assessing the Abdomen

The abdominal cavity, the largest cavity in the body, contains the stomach, small intestine, large intestine, liver, gallbladder, pancreas, spleen, kidneys, urinary bladder, adrenal gland, and major blood vessels. In women, the uterus, fallopian tubes, and ovaries are also located in the abdomen. Not all of these organs can be assessed. For identification and documentation purposes, the abdomen can be divided into four quadrants (Figure 1).

The order of the techniques differs for the abdominal assessment from the other systems. Assessment of the abdomen starts with inspection, then auscultation, percussion, and palpation. The order of assessment differs for this system because palpation and percussion before auscultation may alter the sounds heard on auscultation. Advanced practice professionals perform percussion and deep palpation of the abdomen. Therefore, these techniques will not be discussed here. Before beginning the abdominal assessment, ask the patient to empty his or her bladder because a full bladder may cause discomfort during the examination.

Right Upper Quadrant
- Pylorous
- Duodenum
- Liver
- Right kidney and adrenal gland
- Hepatic flexure of colon
- Head of pancreas

Left Upper Quadrant
- Stomach
- Spleen
- Left kidney and adrenal gland
- Splenic flexure of colon
- Body of pancreas

Right Lower Quadrant
- Cecum
- Appendix
- Right ovary and fallopian tube (female)
- Right ureter and lower kidney pole
- Right spermatic cord (male)

Left Lower Quadrant
- Sigmoid colon
- Left ovary and fallopian tube (female)
- Left ureter and lower kidney pole
- Left spermatic cord (male)

Midline
- Urinary bladder
- Urethra (female)

FIGURE 1. Diagram of abdominal quadrants and outline of underlying organs.

DELEGATION CONSIDERATIONS

Assessment of the patient's abdomen should not be delegated to nursing assistive personnel (NAP) or unlicensed assistive personnel (UAP). However, the NAP or UAP may notice some items while providing care. The nurse must then validate, analyze, document, communicate, and act on these findings, as appropriate. Depending on the state's nurse practice act and the organization's policies and procedures, the licensed practical/vocational nurses (LPN/LVNs) may perform some or all of the parts of assessment of the patient's abdomen. The decision to delegate must be based on careful analysis of the patient's needs and circumstances, as well as the qualifications of the person to whom the task is being delegated. Refer to the Delegation Guidelines in Appendix A.

| EQUIPMENT | • PPE, as indicated | • Examination gown |
| | • Bath blanket or other drape | • Stethoscope |

ASSESSMENT

Complete a health history, focusing on the abdomen. Identify risk factors for altered health by asking about the following:

- History of abdominal pain
- History of indigestion, nausea or vomiting, constipation or diarrhea
- History of food allergies or lactose intolerance
- Appetite and usual food and fluid intake
- Usual bowel and bladder elimination patterns
- History of gastrointestinal disorders
- History of urinary tract disorders
- History of abdominal surgery or trauma
- Amount and type of alcohol ingestion
- For women, menstrual history

NURSING DIAGNOSIS

Determine the related factors for the nursing diagnoses based on the patient's current health status. Appropriate nursing diagnoses may include:

- Constipation
- Acute pain
- Diarrhea

OUTCOME IDENTIFICATION AND PLANNING

The expected outcome to achieve in performing an examination of the abdomen is that the assessment is completed without causing the patient to experience anxiety or discomfort, the findings are documented, and the appropriate referral is made to other health care professionals, as needed, for further evaluation. Other specific outcomes will be formulated, depending on the identified nursing diagnosis.

IMPLEMENTATION

ACTION	RATIONALE
1. Perform hand hygiene and put on PPE, if indicated.	Hand hygiene and PPE prevent the spread of microorganisms. PPE is required based on transmission precautions.
2. Identify the patient.	Identifying the patient ensures the right patient receives the intervention and helps prevent errors.
3. Close the curtains around bed and close the door to the room, if possible. Explain the purpose of the abdominal examination and what you are going to do. Answer any questions.	This ensures the patient's privacy. Explanation relieves anxiety and facilitates cooperation.
4. Help the patient undress, if needed, and provide a patient gown. Assist the patient to a supine position, if possible, and expose the abdomen. Use the bath blanket to cover any exposed area other than the one being assessed.	Having the patient wear a gown facilitates examination of the abdomen. Use of a bath blanket provides for comfort and warmth.
5. Inspect the abdomen for skin color, contour, pulsations, the umbilicus, and other surface characteristics (rashes, lesions, masses, scars).	The umbilicus should be centrally located and may be flat, rounded, or concave. The abdomen should be evenly rounded or symmetric, without visible peristalsis. In thin people, an upper midline pulsation may normally be visible. Abnormal findings include asymmetry (possibly from an enlarged organ or mass), distention (possibly indicating retained gas or air; obesity), swelling of the abdomen (possibly indicating **ascites**) and abdominal masses, or unusual pulsations.

(*continued*)

Skill 3-7 ▶ Assessing the Abdomen *(continued)*

ACTION

6. Auscultate all four quadrants of the abdomen (Figure 1) for bowel sounds. Warm the stethoscope and, using light pressure, place the flat diaphragm on the right lower quadrant of the abdomen, then move to the right upper quadrant (Figure 2), left upper quadrant, and finally left lower quadrant. Listen carefully for bowel sounds (gurgles and clicks), and note their frequency and character.

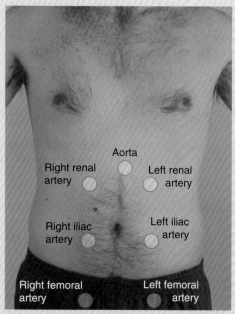

FIGURE 2. Auscultating the abdomen. (From Jensen, S. [2011]. Nursing health assessment. P. 606; Wolters Kluwer Health | Lippincott Williams & Wilkins; Philadelphia, PA.)

7. Auscultate the abdomen for vascular sounds. Using the bell of the stethoscope, auscultate over the abdominal aorta, femoral arteries, and iliac arteries for bruits (Figure 3).

8. Palpate the abdomen lightly in all four quadrants. The pads of the fingers are used to palpate with a light, gentle, dipping motion approximately 1 cm (approx. 0.5 in) (Jensen, 2015). Watch the patient's face for nonverbal signs of pain during palpation. Palpate each quadrant in a systematic manner, noting muscular resistance, tenderness, enlargement of the organs, or masses. (Figure 4). **If the patient complains of pain or discomfort in a particular area of the abdomen, palpate that area last.**

RATIONALE

Performing auscultation before percussion or palpation prevents percussion and palpation techniques from interfering with findings. Bowel sounds usually occur every 5 to 34 seconds. Before documenting bowel sounds as absent, listen for 2 minutes or longer in each abdominal quadrant. Abnormal findings include increased bowel sounds (often heard with diarrhea or in early bowel obstruction), decreased bowel sounds (heard after abdominal surgery or late bowel obstruction), or absent bowel sounds (indicating peritonitis or paralytic ileus). Bowel sounds of high-pitched tinkling or rushes of high-pitched sounds indicate a bowel obstruction.

A bruit may be heard in the presence of stenosis (narrowing) or occlusion of an artery. Bruits may also be caused by abnormal dilation of a vessel.

Palpation provides information about the location, size, tenderness, and condition of the underlying structures. The abdomen should normally be soft, relaxed, and free of tenderness. Abnormal findings include involuntary rigidity, spasm, and pain (which may indicate trauma, peritonitis, infection, tumors, or enlarged or diseased abdominal organs, such as appendicitis).

Aorta
Right renal artery
Left renal artery
Right iliac artery
Left iliac artery
Right femoral artery
Left femoral artery

FIGURE 3. Locations to auscultate for bruits. (*Photo by B. Proud.*)

FIGURE 4. Palpating the abdomen lightly. (*Photo by B. Proud.*)

ACTION	**RATIONALE**
9. Palpate and then auscultate the femoral pulses in the groin. Note the strength of the pulse and grade it as with peripheral pulses (see Skill 3-10). Use the bell of the stethoscope to auscultate the arteries.	This is part of the assessment of the peripheral vascular system in Skill 3-10. However, some health care providers include this assessment here for organizational convenience and time management. This technique assesses flow of blood through the arteries. Auscultation can detect a bruit.

10. Assist the patient into a comfortable position and in replacing the gown. Remove PPE, if used. Perform hand hygiene. Continue with assessments of specific body systems, as appropriate, or indicated. Initiate appropriate referral to other health care providers for further evaluation, as indicated.

Replacing the gown ensures patient comfort. Proper removal of PPE reduces the risk for infection transmission and contamination of other items. Hand hygiene prevents the spread of microorganisms. Additional assessments should be completed, as indicated, to evaluate the patient's health status. Intervention by other health care providers may be indicated to evaluate and treat the patient's health status.

EVALUATION

The expected outcomes have been met when the patient participates in the assessment of the abdomen, the patient verbalizes understanding of the assessment techniques as appropriate, the assessment is completed without the patient experiencing anxiety or discomfort, the findings are documented, and the appropriate referrals are made to the other health care professionals, as needed, for further evaluation.

DOCUMENTATION

Guidelines

Document assessment techniques performed, along with specific findings. Note assessment data related to color of the skin, presence of symmetry/asymmetry, distention, swelling, lesions, rashes, scars, or masses. Note the character of the bowel sounds and if any bruits are present. Note the overall softness or hardness of the abdomen, presence of palpable masses, the presence of pain or tenderness, and unusual pulsations.

Sample Documentation

DocuCare Practice documenting assessment techniques and findings in *Lippincott DocuCare*.

> <u>3/30/20</u> 0930 Patient states, "I have been feeling sick to my stomach for the last 24 hours." Denies any abdominal pain. Abdomen symmetric; soft, slightly distended, umbilicus midline, no scars or pulsations, bowel sounds present in all four quadrants, but decreased.
>
> —B. Gentzler, RN

SPECIAL CONSIDERATIONS

General Considerations
- Warm equipment, such as a stethoscope, before using it to prevent chilling the patient.

Infant and Child Considerations
- Umbilical cord in newborns; dries and falls off within the first few weeks of life.
- In infants, expect a large abdomen in relation to the pelvis.
- The abdomen of a child is normally protuberant.

Older Adult Considerations
- Decreased bowel sounds
- Decreased abdominal tone
- Fat accumulation on the abdomen and hips

Skill 3-8 ▷ Assessing the Female Genitalia

The external female genitalia consist of the mons pubis, labia majora and minora, clitoris, vestibular glands, vaginal vestibule, vaginal orifice, and urethral opening (Figure 1). During the physical assessment, examine the external genitalia by inspection and palpation. The internal pelvic examination is a skill most often performed by an advanced practice professional. Women from some cultures or those who practice certain religions (e.g., Islam) may agree to a physical examination of the genitalia only if it is performed by a female nurse or female practitioner.

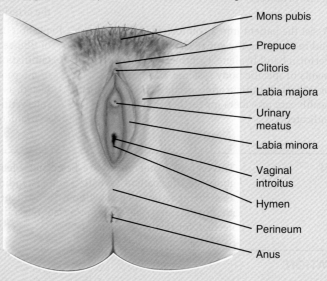

Mons pubis
Prepuce
Clitoris
Labia majora
Urinary meatus
Labia minora
Vaginal introitus
Hymen
Perineum
Anus

FIGURE 1. External female genitalia.

DELEGATION CONSIDERATIONS	Assessment of the patient's genitalia should not be delegated to nursing assistive personnel (NAP) or unlicensed assistive personnel (UAP). However, an NAP or UAP may notice some items while providing care. The nurse must then validate, analyze, document, communicate, and act on these findings, as appropriate. Depending on the state's nurse practice act and the organization's policies and procedures, the licensed practical/vocational nurses (LPN/LVNs) may perform some or all of the parts of assessment of the patient's genitalia. The decision to delegate must be based on careful analysis of the patient's needs and circumstances, as well as the qualifications of the person to whom the task is being delegated. Refer to the Delegation Guidelines in Appendix A.

EQUIPMENT	• PPE, as indicated • Examination gown • Bath blanket or other drape • Gloves

ASSESSMENT

Complete a health history, focusing on the female genital system. Identify risk factors for altered health by asking about the following:

- Menstrual history (age of first and last period, length of flow, type of flow, pain)
- Sexual history (age at which sexual activity began, number and biological sex of partners)
- Pain with intercourse, difficulty achieving orgasm
- Number of pregnancies and live births
- History of sexually transmitted infection
- Use of contraceptives
- Frequency of pelvic examinations and Pap smears
- History of vaginal discharge, itching, or pain on urination
- Use of hormones and tobacco (how long, how much, how many packs/day)

NURSING DIAGNOSIS

Determine the related factors for the nursing diagnoses based on the patient's current health status. Appropriate nursing diagnoses may include:

- Ineffective health maintenance
- Risk for infection
- Sexual dysfunction

| OUTCOME IDENTIFICATION AND PLANNING | The expected outcome to achieve in performing an examination of the female genitalia is that the assessments are completed without causing the patient to experience anxiety or discomfort, the findings are documented, and the appropriate referral is made to other health care professionals, as needed, for further evaluation. Other specific outcomes will be formulated, depending on the identified nursing diagnosis. |

IMPLEMENTATION

ACTION	RATIONALE
1. Perform hand hygiene and put on PPE, if indicated.	Hand hygiene and PPE prevent the spread of microorganisms. PPE is required based on transmission precautions.
2. Identify the patient.	Identifying the patient ensures the right patient receives the intervention and helps prevent errors.
3. Close the curtains around bed and close the door to the room, if possible. Explain the purpose of the examination of genitalia and what you are going to do. Answer any questions.	This ensures the patient's privacy. Explanation relieves anxiety and facilitates cooperation.
4. Help the patient undress, if needed, and provide a patient gown. Assist the patient to a supine position, or lying on her side, if possible. Use the bath blanket to cover any exposed area other than the one being assessed.	Having the patient wear a gown facilitates examination of the genitalia. Use of a bath blanket provides for comfort and warmth.
5. Inspect the external genitalia for color, size of the labia majora and vaginal opening, lesions, and discharge.	The vulva normally has more pigmentation than other skin areas, and the mucous membranes are dark pink and moist. The skin and mucosa should be smooth, without lesions or swelling. The labia should be symmetric without lesions or swelling. Lesions may be the result of infections (e.g., herpes or syphilis). There may normally be a small amount of clear or whitish vaginal discharge.
6. Palpate the labia for masses.	The vulva should be without lumps or masses.
7. Assist the patient to a comfortable position.	This ensures the patient's comfort.
8. Remove PPE, if used. Perform hand hygiene. Continue with assessments of specific body systems, as appropriate, or indicated. Initiate appropriate referral to other health care providers for further evaluation, as indicated.	Proper removal of PPE reduces the risk for infection transmission and contamination of other items. Hand hygiene prevents the spread of microorganisms. Additional assessments should be completed, as indicated, to evaluate the patient's health status. Intervention by other health care providers may be indicated to evaluate and treat the patient's health status.

| EVALUATION | The expected outcomes have been met when the patient participates in the assessment of the genitalia; the patient verbalizes an understanding of the assessment techniques as appropriate; the assessment is completed without the patient experiencing anxiety or discomfort; the findings are documented; and the appropriate referrals are made to the other health care professionals as needed for further evaluation. |

DOCUMENTATION	
Guidelines	Document assessment techniques performed, along with specific findings. Note and record the color, size of the labia majora and vaginal opening, lesions, and presence of any discharge. Document any patient statements of pain and risk factors.

(continued)

Skill 3-8 ▶ Assessing the Female Genitalia *(continued)*

Sample Documentation

<u>1/12/20</u> 1645 Patient denies vaginal itching, pain, lumps, or discharge. Vulva with darker pigmentation than surrounding skin tone; mucous membranes are dark pink and moist. Skin and mucosa smooth, without lesions or swelling. Labia are symmetric without lesions or swelling. No discharge noted. Vulva is without lumps or masses.

—*B. Holmes, RN*

SPECIAL CONSIDERATIONS

Infant and Child Considerations

- In newborns, enlargement of the labia and clitoris and breast enlargement occur, resulting from exposure to maternal hormones in utero and normally seen in the first week after birth, subsiding by the second week after birth.
- Pubic hair and breast development occur at puberty and follow a regular sequence of development.
- Menstruation begins about 2.5 years after puberty begins.
- Irregular menstrual cycle is common for first 2 years.

Older Adult Considerations

- Decreased size of labia
- Decreased amount of pubic hair
- Decreased vaginal secretions

Skill 3-9 ▶ Assessing the Male Genitalia

The external male genitalia (Figure 1) include the penis and scrotum. In addition, the inguinal area may be assessed as part of this assessment. During the physical assessment, the nurse examines the external genitalia by inspection and palpation. Examination of the prostate gland is a skill performed by an advanced practice professional.

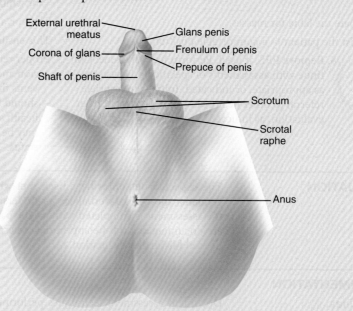

FIGURE 1. External male genitalia. (From Pansky, B., & Gest, T. R. [2013]. *Lippincott's concise illustrated anatomy: Thorax, abdomen & pelvis.* Philadelphia, PA: Wolters Kluwer Health, p. 205, Figure 3.1F.)

| DELEGATION CONSIDERATIONS | The assessment of the patient's genitalia should not be delegated to nursing assistive personnel (NAP) or unlicensed assistive personnel (UAP). However, the NAP or UAP may notice some items while providing care. The nurse must then validate, analyze, document, communicate, and act on these findings, as appropriate. Depending on the state's nurse practice act and the organization's policies and procedures, the licensed practical/vocational nurses (LPN/LVNs) may perform some or all of the parts of assessment of the patient's genitalia. The decision to delegate must be based on careful analysis of the patient's needs and circumstances, as well as the qualifications of the person to whom the task is being delegated. Refer to the Delegation Guidelines in Appendix A. |

EQUIPMENT

- PPE, as indicated
- Bath blanket or other drape
- Examination gown
- Gloves

ASSESSMENT

Complete a health history, focusing on the male genitalia. Identify risk factors for altered health by asking about the following:

- Frequency of digital rectal examinations
- Frequency of testicular self-examination
- Use of contraceptives
- Occupational exposure to chemicals (tire and rubber manufacturing, farming, mechanics)
- Sexual history (age at which sexual activity began, number and biological sex of partners)
- History of sexually transmitted infection
- History of discharge from the penis
- Difficulty with urination (incontinence, hesitancy, frequency, voiding at night)
- History of erectile dysfunction, pain with intercourse

NURSING DIAGNOSIS

Determine the related factors for the nursing diagnoses based on the patient's current health status. Appropriate nursing diagnoses may include:

- Ineffective health maintenance
- Risk for infection
- Sexual dysfunction

OUTCOME IDENTIFICATION AND PLANNING

The expected outcome to achieve in performing an examination of the male genitalia is that the assessments are completed without causing the patient to experience anxiety or discomfort, the findings are documented, and the appropriate referral is made to other health care professionals, as needed, for further evaluation. Other specific outcomes will be formulated, depending on the identified nursing diagnosis.

IMPLEMENTATION

ACTION	RATIONALE
1. Perform hand hygiene and put on PPE, if indicated.	Hand hygiene and PPE prevent the spread of microorganisms. PPE is required based on transmission precautions.
2. Identify the patient.	Identifying the patient ensures the right patient receives the intervention and helps prevent errors.
3. Close the curtains around the bed and close the door to the room, if possible. Explain the purpose of the examination of genitalia and what you are going to do. Answer any questions.	This ensures the patient's privacy. Explanation relieves anxiety and facilitates cooperation.
4. Help the patient undress, if needed, and provide a patient gown. Assist the patient to a supine or sitting position, if possible. Use a bath blanket to cover any exposed area other than the one being assessed.	Having the patient wear a gown facilitates examination of the genitalia. Use of a bath blanket provides for comfort and warmth.

(continued)

Skill 3-9 ▶ Assessing the Male Genitalia *(continued)*

ACTION	RATIONALE
5. Put on gloves. Inspect the external genitalia for size, placement, contour, appearance of the skin, redness, edema, and discharge. If the patient is uncircumcised, retract the foreskin for inspection of the glans penis. Assess the location of the urinary meatus. Inspect the scrotum for symmetry.	Gloves prevent contact with blood and body fluids. The size and shape of the scrotum should be similar bilaterally. It is not unusual for the left testicle to lie lower in the scrotal sac than the right testicle. Normal findings include skin that is free of lesions, and a foreskin (if present) that is intact, uniform in color, and easily retracted. The urinary meatus is normally located in the center of the glans penis and is free of discharge. Abnormal findings include lesions, redness, edema, discharge, and displacement of the urinary meatus or difficulties with voiding. Lesions may be the result of infections (e.g., herpes or syphilis). Edema, redness, or discharge may indicate an infection. Voiding difficulties may result from scarring caused by infections or prostate enlargement.
6. Palpate the scrotum for consistency, nodules, masses, and tenderness.	The consistency of the scrotal contents (i.e., testes) should be similar bilaterally. The scrotum and testes should be free of masses and nontender. Pain may indicate an infection.
7. Inspect the inguinal area. Ask the patient to bear down and look for bulging of the area.	Normally, the inguinal area is free of bulges.
8. Assist the patient to a comfortable position.	This ensures the patient's comfort.
9. Remove PPE, if used. Perform hand hygiene. Continue with assessments of specific body systems, as appropriate, or indicated. Initiate appropriate referral to other health care providers for further evaluation, as indicated.	Proper removal of PPE reduces the risk for infection transmission and contamination of other items. Hand hygiene prevents the spread of microorganisms. Additional assessments should be completed, as indicated, to evaluate the patient's health status. Intervention by other health care providers may be indicated to evaluate and treat the patient's health status.

EVALUATION

The expected outcomes have been met when the patient participates in the assessment of the genitalia; the patient verbalizes understanding of the assessment techniques as appropriate; the assessment is completed without the patient experiencing anxiety or discomfort; the findings are documented; and the appropriate referrals are made to the other health care professionals as needed for further evaluation.

DOCUMENTATION

Guidelines

Document assessment techniques performed, along with specific findings. Note and record the size, placement, contour, appearance of the skin, presence of foreskin, redness, edema, location of urinary meatus, and discharge. Document any patient statements of pain and risk factors.

Sample Documentation

> 09/23/20 1730 Patient denies pain and discharge from penis; denies lumps or changes in scrotum. Patient reports no difficulty with urination. Scrotum of equal size and shape. Skin without lesions, edema, redness; foreskin present and intact, uniform in color, and easily retracted. Urinary meatus located in the center of the glans penis and is free of discharge. Scrotum and testes free of masses and nontender. Inguinal area is free of bulges.
> —B. Holmes, RN

SPECIAL CONSIDERATIONS

Infant and Child Considerations

- In newborns, breast enlargement occurs, resulting from exposure to maternal hormones in utero and normally seen in the first week after birth, subsiding by the second week after birth.
- Development of pubic hair and enlargement of the scrotum, testes, and penis occur at puberty and follow a regular sequence to adult configuration.
- Spontaneous nocturnal emission of seminal fluid occurs at puberty.

Older Adult Considerations

- Decreased penis size
- Decreased pubic hair
- Decreased size and firmness of testes

Skill 3-10

Assessing the Neurologic, Musculoskeletal, and Peripheral Vascular Systems

The following assessment integrates the findings from the neurologic, musculoskeletal, and peripheral vascular systems. In assessing the neurologic system, ask the patient to respond to a series of questions that will enable you to obtain data related to overall cognitive function. In addition, evaluate sensation in different areas of the body as well as selected cranial nerves. Musculoskeletal examination will provide information concerning the condition and functioning of certain muscles and joints throughout the body. The peripheral vascular system assessment will identify the condition of the arteries and veins in the extremities as gained through inspection and palpation of the skin and peripheral pulses.

Musculoskeletal trauma, crush injuries, orthopedic surgery, and external pressure from a cast or tight-fitting bandage can cause damage to blood vessels and nerves. This damage causes localized inflammation and tissue edema, which can lead to significantly diminished perfusion and severe ischemia, with resulting severe and permanent dysfunction of the affected area and/or loss of a limb. Assessment of neurovascular status is an important nursing intervention leading to early identification of neurovascular impairment and timely intervention (Johnston-Walker & Hardcastle, 2011; Turney, Raley Noble, & Chae Kim, 2013). A neurovascular assessment includes assessing for changes in circulation, motor function, and sensation. Box 3-2 outlines the components of a neurovascular assessment.

Box 3-2 | Components of a Neurovascular Assessment

- **Pain:** Extreme pain, especially on passive motion, is a significant sign of probable neurovascular impairment in an extremity. Subjective and objective assessments should be included. Opioid analgesia is unlikely to relieve the pain.
- **Pallor (perfusion):** Comparison between affected and unaffected limb is important. Color and temperature of the extremity: Pale skin, decreased tone, or white color may indicate poor arterial perfusion. Cyanosis may indicate venous stasis. Coolness or decreased temperature may indicate decreased arterial supply. Compare distal to proximal temperature variation in affected limb. Assess capillary refill. Using your thumb and forefinger, squeeze the patient's fingernail or toenail until it appears white. Release the pressure and observe the time it takes for normal color to return. Normally, color returns immediately, in less than 2 to 3 seconds.
- **Peripheral pulses:** Comparison between affected and unaffected limb is important. Assess the consistency of arterial blood flow (pulse presence, rate, quality) up to and past the affected area. Assess capillary refill, especially in patients whose pulses cannot be palpated due to casts or bandages (Johnston-Walker & Hardcastle, 2011; Judge, 2007) and in nonverbal patients.
- **Paraesthesia (sensation):** May be first symptom of changes in sensory nerves to appear. Compare sensation to touch between affected and unaffected limb. Numbness, tingling, or 'pins and needles' sensations may be reported. Evaluate the areas above and below the affected area.
- **Paralysis (movement):** The ability of the patient to move the extremity distal to the injury. Paralysis of an extremity may be the result of prolonged nerve compression or irreversible muscle damage.
- **Pressure:** Comparison between affected and unaffected limb is important. Affected area may become taut and firm to the touch, with surrounding skin appearing shiny. The feeling of tightness or pressure may be present.

Source: Adapted from Hinkle, J. L., & Cheever, K. H. [2018]. *Brunner & Suddarth's textbook of medical-surgical nursing* (14th ed.). Philadelphia, PA: Wolters Kluwer; Johnston-Walker, E., & Hardcastle, J. (2011). Neurovascular assessment in the critically ill patient. *Nursing in Critical Care,* *16*(4), 170–177.

DELEGATION CONSIDERATIONS

The assessment of the patient's neurologic, musculoskeletal, and peripheral vascular systems should not be delegated to nursing assistive personnel (NAP) or unlicensed assistive personnel (UAP). Some items may be noticed while providing care and noted by the NAP or UAP. The nurse must then validate, analyze, document, communicate, and act on these findings, as appropriate. Depending on the state's nurse practice act and the organization's policies and procedures, the licensed practical/vocational nurses (LPN/LVNs) may perform some or all of the parts of assessment of the patient's neurologic, musculoskeletal, and peripheral vascular systems. The decision to delegate must be based on careful analysis of the patient's needs and circumstances, as well as the qualifications of the person to whom the task is being delegated. Refer to the Delegation Guidelines in Appendix A.

(continued)

Skill 3-10 ▶ Assessing the Neurologic, Musculoskeletal, and Peripheral Vascular Systems (continued)

EQUIPMENT

- PPE, as indicated
- Bath blanket or other drape
- Tongue depressor
- Examination gown
- Gloves
- Containers of odorous materials (e.g., coffee or chocolate), as indicated
- Miscellaneous items (e.g., pin, cotton, paper clip)
- Cotton-tipped applicators

ASSESSMENT

Complete a health history, focusing on the neurologic, musculoskeletal, and peripheral vascular systems. Identify risk factors for altered health by asking about the following:

- History of numbness, tingling, or tremors
- History of seizures
- History of headaches or dizziness
- History of trauma to the head or spine
- History of high blood pressure or stroke
- Changes in the ability to hear, see, taste, or smell
- Loss of ability to control bladder and bowel
- History of smoking
- History of chronic alcohol use
- History of diabetes mellitus or cardiovascular disease
- Use of prescription and over-the-counter medications
- Frequency of blood cholesterol tests and results
- History of trauma, arthritis, or neurologic disorder
- History of pain or swelling in the joints or muscles
- Frequency and type of usual exercise
- Dietary intake of calcium
- Changes in color or temperature of the extremities
- History of pain in the legs when sleeping or pain that worsens by walking
- History of blood clots or sores on the legs that do not heal

NURSING DIAGNOSIS

Determine the related factors for the nursing diagnoses based on the patient's current health status. Appropriate nursing diagnoses may include:

- Risk for falls
- Impaired verbal communication
- Impaired physical mobility

OUTCOME IDENTIFICATION AND PLANNING

The expected outcome to achieve in performing an examination of the neurologic, musculoskeletal, and peripheral vascular systems is that the assessments are completed without causing the patient to experience anxiety or discomfort, the findings are documented, and the appropriate referral is made to other health care professionals, as needed, for further evaluation. Other specific outcomes will be formulated, depending on the identified nursing diagnosis.

IMPLEMENTATION

ACTION	RATIONALE

1. Perform hand hygiene and put on PPE, if indicated.

Hand hygiene and PPE prevent the spread of microorganisms. PPE is required based on transmission precautions.

2. Identify the patient.

Identifying the patient ensures the right patient receives the intervention and helps prevent errors.

ACTION

3. Close the curtains around the bed and close the door to the room, if possible. Explain the purpose of the neurologic, musculoskeletal, and peripheral vascular examinations and what you are going to do. Answer any questions.

4. Help the patient undress, if needed, and provide a patient gown. Assist the patient to a supine position, if possible. Use the bath blanket to cover any exposed area other than the one being assessed.

5. Begin with a survey of the patient's overall hygiene and physical appearance.

6. Assess the patient's mental status.

   a. Evaluate level of consciousness. Refer to Chapter 17 for standardized assessment tools to assess level of consciousness.

   b. Evaluate the patient's orientation to person, place, and time.

   c. Assess memory (immediate recall and past memory).

   d. Evaluate the patient's ability to understand spoken and written word.

7. Test cranial nerve (CN) function, as indicated.

   a. Ask the patient to close the eyes, occlude one nostril, and then identify the smell of different substances, such as coffee, chocolate, or alcohol. Repeat with other nostril.

   b. Test visual acuity and pupillary constriction. Refer to previous discussion in the assessment of the head and neck.

   c. Move the patient's eyes through the six cardinal positions of gaze. Refer to previous discussion in the assessment of the head and neck.

   d. Ask the patient to smile, frown, wrinkle the forehead, and puff out cheeks (Figure 1).

RATIONALE

This ensures the patient's privacy. Explanation relieves anxiety and facilitates cooperation.

Having the patient wear a gown facilitates examination of the neurologic, musculoskeletal, and peripheral vascular systems. Use of a bath blanket provides for comfort and warmth.

This provides initial impressions of the patient. Hygiene and appearance can provide clues about the patient's mental state and comfort level.

This helps identify the patient's level of awareness.

The patient should be awake and alert. Patients with altered level of consciousness may be lethargic, stuporous, or comatose.

Memory problems may indicate neurologic impairment.

Evaluation of the patient's ability to understand spoken and written word helps assess for aphasia.

It is not necessary to assess every cranial nerve for every patient. Assessment should be individualized based on the patient's needs and health care setting and circumstances (Jensen, 2015, p. 42).

This action tests the function of CN I (olfactory nerve).

This tests function of CN II and CN III (optic and oculomotor nerves).

This testing evaluates the function of tests CN III, CN IV, and CN VI (oculomotor, trochlear, and abducens nerves).

This maneuver evaluates the motor function of CN VII (facial nerve).

FIGURE 1. Puffing out cheeks.

(*continued*)

Skill 3-10 ▶ Assessing the Neurologic, Musculoskeletal, and Peripheral Vascular Systems *(continued)*

ACTION	RATIONALE
e. Ask the patient to protrude tongue and push against the cheek with the tongue.	This evaluates function of CN XII (hypoglossal nerve).
f. Palpate the jaw muscles. Ask the patient to open and clench jaws. Stroke the patient's face with a cotton ball.	This evaluates function of CN V (trigeminal nerve).
g. Test hearing with the whispered voice test. Refer to previous discussion in the assessment of the head and neck.	This evaluates function of CN VIII (acoustic nerve).
h. Put on gloves. Ask patient to open mouth. While observing soft palate, ask patient to say "ah"; observe upward movement of the soft palate. Test the gag reflex by touching the posterior pharynx with the tongue depressor. Explain to patient that this may be uncomfortable. Ask the patient to swallow. Remove gloves.	Gloves prevent contact with blood and body fluids. An intact gag reflex and swallowing indicate normal functioning of CN IX and X (glossopharyngeal and vagus nerves).
i. Place your hands on the patient's shoulders (Figure 2) while he or she shrugs against resistance. Then place your hand on the patient's left cheek, then the right cheek, and have the patient push against it.	These actions check CN XI (spinal accessory nerve) function and trapezius and sternocleidomastoid muscle strength.
8. Check the patient's ability to move his or her neck. Ask the patient to touch his or her chin to the chest and to each shoulder, then move each ear to the corresponding shoulder (Figure 3), and then tip the head back as far as possible.	These actions assess neck ROM, which is normally smooth and controlled.

FIGURE 2. Assessing function of the spinal accessory nerve (CN XI) and muscular strength. (From Weber, J.R., & Kelley, J.H. [2014]. Health assessment in nursing [5th ed.]. Philadelphia: Wolters Kluwer Health/Lippincott Williams & Wilkins.)

FIGURE 3. Moving each ear to the corresponding shoulder. (From Jensen, S. [2011]. Nursing health assessment. P. 654; Wolters Kluwer Health | Lippincott Williams & Wilkins; Philadelphia, PA.)

ACTION	RATIONALE
9. Inspect the upper extremities. Observe for skin color, presence of lesions, rashes, and muscle mass. Palpate for skin temperature, texture, and presence of masses.	Examination of the upper extremities provides information about the circulatory, integumentary, and musculoskeletal systems.
10. Ask the patient to extend arms forward and then rapidly turn palms up and down.	This maneuver tests proprioception and cerebellar function.
11. Ask the patient to flex upper arm and to resist examiner's opposing force (Figure 4).	This technique assesses the muscle strength of the upper extremities.
12. Inspect and palpate the hands, fingers, wrists (Figure 5), and elbow joints.	Inspection and palpation provide information about abnormalities, tenderness, and ROM.

ACTION	RATIONALE

FIGURE 4. Assessing muscle strength of the upper extremities. (From Jensen, S. [2011]. Nursing health assessment. P. 658; Wolters Kluwer Health | Lippincott Williams & Wilkins; Philadelphia, PA.)

FIGURE 5. Palpating the wrist. (*Photo by B. Proud.*)

13. Ask the patient to bend and straighten the elbow, and flex and extend the wrists and hands.

Tests ROM of elbow joint and wrists.

14. Palpate the skin and the radial and brachial pulses. Assess the pulse rate, quality or amplitude, and rhythm. Test capillary refill (Refer to Box 3-2).

Pulse palpation and capillary refill evaluate the peripheral vascular status of the upper extremities.

15. Have the patient squeeze your index and middle fingers (Figure 6).

This maneuver tests the muscle strength of the hands.

16. Assist the patient to a supine position. Palpate (Figure 7A) and then use the bell of the stethoscope to auscultate the femoral pulses in the groin (Figure 7B), if not done during assessment of the abdomen. Note the strength of the pulse and grade it as with peripheral pulses.

This technique assesses flow of blood through the arteries. Auscultation can detect a bruit.

FIGURE 6. Testing grip. Patient squeezes nurse's index and middle fingers. (*Photo by B. Proud.*)

A

B

FIGURE 7. Palpating (**A**) and auscultating (**B**) the femoral pulses. (*Photos by B. Proud.*)

(*continued*)

Skill 3-10 Assessing the Neurologic, Musculoskeletal, and Peripheral Vascular Systems *(continued)*

ACTION	**RATIONALE**

17. Examine the lower extremities. Inspect the legs and feet for color, lesions, varicosities, hair growth, nail growth, edema, and muscle mass.

Inspection provides information about peripheral vascular function.

18. Assess for pitting edema in the lower extremities by pressing fingers into the skin at the pretibial area and dorsum of the foot (Figure 8A). If an indentation remains in the skin after the fingers have been lifted, pitting edema is present (Figure 8B).

This technique reveals information about excess interstitial fluid. Refer to an edema scale in assessing the amount of edema: 1+ about 2 mm deep to 4+ about 8 mm deep.

FIGURE 8. Assessing for pitting edema in lower extremities. (From Hogan-Quigley, et al. [2012]. Bates' nursing guide to physical examination and history taking. 1st Edition, P. 412; Wolters Kluwer Health | Lippincott Williams & Wilkins; Philadelphia, PA.)

19. Palpate for pulses and skin temperature at the posterior tibial, dorsalis pedis, and popliteal areas. Assess the pulse rate, quality or amplitude, and rhythm. Test capillary refill (Refer to Box 3-2).

Pulses, skin temperature, and capillary refill provide information about the patient's peripheral vascular status.

20. Ask the patient to move one leg laterally with the knee straight to test abduction of the hip. Keeping knee straight, move leg medially to test adduction of the hip. Repeat with other leg.

This maneuver assesses ROM and provides information about joint problems.

21. Ask the patient to raise the thigh against the resistance of your hand (Figure 9); next have the patient push outward against the resistance of your hand; then have the patient pull backward against the resistance of your hand. Repeat on the opposite side.

These measures assess motor strength of the upper and lower legs.

FIGURE 9. Testing motor strength of upper leg. Patient attempts to raise thigh against nurse's resistance. (*Photo by B. Proud.*)

ACTION	RATIONALE

22. Ask the patient to dorsiflex and then plantarflex both feet against opposing resistance (Figure 10).

These measure ankle flexion and dorsiflexion.

A

B

FIGURE 10. A. Testing ankle flexion and dorsiflexion. The patient first pushes the balls of the feet against resistance of the nurse's hands. **B.** Then attempts to pull against nurse's resistance. (*Photos by B. Proud.*)

23. As needed, assist the patient to a standing position. Observe the patient as he or she walks with a regular gait, on the toes, on the heels, and then heel to toe (Figure 11).

This procedure evaluates cerebellar and motor function.

24. Perform the Romberg's test; ask the patient to stand straight with feet together, both eyes closed with arms at side (Figure 12). Wait 20 seconds and observe for patient swaying and ability to maintain balance. Be alert to prevent patient fall or injury related to losing balance during this assessment.

This test checks cerebellar functioning and evaluates balance, equilibrium, and coordination. Slight swaying is normal, but patient should be able to maintain balance.

FIGURE 11. Testing heel to toe walking. (From Jensen, S. [2011]. Nursing health assessment. P. 707; Wolters Kluwer Health | Lippincott Williams & Wilkins; Philadelphia, PA.)

FIGURE 12. Positioning for the Romberg's test. (From Jensen, S. [2011]. Nursing health assessment. P. 707; Wolters Kluwer Health | Lippincott Williams & Wilkins; Philadelphia, PA.)

(*continued*)

Skill 3-10 ▶ Assessing the Neurologic, Musculoskeletal, and Peripheral Vascular Systems *(continued)*

ACTION	**RATIONALE**
25. Assist the patient to a comfortable position.	This ensures the patient's comfort.
26. Remove PPE, if used. Perform hand hygiene. Continue with assessments of specific body systems, as appropriate, or indicated. Initiate appropriate referral to other health care providers for further evaluation, as indicated.	Proper removal of PPE reduces the risk for infection transmission and contamination of other items. Hand hygiene prevents the spread of microorganisms. Additional assessments should be completed, as indicated, to evaluate the patient's health status. Intervention by other health care providers may be indicated to evaluate and treat the patient's health status.

EVALUATION

The expected outcomes have been met when the patient participates in the assessment of the neurologic, musculoskeletal, and peripheral vascular systems; the patient verbalizes understanding of the assessment techniques as appropriate; the assessment is completed without the patient experiencing anxiety or discomfort; the findings are documented; and the appropriate referrals are made to the other health care professionals as needed for further evaluation.

DOCUMENTATION

Guidelines

Document assessment techniques performed, along with specific findings. Note the cognitive responses of the patient, the tested cranial nerves, and sensation and motor responses. Document any patient statements of pain, muscle weakness, or joint abnormality. Record findings, including color, turgor, temperature, pulses, and capillary refill.

Sample Documentation

DocuCare Practice documenting assessment techniques and findings in *Lippincott DocuCare*.

> 4/4/20 Patient alert, oriented, cognitively appropriate. Full ROM of all joints. Muscles soft, firm, nontender, no atrophy. Patient states pain in right calf. Right calf skin paler tone and slightly cooler compared with left calf. Peripheral pulses 72, +2, regular rhythm, equal bilaterally; exception—right posterior tibial and dorsalis pedis pulses +1. Capillary refill right lower extremity sluggish, >3 seconds, +sensation in feet, equal bilaterally.
>
> —S. Moses, RN

SPECIAL CONSIDERATIONS

General Considerations

- Before performing the mental status examination, inform the patient that some of the questions may seem unusual, but that you are attempting to evaluate overall cognitive function.

Infant and Child Considerations

- In an infant, jerky and brief twitching of the extremities may be noted and considered a normal finding.
- The Babinski sign is typically elicited in children aged 24 months and younger (Jensen, 2015).
- The infant's extremities move symmetrically through ROM, but lack full extension.
- Motor control develops in head, neck, trunk, and extremities in sequence.
- Coordination of movement varies according to the developmental level of the young child.

Older Adult Considerations

- Be aware that short-term memory, such as recall of recent events, may diminish with age. Older adults may also experience slowed reaction time as well.
- In the older adult patient, expect to find decreased musculoskeletal function, such as loss of muscle strength.
- Slower gait, with a wider base and flexed hips and knees.
- Keep in mind that older adults may take longer to perform certain actions, such as completing activities for testing coordination.

Enhance Your Understanding

Focusing on Patient Care: Developing Clinical Reasoning

Consider the case scenarios at the beginning of the chapter as you answer the following questions to enhance your understanding and apply what you have learned.

QUESTIONS

1. When obtaining the history from Mr. Lincoln, he reports having a stuffed-up nose, postnasal drip, and a cough that sometimes produces mucus. He has smoked about one and a half packs of cigarettes a day for the past 20 years. Which areas of his physical examination would be most important?

2. Lois Felker, who has a history of type 1 diabetes mellitus, has arrived for her appointment with the health care provider. Due to this patient's diagnosis, what systems will be most important to include in the routine checkup?

3. Bobby Williams is suspected of having appendicitis. Which aspects of the physical examination are significant in relation to this diagnosis?

You can find suggested answers after the Bibliography at the end of this chapter.

Integrated Case Study Connection

The case studies in the back of the book focus on integrating concepts. Refer to the following case studies to enhance your understanding of the concepts and skills in this chapter.

- Basic Case Studies: Abigail Cantonelli, page 1099; James White, page 1102; Naomi Bell, page 1103; Joe LeRoy, page 1108; Kate Townsend, page 1109.
- Intermediate Case Studies: Olivia Greenbaum, page 1113; Victoria Holly, page 1115; Jason Brown, page 1119; Kent Clark, page 1121; Lucille Howard, page 1123; George Patel, page 1126.
- Advanced Case Studies: Cole McKean, page 1128; Damian Wallace, page 1130; Robert Espinoza, page 1132.

Taylor Suite Resources

Explore these additional resources to enhance learning for this chapter:

- NCLEX-Style Questions and other resources on thePoint®, http://thePoint.lww.com/Lynn5e
- *Skill Checklists for Taylor's Clinical Nursing Skills*, 5e
- *Taylor's Video Guide to Clinical Nursing Skills:* Physical Assessment
- *Fundamentals of Nursing:* Chapter 26, Health Assessment
- *Lippincott DocuCare* Fundamentals cases

Bibliography

American Speech-Language Hearing Association. (n.d.). *Hearing screening and testing*. Retrieved http://www.asha.org/public/hearing/Hearing-Testing

Anderson, B., Nix, E., Norman, B., & McPike, H. D. (2014). An evidence based approach to undergraduate physical assessment practicum course development. *Nurse Education in Practice, 14*(3), 242–246.

Centers for Disease Control and Prevention. (n.d. a). *BMI percentile calculator for child and teen*. Retrieved http://nccd.cdc.gov/dnpabmi/calculator.aspx

Centers for Disease Control and Prevention (CDC). (n.d. b). *Immunization schedules*. Retrieved http://www.cdc.gov/vaccines/schedules

Curro Fosbrook, S. (2015). Mental snapshots: Creating an organized plan for health assessment. *Journal of Professional Nursing, 31*(5), 416–423.

Doenges, M. E., Moorhouse, M. F., & Murr, A. C. (2016). *Nursing diagnoses manual: Planning, individualizing, and documenting client care* (5th ed.). Philadelphia, PA: F.A. Davis.

Douglas, C., Osborne, S., Reid, C., Batch, M., Hollingdrake, O., & Gardner, G.; Members of the RBWH Patient Assessment Research Council. (2014). What factors influence nurses' assessment practices? Development of the Barriers to Nurses' use of Physical Assessment Scale. *Journal of Advanced Nursing, 70*(11), 2683–2694.

Douglas, C., Windsor, C., & Lewis, P. (2015). Too much knowledge for a nurse? Use of physical assessment by final-semester nursing students. *Nursing & Health Sciences, 17*(4), 492–499.

Doyle, M., Noonan, B., & O'Connell, E. (2013). Care study: A cardiovascular physical assessment. *British Journal of Cardiac Nursing, 8*(3), 122–126.

Dudek, S. (2014). *Nutrition essentials for nursing practice* (7th ed.). Philadelphia, PA: Wolters Kluwer Health/Lippincott Williams & Wilkins.

Fawcett, T., & Rhynas, S. (2012). Taking a patient history: The role of the nurse. *Nursing Standard, 15*(26), 41–46.

Gentleman, B. (2014). Focused assessment in the care of the older adult. *Critical Care Nursing Clinics of North America, 26*(1), 15–20.

Grossman, S., & Porth, C. M. (2014). *Porth's pathophysiology: Concepts of altered health states* (9th ed.). Philadelphia, PA: Wolters Kluwer.

Henley Haugh, K. (2015). Head-to-toe: Organizing your baseline patient physical assessment. *Nursing, 45*(12), 58–61.

Hickey, J. V. (2014). *The clinical practice of neurological and neurosurgical nursing* (7th ed.). Philadelphia, PA: Wolters Kluwer Health.

Hill, K. E., Tuck, A., Ranner, S., Davies, N., & Bolieiro-Amaral, K. (2014). The use of a nursing oral and nutritional assessment tool to improve patient outcomes – one centre's experience. *Renal Society of Australasia Journal, 10*(1), 6–10.

Hinkle, J. L., & Cheever, K. H. (2018). *Brunner & Suddarth's textbook of medical-surgical nursing* (14th ed.). Philadelphia, PA: Wolters Kluwer.

Hogan-Quigley, B., Palm, M. L., & Bickley, L. (2017). *Bates' nursing guide to physical examination and history taking* (2nd ed.). Philadelphia, PA: Wolters Kluwer.

Iyer, V. N., Mandrekar, J. N., Danielson, R. D., Zubkov, A. Y., Elmer, J. L., & Wijdicks, E. F. (2009). Validity of the FOUR score coma scale in the medical intensive care unit. *Mayo Clinic Proceedings, 84*(8), 694–701.

Jalali, R., & Rezaei, M. (2014). A comparison of the Glasgow Coma Scale Score with Full Outline of Unresponsiveness Scale to predict patients' traumatic brain injury outcomes in intensive care units. *Critical Care Research and Practice, 2014*(2014), 4. Article ID 289803. DOI: 10.1155/2014/289803

Jarvis, C. (2016). *Physical examination and health assessment* (7th ed.). St. Louis, MO: Elsevier.

Jensen, S. (2015). *Nursing health assessment: A best practice approach* (2nd ed.). Philadelphia, PA: Wolters Kluwer Health.

Jensen, G. L., Compher, C., Sullivan, D. H., & Mullin, G. E. (2013). Recognizing malnutrition in adults: Definitions and characteristics, screening, assessment, and team approach. *Journal of Parenteral and Enteral Nutrition, 37*(6), 802–807.

Johnston-Walker, E., & Hardcastle, J. (2011). Neurovascular assessment in the critically ill patient. *Nursing in Critical Care, 16*(4), 170–177.

Judge, N. L. (2007). Neurovascular assessment. *Nursing Standard, 21*(45), 39–44.

Kyle, T., & Carman, S. (2017). *Essentials of pediatric nursing* (3rd ed.). Philadelphia, PA: Wolters Kluwer Health.

McGough, E. L., Logsdon, R. G., Kelly, V. E., & Teri, L. (2013). Functional mobility limitations and falls in assisted living residents with dementia: Physical performance assessment and quantitative gait analysis. *Journal of Geriatric Physical Therapy, 36*(2), 78–86.

Mercy, A. S., Thakur, R., Yaddanapudi, S., & Bhagat, H. (2013). Can FOUR Score replace GCS for assessing neurological status of critically ill patients-An Indian study. *Nursing and Midwifery Research Journal, 9*(2), 63–72.

Miller, S., Owens, L., & Silverman, E. (2015). Physical examination of the adult patient with chronic respiratory disease. *Medsurg Nursing, 24*(3), 195–198.

Moyer, V. A. (2013). Screening for peripheral artery disease and cardiovascular disease risk assessment with the ankle-brachial index in adults: U.S. Preventive Services Task Force recommendation statement. *Annals of Internal Medicine, 159*(5), 342–349.

NANDA International, Inc.: Nursing Diagnoses - Definitions and Classification 2018–2020 © 2017 NANDA International, ISBN 978-1-62623-929-6. Used by arrangement with the Thieme Group, Stuttgart/New York.

National Heart, Lung, and Blood Institute. (n.d.). *Assessing your weight and health risk.* Retrieved https://www.nhlbi.nih.gov/health/educational/lose_wt/risk.htm

National Institutes of Health, National Heart, Lung, and Blood Institute. (2000). NHLBI Obesity Education Initiative. *The practical guide: Identification, evaluation, and treatment of overweight and obesity in adults.* NIH publication no. 00–4084. October 2000. Retrieved www.nhlbi.nih.gov/guidelines/obesity/prctgd_c.pdf

National Institutes of Health (NIH), National Heart, Lung, and Blood Institute (NHLBI). (2012). *How are overweight and obesity diagnosed?* Retrieved http://www.nhlbi.nih.gov/health/health-topics/topics/obe/diagnosis.html

Okamura, K. (2014). Glasgow Coma Scale flow chart: A beginner's guide. *British Journal of Nursing, 23*(20), 1068–1073.

Osborne, S., Douglas, C., Reid, C., Jones, L., & Gardner, G. (2015). The primacy of vital signs – Acute care nurses' and midwives' use of physical assessment skills: A cross sectional study. *International Journal of Nursing Studies, 52*(5), 951–962.

Perry, S. E., Hockenberry, M. J., Lowdermilk, D. L., & Wilson, D. (2014). *Maternal child nursing care* (5th ed.). St. Louis, MO: Elsevier Mosby.

Pichora-Fuller, M. K. (2015). Cognitive decline and hearing health care for older adults. *American Journal of Audiology, 24*(2), 108–111.

Purnell, L. D. (2013). *Transcultural health care: A culturally competent approach* (4th ed.). Philadelphia, PA: F.A. Davis Company.

Roets-Merken, L. M., Zuidema, S. U., Vernooij-Dassen, M. J., & Kempen, G. I. (2014). Screening for hearing, visual and dual sensory impairment in older adults using behavioral cures: A validation study. *International Journal of Nursing Studies, 51*(11), 1434–1440.

Romanelli, L. H., Landsverk, J., Levitt, J. M., et al. (2009). Best practices for mental health in child welfare: Screening, assessment and treatment guidelines. *Child Welfare, 88*(1), 163–188.

Substance Abuse and Mental Health Services Administration (SAMHSA) and the Health Resources and Services Administration (HRSA), SAMHSA-HRSA Center for Integrated Health Solutions (CIHS). (2012). *Screening tools.* Retrieved http://www.integration.samhsa.gov/clinical-practice/screening-tools

Taylor, J. J., & Cohen, B. J. (2013). *Memmler's structure and function of the human body* (10th ed.). Philadelphia, PA: Wolters Kluwer Health.

Taylor, C., Lynn, P., & Bartlett, J. (2019). *Fundamentals of nursing: The art and science of person-centered care* (9th ed.). Philadelphia, PA: Wolters Kluwer.

Turney, J., Raley Noble, D., & Chae Kim, S. (2013). Orthopaedic nurses' knowledge and interrater reliability of neurovascular assessments with 2-point discrimination test. *Orthopaedic Nursing, 32*(3), 167–172.

VHA Center for Engineering & Occupational Safety and Health (CEOSH). (2016). *Safe patient handling and mobility guidebook.* St. Louis, MO: Author. Retrieved http://www.tampavaref.org/safe-patient-handling.htm

Yesavage, J. A. (1986). The use of self-rating depression scales in the elderly. In L. W. Poon (Ed.). *Handbook for clinical memory assessment of older adults.* Washington, DC: American Psychological Association.

SUGGESTED ANSWERS FOR FOCUSING ON PATIENT CARE: DEVELOPING CLINICAL REASONING

1. Assessment of the patient's head and neck, as well as his thorax and lungs, would be most important. Examination of his head and neck will provide additional information related to his nasal symptoms, as well as his cough. Assessment of his thorax and lungs will provide additional information related to his cough and possible effects of smoking.

2. Assessment of integumentary, neurologic, and peripheral vascular systems would be important to include when caring for a patient with diabetes. Major complications of diabetes include retinopathy, nephropathy, and neuropathy. Assessment of these systems would aid in identifying possible complications from diabetes that should be addressed.

3. Assessment of the patient's abdomen would be important to aid in confirming a diagnosis of appendicitis. In particular, you should assess for tenderness, which can indicate peritoneal irritation, such as from appendicitis.

Safety

Focusing on Patient Care

This chapter will help you develop some of the skills related to safety issues that may be necessary to care for the following patients:

Megan Lewis, an 18 month old who has an IV access in her left forearm.

Kevin Mallory, a 35-year-old professional body builder admitted with a severe closed head injury. He is intubated and is constantly reaching for his endotracheal tube.

John Frawley, a 72 year old diagnosed with Alzheimer's disease who continues to try to get out of bed after falling and breaking a hip.

Refer to Focusing on Patient Care: Developing Clinical Reasoning at the end of the chapter to apply what you learn.

Learning Objectives

After completing the chapter, you will be able to accomplish the following:

1. Perform a situational assessment.
2. Implement nursing interventions related to fall prevention.
3. Implement nursing interventions to be used as alternatives to restraints.
4. Identify guidelines for the use of physical restraints.
5. Apply an extremity restraint correctly and safely.
6. Apply a waist restraint correctly and safely.
7. Apply an elbow restraint correctly and safely.
8. Apply a mummy restraint correctly and safely.

Key Terms

restraint: any manual method, physical or mechanical device, material, or equipment that immobilizes or reduces the ability of a patient to move or access to his or her body freely; a drug or medication when it is used as a restriction to manage the patient's behavior or restrict the patient's freedom of movement and is not a standard treatment or dosage for the patient's condition (CMS, 2006, p. 71427).

safety event report: documentation that describes any occurrence that results in injury or has the potential to result in injury, to a patient, employee, or visitor; also called a variance, occurrence, or incident report.

Safety and security are basic human needs. Safety is a paramount concern that underlies all nursing care, and patient safety is a responsibility of all health care providers. It is a focus in all health care facilities as well as in the home, workplace, and community. Nursing strategies that identify potential hazards and promote wellness evolve from an awareness of factors that affect safety in the environment. Fundamentals Review 4-1 outlines patient safety risks related to developmental stage, as well as patient teaching to promote patient safety. Guidelines to promote patient safety are provided by The Joint Commission (TJC). The purpose of the National Patient Safety Goals is to improve patient safety, focusing on problems in health care safety and how to solve them. The National Patient Safety Goals are updated yearly and can be found on The Joint Commission website at: http://www.jointcommission.org/PatientSafety/NationalPatientSafetyGoals.

This chapter covers the skills nurses will need when working with patients to monitor for safety, prevent injury, and to intervene when safety issues arise. The first skill addresses the use of a general patient and environmental survey to identify immediate patient concerns, as well as safety concerns. The next two skills discuss fall prevention and utilizing alternatives to the use of restraints. The remaining skills address how to use several types of physical restraints safely and correctly. A physical restraint is any manual method, physical or mechanical device, material, or equipment that the person cannot remove easily, which immobilizes or reduces the person's freedom of movement or normal access to one's body (CMS, 2006). **Physical restraints should be considered as a last resort after other care alternatives have been unsuccessful.**

Whether or not a specific device is considered a restraint is determined by several factors:

- Intended use of a device, such as physical restriction
- Its involuntary application
- Identified patient need

For example, if a bed rail is used to facilitate a patient's mobility in and out of bed, it is not a restraint. If side rails could potentially restrict a patient's freedom to leave the bed, the rails would be a restraint. If a patient can release or remove a device, it is not a restraint.

When it is necessary to apply a restraint, the nurse should use the least restrictive method and should remove it at the earliest possible time. Consider the laws regulating the use of restraints and facility regulations and policies. Ensure compliance with ordering, assessment, and maintenance procedures. Fundamentals Review 4-2 provides general guidelines for restraint use. Always treat patients with respect and protect their dignity.

Fundamentals Review 4-1

PREVENTING ACCIDENTS AND PROMOTING SAFETY AT VARYING DEVELOPMENTAL STAGES

Developmental Stage/Safety Risks	Teaching Tip	Why Is This Important
Fetus Abnormal growth and development	• Abstain from alcohol and caffeine while pregnant. • Stop smoking or reduce the number of cigarettes smoked per day. • Avoid all drugs, including OTC drugs, unless prescribed by the health care provider. • Avoid exposure to pesticides and certain environmental chemicals. • Avoid exposure to radiation.	Any factors, chemical or physical, can adversely affect the fertilized ovum, embryo, and developing fetus. A fetus is extremely vulnerable to environmental hazards.
Neonate (first 28 days of life) Infection Falls SIDS	• Wash hands frequently. • Never leave an infant unsupervised on a raised surface without side rails. • Use the appropriate infant car seat that is secured in the backseat facing the rear of the car. • Handle the infant securely while supporting the head. • Place infant on the back to sleep.	Physical care for the newborn includes maintaining a patent airway, protecting the baby from infection and injury, and providing optimal nutrition.
Infant Falls Injuries from toys Burns Suffocation or drowning Inhalation or ingestion of foreign bodies	• Supervise the child closely to prevent injury. • Select toys appropriate for developmental level. • Use appropriate safety equipment in the home (e.g., locks for cabinets, gates, electrical outlet covers). • Never leave the child alone in the bathtub. • Childproof the entire house.	Infants progress from rolling over to sitting, crawling, and pulling up to stand. They are very curious and will explore everything in their environment that they can.
Toddler Falls Cuts from sharp objects Burns Suffocation or drowning Inhalation or ingestion of foreign bodies/ poisons	• Have poison control center phone number in readily accessible location. • Use appropriate car seat for the toddler. • Supervise the child closely to prevent injury. • Childproof the house to ensure that poisonous products, drugs, guns, and small objects are out of the toddler's reach. • Never leave the child alone and unsupervised outside. • Keep all hot items on the stove out of the child's reach.	Toddlers accomplish a wide variety of developmental tasks and progress to walking and talking. They become more independent and continue to explore their environment.
Preschooler Falls Cuts Burns Drowning Inhalation or ingestion Guns and weapons	• Teach the child to wear proper safety equipment when riding bicycles or scooters. • Ensure that playing areas are safe. • Begin to teach safety measures to the child. • Do not leave the child alone in the bathtub or near water. • Practice emergency evacuation measures. • Teach about fire safety.	Though more independent, preschoolers still have an immature understanding of dangerous behavior. They may strive to imitate adults and thus attempt dangerous behavior.

(continued)

Fundamentals Review 4-1 continued

PREVENTING ACCIDENTS AND PROMOTING SAFETY AT VARYING DEVELOPMENTAL STAGES

Developmental Stage/Safety Risks	Teaching Tip	Why Is This Important
School-aged child Burns Drowning Broken bones Concussions (TBI) Inhalation or ingestion Guns and weapons Substance abuse	• Teach accident prevention at school and home. • Teach the child to wear safety equipment when playing sports. • Reinforce teaching about symptoms that require immediate medical attention. • Continue immunizations as scheduled. • Provide drug, alcohol, and sexuality education. • Reinforce the use of seat belts and pedestrian safety.	School-aged children have developed more refined muscular coordination, but increasing involvement in sports and play activities increases their risk for injury. TBI can cause disruption in brain function and death. Cognitive maturity improves their ability to understand safety instructions.
Adolescent Motor vehicle accidents Drowning Guns and weapons Inhalation and ingestion	• Teach responsibilities of new freedoms that accompany being a teenager. • Enroll the teen in safety courses (driver education, water safety, emergency care measures). • Emphasize gun safety. • Get physical examination before participating in sports. • Make time to listen to and talk with your adolescent (helps with stress reduction). • Follow healthy lifestyle (nutrition, rest, etc.). • Teach about sexuality, sexually transmitted infections, and birth control. • Encourage the child to report any sexual harassment or abuse of any kind.	Adolescence is a critical period in growth and development. The adolescent needs increasing freedom and responsibility to prepare for adulthood. During this time, the mind has a great ability to acquire and use knowledge. The teen's peer group is a greater influence than parents during this stage.
Adult Stress Domestic violence Motor vehicle accidents Industrial accidents Drug and alcohol abuse	• Practice stress reduction techniques (e.g., meditation, exercise). • Enroll in a defensive driving course. • Evaluate the workplace for safety hazards and utilize safety equipment as prescribed. • Practice moderation when consuming alcohol. • Avoid the use of illegal drugs. • Provide options and referrals to domestic violence victims.	As people progress through the adult years, visible signs of aging become apparent. Lifestyle behaviors and situational or family crises can also impact an adult's overall health and cause stress. Preventive health practices help adults improve the quality and duration of life.
Older Adult Falls Motor vehicle accidents Elder abuse Sensorimotor changes Fires	• Identify safety hazards in the environment. • Modify the environment as necessary. • Attend defensive driving courses on courses designed for older adult drivers. • Encourage regular vision and hearing tests. • Ensure that prescribed eyeglasses and hearing aids are available and functioning. • Wear appropriate footwear. • Have operational smoke detectors in place. • Objectively document and report any signs of neglect and abuse.	Accidental injuries occur more frequently in older adults because of decreased sensory abilities, slower reflexes and reaction times, changes in hearing and vision, and loss of strength and mobility. Collaboration between family and health care providers can ensure a safe, comfortable environment and promote healthy aging.

Fundamentals Review 4-2

GENERAL GUIDELINES FOR RESTRAINT USE

- The patient has the right to be free from restraints that are not medically necessary. Restraints may be used only to protect the patient, staff, or others, and must be discontinued at the earliest possible time. Restraints *must not* be used for the convenience of staff or to punish a patient.
- The patient's family must be involved in the plan of care. They must be consulted when the decision is made to use restraints. The family must be instructed regarding the facility's restraint policy and alternatives to restraints that are available.
- Physical restraints should be considered only after assessment of the patient, environment, and the situation; interventions to relieve discomforting behaviors have been used, precipitating factors have been identified and eliminated, if possible; and consultation with other health care professionals has occurred.
- **Alternatives to restraints and less-restrictive interventions must have been implemented and failed. All alternatives used must be documented.**
- Contradictions to physical restraints should be assessed.

- The benefit gained from using a restraint must outweigh the known risks for that patient.
- The restraints must be ordered by a physician or other licensed independent practitioner who is responsible for the care of the patient. The order can never be for use on an "as needed" basis.
- Once in place, the patient must be monitored and reassessed frequently, based on facility policy and patient status. The patient's vital signs must be assessed and the medical patient must be visually observed every hour or according to facility policy.
- A physician or licensed independent practitioner must reevaluate and assess the patient every 24 hours (in the medical-surgical setting).
- Personal needs must be met. Provide fluids, nutrition, and toileting assistance every 2 hours.
- Skin integrity must be assessed and range-of-motion exercises provided every 2 hours.
- Documentation regarding why, how, where, and for how long the restraints were placed, and patient monitoring is vital.

Source: Modified from Centers for Medicare & Medicaid Services (CMS). (2006). Department of Health and Human Services. 42 CFR Part 482. Conditions of Participation: Patients' Rights. Final Rule; Said, A. A., & Kautz, D. D. (2013). Patient safety. Reducing restraint use for older adults in acute care. *Nursing, 43*(12), 59–61; and Springer, G. (2015). When and how to use restraints. *American Nurse Today, 10*(1), 26–27.

Skill 4-1 ▸ Performing a Situational Assessment

Awareness of the patient's environment and of the patient's situation is an integral part of nursing care. Situational awareness involves knowing and understanding what's happening around you (ESRI, 2008). Situational awareness in nursing includes routine use of a general survey (observation) of the patient, family, and environment, using input from all senses (Cohen, 2013). These observations contribute to an understanding of the current situation and support anticipation of potential problems. Identifying and solving problems is essential to effective and safe nursing practice (Caputi, 2013, p. 4). Integration of situational awareness as part of routine nursing care allows nurses to anticipate patients' needs "by knowing what is going on, why it's happening and what's likely to happen next" (Cohen, 2013, p. 64). Situational awareness promotes a safer patient care environment, reduces risk for falls, and helps the nurse develop care priorities, acting correctly when things go as planned and reacting appropriately when they don't (Cohen, 2013, p. 64; Godlock, Christiansen & Feider, 2016; Struth, 2009).

DELEGATION CONSIDERATIONS

A situational assessment should not be delegated to nursing assistive personnel (NAP) or unlicensed assistive personnel (UAP). However, the NAP or UAP may notice some items while providing care. The nurse must then validate, analyze, document, communicate, and act on these findings, as appropriate. Depending on the state's nurse practice act and the organization's policies and procedures, the licensed practical/vocational nurses (LPN/LVNs) may perform some or all of the parts of a situational assessment. The decision to delegate must be based on careful analysis of the patient's needs and circumstances, as well as the qualifications of the person to whom the task is being delegated. Refer to the Delegation Guidelines in Appendix A.

(continued)

Skill 4-1 ▶ Performing a Situational Assessment *(continued)*

EQUIPMENT	• PPE, as indicated

ASSESSMENT	A situational assessment is completed during every encounter with the patient and periodically at planned intervals throughout the day. Observations should be modified based on the specific patient care setting (e.g., long-term care, school, home health, etc. [NCSBN, n.d.])

NURSING DIAGNOSIS	Determine the related factors for nursing diagnoses based on the patient's current status. Appropriate nursing diagnoses may include: • Risk for falls • Risk for injury • Impaired physical mobility

OUTCOME IDENTIFICATION AND PLANNING	The expected outcome to achieve is that a situational assessment is completed; the patient's needs are met; and the patient remains free from injury.

IMPLEMENTATION

ACTION	**RATIONALE**
1. Perform hand hygiene and put on PPE, if indicated.	Hand hygiene and PPE prevent the spread of microorganisms. PPE is required based on transmission precautions.
2. Identify the patient. Explain the purpose of the assessment to the patient.	Identifying the patient ensures the right patient receives the intervention and helps prevent errors. Explanation helps reduce anxiety and promotes compliance and understanding.
3. Assess for data that suggest a problem with the patient's airway, breathing, or circulation. If a problem is present, identify if it is urgent or nonurgent in nature. Refer to Chapter 3 for specific related assessments.	Problems with the patient's airway, breathing, or circulation may signal a situation requiring immediate action. It is important to determine the importance of information, act on that which is important and disregard that which is not (Caputi, 2015).
4. Assess the patient's level of consciousness, orientation, and speech. Observe the patient's behavior and affect. Refer to Chapter 3 for specific related assessments.	Problems with the patient's level of consciousness, orientation, speech, behavior, or affect may signal a situation requiring immediate action. It is important to determine the importance of information, act on that which is important and disregard that which is not (Caputi, 2015).

FIGURE 1. Observing the patient's behavior and affect. (Photo by Rick Brady. From Eliopoulos, C. [2013]. *Gerontological Nursing* [8th ed.]. Philadelphia: Wolters Kluwer.)

5. Assess the patency of an oxygen delivery device, if in use. Refer to Chapter 14 for specific related assessments.	Properly functioning equipment is required to maintain delivery of oxygen.
6. Survey the patient's environment. Assess the bed position and call bell location. Bed should be in the lowest positon and the call bell (based on specific patient care setting) should be within the patient's reach.	Environmental survey identifies problems that may harm the patient (Cohen, 2013).

ACTION	RATIONALE
7. Assess for clutter and hazards. Remove excess equipment, supplies, furniture, and other objects from rooms and walkways. Pay particular attention to high traffic areas and the route to the bathroom.	All are possible hazards and could cause the patient to fall.
8. Note the presence and location of appropriate emergency equipment, based on individual patient situation.	Emergency equipment must be immediately available if needed.
9. Note the presence and location of appropriate assistive devices and mobility aids, based on individual patient situation. Ensure any devices are within the patient's reach.	Assistive devices should be available for patient use.
10. Assess for the presence of an intravenous access and/or infusion. Assess patency of the device and the insertion site. If an infusion is present, assess the solution and rate. Refer to Chapter 15 for specific related assessments.	Assessment allows for identification of problems and ensures administration of intravenous fluids as prescribed.
11. Assess for the presence of any tubes, such as gastric tubes, chest tubes, surgical drains, or urinary catheters. Assess patency of device and insertion site. Refer to Chapters 8 and 11 to 14 for specific related assessments.	Assessment allows for identification of problems and ensures patency of devices.
12. Provide a bedside commode and/or urinal/bedpan, if appropriate. Ensure that it is near the bed at all times.	This prevents falls related to incontinence or trying to get to the bathroom.
13. Ensure that the bedside table, telephone, and other personal items are within the patient's reach at all times.	This prevents the patient from having to overreach for a device or items, and/or possibly attempt ambulation or transfer unassisted.
14. Consider what further assessments should be completed and additional interventions that may be indicated. Identify problems that need to be reported and whom to contact.	Early detection of problems allows for corresponding interventions to prevent adverse occurrences, supporting improved patient outcomes (Caputi, 2013).
15. Remove PPE, if used. Perform hand hygiene.	Proper removal of PPE reduces the risk for infection transmission and contamination of other items. Hand hygiene prevents transmission of microorganisms.

EVALUATION

The expected outcomes have been met when a situational assessment has been completed; the patient's needs are met; and the patient remains free from injury.

DOCUMENTATION

Guidelines

Document significant assessment findings as directed by facility policy and protocol. Include associated interventions and/or related communication.

SPECIAL CONSIDERATIONS

Home Care Considerations

- Examine the home for objects on the floor, the presence of wires or cords, objects on the steps, and loose or torn carpet. Encourage residents to keep walkways, floors, and stairs clear.
- Assess for adequate lighting, especially at the top and bottom of stairs and pathways from the bedroom to bathroom.
- Assess for the presence of working smoke detectors on every floor of the home, if not in every room. Provide education regarding safe use as appropriate.
- Assess for the presence of firearms in the home. Provide education regarding safe storage as appropriate.
- Assess for the presence of space heaters. Provide education regarding safe use as appropriate.
- If there are children in the home, evaluate the method used to store medications, cleaning products, insecticides, and corrosives. Provide education regarding safe storage as appropriate.

Skill 4-2 ▶ Fall Prevention

Falls are the primary cause of unintentional injuries throughout life, with older adults and children being at highest risk (Robinovitch, Scott, & Feldman, 2014). Fall-related injuries are often serious and are associated with disability, loss of independence, nursing home placement, and death (Aging & Technology Research Center, 2013; NIH, 2013). Falls are caused by and associated with multiple factors. Primary causes of falls include:

- Change in balance or gait disturbance
- Muscle weakness
- Dizziness, syncope, and vertigo
- Cardiovascular changes, such as postural hypotension
- Change in vision or vision impairment
- Physical environment/environmental hazards
- Acute illness
- Neurologic disease, such as dementia or depression
- Language disorders that impair communication
- Polypharmacy

Many of these causes are within the realm of nursing responsibility. Identifying at-risk patients is crucial to planning appropriate interventions to prevent a fall. The combination of an assessment tool with an individualized care/intervention plan sets the stage for best practice (AGS, 2012b; AGS & BGS, 2010; Cox et al., 2015; Quigley, 2015b). A team approach utilizing an interdisciplinary, multifactorial approach to assessment, intervention, and evaluation leads to maximum prevention (Quigley, 2015b; Stubbs et al., 2015; Tomita et al., 2014). Table 4-1 identifies examples of fall

Table 4-1 Recommended Fall Prevention Strategies by Fall Risk Level

LOW FALL RISK	MODERATE FALL RISK	HIGH FALL RISK
Fall Risk Score: 0–5 Points	*Fall Risk Score: 6–10 Points* Color Code: Yellow	*Fall Risk Score: >10 Points* Color Code: Red
Maintain safe unit environment, including: • Remove excess equipment/supplies/furniture from rooms and hallways. • Coil and secure excess electrical and telephone wires. • Clean all spills in patient room or in hallway immediately. Place signage to indicate wet floor danger. • Restrict window openings. The following are examples of basic safety interventions: • Orient patient to surroundings, including bathroom location, use of bed, and location of call bell. • Keep bed in lowest position during use unless impractical (as in ICU nursing or specialty beds). • Keep top two side rails up (excludes box beds). In ICU, keep all side rails up. • Secure locks on beds, stretchers, and wheelchairs. • Keep floors clutter/obstacle free (with attention to path between bed and bathroom/commode). • Place call bell and frequently needed objects within patient reach. Answer call bell promptly. • Encourage patients/families to call for assistance when needed. • Display special instructions for vision and hearing. • Ensure adequate lighting, especially at night. • Use properly fitting nonskid footwear.	• Institute flagging system: yellow card outside room and yellow sticker on medical record. Hill ROM flag (if available), assignment board/electronic board. In addition to measures listed under low fall risk: • Monitor and assist patient in following daily schedules. • Supervise and/or assist bedside sitting, personal hygiene, and toileting, as appropriate. • Reorient confused patients, as necessary. • Establish elimination schedule, including use of bedside commode, if appropriate. • PT (physical therapy) consult if patient has a history of fall and/or mobility impairment. Evaluate need for: • OT (occupational therapy) consult • Slip-resistant chair mat (do *not* use in shower chair) • Use of seat belt, when in wheelchair	• Institute flagging system: red card outside room and red sticker on medical record, assignment board/electronic board: nurse call system flag, if available. In addition to measures listed under moderate and low fall risk: • Remain with patient while toileting. • Observe every 60 minutes unless patient is on activated bed/chair alarm. • If patient requires an air overlay, remove mattress (unless contraindicated by overlay type) or use side rail protectors. • When necessary, transport throughout hospital with assistance of staff or trained caregivers. Consider alternatives, for example, bedside procedure. Notify receiving area of high fall risk. Evaluate need for the following, starting with less restrictive to more restrictive measures in the listed order: • Moving patient to room with best visual access to nursing station • Bed/chair alarm • Specialty fall prevention bed • 24-hour supervision/sitter • Physical restraint/enclosed bed (only if less-restrictive alternatives have been considered and found to be ineffective)

Source: Recommended fall prevention strategies by fall risk level. Reprinted with permission. ©2003, The Johns Hopkins Hospital.

prevention strategies based on fall risk assessment. Fall risk assessment is discussed in the following assessment section. Providing patient education and a safer patient environment can reduce the incidence and severity of falls. The ultimate goal is to reduce the physical and psychological trauma experienced by patients and their significant others.

DELEGATION CONSIDERATIONS

After assessment of fall risk by the RN, activities related to the prevention of falls may be delegated to nursing assistive personnel (NAP) or unlicensed assistive personnel (UAP), as well as to licensed practical/vocational nurses (LPN/LVNs). The decision to delegate must be based on careful analysis of the patient's needs and circumstances, as well as the qualifications of the person to whom the task is being delegated. Refer to the Delegation Guidelines in Appendix A.

EQUIPMENT

- Fall risk assessment tool, if available
- PPE, as indicated
- Additional intervention tools, as appropriate (refer to sample intervention equipment in this skill)

ASSESSMENT

At a minimum, fall risk assessment needs to occur on admission to the facility, during an initial home visit, following a change in the patient's condition, after a fall, and when the patient is transferred. If it is determined that the patient is at risk for falling, regular assessment must continue. Assess the patient and the medical record for factors that increase the patient's risk for falling. Assess for a history of a fall or falls. Once a person falls one time, the chance of falling again increases dramatically regardless of whether the patient is in a hospital, a long-term care facility, or the community (Ayoung-Chee, 2014, as cited in *Severity of Injuries, 2014*). The use of an objective, systematic fall assessment is made easier by the use of a fall assessment tool. The Johns Hopkins Fall Risk Assessment Tool (Figure 1) is an example of a fall assessment tool. The Hendrich II Fall

Fall risk factor category* (NA If comatose, complete paralysis, or completely immobilized)	Points
Age • 70–79 y (2 points) • ≥80 y (3 points)	
Fall history • Fall within 3 months before admission (5 points) • Fall during this hospitalization (11 points)	
Mobility • Ambulates or transfers with unsteady gait and **NO** assistance or assistive devices (2 points) • Ambulates or transfers with assistance or assistive device (2 points) • Visual or auditory impairment affecting mobility (4 points)	
Elimination • Urgency/nocturia (2 points) • Incontinence (5 points)	
Mental status changes • Affecting awareness of environment (2 points) • Affecting awareness of one's physical limitations (4 points)	

Medications: One present (3 points); 2 or more present; or sedated procedure within the past 24 h (5 points)
   Psychotropics (antidepressants, hypnotics, antipsychotics, sedatives, benzodiazepines, some antiemetics)
   Anticonvulsants
   Diuretics/cathartics
   PCS/narcotics/opiates
   Antihypertensives	

Patient care equipment: One present (1 point); ≥ 2 present (2 points) (IV, chest tube, indwelling catheter, SCDs, etc)	
Total points	

*Moderate risk = 6–10 Total points, High risk > 10 Total points

FIGURE 1. Johns Hopkins Fall Risk Assessment Tool. (Reprinted with permission. ©2003, The Johns Hopkins Hospital.)

(continued)

Skill 4-2 ▶ Fall Prevention *(continued)*

Risk Model, another tool to evaluate fall risk factors, can be viewed on thePoint˚. Assess for a history of falls. If the patient has experienced a previous fall, assess the circumstances surrounding the fall and any associated symptoms. Review the patient's medication history and medication record for medications that may increase the risk for falls. Assess for the following additional risk factors for falls (AGS & BGS, 2010; Sitzer, 2016):

- Lower extremity muscle weakness
- Gait or balance deficit
- Mobility impairment
- Restraint use
- Use of an assistive device
- Presence of intravenous therapy
- Impaired activities of daily living (ADLs)
- Age older than 75 years
- Altered elimination
- History of falls
- Administration of high-risk drugs, such as narcotic analgesics, antiepileptics, benzodiazepines, and drugs with anticholinergic effects
- Use of four or more medications
- Depression
- Visual deficit
- Arthritis
- History of cerebrovascular accident
- Cognitive impairment
- Secondary diagnosis/chronic disease

NURSING DIAGNOSIS	Determine the related factors for nursing diagnoses based on the patient's current status. Appropriate nursing diagnoses may include: - Risk for falls - Risk for injury - Impaired physical mobility
OUTCOME IDENTIFICATION AND PLANNING	The expected outcome to achieve is that the patient does not experience a fall and remains free of injury. Other outcomes that may be appropriate include the following: the patient's environment is free from hazards; patient and/or caregiver demonstrates an understanding of appropriate interventions to prevent falls; the patient uses assistive devices correctly; the patient uses safe transfer procedures; and appropriate precautions are implemented related to the use of medications that increase the risk for falls.

IMPLEMENTATION

ACTION	**RATIONALE**
1. Perform hand hygiene and put on PPE, if indicated.	Hand hygiene and PPE prevent the spread of microorganisms. PPE is required based on transmission precautions.
2. Identify the patient. Assess fall risk as outlined above.	Identifying the patient ensures the right patient receives the intervention and helps prevent errors. Fall risk assessment aids in providing appropriate fall prevention interventions for the individual patient.

ACTION

3. Review the results of the fall risk assessment and fall risk factors with the patient and family (Figure 2).

4. Explain the rationale for fall prevention interventions to the patient and family/significant others.

5. Include the patient's family and/or significant others in the plan of care.

6. Provide time for the patient and family to discuss concerns about falling, identify fall risk factors not identified by the risk assessment, confirm their understanding of risk factors and interventions, and to verbalize concerns or questions (Quigley, 2015).

7. Provide adequate lighting. Use a night light during sleeping hours.

8. Remove excess equipment, supplies, furniture, and other objects from rooms and walkways. Pay particular attention to high traffic areas and the route to the bathroom.

9. Orient patient and significant others to new surroundings, including use of the telephone, call bell, patient bed, and room illumination. Indicate the location of the patient's bathroom.

10. Provide a "low bed" to replace regular hospital bed (Figure 3).

RATIONALE

Promotes patient and family engagement, compliance, and understanding.

Explanation helps reduce anxiety and promotes compliance and understanding.

Promotes engagement, continuity of care, understanding, and cooperation.

Promotes engagement, continuity of care, understanding, and cooperation. Active involvement on the part of patients and family members is an important part of identification of fall risk and fall prevention (Sitzer, 2016).

Good lighting reduces accidental tripping over and bumping into objects that may not be seen. Night light provides illumination in an unfamiliar environment.

All are possible hazards.

Knowledge of proper use of equipment relieves anxiety and promotes compliance.

The use of low beds is associated with decreased serious fall-related injuries (Barker et al., 2013). To be considered a "low hospital bed" the frame of the bed must be lower so that the height of the mattress deck off the floor is between 6.5 in and 10.5 in. This low height, as determined by the FDA, reduces the risk of fall-related injuries from bed.

FIGURE 2. Reviewing the results of the fall risk assessment and fall risk factors with the patient. (From Eliopoulos, C. [2014]. Gerontological Nursing [8th ed.]; page 105. Philadelphia, PA: Wolters Kluwer.)

FIGURE 3. Low bed with floor mats. (Reprinted with permission from CHG Hospital Beds, London, ON.)

11. Use floor mats if patient is at risk for serious injury (Figure 3).

Floor mats cushion falls and may prevent serious injury in patients at risk, such as those with osteoporosis (Gray-Micelli, 2012).

(continued)

Skill 4-2 ▸ Fall Prevention *(continued)*

ACTION	RATIONALE
12. Provide nonskid footwear and/or walking shoes (Figure 4).	Nonskid footwear prevents slipping and walking shoes improve balance when ambulating or transferring.

FIGURE 4. Providing nonskid footwear.

ACTION	RATIONALE
13. Institute a toileting regimen and/or continence program, if appropriate.	Toileting on a regular basis decreases risk for falls.
14. Provide a bedside commode and/or urinal/bedpan, if appropriate. Ensure that it is near the bed at all times, if appropriate for individual patient.	This prevents falls related to incontinence or trying to get to the bathroom. It may be necessary to move the bedside commode out of sight to discourage attempts at independent transfer by patients with altered mobility, as appropriate.
15. Ensure that the call bell, bedside table, telephone, and other personal items are within the patient's reach at all times.	This prevents the patient from having to overreach for a device or items, and/or possibly attempt ambulation or transfer unassisted.
16. Confer with primary care provider regarding and encourage appropriate exercise and physical therapy (Figure 5).	Exercise programs, such as muscle strengthening, balance training, and walking plans, decrease falls and fall-related injuries (AGS & BGS, 2010).

FIGURE 5. Encouraging appropriate exercise. (From Hinkle JL and Cheever KH. [2018] *Brunner & Suddarth's Textbook of Medical-Surgical Nursing [14th edition]*. Philadelphia, PA: Wolters Kluwer Health | Lippincott Williams & Wilkins.)

ACTION	**RATIONALE**
17. Confer with primary care provider regarding appropriate mobility aids, such as a cane or walker.	Mobility aids can help improve balance and steady the patient's gait.
18. Confer with primary care provider regarding the use of bone-strengthening medications, such as calcium, vitamin D, and drugs to prevent/treat osteoporosis.	Bone strengthening has been suggested to reduce fracture rates with falls (AGS & BGS, 2010).
19. Encourage the patient to rise or change position slowly and sit for several minutes before standing.	Gradual position changes reduce the risk of falls related to orthostatic hypotension.
20. Evaluate the appropriateness of elastic stockings for lower extremities.	Elastic stockings minimize venous pooling and promote venous return.
21. Review medications for potential hazards.	Certain medications and combinations of medications have been associated with increased risk for falls.
22. Keep the bed in the lowest position. If elevated to provide care (to reduce caregiver strain), ensure that it is lowered when care is completed.	Keeping bed in lowest position reduces the risk of a fall-related injury.
23. Make sure locks on the bed or wheelchair are secured at all times (Figure 6).	Locking prevents the bed or wheelchair from moving out from under the patient.
24. Use bed rails according to facility policy, when appropriate, based on individual patient assessment (Figure 7).	Inappropriate bed-rail use has been associated with patient injury and increased fall risk (Haugh et al., 2014; Keeling, 2013). Side rails may be considered a restraint when used to prevent an ambulatory patient from getting out of bed.

FIGURE 6. Engaging bed locks.

FIGURE 7. Raising side rails on bed at the patient's request.

25. Anticipate patient needs and provide assistance with activities instead of waiting for the patient to ask.	Patients whose needs are met sustain fewer falls.
26. Consider the use of an electronic personal alarm or pressure sensor alarm for the bed or chair (Figure 8).	The alarm helps alert staff to unassisted changes in position by the patient.

FIGURE 8. Patient wearing a personal alarm device.

(continued)

Skill 4-2 ▶ Fall Prevention *(continued)*

ACTION	**RATIONALE**
27. Discuss the possibility of appropriate family member(s) staying with patient.	The presence of a family member provides familiarity and companionship.
28. Consider the use of patient attendant or sitter.	Attendant or sitter can provide companionship and supervision.
29. Increase the frequency of patient observation and surveillance. Utilize 1- or 2-hour nursing rounds, including pain assessment, toileting assistance, patient comfort, making sure personal items are in reach, and meeting patient needs.	Patient care rounds/nursing rounds anticipate and proactively address patient needs (Hicks, 2015; Reimer & Herbener, 2014). Patient care rounds can reduce patient falls (Brosey & March, 2015; Goldsack et al., 2015; Hicks, 2015).
30. Remove PPE, if used. Perform hand hygiene.	Proper removal of PPE reduces the risk for infection transmission and contamination of other items. Hand hygiene prevents transmission of microorganisms.

EVALUATION

The expected outcomes have been met when the patient does not experience a fall and remains uninjured; interventions to minimize risk factors that might precipitate a fall have been implemented; patient's environment is free from hazards; patient and/or caregiver demonstrates an understanding of appropriate interventions to prevent falls; the patient uses assistive devices correctly; the patient uses safe transfer procedures; and appropriate precautions are implemented related to the use of medications that increase the risk for falls.

DOCUMENTATION

Guidelines

Document patient fall risk assessment. Include appropriate interventions to reduce fall risk in nursing care plan. Document patient and family teaching relative to fall risk reduction. Document interventions included in care.

Sample Documentation

> <u>11/1/20</u> 1730 Patient admitted to room 650W; oriented to room. Fall assessment low risk (five patients). Basic safety interventions in place per facility Fall Prevention Guidelines. Will continue to monitor and reevaluate.
>
> —B. Clapp, RN

UNEXPECTED SITUATIONS AND ASSOCIATED INTERVENTIONS

- *Patient experiences a fall:* Immediately assess the patient's condition. Provide care and interventions appropriate for status/injuries. Notify the patient's primary caregiver of the incident and your assessment of the patient. Ensure prompt follow-through for any orders for diagnostic tests, such as x-rays or CT scans, as ordered. Evaluate circumstances of the fall and the patient's environment and institute appropriate measures to prevent further incidents. Document incident, assessments, and interventions in the patient's medical record. Complete a safety event report per facility policy.

SPECIAL CONSIDERATIONS

General Considerations

- For each fall risk factor, identify specific interventions that relate directly to the risk. Some factors can be modified; others require the patient and family or caregiver to compensate (Quigley, 2015).
- If a "low bed" is used, patients who are weak may have trouble getting out of bed safely. Low beds should be raised to the appropriate height for each patient to allow safe transition out of bed (Hester, 2015).
- Empower patients to become active participants in fall prevention. Provide health care interventions that are patient centered to enable patients to be a partner in fall prevention (Sitzer, 2016; Tzeng & Yin, 2015).
- Implement and use injury-prevention strategies and devices to prevent and reduce injuries from falls.
  - Floor matting and compliant flooring provide a cushioned surface that reduces impact, decreasing the likelihood of injury if the patient falls (Hester, 2015).

- Hip protectors reduce impact from falls that could cause hip fracture (Hester, 2015; Santesso et al., 2014).
- Helmets and protective caps protect the head from impact during a fall and are particularly useful and effective in patients at risk for head bleeding secondary to anticoagulants, have liver disease, have elevated coagulation studies or have decreased platelet counts (Hester, 2015).

Infant and Child Considerations

- Many pediatric falls occur in children scoring low on risk assessment scales and may result from a momentary convergence of events, limiting the effectiveness of risk prediction tools (Ryan-Wenger & Dufek, 2013). All hospitalized children may be at risk for falling, reinforcing the need for increased emphasis on fall prevention, and minimization of fall-related injuries (Ryan-Wenger & Dufek, 2013).

Older Adult Considerations

- Encourage older adults to avoid wearing bifocal or multifocal glasses when walking, especially on stairs (NIH, 2013).
- Exercise improves balance and strengthens muscles in older adults (NIH, 2013).
- Exercise programs should be encouraged for older adults. Exercise significantly decreases falls in older adults (Grabiner, 2014; Stubbs et al., 2015).

Home Care Considerations

- Patients are at risk for falls in their home. Assess for risk factors in the home and assess the home environment. Include patient teaching regarding falls as part of the nursing care plan. See Box 4-1 for possible interventions for the home setting.

Box 4-1 | Patient Education for Preventing Falls in the Home

- Talk with your doctor about a plan for an exercise program. Regular exercise helps maintain strength and flexibility, and can help slow bone loss.
- Have regular hearing and vision testing. Always wear glasses and hearing aids, if prescribed. Even small changes in sight and hearing can affect stability.
- Wear low-heeled, rubber-soled shoes. Avoid wearing only socks or shoes with smooth soles.
- Have hand rails on both sides of stairs and make use of them when using the stairs. Try not to carry things when using the steps. When necessary, hold item in one hand and use the hand rail with the other hand.
- Avoid using chairs and tables as ladders to reach items that are too high to reach.
- Keep electrical and telephone cords against the wall and out of walkways.
- Consider rails next to the toilet and in the shower or tub and raised toilet seats.
- Know the possible side effects of medications used. Some can affect coordination and balance.

- Use a cane, walking stick, or walker to help improve stability.
- Keep home temperature at a moderate level. Temperatures too hot or too cold can contribute to dizziness.
- Stand up slowly after eating, lying down, or resting. Standing too quickly can cause fainting or dizziness.
- Make sure there is good lighting, particularly at the stairs.
- Use a night light.
- Remove clutter from walkways inside and outside the house.
- Carpets should be fixed firmly to the floor to prevent slipping. Use no-slip strips on uncarpeted surfaces.
- Use nonskid mats, strips, or carpet on surfaces that get wet.
- Check all medications, including prescriptions, and over-the-counter drugs, herbs, and vitamins, with your health care provider and/or pharmacist to find out if any put you at risk for falling.

Source: Adapted from American Geriatrics Society (AGS). (2012a). Tips for preventing serious falls. Retrieved http://www.healthinaging.org/files/documents/tipsheets/falls_prevention.pdf; American Geriatrics Society (AGS). (2012b). Aging & health A to Z. Retrieved http://www.healthinaging.org/aging-and-health-a-to-z/topic:falls; National Institute on Aging. (2016). Age page: Falls and fractures. Retrieved https://www.nia.nih.gov/health/publication/falls-and-fractures; and Stubbs, B., Brefka, S., & Denkinger, M. D. (2015). What works to prevent falls in community-dwelling older adults? Umbrella review of meta-analyses of randomized controlled trials. *Physical Therapy*, *95*(8), 1095–1110.

EVIDENCE FOR PRACTICE ▶

HOURLY PATIENT ROUNDS
Many factors increase a patient's risk for falling, including cognitive impairments, impaired ability to perform activities ADLs, and impaired elimination. Can nursing interventions that focus on proactive, protective strategies, and patient comfort reduce the risk for falls?

(continued)

Skill 4-2 ▶ Fall Prevention *(continued)*

Related Research

Hicks, D. (2015). Can rounding reduce patient falls in acute care? An integrative literature review. *MEDSURG Nursing, 24*(1), 51–55.

This integrative research review analyzed evidence related to nursing rounds and patient falls in acute care settings. Fourteen studies of the use of rounding as a tool in fall prevention were reviewed. Rounding interventions varied in timing of rounds, type of person performing the rounds, and the use of a prepared script or plan. Interventions included in rounding also varied and included interventions related to pain, personal needs, repositioning, toileting, comfort, and environmental checks. Limitations of the studies included nonrandomized sampling, small sample size, and brief implementation times. The authors suggest hourly rounding is an autonomous intervention that aids in proactive meeting of patient needs and has the potential to decrease patient falls, resulting in improved patient outcomes and reduced costs associated with falls in acute care. The authors noted it is important for the nursing staff to be convinced of the benefits of interventions in order for hourly rounding to be successful.

Relevance for Nursing Practice

Nursing rounds are a simple, easy-to-implement intervention. A protocol that incorporates hourly or once every 2-hour rounds can reduce the frequency of patients' call bell use, increase patient satisfaction with nursing care, and reduce falls, leading to more effective patient-care management, improved patient satisfaction, and improved safety.

Refer to thePoint® for additional research on related nursing topics.

EVIDENCE FOR PRACTICE ▶

ENGAGING PATIENTS IN FALL RISK ASSESSMENT

Providing patient education and a safer patient environment can reduce the incidence and severity of falls (Quigley, 2015; Stubbs et al., 2015; Tomita et al., 2014). How can nurses engage patients and their families in this assessment and intervention process? Can computer-based program applications provide a means for fall risk assessment and fall prevention education?

Related Research

Sitzer, V. (2016). Development of an automated self-assessment of fall-risk questionnaire for hospitalized patients. *Journal of Nursing Care Quality, 31*(1), 46–53.

This study examined the use of a computer-based questionnaire to engage patients in determining their risk for falling. The computer system included hospital information and services, health education videos, entertainment, and feedback modalities, as well as the fall-risk self-assessment and fall prevention education. The questionnaire asked patients if they possessed characteristics known to be associated with falling. Information was provided to patients after completion about additional resources to prevent a fall, such as a fall prevention video. Completion of the SAFR did not replace the assessment of fall risk by nurses. The questionnaire was administered to all patients admitted to a room with a television-enabled computer system. Patient responses were compared with nursing fall risk assessment scores using the Schmid fall risk assessment tool. The questionnaire was found to be a reliable and valid means for patients and nurses to assess risk of falls. The authors concluded that the use of this tool provides patients with a role in fall prevention. Engaging patients in the fall risk assessment process can provide for a more meaningful discussion with patients about risk factors for falling, fall prevention strategies, and the important role patients have in fall prevention.

Relevance for Nursing Practice

Nurses usually determine the fall risk for patients based on knowledge and assessment of fall risk factors. Nurses have a key role to play in engaging patients in their health care. The use of a computer-based questionnaire is one method that can be used to provide patients with information related to fall risk and can facilitate communication between health care providers and patients about fall risk and fall prevention.

Refer to thePoint® for additional research on related nursing topics.

Skill 4-3 ▶ Implementing Alternatives to the Use of Restraints

Restraint-free care is the standard of practice and an indicator of quality care in all health care settings (Touhy & Jett, 2014, p. 210). Physical restraints do not prevent falls, and they increase the possibility of serious injury due to a fall. Restraint use in older adults is associated with falls and injurious falls, pressure injuries, and other adverse outcomes (Bolz et al., 2013). Additional negative outcomes of restraint use include skin breakdown and contractures, incontinence, depression, delirium, anxiety, aspiration and respiratory difficulties, and even death (Taylor et al., 2019). Nurses should identify patients at risk for unsafe behaviors and restraints as early as possible, when interventions are most likely to be successful in preventing problem behaviors (Lach, Leach, & Butcher, 2016). The American Nurses Association (ANA, 2012) has approved a position statement defining the nurses' role in reducing restraint use in health care. Their recommendations are included in Box 4-2. Restraints should be used only after less-restrictive methods have failed. The following skill outlines possible alternatives to restraint use.

Box 4-2 ANA Board of Directors Position Statement: Reduction of Patient Restraint and Seclusion in Health Care Settings

Recommendations: To ensure safe, quality care for all patients in the least restrictive environment, ANA supports nursing efforts to:

1. Educate nurses, nursing students, unlicensed personnel, other members of the interdisciplinary team, and family caregivers on the appropriate use of restraint and seclusion, and on the alternatives to these restrictive interventions;
2. Ensure sufficient nursing staff to monitor and individualize care with the goal of only using restraint when no other viable option is available;
3. Ensure policies and environment support services are in place to provide feasible alternatives to physical and chemical restraints;
4. Move progressively toward a restraint-free environment while providing a therapeutic sanctuary for all;
5. Enforce documentation requirements and education about what should be documented;
6. Explore the ethical implications of restraining patients with nursing students and discuss the need for institutional policy that clarifies when, where, and how patients are to be restrained and monitored while restrained;
7. Be aware of all implications of allowing the application of restraints in health care settings. The nurse administrator should make consultation available to nurses, including ethical consultation about decisions to restrain; and
8. Develop clear policies based on accepted national standards to guide decision making regarding restraints.

DELEGATION CONSIDERATIONS

After assessment by the RN, activities related to the use of alternatives to restraints may be delegated to nursing assistive personnel (NAP) or unlicensed assistive personnel (UAP), as well as to licensed practical/vocational nurses (LPN/LVNs). The decision to delegate must be based on careful analysis of the patient's needs and circumstances, as well as the qualifications of the person to whom the task is being delegated. Refer to the Delegation Guidelines in Appendix A.

EQUIPMENT

- PPE, as indicated
- Additional intervention tools, as appropriate (refer to sample intervention equipment in this skill)

ASSESSMENT

Assess the patient's status. Determine whether the patient's pattern of behavior (wandering, fall risk, interfering with medical devices, resistive to care, danger to self or others) increases the potential need for restraint use. Assess to determine the meaning of the behavior and its cause. Assess for pain. Assess respiratory status, vital signs, blood glucose level, fluid and electrolyte issues, and medications. Assess the patient's functional, mental, and psychological status. Evaluate the patient's environment, including noise level, lighting, floor surfaces, design/suitability of equipment and furniture, visual cues, barriers to mobility, space for privacy, and clothing. Assess and evaluate the effectiveness of restraint alternatives.

NURSING DIAGNOSIS

Determine the related factors for the nursing diagnosis based on the patient's current status. Appropriate nursing diagnoses may include:

- Acute confusion
- Risk for injury
- Risk for other-directed violence

(*continued*)

Skill 4-3 ▶ Implementing Alternatives to the Use of Restraints (continued)

| OUTCOME IDENTIFICATION AND PLANNING | The expected outcome to achieve when implementing alternatives to restraints is that the use of restraints is avoided and the patient and others remain free from injury. |

IMPLEMENTATION

ACTION	RATIONALE
1. Perform hand hygiene and put on PPE, if indicated.	Hand hygiene and PPE prevent the spread of microorganisms. PPE is required based on transmission precautions.
2. Identify the patient.	Identifying the patient ensures the right patient receives the intervention and helps prevent errors.
3. Explain the rationale for interventions to the patient and family/significant others.	Explanation helps reduce anxiety and promotes compliance and understanding.
4. Include the patient's family and/or significant others in the plan of care.	This promotes continuity of care and cooperation.
5. Identify behavior(s) that place the patient at risk for restraint use. Assess the patient's status and environment, as outlined above.	Behaviors, such as interference with therapy or treatment, risk for falls, agitation/restlessness, resistance to care, wandering, and/or cognitive impairment, put the patient at risk for restraint use. Assessment and interpretation of patient behavior identifies unmet physiologic or psychosocial needs, acute changes in mental or physical status, provides for appropriate environments and individualized care, and respects patient's needs and rights.
6. Identify triggers or contributing factors to patient behaviors. Evaluate medication usage for medications that can contribute to cognitive and movement dysfunction and to increased risk for falls.	Removal of contributing factors and/or triggers can decrease need for restraint use. Possible changes in prescribed medications can be addressed to decrease adverse effects and decrease the need for restraint use.
7. Assess the patient's functional, mental, and psychological status and the environment, as outlined above.	Assessment provides a better understanding of the reason for the behavior, leading to individualized interventions that can eliminate restraint use and provide for patient safety.
8. Provide adequate lighting. Use a night light during sleeping hours.	Appropriate lighting can reduce disruptive behavior related to fear in an unfamiliar environment.
9. Consult with primary care provider and other appropriate health care providers regarding the continued need for treatments/therapies and the use of the least invasive method to deliver care.	Exploring the possibility of administering treatment in a less intrusive manner or discontinuing treatment no longer needed can remove the stimulus for behavior that increases risk for the use of restraints.
10. Assess the patient for pain and discomfort. Provide appropriate pharmacologic and nonpharmacologic interventions. (Refer to Chapter 10)	Unrelieved pain can contribute to behaviors that increase the risk for the use of restraints.
11. Ask a family member or significant other to stay with the patient.	Having someone stay with the patient provides companionship and familiarity.
12. Reduce unnecessary environmental stimulation and noise.	Increased stimulation can contribute to behaviors that increase the risk for the use of restraints.
13. Provide simple, clear, and direct explanations for treatments and care. Repeat to reinforce, as needed.	Explanation helps reduce anxiety and promotes compliance and understanding.
14. Distract and redirect using a calm voice.	Distraction and redirection can reduce or remove behaviors that increase risk for the use of restraints.

ACTION	**RATIONALE**
15. Increase the frequency of patient observation and surveillance; 1- or 2-hour nursing rounds, including pain assessment, toileting assistance, patient comfort, keeping personal items in reach, and meeting patient needs.	Patient care rounds/nursing rounds improve identification of unmet needs, which can decrease behaviors that increase risk for the use of restraints.
16. Implement fall precaution interventions. Refer to Skill 4-2.	Behaviors that increase risk for the use of restraints also increase the risk for falls.
17. Camouflage tube and other treatment sites with clothing, elastic sleeves, or bandaging.	Camouflaging tubes and other treatment sites removes stimulus that can trigger behaviors that increase risk for the use of restraints.
18. Ensure the use of glasses and hearing aids, if necessary.	Glasses and hearing aids allow for correct interpretation of the environment and activities to reduce confusion.
19. Consider relocation to a room close to the nursing station.	Relocation close to the nursing station provides the opportunity for increased frequency of observation.
20. Encourage daily exercise/provide exercise and activities or relaxation techniques.	Activity provides an outlet for energy and stimulation, decreasing behaviors associated with increased risk for the use of restraints.
21. Make the environment as homelike as possible; provide familiar objects.	Familiarity provides reassurance and comfort, decreasing apprehension and reducing behaviors associated with increased risk for the use of restraints.
22. Allow restless patients to walk after ensuring that the environment is safe. Use a large plant or a piece of furniture as a barrier to limit wandering from the designated area.	Activity provides an outlet for energy and stimulation, decreasing behaviors associated with increased risk for the use of restraints.
23. Consider the use of a patient attendant or sitter.	An attendant or sitter provides companionship and supervision.
24. Remove PPE, if used. Perform hand hygiene.	Proper removal of PPE reduces the risk for infection transmission and contamination of other items. Hand hygiene prevents transmission of microorganisms.

EVALUATION

The expected outcomes have been met when the use of restraints is avoided and the patient and others remain free from injury.

DOCUMENTATION

Guidelines

Document patient assessment. Include appropriate interventions to reduce the need for restraints in nursing care plan. Document patient and family teaching relative to the use of interventions. Document interventions included in care.

Sample Documentation

<u>1/1/20</u> 2330 Patient pulling IV tubing and attempting to remove dressing at insertion site left antecubital. NPO status; IV necessary for hydration and medication. Explanation regarding IV access reinforced with patient and wife. IV site covered with gauze and tubing placed under top bed linen to minimize appearance. Wife provided CD of favorite music and a puzzle. Rounding increased to every 30 minutes when family not present.

—B. Clapp, RN

UNEXPECTED SITUATIONS AND ASSOCIATED INTERVENTIONS

• *Interventions to distract no longer effective. Patient continues to pull at IV site and tubing:* Reevaluate need for IV fluid infusion. Consult with primary care provider regarding possibility of converting to intermittent access. Reevaluate patient and environment; attempt additional/different interventions as outlined above.

(continued)

Skill 4-3 ▶ Implementing Alternatives to the Use of Restraints *(continued)*

SPECIAL CONSIDERATIONS

- An alternative approach for temporary restraint is therapeutic holding, which makes use of a secure, comfortable, temporary holding position that provides close physical contact with the parent or caregiver for 30 minutes or less (Perry et al., 2014).

EVIDENCE FOR PRACTICE ▶

MINIMIZING RESTRAINT USE

These resources summarize current best evidence on the topic of interventions to be used as alternatives to the use of restraints, as well as minimizing and eliminating the use of restraints.

- American Nurses Association (ANA). (2012). *Reduction of patient restraint and seclusion in health care settings.* Retrieved http://www.nursingworld.org/restraintposition.
- Centers for Medicare & Medicaid Services (CMS). (2006). Department of Health and Human Services. Federal Register. 42 CFR Part 482. *Conditions of participation: Patients' rights. Final rule.* Retrieved http://www.cms.gov/Regulations-and-Guidance/Legislation/CFCsAndCoPs/downloads/finalpatientrightsrule.pdf.
- Cotter, V. T., & Evans, L. K. (n.d.). The Hartford Institute for Geriatric Nursing. Avoiding restraints in patients with dementia. Try this. Dementia. Issue-D1. Retrieved https://consult-geri.org/try-this/dementia/issue-d1.
- March, P., & Caple, C. (2014). Evidence-based care sheet. Restraint and seclusion: Minimizing use in psychiatric facilities. Glendale, CA: Cinahl Information Systems.
- Purcell Kirk, A., McGlinsey, A., Beckett, A., Rudd, P., & Arbour, R. (2015). Restraint reduction, restraint elimination, and best practice. *Clinical Nurse Specialist, 29*(6), 321–328.
- Registered Nurses' Association of Ontario (RNAO). (2012). International affairs & best practice guidelines. Promoting safety: Alternative approaches to the use of restraints. Retrieved http://rnao.ca/bpg/guidelines/promoting-safety-alternative-approaches-use-restraints.
- Rutledge, D. N., & March, P. (2014). Evidence-based care sheet. Restraint: Minimizing use in acute non-psychiatric care. Glendale, CA: Cinahl Information Systems.

Refer to thePoint° for additional research on related nursing topics.

Skill 4-4 ▶ Applying an Extremity Restraint

Cloth extremity restraints immobilize one or more extremities. They may be indicated after other measures have failed to prevent a patient from removing therapeutic devices, such as intravenous (IV) access devices, endotracheal tubes, oxygen, or other treatment interventions. **Restraints should be used only after less-restrictive methods have failed. Ensure compliance with ordering, assessment, and maintenance procedures. Restraints must be applied safely and appropriately to reduce risks of injury.** An extremity restraint may be applied to the hands, wrists, or ankles. Review the general guidelines for using restraints in the chapter introduction and in Fundamentals Review 4-2 and Box 4-2 in Skill 4-3. See also Evidence for Practice after Skill 4-3 for best evidence on the topic of interventions to be used as alternatives to the use of restraints, as well as minimizing and eliminating the use of restraints.

DELEGATION CONSIDERATIONS

After assessment of the patient by the RN, the application of an extremity restraint may be delegated to nursing assistive personnel (NAP) or unlicensed assistive personnel (UAP), as well as to licensed practical/vocational nurses (LPN/LVNs). The decision to delegate must be based on careful analysis of the patient's needs and circumstances, as well as the qualifications of the person to whom the task is being delegated. Refer to the Delegation Guidelines in Appendix A.

EQUIPMENT

- Appropriate cloth restraint for the extremity that is to be immobilized
- Padding, if necessary, for bony prominences
- PPE, as indicated

ASSESSMENT

Assess both the patient's physical condition and the potential for injury to self or others. A confused patient who might remove devices needed to sustain life is considered at risk for injury to self and may require the use of restraints. Assess the patient's behavior, including the presence of confusion, agitation, and combativeness, as well as the patient's ability to understand and follow directions. Evaluate the appropriateness of the least restrictive restraint device. For example, if the patient has had a stroke and cannot move the left arm, a restraint may be needed only on the right arm. Inspect the extremity where the restraint will be applied. Establish baseline skin condition for comparison at future assessments while the restraint is in place. Consider using another form of restraint if the restraint may cause further injury at the site. Before application, assess for adequate circulation in the extremity to which the restraint is to be applied, including capillary refill and proximal pulses.

NURSING DIAGNOSIS

Determine the related factors for nursing diagnoses based on the patient's current status. Appropriate nursing diagnoses may include:

- Risk for injury
- Risk for impaired skin integrity
- Acute confusion

OUTCOME IDENTIFICATION AND PLANNING

The expected outcome to achieve is that the patient is constrained by the restraint, remains free from injury, and the restraint does not interfere with therapeutic devices. Other outcomes that may be appropriate include the following: the patient does not experience impaired skin integrity; the patient does not injure himself or herself due to the restraints; and the patient's family will demonstrate an understanding about the use of the restraint and their role in the patient's care.

IMPLEMENTATION

ACTION	RATIONALE
1. Determine the need for restraints. Assess the patient's physical condition, behavior, and mental status. (Refer to Fundamentals Review 4-2 at the beginning of the chapter and Box 4-2 in Skill 4-3.)	Restraints should be used only as a last resort when alternative measures have failed and the patient is at increased risk for harming self or others.
2. Confirm facility policy for the application of restraints. Secure an order from the primary care provider, or validate that the order has been obtained within the required time frame.	Policy protects the patient and the nurse and specifies guidelines for application as well as the type of restraint and duration. Each order for restraint or seclusion used for the management of violent or self-destructive behavior that jeopardizes the immediate physical safety of the patient, a staff member, or others may only be renewed in accordance with the following limits for up to a total of 24 hours: (A) 4 hours for adults 18 years of age or older; (B) 2 hours for children and adolescents 9 to 17 years of age; or (C) 1 hour for children under 9 years of age. After 24 hours, before writing a new order for the use of restraint or seclusion for the management of violent or self-destructive behavior, a physician or other licensed independent practitioner who is responsible for the care of the patient must see and assess the patient (CMS, 2006).
3. Perform hand hygiene and put on PPE, if indicated.	Hand hygiene and PPE prevent the spread of microorganisms. PPE is required based on transmission precautions.
4. Identify the patient.	Identifying the patient ensures the right patient receives the intervention and helps prevent errors.

(continued)

Skill 4-4 ▶ Applying an Extremity Restraint *(continued)*

ACTION	**RATIONALE**
5. Explain the reason for restraint use to patient and family. Clarify how care will be given and how needs will be met. Explain that restraint is a temporary measure.	Explanation to the patient and family may lessen confusion and anger and provide reassurance. A clearly stated facility policy on the application of restraints should be available for the patient and family to read. In a long-term care facility, the family must give consent before a restraint is applied.
6. Include the patient's family and/or significant others in the plan of care.	This promotes continuity of care and cooperation.
7. Apply restraint according to the manufacturer's directions:	Proper application prevents injury.
a. Choose the least restrictive type of device that allows the greatest possible degree of mobility.	This provides minimal restriction.
b. Pad bony prominences.	Padding helps prevent skin injury.
c. Wrap the restraint around the extremity with the soft part in contact with the skin (Figure 1). If a hand mitt is being used, pull over the hand with cushion to the palmar aspect of the hand (Figure 2).	Prevents excess pressure on the extremity.

FIGURE 1. Wrapping the restraint around the extremity with the soft part in contact with the skin.

FIGURE 2. Using a hand mitt, with cushion to the palmar aspect of hand.

8. Secure in place with the Velcro straps or other mechanism, depending on specific restraint device (Figure 3). Depending on the characteristics of the specific restraint, it may be necessary to tie a knot in the restraint ties, to ensure the restraint remains secure on the extremity.	Proper application secures the restraint and ensures that there is no interference with the patient's circulation and potential alteration in neurovascular status.
9. **Ensure that two fingers can be inserted between the restraint and patient's extremity (Figure 4).**	Proper application ensures that nothing interferes with the patient's circulation and potential alteration in the neurovascular status.

FIGURE 3. Securing restraint on extremity.

FIGURE 4. Ensuring that two fingers can be inserted between the restraint and the patient's extremity.

ACTION	RATIONALE

10. Maintain restrained extremity in normal anatomic position. **Use a quick-release knot to tie the restraint to the bed frame, not side rail (Figure 5). The restraint may also be attached to a chair frame. The site should not be readily accessible to the patient.**

Maintaining a normal position lessens the possibility of an injury. A quick-release knot ensures that the restraint will not tighten when pulled and can be removed quickly in an emergency. Securing the restraint to a side rail may injure the patient when the side rail is lowered. Tying the restraint out of the patient's reach promotes security.

FIGURE 5. Securing restraint to bed frame.

11. Remove PPE, if used. Perform hand hygiene.

Proper removal of PPE reduces the risk for infection transmission and contamination of other items. Hand hygiene prevents transmission of microorganisms.

12. Assess the patient at least every hour or according to facility policy. Assessment should include the placement of the restraint, neurovascular assessment of the affected extremity, and skin integrity. In addition, assess for signs of sensory deprivation, such as increased sleeping, daydreaming, anxiety, panic, and hallucinations. Monitor the patient's vital signs.

Improperly applied restraints may cause skin tears, abrasions, or bruises. Decreased circulation may result in paleness, coolness, decreased sensation, tingling, numbness, or pain in extremity. The use of restraints may decrease environmental stimulation and result in sensory deprivation. Monitoring vital signs helps determine how the patient is responding to the restraint (Springer, 2015).

13. **Remove the restraint at least every 2 hours, or according to facility policy and patient need.** Perform range-of-motion (ROM) exercises.

Removal allows you to assess the patient and reevaluate the need for a restraint. It also allows interventions for toileting, provision of nutrition and liquids, exercise, and change of position. Exercise increases circulation in the restrained extremity.

14. Evaluate the patient for continued need of restraint. Reapply restraint only if continued need is evident and order is still valid.

Continued need must be documented for reapplication.

15. Reassure the patient at regular intervals. Provide continued explanation of rationale for interventions, reorientation if necessary, and plan of care. **Keep the call bell within the patient's easy reach.**

Reassurance demonstrates caring and provides an opportunity for sensory stimulation as well as ongoing assessment and evaluation. Patient can use the call bell to summon assistance quickly.

EVALUATION

The expected outcomes have been met when the patient remains free from injury to self or others, circulation to extremity remains adequate, skin integrity is not impaired under the restraint, and patient and family are aware of rationale for restraints.

DOCUMENTATION

Guidelines

Document alternative measures attempted before application of the restraint. Document patient assessment before application. Record patient and family education and understanding regarding restraint use. Document family consent, if necessary, according to facility policy. Document reason for restraining patient, date and time of application, type of restraint, times when removed, and result and frequency of nursing assessment.

(continued)

Skill 4-4 ▶ Applying an Extremity Restraint *(continued)*

Sample Documentation

> 7/10/20 0830 Patient disoriented and combative. Attempting to remove tracheostomy and indwelling urinary catheter. Sitting at bedside, patient continued to tug at catheter and pull on tracheostomy. Family unwilling to sit with patient. Wrist restraints applied bilaterally as ordered.
>
> —K. Urhahn, RN
>
> 7/10/20 1030 Patient continues to be disoriented and combative. Wrist restraints removed for 30 minutes during patient's bath; skin intact, hands warm, even skin tone, + radial pulses, + movement; passive and active range of motion completed. Wrist restraints reapplied.
>
> —K. Urhahn, RN

UNEXPECTED SITUATIONS AND ASSOCIATED INTERVENTIONS

- *Patient has an IV catheter in the right wrist and is trying to remove the drain from the wound:* The left wrist may have a cloth restraint applied. Due to the IV in the right wrist, alternative forms of restraints should be tried, such as a cloth mitt or an elbow restraint.
- *Patient cannot move left arm:* Do not apply the restraint to an extremity that is immobile. If the patient cannot move the extremity, there is no need to apply a restraint. Restraint may be applied to right arm after obtaining an order from the primary care provider.

SPECIAL CONSIDERATIONS

- Do not position patient with wrist restraints flat in a supine position due to an increased risk for aspiration (Springer, 2015).
- Check restraint for correct size before applying. Extremity restraints are available in different sizes. If restraint is too large, patient may free the extremity. If restraint is too small, circulation may be affected.
- Consider keeping a pair of scissors with emergency supplies in case the restraints cannot be untied quickly.

EVIDENCE FOR PRACTICE ▶

MINIMIZING RESTRAINT USE

Several resources summarize the current best evidence on the topic of interventions to be used as alternatives to the use of restraints, as well as minimizing and eliminating the use of restraints. Refer to the Evidence for Practice placed after Skill 4-3.

Refer to thePoint® for additional research on related nursing topics.

Skill 4-5 ▶ Applying a Waist Restraint

Waist restraints are a form of restraint that is applied to the patient's torso. It is applied over the patient's clothes, gown, or pajamas. When using a waist restraint, patients can move their extremities, but cannot get out of the chair or bed. **Restraints should be used only after less-restrictive methods have failed. Ensure compliance with ordering, assessment, and maintenance procedures. Historically, vest or jacket restraints were used to prevent similar patient movement, but their use has significantly decreased due to concerns for the potential risk for asphyxiation with these devices. However, research suggests that waist restraints pose the same potential risk for asphyxial death as vest restraints** (Capezuti et al., 2008). **Health care providers need to be aware of the potential outcome of using this device and weigh it against possible benefit from its use. Review the general guidelines for using restraints in the chapter introduction and Fundamentals Review 4-2 and Box 4-2 in Skill 4-3. See also Evidence for Practice in Skill 4-3 for best evidence on the topic of interventions to be used as alternatives to the use of restraints, as well as minimizing and eliminating the use of restraints.**

DELEGATION CONSIDERATIONS	After assessment of the patient by the RN, the application of a waist restraint may be delegated to nursing assistive personnel (NAP) or unlicensed assistive personnel (UAP), as well as to licensed practical/vocational nurses (LPN/LVNs). The decision to delegate must be based on careful analysis of the patient's needs and circumstances, as well as the qualifications of the person to whom the task is being delegated. Refer to the Delegation Guidelines in Appendix A.

EQUIPMENT	• Waist restraint • Additional padding as needed • PPE, as indicated

ASSESSMENT	Assess the patient's physical condition and for the potential for injury to self or others. A confused patient who is being treated with devices needed to sustain life, such as pulmonary intubation, might attempt to ambulate and is considered at risk for injury to self, and may require the use of restraints. Assess the patient's behavior, including the presence of confusion, agitation, combativeness, and ability to understand and follow directions. Evaluate the appropriateness of the least restrictive restraint device. Inspect the patient's torso for any wounds or therapeutic devices that may be affected by the waist restraint. Consider using another form of restraint if the restraint may cause further injury at the site. Assess the patient's respiratory effort. If applied incorrectly, the waist restraint can restrict the patient's ability to breathe.

NURSING DIAGNOSIS	Determine the related factors for nursing diagnoses based on the patient's current status. Appropriate nursing diagnoses may include: • Risk for injury • Wandering • Acute confusion

OUTCOME IDENTIFICATION AND PLANNING	The expected outcome to achieve is that the patient is constrained by the restraint, remains free from injury, and the restraint does not interfere with therapeutic devices. Other outcomes that may be appropriate include the following: the patient does not experience impaired skin integrity; the patient does not injure himself or herself due to the restraints; and the patient's family will demonstrate an understanding about the use of the restraint and their role in the patient's care.

IMPLEMENTATION

ACTION	RATIONALE
1. Determine the need for restraints. Assess the patient's physical condition, behavior, and mental status. (Refer to Fundamentals Review 4-2 at the beginning of the chapter and Box 4-2 in Skill 4-3.)	Restraints should be used only as a last resort when alternative measures have failed and the patient is at increased risk for harming self or others.
2. Confirm facility policy for application of restraints. **Secure an order from the primary care provider, or validate that the order has been obtained within the required time frame.**	Policy protects the patient and the nurse and specifies guidelines for application as well as type of restraint and duration. **Each order for restraint or seclusion used for the management of violent or self-destructive behavior that jeopardizes the immediate physical safety of the patient, a staff member, or others may only be renewed in accordance with the following limits for up to a total of 24 hours: (A) 4 hours for adults 18 years of age or older; (B) 2 hours for children and adolescents 9 to 17 years of age; or (C) 1 hour for children under 9 years of age. After 24 hours, before writing a new order for the use of restraint or seclusion for the management of violent or self-destructive behavior, a physician or other licensed independent practitioner who is responsible for the care of the patient must see and assess the patient (CMS, 2006).**

(continued)

Skill 4-5 ▶ Applying a Waist Restraint *(continued)*

ACTION	RATIONALE

3. Perform hand hygiene and put on PPE, if indicated.

Hand hygiene and PPE prevent the spread of microorganisms. PPE is required based on transmission precautions.

4. Identify the patient.

Identifying the patient ensures the right patient receives the intervention and helps prevent errors.

5. Explain reason for the use of restraint to patient and family. Clarify how care will be given and how needs will be met. Explain that restraint is a temporary measure.

Explanation to patient and family may lessen confusion and anger and provide reassurance. A clearly stated facility policy on the application of restraints should be available for patient and family to read. In a long-term care facility, the family must give consent before a restraint is applied.

6. Include the patient's family and/or significant others in the plan of care.

This promotes continuity of care and cooperation.

7. Apply restraint according to the manufacturer's directions.

Proper application prevents injury. Proper application ensures that there is no interference with patient's respiration.

a. Choose the correct size of the least restrictive type of device that allows the greatest possible degree of mobility.

This provides minimal restriction.

b. Pad bony prominences that may be affected by the waist restraint.

Padding helps prevent injury.

c. Assist patient to a sitting position, if not contraindicated.

This will assist you in helping the patient into the waist restraint.

d. Place waist restraint on patient over gown. Bring ties through slots in restraint. Position slots at patient's back (Figure 1).

Placing the waist restraint over the gown protects the patient's skin. Positioning the slots with the ties at the back keeps them out of the patient's vision.

e. Pull the ties secure. **Ensure that the restraint is not too tight and has no wrinkles.**

Securing too tightly could impede breathing. Wrinkles in the restraint may lead to skin impairment.

f. **Insert fist between restraint and patient to ensure that breathing is not constricted. Assess respirations after restraint is applied.**

This prevents impaired respirations.

8. **Use a quick-release knot to tie the restraint to the bed frame, not side rail.** (Refer to Figure 5 in Skill 4-4) If patient is in a wheelchair, lock the wheels and place the ties under the arm rests and tie behind the chair (Figure 2). Site should not be readily accessible to the patient.

A quick-release knot ensures that the restraint will not tighten when pulled and can be removed quickly in an emergency. Securing the restraint to a side rail may injure the patient when the side rail is lowered. Tying the restraint out of patient's reach promotes security.

9. Remove PPE, if used. Perform hand hygiene.

Proper removal of PPE reduces the risk for infection transmission and contamination of other items. Hand hygiene prevents transmission of microorganisms.

FIGURE 1. Positioning waist restraint.

FIGURE 2. Restraint secured behind chair, out of the patient's reach.

ACTION	**RATIONALE**
10. Assess the patient at least every hour or according to facility policy. An assessment should include the placement of the restraint, respirations, and skin integrity. Assess for signs of sensory deprivation, such as increased sleeping, daydreaming, anxiety, panic, and hallucinations. Monitor the patient's vital signs.	Improperly applied restraints may cause difficulty breathing, skin tears, abrasions, or bruises. Decreased circulation can result in impaired skin integrity. The use of restraints may decrease environmental stimulation and result in sensory deprivation. Monitoring vital signs helps determine how the patient is responding to the restraint (Springer, 2015).
11. **Remove restraint at least every 2 hours or according to facility policy and patient need.** Perform ROM exercises.	Removal allows you to assess patient and reevaluate need for restraint. Allows interventions for toileting, provision of nutrition and liquids, exercise, and change of position. Exercise increases circulation in restrained extremity.
12. Evaluate patient for continued need of restraint. Reapply restraint only if continued need is evident and order is still valid.	Continued need must be documented for reapplication.
13. Reassure patient at regular intervals. Provide continued explanation of rationale for interventions, reorientation if necessary, and plan of care. **Keep call bell within easy reach of patient.**	Reassurance demonstrates caring and provides an opportunity for sensory situation as well as ongoing assessment and evaluation. Patient can use call bell to summon assistance quickly.

EVALUATION

The expected outcomes have been met when the patient remains free from injury; the restraints prevent injury to the patient or others; respirations are easy and effortless; skin integrity is maintained under the restraint; and the patient and family demonstrate understanding of the rationale for using the restraints.

DOCUMENTATION

Guidelines

Document alternative measures attempted before applying restraint. Document patient assessment before application. Record patient and family education and understanding regarding restraint use. Document family consent, if necessary, according to facility policy. Document reason for restraining patient, date and time of application, type of restraint, times when removed, and result and frequency of nursing assessment.

Sample Documentation

9/30/20 2130 Patient continues to attempt to get out of bed without assistance. Waist restraint applied at night, as ordered, when family leaves. Bed height low; side rails up × 2.
—B. Clapp, RN

9/30/20 2300 Waist restraint removed; skin intact; patient ambulated to restroom with assistance. Patient requested to ambulate to kitchen for snack; patient assisted to kitchen; graham crackers and milk obtained. Patient returned to bed and waist restraint reapplied after snack.
—B. Clapp, RN

UNEXPECTED SITUATIONS AND ASSOCIATED INTERVENTIONS

- *Patient slides down and neck is caught in restraint:* Immediately release restraint. Determine alternate methods for restraining.
- *Patient slides down and out of restraint:* Immediately release restraint. Ensure restraint is properly applied. Determine alternate methods for restraining.
- *Patient is exhibiting signs of respiratory distress:* Release restraint. Restraint may be applied too tightly and cause difficulty with chest expansion. Ensure restraint is properly applied. Determine alternate methods for restraining.

SPECIAL CONSIDERATIONS

- Consider keeping a pair of scissors with emergency supplies in case the restraints cannot be untied quickly.

EVIDENCE FOR PRACTICE ▶

MINIMIZING RESTRAINT USE
Several resources summarize current best evidence on the topic of interventions to be used as alternatives to the use of restraints, as well as minimizing and eliminating the use of restraints. Refer to the Evidence for Practice after Skill 4-3.
Refer to thePoint® for additional research on related nursing topics.

Skill 4-6 ▶ Applying an Elbow Restraint

Elbow restraints are generally used on infants and children, but may be used with adults. They prevent the patient from bending the elbows and reaching incisions or therapeutic devices. The patient can move all joints and extremities except the elbow. **Restraints should be used only after less-restrictive methods have failed.** Ensure compliance with ordering, assessment, and maintenance procedures. Review the general guidelines for using restraints in the chapter introduction and Fundamentals Review 4-2 and Box 4-2 in Skill 4-3. See also Evidence for Practice in Skill 4-3 for best evidence on the topic of interventions to be used as alternatives to the use of restraints, as well as minimizing and eliminating the use of restraints.

DELEGATION CONSIDERATIONS	After assessment of the patient by the RN, the application of an elbow restraint may be delegated to nursing assistive personnel (NAP) or unlicensed assistive personnel (UAP), as well as to licensed practical/vocational nurses (LPN/LVNs). The decision to delegate must be based on careful analysis of the patient's needs and circumstances, as well as the qualifications of the person to whom the task is being delegated. Refer to the Delegation Guidelines in Appendix A.
EQUIPMENT	• Elbow restraint • Padding, as necessary • PPE, as indicated
ASSESSMENT	Assess the patient's physical condition and for the potential for injury to self or others. A confused patient who might remove devices needed to sustain life is considered at risk for injury to self and may require the use of restraints. Assess the patient's behavior, including the presence of confusion, agitation, combativeness, and ability to understand and follow directions. Evaluate the appropriateness of the least restrictive restraint device. Inspect the arm where the restraint will be applied. Baseline skin condition should be established for comparison at future assessments while the restraint is in place. Consider using another form of restraint if the restraint may cause further injury at the site. Assess capillary refill and proximal pulses in the arm to which the restraint is to be applied. This helps to determine the circulation in the extremity before applying the restraint. The restraint should not interfere with circulation. Measure the distance from the patient's shoulder to wrist to determine the appropriate size of elbow restraint to apply.
NURSING DIAGNOSIS	Determine the related factors for nursing diagnoses based on the patient's current status. Appropriate nursing diagnoses may include: • Risk for injury • Acute confusion • Risk for impaired skin integrity
OUTCOME IDENTIFICATION AND PLANNING	The expected outcome to achieve when applying an elbow restraint is that the patient is constrained by the restraint, remains free from injury, and the restraint does not interfere with therapeutic devices. Other outcomes that may be appropriate include the following: the patient does not experience impaired skin integrity; and the patient's family demonstrates an understanding about the use of the restraint and its role in the patient's care.

IMPLEMENTATION

ACTION	**RATIONALE**
1. Determine the need for restraints. Assess the patient's physical condition, behavior, and mental status. (Refer to Fundamentals Review 4-2 at the beginning of the chapter and Box 4-2 in Skill 4-3.)	Restraints should be used only as a last resort when alternative measures have failed and the patient is at increased risk for harming self or others.

ACTION

2. Confirm facility policy for application of restraints. **Secure an order from the primary care provider, or validate that the order has been obtained within the required time frame.**

3. Perform hand hygiene and put on PPE, if indicated.

4. Identify the patient.

5. Explain the reason for use to the patient and family. Clarify how care will be given and how needs will be met. Explain that the restraint is a temporary measure.

6. Apply the restraint according to manufacturer's directions:

   a. Choose the correct size of the least restrictive type of device that allows the greatest possible degree of mobility.

   b. Pad bony prominences that may be affected by the restraint.

   c. Spread elbow restraint out flat. Place the middle of the elbow restraint behind the patient's elbow. **The restraint should not extend below the wrist or place pressure on the axilla.**

   d. **Wrap the restraint snugly around the patient's arm, but make sure that two fingers can easily fit under the restraint.**

RATIONALE

Policy protects the patient and the nurse and specifies guidelines for application as well as the type of restraint and duration of use. **Each order for restraint or seclusion used for the management of violent or self-destructive behavior that jeopardizes the immediate physical safety of the patient, a staff member, or others may only be renewed in accordance with the following limits for up to a total of 24 hours: (A) 4 hours for adults 18 years of age or older; (B) 2 hours for children and adolescents 9 to 17 years of age; or (C) 1 hour for children under 9 years of age. After 24 hours, before writing a new order for the use of restraint or seclusion for the management of violent or self-destructive behavior, a physician or other licensed independent practitioner who is responsible for the care of the patient must see and assess the patient** (CMS, 2006).

Hand hygiene and PPE prevent the spread of microorganisms. PPE is required based on transmission precautions.

Identifying the patient ensures the right patient receives the intervention and helps prevent errors.

Explanation to patient and family may lessen confusion and anger and provide reassurance. A clearly stated facility policy on application of restraints should be available for the patient and family to read. In a long-term care facility, the family must give consent before a restraint is applied.

Proper application prevents injury. Proper application ensures that there is no interference with patient's circulation.

This provides minimal restriction.

Padding helps prevent injury.

Elbow restraint should be placed in the middle of the arm to ensure that the patient cannot bend the elbow. The patient should be able to move the wrist. Pressure on the axilla may lead to skin impairment.

Wrapping snugly ensures that the patient will not be able to remove the device. Being able to insert two fingers helps to prevent impaired circulation and potential alterations in neurovascular status.

(continued)

Skill 4-6 ▶ Applying an Elbow Restraint *(continued)*

ACTION	RATIONALE
e. Secure Velcro straps around the restraint (Figure 1).	Velcro straps will hold the restraint in place and prevent removal of the restraint.

FIGURE 1. Child with elbow restraint secured in place.

ACTION	RATIONALE
f. Apply the restraint to the opposite arm if the patient can move the arm.	Bilateral elbow restraints are needed if the patient can move both arms.
g. Thread Velcro strap from one elbow restraint across the back and into the loop on the opposite elbow restraint.	Strap across the back prevents the patient from wiggling out of elbow restraints.
7. **Assess circulation to fingers and hand.**	Circulation should not be impaired by the elbow restraint.
8. Remove PPE, if used. Perform hand hygiene.	Proper removal of PPE reduces the risk for infection transmission and contamination of other items. Hand hygiene prevents transmission of microorganisms.
9. Assess the patient at least every hour or according to facility policy. An assessment should include the placement of the restraint, neurovascular assessment, and skin integrity. Assess for signs of sensory deprivation, such as increased sleeping, daydreaming, anxiety, inconsolable crying, and panic. Monitor the patient's vital signs.	Improperly applied restraints may cause alterations in circulation, skin tears, abrasions, or bruises. Decreased circulation may result in impaired skin integrity. The use of restraints may decrease environmental stimulation and result in sensory deprivation. Monitoring vital signs helps determine how the patient is responding to the restraint (Springer, 2015).
10. **Remove the restraint at least every 2 hours or according to facility policy and patient need. Remove the restraint at least every 2 hours for children ages 9 to 17 years and at least every 1 hour for children under age 9, or according to facility policy and patient need. Perform ROM exercises.**	Removal allows you to assess patient and reevaluate the need for a restraint. Allows interventions for toileting; provision of nutrition and liquids, and exercise; and change of position. Exercise increases circulation in restrained extremity.
11. Evaluate the patient for continued need of restraint. Reapply the restraint only if continued need is evident.	Continued need must be documented for reapplication.
12. Reassure the patient at regular intervals. **Keep call bell within easy reach of the patient.**	Reassurance demonstrates caring and provides opportunity for sensory situation as well as ongoing assessment and evaluation. Parent or child old enough to use a call bell can use it to summon assistance quickly.

EVALUATION

The expected outcome has been met when the restraint prevents injury to self or others. In addition, the patient cannot bend the elbow; skin integrity is maintained under the restraint; and the family demonstrates an understanding of the rationale for the elbow restraint.

DOCUMENTATION

Guidelines

Document alternative measures attempted before applying restraint. Document patient assessment before application. Record patient and family education regarding restraint use and their understanding. Document family consent, if necessary, according to facility policy. Document the reason for restraining patient, date and time of application, type of restraint, times when removed, and result and frequency of nursing assessment.

Sample Documentation

9/1/20 0800 Elbow restraints removed while AM care performed (45 minutes). Skin warm, dry, even tone; + radial and brachial pulses, equal bilaterally, capillary refill <3 seconds. Patient moving arms appropriately. Continues to pick at colostomy bag. Distraction techniques used to no avail. Child removes abdominal binder when applied.

—*B. Clapp, RN*

9/1/20 0855 Skin intact and warm. Elbow restraints reapplied. Will remove when family arrives at bedside or every 2 hours as per policy.

—*B. Clapp, RN*

UNEXPECTED SITUATIONS AND ASSOCIATED INTERVENTIONS

- *Skin breakdown is noted on elbows:* Ensure that restraints are being removed routinely for at least 30 minutes and a skin inspection is done. If restraints are still needed, a padded dressing should be applied under the elbow restraint. Ensure restraint is properly applied. Determine possible alternate methods for restraining.
- *Patient reports discomfort and pain or cries when elbow is moved:* Restraints need to be removed more frequently, with active and/or passive ROM. If elbow is not moved, it will become stiff and painful. Ensure restraint is properly applied. Determine possible alternate methods for restraining.
- *Application of elbow restraint does not control the patient's body movement to allow for needed examination or treatment:* Reassess situation and consider more restrictive type of restraint.

EVIDENCE FOR PRACTICE ▶

MINIMIZING RESTRAINT USE
Several resources summarize current best evidence on the topic of interventions to be used as alternatives to the use of restraints, as well as minimizing and eliminating the use of restraints. Refer to the Evidence for Practice after Skill 4-3.

Refer to thePoint® for additional research on related nursing topics.

Skill 4-7 ▶ Applying a Mummy Restraint

A mummy restraint is appropriate for short-term restraint of an infant or small child to control the child's movements during examination or to provide care for the head and neck. **Restraints should be used only after less-restrictive methods have failed.** Ensure compliance with ordering, assessment, and maintenance procedures. Review the general guidelines for using restraints in the chapter introduction and Fundamentals Review 4-2 and Box 4-2 in Skill 4-3. See also Evidence for Practice after Skill 4-3 for best evidence on the topic of interventions to be used as alternatives to the use of restraints, as well as minimizing and eliminating the use of restraints.

DELEGATION CONSIDERATIONS

After assessment of the patient by the RN, the application of a mummy restraint may be delegated to the nursing assistive personnel (NAP) or unlicensed assistive personnel (UAP), as well as to licensed practical/vocational nurses (LPN/LVNs). The decision to delegate must be based on careful analysis of the patient's needs and circumstances, as well as the qualifications of the person to whom the task is being delegated. Refer to the Delegation Guidelines in Appendix A.

EQUIPMENT

- Small blanket or sheet
- PPE, as indicated

(*continued*)

Skill 4-7 ▶ Applying a Mummy Restraint *(continued)*

ASSESSMENT	Assess the patient's behavior and need for a restraint. Assess for wounds or therapeutic devices that may be affected by the restraint. Evaluate the appropriateness of the least restrictive restraint device. Another form of restraint may be more appropriate to prevent injury.
NURSING DIAGNOSIS	Determine the related factors for nursing diagnoses based on the patient's current status. Appropriate nursing diagnoses may include: • Risk for injury • Anxiety • Impaired physical mobility
OUTCOME IDENTIFICATION AND PLANNING	The expected outcome to achieve is that the patient is constrained by the restraint, remains free from injury, and that the restraint does not interfere with therapeutic devices. Other outcomes that may be appropriate include the following: examination and/or treatment is provided without incident and the patient's family will demonstrate an understanding about the use of the restraint and its role in the patient's care.

IMPLEMENTATION

ACTION	RATIONALE
1. Determine the need for restraints. Assess the patient's physical condition, behavior, and mental status. (Refer to Fundamentals Review 4-2 at the beginning of the chapter and Box 4-2 in Skill 4-3.)	Restraints should be used only as a last resort when alternative measures have failed, and the patient is at increased risk for harming self or others.
2. Confirm facility policy for application of restraints. Secure an order from the primary care provider, or validate that the order has been obtained within the required time frame.	Policy protects the patient and the nurse and specifies guidelines for application as well as the type of restraint and duration. Each order for restraint or seclusion used for the management of violent or self-destructive behavior that jeopardizes the immediate physical safety of the patient, a staff member, or others may only be renewed in accordance with the following limits for up to a total of 24 hours: (A) 4 hours for adults 18 years of age or older; (B) 2 hours for children and adolescents 9 to 17 years of age; or (C) 1 hour for children under 9 years of age. After 24 hours, before writing a new order for the use of restraint or seclusion for the management of violent or self-destructive behavior, a physician or other licensed independent practitioner who is responsible for the care of the patient must see and assess the patient (CMS, 2006).
3. Perform hand hygiene and put on PPE, if indicated.	Hand hygiene and PPE prevent the spread of microorganisms. PPE is required based on transmission precautions.
4. Identify the patient.	Identifying the patient ensures the right patient receives the intervention and helps prevent errors.
5. Explain the reason for use to the patient and family. Clarify how care will be given and how needs will be met. Explain that restraint is a temporary measure.	Explanation to the patient and family may lessen confusion and anger and provide reassurance. A clearly stated facility policy on application of restraints should be available for patient and family to read. In a long-term care facility, the family must give consent before a restraint is applied.
6. Open the blanket or sheet. Place the child on the blanket, with the edge of the blanket at or above neck level.	This positions the child correctly on the blanket.

ACTION

7. Position the child's right arm alongside the child's body. Left arm should not be constrained at this time. Pull the right side of the blanket tightly over the child's right shoulder and chest. Secure under the left side of the child's body (Figure 1).

8. Position the left arm alongside the child's body. Pull the left side of the blanket tightly over the child's left shoulder and chest. Secure under the right side of the child's body (Figure 2).

9. Fold the lower part of the blanket up and pull over the child's body. Secure under the child's body on each side or with safety pins (Figure 3).

RATIONALE

Wrapping snugly ensures that the child will not be able to wiggle out.

Wrapping snugly ensures that the child will not be able to wiggle out.

This ensures that the child will not be able to wiggle out.

FIGURE 1. Pulling blanket over right shoulder and chest and securing under patient's left side.

FIGURE 2. Securing blanket under right side of body.

FIGURE 3. Securing lower corner of blanket under each side of patient's body.

10. Stay with the child while the mummy wrap is in place. Reassure the child and parents at regular intervals. Once examination or treatment is completed, unwrap the child.

11. Remove PPE, if used. Perform hand hygiene.

Remaining with the child prevents injury. Reassurance demonstrates caring and provides opportunity for ongoing assessment and evaluation.

Proper removal of PPE reduces the risk for infection transmission and contamination of other items. Hand hygiene prevents transmission of microorganisms.

EVALUATION

The expected outcome has been met when the restraint prevents injury to self or others. In addition, the examination or treatment is provided without incident; and the family demonstrates an understanding of the rationale for the mummy restraint.

DOCUMENTATION

Guidelines

Document alternative measures attempted before applying a restraint. Document patient assessment before application. Record patient and family education and understanding regarding restraint use. Document family consent, if necessary, according to facility policy. Document reason for restraining patient, date and time of application, type of restraint, times when removed, and result and frequency of nursing assessment.

Sample Documentation

6/9/20 0230 Patient requires suturing of forehead. Parent attempted to hold child for procedure without success. Need to restrain child explained to parents. Mummy restraint applied with parents' consent. Restraint removed after 20 minutes; sutures intact. Wound care instructions (verbal and written) provided to parents; parents verbalize understanding.
—D. Dunn, RN

(continued)

Skill 4-7 ▶ Applying a Mummy Restraint *(continued)*

UNEXPECTED SITUATIONS AND ASSOCIATED INTERVENTIONS	• *Application of mummy wrap does not control the infant's or child's body movement to allow for needed examination or treatment:* Reassess situation and consider more restrictive type of restraint.
SPECIAL CONSIDERATIONS	• An alternative approach for temporary restraint is therapeutic holding, which makes use of a secure, comfortable, temporary holding position that provides close physical contact with the parent or caregiver for 30 minutes or less (Perry et al., 2014).

EVIDENCE FOR PRACTICE ▶	**MINIMIZING RESTRAINT USE** Several resources summarize current best evidence on the topic of interventions to be used as alternatives to the use of restraints, as well as minimizing and eliminating the use of restraints. Refer to the Evidence for Practice after Skill 4-3. Refer to thePoint° for additional research on related nursing topics.

Enhance Your Understanding

Focusing on Patient Care: Developing Clinical Reasoning

Consider the case scenarios at the beginning of the chapter as you answer the following questions to enhance your understanding and apply what you have learned.

QUESTIONS

1. Megan Lewis, an 18 month old with an IV access in her left forearm, is continually picking at the IV and dressing. What interventions would be appropriate as alternatives to restraints? If unsuccessful, what restraint(s) would be appropriate for Megan?

2. Kevin Mallory, a 35-year-old body builder with a closed head injury, is extremely strong. The fear is that he will rip the cloth restraints and extubate himself. What other type of restraints could be tried?

3. John Frawley, a 72-year-old patient with Alzheimer's disease, continually tries to get out of bed without assistance. He has an unsteady gait and has one broken hip due to a fall. What are the appropriate interventions to try with Mr. Frawley?

You can find suggested answers after the Bibliography at the end of this chapter.

Integrated Case Study Connection

The case studies in the back of the book focus on integrating concepts. Refer to the following case studies to enhance your understanding of the concepts and skills in this chapter.

Taylor Suite Resources

Explore these additional resources to enhance learning for this chapter:

• NCLEX-Style Questions and other resources on thePoint°, http://thePoint.lww.com/Lynn5e
• Skill Checklists for *Taylor's Clinical Nursing Skills*, 5e
• *Fundamentals of Nursing:* Chapter 27, Safety, Security, and Emergency Preparedness

Bibliography

Aging & Technology Research Center. (2013). School of Public Health and Health Professions. University at Buffalo. The State University of New York. Home safety self assessment tool (HSSAT). Retrieved http://aging-research.buffalo.edu/hssat

American Geriatrics Society (AGS). (2012a). Tips for preventing serious falls. Retrieved http://www.healthinaging.org/files/documents/tipsheets/falls_prevention.pdf

American Geriatrics Society (AGS). (2012b). Aging & health A to Z. Retrieved http://www.healthinaging.org/aging-and-health-a-to-z/topic:falls

American Geriatrics Society and British Geriatrics Society. (2010). 2010 AGS/BGS Clinical practice guideline: Prevention of falls in older persons. Retrieved http://www.medcats.com/FALLS/frameset.htm

American Nurses Association (ANA). (2012). Reduction of patient restraint and seclusion in health care settings. Retrieved https://www.nursingworld.org/~4ad4a8/globalassets/docs/ana/reduction-of-patient-restraint-and-seclusion-in-health-care-settings.pdf

Bak, J., Zoffmann, V., Sestoft, D. M., Almivk, R., Philos, D., & Brandt-Christensen, M. (2014). Mechanical restraint in psychiatry: Preventive factors in theory and practice. A Danish-Norwegian Association study. *Perspectives in Psychiatric Care, 50*(3), 155–166.

Barker, A., Kamar, J., Tyndall, T., & Hill, K. (2013). Reducing serious fall-related injuries in acute hospitals: Are low-low beds a critical success factor? *Journal of Advanced Nursing, 69*(1), 112–121.

Bolz, M., Capezuti, E., Wagner, L., Rosenberg, M. C., & Secic, M. (2013). Patient safety in medical-surgical units: Can nurse certification make a difference? *Medsurg Nursing, 22*(1), 26–37.

Brosey, L. A., & March, K. S. (2015). Effectiveness of structured hourly nurse rounding on patient satisfaction and clinical outcomes. *Journal of Nursing Care Quality, 30*(2), 153–159.

Capezuti, E., Brush, B., Won, R., et al. (2008). Least restrictive or least understood? Waist restraints, provider practices, and risk of harm. *Journal of Aging & Social Policy, 20*(3), 305–322.

Caputi, L. (2013). A practical approach to teaching clinical reasoning. Retrieved http://contemporaryforums.com/conf_downloads/070713(2)-PCB-Caputi.pdf

Caputi, L. (2015). Focus on thinking. Retrieved http://www.lindacaputi.com/userfiles/Tools%20for%20Implementing%20Clinical%20Reasoning.pdf

Centers for Disease Control and Prevention (CDC). (2015). Costs of falls among older adults. Retrieved http://www.cdc.gov/HomeandRecreationalSafety/Falls/fallcost.html

Centers for Disease Control and Prevention (CDC). (2016a). Health alert network (HAN). Retrieved http://www.bt.cdc.gov/HAN

Centers for Disease Control and Prevention (CDC). (2016b). Injury prevention & control. Retrieved http://www.cdc.gov/injury

Centers for Medicare & Medicaid Services (CMS). (2006). Department of Health and Human Services. Federal Register. 42 CFR Part 482. Conditions of participation: Patients' rights. Final rule. Retrieved http://www.cms.gov/Regulations-and-Guidance/Legislation/CFCsAndCoPs/downloads/finalpatientrightsrule.pdf

Cohen, N. L. (2013). Using the ABCs of situational awareness for patient safety. *Nursing, 43*(4), 64–65.

Cosper, P., Morelock, V., & Provine, B. (2015). Please release me. Restraint reduction initiative in a health care system. *Journal of Nursing Care Quality, 30*(1), 16–23.

Cotter, V. T., & Evans, L. K. (n.d.). The Hartford Institute for Geriatric Nursing. Avoiding restraints in patients with dementia. Try this. Dementia. Issue-D1. Retrieved https://consultgeri.org/try-this/dementia/issue-d1

Cox, J., Thomas-Gawkins, C., Pajarillo, E., DeGennaro, S., Cadmus, E., & Martinez, M. (2015). Factors associated with falls in hospitalized adult patients. *Applied Nursing Research, 28*(2), 78–82.

Degelau, J., Belz, M., Bungum, L., et al. (2012). *Institute for Clinical Systems Improvement (ICSI). Prevention of falls (acute care).* Health care protocol. Bloomington, MN: Institute for Clinical Systems Improvement (ICSI). Facility for Healthcare Research and Quality (AHRQ). Retrieved http://guideline.gov/content.aspx?id = 36906#Section420

Doenges, M. E., Moorhouse, M. F., & Murr, A. C. (2016). *Nursing diagnoses manual. Planning, individualizing, and documenting client care* (5th ed.). Philadelphia, PA: F.A. Davis.

Eliopoulos, C. (2014). *Gerontological nursing* (8th ed.). Philadelphia, PA: Wolters Kluwer.

Enns, E., Rhemtulla, R., Ewa, V., Fruetel, K., & Holroyd-Leduc, J. M. (2014). A controlled quality improvement trial to reduce the use of physical restraints in older hospitalized adults. *Journal of the American Geriatrics Society, 62*(3), 541–545.

ESRI. (2008). *Public safety and homeland security situational awareness. An ESRI white paper.* Redlands, CA: Author. Retrieved https://www.esri.com/library/whitepapers/pdfs/situational-awareness.pdf

Fabry, D. (2015). Hourly rounding: Perspectives and perceptions of the frontline nursing staff. *Journal of Nursing Management, 23*(2), 200–210.

Facility for Healthcare Research and Quality (AHRQ). (2014). Patient safety network. Patient safety primer. Safety culture. Retrieved https://psnet.ahrq.gov/primers/primer/5/safety-culture

Gerace, A., Mosel, K., Oster, C., & Muir-Cochrane, E. (2013). Restraint use in acute and extended mental health services for older persons. *International Journal of Mental Health Nursing, 22*(6), 545–557.

Godlock, G., Christiansen, M., & Feider, L. (2016). Implementation of an evidence-based patient safety team to prevent falls in inpatient medical units. *MEDSURG Nursing, 25*(1), 17–23.

Goldsack, J., Bergey, M., Mascioli, S., & Cunningham, J. (2015). Hourly rounding and patient falls: What factors boost success? *Nursing, 45*(2), 25–30.

Grabiner, M. D. (2014). Exercise-based fall prevention programmes decrease fall-related injuries. *Evidence Based Nursing, 17*(4), 125.

Gray-Micelli, D. (2012). Hartford Institute for Geriatric Nursing. FALLS. Nursing standard of practice protocol: Fall prevention. Retrieved https://consultgeri.org/geriatric-topics/falls

Haugh, J., Ó Flatharta, T., Griffin, T. P., & O'Keeffe, S. T. (2014). High frequency of potential entrapment gaps in beds in an acute hospital. *Age and Ageing, 43*(6), 862–865.

Hendrich, A. (2007). Predicting patient falls. *American Journal of Nursing, 107*(11), 50–58.

Hester, A. L. (2015). Preventing injuries from patient falls. *American Nurse Today, 10*(7), 36–37.

Hicks, D. (2015). Can rounding reduce patient falls in acute care? An integrative literature review. *MEDSURG Nursing, 24*(1), 51–55.

Hinkle, J. L., & Cheever, K. H. (2018). *Brunner & Suddarth's textbook of medical-surgical nursing* (14th ed.). Philadelphia, PA: Wolters Kluwer.

Hoffman, H., & Hahn, S. (2014). Characteristics of nursing home residents and physical restraint: A systematic literature review. *Journal of Clinical Nursing, 23*(21/22), 3012–3024.

The Joint Commission (TJC). (2018). National patient safety goals. Hospital: 2016. Retrieved https://www.jointcommission.org/hap_2017_npsgs

Keall, M. D., Pierse, N., Howden-Chapman, P., et al. (2015). Home modifications to reduce injuries for falls in the Home Injury Prevention Intervention (HIPI) study: A cluster-randomised controlled trial. *The Lancet, 385*(9964), 231–238.

Keeling, C. (2014). Practical and ethical use of bed rails. *Nursing & Residential Care, 15*(4), 230–233.

Kyle, T., & Carman, S. (2017). *Essentials of pediatric nursing* (3rd ed.). Philadelphia, PA: Wolters Kluwer Health.

Lach, H. W. (2012). The Hartford Institute for Geriatric Nursing. Try this series. Dementia. Home safety inventory for older adults with dementia. Issue-D12. Retrieved https://consultgeri.org/try-this/dementia/issue-d12

Lach, H. W., Leach, K. M., & Butcher, H. K. (2016). Changing the practice of physical restraint use in acute care. *Journal of Gerontological Nursing, 42*(2), 17–26.

March, P., & Caple, C. (2014). *Evidence-based care sheet. Restraint and seclusion: Minimizing use in psychiatric facilities.* Glendale, CA: Cinahl Information Systems.

Möhler, R., & Meyer, G. (2014). Attitudes of nurses towards the use of physical restraints in geriatric care: A systematic review of qualitative and quantitative studies. *International Journal of Nursing Studies, 51*(2), 274–288.

NANDA International, Inc.: Nursing Diagnoses - Definitions and Classification 2018–2020 © 2017 NANDA International, ISBN 978-1-62623-929-6. Used by arrangement with the Thieme Group, Stuttgart/New York.

National Council of State Boards of Nursing (NCSBN). (n.d.). Transition to practice. Patient-centered care module. 60 second assessment tool. Retrieved https://www.ncsbn.org/687.htm

National Institute of Health (NIH). NIH Senior Health. (2013). Falls and older adults. Retrieved http://nihseniorhealth.gov/falls/aboutfalls/01.html

National Institute on Aging. (2016). Age page: Falls and fractures. Retrieved https://www.nia.nih.gov/health/publication/falls-and-fractures

National Safety Council. (2016). Safety knowledge. Safety at home. Top causes of unintentional injury and death in homes and communities. Retrieved http://www.nsc.org/learn/safety-knowledge/Pages/safety-at-home.aspx?var = mnm

Perry, S. E., Hockenberry, M. J., Lowdermilk, D. L., & Wilson, D. (2014). *Maternal child nursing care* (5th ed.). St. Louis, MO: Elsevier Mosby.

Public Health Facility of Canada. (2011). The safe living guide – A guide to home safety for seniors. Retrieved http://www.phac-aspc.gc.ca/seniors-aines/publications/public/injury-blessure/safelive-securite/index-eng.php

Purcell Kirk, A., McGlinsey, A., Beckett, A., Rudd, P., & Arbour, R. (2015). Restraint reduction, restraint elimination, and best practice. *Clinical Nurse Specialist: The Journal for Advanced Nursing Practice, 29*(6), 321–328.

Purnell, L. D. (2013). *Transcultural health care. A culturally competent approach* (4th ed.). Philadelphia, PA: F.A. Davis Company.

Quigley, P. (2015a). Taking appropriate precautions against falls. *American Nurse Today, 10*(7), 32–33.

Quigley, P. (2015b). Tailoring falls-prevention interventions to each patient. *American Nurse Today* (Supplement), 8–10.

Registered Nurses' Association of Ontario (RNAO). (2012). International affairs & best practice guidelines. Promoting safety: Alternative approaches to the use of restraints. Retrieved http://rnao.ca/bpg/guidelines/promoting-safety-alternative-approaches-use-restraints

Reimer, N., & Herbener, L. (2014). Round and round we go: Rounding strategies to impact exemplary professional practice. *Clinical Journal of Oncology Nursing, 18*(6), 654–660.

Restraint use cut in half. (2010). *Nursing, 40*(10), 20.

Robinovitch, S. N., Scott, V., & Feldman, F. (2015). Home-safety modifications to reduce injuries from falls. *The Lancet, 385*(9964), 205–206.

Rutledge, D. N., & March, P. D. (2011a). *Evidence-based care sheet. Restraint: Minimizing use in acute, nonpsychiatric care.* Glendale, CA: Cinahl Information Systems.

Rutledge, D. N., & March, P. D. (2011b). *Evidence-based care sheet. Restraint: Minimizing usage in skilled nursing facilities.* Glendale, CA: Cinahl Information Systems.

Rutledge, D. N., & March, P. (2014). *Evidence-based care sheet. Restraint: Minimizing use in acute non-psychiatric care.* Glendale, CA: Cinahl Information Systems.

Ryan-Wenger, N. A., & Dufek, J. S. (2013). An interdisciplinary momentary confluence of events model to explain, minimize, and prevent pediatric patient falls and fall-related injuries. *Journal for Specialists in Pediatric Nursing, 18*(1), 4–12.

Said, A. A., & Kautz, D. D. (2013). Patient safety. Reducing restraint use for older adults in acute care. *Nursing, 43*(12), 59–61.

Santesso, N., Carrasco-Labra, A., & Brignardello-Peterson, R. (2014). Hip protectors for preventing hip fractures in older people. *Cochrane Database of Systematic Reviews, Issue3.* Art. No.: CD001255.

Severity of injuries makes fall prevention a priority. (2014). *PPS Alert for Long-Term Care, 17*(4), 4–6.

Sitzer, V. (2016). Development of an automated self-assessment of fall-risk questionnaire for hospitalized patients. *Journal of Nursing Care Quality,* *31*(1), 46–53.

Springer, G. (2015). When and how to use restraints. *American Nurse Today, 10*(1), 26–27.

Stinson, K. J. (2016). Practice issues with use of physical restraints in critical care units. *American Journal of Critical Care, 25*(1), 21–26.

Struth, D. (2009). TCAB in the curriculum. *American Journal of Nursing, 109*(11), 55–58.

Stubbs, B., Brefka, S., & Denkinger, M. D. (2015). What works to prevent falls in community-dwelling

older adults? Umbrella review of meta-analyses of randomized controlled trials. *Physical Therapy, 95*(8), 1095–1110.

Taylor, C., Lynn, P., & Bartlett, J. (2019). *Fundamentals of nursing: The art and science of person-centered care* (9th ed.). Philadelphia, PA: Wolters Kluwer.

Tomita, M. R., Saharan, S., Rajendran, S., Mochajski, S. M., & Schweitzer, J. A. (2014). Psychometrics of the Home Safety Self-Assessment Tool (HSSAT) to prevent falls in community-swelling older adults. *The American Journal of Occupational Therapy, 68*(6), 711–718.

Touhy, T. A., & Jett, K. F. (2014). *Ebersole and Hess' gerontological nursing & healthy aging* (4th ed.). St. Louis, MO: Elsevier Mosby.

Tzeng, H. M., & Yin, C. Y. (2015). Patient engagement in hospital fall prevention. *Nursing Economics, 33*(6), 326–334.

U.S. Food and Drug Administration (FDA). (2016). Bed rail safety. Retrieved http://www.fda.gov/MedicalDevices/ProductsandMedicalProcedures/HomeHealthandConsumer/ConsumerProducts/BedRailSafety/default.htm

SUGGESTED ANSWERS FOR FOCUSING ON PATIENT CARE: DEVELOPING CLINICAL REASONING

1. Nursing interventions for Megan should include the use of distraction, such as play, toys, music, games, and so forth. (Refer to Skill 4-3.) Megan's parent should be encouraged to stay with her to provide supervision and distraction, also. Cover the IV access site with a dressing and gauze, or other cover, such as the I.V. House dressing. If all other alternatives to restraints are attempted, and it is necessary to maintain the IV infusion, an elbow restraint (Skill 4-6) or hand mitt (Skill 4-4) would be the least restrictive restraints to prevent dislodgement of Megan's IV access.

2. You must implement as many alternatives to restraints as possible for Mr. Mallory. Refer to Skill 4-3. In addition, consult with the primary care provider to discuss a possible time frame for extubation. Increase frequency of monitoring, repeat explanations, and provide distraction as part of the nursing care plan for this patient. Elbow restraints (Skill 4-6) would be a possible solution if it is determined that restraints are required.

3. Fall prevention is best achieved through the implementation of multiple strategies. Begin by assessing the patient's motivation for attempting activity unassisted. Provide reassurance and explanations related to care. If possible, Mr. Frawley could be moved to a room closer to the nursing station to allow increased monitoring. Additional nursing interventions to try could include asking family members to stay with Mr. Frawley, providing distraction based on information from the family regarding favorite activities, more frequent rounding to ensure that his toileting needs are met, as well as need for hydration. Provide a low bed for the patient, as well as floor mats, to reduce the risk for serious injury if Mr. Frawley should fall. Refer to Skill 4-2 for additional intervention suggestions.

Medications

Focusing on Patient Care

This chapter will help you develop the skills needed to administer medications safely to the following patients:

Cooper Jackson, age 2, does not want to take his ordered oral antibiotic.

Erika Jenkins, age 20, is extremely afraid of needles and is at the clinic for her birth-control injection.

Jonah Dinerman, age 63, was recently diagnosed with diabetes and needs to be taught how to give himself insulin injections.

Refer to Focusing on Patient Care: Developing Clinical Reasoning at the end of the chapter to apply what you learn.

Learning Objectives

After completing the chapter, you will be able to accomplish the following:

1. Prepare medications for administration in a safe manner.
2. Administer oral medications.
3. Administer medications via a gastric tube.
4. Remove medication from an ampule.
5. Remove medication from a vial.
6. Mix medications from two vials in one syringe.
7. Identify appropriate needle size and angle of insertion for intradermal, subcutaneous, and intramuscular injections.
8. Locate appropriate sites for intradermal injection.
9. Administer an intradermal injection.
10. Locate appropriate sites for a subcutaneous injection.
11. Administer a subcutaneous injection.
12. Locate appropriate sites for an intramuscular injection.
13. Administer an intramuscular injection.
14. Apply an insulin pump.
15. Administer medications by intravenous bolus or push through a continuous intravenous infusion.
16. Administer medications by intravenous bolus or push through a medication or drug-infusion lock.
17. Administer a piggyback, intermittent, intravenous infusion of medication.
18. Apply a transdermal patch.
19. Administer eye drops.
20. Administer eye irrigation.

21. Administer ear drops.
22. Administer ear irrigation.
23. Administer a nasal spray.
24. Administer a vaginal cream.
25. Administer a rectal suppository.
26. Administer medication via a metered-dose inhaler.
27. Administer medication via a dry-powder inhaler.
28. Administer medication via a small-volume nebulizer.

Key Terms

adverse drug reaction: undesirable effect other than the intended therapeutic effect of a drug; also known as adverse effects

ampule: a glass flask that contains a single dose of medication for parenteral administration

inhalation: route to administer medications directly into the lungs or airway passages

intradermal injection: injection placed just below the epidermis

intramuscular injection: injection placed into muscular tissue

intravenous (IV) route: route to administer medications directly into the vein or venous system

metered-dose inhaler (MDI): device to deliver a controlled dose of medication for inhalation

nebulizer: instrument that produces a fine spray or mist; passing air through a liquid medication to produce fine particles for inhalation

needle gauge: measurement of the diameter of a needle

subcutaneous injection: injection placed between the epidermis and muscle, into the subcutaneous tissue

suppository: oval or cone-shaped substance that is inserted into a body cavity, melting at body temperature

vial: a glass bottle with a self-sealing stopper through which medication is removed

Medication administration is a core nursing function that involves skillful technique and consideration of the patient's development, health status, and safety. The nurse administering medications needs to have knowledge of drugs, including drug names, preparations, classifications, adverse effects, and physiologic factors that affect drug action (Fundamentals Review 5-1).

Use of the three checks and the rights of medication administration when administering medications can assist with safe administration of medications. The use of technology, such as bar-code labeling, does not relieve the nurse of responsibility for ensuring safe medication administration. Check the label on the medication package or container three times during medication preparation and administration (Fundamentals Review 5-2).

The rights of medication administration (Fundamentals Review 5-3) can help to ensure accuracy when administering medications. However, the Institute for Safe Medication Practices (2007) reiterated a position taken in 1999 that the rights of medication administration "are merely broadly stated goals or desired outcomes of safe medication practices" (para. 1). The rights themselves do not ensure medication safety. The nurse assumes individual accountability for safe drug administration by collaborating with the interprofessional team and engaging in behavior that follows standards of practice and behaviors prescribed by the institution to achieve the goals of the rights (Adhikari, Tocher, Smith, Corcoran, & MacArthur, 2014; Frandsen & Pennington, 2014). Suggested rights of administration vary slightly between references, spanning from the classic 5 rights (Rights 1 through 5 in Fundamentals Review 5-3) to up to 10 or 11 rights of medication administration common in the literature (Frandsen & Pennington; Kee, Hayes, & McCuistion, 2015; Smeulers, Verweij, & Maaskant, 2015).

Nursing responsibilities for drug administration are summarized in Fundamentals Review 5-4. This chapter covers skills that the nurse needs to administer medications safely via multiple routes. Proper use of equipment and proper technique are imperative. Fundamentals Review 5-5 and Figure 5-1 review important guidelines related to administering parenteral medications. Nurses should be aware of the higher risk of making an error when their workflow is disrupted from either a distraction or interruption; effective reduction and management of distractions and interruptions is critical to safe medication administration and increased patient safety (Bravo, Cochran, & Barrett, 2016; Williams, King, Thompson, & Champagne, 2014).

When administering medication, consider factors that may affect drug action, such as age-related considerations. For example, physiologic changes associated with the aging process, including decreased gastric motility, muscle mass, acid production, and blood flow affect drug action. Older adults may also be more susceptible to certain **adverse drug reactions**. Drug interactions in older adults are a very real and dangerous problem because older adults are more likely to take multiple drugs simultaneously and because of age-related declines in hepatic and renal function (Adams, Holland & Urban, 2017).

Fundamentals Review 5-1

KNOW YOUR MEDICATIONS

Before administering any medication, know the following:

- Mode of action and purpose of medication (making sure that this medication is appropriate for the patient's diagnosis)
- Adverse effects of and contraindications for the medication

- Antagonist of medication (as appropriate)
- Safe dosage range for medication
- Potential interactions with other medications
- Precautions to take before administration
- Proper administration technique

Fundamentals Review 5-2

THE THREE CHECKS

"Three Checks" denotes that the label on the medication package or container should be checked three times during medication preparation and administration.

1. Read the Electronic Medication Administration Record (eMAR) or Medication Administration Record (MAR) and select the proper medication from the patient's medication drawer or medication supply system. This is the *first check* of the medication label.
2. After retrieving the medication from the drawer, compare the medication label with the eMAR/MAR. Note: Compare with the eMAR/MAR immediately before

pouring from a multidose container. This is the *second check* of the medication label.
3. The *third check* can be performed in one of two ways, depending on facility policy:
   - Most commonly, at the bedside, recheck the labels with the eMAR/MAR after identifying the patient and before administration.
   - When all medications for one patient have been prepared, recheck the labels with the eMAR/MAR before taking the medication to the patient.

Fundamentals Review 5-3

RIGHTS OF MEDICATION ADMINISTRATION

The "Rights of Medication Administration" can help to ensure accuracy when administering medications. To prevent medication errors, always ensure that the:

1. **Right medication** is given to the
2. **Right patient** in the
3. **Right dosage** (in the right form) through the
4. **Right route** at the
5. **Right time** for the
6. **Right reason** based on the

7. **Right (appropriate) assessment** data using the
8. **Right documentation** and monitoring for the
9. **Right response** by the patient.

Additional rights have been suggested to include (10) the **right to education**, ensuring patients receive accurate and thorough information about the medication, and (11) the **right to refuse**, acknowledging that patients can and do refuse to take a medication.

Fundamentals Review 5-4

NURSING RESPONSIBILITIES FOR ADMINISTERING DRUGS

- Assessing the patient and understanding clearly why the patient is receiving a particular medication
- Preparing the medication to be administered (checking labels, preparing injections, observing proper asepsis techniques with needles and syringes)
- Calculating accurate dosages
- Validating medication calculations with another nurse

- Administering the medication (e.g., proper injection techniques, aids to help swallowing, topical methods, and so on)
- Documenting the medications given
- Monitoring the patient's reaction and evaluating the patient's response
- Educating the patient regarding his or her medications and medication regimen

Fundamentals Review 5-5

NEEDLE/SYRINGE SELECTION

- The route of administration directs the choice of needle length. Refer to the discussion related to each particular route for specific guidelines regarding needle length.
- When looking at a needle package, the first number is the needle gauge or diameter of the needle (e.g., 18, 20) and the second number is the length in inches (e.g., 1, 1.5).
- As the gauge number becomes larger, the size of the needle becomes smaller; for instance, a 24-gauge needle is smaller than an 18-gauge needle.
- When giving an injection, the viscosity of the medication directs the choice of gauge (diameter). A thicker

medication, such as a hormone, is given through a needle with a larger gauge, such as a 20-gauge. A thinner-consistency medication, such as morphine, is given through a needle with a smaller gauge, such as a 24-gauge.

- The amount of medication to be administered directs the choice of the size of the syringe. Smaller syringes should be used as needed for precise dosing because they provide smaller increments of measurement—never estimate a dose. For example, a 1-mL syringe provides increments of 0.02 mL, but a 5-mL syringe allows for precise measures only down to 0.2 mL.

Needle package showing first number (gauge or diameter of the needle) and second number (length of the needle in inches).

Different needle sizes. An 18-gauge needle (*top*) and a 24-gauge needle (*bottom*).

FIGURE 5-1. Comparison of insertion angles for intramuscular, subcutaneous, and intradermal injections.

 Skill 5-1 ▶ **Administering Oral Medications**

Drugs given orally are intended for absorption in the stomach and small intestine. The oral route is the most commonly used route of administration and is usually the most convenient and comfortable route for the patient. After oral administration, drug action has a slower onset and a more prolonged, but less potent, effect compared to other routes of administration.

DELEGATION CONSIDERATIONS	The administration of oral medications is not delegated to nursing assistive personnel (NAP) or to unlicensed assistive personnel (UAP) in the acute care setting. The administration of specified oral medications to stable patients in some long-term care settings may be delegated to NAP or UAP who have received appropriate training. Depending on the state's nurse practice act and the organization's policies and procedures, the administration of oral medications may be delegated to licensed practical/vocational nurses (LPN/LVNs). The decision to delegate must be based on careful analysis of the patient's needs and circumstances, as well as the qualifications of the person to whom the task is being delegated. Refer to the Delegation Guidelines in Appendix A.
EQUIPMENT	• Medication in disposable cup or oral syringe • Liquid (e.g., water, juice) with straw, if not contraindicated • Electronic Medication Administration Record (eMAR) or Medication Administration Record (MAR) • PPE, as indicated
ASSESSMENT	Assess the appropriateness of the drug for the patient. Review medical history, allergy, assessment, and laboratory data that may influence drug administration. Assess the patient's ability to swallow medications; check the gag reflex, if indicated. If the patient cannot swallow, is unconscious or NPO, does not have gag reflex, or is experiencing nausea or vomiting, withhold the medication, notify the primary health care provider, and complete proper documentation. Assess the patient's knowledge of the medication. If the patient has a knowledge deficit about the medication, this may be the appropriate time to begin education about the medication. If the medication may affect the patient's vital signs, assess them before administration. If the medication is for pain relief, assess the patient's pain level before and after administration. Verify the patient's name as well as the dose, route, and time of administration.
NURSING DIAGNOSIS	Determine related factors for the nursing diagnoses based on the patient's current status. Appropriate nursing diagnoses may include: • Impaired swallowing • Deficient knowledge • Risk for aspiration

(*continued*)

Skill 5-1 ▶ Administering Oral Medications *(continued)*

OUTCOME IDENTIFICATION AND PLANNING

The expected outcomes to achieve when administering an oral medication include that the medication is successfully administered via the oral route; the patient will experience the desired effect from the medication; the patient will not aspirate; the patient experiences decreased anxiety; the patient does not experience adverse effects; and the patient understands and complies with the medication regimen.

IMPLEMENTATION

ACTION	RATIONALE
1. Gather equipment. Check each medication order against the original in the medical record, according to facility policy. Clarify any inconsistencies. Check the patient's medical record for allergies.	This comparison helps to identify errors that may have occurred when orders were transcribed. The primary care provider's order or prescription is the legal record of medication orders for each facility.
2. Know the actions, special nursing considerations, safe dose ranges, purpose of administration, and potential adverse effects of the medications to be administered. Consider the appropriateness of the medication for this patient.	This knowledge aids the nurse in evaluating the therapeutic effect of the medication in relation to the patient's disorder and can also be used to educate the patient about the medication.
3. Perform hand hygiene.	Hand hygiene prevents the spread of microorganisms.
4. Move the medication supply system to the outside of the patient's room or prepare for administration at the medication supply system in the medication area. Alternatively, access the medication administration supply system at or inside the patient's room.	Organization facilitates error-free administration and saves time.
5. Unlock the medication supply system or drawer. Enter pass code into the computer and scan employee identification, if required.	Locking the medication supply system or drawer safeguards each patient's medication supply. Facility accrediting organizations require medication supply systems to be locked when not in use. Entering pass code and scanning ID allows only authorized users into the computer system and identifies the user for documentation by the computer.
6. **Prepare medications for one patient at a time.**	This prevents errors in medication administration.
7. Read the eMAR/MAR and select the proper medication from the medication supply system or patient's medication drawer.	This is the *first* check of the medication label.
8. Compare the medication label with the eMAR/MAR (Figure 1). Check expiration dates and perform calculations, if necessary. Scan the bar code on the package, if required.	This is the *second* check of the label. Verify calculations with another nurse to ensure safety, if necessary.

FIGURE 1. Comparing medication label with eMAR.

ACTION

9. Prepare the required medications:

   a. *Unit dose packages:* **Do not open the wrapper until at the bedside.** Keep opioids and medications that require special nursing assessments separate from other medication packages.

   b. *Multidose containers:* When removing tablets or capsules from a multidose bottle, pour the necessary number into the bottle cap and then place the tablets or capsules in a medication cup. Break only scored tablets, if necessary, to obtain the proper dosage. Do not touch tablets or capsules with hands.

   c. *Liquid medication in multidose bottle:* When pouring liquid medications out of a multidose bottle, hold the bottle so the label is against the palm. Use the appropriate measuring device when pouring liquids, and read the amount of medication at the bottom of the meniscus at eye level (Figure 2). Wipe the lip of the bottle with a paper towel.

RATIONALE

Wrapper is kept intact because the label is needed for an additional safety check. Special assessments may be required before giving certain medications. These may include assessing vital signs and checking laboratory test results.

Pouring medication into the cap allows for easy return of excess medication to the bottle. Pouring tablets or capsules into your hand is unsanitary.

Liquid that may drip onto the label makes the label difficult to read. Accuracy is possible when the appropriate measuring device is used and then read accurately.

FIGURE 2. Measuring at eye level. (*Photo by B. Proud.*)

10. **Depending on facility policy, the third check of the label may occur at this point. If so, when all medications for one patient have been prepared, recheck the labels with the eMAR/MAR before taking the medications to the patient. However, many facilities require the third check to occur at the bedside, after identifying the patient.**

11. Replace any multidose containers in the patient's drawer or medication supply system. **Lock the medication supply system before leaving it.**

12. Transport medications to the patient's bedside carefully, and keep the medications in sight at all times.

13. **Ensure that the patient receives the medications at the correct time.**

 14. Perform hand hygiene and put on PPE, if indicated.

This *third* check ensures accuracy and helps to prevent errors. *Note:* Many facilities require the third check to occur at the bedside, after identifying the patient and before administration.

Locking the medication supply system or drawer safeguards the patient's medication supply. Facility accrediting organizations require medication supply systems to be locked when not in use.

Careful handling and close observation prevent accidental or deliberate disarrangement of medications.

Check facility policy, which may allow for administration within a period of 30 minutes before or 30 minutes after the designated time.

Hand hygiene and PPE prevent the spread of microorganisms. PPE is required based on transmission precautions.

(*continued*)

Skill 5-1 ▶ Administering Oral Medications *(continued)*

ACTION	**RATIONALE**

15. Identify the patient. Compare the information with the eMAR/MAR. The patient should be identified using at least two of the following methods (The Joint Commission, 2018):

Identifying the patient ensures the right patient receives the medications and helps prevent errors. The patient's room number or physical location is not used as an identifier (The Joint Commission, 2018). Replace the identification band if it is missing or inaccurate in any way.

a. Check the name on the patient's identification band (Figure 3).

b. Check the identification number on the patient's identification band.

c. Check the birth date on the patient's identification band.

d. Ask the patient to state his or her name and birth date, based on facility policy.

This requires a response from the patient, but illness and strange surroundings often cause patients to be confused.

16. Complete necessary assessments before administering medications. Check the patient's allergy bracelet or ask the patient about allergies. Explain the purpose and action of each medication to the patient.

Assessment is a prerequisite to administration of medications.

17. Scan the patient's bar code on the identification band, if required (Figure 4).

The bar code provides an additional check to ensure that the medication is given to the right patient.

FIGURE 3. Comparing patient's name and identification number with eMAR.

FIGURE 4. Scanning bar code on patient's identification bracelet. (*Photo by B. Proud.*)

18. Based on facility policy, the third check of the medication label may occur at this point. If so, recheck the label with the eMAR/MAR before administering the medications to the patient.

Many facilities require the *third* check to occur at the bedside, after identifying the patient and before administration. If facility policy directs the *third* check at this time, this *third* check ensures accuracy and helps prevent errors.

19. Assist the patient to an upright or lateral (side-lying) position.

Swallowing is facilitated by proper positioning. An upright or side-lying position protects the patient from aspiration.

20. Administer medications:

a. Offer water or other permitted fluids with pills, capsules, tablets, and some liquid medications.

Liquids facilitate swallowing of solid drugs. Some liquid drugs are intended to adhere to the pharyngeal area, in which case liquid is not offered with the medication.

b. Ask whether the patient prefers to take the medications by hand or in a cup.

This encourages the patient's participation in taking the medications.

ACTION	**RATIONALE**
21. Remain with the patient until each medication is swallowed. Never leave medication at the patient's bedside (Figure 5).	Unless you have seen the patient swallow the drug, the drug cannot be recorded as administered. The patient's health record is a legal record. Medications can be left at the bedside only with a prescriber's order.

FIGURE 5. Remaining with patient until each medication is swallowed.

22. Assist the patient to a comfortable position. Remove PPE, if used. Perform hand hygiene.	Promotes patient comfort. Proper removal of PPE prevents transmission of microorganisms. Hand hygiene deters the spread of microorganisms.
23. Document the administration of the medication immediately after administration. See Documentation section below.	Timely documentation helps to ensure patient safety.
24. Evaluate the patient's response to the medication within the appropriate time frame.	The patient needs to be evaluated for therapeutic and adverse effects from the medication.

EVALUATION

The expected outcomes have been met when the patient swallows the medication, does not aspirate, verbalizes an understanding of the medication, experiences the desired effect from the medication, and does not experience adverse effects.

DOCUMENTATION

Guidelines

Record each medication immediately after it is administered on the eMAR/MAR or health record using the required format. Include the date and time of administration (Figure 6). If using a barcode system, medication administration is automatically recorded when the bar code is scanned.

FIGURE 6. Recording each medication administered on eMAR.

(continued)

Skill 5-1 ▶ Administering Oral Medications *(continued)*

PRN medications require documentation of the reason for administration. Prompt recording avoids the possibility of accidentally repeating the administration of the drug. If the drug was refused or omitted, record this in the appropriate area on the medication record and notify the primary care provider. This verifies the reason medication was omitted and ensures that health care personnel providing care for the patient are aware of the occurrence. Recording administration of an opioid may require additional documentation on a controlled-substance record, stating drug count and other specific information. A record of fluid intake and output measurement is required.

Sample Documentation

DocuCare Practice documenting medication administration in *Lippincott DocuCare.*

8/6/20 0835 Patient states he is having constant stabbing leg pains. Rates pain as an 8/10. Percocet 2 tabs administered.

—K. Sanders, RN

8/6/20 0905 Patient resting comfortably. Rates leg pain as a 1/10.

—K. Sanders, RN

8/6/20 1300 Patient states he does not want pain medication, despite return of leg pain. States, "It made me feel woozy last time." Feelings discussed with patient. Patient agrees to take Percocet 1 tab at this time.

—K. Sanders, RN

8/6/20 1320 Percocet, 1 tablet given PO.

—K. Sanders, RN

UNEXPECTED SITUATIONS AND ASSOCIATED INTERVENTIONS

- *Patient states that it feels like medication is lodged in throat:* Offer patient more fluids to drink. If allowed, offer the patient bread or crackers to help move the medication to the stomach.
- *It is unclear whether the patient swallowed the medication:* Check in the patient's mouth, under tongue, and between cheek and gum. Patients with altered cognition may not be aware that the medication was not swallowed. Also, patients may "cheek" medications to avoid taking the medication or to save it for later use.
- *Patient vomits immediately or shortly after receiving oral medication:* Assess vomit, looking for pills or fragments. Do not re-administer medication without notifying the primary health care provider. If a whole pill is seen and can be identified, the primary health care provider may ask that the medication be administered again. If a pill is not seen or medications cannot be identified, do not re-administer the medication in order to prevent the patient from receiving too large a dose.
- *Child refuses to take oral medications:* Some medications may be mixed in a small amount of food, such as pudding or ice cream. Do not add the medication to liquids because the medication may alter the taste of liquids; if child then refuses to drink the rest of the liquid, you will not know how much of the medication was ingested. Use creativity when devising ways to administer medications to a child. See the section below, Infant and Child Considerations, for suggestions.
- *Capsule or tablet falls to the floor during administration:* Discard and obtain a new dose for administration. This prevents contamination and transmission of microorganisms.
- *Patient refuses medication:* Explore the reason for the patient's refusal. Review the rationale for use of the drug, explain the risk of refusal, and any other information that may be appropriate. If you are unable to administer the medication despite education and discussion, document the omission and any education and/or explanation provided related to attempts to facilitate administration according to facility policy. The primary care provider should be informed of the refusal when the omission poses a specific threat to the patient (Kee et al., 2015).

SPECIAL CONSIDERATIONS

General Considerations

- Some liquid medication preparations, such as suspensions and emulsions, require agitation to ensure even distribution of medication in the solution. Be familiar with the specific requirements for medications you are administering.

- Place medications intended for sublingual absorption under the patient's tongue. Instruct the patient to allow the medication to dissolve completely. Reinforce the importance of not swallowing the medication tablet.
- Some oral medications are provided in powdered forms. Verify the correct liquid in which to dissolve the medication for administration. This information is usually included on the package. Verify any unclear instructions with a pharmacist or medication reference. If there is more than one possible liquid in which to dissolve the medication, include the patient in the decision process; patients may find one choice more palatable than another.
- Ongoing assessment is an important part of nursing care for both evaluation of patient response to administered medications and early detection of adverse drug reactions. If an adverse effect is suspected, withhold further medication doses and notify the patient's primary care provider. Additional intervention is based on type of reaction and patient assessment.
- If the patient questions a medication order or states the medication is different from the usual dose, always recheck and clarify with the original order and/or primary care provider before giving the medication.
- If the patient's level of consciousness is altered or his or her swallowing is impaired, check with the primary care provider to clarify the route of administration or alternative forms of medication. This may also be a solution for a pediatric or a confused patient who is refusing to take a medication.
- Patients with poor vision can request large-type labels on medication containers. A magnifying lens also may be helpful.
- Provide written medication information to reinforce discussion and education in the appropriate language, if the patient is literate. If the patient is unable to read, provide written information to family or significant other, if appropriate. Written information should be at a 5th-grade level to ensure ease of understanding.
- If the patient has difficulty swallowing tablets, it may be appropriate to crush the medication to facilitate administration. However, not all medications can be crushed or altered; long-acting and slow-release drugs are examples of medications that cannot be crushed. Therefore, it is important to consult a medication reference and/or pharmacist. If the medication can be crushed, use a pill-crusher or mortar and pestle to grind the tablet into a powder. Crush each pill one at a time. Dissolve the powder with water or other recommended liquid in a liquid medication cup, keeping each medication separate from the others. Keep the package label with the medication cup for future comparison of information. Combine the crushed medication with a small amount of soft food, such as applesauce or pudding, to facilitate administration.

Infant and Child Considerations

- Special devices, such as oral syringes and calibrated nipples, are available in a pharmacy to ensure accurate dose calculations for young children and infants.
- Some creative ways to administer medications to children include the following: have a "tea party" with medicine cups; place oral syringe (without needle) or dropper in the space between the cheek and gum and slowly administer the medication; save a special treat for after the medication administration (e.g., movie, playroom time, or a special food, if allowed).
- If a medication has an objectionable taste, warn the child if he or she is old enough to understand. Failing to warn the child is likely to decrease the child's trust in the nurse. Do not lie to a child about medication administration.
- Caution caregivers to remove and dispose of plastic syringe caps present on the end of syringes before drug administration to reduce the risk of choking. Companies manufacture syringes labeled "oral use" without the caps on them and should be considered for use (Grissinger, 2014; ISMP, 2012b).

Older Adult Considerations

- Older adults with arthritis may have difficulty opening childproof caps. On request, the pharmacist can substitute a cap that is easier to open. A rubber band twisted around the cap may provide a more secure grip for older adults.
- Consider large-print written medication information, when appropriate.
- Physiologic changes associated with the aging process, including decreased gastric motility, muscle mass, acid production, and blood flow, can affect patient's response to medication, including drug absorption and increased risk of adverse effects. Older adults are more likely to take multiple drugs, so drug interactions in the older adult are a very real and dangerous problem (Adams et al., 2017).

(continued)

Skill 5-1 ▶ Administering Oral Medications *(continued)*

Home Care Considerations

- Encourage the patient to discard expired prescription medications based on label instructions or community guidelines.
- Discuss safe storage of medications when there are children and pets in the home environment.
- Discuss with parents the difference in over-the-counter medications made for infants and medications made for children. Many times parents do not realize that there are different strengths to the actual medications, leading to under- or overdosing.
- Encourage patients to carry a card listing all medications they take, including dosage and frequency, in case of an emergency.
- Discuss the importance of using an appropriate measuring device for liquid medications. Caution patients not to use eating utensils for measuring medications; use a liquid medication cup, oral syringe, or measuring spoon to provide accurate dosing.

EVIDENCE FOR PRACTICE ▶

MEDICATION ERRORS

Medication errors occur frequently and are a serious problem in health care. Medication errors may have serious consequences. Health care providers, including nurses, have a responsibility to prevent medication errors. What nursing practices may help improve the medication administration process?

Related Research

Niemann, D., Bertsche, A., Meyrath, D., et al. (2015). A prospective three-step intervention study to prevent medication errors in drug handling in paediatric care. *Journal of Clinical Nursing, 24*(1/2), 101–114.

This study investigated errors in drug handling by pediatric nurses on one unit of a university children's hospital. Medication errors on the unit were tracked before the intervention to provide a baseline. Errors were tracked again after the three steps of the intervention were completed. Four pharmacists, trained to monitor and document drug-handling processes using a developed checklist, monitored drug handling during morning medication administration for 20 working days. Each error on the checklist was assessed in an independent survey by an expert panel and assigned a clinical relevance value. Following baseline monitoring, nurse participants completed a survey to detect their knowledge regarding drug handling. Each nurse then participated in three education interventions, with content based on individual responses to the questionnaire. Nursing education targeting different causes of errors included a three-page handout addressing knowledge deficits; an hour-long training course addressing errors caused by rule violations and slips; and a comprehensive reference book addressing knowledge-, memory-, and rule-based errors. A total of 37 nurses, including 14 student nurses, agreed to participate, and 83% of the licensed participants specialized in pediatric care. Medications were administered to a total of 195 patients during the four monitoring periods, with a total of 1,920 drug-handling processes. The number of patients subjected to at least one medication error in drug handling decreased from 88% at baseline to 49% after the third intervention. The overall frequency of errors decreased form 91% to 26%. The authors concluded that interventions targeting the different causes of errors is an effective means to reduce medication errors and must be multifactorial.

Relevance to Nursing Practice

Medication administration is an important nursing responsibility. Nurses need to be aware of the factors that contribute to medication errors and work to reduce these factors in their practice. Nurses have a responsibility to be familiar with, and conform to, facility policies, as well as to maintain professional competency in regard to current and best practice guidelines.

Refer to thePoint® for additional research on related nursing topics.

Skill 5-2 ▶ Administering Medications via a Gastric Tube

Patients with a gastrointestinal tube (nasogastric, nasointestinal, percutaneous endoscopic gastrostomy [PEG], or jejunostomy [J] tube) often receive medication through the tube. Care of the patient with an enteral feeding tube is described in Chapter 11. Use liquid medications, when possible, because they are readily absorbed and less likely to cause tube occlusions. Dilute thick suspensions as recommended (Bankhead et al., 2009; Best & Wilson, 2011). Certain solid dosage medications can be crushed and combined with liquid. Crush each pill, one at a time, grinding to a fine powder and mix with 15 to 30 mL of water before delivery through the tube, keeping each medication separate from the others and flushing with water between each medication. The medications may not be physically or chemically compatible; mixing them can lead to tube obstruction or altered therapeutic actions (Bankhead et al.; Best & Wilson). Some sources recommend sterile water for medication administration, as the chemical contaminants in tap water can potentiate drug–drug interactions (Bankhead et al.). In addition, sterile water should be used for tube flushes in immunocompromised or critically ill patients (Bankhead et al.; Allen, 2015).

Certain capsules may be opened, emptied into liquid, and administered through the tube (Williams, 2008). **Not all medications can be crushed or altered; long-acting and slow-release drugs are examples of medications that cannot be crushed.** Check manufacturer's recommendations and/or with a pharmacist to verify. In addition, the absorption (e.g., phenytoin) and/or effect (carbidopa/levodopa) of some medications are altered when co-administered with enteral feeding formulas (Zhu & Zhou, 2013). Nurses must know procedures for and the latest evidence on drug administration by nasogastric and gastric tubes (Zhu & Zhou). Once prepared, keep the package label with the medication cup for future comparison of information.

DELEGATION CONSIDERATIONS

The administration of medications via a gastric tube is not delegated to nursing assistive personnel (NAP) or to unlicensed assistive personnel (UAP). Depending on the state's nurse practice act and the organization's policies and procedures, the administration of medications via a gastric tube may be delegated to licensed practical/vocational nurses (LPN/LVNs). The decision to delegate must be based on careful analysis of the patient's needs and circumstances, as well as the qualifications of the person to whom the task is being delegated. Refer to the Delegation Guidelines in Appendix A.

EQUIPMENT

- Irrigation set (60-mL syringe and irrigation container)
- Medications
- Tap water or sterile water (or normal saline), for irrigation, depending on facility policy
- Gloves
- Additional PPE, as indicated

ASSESSMENT

Assess the appropriateness of the drug for the patient. Review medical history, allergy, assessment, and laboratory data that may influence drug administration. Research each medication to be given, especially for mode of action, side effects, nursing implications, ability to be crushed, and whether the medication should be given with or without food. Verify patient name, dose, route, and time of administration. Assess patient's knowledge of the medication and the reason for its administration. If the patient has a knowledge deficit about the medication, this may be the appropriate time to begin educating the patient about the medication. Auscultate the abdomen for evidence of bowel sounds. Palpate the abdomen for tenderness and distention. Ascertain the time of the patient's last bowel movement and measure abdominal girth, if appropriate. If the medication may affect the patient's vital signs, assess them before administration. If the medication is for pain relief, assess the patient's pain level before and after administration.

(continued)

Skill 5-2 ▶ Administering Medications via a Gastric Tube *(continued)*

NURSING DIAGNOSIS	Determine the related factors for the nursing diagnoses based on the patient's current status. Possible nursing diagnoses may include:

- Deficient knowledge
- Risk for aspiration
- Risk for injury

OUTCOME IDENTIFICATION AND PLANNING	The expected outcome to achieve is that the patient receives the medication via the tube and experiences the intended effect of the medication. In addition, the patient verbalizes knowledge of the medications given; the patient remains free from adverse effects and injury; and the gastric tube remains patent.

IMPLEMENTATION

ACTION	RATIONALE
1. Gather equipment. Check each medication order against the original in the medical record, according to facility policy. Clarify any inconsistencies. Check the patient's health record for allergies.	This comparison helps to identify errors that may have occurred when orders were transcribed. The primary care provider's order or prescription is the legal record of medication orders for each facility.
2. Know the actions, special nursing considerations, safe dose ranges, purpose of administration, and adverse effects of the medications to be administered. Consider the appropriateness of the medication for this patient.	This knowledge aids the nurse in evaluating the therapeutic effect of the medication in relation to the patient's disorder and can also be used to educate the patient about the medication.
3. Perform hand hygiene.	Hand hygiene prevents the spread of microorganisms.
4. Move the medication supply system to the outside of the patient's room or prepare for administration at the medication supply system in the medication area. Alternatively, access the medication administration supply system at or inside the patient's room.	Organization facilitates error-free administration and saves time.
5. Unlock the medication supply system or drawer. Enter pass code into the computer and scan employee identification, if required.	Locking the medication supply system or drawer safeguards each patient's medication supply. Facility accrediting organizations require medication supply systems to be locked when not in use. Entering pass code and scanning ID allows only authorized users into the computer system and identifies the user for documentation by the computer.
6. **Prepare medications for one patient at a time.**	This prevents errors in medication administration.
7. Read the eMAR/MAR and select the proper medication from the medication supply system or patient's medication drawer.	This is the *first* check of the label.
8. Compare the label with the eMAR/MAR. Check expiration dates and perform calculations, if necessary. Scan the bar code on the package, if required.	This is the *second* check of the label. Verify calculations with another nurse to ensure safety, if necessary.
9. Check to see if medications to be administered come in a liquid form. **If pills or capsules are to be given, check with pharmacy or drug reference to verify the ability to crush tablets or open capsules.**	To prevent the tube from becoming clogged, all medications should be given in liquid form whenever possible. Medications in extended-release formulations should not be crushed before administration.

ACTION	RATIONALE

10. Prepare medication.

  Pills: Using a pill crusher, crush each pill one at a time. Dissolve the powder with water or other recommended liquid in a liquid medication cup, keeping each medication separate from the others. Keep the package label with the medication cup, for future comparison of information.

Some medications require dissolution in liquid other than water. The medications may not be physically or chemically compatible; mixing them can lead to tube obstruction or altered therapeutic actions (Bankhead et al., 2009; Best & Wilson, 2011). The label is needed for an additional safety check. Some medications require pre-administration assessments.

  Liquid: When pouring liquid medications from a multidose bottle, hold the bottle with the label against the palm. Use the appropriate measuring device when pouring liquids, and read the amount of medication at the bottom of the meniscus at eye level (Refer to Step 9c in Skill 5-1). Wipe the lip of the bottle with a paper towel.

Liquid that may drip onto the label makes the label difficult to read. Accuracy is possible when the appropriate measuring device is used and then read accurately.

11. **Depending on facility policy, the third check of the label may occur at this point. If so, when all medications for one patient have been prepared, recheck the labels with the eMAR/MAR before taking the medications to the patient. However, many facilities require the third check to occur at the bedside, after identifying the patient.**

This *third* check ensures accuracy and helps to prevent errors. *Note:* Many facilities require the *third* check to occur at the bedside, after identifying the patient and before administration.

12. Replace any multidose containers in the patient's drawer or medication supply system.

Proper storage safeguards medications.

13. **Lock the medication supply system before leaving it.**

Locking the medication supply system or drawer safeguards the patient's medication supply. Facility accrediting organizations require medication supply systems to be locked when not in use.

14. Transport medications to the patient's bedside carefully, and keep the medications in sight at all times.

Careful handling and close observation prevent accidental or deliberate disarrangement of medications.

15. **Ensure that the patient receives the medications at the correct time.**

Check facility policy, which may allow for administration within a period of 30 minutes before or 30 minutes after the designated time.

 16. Perform hand hygiene and put on PPE, if indicated.

Hand hygiene and PPE prevent the spread of microorganisms. PPE is required based on transmission precautions.

 17. **Identify the patient. Compare the information with the eMAR/MAR. The patient should be identified using at least two of the following methods (The Joint Commission, 2018):**

Identifying the patient ensures the right patient receives the medications and helps prevent errors. The patient's room number or physical location is not used as an identifier (The Joint Commission, 2018). Replace the identification band if it is missing or inaccurate in any way.

  a. Check the name on the patient's identification band.

  b. Check the identification number on the patient's identification band.

This requires a response from the patient, but illness and strange surroundings often cause patients to be confused.

  c. Check the birth date on the patient's identification band.

  d. Ask the patient to state his or her name and birth date, based on facility policy.

18. **Complete necessary assessments before administering medications. Check the patient's allergy bracelet or ask the patient about allergies. Explain what you are going to do, and the reason for doing it, to the patient.**

Assessment is a prerequisite to administration of medications. Explanation relieves anxiety and facilitates cooperation.

(continued)

Skill 5-2 ▶ Administering Medications via a Gastric Tube *(continued)*

ACTION	RATIONALE
19. Scan the patient's bar code on the identification band, if required (Figure 1).	This provides an additional check to ensure that the medication is given to the right patient.
20. **Based on facility policy, the third check of the label may occur at this point. If so, recheck the labels with the eMAR/MAR before administering the medications to the patient.**	Many facilities require the *third* check to occur at the bedside, after identifying the patient and before administration. If facility policy directs the *third* check at this time, this *third* check ensures accuracy and helps to prevent errors.
21. Assist the patient to the high-Fowler's position, unless contraindicated.	This reduces the risk of aspiration.
22. Put on gloves.	Gloves prevent contact with mucous membranes and body fluids.
23. If patient is receiving continuous tube feedings, pause the tube-feeding pump (Figure 2).	If the pump is not stopped, tube feeding will flow out of the tube and onto the patient.

FIGURE 1. Scanning bar code on the patient's identification bracelet. (*Photo by B. Proud.*)

FIGURE 2. Pausing feeding pump. (*Photo by B. Proud.*)

24. Pour the water into the irrigation container. Measure 30 mL of water. Apply clamp on feeding tube, if present. Alternatively, pinch gastric tube below port with fingers, or position stopcock to correct direction. Open port on gastric tube delegated to medication administration (Figure 3) or disconnect tubing for feeding from gastric tube and place cap on end of feeding tubing.	Fluid is ready for flushing of the tube. Applying clamp, folding the tube over, and clamping, or the correct positioning of the stopcock prevents any backflow of gastric drainage. Covering end of feeding tubing prevents contamination.

FIGURE 3. Pinching gastric tubing to prevent backflow of gastric drainage and opening medication administration port. (*Photo by B. Proud.*)

ACTION

25. **Check tube placement, depending on type of tube and facility policy.** Refer to Chapter 11.

26. Note the amount of any residual. Refer to Chapter 11. Replace residual back into stomach, based on facility policy.

27. Apply clamp on feeding tube, if present. Alternatively, pinch the gastric tube below port with fingers, or position stop-cock to correct direction. Remove 60-mL syringe from gastric tube. Remove the plunger of the syringe. Reinsert the syringe in the gastric tube without the plunger. Pour 30 mL of water into the syringe (Figure 4). **Unclamp the tube and allow the water to enter the stomach via gravity infusion.**

28. Administer the first dose of medication by pouring it into the syringe (Figure 5). Follow with a 5- to 10-mL water flush between medication doses. Follow the last dose of medication with 30 to 60 mL of water flush.

FIGURE 4. Pouring water into syringe inserted in gastric tube. (*Photo by B. Proud.*)

29. Clamp the tube, remove the syringe, and replace the feeding tubing. If a stopcock is used, position it to correct direction. If a tube medication port was used, cap the port. Unclamp the gastric tube and restart tube feeding, if appropriate for medications administered.

30. Remove gloves. Assist the patient to a comfortable position. If receiving a tube feeding, the head of the bed must remain elevated at least 30 degrees.

31. Remove additional PPE, if used. Perform hand hygiene.

32. Document the administration of the medication immediately after administration. See Documentation section below.

33. Evaluate the patient's response to the medication within the appropriate time frame.

RATIONALE

Tube placement must be confirmed before administering anything through the tube to avoid inadvertent instillation in the respiratory tract.

Research findings are inconclusive on the benefit of returning gastric volumes to the stomach or intestine to avoid fluid or electrolyte imbalance, which has been accepted practice. Consult facility policy concerning this practice.

Clamping prevents backflow of gastric drainage. Flushing the tube ensures that all the residual is cleared from the tube.

Flushing between medications prevents any possible interactions between the medications. Flushing at the end maintains tube patency, prevents blockage by medication particles, and ensures all doses enter the stomach.

FIGURE 5. Pouring medication into syringe inserted in gastric tube. (*Photo by B. Proud.*)

Some medications require the holding of the tube feeding for a certain period of time after administration. Consult a drug reference or a pharmacist.

Ensures patient comfort. Keeping the head of the bed elevated helps prevent aspiration.

Proper removal of PPE reduces the risk for infection transmission and contamination of other items. Hand hygiene prevents the spread of microorganisms.

Timely documentation helps to ensure patient safety.

The patient needs to be evaluated for therapeutic and adverse effects from the medication.

(continued)

Skill 5-2 ▶ Administering Medications via a Gastric Tube *(continued)*

EVALUATION	The expected outcome has been met when the patient receives the prescribed medications and experiences the intended effects of the medications administered. In addition, the patient demonstrates a patent and functioning gastric tube, verbalizes knowledge of the medications given, and remains free from adverse effects and injury.

DOCUMENTATION *Guidelines*	Document the administration of the medication immediately after administration, including date, time, dose, and route of administration on the eMAR/MAR or record using the required format. If using a bar-code system, medication administration is automatically recorded when the bar code is scanned. PRN medications require documentation of the reason for administration. Prompt recording avoids the possibility of accidentally repeating the administration of the drug. Record the amount of gastric residual, if appropriate. Record the amount of liquid given on the intake and output record. If the drug was refused or omitted, record this in the appropriate area on the medication record and notify the primary care provider. This verifies the reason medication was omitted and ensures that health care personnel providing care for the patient are aware of the occurrence.

UNEXPECTED SITUATIONS AND ASSOCIATED INTERVENTIONS	• *Medication enters tube and then tube becomes clogged:* Attach a 60-mL syringe onto end of tube. Pull back and then lightly apply pressure to plunger in a repetitive motion. This may dislodge the medication. Try using warm water or air and gentle pressure to remove the clog. Carbonated sodas, such as colas, and meat tenderizers have not been shown effective in removing clogs in feeding tubes. Never use a stylet to unclog tubes. If the medication does not move through the tube, notify the primary care provider. The tube may have to be replaced.

SPECIAL CONSIDERATIONS	• If medications are being administered via an NG tube that is attached to suction, the tube should remain clamped, off suction, for a period of time after medication administration. This allows for medication absorption before returning to suction. Check facility policy and drug reference for specific drug requirements. • If necessary to use plunger in irrigation syringe to administer medications, instill gently and slowly. Gravity administration is considered best to avoid excess pressure. • Give medications separately and flush with water between each drug. Some medications may interact with each other or become less effective if mixed with other drugs. • If the patient is receiving tube feedings, review information about the drugs to be administered. Absorption of some drugs, such as phenytoin, is affected by tube feeding formulas. Discontinue a continuous tube feeding and leave the tube clamped for the required period of time before and after the medication has been given, according to the reference and facility protocol. • Ongoing assessment is an important part of nursing care for both evaluation of patient response to administered medications and early detection of adverse drug reactions. If an adverse effect is suspected, withhold further medication doses and notify the patient's primary care provider. Additional intervention is based on type of reaction and patient assessment.

Skill 5-3 ▶ Removing Medication From an Ampule

	An **ampule** is a glass flask that contains a single dose of medication for parenteral administration. Because there is no way to prevent contamination of any unused portion of medication after the ampule is opened, discard any remaining medication if not all the medication is used for the prescribed dose. You must break the thin neck of the ampule to remove the medication.

DELEGATION CONSIDERATIONS	The preparation of medication from an ampule is not delegated to nursing assistive personnel (NAP) or to unlicensed assistive personnel (UAP). Depending on the state's nurse practice act and

the organization's policies and procedures, the preparation of medication from an ampule may be delegated to a licensed practical/vocational nurse (LPN/LVN). The decision to delegate must be based on careful analysis of the patient's needs and circumstances, as well as the qualifications of the person to whom the task is being delegated. Refer to the Delegation Guidelines in Appendix A.

EQUIPMENT	<ul><li>Sterile syringe and filter needle</li><li>Ampule of medication</li><li>Antimicrobial swab</li><li>Small, sterile gauze pad</li></ul>	<ul><li>Electronic Medication Administration Record (eMAR) or Medication Administration Record (MAR)</li></ul>

ASSESSMENT

Assess the appropriateness of the drug for the patient. Review medical history, allergy, assessment, and laboratory data that may influence drug administration. Assess the medication in the ampule for any particles or discoloration. Assess the ampule for any cracks or chips. Check expiration date before administering the medication. Verify patient name, dose, route, and time of administration.

NURSING DIAGNOSIS

Determine related factors for the nursing diagnoses based on the patient's current status. Appropriate nursing diagnoses may include:

- Risk for infection
- Deficient knowledge
- Risk for injury

OUTCOME IDENTIFICATION AND PLANNING

The expected outcome to achieve when removing medication from an ampule is that the medication is removed in a sterile manner; the medication is free from glass shards and contamination; and the proper dose prepared.

IMPLEMENTATION

ACTION	**RATIONALE**
1. Gather equipment. Check the medication order against the original order in the medical record, according to facility policy. Clarify any inconsistencies. Check the patient's health record for allergies.	This comparison helps to identify errors that may have occurred when orders were transcribed. The primary care provider's order or prescription is the legal record of medication orders for each facility.
2. Know the actions, special nursing considerations, safe dose ranges, purpose of administration, and adverse effects of the medications to be administered. Consider the appropriateness of the medication for this patient.	This knowledge aids the nurse in evaluating the therapeutic effect of the medication in relation to the patient's disorder and can also be used to educate the patient about the medication.
3. Perform hand hygiene.	Hand hygiene prevents the spread of microorganisms.
4. Move the medication supply system to the outside of the patient's room or prepare for administration at the medication supply system in the medication area. Alternatively, access the medication administration supply system at or inside the patient's room.	Organization facilitates error-free administration and saves time.
5. Unlock the medication supply system or drawer. Enter pass code and scan employee identification, if required.	Locking the medication supply system or drawer safeguards each patient's medication supply. Facility accrediting organizations require medication supply systems to be locked when not in use. Entering pass code and scanning ID allows only authorized users into the computer system and identifies the user for documentation by the computer.

(continued)

Skill 5-3 Removing Medication From an Ampule *(continued)*

ACTION	RATIONALE
6. **Prepare medications for one patient at a time.**	This prevents errors in medication administration.
7. Read the eMAR/MAR and select the proper medication from the medication supply system or the patient's medication drawer.	This is the *first* check of the label.
8. Compare the label with the eMAR/MAR. Check expiration dates and perform calculations, if necessary. Scan the bar code on the package, if required.	This is the *second* check of the label. Verify calculations with another nurse to ensure safety, if necessary.
9. Tap the stem of the ampule (Figure 1) or twist your wrist quickly (Figure 2) while holding the ampule vertically.	This facilitates movement of medication in the stem to the body of the ampule.

FIGURE 1. Tapping stem of the ampule.

FIGURE 2. Twisting wrist quickly while holding ampule vertically.

10. Using the antimicrobial swab, scrub the neck of the ampule (Dolan et al, 2016). Wrap a small sterile gauze pad around the neck of the ampule.	Scrubbing the neck is necessary to reduce the risk of contamination (Dolan et al., 2016). Wrapping the neck of the ampule with gauze protects your fingers from the glass as the ampule is broken.
11. Breaking away from your body, use a snapping motion to break off the top of the ampule along the scored line at its neck (Figure 3). **Always break away from your body.**	This protects your face and fingers from any shattered glass fragments.

FIGURE 3. Using a snapping motion to break top of ampule.

ACTION	RATIONALE

12. Attach filter needle to syringe. Remove the cap from the filter needle by pulling it straight off.

Use of a filter needle prevents the accidental withdrawing of small glass particles with the medication. Pulling the cap off in a straight manner prevents accidental needlestick.

13. Withdraw medication in the amount ordered plus a small amount more (approximately 30% more). **Do not inject air into the solution. While inserting the filter needle into the ampule, be careful not to touch the rim.** Use either of the following methods to withdraw the medication:

By withdrawing an additional small amount of medication, any air bubbles in the syringe can be displaced once the syringe is removed while allowing ample medication to remain in the syringe. The contents of the ampule are not under pressure; therefore, air is unnecessary and will cause the contents to overflow. The rim of the ampule is considered contaminated.

  a. Insert the tip of the needle into the ampule, which is upright on a flat surface, and withdraw fluid into the syringe (Figure 4). **Touch the plunger only at the knob.**

Handling the plunger only at the knob will keep the shaft of the plunger sterile.

  b. Insert the tip of the needle into the ampule and invert the ampule. Keep the needle centered and not touching the sides of the ampule. Withdraw fluid into syringe (Figure 5). **Touch the plunger only at the knob.**

Surface tension holds the fluids in the ampule when inverted. If the needle touches the sides or is removed and then reinserted into the ampule, surface tension is broken, and fluid runs out. Handling the plunger only at the knob will keep the shaft of the plunger sterile.

FIGURE 4. Withdrawing medication from upright ampule. (*Photo by B. Proud.*)

FIGURE 5. Withdrawing medication from inverted ampule. (*Photo by B. Proud.*)

14. Wait until the needle has been withdrawn to tap the syringe and expel the air carefully by pushing on the plunger. **Check the amount of medication in the syringe with the medication dose and discard any surplus, according to facility policy.**

Ejecting air into the solution increases pressure in the ampule and can force the medication to spill out over the ampule. Ampules may have overfill. Careful measurement ensures that the correct dose is withdrawn.

15. **Depending on facility policy, the third check of the label may occur at this point. If so, when all medications for one patient have been prepared, recheck the labels with the eMAR/MAR before taking the medications to the patient. However, many facilities require the third check to occur at the bedside, after identifying the patient.**

This *third* check ensures accuracy and helps to prevent errors. *Note:* Many facilities require the *third* check to occur at the bedside, after identifying the patient and before administration.

16. **Engage safety guard on filter needle and remove the needle. Discard the filter needle in a suitable container. Attach appropriate administration device to syringe.**

The filter needle used to draw up medication should not be used to administer the medication. This will prevent any glass shards from entering the patient during administration.

17. Discard the ampule in a suitable container.

Any medication that has not been removed from the ampule must be discarded because sterility of contents cannot be maintained in an opened ampule.

(*continued*)

Skill 5-3 ▶ Removing Medication From an Ampule *(continued)*

ACTION	RATIONALE
18. Lock the medication supply system before leaving it.	Locking the medication supply system safeguards the patient's medication supply. Facility accrediting organizations require medication supply systems to be locked when not in use.
19. Perform hand hygiene.	Hand hygiene deters the spread of microorganisms.
20. Proceed with administration, based on prescribed route.	See appropriate skill for prescribed route.

EVALUATION

The expected outcomes have been met when the medication is removed from the ampule in a sterile manner, is free from glass shards, and the proper dose is prepared.

DOCUMENTATION

Guidelines

It is not necessary to record the removal of the medication from the ampule. Prompt recording of administration of the medication is required immediately after it is administered.

UNEXPECTED SITUATIONS AND ASSOCIATED INTERVENTIONS

- *You cut yourself while trying to open the ampule:* Discard ampule and medication in case contamination has occurred. Clean and bandage the wound and obtain a new ampule. Report incident according to facility policy.
- *All of medication was not removed from the stem and insufficient medication remains in body of ampule:* Discard ampule and drawn medication. Obtain a new ampule and start over. Medication in original ampule stem is considered contaminated once neck of ampule has been placed on a nonsterile surface.
- *You inject air into inverted ampule, spraying medication:* Wash hands to remove any medication. If any medication has gotten into eyes, perform eye irrigation. Obtain a new ampule for medication dose. Report injury, if appropriate, according to facility policy.
- *Plunger becomes contaminated before inserted into ampule:* Discard needle and syringe and start over. If plunger is contaminated after medication is drawn into the syringe, it is not necessary to discard and start over. The contaminated plunger will enter the barrel of the syringe when pushing the medication out and will not come in contact with the medication and will not contaminate the medication.

SPECIAL CONSIDERATIONS

- When mixing medications in one syringe, preparation of medications in one syringe depends on how the medication is supplied. When preparing medications from an ampule and a vial, prepare the medication in the vial first. Draw up the medication in the ampule after the medication in the vial.

Skill 5-4 ▶ Removing Medication From a Vial

A **vial** is a glass bottle with a self-sealing stopper through which medication is removed. For safety in transporting and storing, the vial top is usually covered with a metal or plastic cap that can be removed easily. The self-sealing stopper that is then exposed is the means of entrance into the vial. Single-dose vials are used once, and then discarded, regardless of the amount of the drug that is used from the vial. Multidose vials contain several doses of medication and can be used multiple times. The Centers for Disease Control and Prevention (CDC) recommends that medications packaged as multiuse vials be assigned to a single patient whenever possible (CDC, n.d.b). In addition, it is recommended that the top of the vial be cleaned before each entry, and that a new sterile needle and syringe are used for each entry (CDC, 2011).

The medication contained in a vial can be in liquid or powder form. Powdered forms must be dissolved in an appropriate diluent before administration. The following skill reviews removing liquid medication from a vial. Refer to the accompanying Skill Variation for steps to reconstitute powdered medication.

DELEGATION CONSIDERATIONS	The preparation of medication from a vial is not delegated to nursing assistive personnel (NAP) or to unlicensed assistive personnel (UAP). Depending on the state's nurse practice act and the organization's policies and procedures, the preparation of medication from a vial may be delegated to licensed practical/vocational nurses (LPN/LVNs). The decision to delegate must be based on careful analysis of the patient's needs and circumstances, as well as the qualifications of the person to whom the task is being delegated. Refer to the Delegation Guidelines in Appendix A.
EQUIPMENT	• Sterile syringe and needle or blunt cannula (size depends on medication being administered) • Vial of medication • Antimicrobial swab • Second needle (optional) • Filter needle (optional) • Electronic Medication Administration Record (eMAR) or Medication Administration Record (MAR)
ASSESSMENT	Assess the appropriateness of the drug for the patient. Review assessment and laboratory data that may influence drug administration. Assess the medication in the vial for any discoloration or particles. Check expiration date before administering medication. Verify patient name, dose, route, and time of administration.
NURSING DIAGNOSIS	Determine related factors for the nursing diagnoses based on the patient's current status. Appropriate nursing diagnoses include: • Risk for infection • Deficient knowledge • Risk for injury
OUTCOME IDENTIFICATION AND PLANNING	The expected outcome to achieve when removing medication from a vial is withdrawal of the medication into a syringe in a sterile manner; the medication is free from contamination; and the proper dose is prepared.

IMPLEMENTATION

ACTION	**RATIONALE**
1. Gather equipment. Check the medication order against the original order in the medical record, according to facility policy. Clarify any inconsistencies. Check the patient's health record for allergies.	This comparison helps to identify errors that may have occurred when orders were transcribed. The primary care provider's order or prescription is the legal record of medication orders for each facility.
2. Know the actions, special nursing considerations, safe dose ranges, purpose of administration, and adverse effects of the medications to be administered. Consider the appropriateness of the medication for this patient.	This knowledge aids the nurse in evaluating the therapeutic effect of the medication in relation to the patient's disorder and can also be used to educate the patient about the medication.
3. Perform hand hygiene.	Hand hygiene deters the spread of microorganisms.
4. Move the medication supply system to the outside of the patient's room or prepare for administration at the medication supply system in the medication area. Alternatively, access the medication administration supply system at or inside the patient's room.	Organization facilitates error-free administration and saves time.

(continued)

Skill 5-4 ▶ Removing Medication From a Vial (continued)

ACTION	RATIONALE
5. Unlock the medication supply system or drawer. Enter pass code and scan employee identification, if required.	Locking the medication supply system or drawer safeguards each patient's medication supply. Facility accrediting organizations require medication supply systems to be locked when not in use. Entering pass code and scanning ID allows only authorized users into the system and identifies the user for documentation by the computer.
6. **Prepare medications for one patient at a time.**	This prevents errors in medication administration.
7. Read the eMAR/MAR and select the proper medication from the medication supply system or the patient's medication drawer.	This is the *first* check of the label.
8. Compare the label with the eMAR/MAR. Check expiration dates and perform calculations, if necessary. Scan the bar code on the package, if required.	This is the *second* check of the label. Verify calculations with another nurse to ensure safety, if necessary.
9. Remove the metal or plastic cap on the vial that protects the self-sealing stopper.	Cap needs to be removed to access medication in the vial.
10. **Scrub the self-sealing stopper top with the antimicrobial swab and allow to dry.**	Antimicrobial swab removes surface microbial contamination. Allowing the antimicrobial solution to dry completely (15 to 30 seconds) ensures complete antimicrobial effectiveness (Harper, 2014). Drying also prevents antimicrobial solution from entering the vial on the needle.
11. Remove the cap from the needle or blunt cannula by pulling it straight off. **If the vial in use is a multidose vial, touch the plunger only at the knob and draw back an amount of air into the syringe that is equal to the specific dose of medication to be withdrawn. If the vial in use is a single-use vial, there is no need to draw air into the syringe.**	Pulling the cap off in a straight manner prevents accidental needlestick injury. Handling the plunger only at the knob will keep the shaft of the plunger sterile. Because a vial is a sealed container, injection of an equal amount of air (before fluid is removed) is required to prevent the formation of a partial vacuum. If not enough air is injected, the negative pressure makes it difficult to withdraw the medication after repeated use.
12. Hold the vial on a flat surface. Pierce the self-sealing stopper in the center with the needle tip and inject the measured air into the space above the solution (Figure 1). **Do not inject air into the solution.** If the vial in use is a single-use vial, there is no need to inject air into the vial.	Air bubbled through the solution could result in withdrawal of an inaccurate amount of medication.

FIGURE 1. Injecting air with vial upright.

ACTION

13. Invert the vial. **Keep the tip of the needle or blunt cannula below the fluid level (Figure 2).**

14. Hold the vial in one hand and use the other to withdraw the medication. **Touch the plunger only at the knob. Draw up the prescribed amount of medication while holding the syringe vertically and at eye level (Figure 3).**

FIGURE 2. Positioning needle tip in solution.

15. If any air bubbles accumulate in the syringe, tap the barrel of the syringe sharply and move the needle past the fluid into the air space to re-inject the air bubble into the vial. Return the needle tip to the solution and continue withdrawal of the medication.

16. After the correct dose is withdrawn, remove the needle from the vial and carefully replace the cap over the needle. Some facilities require changing the needle, if one was used to withdraw the medication, before administering the medication.

17. **Check the amount of medication in the syringe with the medication dose and discard any surplus.**

18. **Depending on facility policy, the third check of the label may occur at this point. If so, when all medications for one patient have been prepared, recheck the labels with the eMAR/MAR before taking the medications to the patient. However, many facilities require the third check to occur at the bedside, after identifying the patient.**

RATIONALE

This prevents air from being aspirated into the syringe.

Handling the plunger only at the knob will keep the shaft of the plunger sterile. Holding the syringe at eye level facilitates accurate reading, and the vertical position makes removal of air bubbles from the syringe easy.

FIGURE 3. Withdrawing medication at eye level.

Removal of air bubbles is necessary to ensure an accurate dose of medication.

Capping prevents contamination of the needle and protects against accidental needlesticks. A one-handed recap method may be used as long as care is taken not to contaminate the needle during the process. Changing the needle may be necessary because passing the needle through the stopper on the vial may dull the needle. In addition, it ensures the tip of the needle is free from medication residue, significantly reducing pain intensity associated with the injection (Ağaç & Günes, 2010).

Careful measurement ensures that the correct dose is withdrawn.

This *third* check ensures accuracy and helps to prevent errors. *Note:* Many facilities require the *third* check to occur at the bedside, after identifying the patient and before administration.

(*continued*)

Skill 5-4 ▶ Removing Medication From a Vial *(continued)*

ACTION	**RATIONALE**
19. If a multidose vial is being used, label the vial with the date and time opened and the beyond-use date (see Special Considerations), and store the vial containing the remaining medication according to facility policy. Limit the use of multiple-dose vials and dedicate them to a single patient whenever possible (CDC, n.d.b).	Because the vial is sealed, the medication inside remains sterile and can be used for future injections. Labeling the opened vials with a date, time, and beyond-use date limits its use after a specific time period. Limiting use of multiple-dose vials and dedicating their use to a single patient when possible limits risk of contamination and transfer of microorganisms (CDC, n.d.b; Dolan et al., 2016).
20. Lock the medication supply system before leaving it.	Locking the medication supply system or drawer safeguards the patient's medication supply. Facility accrediting organizations require medication supply systems to be locked when not in use.
21. Perform hand hygiene.	Hand hygiene deters the spread of microorganisms.
22. Proceed with administration, based on prescribed route.	See appropriate skill for prescribed route.

EVALUATION

The expected outcomes have been met when the medication was withdrawn into the syringe in a sterile manner and is free from contamination, and the proper dose is prepared.

DOCUMENTATION

Guidelines

It is not necessary to record the removal of the medication from a vial. Prompt recording of administration of the medication is required immediately after it is administered.

UNEXPECTED SITUATIONS AND ASSOCIATED INTERVENTIONS

- *A piece of self-sealing stopper is noticed floating in the medication in the syringe:* Discard the syringe, needle, and vial. Obtain a new vial, syringe, and needle and prepare dose as ordered.
- *As the needle attached to the syringe filled with air is inserted into vial, the plunger is immediately pulled down:* If possible to withdraw medication, continue steps as explained above. If such a vacuum has formed that this is impossible, remove syringe and inject more air into the vial.
- *Plunger is contaminated before injecting air into vial:* Discard needle and syringe and start over.
- *Plunger is contaminated after medication is drawn into syringe:* It is not necessary to discard needle and syringe and start over. The contaminated plunger will enter the barrel of the syringe when pushing the medication out and will not come in contact with the medication, and therefore will not contaminate the medication.

SPECIAL CONSIDERATIONS

- When mixing medications in one syringe, preparation of medications in one syringe depends on how the medication is supplied. When using a single-dose vial and a multidose vial, inject air into the multidose vial and draw the medication in the multidose vial into the syringe first. This prevents the contents of the multidose vial from being contaminated with the medication in the single-dose vial. The steps to follow when preparing medications from two multidose vials in one syringe are outlined in Skill 5-5.
- Vials used to draw two or more medications into a single syringe must be discarded after use (Dolan et al., 2016).
- Do not administer medication from a single-dose vial to multiple patients (CDC, n.d.b).
- Limit the use of multiple-dose vials and dedicate them to a single patient whenever possible (CDC, n.d.b).
- Multiple-dose vials must be labeled with a beyond-use date when first opened, as indicated by facility policy (Dolan et al., 2016).

Skill Variation > Reconstituting Powdered Medication in a Vial

Drugs that are unstable in liquid form are often provided in a dry powder form. The powder must be mixed with the correct amount of appropriate solution (diluent) to prepare the medication for administration. Verify the correct amount and correct solution type for the specific medication prescribed. This information is found on the vial label, package insert, in a drug reference, an on-line pharmacy source, or from the pharmacist. To reconstitute powdered medication:

1. Gather equipment. Check the medication order against the original order in the medical record, according to facility policy.
2. Know the actions, special nursing considerations, safe dose ranges, purpose of administration, and adverse effects of the medications to be administered. Consider the appropriateness of the medication for this patient.

3. Perform hand hygiene.

4. Move the medication supply system to the outside of the patient's room or prepare for administration at the medication supply system in the medication area. Alternatively, access the medication administration supply system at or inside the patient's room.
5. Unlock the medication supply system or drawer. Enter pass code and scan employee identification, if required.
6. **Prepare medications for one patient at a time.**
7. Read the eMAR/MAR and select the proper medication and diluent from medication supply system or from the patient's medication drawer. This is the *first* check of the medication label.
8. Compare the labels with the eMAR/MAR. This is the *second* check of the medication label. Check expiration dates and perform calculations, check medication calculation with another nurse. Scan the bar code on the package, if required.

9. Remove the metal or plastic cap on the medication vial and diluent vial that protects the self-sealing stoppers.
10. Scrub the self-sealing tops on both the diluent and powdered medication vials with the antimicrobial swab and allow to dry.
11. **Draw up the appropriate amount of diluent into the syringe.**
12. Insert the needle or blunt cannula through the center of the self-sealing stopper on the powdered medication vial.
13. Inject the diluent into the powdered medication vial.
14. Remove the needle or blunt cannula from the vial and replace cap.
15. **Gently agitate the vial to mix the powdered medication and the diluent completely. Do not shake the vial.**
16. **Draw up the prescribed amount of medication while holding the syringe vertically and at eye level.**
17. After the correct dose is withdrawn, remove the needle from the vial and carefully replace the cap over the needle. Some facilities require changing the needle, if one was used to withdraw the medication, before administering the medication.
18. **Check the amount of medication in the syringe with the medication dose and discard any surplus.**
19. **Depending on facility policy, the *third* check of the label may occur at this point. If so, recheck the label with the eMAR/MAR before taking the medications to the patient. However, many facilities require the third check to occur at the bedside, after identifying the patient.**
20. **Lock the medication supply system before leaving it.**

21. Perform hand hygiene.

22. Proceed with administration, based on prescribed route.

Skill 5-5 > Mixing Medications From Two Vials in One Syringe

Preparation of medications in one syringe depends on how the medication is supplied. When using two multidose vials, air is injected into both vials before withdrawing the first medication, to prevent the accidental injection of medication into the second vial. When using a single-dose vial and a multidose vial, air is injected into the multidose vial and the medication in the multidose vial is drawn into the syringe first. This prevents the contents of the multidose vial from being contaminated with the medication in the single-dose vial. The CDC recommends that medications packaged as multiuse vials be assigned to a single patient whenever possible (CDC, n.d.b). In addition, it is recommended that the top of the vial be cleaned before each entry, and that a new sterile needle and syringe are used before each entry (CDC, 2011).

(continued)

Skill 5-5 ▶ Mixing Medications From Two Vials in One Syringe *(continued)*

When considering mixing two medications in one syringe, you must ensure that the two drugs are compatible. Be aware of drug incompatibilities when preparing medications in one syringe. Certain medications are incompatible with other drugs in the same syringe. Other drugs have limited compatibility and should be administered within 15 minutes of preparation. Mixing more than two drugs in one syringe is not recommended. If it must be done, contact the pharmacist to determine the compatibility of the three drugs, as well as the compatibility of their pH values and the preservatives that may be present in each drug. A drug-compatibility table should be available to nurses who are preparing medications.

Insulin, with many types available for use, is an example of a medication that may be combined together in one syringe for injection. Insulins vary in their onset and duration of action and are classified as rapid acting, short acting, intermediate acting, and long acting (Frandsen & Pennington, 2014). Before administering any insulin, be aware of the onset time, peak, and duration of effects, and ensure that proper food is available. Be aware that some insulins, such as glargine and detemir, cannot be mixed with other insulins. Refer to a drug reference for a listing of the different types of insulin and action specific to each type.

Insulin is used as the sample medication in the steps outlined below for mixing two medications in one syringe. Insulin is typically available in multidose vials, and dosages are calculated in units. The scale commonly used is U100, which is based on 100 units of insulin contained in 1 mL of solution. An insulin syringe is also calibrated in units. Insulin is also available in injection pens, which eliminate the need to prepare two medications in one syringe. Insulin injection pens are prefilled devices that combine the insulin container and syringe. Patients attach a needle for each administration, dial a dose of insulin, and depress a plunger to administer the dose. Use of an insulin injection pen is outlined in the Skill Variation in Skill 5-7 on page 211.

DELEGATION CONSIDERATIONS	The preparation of medication from two vials is not delegated to nursing assistive personnel (NAP) or to unlicensed assistive personnel (UAP). Depending on the state's nurse practice act and the organization's policies and procedures, the preparation of medication from two vials may be delegated to licensed practical/vocational nurses (LPN/LVNs). The decision to delegate must be based on careful analysis of the patient's needs and circumstances, as well as the qualifications of the person to whom the task is being delegated. Refer to the Delegation Guidelines in Appendix A.
EQUIPMENT	The preparation of two types of insulin in one syringe is used as the example in the following procedure. • Two vials of medication (insulin in this example) • Sterile syringe (insulin syringe in this example) • Antimicrobial swabs • Electronic Medication Administration Record (eMAR) or Medication Administration Record (MAR)
ASSESSMENT	Assess the appropriateness of the drug for the patient. Review medical history, allergy, assessment, and laboratory data that may influence drug administration. Determine the compatibility of the two medications. Not all insulin can be mixed together. Assess the contents of each vial of insulin. It is very important to be familiar with the particular drug's properties to be able to assess the quality of the medication in the vial before withdrawal. Unmodified preparations of insulin typically appear as clear substances, so they should be without particles or foreign matter. Modified preparations of insulin are typically suspensions, so they do not appear as clear substances. Check the expiration date before administering the medication. Check the patient's blood glucose level, if appropriate, before administering the insulin. Verify patient name, dose, route, and time of administration.
NURSING DIAGNOSIS	Determine related factors for the nursing diagnoses based on the patient's current status. Appropriate nursing diagnoses include: • Risk for infection • Deficient knowledge • Risk for unstable blood glucose level

OUTCOME IDENTIFICATION AND PLANNING

The expected outcome to achieve when mixing two different types of medication in one syringe is the accurate withdrawal of the medication into a syringe in a sterile manner; the medication is free from contamination; and the proper dose is prepared.

IMPLEMENTATION

ACTION	RATIONALE
1. Gather equipment. Check medication order against the original order in the medical record, according to facility policy.	This comparison helps to identify errors that may have occurred when orders were transcribed. The primary care provider's order or prescription is the legal record of medication orders for each facility.
2. Know the actions, special nursing considerations, safe dose ranges, purpose of administration, and adverse effects of the medications to be administered. Consider the appropriateness of the medication for this patient.	This knowledge aids the nurse in evaluating the therapeutic effect of the medication in relation to the patient's disorder and can also be used to educate the patient about the medication.
3. Perform hand hygiene.	Hand hygiene prevents the spread of microorganisms.
4. Move the medication supply system to the outside of the patient's room or prepare for administration at the medication supply system in the medication area. Alternatively, access the medication administration supply system at or inside the patient's room.	Organization facilitates error-free administration and saves time.
5. Unlock the medication supply system or drawer. Enter pass code and scan employee identification, if required.	Locking the supply system or drawer safeguards each patient's medication supply. Facility accrediting organizations require medication supply systems to be locked when not in use. Entering pass code and scanning ID allows only authorized users into the system and identifies the user for documentation by the computer.
6. Prepare medications for one patient at a time.	This prevents errors in medication administration.
7. Read the eMAR/MAR and select the proper medications from the medication supply system or the patient's medication drawer.	This is the *first* check of the label.
8. Compare the labels with the eMAR/MAR. Check expiration dates and perform dosage calculations, if necessary. Scan the bar code on the package, if required.	This is the *second* check of the labels. Verify calculations with another nurse to ensure safety, if necessary.
9. If necessary, remove the cap that protects the self-sealing stopper on each vial.	The cap protects the self-sealing top.
10. If medication is a suspension (e.g., a modified insulin, such as NPH insulin), roll and agitate the vial to mix it well.	There is controversy regarding how to mix insulin in suspension. Some sources advise rolling the vial; others advise shaking the vial. Consult facility policy. Regardless of the method used, it is essential that the suspension be mixed well to avoid administering an inconsistent dose.
11. Scrub the self-sealing stopper top with the antimicrobial swab and allow to dry.	Antimicrobial swab removes surface microbial contamination. Allowing the antimicrobial solution to dry completely (15 to 30 seconds) ensures complete antimicrobial effectiveness (Harper, 2014). Drying also prevents antimicrobial solution from entering the vial on the needle.
12. Remove cap from needle by pulling it straight off. Touch the plunger only at the knob. Draw back an amount of air into the syringe that is equal to the dose of modified insulin to be withdrawn.	Pulling the cap off in a straight manner prevents accidental needlestick. Handling the plunger only by the knob ensures sterility of the shaft of the plunger. Before fluid is removed, injection of an equal amount of air is required to prevent the formation of a partial vacuum, because a vial is a sealed container. If not enough air is injected, the negative pressure makes it difficult to withdraw the medication with repeated use.

(*continued*)

Skill 5-5 ▶ Mixing Medications From Two Vials in One Syringe   *(continued)*

ACTION	RATIONALE
13. Hold the modified vial on a flat surface. Pierce the self-sealing stopper in the center with the needle tip and inject the measured air into the space above the solution (Figure 1). Do not inject air into the solution. Withdraw the needle.	Unmodified insulin should never be contaminated with modified insulin. Placing air in the modified insulin first without allowing the needle to contact the insulin ensures that the second vial-entered (unmodified) insulin is not contaminated by the medication in the other vial. Air bubbled through the solution could result in withdrawal of an inaccurate amount of medication.
14. Draw back an amount of air into the syringe that is equal to the dose of unmodified insulin to be withdrawn.	A vial is a sealed container. Therefore, injection of an equal amount of air (before fluid is removed) is required to prevent the formation of a partial vacuum. If not enough air is injected, the negative pressure makes it difficult to withdraw the medication.
15. Hold the unmodified vial on a flat surface. Pierce the self-sealing stopper in the center with the needle tip and inject the measured air into the space above the solution (Figure 2). Do not inject air into the solution. Keep the needle in the vial.	Air bubbled through the solution could result in withdrawal of an inaccurate amount of medication.

FIGURE 1. Injecting air into modified insulin preparation.

FIGURE 2. Injecting air into unmodified insulin vial.

16. Invert the vial of unmodified insulin. Hold the vial in one hand and use the other to withdraw the medication. **Touch the plunger only at the knob. Draw up the prescribed amount of medication while holding the syringe at eye level and vertically (Figure 3). Turn the vial over and then remove the needle from the vial.**	Holding the syringe at eye level facilitates accurate reading, and the vertical position allows easy removal of air bubbles from the syringe. First dose is prepared and is not contaminated by insulin that contains modifiers.
17. Check that there are no air bubbles in the syringe.	The presence of air in the syringe would result in an inaccurate dose of medication.
18. **Check the amount of medication in the syringe with the medication dose and discard any surplus.**	Careful measurement ensures that correct dose is withdrawn.
19. **Recheck the vial label with the eMAR/MAR.**	This is the *third* check to ensure accuracy and to prevent errors. It must be checked now for the first medication in the syringe, as it is not possible to ensure accuracy once a second drug is in the syringe.
20. Calculate the endpoint on the syringe for the combined insulin amount by adding the number of units for each dose together.	Allows for accurate withdrawal of the second dose.

ACTION

21. Insert the needle into the modified vial and invert it, taking care not to push the plunger and inject medication from the syringe into the vial. Invert vial of modified insulin. Hold the vial in one hand and use the other to withdraw the medication. **Touch the plunger only at the knob. Draw up the prescribed amount of medication while holding the syringe at eye level and vertically (Figure 4). Take care to withdraw only the prescribed amount. Turn the vial over and then remove the needle from the vial. Carefully recap the needle. Carefully replace the cap over the needle.**

FIGURE 3. Withdrawing prescribed amount of unmodified insulin.

22. **Check the amount of medication in the syringe with the medication dose.**

23. **Depending on facility policy, the third check of the label may occur at this point. If so, recheck the label with the MAR before taking the medications to the patient. However, many facilities require the third check to occur at the bedside, after identifying the patient.**

24. **Label the vials with the date and time opened and beyond-use date, and store the vials containing the remaining medication, according to facility policy.**

25. **Lock the medication supply system before leaving it.**

  26. Perform hand hygiene.

27. Proceed with administration, based on prescribed route.

RATIONALE

Previous addition of air eliminates need to create positive pressure. Holding the syringe at eye level facilitates accurate reading. Capping the needle prevents contamination and protects the nurse against accidental needlesticks. A one-handed recap method may be used as long as care is taken to ensure that the needle remains sterile.

FIGURE 4. Withdrawing modified insulin.

Careful measurement ensures that correct dose is withdrawn.

This *third* check ensures accuracy and helps to prevent errors. *Note:* Many facilities require the *third* check to occur at the bedside, after identifying the patient and before administration.

Because the vial is sealed, the medication inside remains sterile and can be used for future injections. Labeling the opened vials with a date and time limits its use after a specific time period. The CDC recommends that medications packaged as multiuse vials be assigned to a single patient whenever possible (CDC, n.d.b; Dolan et al., 2016).

Locking the medication supply system or drawer safeguards the patient's medication supply. Facility accrediting organizations require medication supply systems to be locked when not in use.

Hand hygiene deters the spread of microorganisms.

See appropriate skill for prescribed route.

(continued)

Skill 5-5 ▶ Mixing Medications From Two Vials in One Syringe (continued)

EVALUATION	The expected outcomes have been met when the medication is withdrawn into the syringe in a sterile manner and is free from contamination and the proper dose is prepared.

DOCUMENTATION

Guidelines

It is not necessary to record the removal of the medication from the vials. Prompt recording of administration of the medication is required immediately after it is administered.

UNEXPECTED SITUATIONS AND ASSOCIATED INTERVENTIONS

- *You contaminate the plunger before injecting air into the insulin vial:* Discard the needle and syringe and start over.
- *The plunger is contaminated after medication is drawn into the syringe:* It is not necessary to discard and start over. The contaminated plunger will enter the barrel of the syringe when pushing the medication out and will not contaminate the medication.
- *You allow modified insulin to come in contact with the needle before entering the unmodified insulin vial:* Discard needle and syringe and start over.
- *You notice that the combined amount is not the ordered amount (e.g., you have less or more units in combined syringe than ordered):* Discard syringe and start over. There is no way to know for sure which dosage is wrong or which medication should be expelled.
- *You inject medication from the first vial (in syringe) into the second vial:* Discard vial and syringe and start over.

SPECIAL CONSIDERATIONS

General Considerations

- A patient with diabetes who is visually impaired may find it helpful to use a magnifying apparatus that fits around the syringe.
- Before attempting to explain or demonstrate devices that help low-vision diabetic patients to prepare their medication, attempt to use the device yourself under similar circumstances. To detect any difficulties the patient may experience, practice using the aid with your eyes closed or in a poorly lit room.

Infant and Child Considerations

- School-age children are generally able to prepare and administer their own injections, such as insulin, with supervision (Kyle & Carman, 2017). Parents/significant others and the child should be involved in teaching.

Skill 5-6 ▶ Administering an Intradermal Injection

Intradermal injections are administered into the dermis, just below the epidermis. The intradermal route has the longest absorption time of all parenteral routes. For this reason, intradermal injections are used for sensitivity tests, such as tuberculin and allergy tests, and local anesthesia. The advantage of the intradermal route for these tests is that the body's reaction to substances is easily visible, and degrees of reaction are discernible by comparative study.

Sites commonly used are the inner surface of the forearm and the upper back, under the scapula. Equipment used for an intradermal injection includes a tuberculin syringe calibrated in tenths and hundredths of a milliliter and a 0.25- to 0.5-in, 25- or 27-gauge needle. The dosage given intradermally is small, usually less than 0.5 mL. The angle of administration for an intradermal injection is 5 to 15 degrees (see Figure 5-1 in the chapter opener).

DELEGATION CONSIDERATIONS

The administration of an intradermal injection is not delegated to nursing assistive personnel (NAP) or to unlicensed assistive personnel (UAP). Depending on the state's nurse practice act and the organization's policies and procedures, the administration of an intradermal injection may be delegated to licensed practical/vocational nurses (LPN/LVNs). The decision to delegate must be based on careful analysis of the patient's needs and circumstances, as well as the qualifications of the person to whom the task is being delegated. Refer to the Delegation Guidelines in Appendix A.

EQUIPMENT	
	• Prescribed medication • Sterile syringe, usually a tuberculin syringe calibrated in tenths and hundredths, and a needle, ¼- to ½-in, 25- or 27-gauge • Antimicrobial swab • Disposable gloves • Small gauze square • Electronic Medication Administration Record (eMAR) or Medication Administration Record (MAR) • PPE, as indicated

ASSESSMENT	
	Assess the appropriateness of the drug for the patient. Review medical history, allergy, assessment, and laboratory data that may influence drug administration. Check expiration date before administering medication. Assess the site on the patient where the injection is to be given. Avoid areas of broken or open skin. Avoid areas that are highly pigmented, and those that have lesions, bruises, or scars and are hairy. Assess the patient's knowledge of the medication. This may provide an opportune time for patient education. Verify the patient's name, dose, route, and time of administration.

NURSING DIAGNOSIS	
	Determine related factors for the nursing diagnoses based on the patient's current status. Appropriate nursing diagnoses may include: • Deficient knowledge • Risk for injury • Risk for infection

OUTCOME IDENTIFICATION AND PLANNING	
	The expected outcome to achieve when administering an intradermal injection is that the medication is injected and a wheal appears at the injection site. Other outcomes that may be appropriate include the following: the patient refrains from rubbing the site; the patient does not experience adverse effects; and the patient understands and complies with the medication regimen.

IMPLEMENTATION

ACTION	RATIONALE
1. Gather equipment. Check each medication order against the original order in the medical record according to facility policy. Clarify any inconsistencies. Check the patient's health record for allergies.	This comparison helps to identify errors that may have occurred when orders were transcribed. The primary care provider's order or prescription is the legal record of medication orders for each facility.
2. Know the actions, special nursing considerations, safe dose ranges, purpose of administration, and adverse effects of the medications to be administered. Consider the appropriateness of the medication for this patient.	This knowledge aids the nurse in evaluating the therapeutic effect of the medication in relation to the patient's disorder and can also be used to educate the patient about the medication.
3. Perform hand hygiene.	Hand hygiene deters the spread of microorganisms.
4. Move the medication supply system to the outside of the patient's room or prepare for administration at the medication supply system in the medication area. Alternatively, access the medication administration supply system at or inside the patient's room.	Organization facilitates error-free administration and saves time.
5. Unlock the medication supply system or drawer. Enter pass code and scan employee identification, if required.	Locking the medication supply system or drawer safeguards each patient's medication supply. Facility accrediting organizations require medication supply systems to be locked when not in use. Entering pass code and scanning ID allows only authorized users into the system and identifies the user for documentation by the computer.

(continued)

Skill 5-6 ▸ Administering an Intradermal Injection (continued)

ACTION	RATIONALE
6. Prepare medications for one patient at a time.	This prevents errors in medication administration.
7. Read the eMAR/MAR and select the proper medication from the medication supply system or the patient's medication drawer.	This is the *first* check of the label.
8. Compare the label with the eMAR/MAR. Check expiration dates and perform calculations, if necessary. Scan the bar code on the package, if required.	This is the *second* check of the label. Verify calculations with another nurse to ensure safety.
9. If necessary, withdraw the medication from an ampule or vial as described in Skills 5-3 and 5-4.	
10. **Depending on facility policy, the third check of the label may occur at this point. If so, when all medications for one patient have been prepared, recheck the labels with the eMAR/MAR before taking the medications to the patient. However, many facilities require the third check to occur at the bedside, after identifying the patient.**	This *third* check ensures accuracy and helps to prevent errors. *Note:* Many facilities require the *third* check to occur at the bedside, after identifying the patient and before administration.
11. **Lock the medication supply system before leaving it.**	Locking the medication supply system or drawer safeguards the patient's medication supply. Facility accrediting organizations require medication supply systems to be locked when not in use.
12. Transport medications to the patient's bedside carefully, and keep the medications in sight at all times.	Careful handling and close observation prevent accidental or deliberate disarrangement of medications.
13. **Ensure that the patient receives the medications at the correct time.**	Check facility policy, which may allow for administration within a period of 30 minutes before or 30 minutes after the designated time.
14. Perform hand hygiene and put on PPE, if indicated.	Hand hygiene and PPE prevent the spread of microorganisms. PPE is required based on transmission precautions.
15. **Identify the patient. Compare the information with the eMAR/MAR. The patient should be identified using at least two of the following methods (The Joint Commission, 2018):**	Identifying the patient ensures the right patient receives the medications and helps prevent errors. The patient's room number or physical location is not used as an identifier (The Joint Commission, 2018). Replace the identification band if it is missing or inaccurate in any way.
a. Check the name on the patient's identification band.	This requires a response from the patient, but illness and strange surroundings often cause patients to be confused.
b. Check the identification number on the patient's identification band.	
c. Check the birth date on the patient's identification band.	
d. Ask the patient to state his or her name and birth date, based on facility policy.	
16. Close the door to the room or pull the bedside curtain.	This provides patient privacy.
17. **Complete necessary assessments before administering medications. Check allergy bracelet or ask the patient about allergies. Explain the purpose and action of the medication to the patient.**	Assessment is a prerequisite to administration of medications. Explanation provides rationale, increases knowledge, and reduces anxiety.
18. Scan the patient's bar code on the identification band, if required.	Provides an additional check to ensure that the medication is given to the right patient.
19. **Based on facility policy, the third check of the label may occur at this point. If so, recheck the labels with the eMAR/MAR before administering the medications to the patient.**	Many facilities require the *third* check to occur at the bedside, after identifying the patient and before administration. If facility policy directs the *third* check at this time, this *third* check ensures accuracy and helps to prevent errors.
20. Put on clean gloves.	Gloves help prevent exposure to contaminants.

ACTION	RATIONALE
21. Select an appropriate administration site. Assist the patient to the appropriate position for the site chosen. Drape, as needed, to expose only site area to be used.	Appropriate site prevents injury and allows for accurate reading of the test site at the appropriate time. Draping provides privacy and warmth.
22. Cleanse the site with an antimicrobial swab while wiping with a firm, circular motion and moving outward from the injection site. Allow the skin to dry.	Pathogens on the skin can be forced into the tissues by the needle. Moving from the center outward prevents contamination of the site. Allowing the antimicrobial solution to dry completely (15 to 30 seconds) ensures complete antimicrobial effectiveness (Harper, 2014), and prevents introducing alcohol into the tissue, which can be irritating and uncomfortable.
23. Remove the needle cap with the nondominant hand by pulling it straight off.	This technique lessens the risk of an accidental needlestick.
24. Use the nondominant hand to spread the skin taut over the injection site (Figure 1).	Taut skin provides an easy entrance into intradermal tissue.
25. Hold the syringe in the dominant hand, between the thumb and forefinger with the bevel of the needle up.	Using the dominant hand allows for easy, appropriate handling of the syringe. Having the bevel up allows for smooth piercing of the skin and introduction of medication into the dermis.
26. Hold the syringe at a 5- to 15-degree angle from the site. Place the needle almost flat against the patient's skin (Figure 2), bevel side up, and insert the needle into the skin. Insert the needle only about ⅛ in with entire bevel under the skin.	The dermis is entered when the needle is held as nearly parallel to the skin as possible and is inserted about ⅛ in.

FIGURE 1. Spreading skin taut over injection site.

FIGURE 2. Inserting needle almost flat against the skin.

ACTION	RATIONALE
27. Once the needle is in place, steady the lower end of the syringe. Slide your dominant hand to the end of the plunger.	Prevents injury and inadvertent advancement or withdrawal of needle.
28. Slowly inject the agent while watching for a small wheal to appear (Figure 3).	The appearance of a wheal indicates the medication is in the dermis.

FIGURE 3. Observing for wheal while injecting medication.

(continued)

Skill 5-6 ▶ Administering an Intradermal Injection *(continued)*

ACTION	RATIONALE
29. Withdraw the needle quickly at the same angle that it was inserted. Do not recap the used needle. Engage the safety shield or needle guard.	Withdrawing the needle quickly and at the angle at which it entered the skin minimizes tissue damage and discomfort for the patient. Safety shield or needle guard prevents accidental needlestick injury.
30. **Do not massage the area after removing needle. Tell the patient not to rub or scratch the site. If necessary, gently blot the site with a dry gauze square. Do not apply pressure or rub the site.**	Massaging or rubbing the area where an intradermal injection is given may spread the medication to underlying subcutaneous tissue.
31. Assist the patient to a position of comfort.	This provides for the well-being of the patient.
32. Discard the needle and syringe in the appropriate receptacle.	Proper disposal of the needle prevents injury.
33. Remove gloves and additional PPE, if used. Perform hand hygiene.	Proper removal of PPE reduces the risk for infection transmission and contamination of other items. Hand hygiene prevents the spread of microorganisms.
34. Document the administration of the medication immediately after administration. See Documentation section below.	Timely documentation helps to ensure patient safety.
35. Evaluate the patient's response to the medication within the appropriate time frame.	The patient needs to be evaluated for therapeutic and adverse effects from the medication.
36. Observe the area for signs of a reaction at determined intervals after administration. Inform the patient of the need for inspection.	With many intradermal injections, you need to look for a localized reaction in the area of the injection at the appropriate interval(s) determined by the type of medication and purpose. Explaining this to the patient increases compliance.

EVALUATION

The expected outcomes have been met when you note a wheal at the injection site; the patient refrains from rubbing the site; the patient did not experience adverse effects; and the patient verbalizes an understanding of, and complies with, the medication regimen.

DOCUMENTATION

Guidelines

Record each medication administered on the eMAR/MAR or health record using the required format, including date, time, and the site of administration, immediately after administration. Some facilities recommend circling the injection site with ink. Circling the injection site easily identifies the intradermal injection site and allows for future careful observation of the exact area. If using a bar-code system, medication administration is automatically recorded when the bar code is scanned. PRN medications require documentation of the reason for administration. Prompt recording avoids the possibility of accidentally repeating the administration of the drug. If the drug was refused or omitted, record this in the appropriate area on the medication record and notify the primary care provider. This verifies the reason medication was omitted and ensures that health care personnel providing care for the patient are aware of the occurrence.

UNEXPECTED SITUATIONS AND ASSOCIATED INTERVENTIONS

- *You do not note a wheal or blister at the injection site:* Medication has been injected subcutaneously. Document according to facility policy and inform the primary care provider. You may need to obtain an order to repeat the procedure.
- *Medication leaks out of the injection site before the needle is withdrawn:* Needle was inserted less than ⅛ in. Document according to facility policy and inform the primary care provider. You may need to obtain an order to repeat the procedure.
- *You stick yourself with the needle before injection:* Discard needle and syringe appropriately. Follow facility policy regarding needlestick injury. Prepare new syringe with medication and administer to patient. Complete appropriate paperwork and follow facility's policy regarding accidental needlestick injuries.
- *You stick yourself with the needle after injection:* Discard needle and syringe appropriately. Follow facility policy regarding needlestick injury. Complete appropriate paperwork and follow facility's policy regarding accidental needlestick injuries.

**SPECIAL
CONSIDERATIONS**

- Fluzone Intradermal is the only vaccine in the United States administered by the intradermal route and is available for patients 18 to 64 years of age (CDC, 2015a; Sanofi Pasteur, 2016). The site of administration for this vaccine is the deltoid region of the upper arm, and the needle is inserted perpendicular to the skin (CDC, 2015a). **This vaccine should not be administered into the forearm or other site used to administer other intradermal medications.** The prefilled microinjection syringe administers a 0.1-mL dose into the dermal layer of the skin via a 30-gauge, 1.5-mL microneedle (CDC, 2015a). **No other influenza vaccine formulations should be administered by the intradermal route** (CDC, 2015a). Follow manufacturer directions for appropriate administration.
- Ongoing assessment is an important part of nursing care for both evaluation of patient response to administered medications and early detection of adverse reactions. If an adverse effect is suspected, withhold further medication doses and notify the patient's primary care provider. Additional intervention is based on type of reaction and patient assessment.
- Some facilities recommend administering intradermal injections with the bevel down instead of the bevel up. Check facility policy.

  Skill 5-7 ▶ **Administering a Subcutaneous Injection**

Subcutaneous injections are administered into the adipose tissue layer just below the epidermis and dermis. This tissue has few blood vessels, so drugs administered here have a slow, sustained rate of absorption into the capillaries. Various sites may be used for subcutaneous injections, including the outer aspect of the upper arm, the abdomen (from below the costal margin to the iliac crests), the anterior aspects of the thigh, the upper back, and the upper ventral- or dorsogluteal area. Figure 1 displays the sites on the body where subcutaneous injections can be given. Absorption rates differ among the various sites. Injections in the abdomen are absorbed most rapidly; ones in the arms are absorbed somewhat more slowly; those in the thighs, even more slowly; and those in the ventral or dorsogluteal areas have the slowest absorption (American Diabetes Association [ADA], 2015).

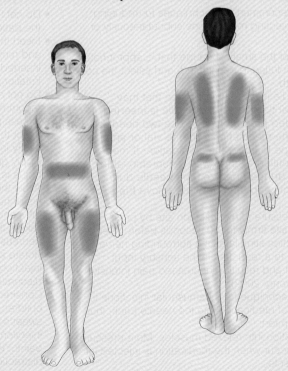

FIGURE 1. Body sites where subcutaneous injections can be given.

(continued)

Skill 5-7 ▶ Administering a Subcutaneous Injection *(continued)*

It is important to choose the right equipment to ensure depositing the medication into the intended subcutaneous tissue and not the underlying muscle. Equipment used for a subcutaneous injection includes a syringe of appropriate volume for the amount of drug being administered. An insulin injection pen may be used for subcutaneous injection of insulin (see the accompanying Skill Variation for technique). A 25- to 30-gauge, ⅜- to 1-in needle can be used; ⅜- and ⅝-in needles are most commonly used for subcutaneous injections. Choose the needle length based on the amount of subcutaneous tissue present, which is based on the patient's body weight and build (Annersten & Willman, 2005). Some medications are packaged in prefilled cartridges with a needle attached. Confirm that the provided needle is appropriate for the patient before use. If not, the medication will have to be transferred to another syringe and the appropriate needle attached.

Subcutaneous injections are administered at a 45- or 90-degree angle, with the 45-degree angle used only for patients with a limited amount of subcutaneous tissue. Choose the angle of needle insertion based on the amount of subcutaneous tissue present and the length of the needle. In general, insert the shorter, ⅜-in needle, at a 90-degree angle (common on prefilled and insulin syringes). The longer, ⅝-in needle, may be inserted at a 45-degree angle. Figure 5-1 in the chapter opener shows the angles of insertion for subcutaneous injections.

Recommendations differ regarding pinching a skin fold for administration. Forming a skin fold is advised for thinner patients and when a longer needle is used to lift the adipose tissue away from underlying muscle and tissue. If pinching to form a skin fold is used, once the needle is inserted, release the skin and stabilize the base of the needle to avoid injecting into the compressed tissue.

Usually, no more than 1 mL of solution is given subcutaneously. Giving larger amounts adds to the patient's discomfort and may predispose to poor absorption. It is necessary to rotate sites or areas for injection if the patient is to receive frequent injections. This helps to prevent buildup of fibrous tissue and permits complete absorption of the medication. Further information regarding insulin administration and rotation of injection sites can be found in the General Considerations at the end of this skill.

Box 5-1 discusses techniques for reducing discomfort when injecting medications subcutaneously or intramuscularly.

Box 5-1 ▶ Reducing Discomfort in Subcutaneous and Intramuscular Administrations

The following are recommended techniques for reducing discomfort when injecting medications subcutaneously or intramuscularly:

- Select a needle of the smallest gauge that is appropriate for the site and solution to be injected, and select the correct needle length.
- Be sure the needle is free of medication that may irritate superficial tissues as the needle is inserted. The recommended procedure is to use two needles—one to remove the medication from the vial or ampule and a second one to inject the medication. If medication is in a prefilled syringe with a nonremovable needle and has dripped back on the needle during preparation, gently tap the barrel to remove the excess solution.
- Apply manual pressure at the insertion site by pressing the insertion site firmly for 10 seconds before needle insertion. This action stimulates the surrounding nerve endings, leading to a reduction in the sensory input from the injection and resulting decreased pain intensity (Chung, Ng, & Wong, 2002).
- Use the Z-track technique for intramuscular injections to prevent leakage of medication into the needle track, thus minimizing discomfort.
- Inject the medication into relaxed muscles. More pressure and discomfort occur when the medication is injected into a contracted muscle.

- Do not inject areas that feel hard on palpation or tender to the patient.
- Insert the needle with a dart-like motion without hesitation, and remove it quickly at the same angle at which it was inserted. These techniques reduce discomfort and tissue irritation.
- Do not administer more solution in one injection than is recommended for the site. Injecting more solution creates excess pressure in the area and increases discomfort.
- Inject the solution slowly so that it may be dispersed more easily into the surrounding tissue (10 seconds per 1 mL).
- Apply gentle pressure after injection, unless this technique is contraindicated.
- Allow the patient who is fearful of injections to talk about his or her fears. Answer the patient's questions truthfully, and explain the nature and purpose of the injection. Taking the time to offer support often allays fears and decreases discomfort.
- Rotate sites when the patient is to receive repeated injections. Injections in the same site may cause undue discomfort, irritation, or abscesses in tissues.
- Consider nonpharmacologic methods for infants and children, such as breastfeeding, the administration of sweet solutions, front-to-front upright holding, rapid injection without aspiration, administration of the most painful vaccine last, tactile stimulation, and other distractions (Harrison et al., 2014; Taddio et al., 2010).

DELEGATION CONSIDERATIONS

The administration of a subcutaneous injection is not delegated to nursing assistive personnel (NAP) or to unlicensed assistive personnel (UAP). Depending on the state's nurse practice act and the organization's policies and procedures, the administration of a subcutaneous injection may be delegated to licensed practical/vocational nurses (LPN/LVNs). The decision to delegate must be based on careful analysis of the patient's needs and circumstances, as well as the qualifications of the person to whom the task is being delegated. Refer to the Delegation Guidelines in Appendix A.

EQUIPMENT

- Prescribed medication
- Sterile syringe and needle. Needle size depends on the medication to be administered and patient body type (see previous discussion).
- Antimicrobial swab
- Nonlatex, disposable gloves
- Small gauze square
- Electronic Medication Administration Record (eMAR) or Medication Administration Record (MAR)
- PPE, as indicated

ASSESSMENT

Assess the appropriateness of the drug for the patient. Review medical history, allergy, assessment, and laboratory data that may influence drug administration. Check expiration date before administering medication. Assess the site on the patient where the injection is to be given. Avoid sites that are bruised, tender, hard, swollen, inflamed, or scarred. These conditions could affect absorption (ADA, 2015; Gelder, 2014). Assess the patient's knowledge of the medication. If the patient has deficient knowledge about the medication, this may be the appropriate time to begin education about it. If the medication may affect the patient's vital signs, assess them before administration. If the medication is for pain relief, assess the patient's pain before and after administration. Verify patient name, dose, route, and time of administration.

NURSING DIAGNOSIS

Determine related factors for the nursing diagnoses based on the patient's current status. Appropriate nursing diagnoses may include:

- Deficient knowledge
- Risk for injury
- Risk for infection

OUTCOME IDENTIFICATION AND PLANNING

The expected outcome to achieve is that the patient receives the medication via the subcutaneous route and experiences the intended effect of the medication. Other outcomes that may be appropriate include the following: the patient does not experience adverse effects; and the patient understands and complies with the medication regimen.

IMPLEMENTATION

ACTION	RATIONALE
1. Gather equipment. Check each medication order against the original order in the medical record, according to facility policy. Clarify any inconsistencies. Check the patient's health record for allergies.	This comparison helps to identify errors that may have occurred when orders were transcribed. The primary care provider's order or prescription is the legal record of medication orders for each facility.
2. Know the actions, special nursing considerations, safe dose ranges, purpose of administration, and adverse effects of the medications to be administered. Consider the appropriateness of the medication for this patient.	This knowledge aids the nurse in evaluating the therapeutic effect of the medication in relation to the patient's disorder and can also be used to educate the patient about the medication.
3. Perform hand hygiene.	Hand hygiene prevents the spread of microorganisms.

(continued)

Skill 5-7 ▶ Administering a Subcutaneous Injection *(continued)*

ACTION	RATIONALE
4. Move the medication supply system to the outside of the patient's room or prepare for administration at the medication supply system in the medication area. Alternatively, access the medication administration supply system at or inside the patient's room.	Organization facilitates error-free administration and saves time.
5. Unlock the medication supply system or drawer. Enter pass code and scan employee identification, if required.	Locking the medication supply system or drawer safeguards each patient's medication supply. Facility accrediting organizations require medication supply systems to be locked when not in use. Entering pass code and scanning ID allows only authorized users into the computer system and identifies the user for documentation by the computer.
6. **Prepare medications for one patient at a time.**	This prevents errors in medication administration.
7. Read the eMAR/MAR and select the proper medication from the medication supply system or the patient's medication drawer.	This is the *first* check of the label.
8. Compare the medication label with the eMAR/MAR. Check expiration dates and perform calculations, if necessary. Scan the bar code on the package, if required.	This is the *second* check of the label. Verify calculations with another nurse to ensure safety, if necessary.
9. If necessary, withdraw medication from an ampule or vial as described in Skills 5-3 and 5-4.	
10. **Depending on facility policy, the third check of the label may occur at this point. If so, when all medications for one patient have been prepared, recheck the labels with the eMAR/MAR before taking the medications to the patient. However, many facilities require the third check to occur at the bedside, after identifying the patient.**	This *third* check ensures accuracy and helps to prevent errors. *Note:* Many facilities require the *third* check to occur at the bedside, after identifying the patient and before administration.
11. **Lock the medication supply system before leaving it.**	Locking the medication supply system or drawer safeguards the patient's medication supply. Facility accrediting organizations require medication supply systems to be locked when not in use.
12. Transport medications to the patient's bedside carefully, and keep the medications in sight at all times.	Careful handling and close observation prevent accidental or deliberate disarrangement of medications.
13. **Ensure that the patient receives the medications at the correct time.**	Check facility policy, which may allow for administration within a period of 30 minutes before or 30 minutes after the designated time.
14. Perform hand hygiene and put on PPE, if indicated.	Hand hygiene and PPE prevent the spread of microorganisms. PPE is required based on transmission precautions.
15. **Identify the patient. Compare the information with the eMAR/MAR. The patient should be identified using at least two of the following methods (The Joint Commission, 2018):**	Identifying the patient ensures the right patient receives the medications and helps prevent errors. The patient's room number or physical location is not used as an identifier (The Joint Commission, 2018). Replace the identification band if it is missing or inaccurate in any way.
a. Check the name on the patient's identification band.	
b. Check the identification number on the patient's identification band.	
c. Check the birth date on the patient's identification band.	
d. Ask the patient to state his or her name and birth date, based on facility policy.	This requires a response from the patient, but illness and strange surroundings often cause patients to be confused.

ACTION	RATIONALE

16. Close the door to the room or pull the bedside curtain.

This provides patient privacy.

17. **Complete necessary assessments before administering medications. Check the patient's allergy bracelet or ask the patient about allergies.** Explain the purpose and action of the medication to the patient.

Assessment is a prerequisite to administration of medications. Explanation provides rationale, increases knowledge, and reduces anxiety.

18. Scan the patient's bar code on the identification band, if required (Figure 2).

Scanning provides an additional check to ensure that the medication is given to the right patient.

FIGURE 2. Scanning bar code on the patient's identification bracelet. (*Photo by B. Proud.*)

19. **Based on facility policy, the third check of the label may occur at this point. If so, recheck the labels with the eMAR/MAR before administering the medications to the patient.**

Many facilities require the *third* check to occur at the bedside, after identifying the patient and before administration. If facility policy directs the *third* check at this time, this *third* check ensures accuracy and helps to prevent errors.

20. Put on clean gloves.

Gloves help prevent exposure to contaminants.

21. Select an appropriate administration site.

Appropriate site prevents injury and allows for accurate reading of the test site at the appropriate time.

22. Assist the patient to the appropriate position for the site chosen. Drape, as needed, to expose only site area to be used.

Appropriate site prevents injury. Draping helps maintain the patient's privacy.

23. Identify the appropriate landmarks for the site chosen.

Good visualization is necessary to establish the correct site location and to avoid tissue damage.

24. Cleanse the area around the injection site with an antimicrobial swab. Use a firm, circular motion while moving outward from the injection site (Figure 3). Allow the area to dry.

Pathogens on the skin can be forced into the tissues by the needle. Moving from the center outward prevents contamination of the site. Allowing the antimicrobial solution to dry completely (15 to 30 seconds) ensures complete antimicrobial effectiveness (Harper, 2014), and prevents introducing alcohol into the tissue, which can be irritating and uncomfortable.

FIGURE 3. Cleaning injection site.

(*continued*)

Skill 5-7 ▶ Administering a Subcutaneous Injection *(continued)*

ACTION	**RATIONALE**
25. Remove the needle cap with the nondominant hand, pulling it straight off.	The cap protects the needle from contact with microorganisms. This technique lessens the risk of an accidental needlestick.
26. Create a skin fold, if necessary, by pinching the area surrounding the injection site. Alternatively, spread the skin taut at the site, based on assessment of the patient and needle length used for the injection (Figure 4).	Decision to create a skin fold is based on the nurse's assessment of the patient and needle length used. Recommendations differ regarding pinching a skin fold for administration. Pinching is advised for thinner patients and when a longer needle is used to lift the adipose tissue away from underlying muscle and tissue (Gelder, 2014; Sexson et al., 2016). If skin is pulled taut, it may provide less painful entry into the subcutaneous tissue.
27. Hold the syringe in the dominant hand between the thumb and forefinger. Inject the needle quickly at a 45- or 90-degree angle, depending on the amount of underlying subcutaneous tissue. (Figure 5).	Inserting the needle quickly causes less pain to the patient. For a person with a limited amount of subcutaneous tissue, insert the needle at a 45-degree angle.

FIGURE 4. Pinching the area surrounding the injection site to create a skin fold, if necessary.

FIGURE 5. Inserting needle.

28. If pinching is used, once the needle is inserted, release the skin and stabilize the base of the needle to avoid injecting into the compressed tissue. Slide your dominant hand to the end of the plunger. Avoid moving the syringe.	Injecting the solution into compressed tissues results in pressure against nerve fibers and creates discomfort. Stabilizing the base of the needle secures the syringe. Moving the syringe could cause damage to the tissues and inadvertent administration into an incorrect area.
29. Inject the medication slowly (at a rate of 10 sec/mL).	Rapid injection of the solution creates pressure in the tissues, resulting in discomfort.
30. Withdraw the needle quickly at the same angle at which it was inserted, while supporting the surrounding tissue with your nondominant hand.	Slow withdrawal of the needle pulls the tissues and causes discomfort. Applying counter traction around the injection site helps to prevent pulling on the tissue as the needle is withdrawn. Removing the needle at the same angle at which it was inserted minimizes tissue damage and discomfort for the patient.
31. Do not recap the used needle. Engage the safety shield or needle guard.	Safety shield or needle guard prevents accidental needlestick.
32. If blood or clear fluid appears at the site after withdrawing the needle, use a gauze square to apply gentle pressure to the site. **Do not massage the site.**	Massaging the site can damage underlying tissue and increase the absorption of the medication. Massaging after heparin administration can contribute to hematoma formation.
33. Assist the patient to a position of comfort.	This provides for the well-being of the patient.

ACTION	**RATIONALE**
34. Discard the needle and syringe in the appropriate receptacle.	Proper disposal of the needle prevents injury.
35. Remove gloves and additional PPE, if used. Perform hand hygiene.	Proper removal of PPE reduces the risk for infection transmission and contamination of other items. Hand hygiene prevents the spread of microorganisms.
36. Document the administration of the medication immediately after administration.	Timely documentation helps to ensure patient safety.
37. Evaluate the patient's response to the medication within the appropriate time frame for the particular medication.	The patient needs to be evaluated for therapeutic and adverse effects from the medication.

EVALUATION

The expected outcomes have been met when the patient receives the medication via the subcutaneous route and experiences the intended effect of the medication; the patient does not experience adverse effects; and the patient understands and complies with the medication regimen.

DOCUMENTATION

Guidelines

Record each medication given on the eMAR/MAR or health record using the required format immediately after administration, including date, dose, time, and the site of administration. If using a bar-code system, medication administration is automatically recorded when the bar code is scanned. PRN medications require documentation of the reason for administration. Prompt recording avoids the possibility of accidentally repeating the administration of the drug. If the drug was refused or omitted, record this in the appropriate area on the medication record and notify the primary care provider. This verifies the reason medication was omitted and ensures that health care personnel providing care for the patient are aware of the occurrence.

UNEXPECTED SITUATIONS AND ASSOCIATED INTERVENTIONS

- *When skin fold is released, needle pulls out of skin:* Engage safety shield or needle guard. Appropriately discard needle. Attach new needle to syringe and administer injection.
- *Patient refuses to let you administer medication in a different location:* Explain the rationale behind rotating injection sites. Discuss other available injection sites with the patient. If the patient will still not allow injection in another area, administer medication to patient, document patient's refusal of rotation of injection site and discussion, and notify primary care provider.
- *You stick yourself with the needle before injection:* Discard needle and syringe appropriately. Follow facility policy regarding needlestick injury. Prepare new syringe with medication and administer to patient. Complete appropriate paperwork and follow facility's policy regarding accidental needlestick injuries.
- *You stick yourself with the needle after injection:* Discard needle and syringe appropriately. Complete appropriate paperwork and follow facility's policy regarding accidental needlestick injuries.
- *During injection, patient pulls away from the needle before the medication is delivered fully:* Remove and appropriately discard needle. Attach a new needle to syringe and administer remaining medication at a different site. Document events and interventions according to facility policy.

SPECIAL CONSIDERATIONS

General Considerations

- Ongoing assessment is an important part of nursing care for both evaluation of patient response to administered medications and early detection of adverse drug reactions. If an adverse effect is suspected, withhold further medication doses and notify the patient's primary care provider. Additional intervention is based on type of reaction and patient assessment.

Skill 5-7 ▶ Administering a Subcutaneous Injection *(continued)*

- Because absorption rates vary from site to site, it is recommended that patients administering their own insulin use the same area of the body at the same time every day to ensure more consistent absorption and prevent tissue changes from repeated use of the same site (Frandsen & Pennington, 2014; ADA, 2015). For instance, every morning the patient may use the abdomen for insulin injection, and every evening before dinner, the patient may inject the insulin into the arms or thighs. Keep in mind that the best absorption occurs in the abdomen. In each case, the injections should be given an inch away from the previous injection site so that the same area will not be used again in the same month. A small spot bandage or piece of tape can be used to mark the first injection site, with subsequent injections rotated in a circle around that site. After this area has been used, an adjacent site, an inch away, can be selected, using the same rotation format. A marked diagram incorporated into the patient's plan of care is also helpful for noting alternative sites. Do not rely on memory. The patient cannot always recall the site of the previous injection, thus the site of administration should be recorded; when the patient is receiving care from a health care provider, the site of administration must be recorded in the patient's health record.
- Heparin is administered subcutaneously. The abdomen is the most commonly used administration site. Avoid the area 2 in around the umbilicus and the belt line.
- Certain medications have specific manufacturer-recommended administration requirements. For example, enoxaparin (low–molecular-weight heparin) should be administered alternating between the left and right anterolateral and left and right posterolateral abdominal wall ("love handles") (Sanofi Aventis, 2013, 2016) (Figure 6). To administer the medication, pinch the tissue gently to form a skin fold and insert the needle at a 90-degree angle (Sanofi Aventis, 2016). In addition, enoxaparin is packaged in a prefilled syringe with an air bubble. Do not expel the air bubble before administration.

Anterior view   Posterior view

FIGURE 6. Sites for administration of enoxaparin.

Infant and Child Considerations
- Do not tell a child that an injection will not hurt. Describe the feel of the injection as a pinch or a sting. A child who believes you have been dishonest with him/her is less likely to cooperate with future procedures.

Older Adult Considerations
- Many older adults have less adipose tissue. Adjust the needle length and insertion angle accordingly. (Refer to discussion earlier in Skill.) You do not want to inadvertently give a subcutaneous medication intramuscularly.

Home Care Considerations
- Reuse of syringes in the home setting is not recommended.
- The use of antimicrobial swabs to clean the injection site in home environments may be unnecessary; patients may use soap and water to clean the site if the area is visibly soiled (Sexson et al., 2016).
- Because absorption rates vary from site to site, it is recommended that patients administering their own insulin use the same area of the body at the same time every day to ensure more consistent absorption and prevent tissue changes from repeated use of the same site (Frandsen & Pennington, 2014; ADA, 2015). Refer to the information discussed in the "General Considerations" section of this Skill.
- Encourage patients to consult the policies of their local government regarding contaminated and sharps waste disposal. Depending on local requirements, patients may dispose of needles and syringes in a hard, plastic container. Liquid detergent or liquid fabric softener containers are good choices. Never use glass containers.

Skill Variation | Using an Insulin Injection Pen to Administer Insulin via the Subcutaneous Route

Prepare medication as outlined in steps 1–23 above (Skill 5-7).

1. Remove the pen cap.
2. Insert an insulin cartridge into the pen, if necessary, following the manufacturer's directions.
3. If administering an insulin suspension, gently roll the pen 10 times and invert the pen 10 times to mix the insulin.
4. Scrub the self-sealing seal end of the pen cartridge holder with an antimicrobial swab.
5. Remove the protective paper tab from the needle.
6. Screw the needle onto the reservoir.
7. Remove the outer and inner needle caps. (Patients at home should reserve the outer shield for later use.)
8. Dial the dose selector to 2 units to prime the pen (perform an "air shot") to get rid of air and make certain the pen is working properly.
9. Hold the pen upright and tap to force any air bubbles to the top.
10. Hold the pen upright and press the injection button or plunger firmly. Watch for a drop of insulin at the needle tip.
11. Check the drug reservoir to make sure sufficient insulin is available for the dose.
12. Check that the dose selector is at "0," then dial the units of insulin for the dose.
13. Put on gloves.
14. Clean the injection site. If the pen needle is longer than 5 mm, gently pinch the skin at the injection site to form a skin fold (Becton, Dickinson and Company, 2016a).
15. Hold the pen in the palm of the hand, perpendicular to the forearm, with the thumb at the injection button end of the pen. Use the thumb for injection (Figure A).
16. Administer the subcutaneous injection. Press the injection button on the pen all the way in. Keep the button depressed and count to 10 before removing from the skin.
17. The safety shield automatically covers the needle when needle is removed from the skin. Remove the needle

FIGURE A. Patient using insulin pen. (*Photo by B. Proud.*)

from the pen; a second safety shield automatically covers the back end of the needle when removed from the pen. Dispose of the needle in a sharps container.

18. Alternatively, patients at home should replace the reserved outer shield on the needle before removing the needle from the pen. Other needle removal devices and procedures exist; patients should follow the instructions provided by their health care provider related to their specific insulin pen.
19. Remove gloves and additional PPE, if used.

 20. Perform hand hygiene.

21. Document administration on the eMAR/MAR, including the injection site.

Source: Adapted from Becton, Dickinson and Company. (2016a). How to inject with a pen. Retrieved https://www.bd.com/en-us/company/video-gallery?video=4592430149001; Becton, Dickinson and Company. (2016b). Safety needles. Retrieved http://www.bd.com/hypodermic/products/autoshield/duo

 ## Skill 5-8 | Administering an Intramuscular Injection

Intramuscular injections deliver medication through the skin and subcutaneous tissues into certain muscles. Muscles have a larger and a greater number of blood vessels than subcutaneous tissue, allowing faster onset of action than with subcutaneous injections. An intramuscular injection is chosen when a reasonably rapid systemic uptake of the drug is needed by the body and when a relatively prolonged action is required. Some medications administered intramuscularly are formulated to have a longer duration of effect. The deposit of medication creates a depot at the injection site, designed to deliver slow, sustained release over hours, days, or weeks.

(continued)

Skill 5-8 ▶ Administering an Intramuscular Injection *(continued)*

It is important to choose the right needle length for a particular intramuscular injection. Needle length should be based on the individual patient. (See Table 5-1 for intramuscular needle length recommendations.) Patients who are obese may require a longer needle, and emaciated patients may require a shorter needle. Appropriate gauge is determined by the medication being administered. In general, biologic agents and medications in aqueous solutions should be administered with a 20- to 25-gauge needle. Medications in oil-based solutions should be administered with an 18- to 25-gauge needle. Many medications come in prefilled syringe units. If a needle is provided on the prefilled unit, ensure that the needle on the unit is the appropriate length for the patient and situation.

To avoid complications, the nurse must be able to identify anatomic landmarks and site boundaries. See Figure 1 for a depiction of anatomic landmarks and site boundaries for potential intramuscular injection sites. Consider the age of the patient, medication type, and medication volume when selecting an intramuscular injection site. (See Table 5-2 for information related to intramuscular site selection.) Rotate the sites used to administer intramuscular medications when therapy requires repeated injections. Depending on the site selected, it may be necessary to reposition the patient (refer to Table 5-3).

Table 5-1 Intramuscular Injection Needle Length

SITE/AGE	NEEDLE LENGTH
Vastus lateralis	5⁄8″ to 1¼″
Deltoid (children)	5⁄8″ to 1¼″
Deltoid (adults)	1″ to 1½″
Ventrogluteal (adults)	1½″

Note: Biological sex and weight are directly related to needle length choice; the size of the muscle, the adipose tissue thickness at the injection site, the volume of medication to be administered, and the injection technique also need to be considered.

Source: Adapted from Centers for Disease Control and Prevention (CDC). (2015a). Chapter 6. Vaccine administration. *The pink book.* Retrieved https://www.cdc.gov/vaccines/pubs/pinkbook/vac-admin.html; Centers for Disease Control and Prevention (CDC). (2015b). In J. Hamborsky, A. Kroger, & S. Wolfe (Eds.). *Epidemiology and prevention of vaccine-preventable diseases* (13th ed.). Washington, DC: Public Health Foundation. Retrieved http://www.cdc.gov/vaccines/pubs/pinkbook/index.html; and Nicoll, L., & Hesby, A. (2002). Intramuscular injection: An integrative research review and guideline for evidence-based practice. *Applied Nursing Research, 16*(2), 149–162.

Table 5-2 Intramuscular Site Selection

AGE OF PATIENT	RECOMMENDED SITE
Infants	Vastus lateralis
Toddlers (1–2 years)	Vastus lateralis (preferred) or deltoid
Child/Adolescent (3–18 years)	Deltoid (preferred) or vastus lateralis
Adults	Deltoid (vaccines) or ventrogluteal (general IM injections)

Source: Adapted from Centers for Disease Control and Prevention (CDC). (2015a). Chapter 6. Vaccine administration. *The pink book.* Retrieved https://www.cdc.gov/vaccines/pubs/pinkbook/vac-admin.html; and Nicoll, L., & Hesby, A. (2002). Intramuscular injection: An integrative research review and guideline for evidence-based practice. *Applied Nursing Research, 16*(2), 149–162.

Table 5-3 Patient Positioning

INJECTION SITE	PATIENT POSITION
Deltoid	Patient may sit or stand. A child may be held in an adult's lap.
Ventrogluteal	Patient may stand, sit, lie laterally, and lie supine.
Vastus lateralis	Patient may sit or lie supine. Infants and young children may lie supine or be held in an adult's lap.

Source: Adapted from Centers for Disease Control and Prevention (CDC). (2015a). Chapter 6. Vaccine administration. *The pink book.* Retrieved https://www.cdc.gov/vaccines/pubs/pinkbook/vac-admin.html.

FIGURE 1. Sites for intramuscular injections. Descriptions for locating sites are given in the text. (**A**) Ventrogluteal site is located by placing palm on greater trochanter and index finger toward the anterosuperior iliac spine. (**B**) Vastus lateralis site is identified by dividing the thigh into thirds, horizontally and vertically. (**C**) Deltoid muscle site is located by palpating lower edge of acromion process.

Administer the intramuscular injection so that the needle is perpendicular to the patient's body. This ensures it is given using an injection angle between 72 and 90 degrees, with the goal of 90 degrees (CDC, 2015b; Katsma & Katsma, 2000). Figure 5-1 in the chapter opener on page 179 shows the angle of insertion for intramuscular injections.

The medication volume that can be administered intramuscularly varies based on the intended site. In general, 1 to 5 mL is the accepted volume range, with a limitation of 1 mL of solution at the deltoid site. However, up to 2 mL may be administered at the deltoid site, depending on the size of the muscle (Hunt, 2008). The less-developed muscles of children and older people limit the intramuscular injection to 1 to 2 mL.

Many of the drugs given intramuscularly can cause irritation to subcutaneous tissues when backflow into the tissues occurs along the injection track. Therefore, the Z-track technique is

(*continued*)

Skill 5-8 ▶ Administering an Intramuscular Injection *(continued)*

recommended for all intramuscular injections (particularly nonvaccine injections) to ensure that medication does not leak back along the needle track and into the subcutaneous tissue (Nicoll & Hesby, 2002; Zimmerman, 2010). This technique reduces pain and discomfort, particularly for patients receiving injections over an extended period. The Z-track method is also suggested for older adults who have decreased muscle mass. Some medications, such as iron, are best given via the Z-track method due to the irritation and discoloration associated with the medication. The decision regarding stretching or pinching the skin, or using the Z-track method is based on the individual patient and nursing judgment.

Aspiration, or pulling back on the plunger to check that a blood vessel has been entered, is not necessary and has not proved to be a reliable indicator of needle placement. Despite a tradition of aspiration, if correct technique is used, the likelihood of injecting into a blood vessel is small and there is no scientific evidence to support aspiration (Davidson & Rourke, 2013; Sisson, 2015). The World Health Organization (WHO) (2016) and CDC (2015b) continue to recommend no aspiration for intramuscular injections. In addition, aspiration causes increased pain when performed over the standard 5 to 10 seconds (Sisson). Some literature suggests that aspiration may be indicated when administering certain medications (nonvaccines, such as the antibiotic penicillin), at certain dosages and certain rates, but more research needs to be done on this topic in the adult setting (CDC, 2015b; Thomas, Mraz, & Rajcan, 2015). Consult facility policy and manufacturer recommendations to ensure safe administration.

Refer to Box 5-1 in Skill 5-7 on page 212 for techniques for reducing discomfort when injecting medications subcutaneously or intramuscularly.

The following skill outlines administration of an intramuscular injection using the Z-track technique. If, based on assessment of the particular circumstances for an individual patient, the nurse decides not to use the Z-track technique, the skin should be stretched flat between two fingers and held taut for needle insertion.

DELEGATION CONSIDERATIONS	The administration of an intramuscular injection is not delegated to nursing assistive personnel (NAP) or to unlicensed assistive personnel (UAP). Depending on the state's nurse practice act and the organization's policies and procedures, the administration of an intramuscular injection may be delegated to licensed practical/vocational nurses (LPN/LVNs). The decision to delegate must be based on careful analysis of the patient's needs and circumstances, as well as the qualifications of the person to whom the task is being delegated. Refer to the Delegation Guidelines in Appendix A.
EQUIPMENT	• Gloves • Additional PPE, as indicated • Medication • Sterile syringe and needle of appropriate size and gauge • Antimicrobial swab • Small gauze square • Electronic Medication Administration Record (eMAR) or Medication Administration Record (MAR)
ASSESSMENT	Assess the appropriateness of the drug for the patient. Review medical history, allergy, assessment, and laboratory data that may influence drug administration. Check the expiration date before administering the medication. Assess the site on the patient where the injection is to be given. Avoid any site that is bruised, tender, hard, swollen, inflamed, or scarred. Assess the patient's knowledge of the medication. If the patient has deficient knowledge about the medication, this may be the appropriate time to begin education about it. If the medication may affect the patient's vital signs, assess them before administration. If the medication is intended for pain relief, assess the patient's pain before and after administration. Verify patient name, dose, route, and time of administration.
NURSING DIAGNOSIS	Determine related factors for the nursing diagnoses based on the patient's current status. Appropriate diagnoses may include: • Deficient knowledge • Risk for injury • Risk for infection

OUTCOME IDENTIFICATION AND PLANNING

The expected outcome to achieve when administering an intramuscular injection is that the patient receives the medication via the intramuscular route and experiences the intended effect of the medication; the patient does not experience adverse effects; and the patient understands and complies with the medication regimen.

IMPLEMENTATION

ACTION	RATIONALE
1. Gather equipment. Check each medication order against the original order in the health record according to facility policy. Clarify any inconsistencies. Check the patient's health record for allergies.	This comparison helps to identify errors that may have occurred when orders were transcribed. The primary care provider's order or prescription is the legal record of medication orders for each facility.
2. Know the actions, special nursing considerations, safe dose ranges, purpose of administration, and adverse effects of the medications to be administered. Consider the appropriateness of the medication for this patient.	This knowledge aids the nurse in evaluating the therapeutic effect of the medication in relation to the patient's disorder and can also be used to educate the patient about the medication.
3. Perform hand hygiene.	Hand hygiene prevents the spread of microorganisms.
4. Move the medication supply system to the outside of the patient's room or prepare for administration at the medication supply system in the medication area. Alternatively, access the medication administration supply system at or inside the patient's room.	Organization facilitates error-free administration and saves time.
5. Unlock the medication supply system or drawer. Enter pass code and scan employee identification, if required.	Locking the medication supply system or drawer safeguards each patient's medication supply. Facility accrediting organizations require medication supply systems to be locked when not in use. Entering pass code and scanning ID allows only authorized users into the system and identifies the user for documentation by the computer.
6. **Prepare medications for one patient at a time.**	This prevents errors in medication administration.
7. Read the eMAR/MAR and select the proper medication from medication supply system or the patient's medication drawer.	This is the *first* check of the label.
8. Compare the label with the eMAR/MAR. Check expiration dates and perform calculations, if necessary. Scan the bar code on the package, if required.	This is the *second* check of the label. Verify calculations with another nurse to ensure safety, if necessary.
9. If necessary, withdraw medication from an ampule or vial as described in Skills 5-3 and 5-4.	
10. **Depending on facility policy, the third check of the label may occur at this point. If so, when all medications for one patient have been prepared, recheck the labels with the eMAR/MAR before taking the medications to the patient. However, many facilities require the third check to occur at the bedside, after identifying the patient.**	This *third* check ensures accuracy and helps to prevent errors. *Note:* Many facilities require the *third* check to occur at the bedside, after identifying the patient and before administration.
11. **Lock the medication supply system before leaving it.**	Locking the medication supply system or drawer safeguards the patient's medication supply. Facility accrediting organizations require medication supply systems to be locked when not in use.
12. Transport medications to the patient's bedside carefully, and keep the medications in sight at all times.	Careful handling and close observation prevent accidental or deliberate disarrangement of medications.

(continued)

Skill 5-8 ▶ Administering an Intramuscular Injection *(continued)*

ACTION	RATIONALE

13. Ensure that the patient receives the medications at the correct time.

Check facility policy, which may allow for administration within a period of 30 minutes before or 30 minutes after the designated time.

14. Perform hand hygiene and put on PPE, if indicated.

Hand hygiene and PPE prevent the spread of microorganisms. PPE is required based on transmission precautions.

15. Identify the patient. Compare the information with the eMAR/MAR. The patient should be identified using at least two of the following methods (The Joint Commission, 2018):

Identifying the patient ensures the right patient receives the medications and helps prevent errors. The patient's room number or physical location is not used as an identifier (The Joint Commission, 2018). Replace the identification band if it is missing or inaccurate in any way.

   a. Check the name on the patient's identification band.

   b. Check the identification number on the patient's identification band.

   c. Check the birth date on the patient's identification band.

   d. Ask the patient to state his or her name and birth date, based on facility policy.

This requires a response from the patient, but illness and strange surroundings often cause patients to be confused.

16. Close the door to the room or pull the bedside curtain.

This provides patient privacy.

17. Complete necessary assessments before administering medications. Check the patient's allergy bracelet or ask the patient about allergies. Explain the purpose and action of the medication to the patient.

Assessment is a prerequisite to administration of medications. Explanation provides rationale, increases knowledge, and reduces anxiety.

18. Scan the patient's bar code on the identification band, if required (Figure 2).

Provides an additional check to ensure that the medication is given to the right patient.

FIGURE 2. Scanning bar code on the patient's identification bracelet. (*Photo by B. Proud.*)

19. Based on facility policy, the third check of the label may occur at this point. If so, recheck the labels with the eMAR/MAR before administering the medications to the patient.

Many facilities require the *third* check to occur at the bedside, after identifying the patient and before administration. If facility policy directs the *third* check at this time, this *third* check ensures accuracy and helps to prevent errors.

20. Put on clean gloves.

Gloves help prevent exposure to contaminants.

21. Select an appropriate administration site.

Selecting the appropriate site prevents injury.

22. Assist the patient to the appropriate position for the site chosen. See Table 5-3. Drape, as needed, to expose only the site area being used.

Appropriate positioning for the site chosen prevents injury. Draping helps maintain the patient's privacy.

ACTION

RATIONALE

23. **Identify the appropriate landmarks for the site chosen (Figure 3).**

Good visualization is necessary to establish the correct site location and to avoid tissue damage.

FIGURE 3. Identifying the appropriate landmarks.

24. Cleanse the area around the injection site with an antimicrobial swab. Use a firm, circular motion while moving outward from the injection site. Allow the area to dry.

Pathogens on the skin can be forced into the tissues by the needle. Moving from the center outward prevents contamination of the site. Allowing the antimicrobial solution to dry completely (15 to 30 seconds) ensures complete antimicrobial effectiveness (Harper, 2014), and prevents introducing alcohol into the tissue, which can be irritating and uncomfortable.

25. Remove the needle cap by pulling it straight off. Hold the syringe in your dominant hand between the thumb and forefinger.

This technique lessens the risk of an accidental needlestick and also prevents inadvertently unscrewing the needle from the barrel of the syringe.

26. Displace the skin in a Z-track manner. Pull the skin and underlying tissue down or to one side about 1 in (2.5 cm) with your nondominant hand and hold the skin and tissue in this position (Figure 4). Hand and fingers should remain in the appropriate position for the site chosen to continue accurate identification of landmarks and ensure safe injection technique. Alternatively, if, based on assessment of the particular circumstances for an individual patient, the nurse decides not to use the Z-Track technique, the skin should be stretched flat between two fingers and held taut for needle insertion.

Z-track technique is recommended for all intramuscular injections to ensure medication does not leak back along the needle track and into the subcutaneous tissue (Nicoll & Hesby, 2002; Zimmerman, 2010). This technique reduces pain and discomfort, particularly for patients receiving injections over an extended period. The Z-track method is also suggested for older adults who have decreased muscle mass. Some agents, such as iron, are best given via the Z-track method due to the irritation and discoloration associated with this agent.

A   **B**   **C**   **D**

FIGURE 4. Z-track or zigzag technique is recommended for intramuscular injections. (**A**) Normal skin and tissues. (**B**) Moving skin to one side. (**C**) Needle is inserted at a 90-degree angle. (**D**) Once needle is withdrawn, displaced tissue is allowed to return to its normal position, preventing solution from escaping from muscle tissue. Hand and finger positioning is adjusted for the specific administration site for accurate identification of landmarks and use of safe injection technique.

(continued)

Skill 5-8 ▶ Administering an Intramuscular Injection *(continued)*

ACTION	RATIONALE
27. Quickly dart the needle into the tissue so that the needle is perpendicular to the patient's body, with the goal of an angle of 90 degrees (Figure 5).	A quick injection is less painful. Inserting the needle at a 90-degree angle is the goal; actual administration using a 72- to 90-degree angle facilitates entry into muscle tissue.
28. As soon as the needle is in place, use the thumb and forefinger of your nondominant hand to hold the lower end of the syringe, taking care to maintain the displacement of the skin and tissue. Slide your dominant hand to the end of the plunger. Inject the solution slowly (10 sec/mL of medication).	Moving the syringe could cause damage to the tissues and inadvertent administration into an incorrect area. Rapid injection of the solution creates pressure in the tissues, resulting in discomfort. Aspiration, or pulling back on the plunger to check that a blood vessel has been entered, is not necessary and has not proved to be a reliable indicator of needle placement (Davidson & Rourke, 2013; Sisson, 2015). Some literature suggests that aspiration may be indicated when administering certain medications, at certain dosages, at certain rates, but more research needs to be done on this topic in the adult setting (CDC, 2015b; Thomas, Mraz, & Rajcan, 2015). Consult facility policy and manufacturer recommendations to ensure safe administration.
29. Once the medication has been instilled, wait 10 seconds before withdrawing the needle.	Allows medication to begin to diffuse into the surrounding muscle tissue (Nicoll & Hesby, 2002).
30. Withdraw the needle smoothly and steadily at the same angle at which it was inserted, supporting tissue around the injection site with your nondominant hand. **Remove the hand holding the displaced skin and tissue only after removal of the needle.**	Slow withdrawal of the needle pulls the tissues and causes discomfort. Applying counter traction around the injection site helps to prevent pulling on the tissue as the needle is withdrawn. Removing the needle at the same angle at which it was inserted minimizes tissue damage and discomfort for the patient. Allowing displaced skin and tissue to move back into place while needle is still inserted causes damage to the tissues
31. Do not recap the used needle. Engage the safety shield or needle guard, if present.	Safety shield or needle guard prevents accidental needlestick.
32. Apply gentle pressure at the site with a dry gauze (Figure 6). **Do not massage the site.**	Light pressure causes less trauma and irritation to the tissues. Massaging can force medication into subcutaneous tissues and increase discomfort.

FIGURE 5. Darting needle into tissue.

FIGURE 6. Applying gentle pressure at injection site.

33. Assist the patient to a position of comfort.	This provides for the well-being of the patient.
34. Discard the needle and syringe in the appropriate receptacle.	Proper disposal of the needle prevents injury.

ACTION	**RATIONALE**

 35. Remove gloves and additional PPE, if used. Perform hand hygiene.

Proper removal of PPE reduces the risk for infection transmission and contamination of other items. Hand hygiene prevents the spread of microorganisms.

36. Document the administration of the medication immediately after administration. See Documentation section below.

Timely documentation helps to ensure patient safety.

37. Evaluate the patient's response to the medication within the appropriate time frame. Assess site, if possible, within 2 to 4 hours after administration.

The patient needs to be evaluated for therapeutic and adverse effects from the medication. Visualization of the site allows for assessment of any untoward effects.

EVALUATION

The expected outcomes have been met when the patient receives the medication via the intramuscular route and experiences the intended effect of the medication; the patient does not experience adverse effects; and the patient understands and complies with the medication regimen.

DOCUMENTATION

Guidelines

Record each medication given on the eMAR/MAR or record using the required format, including date, time, and the site of administration, immediately after administration. If using a bar-code system, medication administration is automatically recorded when the bar code is scanned. PRN medications require documentation of the reason for administration. Prompt recording avoids the possibility of accidentally repeating the administration of the drug. If the drug was refused or omitted, record this in the appropriate area on the medication record and notify the primary care provider. This verifies the reason medication was omitted and ensures that health care personnel providing care for the patient are aware of the occurrence.

UNEXPECTED SITUATIONS AND ASSOCIATED INTERVENTIONS

- *You stick yourself with the needle before injection:* Discard needle and syringe appropriately. Follow facility policy regarding needlestick injury. Prepare new syringe with medication and administer to patient. Complete appropriate paperwork and follow facility's policy regarding accidental needlesticks.
- *You stick yourself with the needle after injection:* Discard needle and syringe appropriately. Follow facility policy regarding needlestick injury. Complete appropriate paperwork and follow facility's policy regarding accidental needlesticks.
- *During injection, the patient pulls away from the needle before the medication is delivered fully:* Remove and appropriately discard needle. Attach a new needle to syringe and administer remaining medication at a different site. Document events and interventions, according to facility policy.
- *While injecting the needle into the patient, you hit patient's bone:* Withdraw and discard the needle. Apply a new needle to the syringe and administer in an alternate site. Document incident in patient's medical record. Notify primary care provider. Complete appropriate paperwork related to special events, according to facility policy.

SPECIAL CONSIDERATIONS

General Considerations

- Ongoing assessment is an important part of nursing care for both evaluation of patient response to administered medications and early detection of adverse drug reactions. If an adverse effect is suspected, withhold further medication doses and notify the patient's primary care provider. Additional intervention is based on the type of reaction and patient assessment.
- The deltoid is the recommended site for vaccines for adults (CDC, 2015a).
- The ventrogluteal site is recommended for general IM injections in adults.

(continued)

Skill 5-8 ▶ Administering an Intramuscular Injection *(continued)*

Infant and Child Considerations

- The vastus lateralis is the preferred site for intramuscular injections in infants and young children (CDC, 2015a).
- The deltoid is the preferred site for children 3 through 18 years (CDC, 2015a).

Older Adult Considerations

- Muscle mass atrophies as a person ages. Take care to evaluate the patient's muscle mass and body composition. Use appropriate needle length and gauge for patient's body composition. Choose appropriate site based on the patient's body composition.

Home Care Considerations

- The use of antimicrobial swabs to clean the injection site in home environments may be unnecessary; patients may use soap and water to clean the site if the area is visibly soiled (Sexson et al., 2016).
- Encourage patients to consult the policies of their local government regarding contaminated and sharps waste disposal. Depending on local requirements, patients may dispose of needles and syringes in a hard, plastic container. Liquid detergent or liquid fabric softener containers are good choices. Never use glass containers.
- Reuse of syringes in the home setting is not recommended.

Skill 5-9 ▶ Administering a Continuous Subcutaneous Infusion: Applying an Insulin Pump

Some medications, such as insulin and morphine, may be administered continuously via the subcutaneous route. Continuous subcutaneous insulin infusion (CSII or insulin pump) allows for multiple preset rates of insulin delivery. This system uses a small, computerized reservoir that delivers insulin through infusion tubing to a small plastic cannula or needle or a wireless patch-pump system, that has no infusion set attached, inserted into the subcutaneous tissue (Phillips, 2016). The pump can be programmed to deliver multiple preset rates of insulin. The settings can be adjusted for exercise and illness, and bolus dose delivery can be timed in relation to meals. It is recommended that the site is changed every 2 to 3 days to prevent tissue damage or absorption problems (American Association of Diabetes Educators, 2014). Advantages of continuous subcutaneous medication infusion include the longer rate of absorption via the subcutaneous route and convenience for the patient. There are many different manufacturers of insulin pumps. Nurses need to be familiar with the particular pump in use by their patient and to refer to the specific manufacturer's recommendations for use. The following skill outlines steps in applying an insulin pump utilizing infusion tubing and a small needle-insertion device.

DELEGATION CONSIDERATIONS

The administration of a continuous subcutaneous infusion using an insulin pump is not delegated to nursing assistive personnel (NAP) or to unlicensed assistive personnel (UAP). Depending on the state's nurse practice act and the organization's policies and procedures, the management of an insulin pump in some settings may be delegated to licensed practical/vocational nurses (LPN/LVNs) who have received appropriate training. The decision to delegate must be based on careful analysis of the patient's needs and circumstances, as well as the qualifications of the person to whom the task is being delegated. Refer to the Delegation Guidelines in Appendix A.

EQUIPMENT

- Insulin pump
- Pump syringe and vial of insulin or prefilled cartridge, as ordered
- Sterile infusion set
- Insertion (triggering) device
- Needle (24- or 22-gauge, or blunt-ended needle)
- Antimicrobial swabs
- Sterile nonocclusive dressing
- Electronic Medication Administration Record (eMAR) or Medication Administration Record (MAR)
- Disposable gloves
- Additional PPE, as indicated

ASSESSMENT	Assess the appropriateness of the drug for the patient. Review medical history, allergy, assessment, and laboratory data that may influence drug administration. Check the expiration date before administering the medication. Assess the infusion site. Typical infusion sites include those areas used for subcutaneous insulin injection. Assess the area where the pump is to be applied. Do not place the pump on skin that is irritated or not intact. Assess the patient's knowledge of the medication. If the patient has a knowledge deficit about the medication, this may be the appropriate time to begin education about it. Assess the patient's blood glucose level as appropriate or as ordered. Verify patient name, dose, route, and time of administration.
NURSING DIAGNOSIS	Determine related factors for the nursing diagnoses based on the patient's current status. Appropriate nursing diagnoses may include: • Deficient knowledge • Risk for unstable blood glucose level • Risk for infection
OUTCOME IDENTIFICATION AND PLANNING	The expected outcome is that the device is applied successfully, the medication is administered correctly, and the patient experiences the intended effect of the medication. Other outcomes that may be appropriate include the following: the patient understands the rationale for the pump use and mechanism of action; the patient's skin remains intact; pump is applied using aseptic technique; and the patient does not experience unstable blood glucose levels or adverse effect.

IMPLEMENTATION

ACTION	RATIONALE
1. Gather equipment. Check each medication order against the original order in the health record, according to facility policy. Clarify any inconsistencies. Check the patient's health record for allergies.	This comparison helps to identify errors that may have occurred when orders were transcribed. The primary care provider's order or prescription is the legal record of medication orders.
2. Know the actions, special nursing considerations, safe dose ranges, purpose of administration, and adverse effects of the medications to be administered. Consider the appropriateness of the medication for this patient.	This knowledge aids the nurse in evaluating the therapeutic effect of the medication in relation to the patient's disorder and can also be used to educate the patient about the medication.
3. Perform hand hygiene.	Hand hygiene prevents the spread of microorganisms.
4. Move the medication supply system to the outside of the patient's room or prepare for administration at the medication supply system in the medication area. Alternatively, access the medication administration supply system at or inside the patient's room.	Organization facilitates error-free administration and saves time.
5. Unlock the medication supply system or drawer. Enter pass code and scan employee identification, if required.	Locking the medication supply system or drawer safeguards each patient's medication supply. Facility accrediting organizations require medication supply systems to be locked when not in use. Entering pass code and scanning ID allows only authorized users into the system and identifies the user for documentation by the computer.
6. **Prepare medications for one patient at a time.**	This prevents errors in medication administration.
7. Read the eMAR/MAR and select the proper medication from medication supply system or the patient's medication drawer.	This is the *first* check of the label.

(continued)

Skill 5-9 ▶ Administering a Continuous Subcutaneous Infusion: Applying an Insulin Pump *(continued)*

ACTION	RATIONALE
8. Compare the label with the eMAR/MAR. Check expiration dates and perform calculations, if necessary. Scan the bar code on the package, if required.	This is the *second* check of the label. Verify calculations with another nurse to ensure safety, if necessary.
9. Attach a blunt-ended needle or a small-gauge needle to a syringe. Follow Skill 5-4 to prepare insulin from a vial, if necessary. Prepare enough insulin to last the patient 2 to 3 days, plus 30 units for priming tubing. If using a prepackaged insulin syringe or cartridge, remove from packaging.	Patient will wear pump for up to 3 days without changing syringe or tubing.
10. **Depending on facility policy, the third check of the label may occur at this point. If so, when all medications for one patient have been prepared, recheck the labels with the eMAR/MAR before taking the medications to the patient. However, many facilities require the third check to occur at the bedside, after identifying the patient.**	This *third* check ensures accuracy and helps to prevent errors. *Note:* Many facilities require the *third* check to occur at the bedside, after identifying the patient and before administration.
11. **Lock the medication supply system before leaving it.**	Locking the medication supply system or drawer safeguards the patient's medication supply. Facility accrediting organizations require medication supply systems to be locked when not in use.
12. Transport medications to the patient's bedside carefully, and keep the medications in sight at all times.	Careful handling and close observation prevent accidental or deliberate disarrangement of medications.
13. **Ensure that the patient receives the medications at the correct time.**	Check facility policy, which may allow for administration within a period of 30 minutes before or 30 minutes after the designated time.
14. Perform hand hygiene and put on PPE, if indicated.	Hand hygiene and PPE prevent the spread of microorganisms. PPE is required based on transmission precautions.
15. **Identify the patient. Compare the information with the eMAR/MAR. The patient should be identified using at least two of the following methods** (The Joint Commission, 2018):	Identifying the patient ensures the right patient receives the medications and helps prevent errors. The patient's room number or physical location is not used as an identifier (The Joint Commission, 2018). Replace the identification band if it is missing or inaccurate in any way.
a. Check the name on the patient's identification band.	This requires a response from the patient, but illness and strange surroundings often cause patients to be confused.
b. Check the identification number on the patient's identification band.	
c. Check the birth date on the patient's identification band.	
d. Ask the patient to state his or her name and birth date, based on facility policy.	
16. Close the door to the room or pull the bedside curtain.	This provides patient privacy.
17. **Complete necessary assessments before administering medications. Check the patient's allergy bracelet or ask the patient about allergies. Explain the purpose and action of the medication to the patient.**	Assessment is a prerequisite to administration of medications. Explanation provides rationale, increases knowledge, and reduces anxiety.

ACTION	**RATIONALE**

18. Scan the patient's bar code on the identification band, if required (Figure 1).

Provides an additional check to ensure that the medication is given to the right patient.

FIGURE 1. Scanning bar code on patient's identification bracelet. (*Photo by B. Proud.*)

19. Based on facility policy, the third check of the label may occur at this point. If so, recheck the labels with the eMAR/MAR before administering the medications to the patient.

Many facilities require the *third* check to occur at the bedside, after identifying the patient and before administration. If facility policy directs the *third* check at this time, this *third* check ensures accuracy and helps to prevent errors.

 20. Perform hand hygiene. Put on gloves.

Hand hygiene prevents the spread of microorganisms. Gloves prevent contact with blood and body fluids.

21. Remove the cap from the syringe or insulin cartridge (Figure 2). Attach sterile tubing to the syringe or insulin cartridge. Open the pump and place the syringe or cartridge in compartment according to manufacturer's directions (Figure 3). Close the pump.

Tubing must be attached correctly and syringe must be placed in pump correctly for insulin delivery.

FIGURE 2. Removing cap from syringe or insulin cartridge.

FIGURE 3. Placing syringe or cartridge in compartment according to manufacturer's directions.

(*continued*)

Skill 5-9 ▶ Administering a Continuous Subcutaneous Infusion: Applying an Insulin Pump *(continued)*

ACTION	RATIONALE
22. Initiate priming of the tubing, according to manufacturer's directions. Program the pump according to manufacturer's recommendations following primary care provider's orders (Figure 4). **Check for any bubbles in the tubing.**	Removing all the air from the tubing and correct programming of pump ensures the patient receives the correct dose of insulin.
23. Activate the delivery device. Place the needle between prongs of the insertion device with the sharp edge facing out. Push insertion set down until a click is heard.	To ensure correct placement of insulin pump needle, an insertion device must be used.
24. Select an appropriate administration site.	Appropriate site prevents injury.
25. Assist the patient to the appropriate position for the site chosen. Drape, as needed, to expose only site area to be used.	Appropriate site prevents injury. Draping maintains privacy and warmth.
26. **Identify the appropriate landmarks for the site chosen.**	Good visualization is necessary to establish the correct site location and to avoid tissue damage.
27. Cleanse area around injection site with antimicrobial swab (Figure 5). Use a firm, circular motion while moving outward from insertion site. Allow antiseptic to dry.	Pathogens on the skin can be forced into the tissues by the needle. Moving from the center outward prevents contamination of the site. Allowing the antimicrobial solution to dry completely (15 to 30 seconds) ensures complete antimicrobial effectiveness (Harper, 2014), and prevents introducing alcohol into the tissue, which can be irritating and uncomfortable.

FIGURE 4. Programming pump according to manufacturer's recommendations following primary care provider's orders.

FIGURE 5. Cleansing area around injection site with antimicrobial swab.

ACTION	RATIONALE
28. Remove paper from adhesive backing. Remove the needle guard. Pinch skin at insertion site, press insertion device on site, and press release button to insert needle. Remove triggering device. Alternatively, if a needle was used to introduce a subcutaneous catheter and then withdrawn, engage the safety shield or needle guard.	To ensure delivery of insulin into subcutaneous tissue, a skin fold is made with a pinch *before* insertion of the medication. Safety shield or needle guard prevents accidental needlestick.
29. Apply sterile occlusive dressing over the insertion site, if not part of the insertion device. Attach the pump to patient's clothing, as desired (Figure 6).	Dressing prevents contamination of site. Pump can be dislodged easily if not attached securely to patient.
30. Assist the patient to a position of comfort.	This provides for the well-being of the patient.
31. If a needle was used to introduce a subcutaneous catheter and then withdrawn, discard the needle and syringe in the appropriate receptacle.	Proper disposal of the needle prevents injury.

ACTION	RATIONALE

FIGURE 6. Insulin pump in place.

32. Remove gloves and additional PPE, if used. Perform hand hygiene.

Proper removal of PPE reduces the risk for infection transmission and contamination of other items. Hand hygiene prevents the spread of microorganisms.

33. Document the administration of the medication immediately after administration. See Documentation section below.

Timely documentation helps to ensure patient safety.

34. Evaluate the patient's response to the medication within the appropriate time frame. Monitor the patient's blood glucose levels, as appropriate, or as ordered.

Patient needs to be evaluated to ensure that the pump is delivering the drug appropriately. The patient needs to be evaluated for therapeutic and adverse effects from the medication.

EVALUATION

The expected outcomes have been met when the device has been applied successfully; the medication is administered correctly; the patient experiences the intended effect of the medication; the patient understands the rationale for the pump use and mechanism of action; the patient's skin remains intact; and the patient does not experience unstable blood glucose levels or adverse effect.

DOCUMENTATION

Guidelines

Document the application of the pump, the type of insulin used, pump settings, insertion site, and any teaching done with the patient on the eMAR/MAR or record using the required format, including date, time, and the site of administration, immediately after administration. If using a bar-code system, medication administration is automatically recorded when the bar code is scanned. PRN medications require documentation of the reason for administration. Prompt recording avoids the possibility of accidentally repeating the administration of the drug. If the drug was refused or omitted, record this in the appropriate area on the medication record and notify the primary care provider. This verifies the reason medication was omitted and ensures that health care personnel providing care for the patient are aware of the occurrence.

Sample Documentation

> 9/22/20 1000 Insulin pump inserted by patient on left upper quadrant of abdomen with minimal assistance. Pump filled with 300 units (3 mL) of lispro insulin. Rate set at 1 unit per hour. Patient verbalizes desire to apply pump without assistance when site next changed.
>
> —B. Clapp, RN

(*continued*)

Skill 5-9 ▶ Administering a Continuous Subcutaneous Infusion: Applying an Insulin Pump *(continued)*

UNEXPECTED SITUATIONS AND ASSOCIATED INTERVENTIONS

- *After the pump is attached to the patient, a large amount of air is noted in tubing:* Remove the pump from patient. Obtain new sterile tubing with insertion needle. Prime the tubing and reinsert.
- *Patient must rotate site more frequently than every 2 to 3 days due to insulin usage:* Check manufacturer's recommendations. Most pumps are initially set in a smaller mode but can be changed for a larger amount of insulin delivery.
- *Patient is refusing to rotate site at least every 3 days:* Inform the patient that absorption of medication decreases after 3 days, which may increase his or her need for insulin. Rotating sites prevents this decrease in absorption from developing. In addition, site rotation reduces risk of infection at the site.
- *You note that the insertion site is now erythematous:* Remove the stylet, obtain a new pump setup, and insert at a different site at least 1 in from old site.
- *Occlusive dressing will not stick due to perspiration:* Apply deodorant around insertion site but not over insertion site. Alternatively, apply skin barrier around insertion site but not over insertion site.

SPECIAL CONSIDERATIONS

General Considerations

- Assess infusion site areas routinely for inflammation, allergic reactions, infection, and lipodystrophy.
- Good hygiene and frequent catheter site changes reduce the risk of site complications. Change catheter site every 2 to 3 days.
- Contact dermatitis is sometimes a problem at the catheter site area. The primary care provider may order topical antibiotics, aloe, vitamin E, or corticosteroids to treat a contact dermatitis.
- Insulin self-administered by the patient through the insulin pump should be communicated to the nurse at the time of administration. This allows for accurate documentation of insulin requirements.
- Ongoing assessment is an important part of nursing care for both evaluation of patient response to administered medications and early detection of adverse reactions. If an adverse effect is suspected, withhold further medication doses and notify the patient's primary care provider. Additional intervention is based on type of reaction and patient assessment.

Home Care Considerations

- Encourage patients to consult the policies of their local government regarding contaminated and sharps waste disposal. Depending on local requirements, patients may dispose of needles and syringes in a hard, plastic container. Liquid detergent or liquid fabric softener containers are good choices. Never use glass containers.

EVIDENCE FOR PRACTICE ▶

CONTINUOUS SUBCUTANEOUS INSULIN INFUSION (CSII)

American Association of Diabetes Educators (AADE). (2014). AADE White paper. Continuous subcutaneous insulin infusion (CSII). Retrieved https://www.diabeteseducator.org/docs/default-source/legacy-docs/_resources/pdf/publications/csii_pentulimate.pdf?sfvrsn=2

This white paper outlines critical topics to be covered when teaching patients and families or significant other about insulin pump therapy. These guidelines are directed to diabetes nurse educators, but provide best-practice guidelines for all nurses caring for patients with diabetes considering or using continuous subcutaneous insulin infusion (CSII).

Refer to thePoint® for additional research on related nursing topics.

Skill 5-10 ▶ Administering Medications by Intravenous Bolus or Push Through an Intravenous Infusion

A medication can be administered via the **intravenous (IV) route** as an IV bolus or push through a venous access device being used for continuous infusion of fluid. This involves a single injection of a concentrated solution directly into an IV access. Drugs given by IV push are used for intermittent dosing or to treat emergencies. The drug is administered at the rate recommended by the manufacturer, supported by evidence in peer-reviewed biomedical literature, or in accordance with approved institutional guidelines (Institute for Safe Medication Practices, 2015, p. 13). Confirm exact administration times by consulting a drug reference, package insert, or a pharmacist.

DELEGATION CONSIDERATIONS

The administration of medications by intravenous bolus is not delegated to nursing assistive personnel (NAP) or to unlicensed assistive personnel (UAP). Depending on the state's nurse practice act and the organization's policies and procedures, the administration of specified intravenous medications in some settings may be delegated to licensed practical/vocational nurses (LPN/LVNs) who have received appropriate training. The decision to delegate must be based on careful analysis of the patient's needs and circumstances, as well as the qualifications of the person to whom the task is being delegated. Refer to the Delegation Guidelines in Appendix A.

EQUIPMENT

- Antimicrobial swab
- Watch or clock with second hand
- Disposable gloves
- Additional PPE, as indicated
- Prescribed medication
- 2 – Normal saline flushes prepared in a syringe (3 to 10 mL) according to facility policy
- Passive disinfection caps (based on facility policy)
- Syringe with a needleless device or 23- to 25-gauge, 1-in needle (follow facility policy)
- Electronic Medication Administration Record (eMAR) or Medication Administration Record (MAR)

ASSESSMENT

Assess the appropriateness of the drug for the patient. Review medical history, allergy, assessment, and laboratory data that may influence drug administration. Check the expiration date before administering the medication. Assess the compatibility of the ordered medication and the IV fluid. Assess the patient's IV site for signs of any complications. (Refer to Fundamentals Review 15-3 and Box 15-3 in Chapter 15 on pages 887 and 907). Assess the patient's knowledge of the medication. If the patient has a knowledge deficit about the medication, this may be the appropriate time to begin education about the medication. If the medication may affect the patient's vital signs, assess them before administration. If the medication is for pain relief, assess the patient's pain before and after administration. Verify the patient's name, dose, route, and time of administration.

NURSING DIAGNOSIS

Determine related factors for the nursing diagnoses based on the patient's current status. Appropriate nursing diagnoses may include:

- Risk for injury
- Risk for allergy reaction
- Risk for infection

OUTCOME IDENTIFICATION AND PLANNING

The expected outcome to achieve is that the medication is given safely via the IV route and the patient experiences the intended effect of the medication. Other outcomes that may be appropriate include the following: the patient experiences no adverse effects; and the patient understands and complies with the medication regimen.

(continued)

Skill 5-10 ▶ Administering Medications by Intravenous Bolus or Push Through an Intravenous Infusion *(continued)*

IMPLEMENTATION

ACTION	RATIONALE
1. Gather equipment. Check medication order against the original order in the medical record, according to facility policy. Clarify any inconsistencies. Check the patient's health record for allergies. Check a drug resource to clarify whether the medication needs to be diluted before administration. Check the administration rate.	This comparison helps to identify errors that may have occurred when orders were transcribed. The primary care provider's order or prescription is the legal record of medication orders for each facility. Compatibility of medication and solution prevents complications. Delivers the correct dose of medication as prescribed.
2. Know the actions, special nursing considerations, safe dose ranges, purpose of administration, and adverse effects of the medications to be administered. Consider the appropriateness of the medication for this patient.	This knowledge aids the nurse in evaluating the therapeutic effect of the medication in relation to the patient's disorder and can also be used to educate the patient about the medication.
3. Perform hand hygiene.	Hand hygiene prevents the spread of microorganisms.
4. Move the medication supply system to the outside of the patient's room or prepare for administration at the medication supply system in the medication area. Alternatively, access the medication administration supply system at or inside the patient's room.	Organization facilitates error-free administration and saves time.
5. Unlock the medication supply system or drawer. Enter pass code and scan employee identification, if required.	Locking the medication supply system or drawer safeguards each patient's medication supply. Facility accrediting organizations require medication supply systems to be locked when not in use. Entering pass code and scanning ID allows only authorized users into the system and identifies the user for documentation by the computer.
6. **Prepare medication for one patient at a time.**	This prevents errors in medication administration.
7. Read the eMAR/MAR and select the proper medication from the medication supply system or the patient's medication drawer.	This is the *first* check of the label.
8. Compare the label with the eMAR/MAR. Check expiration dates and perform calculations, if necessary. Scan the bar code on the package, if required.	This is the *second* check of the label. Verify calculations with another nurse to ensure safety, if necessary.
9. If necessary, withdraw medication from an ampule or vial as described in Skills 5-3 and 5-4.	
10. **Depending on facility policy, the third check of the label may occur at this point. If so, when all medications for one patient have been prepared, recheck the labels with the eMAR/MAR before taking the medications to the patient. However, many facilities require the third check to occur at the bedside, after identifying the patient.**	This *third* check ensures accuracy and helps to prevent errors. *Note:* Many facilities require the *third* check to occur at the bedside, after identifying the patient and before administration.
11. **Lock the medication supply system before leaving it.**	Locking the medication supply system or drawer safeguards the patient's medication supply. Facility accrediting organizations require medication supply systems to be locked when not in use.
12. Transport medications and equipment to the patient's bedside carefully, and keep the medications in sight at all times.	Careful handling and close observation prevent accidental or deliberate disarrangement of medications. Having equipment available saves time and facilitates performance of the task.
13. **Ensure that the patient receives the medications at the correct time.**	Check facility policy, which may allow for administration within a period of 30 minutes before or 30 minutes after the designated time.

ACTION	RATIONALE

14. Perform hand hygiene and put on PPE, if indicated.

Hand hygiene and PPE prevent the spread of microorganisms. PPE is required based on transmission precautions.

15. **Identify the patient. Compare the information with the eMAR/MAR. The patient should be identified using at least two of the following methods (The Joint Commission, 2018):**

Identifying the patient ensures the right patient receives the medications and helps prevent errors. The patient's room number or physical location is not used as an identifier (The Joint Commission, 2018). Replace the identification band if it is missing or inaccurate in any way.

a. Check the name on the patient's identification band.

b. Check the identification number on the patient's identification band.

c. Check the birth date on the patient's identification band.

d. Ask the patient to state his or her name and birth date, based on facility policy.

This requires a response from the patient, but illness and strange surroundings often cause patients to be confused.

16. Close the door to the room or pull the bedside curtain.

This provides patient privacy.

17. **Complete necessary assessments before administering medications. Check the patient's allergy bracelet or ask the patient about allergies. Explain the purpose and action of the medication to the patient.**

Assessment is a prerequisite to administration of medications. Explanation provides rationale, increases knowledge, and reduces anxiety.

18. Scan the patient's bar code on the identification band, if required.

Provides an additional check to ensure that the medication is given to the right patient.

19. **Based on facility policy, the third check of the label may occur at this point. If so, recheck the label with the eMAR/MAR before administering the medications to the patient.**

Many facilities require the *third* check to occur at the bedside, after identifying the patient and before administration. If facility policy directs the *third* check at this time, this *third* check ensures accuracy and helps to prevent errors.

20. Assess IV site for presence of inflammation or infiltration or other signs of complications.

IV medication must be given directly into a vein for safe administration.

21. If IV infusion is being administered via an infusion pump, pause the pump.

Pausing prevents infusion of fluid during bolus administration and activation of pump occlusion alarms.

22. Put on clean gloves.

Gloves prevent contact with blood and body fluids.

23. Select injection port on the administration set that is closest to the patient. Close the clamp on the administration set immediately above the injection port (Figure 1). Do not disconnect the administration set from the venous access device hub (INS, 2016a).

Using port closest to the needle insertion site minimizes dilution of medication. Closing of clamp immediately above access port ensures medication is administered to the patient and prevents medication from backing up tubing.

FIGURE 1. Closing the clamp on the administration set.

(continued)

Skill 5-10 ▶ Administering Medications by Intravenous Bolus or Push Through an Intravenous Infusion *(continued)*

ACTION	RATIONALE
24. Remove the passive disinfection cap from the needleless connector or end cap on the infusion set injection port (Figure 2). Alternatively, if a passive disinfection cap is not in place, use an antimicrobial swab to vigorously scrub the needleless connector or end cap on the injection port and allow to dry.	Passive disinfection caps contain an antiseptic-impregnated sponge that dispenses the antiseptic over the connector's top and threads, and protects the hub from contamination by touch or airborne sources (Stango Runyan, Stern, Macri, & Vacca, 2014). Venous access device entry points, end-caps, and needleless connectors must be vigorously scrubbed and disinfected prior to each access to reduce the risk for introduction of microorganisms and prevent venous access device-related infection (Frimpong, Caguioa, & Octavo, 2015; Harper, 2014; INS, 2016b; The Joint Commission, 2018; Loveday et al., 2014). Friction is needed to physically remove microorganisms from the top, sides, and threads of the needleless connector or end cap. Allow the antiseptic to dry completely (15 to 30 seconds) to ensure complete effectiveness (Harper).
25. Uncap saline flush syringe. Insert the saline flush syringe into the needleless connector or end cap on the injection port on the administration tubing (Figure 3).	Assessing patency of venous access device is necessary to ensure intravenous administration of the medication.

FIGURE 2. Removing the passive disinfection cap.

FIGURE 3. Inserting the saline flush syringe into the injection port.

26. Pull back on the syringe plunger to aspirate the catheter for positive blood return (Figure 4). If positive, instill the solution over 1 minute or flush the line according to facility policy. Remove syringe.	Positive blood return confirms patency before administration of medications and solutions (INS, 2016b). Flushing without incident ensures patency of the IV line and administration of medication into the bloodstream.

FIGURE 4. Pulling back on plunger to check blood return.

ACTION

27. Use an antimicrobial swab to vigorously scrub the needleless connector or end cap on the injection port and allow to dry.

28. Uncap the medication syringe. Insert the medication syringe into the needleless connector or end cap on the injection port. Using a watch or clock with a second-hand to time the rate, **inject the medication at the recommended rate (Figure 5).**

29. While administering the medication, observe the infusion site and assess patient for any adverse reaction. If signs of adverse reaction occur, stop infusion immediately and notify the primary health provider.

30. Detach the medication syringe. Use a new antimicrobial swab to vigorously scrub the needleless connector or end cap on the injection port, and allow to dry. Uncap the second saline flush syringe. Insert the saline flush syringe into the needleless connector or end cap on injection port. Instill the flush solution at the same rate as the administered medication (INS, 2016a).

31. Remove the flush syringe. Unclamp the administration set above the injection port.

RATIONALE

Venous access device entry points, end-caps, and needleless connectors must be vigorously scrubbed and disinfected prior to each access to reduce the risk for introduction of microorganisms and prevent venous access device-related infection (Frimpong et al., 2015; Harper, 2014; INS, 2016b; The Joint Commission, 2018; Loveday et al., 2014). Friction is needed to physically remove microorganisms from the top, sides, and threads of the needleless connector or end cap. Allow the antiseptic to dry completely (15 to 30 seconds) to ensure complete effectiveness (Harper, 2014).

This delivers the correct amount of medication at the proper interval.

FIGURE 5. Injecting medication at the recommended rate.

Signs of adverse reaction, such as peripheral IV infiltration, rash or itching, or pain at the infusion, necessitate stopping of administration of the drug (INS, 2016a).

Venous access device entry points, end-caps, and needleless connectors must be vigorously scrubbed and disinfected prior to each access to reduce the risk for introduction of microorganisms and prevent venous access device-related infection (Frimpong et al., 2015; Harper, 2014; INS, 2016b; The Joint Commission, 2018; Loveday et al., 2014). Friction is needed to physically remove microorganisms from the top, sides, and threads of the needleless connector or end cap. Allow the antiseptic to dry completely (15 to 30 seconds) to ensure complete effectiveness (Harper). Flushing after medication administration ensure the entire drug dose has been cleared from the extension tubing on the venous access device or from the infusion system and prevents precipitation due to solution/medication incompatibility (INS, 2016a).

Clamping prevents air from entering the extension set on a capped venous access device. Unclamping the administration set allows for resumption of the continuous intravenous infusion.

(continued)

Skill 5-10 ▶ Administering Medications by Intravenous Bolus or Push Through an Intravenous Infusion *(continued)*

ACTION

32. Using an antimicrobial swab, vigorously scrub the needleless connector or end cap on the extension tubing and allow to dry. Attach a passive disinfection cap to the needleless connector or end cap on the extension tubing or the injection port on the administration set (Figure 6).

33. Restart the infusion pump and check IV fluid infusion rate.

34. Discard the syringe in the appropriate receptacle.

35. Remove gloves and additional PPE, if used. Perform hand hygiene.

36. Document the administration of the medication immediately after administration. See Documentation section below.

37. Evaluate the patient's response to the medication within the appropriate time frame.

RATIONALE

Venous access device entry points, end-caps, and needleless connectors must be vigorously scrubbed and disinfected prior to each access to reduce the risk for introduction of microorganisms and prevent venous access device-related infection (Frimpong et al., 2015; Harper, 2014; INS, 2016b; The Joint Commission, 2018; Loveday et al., 2014). Friction is needed to physically remove microorganisms from the top, sides, and threads of the needleless connector or end cap. Allow the antiseptic to dry completely (15 to 30 seconds) to ensure complete effectiveness (Harper, 2014). Passive disinfection caps contain an antiseptic-impregnated sponge that dispenses the antiseptic over the connector's top and threads, and protect the hub from contamination by touch or airborne sources (Stango et al., 2014).

FIGURE 6. Attaching a passive disinfection cap.

Restarting infusion pump resumes prescribed continuous infusion of fluid. Checking IV fluid infusion rate assures accuracy in administration.

Proper disposal prevents injury and spread of microorganisms.

Proper removal of PPE reduces the risk for infection transmission and contamination of other items. Hand hygiene prevents the spread of microorganisms.

Timely documentation helps to ensure patient safety.

The patient needs to be evaluated for therapeutic and adverse effects from the medication.

EVALUATION

The expected outcomes have been met when the medication has been given safely via the IV route and the patient experiences the intended effect of the medication; the patient experiences no adverse effects; and the patient understands and complies with the medication regimen.

DOCUMENTATION

Guidelines

Document the administration of the medication immediately after administration, including date, time, dose, route of administration, site of administration, and rate of administration on the eMAR/MAR or record using the required format. If using a bar-code system, medication administration is automatically recorded when the bar code is scanned. PRN medications require documentation of the reason for administration. Prompt recording avoids the possibility of accidentally repeating the administration of the drug. If the drug was refused or omitted, record this in the appropriate area on the medication record and notify the primary care provider. This verifies the reason medication was omitted and ensures that health care personnel providing care for the patient are aware of the occurrence.

UNEXPECTED SITUATIONS AND ASSOCIATED INTERVENTIONS

- *Upon assessing the IV site before administering medication, no blood return is aspirated:* If IV appears patent, without signs of infiltration, and IV fluid infuses without difficulty, proceed with administration. Observe closely for signs and symptoms of infiltration during and after administration.
- *Upon assessing the patient's IV site before administering medication, you note that IV has infiltrated:* Stop IV fluid and remove IV from extremity. Restart IV in a different location. Continue to monitor new IV site as medication is administered.
- *While administering medication, you note a cloudy, white substance forming in the IV tubing:* Stop administering medication. Clamp IV at the site nearest to the patient. Change administration tubing and restart infusion. Check literature or consult pharmacist regarding compatibility of medication and IV fluid.
- *While you are administering the medication, the patient begins to complain of pain at the IV site:* Stop medication. Assess IV site for any signs of infiltration or phlebitis. Flush the IV with normal saline to check for patency. If the IV site appears within normal limits, resume medication administration at a slower rate.

SPECIAL CONSIDERATIONS

- Do not withdraw IV push medications from commercially available, cartridge-type syringes into another syringe for administration. Using the cartridge as a vial can lead to contamination and/or dosing errors, drug mix-ups, and other medication errors (ISMP, 2015, p. 11).
- Do not dilute or reconstitute IV push medications by drawing up the contents into a commercially available, prefilled flush syringe of 0.9% sodium chloride. These devices have been approved for flushing of vascular access devices, but have not been approved for the reconstitution, dilution, and/or subsequent administration of IV push medications (ISMP, 2015, p. 11).
- Appropriately label all clinician-prepared syringes of IV push medications or solutions, unless the medication or solution is prepared at the patient's bedside and is immediately administered to the patient (ISMP, 2015, p. 12).
- If the IV is a small gauge (22- to 24-gauge) placed in a small vein, a blood return may not occur even if IV is intact. Also, the patient may complain of stinging and pain at the site while medication is being administered due to irritation of vein. Slowing the rate of administration may relieve discomfort.
- Ongoing assessment is an important part of nursing care for both evaluation of patient response to administered medications and early detection of adverse drug reactions. If an adverse effect is suspected, withhold further medication doses and notify the patient's primary care provider. Additional intervention is based on type of reaction and patient assessment.

EVIDENCE FOR PRACTICE ▶

INFUSION NURSING STANDARDS OF PRACTICE

Infusion Nurses Society (INS). (2016b). Infusion therapy. Standards of practice. *Journal of Infusion Nursing, 39*(Suppl 1), S1–S159.

The Infusion Nurses Society is recognized as the global authority in infusion therapy. The *Infusion Nursing Standards of Practice* is an evidence-based document, providing guidelines for nurses related to infusion therapy for use in all patient settings and addressing all patient populations.

Refer to thePoint for additional research on related nursing topics.

(continued)

Skill 5-10 ▶ Administering Medications by Intravenous Bolus or Push Through an Intravenous Infusion *(continued)*

EVIDENCE FOR PRACTICE ▶	**INFUSION NURSING POLICIES AND PROCEDURES FOR INFUSION THERAPY**

Infusion Nurses Society (INS). (2016a). *Policies and procedures for infusion therapy* (5th ed.). Norwood, MA: Author.

The Infusion Nurses Society is recognized as the global authority in infusion therapy. The *Infusion Nursing Standards of Practice* is an evidence-based document, providing policies and step-by-step procedures for nurses related to infusion therapy for use in all patient settings and addressing all patient populations.

Refer to thePoint® for additional research on related nursing topics.

Skill 5-11 ▶ Administering Medications by Intravenous Bolus or Push Through a Medication or Drug-Infusion Lock

A medication or drug-infusion lock, also known as an intermittent peripheral venous access device or saline lock, is used for patients who require intermittent IV medication, but not a continuous IV infusion. This device consists of a catheter connected to a short length of tubing capped with a sealed injection port. After the catheter is in place in the patient's vein, the catheter and tubing are anchored to the patient's arm so that the catheter remains in place until the patient no longer requires the repeated medication intravenously.

The device is kept patent (working) by flushing with small amounts of saline pushed through the device on a routine basis. Using saline eliminates any possible systemic effects on coagulation, development of a heparin allergy, and drug incompatibility, which may occur when a heparin solution is used. The nurse must confirm IV placement before administration of medication. It is important to flush the drug-infusion lock before and after the medication is administered to clear the vein of any medication and to prevent clot formation in the device. If infiltration or phlebitis occurs, the lock is removed and replaced in a new site. Refer to Chapter 15 for a more detailed discussion of intravenous access devices and associated nursing skills.

DELEGATION CONSIDERATIONS

The administration of medications through an intermittent peripheral venous access device is not delegated to nursing assistive personnel (NAP) or to unlicensed assistive personnel (UAP). Depending on the state's nurse practice act and the organization's policies and procedures, the administration of specified IV medications in some settings may be delegated to licensed practical/vocational nurses (LPN/LVNs) who have received appropriate training. The decision to delegate must be based on careful analysis of the patient's needs and circumstances, as well as the qualifications of the person to whom the task is being delegated. Refer to the Delegation Guidelines in Appendix A.

EQUIPMENT

- Prescribed medication
- 2 – Normal saline flushes prepared in a syringe (3 to 10 mL) according to facility policy
- Antimicrobial swabs
- Passive disinfection caps (based on facility policy)
- Syringe with a needleless device or 23- to 25-gauge, 1-in needle (follow facility policy)
- Watch or clock with a second hand
- Disposable gloves
- Electronic Medication Administration Record (eMAR) or Medication Administration Record (MAR)
- Additional PPE, as indicated

ASSESSMENT

Assess the appropriateness of the drug for the patient. Review medical history, allergy, assessment, and laboratory data that may influence drug administration. Check the expiration date before administering the medication. Assess the patient's IV site for signs of any complications. (Refer to Fundamentals Review 15-3 and Box 15-3 in Chapter 15 on pages 887 and 907). Assess the patient's knowledge of the medication. If the patient has a knowledge deficit about the medication, this may be the appropriate time to begin education about the medication. If the medication may affect the patient's vital signs, assess them before administration. If the medication is for pain relief, assess the patient's pain before and after administration. Verify the patient's name, dose, route, and time of administration.

NURSING DIAGNOSIS

Determine related factors for the nursing diagnoses based on the patient's current status. Appropriate nursing diagnoses may include:

- Risk for allergy reaction
- Risk for infection
- Risk for injury

OUTCOME IDENTIFICATION AND PLANNING

The expected outcome to achieve when administering medication via a medication or drug-infusion lock is that the medication is delivered via the IV route and the patient experiences the intended effect of the medication. Other outcomes that may be appropriate include the following: the patient experiences no adverse effects; and the patient understands and complies with the medication regimen.

IMPLEMENTATION

ACTION	RATIONALE
1. Gather equipment. Check the medication order against the original order in the health record, according to facility policy. Clarify any inconsistencies. Check the patient's health record for allergies. Check a drug resource to clarify whether medication needs to be diluted before bolus administration. Verify the recommended administration rate.	This comparison helps to identify errors that may have occurred when orders were transcribed. The primary care provider's order or prescription is the legal record of medication orders for each facility. Recommended administration rate delivers the correct dose of medication as prescribed.
2. Know the actions, special nursing considerations, safe dose ranges, purpose of administration, and adverse effects of the medications to be administered. Consider the appropriateness of the medication for this patient.	This knowledge aids the nurse in evaluating the therapeutic effect of the medication in relation to the patient's disorder and can also be used to educate the patient about the medication.
3. Perform hand hygiene.	Hand hygiene prevents the spread of microorganisms.
4. Move the medication supply system to the outside of the patient's room or prepare for administration at the medication supply system in the medication area. Alternatively, access the medication administration supply system at or inside the patient's room.	Organization facilitates error-free administration and saves time.
5. Unlock the medication supply system or drawer. Enter pass code and scan employee identification, if required.	Locking the medication supply system or drawer safeguards each patient's medication supply. Facility accrediting organizations require medication supply systems to be locked when not in use. Entering pass code and scanning ID allows only authorized users into the system and identifies the user for documentation by the computer.
6. Prepare medication for one patient at a time.	This prevents errors in medication administration.

(continued)

Skill 5-11 ▶ Administering Medications by Intravenous Bolus or Push Through a Medication or Drug-Infusion Lock *(continued)*

ACTION	**RATIONALE**
7. Read the eMAR/MAR and select the proper medication from medication supply system or the patient's medication drawer.	This is the *first* check of the label.
8. Compare the label with the eMAR/MAR. Check expiration dates and perform calculations, if necessary. Scan the bar code on the package, if required.	This is the *second* check of the label. Verify calculations with another nurse to ensure safety, if necessary.
9. If necessary, withdraw medication from an ampule or vial as described in Skills 5-3 and 5-4.	Allows administration of medication.
10. **Depending on facility policy, the third check of the label may occur at this point. If so, when all medications for one patient have been prepared, recheck the labels with the eMAR/MAR before taking the medications to the patient. However, many facilities require the third check to occur at the bedside, after identifying the patient.**	This *third* check ensures accuracy and helps to prevent errors. *Note:* Many facilities require the *third* check to occur at the bedside, after identifying the patient and before administration.
11. **Lock the medication supply system before leaving it.**	Locking the medication supply system or drawer safeguards the patient's medication supply. Facility accrediting organizations require medication supply systems to be locked when not in use.
12. Transport medications and equipment to the patient's bedside carefully, and keep the medications in sight at all times.	Careful handling and close observation prevent accidental or deliberate disarrangement of medications. Having equipment available saves time and facilitates performance of the task.
13. **Ensure that the patient receives the medications at the correct time.**	Check facility policy, which may allow for administration within a period of 30 minutes before or 30 minutes after the designated time.
14. Perform hand hygiene and put on PPE, if indicated.	Hand hygiene and PPE prevent the spread of microorganisms. PPE is required based on transmission precautions.
15. **Identify the patient. Compare the information with the eMAR/MAR. The patient should be identified using at least two of the following methods (The Joint Commission, 2018):**	Identifying the patient ensures the right patient receives the medications and helps prevent errors. The patient's room number or physical location is not used as an identifier (The Joint Commission, 2018). Replace the identification band if it is missing or inaccurate in any way.
a. Check the name on the patient's identification band.	This requires a response from the patient, but illness and strange surroundings often cause patients to be confused.
b. Check the identification number on the patient's identification band.	
c. Check the birth date on the patient's identification band.	
d. Ask the patient to state his or her name and birth date, based on facility policy.	
16. Close the door to the room or pull the bedside curtain.	This provides patient privacy.
17. **Complete necessary assessments before administering medications. Check the patient's allergy bracelet or ask the patient about allergies. Explain the purpose and action of the medication to the patient.**	Assessment is a prerequisite to administration of medications. Explanation provides rationale, increases knowledge, and reduces anxiety.
18. Scan the patient's bar code on the identification band, if required (Figure 1).	Scanning provides an additional check to ensure that the medication is given to the right patient.
19. **Based on facility policy, the third check of the label may occur at this point. If so, recheck the labels with the eMAR/MAR before administering the medications to the patient.**	Many facilities require the *third* check to occur at the bedside, after identifying the patient and before administration. If facility policy directs the *third* check at this time, this *third* check ensures accuracy and helps to prevent errors.

ACTION	**RATIONALE**
20. Assess IV site for presence of inflammation or infiltration.	IV medication must be given directly into a vein for safe administration.

FIGURE 1. Scanning bar code on patient's identification bracelet.

ACTION	**RATIONALE**
21. Put on clean gloves.	Gloves protect the nurse's hands from contact with the patient's blood.
22. Remove the passive disinfection cap from the needleless connector or access port of the medication lock (Figure 2). Alternatively, if a passive disinfection cap is not in place, use an antimicrobial swab to vigorously scrub the needleless connector or access port of the medication lock and allow to dry.	Passive disinfection caps contain an antiseptic-impregnated sponge that dispenses the antiseptic over the connector's top and threads, and protects the hub from contamination by touch or airborne sources (Stango et al., 2014). Venous access device entry points, end-caps, and needleless connectors must be vigorously scrubbed and disinfected prior to each access to reduce the risk for introduction of microorganisms and prevent venous access device-related infection (Frimpong et al., 2015; Harper, 2014; INS, 2016b; The Joint Commission, 2018; Loveday, 2014). Friction is needed to physically remove microorganisms from the top, sides, and threads of the needleless connector or end cap. Allow the antiseptic to dry completely (15 to 30 seconds) to ensure complete effectiveness (Harper).
23. Uncap saline flush syringe. Stabilize the port with your nondominant hand and insert the saline flush syringe into the needleless connector or end cap on the access port of the medication lock (Figure 3).	Assessing patency of venous access device is necessary to ensure intravenous administration of the medication.

FIGURE 2. Removing the passive disinfection cap from the access port.

FIGURE 3. Inserting the saline flush syringe into the access port.

(continued)

Skill 5-11 ▶ Administering Medications by Intravenous Bolus or Push Through a Medication or Drug-Infusion Lock *(continued)*

ACTION	RATIONALE

ACTION

24. Release the clamp on the extension tubing of the medication lock (Figure 4). Pull back on the syringe plunger to aspirate the catheter for positive blood return (Figure 5). If positive, instill the solution over 1 minute or flush the line according to facility policy. Observe the insertion site while inserting the saline. Remove syringe.

FIGURE 4. Releasing the clamp on the extension tubing.

25. Use an antimicrobial swab to vigorously scrub the needleless connector or end cap on the access port of the medication lock and allow to dry.

26. Uncap the medication syringe. Insert the medication syringe into the needleless connector or end cap on the access port of the medication lock. Using a watch or clock with a second-hand to time the rate, **inject the medication at the recommended rate (Figure 6). Do not force the injection if resistance is felt.**

RATIONALE

Positive blood return confirms patency before administration of medications and solutions (INS, 2016b). Flushing without incident ensures patency of the IV line and administration of medication into the bloodstream. Puffiness, pain, or swelling as the site is flushed could indicate infiltration of the catheter.

FIGURE 5. Pulling back on the plunger to aspirate for a blood return.

Venous access device entry points, end-caps, and needleless connectors must be vigorously scrubbed and disinfected prior to each access to reduce the risk for introduction of microorganisms and prevent venous access device-related infection (Frimpong et al., 2015; Harper, 2014; INS, 2016b; The Joint Commission, 2018; Loveday, 2014). Friction is needed to physically remove microorganisms from the top, sides, and threads of the needleless connector or end cap. Allow the antiseptic to dry completely (15 to 30 seconds) to ensure complete effectiveness (Harper).

This delivers the correct amount of medication at the proper interval. Easy installation of medication usually indicates that the lock is still patent and in the vein. If force is used against resistance, a clot may break away and cause a blockage elsewhere in the body.

FIGURE 6. Injecting the medication at the recommended rate.

ACTION	RATIONALE
27. While administering the medication, observe the infusion site and assess patient for any adverse reaction. If signs of adverse reaction occur, stop infusion immediately and notify the primary health provider.	Signs of adverse reaction, such as peripheral IV infiltration, rash or itching, or pain at the infusion, necessitate stopping of administration of the drug (INS, 2016a).
28. Remove the medication syringe from the access port. Use a new antimicrobial swab to vigorously scrub the needleless connector or end cap on the access port and allow to dry. Stabilize the port with your nondominant hand. Uncap the second saline flush syringe. Insert the saline flush syringe into the needleless connector or end cap on the access port. Instill the flush solution at the same rate as the administered medication (INS, 2016a).	Venous access device entry points, end-caps, and needleless connectors must be vigorously scrubbed and disinfected prior to each access to reduce the risk for introduction of microorganisms and prevent venous access device-related infection (Frimpong et al., 2015; Harper, 2014; INS, 2016b; The Joint Commission, 2018; Loveday, 2014). Friction is needed to physically remove microorganisms from the top, sides, and threads of the needleless connector or end cap. Allow the antiseptic to dry completely (15 to 30 seconds) to ensure complete effectiveness (Harper). Flushing after medication administration ensure the entire drug dose has been cleared from the extension tubing on the venous access device or from the infusion system and prevents precipitation due to solution/medication incompatibility (INS, 2016a).
29. If the medication lock is capped with positive pressure valve/device, remove syringe, and then clamp the extension tubing (Figure 7). Alternatively, to gain positive pressure if positive pressure valve/device is not present, clamp the extension tubing as you are still flushing the last of the saline into the medication lock. Remove syringe.	Positive pressure prevents blood from backing into the catheter and causing the medication lock to clot off.
30. Using an antimicrobial swab, vigorously scrub the needleless connector or end cap on the access port of the medication lock and allow to dry. Attach a passive disinfection cap to the needleless connector or end cap on the access port of the medication lock (Figure 8).	Venous access device entry points, end-caps, and needleless connectors must be vigorously scrubbed and disinfected prior to each access to reduce the risk for introduction of microorganisms and prevent venous access device-related infection (Frimpong et al., 2015; Harper, 2014; INS, 2016b; The Joint Commission, 2018; Loveday et al., 2014). Friction is needed to physically remove microorganisms from the top, sides, and threads of the needleless connector or end cap. Allow the antiseptic to dry completely (15 to 30 seconds) to ensure complete effectiveness (Harper, 2014). Passive disinfection caps contain an antiseptic-impregnated sponge that dispenses the antiseptic over the connector's top and threads, and protect the hub from contamination by touch or airborne sources (Stango et al., 2014).

FIGURE 7. Clamping the extension tubing.

FIGURE 8. Attaching a passive disinfection cap to the access port.

(*continued*)

Skill 5-11 ▶ Administering Medications by Intravenous Bolus or Push Through a Medication or Drug-Infusion Lock *(continued)*

ACTION	RATIONALE
31. Discard the syringe in the appropriate receptacle.	Proper disposal prevents injury and the spread of microorganisms.
32. Remove gloves and additional PPE, if used. Perform hand hygiene.	Proper removal of PPE reduces the risk for infection transmission and contamination of other items. Hand hygiene prevents the spread of microorganisms.
33. Document the administration of the medication immediately after administration. See Documentation section below.	Timely documentation helps to ensure patient safety.
34. Evaluate the patient's response to the medication within an appropriate time frame.	The patient needs to be evaluated for therapeutic and adverse effects from the medication.

EVALUATION

The expected outcomes have been met when the medication is delivered via the IV route; the patient experiences the intended effect of the medication; the patient experiences no adverse effects; and the patient understands and complies with the medication regimen.

DOCUMENTATION

Guidelines

Document the administration of the medication and saline flush, including date, time, dose, route of administration, site of administration, and rate of administration on the eMAR/MAR or record using the required format, immediately after administration. If using a bar-code system, medication administration is automatically recorded when the bar code is scanned. PRN medications require documentation of the reason for administration. Prompt recording avoids the possibility of accidentally repeating the administration of the drug. If the drug was refused or omitted, record this in the appropriate area on the medication record and notify the primary care provider. This verifies the reason medication was omitted and ensures that the health care personnel providing care for the patient are aware of the occurrence.

UNEXPECTED SITUATIONS AND ASSOCIATED INTERVENTIONS

- *Upon assessing the medication lock site before administering the medication, you note that the medication lock has infiltrated:* Remove the medication lock from the extremity. Restart peripheral venous access in a different location. Continue to monitor the new site as medication is administered.
- *While you are administering medication, the patient begins to complain of pain at the site:* Stop the medication. Assess the medication lock site for signs of infiltration and phlebitis. Flush the medication lock with normal saline again to recheck patency. If the IV site appears within normal limits, resume medication administration at a slower rate. If pain persists, stop, remove medication lock and restart in a different location.
- *As you are attempting to access the lock, the syringe tip touches the patient's arm:* Discard syringe. Prepare a new dose for administration.
- *No blood return is noted upon aspiration:* If the medication lock appears patent, without signs of infiltration, and normal saline fluid infuses without difficulty, proceed with administration. Observe closely for signs and symptoms of infiltration during and after administration.

SPECIAL CONSIDERATIONS

General Considerations

- Vascular access devices should also be "locked" after completion of the flush solution at each use to decrease the risk of occlusion and catheter-related bloodstream infection (INS, 2016b). According to the guidelines from the INS (2016b), short peripheral catheters are locked with normal saline solution. If the device is not in use, periodic flushing according to facility policy is required to keep the catheter patent.

- Previously, recommendations suggested routine rotation of insertions sites at various intervals, usually 72 to 96 hours. Current research and guidelines support maintaining peripheral IV access devices until no longer clinically indicated or until a complication develops (Bolton, 2015; INS, 2016a; Loveday et al., 2014; Tuffaha et al., 2014). Nurses should use clinical assessment and judgment in deciding when to replace or discontinue a peripheral IV catheter.
- The clinical need for the IV catheter should be assessed on a daily basis (INS, 2016a). Assessment is based on the patient's overall condition, access site, skin and wound integrity, length and type of therapy, and the integrity of the device, dressing and stabilization device (Helton et al., 2016). The device insertion site and dressing should be assessed every 4 hours at a minimum (INS, 2016a).
- Ongoing assessment is an important part of nursing care to evaluate patient response to administered medications and early detection of adverse reactions. If an adverse effect is suspected, withhold further medication doses and notify the patient's primary health care provider. Additional intervention is based on type of reaction and patient assessment.

Infant and Child Considerations

- If the volume of medication being administered is small (less than 1.0 mL), always include the amount of flush solution as part of the total amount to be injected and take this into account when determining how fast to push a medication. For example, if the medication is to be injected at a rate of 1.0 mL per minute and the total amount of solution to be injected is 2.25 mL (0.25-mL medication volume plus 2.0-mL saline flush solution volume equals 2.25 mL), then the medication would be injected over a period of 2 minutes 15 seconds.

EVIDENCE FOR PRACTICE ▶

INFUSION NURSING STANDARDS OF PRACTICE

Infusion Nurses Society (INS). (2016b). Infusion therapy. Standards of practice. *Journal of Infusion Nursing*, *39*(Suppl 1), S1–S159.

Refer to details in Skill 5-10, Evidence for Practice, and refer to thePoint˚ for additional research on related nursing topics.

EVIDENCE FOR PRACTICE ▶

INFUSION NURSING POLICIES AND PROCEDURES FOR INFUSION THERAPY

Infusion Nurses Society (INS). (2016a). *Policies and procedures for infusion therapy* (5th ed.). Norwood, MA: Author.

Refer to details in Skill 5-10, Evidence for Practice, and refer to thePoint˚ for additional research on related nursing topics.

 Skill 5-12 ▶ **Administering a Piggyback Intermittent Intravenous Infusion of Medication**

Medications can be administered by intermittent intravenous infusion. The drug is mixed with a small amount of the IV solution, such as 50 to 100 mL, and administered over a short period at the prescribed interval (e.g., every 8 hours). The administration is most often performed using an electronic infusion device (IV or infusion pump), which requires the nurse to program the infusion rate into the pump. Smart pumps are intravenous infusion devices that are used to administer intermittent infusions and provide computerized dose error-reduction software with IV therapy libraries and corresponding administration rate limits (Harding, 2013). Smart pumps are used in

(continued)

Skill 5-12

Administering a Piggyback Intermittent Intravenous Infusion of Medication   *(continued)*

the majority (77%) of hospital settings in the United States (Pedersen, Schneider & Scheckelhoff, 2013). Administration of an intermittent infusion may also be achieved by gravity infusion, which requires the nurse to calculate the infusion rate in drops per minute. The best practice, however, is to use an electronic infusion device.

Although newer infusion pumps allow for more flexibly (including concurrent programming of primary and secondary/piggyback lines), some intravenous piggyback delivery systems still require the container with the intermittent or additive solution to be placed higher than the primary solution container. An extension hook provided by the manufacturer provides for easy lowering of the main IV container. The port on the primary IV line has a back-check valve that automatically stops the flow of the primary solution, allowing the secondary or piggyback solution to flow when connected. Because manufacturers' designs vary, it is important to check the directions carefully for the systems used in the facility.

DELEGATION CONSIDERATIONS	The administration of medications by intermittent IV infusion is not delegated to nursing assistive personnel (NAP) or to unlicensed assistive personnel (UAP). Depending on the state's nurse practice act and the organization's policies and procedures, the administration of specified IV medications in some settings may be delegated to licensed practical/vocational nurses (LPN/LVNs) who have received appropriate training. The decision to delegate must be based on careful analysis of the patient's needs and circumstances, as well as the qualifications of the person to whom the task is being delegated. Refer to the Delegation Guidelines in Appendix A.
EQUIPMENT	• Medication prepared in labeled small-volume bag • Short secondary infusion tubing • Infusion pump • Antimicrobial swab • Needleless connector, if required, based on facility procedure • Metal or plastic hook • IV pole • Watch or clock with a second hand (gravity infusion) • Date label for tubing • Electronic Medication Administration Record (eMAR) or Medication Administration Record (MAR) • PPE, as indicated
ASSESSMENT	Assess the appropriateness of the drug for the patient. Review medical history, allergy, assessment, and laboratory data that may influence drug administration. Check the expiration date before administering the medication. **Assess the compatibility of the ordered medication, diluent, and the infusing IV fluid.** Assess the patient's IV site for signs of any complications. (Refer to Fundamentals Review 15-3 and Box 15-3 in Chapter 15 on pages 887 and 907). Assess the patient's knowledge of the medication. If the patient has a knowledge deficit about the medication, this may be the appropriate time to begin education about the medication. If the medication may affect the patient's vital signs, assess them before administration. Verify patient name, dose, route, and time of administration.
NURSING DIAGNOSIS	Determine related factors for the nursing diagnoses based on the patient's current status. Appropriate nursing diagnoses include: • Risk for allergy reaction • Risk for injury • Risk for infection
OUTCOME IDENTIFICATION AND PLANNING	The expected outcome to achieve is that the medication is delivered via the intravenous route and the patient experiences the intended effect of the medication. Other outcomes that may be appropriate include the following: the patient experiences no adverse effects; and the patient understands and complies with the medication regimen.

IMPLEMENTATION

ACTION	RATIONALE
1. Gather equipment. Check each medication order against the original order in the health record, according to facility policy. Clarify any inconsistencies. Check the patient's health record for allergies.	This comparison helps to identify errors that may have occurred when orders were transcribed. The primary care provider's order or prescription is the legal record of medication orders for each facility.
2. Know the actions, special nursing considerations, safe dose ranges, purpose of administration, and adverse effects of the medications to be administered. Consider the appropriateness of the medication for this patient. **Assess the compatibility of the ordered medication, diluent, and the infusing IV fluid.**	This knowledge aids the nurse in evaluating the therapeutic effect of the medication in relation to the patient's disorder and can also be used to educate the patient about the medication. Compatibility of medication and solutions prevents complications.
3. Perform hand hygiene.	Hand hygiene prevents the spread of microorganisms.
4. Move the medication supply system to the outside of the patient's room or prepare for administration at the medication supply system in the medication area. Alternatively, access the medication administration supply system at or inside the patient's room.	Organization facilitates error-free administration and saves time.
5. Unlock the medication supply system or drawer. Enter pass code and scan employee identification, if required.	Locking the medication supply system or drawer safeguards each patient's medication supply. Facility accrediting organizations require medication supply systems to be locked when not in use. Entering pass code and scanning ID allows only authorized users into the system and identifies the user for documentation by the computer.
6. **Prepare medications for one patient at a time.**	This prevents errors in medication administration.
7. Read the eMAR/MAR and select the proper medication from the medication supply system or the patient's medication drawer.	This is the *first* check of the label.
8. Compare the label with the eMAR/MAR. Check expiration dates. Confirm the prescribed or appropriate infusion rate. Calculate the drip rate if using a gravity system. Scan the bar code on the package, if required.	This is the *second* check of the label. Verify calculations with another nurse to ensure safety, if necessary. Infusing medication at an appropriate rate prevents injury.
9. **Depending on facility policy, the third check of the label may occur at this point. If so, when all medications for one patient have been prepared, recheck the labels with the eMAR/MAR before taking the medications to the patient. However, many facilities require the third check to occur at the bedside, after identifying the patient.**	This *third* check ensures accuracy and helps to prevent errors. *Note:* Many facilities require the *third* check to occur at the bedside, after identifying the patient and before administration.
10. **Lock the medication supply system before leaving it.**	Locking the medication supply system or drawer safeguards the patient's medication supply. Facility accrediting organizations require medication supply systems to be locked when not in use.
11. Transport medications to the patient's bedside carefully, and keep the medications in sight at all times.	Careful handling and close observation prevent accidental or deliberate disarrangement of medications.
12. **Ensure that the patient receives the medications at the correct time.**	Check facility policy, which may allow for administration within a period of 30 minutes before or 30 minutes after the designated time.
13. Perform hand hygiene and put on PPE, if indicated.	Hand hygiene and PPE prevent the spread of microorganisms. PPE is required based on transmission precautions.

(continued)

Skill 5-12 ▶ Administering a Piggyback Intermittent Intravenous Infusion of Medication *(continued)*

ACTION	RATIONALE

 14. **Identify the patient. Compare the information with the eMAR/MAR. The patient should be identified using at least two of the following methods** (The Joint Commission, 2018):

Identifying the patient ensures the right patient receives the medications and helps prevent errors. The patient's room number or physical location is not used as an identifier (The Joint Commission, 2018). Replace the identification band if it is missing or inaccurate in any way.

    a. Check the name on the patient's identification band.

    b. Check the identification number on the patient's identification band.

    c. Check the birth date on the patient's identification band.

    d. Ask the patient to state his or her name and birth date, based on facility policy.

This requires a response from the patient, but illness and strange surroundings often cause patients to be confused.

15. Close the door to the room or pull the bedside curtain.

This provides patient privacy.

16. **Complete necessary assessments before administering medications. Check the patient's allergy bracelet or ask the patient about allergies. Explain the purpose and action of the medication to the patient.**

Assessment is a prerequisite to administration of medications. Explanation provides rationale, increases knowledge, and reduces anxiety.

17. Scan the patient's bar code on the identification band, if required.

Scanning provides an additional check to ensure that the medication is given to the right patient.

18. **Based on facility policy, the third check of the label may occur at this point. If so, recheck the labels with the eMAR/MAR before administering the medications to the patient.**

Many facilities require the *third* check to occur at the bedside, after identifying the patient and before administration. If facility policy directs the *third* check at this time, this *third* check ensures accuracy and helps to prevent errors.

19. Assess the IV site for the presence of complications.

IV medication must be given directly into a vein for safe administration.

20. Close the clamp on the short secondary infusion tubing. Using aseptic technique, remove the cap on the tubing spike and the cap on the port of the medication container, taking care to avoid contaminating either end.

Closing the clamp prevents fluid from entering the system until the nurse is ready. Maintaining sterility of the tubing and the medication port prevents contamination.

21. Attach infusion tubing to the medication container by inserting the tubing spike into the port with a firm push and twisting motion, taking care to avoid contaminating either end.

Maintaining sterility of tubing and medication port prevents contamination.

22. Hang piggyback container on IV pole, positioning it higher than primary IV according to manufacturer's recommendations (Figure 1). If necessary for the particular infusion pump in use, use the metal or plastic hook to lower primary IV fluid container. If using gravity infusion, primary IV fluid container must be lowered.

Position of containers influences the flow of IV fluid into the primary setup.

FIGURE 1. Positioning piggyback container on IV pole. *(Photo by B. Proud.)*

ACTION	RATIONALE
23. Place label on administration tubing with the current date.	Label identifies the date of first use of the tubing. Intermittent administration sets disconnected after use should be replaced every 24 hours; repeated disconnection and reconnection increases risk of contamination at the spike end, catheter hub, needleless connector, and the end of the administration set, potentially increasing the risk for catheter-related bloodstream infection (INS, 2016b)
24. Squeeze drip chamber on administration tubing and release. Fill chamber to the line or about half full. Open clamp on administration tubing and prime tubing. Close clamp. Place needleless connector on the end of the tubing, using sterile technique, if required.	This removes air from tubing and preserves the sterility of the setup.
25. Remove the passive disinfection cap from the needleless connector or end cap on the infusion set injection port. Alternatively, if a passive disinfection cap is not in place, use an antimicrobial swab to vigorously scrub the access port or stopcock on the administration set above where the tubing enters the infusion pump or above the roller clamp on the primary IV infusion tubing (gravity infusion) (Figure 2).	Passive disinfection caps contain an antiseptic-impregnated sponge that dispenses the antiseptic over the connector's top and threads, and protects the hub from contamination by touch or airborne sources (Stango et al., 2014). Venous access device entry points, end-caps, and needleless connectors must be vigorously scrubbed and disinfected prior to each access to reduce the risk for introduction of microorganisms and prevent venous access device-related infection (Frimpong et al., 2015; Harper, 2014; INS, 2016b; The Joint Commission, 2018; Loveday et al., 2014). Friction is needed to physically remove microorganisms from the top, sides, and threads of the needleless connector or end cap. Allow the antiseptic to dry completely (15 to 30 seconds) to ensure complete effectiveness (Harper, 2014). Backflow valve in the primary line secondary port stops flow of primary infusion while piggyback solution is infusing. Once completed, backflow valves open and flow of primary solution resumes.
26. Connect piggyback setup to the access port or stopcock (Figure 3). If using, turn the stopcock to the open position.	Needleless systems and stopcock setup eliminate the need for a needle and are recommended by the CDC.

FIGURE 2. Vigorously scrubbing the access port. (*Photo by B. Proud.*)

FIGURE 3. Connecting piggyback administration set to access port. (*Photo by B. Proud.*)

(*continued*)

Skill 5-12 ▶ Administering a Piggyback Intermittent Intravenous Infusion of Medication *(continued)*

ACTION	RATIONALE
27. Open clamp on the secondary infusion tubing. Set rate for secondary infusion on infusion pump and begin infusion (Figure 4). If using gravity infusion, use the roller clamp on the primary infusion tubing to regulate the flow at the prescribed delivery rate (Figure 5). Monitor medication infusion at periodic intervals.	Backflow valve in the primary line secondary port stops flow of primary infusion while piggyback solution is infusing. Once completed, backflow valves open and flow of primary solution resumes. It is important to verify the safe administration rate for each drug to prevent adverse effects.

FIGURE 4. Setting rate for secondary infusion on infusion pump. (*Photo by B. Proud.*)

FIGURE 5. Using roller clamp on primary infusion tubing to regulate gravity flow. (*Photo by B. Proud.*)

28. Clamp tubing on piggyback set when solution is infused. Follow facility policy regarding disposal of equipment.	Most facilities allow the reuse of tubing, reducing the risk for contamination. The frequency of administration set tubing changes varies. Refer to Box 15-2 in Skill 15-2 for recommended administration set change guidelines.
29. Raise primary IV fluid container to original height. **Check primary infusion rate on infusion pump. If using gravity infusion, readjust flow rate of primary IV.**	Most infusion pumps automatically restart primary infusion at previous rate after secondary infusion is completed. If using gravity infusion, piggyback medication administration may interrupt normal flow rate of primary IV. Rate readjustment may be necessary.
30. Remove PPE, if used. Perform hand hygiene.	Proper removal of PPE reduces the risk for infection transmission and contamination of other items. Hand hygiene prevents the spread of microorganisms.
31. Document the administration of the medication immediately after administration. See Documentation section below. Document the volume of fluid administered on the intake and output record, if necessary.	Timely documentation helps to ensure patient safety.
32. Evaluate the patient's response to the medication within an appropriate time frame. Monitor IV site at periodic intervals.	The patient needs to be evaluated for therapeutic and adverse effects from the medication.

EVALUATION

The expected outcomes have been met when the medication is delivered via the intravenous route; the patient experiences the intended effect of the medication; the patient experiences no adverse effects; and the patient understands and complies with the medication regimen.

DOCUMENTATION

Guidelines

Document the administration of the medication immediately after administration, including date, time, dose, route of administration, site of administration, and rate of administration on the eMAR/MAR or record using the required format. If using a bar-code system, medication administration is automatically recorded when the bar code is scanned. PRN medications require documentation of the reason for administration. Prompt recording avoids the possibility of accidentally repeating the administration of the drug. If the drug was refused or omitted, record this in the appropriate area on the medication record and notify the primary care provider. This verifies the reason medication was omitted and ensures that health care personnel providing care for the patient are aware of the occurrence. Document the volume of fluid administered on the intake and output record, if necessary.

UNEXPECTED SITUATIONS AND ASSOCIATED INTERVENTIONS	• *Upon assessing the IV site before administering medication, you note that the IV has infiltrated:* Stop IV fluid and remove the IV from the extremity. Restart the IV in a different location. Continue to monitor the new IV site as medication is administered. • *While administering medication, you note a cloudy, white substance forming in the IV tubing:* Stop the IV from flowing and stop administering the medication to prevent precipitate from entering the patient's circulation. Clamp the IV at the site nearest to the patient. Replace tubing on primary and secondary infusions. Check the literature regarding incompatibilities of medications before administering. Medication infusion may require a second IV site or administration through an access port closer to the IV site and flushing of tubing before and after administration. • *While you are administering medication, the patient begins to complain of pain at the IV site:* Stop the medication. Assess the IV site for any signs of complications. Flush the IV with normal saline to check for patency. If the IV site appears within normal limits, resume medication administration at a slower rate.
SPECIAL CONSIDERATIONS *General Considerations*	• An alternate way to prime the secondary tubing, particularly if administration set is in place from a previous infusion, is to "backfill" the secondary tubing. Attach the medication bag to the secondary infusion tubing. Lower the medication bag below the main IV solution container and open the clamp on the secondary infusion tubing. This allows the primary IV solution to flow up the secondary tubing to the drip chamber, "backfilling" the tubing. Allow the solution to enter the drip chamber until the drip chamber is half full. Close the clamp on the secondary tubing and hang the medication container on the IV pole. Proceed with administration by lowering the primary IV container, as described above. This "backfill" method keeps the infusion system intact, preventing both introduction of microorganisms and loss of medication when the tubing is primed. Check facility policy regarding the use of "backfilling." • Intermittent administration sets disconnected after use should be replaced every 24 hours; repeated disconnection and reconnection increases risk of contamination at the spike end, catheter hub, needleless connector, and the end of the administration set, potentially increasing the risk for catheter-related bloodstream infection (INS, 2016b). • Ongoing assessment is an important part of nursing care for both evaluation of patient response to administered medications and early detection of adverse reactions. If an adverse effect is suspected, withhold further medication doses and notify the patient's primary care provider. Additional intervention is based on type of reaction and patient assessment.
Infant and Child Considerations	• Infants and small children with fluid restrictions may not tolerate the added IV fluid needed for administration with piggyback systems. For these children, consider using the mini-infusion pump (see Skill 5-13).

EVIDENCE FOR PRACTICE ▶	**INFUSION NURSING STANDARDS OF PRACTICE** Infusion Nurses Society (INS). (2016b). Infusion therapy. Standards of practice. *Journal of Infusion Nursing, 39*(Suppl 1), S1–S159. Refer to details in Skill 5-10, Evidence for Practice, and refer to thePoint® for additional research on related nursing topics.

(*continued*)

Skill 5-12 ▶ Administering a Piggyback Intermittent Intravenous Infusion of Medication   *(continued)*

EVIDENCE FOR PRACTICE ▶	**INFUSION NURSING POLICIES AND PROCEDURES FOR INFUSION THERAPY**

Infusion Nurses Society (INS). (2016a). *Policies and procedures for infusion therapy* (5th ed.). Norwood, MA: Author.

Refer to details in Skill 5-10, Evidence for Practice, and refer to thePoint° for additional research on related nursing topics.

Skill 5-13 ▶ Administering an Intermittent Intravenous Infusion of Medication via a Mini-Infusion Pump

Medications can be administered by intermittent intravenous infusion. The mini-infusion pump (syringe pump) for intermittent infusion is battery- or electrical-operated and allows medication mixed in a syringe to be connected to the primary line and delivered by mechanical pressure applied to the syringe plunger. Mini-infusion pumps may use a smart pump design; smart pumps are intravenous infusion devices that are used to administer intermittent infusions and provide computerized dose error-reduction software with IV therapy libraries and corresponding administration rate limits (Harding, 2013). Smart pumps are used in the majority (77%) of hospital settings in the United States (Pedersen et al., 2013).

DELEGATION CONSIDERATIONS

The administration of medications by intermittent IV infusion is not delegated to nursing assistive personnel (NAP) or to unlicensed assistive personnel (UAP). Depending on the state's nurse practice act and the organization's policies and procedures, the administration of specified IV medications in some settings may be delegated to licensed practical/vocational nurses (LPN/LVNs) who have received appropriate training. The decision to delegate must be based on careful analysis of the patient's needs and circumstances, as well as the qualifications of the person to whom the task is being delegated. Refer to the Delegation Guidelines in Appendix A.

EQUIPMENT

- Medication prepared in labeled syringe
- Mini-infusion pump and tubing
- Needleless connector, if required, based on facility system
- Antimicrobial swab
- Date label for tubing
- Electronic Medication Administration Record (eMAR) or Medication Administration Record (MAR)
- PPE, as indicated

ASSESSMENT

Assess the appropriateness of the drug for the patient. Review medical history, allergy, assessment, and laboratory data that may influence drug administration. Check the expiration date before administering medication. **Assess the compatibility of the ordered medication, diluent, and the infusing IV fluid.** Assess the patient's IV site for signs of any complications. (Refer to Fundamentals Review 15-3 and Box 15-3 in Chapter 15 on pages 887 and 907). Assess the patient's knowledge of the medication. If the patient has a knowledge deficit about the medication, this may be the appropriate time to begin education about the medication. If the medication may affect the patient's vital signs, assess them before administration. Verify patient name, dose, route, and time of administration. Assess the patient's knowledge of the medication.

NURSING DIAGNOSIS

Determine related factors for the nursing diagnoses based on the patient's current status. Appropriate nursing diagnoses include:

- Risk for allergy reaction
- Risk for injury
- Risk for infection

OUTCOME IDENTIFICATION AND PLANNING

The expected outcome is that the medication is delivered via the IV route and the patient experiences the intended effect of the medication. Other outcomes that may be appropriate include the following: the patient experiences no adverse effects; and the patient understands and complies with the medication regimen.

IMPLEMENTATION

ACTION	RATIONALE
1. Gather equipment. Check each medication order against the original order in the health record according to facility policy. Clarify any inconsistencies. Check the patient's health record for allergies.	This comparison helps to identify errors that may have occurred when orders were transcribed. The primary care provider's order or prescription is the legal record of medication orders for each facility. Compatibility of medication and solution prevents complications.
2. Know the actions, special nursing considerations, safe dose ranges, purpose of administration, and adverse effects of the medications to be administered. Consider the appropriateness of the medication for this patient. **Assess the compatibility of the ordered medication, diluent, and the infusing IV fluid.**	This knowledge aids the nurse in evaluating the therapeutic effect of the medication in relation to the patient's disorder and can also be used to educate the patient about the medication. Compatibility of medication and solutions prevents complications.
3. Perform hand hygiene.	Hand hygiene prevents the spread of microorganisms.
4. Move the medication supply system to the outside of the patient's room or prepare for administration at the medication supply system in the medication area. Alternatively, access the medication administration supply system at or inside the patient's room.	Organization facilitates error-free administration and saves time.
5. Unlock the medication supply system or drawer. Enter pass code and scan employee identification, if required.	Locking the medication supply system or drawer safeguards each patient's medication supply. Facility accrediting organizations require medication supply systems to be locked when not in use. Entering pass code and scanning ID allows only authorized users into the system and identifies the user for documentation by the computer.
6. **Prepare medications for one patient at a time.**	This prevents errors in medication administration.
7. Read the eMAR/MAR and select the proper medication from the medication supply system or the patient's medication drawer.	This is the *first* check of the label.
8. Compare the label with the eMAR/MAR. Check expiration dates. Confirm the prescribed or appropriate infusion rate. Scan the bar code on the package, if required.	This is the *second* check of the label. Verify calculations with another nurse to ensure safety, if necessary. Infusing medication at appropriate rate prevents injury.
9. **Depending on facility policy, the third check of the label may occur at this point. If so, when all medications for one patient have been prepared, recheck the labels with the eMAR/MAR before taking the medications to the patient. However, many facilities require the third check to occur at the bedside, after identifying the patient.**	This *third* check ensures accuracy and helps to prevent errors. *Note:* Many facilities require the *third* check to occur at the bedside, after identifying the patient and before administration.
10. **Lock the medication supply system before leaving it.**	Locking the medication supply system or drawer safeguards the patient's medication supply. Facility accrediting organizations require medication supply systems to be locked when not in use.

(*continued*)

Skill 5-13 ▸ Administering an Intermittent Intravenous Infusion of Medication via a Mini-Infusion Pump *(continued)*

ACTION	RATIONALE
11. Transport medications to the patient's bedside carefully, and keep the medications in sight at all times.	Careful handling and close observation prevent accidental or deliberate disarrangement of medications.
12. **Ensure that the patient receives the medications at the correct time.**	Check facility policy, which may allow for administration within a period of 30 minutes before or 30 minutes after the designated time.
13. Perform hand hygiene and put on PPE, if indicated.	Hand hygiene and PPE prevent the spread of microorganisms. PPE is required based on transmission precautions.
14. **Identify the patient. Compare the information with the eMAR/MAR. The patient should be identified using at least two of the following methods (The Joint Commission, 2018):**	Identifying the patient ensures the right patient receives the medications and helps prevent errors. The patient's room number or physical location is not used as an identifier (The Joint Commission, 2018). Replace the identification band if it is missing or inaccurate in any way.
a. Check the name on the patient's identification band.	This requires a response from the patient, but illness and strange surroundings often cause patients to be confused.
b. Check the identification number on the patient's identification band.	
c. Check the birth date on the patient's identification band.	
d. Ask the patient to state his or her name and birth date, based on facility policy.	
15. Close the door to the room or pull the bedside curtain.	Provides patient privacy.
16. **Complete necessary assessments before administering medications. Check the patient's allergy bracelet or ask the patient about allergies. Explain the purpose and action of the medication to the patient.**	Assessment is a prerequisite to administration of medications. Explanation provides rationale, increases knowledge, and reduces anxiety.
17. Scan the patient's bar code on the identification band, if required.	Provides an additional check to ensure that the medication is given to the right patient.
18. **Based on facility policy, the third check of the label may occur at this point. If so, recheck the labels with the eMAR/MAR before administering the medications to the patient.**	Many facilities require the *third* check to occur at the bedside, after identifying the patient and before administration. If facility policy directs the *third* check at this time, this *third* check ensures accuracy and helps to prevent errors.
19. Assess the IV site for the presence of complications.	IV medication must be given directly into a vein for safe administration.
20. Using aseptic technique, remove the cap on the administration tubing and the cap on the medication syringe, taking care not to contaminate either end.	Maintaining sterility of tubing and medication port prevents contamination.
21. Attach administration tubing to the syringe, taking care not to contaminate either end.	Maintaining sterility of tubing and medication port prevents contamination.
22. Place label on tubing with current date.	Label identifies the date of first use of the tubing. Intermittent administration sets disconnected after use should be replaced every 24 hours; repeated disconnection and reconnection increases risk of contamination at the spike end, catheter hub, needleless connector and the end of the administration set, potential increasing the risk for catheter-related bloodstream infection (INS, 2016b).
23. Fill administration tubing (prime) with medication by applying gentle pressure to syringe plunger. Place needleless connector on the end of the tubing, if required, using sterile technique.	This removes air from tubing and maintains sterility.

ACTION	**RATIONALE**
24. Insert syringe into mini-infusion pump according to manufacturer's directions (Figure 1).	Syringe must fit securely in pump apparatus for proper operation.
25. Remove the passive disinfection cap from the needleless connector or end cap on the access port on the primary IV infusion tubing, closest to the IV insertion site (Figure 2). Alternatively, if a passive disinfection cap is not in place, use an antimicrobial swab to vigorously scrub the access port or stopcock above the roller clamp on the primary IV infusion tubing, usually the port closest to the IV insertion site.	Passive disinfection caps contain an antiseptic-impregnated sponge that dispenses the antiseptic over the connector's top and threads, and protects the hub from contamination by touch or airborne sources (Stango et al., 2014). Venous access device entry points, end-caps, and needleless connectors must be vigorously scrubbed and disinfected prior to each access to reduce the risk for introduction of microorganisms and prevent venous access device-related infection (Frimpong et al., 2015; Harper, 2014; INS, 2016b; The Joint Commission, 2018; Loveday et al., 2014). Friction is needed to physically remove microorganisms from the top, sides, and threads of the needleless connector or end cap. Allow the antiseptic to dry completely (15 to 30 seconds) to ensure complete effectiveness (Harper, 2014). Proper connection allows IV medication to flow into the primary line.
26. Connect the secondary infusion to the primary infusion at the access port (Figure 3).	Allows for delivery of medication.
27. Program the mini-infusion pump to the appropriate rate and begin infusion (Figure 4). Set the alarm if recommended by the manufacturer.	Pump delivers medication at a controlled rate. Alarm is recommended for use with IV lock apparatus.

FIGURE 1. Inserting syringe into mini-infusion pump.

FIGURE 2. Removing the passive disinfection cap from the access port closest to IV insertion site.

FIGURE 3. Connecting secondary infusion tubing the access port.

FIGURE 4. Programming mini-infusion pump.

(*continued*)

Skill 5-13 ▶ Administering an Intermittent Intravenous Infusion of Medication via a Mini-Infusion Pump *(continued)*

ACTION	**RATIONALE**
28. Clamp tubing on secondary IV infusion administration set when solution is infused. Follow facility policy regarding disposal of equipment.	Most facilities allow the reuse of tubing, reducing the risk for contamination. The frequency of administration set tubing changes varies. Refer to Box 15-2 in Skill 15-2 for recommended administration set change guidelines.
29. Check rate of primary infusion.	Administration of secondary infusion may interfere with primary infusion rate.
30. Remove PPE, if used. Perform hand hygiene.	Proper removal of PPE reduces the risk for infection transmission and contamination of other items. Hand hygiene prevents the spread of microorganisms.
31. Document the administration of the medication immediately after administration. See Documentation section below. Document the volume of fluid administered on the intake and output record, if necessary.	Timely documentation helps to ensure patient safety.
32. Evaluate the patient's response to the medication within appropriate time frame. Monitor IV site at periodic intervals.	The patient needs to be evaluated for therapeutic and adverse effects from the medication.

EVALUATION

The expected outcomes have been met when the medication has been delivered via the IV route; the patient experiences the intended effect of the medication; the patient experiences no adverse effects; and the patient understands and complies with the medication regimen.

DOCUMENTATION

Guidelines

Document the administration of the medication immediately after administration, including date, time, dose, route of administration, site of administration, and rate of administration on the eMAR/MAR or record using the required format. If using a bar-code system, medication administration is automatically recorded when the bar code is scanned. PRN medications require documentation of the reason for administration. Prompt recording avoids the possibility of accidentally repeating the administration of the drug. If the drug was refused or omitted, record this in the appropriate area on the medication record and notify the primary care provider. This verifies the reason medication was omitted and ensures that health care personnel providing care for the patient are aware of the occurrence. Document the volume of fluid administered on the intake and output record, if necessary.

UNEXPECTED SITUATIONS AND ASSOCIATED INTERVENTIONS

- *Upon assessing the IV site before administering medication, you note that the IV has infiltrated:* Stop IV fluid and remove the IV from the extremity. Restart the IV in a different location. Continue to monitor the new IV site as medication is administered.
- *While administering medication, you note a cloudy, white substance forming in the IV tubing:* Stop the IV from flowing and stop administering the medication to prevent precipitate from entering the patient's circulation. Clamp the IV at the site nearest to the patient. Replace tubing on primary and secondary infusions. Check the literature regarding incompatibilities of medications before administering. Medication infusion may require a second IV site or flushing of tubing before and after administration.
- *While you are administering medication, the patient begins to complain of pain at the IV site:* Stop the medication. Assess the IV site for any signs of complications. Flush the IV with normal saline to check for patency. If the IV site appears within normal limits, resume medication administration at a slower rate and continue to monitor.

SPECIAL CONSIDERATIONS

General Considerations

- Intermittent administration sets disconnected after use should be replaced every 24 hours; repeated disconnection and reconnection increases risk of contamination at the spike end, catheter hub, needleless connector and the end of the administration set, potential increasing the risk for catheter-related bloodstream infection (INS, 2016b)
- Ongoing assessment is an important part of nursing care for both evaluation of patient response to administered medications and early detection of adverse drug reactions. If an adverse effect is suspected, withhold further medication doses and notify the patient's primary care provider. Additional intervention is based on type of reaction and patient assessment.

Infant and Child Considerations

- Infants and small children with fluid restrictions may not tolerate the added IV fluid needed for administration with piggyback systems. The mini-infusion pump should be considered for use with these children.

EVIDENCE FOR PRACTICE ▶

INFUSION NURSING STANDARDS OF PRACTICE
Infusion Nurses Society (INS). (2016b). Infusion therapy. Standards of practice. *Journal of Infusion Nursing, 39*(Suppl 1), S1–S159.

Refer to details in Skill 5-10, Evidence for Practice, and refer to thePoint° for additional research on related nursing topics.

EVIDENCE FOR PRACTICE ▶

INFUSION NURSING POLICIES AND PROCEDURES FOR INFUSION THERAPY
Infusion Nurses Society (INS). (2016a). *Policies and procedures for infusion therapy* (5th ed.). Norwood, MA: Author.

Refer to details in Skill 5-10, Evidence for Practice, and refer to thePoint° for additional research on related nursing topics.

Skill 5-14 ▶ Applying a Transdermal Patch

The transdermal route is being used more frequently to deliver medication. A disk or patch that contains medication intended for daily use or longer is applied to the patient's skin. Medications delivered via a transdermal patch have a slow onset of action. Transdermal patches are commonly used to deliver hormones, opioid analgesics, cardiac medications, and nicotine. Medication errors have occurred when patients apply multiple patches at once or fail to remove the overlay on the patch that exposes the skin to the medication. Opioid analgesic patches are associated with the most adverse drug reactions. Clear patches have a cosmetic advantage, but they can be difficult to find on the patient's skin when they need to be removed or replaced.

DELEGATION CONSIDERATIONS

The administration of medication via a transdermal patch is not delegated to nursing assistive personnel (NAP) or to unlicensed assistive personnel (UAP). Depending on the state's nurse practice act and the organization's policies and procedures, the administration of a transdermal patch may be delegated to licensed practical/vocational nurses (LPN/LVNs). The decision to delegate must be based on careful analysis of the patient's needs and circumstances, as well as the qualifications of the person to whom the task is being delegated. Refer to the Delegation Guidelines in Appendix A.

(continued)

Skill 5-14 ▶ Applying a Transdermal Patch *(continued)*

EQUIPMENT

- Medication patch
- Disposable gloves
- Scissors (optional)
- Disposable washcloth or washcloth, soap, and water
- Electronic Medication Administration Record (eMAR) or Medication Administration Record (MAR)
- Additional PPE, as indicated

ASSESSMENT

Assess the appropriateness of the drug for the patient. Review medical history, allergy, assessment, and laboratory data that may influence drug administration. Check the expiration date before administering the medication. Assess the skin at the location where the patch will be applied. Many patches have different and specific instructions for where the patch is to be placed. For example, transdermal patches that contain estrogen cannot be placed on breast tissue. Check the manufacturer's instructions for the appropriate location for the patch. The site should be clean, dry, and free of hair. Do not place transdermal patches on irritated or broken skin. Assess the patient for any old patches. Do not place a new transdermal patch until old patches have been removed. Verify the application frequency for the specific medication. Assess the patient's knowledge of the medication. If the patient has a knowledge deficit about the medication, this may be the appropriate time to begin education about the medication. If the medication may affect the patient's vital signs, assess them before administration. If the medication is for pain relief, assess the patient's pain before and after administration. Verify patient name, dose, route, and time of administration.

NURSING DIAGNOSIS

Determine related factors for the nursing diagnoses based on the patient's current status. Appropriate nursing diagnoses may include:

- Risk for allergy reaction
- Risk for impaired skin integrity
- Deficient knowledge

OUTCOME IDENTIFICATION AND PLANNING

The expected outcome is that the medication is delivered via the transdermal route and the patient experiences the intended effect of the medication. Other outcomes that may be appropriate include the following: the patient experiences no adverse effect; the patient's skin remains free from alterations in integrity; and the patient understands and complies with the medication regimen.

IMPLEMENTATION

ACTION	RATIONALE
1. Gather equipment. Check medication order against the original order in the patient's health record, according to facility policy. Clarify any inconsistencies. Check the patient's health record for allergies.	This comparison helps to identify errors that may have occurred when orders were transcribed. The primary care provider's order or prescription is the legal record of medication orders for each facility.
2. Know the actions, special nursing considerations, safe dose ranges, purpose of administration, and adverse effects of the medications to be administered. Consider the appropriateness of the medication for this patient.	This knowledge aids the nurse in evaluating the therapeutic effect of the medication in relation to the patient's disorder and can also be used to educate the patient about the medication.
3. Perform hand hygiene.	Hand hygiene prevents the spread of microorganisms.
4. Move the medication supply system to the outside of the patient's room or prepare for administration at the medication supply system in the medication area. Alternatively, access the medication administration supply system at or inside the patient's room.	Organization facilitates error-free administration and saves time.

ACTION	**RATIONALE**
5. Unlock the medication supply system or drawer. Enter pass code and scan employee identification, if required.	Locking the medication supply system or drawer safeguards each patient's medication supply. Facility accrediting organizations require medication supply systems to be locked when not in use. Entering pass code and scanning ID allows only authorized users into the system and identifies the user for documentation by the computer.
6. Prepare medications for one patient at a time.	This prevents errors in medication administration.
7. Read the eMAR/MAR and select the proper medication from medication supply system or the patient's medication drawer.	This is the *first* check of the label.
8. Compare the label with the eMAR/MAR. Check expiration dates and perform calculations, if necessary. Scan the bar code on the package, if required.	This is the *second* check of the label. Verify calculations with another nurse to ensure safety, if necessary.
9. Depending on facility policy, the third check of the label may occur at this point. If so, when all medications for one patient have been prepared, recheck the labels with the eMAR/MAR before taking the medications to the patient. However, many facilities require the third check to occur at the bedside, after identifying the patient.	This *third* check ensures accuracy and helps to prevent errors. *Note:* Many facilities require the *third* check to occur at the bedside, after identifying the patient and before administration.
10. Lock the medication supply system before leaving it.	Locking the medication supply system or drawer safeguards the patient's medication supply. Facility accrediting organizations require medication supply systems to be locked when not in use.
11. Transport medications to the patient's bedside carefully, and keep the medications in sight at all times.	Careful handling and close observation prevent accidental or deliberate disarrangement of medications.
12. Ensure that the patient receives the medications at the correct time.	Check facility policy, which may allow for administration within a period of 30 minutes before or 30 minutes after the designated time.
13. Perform hand hygiene and put on PPE, if indicated.	Hand hygiene and PPE prevent the spread of microorganisms. PPE is required based on transmission precautions.
14. Identify the patient. Compare the information with the eMAR/MAR. The patient should be identified using at least two of the following methods (The Joint Commission, 2018):	Identifying the patient ensures the right patient receives the medications and helps prevent errors. The patient's room number or physical location is not used as an identifier (The Joint Commission, 2018). Replace the identification band if it is missing or inaccurate in any way.
a. Check the name on the patient's identification band. b. Check the identification number on the patient's identification band. c. Check the birth date on the patient's identification band. d. Ask the patient to state his or her name and birth date, based on facility policy.	This requires a response from the patient, but illness and strange surroundings often cause patients to be confused.
15. Complete necessary assessments before administering medications. Check the patient's allergy bracelet or ask the patient about allergies. Explain the purpose and action of each medication to the patient.	Assessment is a prerequisite to administration of medications.

(continued)

Skill 5-14 ▶ Applying a Transdermal Patch *(continued)*

ACTION	RATIONALE

16. Scan the patient's bar code on the identification band, if required (Figure 1).

This provides an additional check to ensure that the medication is given to the right patient.

FIGURE 1. Scanning bar code on patient's identification bracelet.

17. **Based on facility policy, the third check of the label may occur at this point. If so, recheck the labels with the eMAR/MAR before administering the medications to the patient.**

Many facilities require the *third* check to occur at the bedside, after identifying the patient and before administration. If facility policy directs the *third* check at this time, this *third* check ensures accuracy and helps to prevent errors.

18. Put on gloves.

Gloves protect the nurse when handling the medication on the transdermal patch.

19. Assess the patient's skin where patch is to be placed, looking for any signs of irritation or breakdown. Site should be clean, dry, and free of hair. Rotate application sites.

Transdermal patches should not be placed on skin that is irritated or broken down. Hair can prevent the patch from sticking to the skin. Rotating sites reduces risk for skin irritation.

20. **Remove any old transdermal patches of the same kind from the patient's skin.** Fold the old patch in half with the adhesive sides sticking together and discard according to facility policy. Gently wash the area where the old patch was with a disposable washcloth or soap and water.

Leaving old patches on a patient while applying new ones may lead to delivery of a toxic level of the drug. Folding sides together prevents accidental contact with remaining medication. Washing area with soap and water removes all traces of medication in that area.

21. Remove the patch from its protective covering. Remove the covering on the patch without touching the medication surface (Figure 2). Apply the patch to the patient's skin (Figure 3). Use the palm of your hand to press firmly for about 10 seconds. Do not massage.

Touching the adhesive side may alter the amount of medication left on the patch. Pressing firmly for 10 seconds ensures that the patch stays on the patient's skin. Massaging the site may increase absorption of the medication.

FIGURE 2. Removing covering on patch.

FIGURE 3. Applying patch to patient's skin.

ACTION	**RATIONALE**
22. Depending on facility policy, initial and write the date and time of administration on a piece of medical tape. Apply the tape to the patient's skin in close proximity to the patch. **Do not write directly on the medication patch.**	Most manufacturers recommend against writing on patches due to insufficient data on the practice. Writing on the patch could damage or tear it. Moreover, if ink is used, it may leach through and come into contact with the medication, and it is not known whether ink might interact with a given medication or impede its delivery (Durand et al., 2012).
23. Remove gloves and additional PPE, if used. Perform hand hygiene.	Proper removal of PPE reduces the risk for infection transmission and contamination of other items. Hand hygiene prevents the spread of microorganisms.
24. Document the administration of the medication immediately after administration. See Documentation section below.	Timely documentation helps to ensure patient safety.
25. Evaluate the patient's response to the medication within the appropriate time frame.	The patient needs to be evaluated for therapeutic and adverse effects from the medication.

EVALUATION

The expected outcomes have been met when medication is delivered via the transdermal route; the patient experiences the intended effect of the medication; the patient experiences no adverse effect; the patient's skin remains free from alterations in integrity; and the patient understands and complies with the medication regimen.

DOCUMENTATION

Guidelines

Document the administration of the medication immediately after administration, including date, time, dose, route of administration, and site of administration on the eMAR/MAR or record using the required format. If using a bar-code system, medication administration is automatically recorded when the bar code is scanned. PRN medications require documentation of the reason for administration. Prompt recording avoids the possibility of accidentally repeating the administration of the drug. If the drug was refused or omitted, record this in the appropriate area on the medication record and notify the primary care provider. This verifies the reason the medication was omitted and ensures that health care personnel providing care for the patient are aware of the occurrence.

UNEXPECTED SITUATIONS AND ASSOCIATED INTERVENTIONS

- *You did not wear gloves while applying the transdermal patch:* Immediately perform good hand hygiene using soap and water to remove any medication that may be on the skin. You may feel the effects of the medication if any came into contact with your skin.
- *You find more than one old transdermal patch while applying a new transdermal patch:* Remove all old patches of the same kind; remember that more than one medication may be delivered via a transdermal patch. Check orders in the health record to ensure that the patient is still receiving the medication. Failure to remove old transdermal patches is considered a medication error and special event. Notify the primary care provider of potential medication overdose. Follow facility policy regarding documentation for special events.
- *When removing an old transdermal patch, you note the skin underneath is erythematosus and swollen:* Wash skin with soap and water and assess the patient for any latex or adhesive allergies. Discuss with the patient whether the patch site has been rotated. Notify the primary care provider before applying a new patch.

SPECIAL CONSIDERATIONS

General Considerations

- Transdermal drug products have specific application sites, application intervals, and considerations. It is important to be knowledgeable about the specific drug administered. For example, fentanyl may be applied to the chest, back, flank, and upper arm; it is reapplied every 3 days; and patients may experience increased absorption with increased body temperature (Janssen

(continued)

Skill 5-14 ▶ Applying a Transdermal Patch *(continued)*

Pharmaceuticals, Inc., 2009, 2015). Fentanyl iontophoretic transdermal system (Ionsys®) is used only in a hospital setting and must be discontinued prior to discharge; it may be applied to the chest or upper outer arm; it is reapplied every 24 hours or after 80 doses have been delivered; it contains metal parts, so it should be removed before MRI, cardioversion, or defibrillation (The Medicines Company, 2016). Nitroglycerin transdermal may be placed on any hairless surface, except on extremities below the knees or elbows, with the chest being the preferred site; it is reapplied every 12 to 14 hours; patients should have a nitrate-free interval each day of 10 to 12 hours to ensure nitrate tolerance does not develop (Ball & Smith, 2008).

- Apply the patch at the same time of the day, according to the order/prescription and medication specifications.
- Check for dislodgement of the patch if the patient is active. Refer to manufacturer information about the patch or consult with the pharmacist to determine reapplication schedule and procedure.
- Aluminum backing on a patch necessitates precautions if defibrillation is required. Burns and smoke may result. In addition, these patches should be removed before an MRI is performed to avoid burning of the skin.
- Assess for any skin irritation at the application site. If necessary, remove the patch, wash the area carefully with soap and water, and allow skin to air dry. Apply a new patch at a different site. Assess the potential for adverse reaction.
- Ongoing assessment is an important part of nursing care to evaluate patient response to administered medications and early detection of adverse drug reactions. If an adverse effect is suspected, withhold further medication doses and notify the patient's primary care provider. Additional intervention is based on type of reaction and patient assessment.

Home Care Considerations

- Some manufacturers recommend that patients wearing patches avoid external heat sources (e.g., heating pads, electric blankets, heat lamps, saunas, hot tubs, sunlight), as heat may promote drug absorption through the skin. Consult specific information from the manufacturer related to a particular medication.
- Caregivers and patients should be sure to remove an old transdermal medication before applying a new one, as many patches have residual drug content even after the recommended application time.
- Instruct patients and caregivers to rotate application sites to decrease the risk of skin irritation.
- Instruct patients and caregivers to wash their hands thoroughly after the application of a transdermal medication to avoid inadvertent eye contact.
- Instruct patients and caregivers to discard used transdermal medications according to manufacturer's instructions and out of reach of children, to avoid inadvertent exposure by children and pets (Durand et al., 2012).

Skill 5-15 ▶ Administering Eye Drops

Eye drops are instilled for their local effects, such as for pupil dilation or constriction when examining the eye, for infection treatment, or for controlling intraocular pressure (e.g., for patients with glaucoma). The type and amount of solution administered depends on the purpose of the instillation.

The eye is a delicate organ, highly susceptible to infection and injury. Although the eye is never free of microorganisms, the secretions of the conjunctiva protect against many pathogens. For maximal safety for the patient, the equipment, solutions, and ointments introduced into the conjunctival sac should be sterile. If this is not possible, follow careful guidelines for medical asepsis.

Refer to the accompanying Skill Variation for the steps to administer eye ointment.

DELEGATION CONSIDERATIONS

The administration of medication via drops in the eye is not delegated to nursing assistive personnel (NAP) or to unlicensed assistive personnel (UAP). Depending on the state's nurse practice act and the organization's policies and procedures, the administration of eye drops may be delegated to licensed practical/vocational nurses (LPN/LVNs). The decision to delegate must be based on careful analysis of the patient's needs and circumstances, as well as the qualifications of the person to whom the task is being delegated. Refer to the Delegation Guidelines in Appendix A.

EQUIPMENT	
• Gloves • Additional PPE, as indicated • Eye drop medication • Tissues • Normal saline solution	• Disposable washcloth, washcloth, cotton balls, or gauze squares • Electronic Medication Administration Record (eMAR) or Medication Administration Record (MAR)

ASSESSMENT

Assess the appropriateness of the drug for the patient. Review medical history, allergy, assessment, and laboratory data that may influence drug administration. Check the expiration date before administering the medication. Assess the affected eye for any drainage, erythema, or swelling. Assess the patient's knowledge of the medication. If the patient has a knowledge deficit about the medication, this may be the appropriate time to begin education about the medication. Verify patient name, dose, route, and time of administration.

NURSING DIAGNOSIS

Determine related factors for the nursing diagnoses based on the patient's current status. Appropriate nursing diagnoses may include:

• Risk for allergy response
• Deficient knowledge
• Risk for injury

OUTCOME IDENTIFICATION AND PLANNING

The expected outcome to achieve when administering eye drops is that the medication is delivered successfully into the eye and the patient experiences the intended effect of the medication. Other outcomes that may be appropriate include the following: the patient experiences no allergy response; the patient does not exhibit systemic effects of the medication; the patient's eye remains free from injury; and patient understands the rationale for medication administration.

IMPLEMENTATION

ACTION	RATIONALE
1. Gather equipment. Check medication order against the original order in the health record, according to facility policy. Clarify any inconsistencies. Check the patient's health record for allergies.	This comparison helps to identify errors that may have occurred when orders were transcribed. The primary care provider's order or prescription is the legal record of medication orders for each facility.
2. Know the actions, special nursing considerations, safe dose ranges, purpose of administration, and adverse effects of the medications to be administered. Consider the appropriateness of the medication for this patient.	This knowledge aids the nurse in evaluating the therapeutic effect of the medication in relation to the patient's disorder and can also be used to educate the patient about the medication.
3. Perform hand hygiene.	Hand hygiene prevents the spread of microorganisms.
4. Move the medication supply system to the outside of the patient's room or prepare for administration at the medication supply system in the medication area. Alternatively, access the medication administration supply system at or inside the patient's room.	Organization facilitates error-free administration and saves time.
5. Unlock the medication supply system or drawer. Enter pass code and scan employee identification, if required.	Locking the medication supply system or drawer safeguards each patient's medication supply. Facility accrediting organizations require medication supply systems to be locked when not in use. Entering pass code and scanning ID allows only authorized users into the system and identifies the user for documentation by the computer.
6. **Prepare medications for one patient at a time.**	This prevents errors in medication administration.

(continued)

Skill 5-15 ▶ Administering Eye Drops *(continued)*

ACTION	**RATIONALE**
7. Read the eMAR/MAR and select the proper medication from the patient's medication drawer or medication supply system.	This is the *first* check of the label.
8. Compare the label with the eMAR/MAR. Check expiration dates and perform calculations, if necessary. Scan the bar code on the package, if required.	This is the *second* check of the label. Verify calculations with another nurse to ensure safety, if necessary.
9. **Depending on facility policy, the third check of the label may occur at this point. If so, when all medications for one patient have been prepared, recheck the labels with the eMAR/MAR before taking the medications to the patient. However, many facilities require the third check to occur at the bedside, after identifying the patient.**	This *third* check ensures accuracy and helps to prevent errors. *Note:* Many facilities require the *third* check to occur at the bedside, after identifying the patient and before administration.
10. **Lock the medication supply system before leaving it.**	Locking the medication supply system or drawer safeguards the patient's medication supply. Facility accrediting organizations require medication supply systems to be locked when not in use.
11. Transport medications to the patient's bedside carefully, and keep the medications in sight at all times.	Careful handling and close observation prevent accidental or deliberate disarrangement of medications.
12. **Ensure that the patient receives the medications at the correct time.**	Check facility policy, which may allow for administration within a period of 30 minutes before or 30 minutes after the designated time.
13. Perform hand hygiene and put on PPE, if indicated.	Hand hygiene and PPE prevent the spread of microorganisms. PPE is required based on transmission precautions.
14. **Identify the patient. Compare the information with the eMAR/MAR. The patient should be identified using at least two of the following methods (The Joint Commission, 2018):**	Identifying the patient ensures the right patient receives the medications and helps prevent errors. The patient's room number or physical location is not used as an identifier (The Joint Commission, 2018). Replace the identification band if it is missing or inaccurate in any way.
a. Check the name on the patient's identification band.	This requires a response from the patient, but illness and strange surroundings often cause patients to be confused.
b. Check the identification number on the patient's identification band.	
c. Check the birth date on the patient's identification band.	
d. Ask the patient to state his or her name and birth date, based on facility policy.	
15. **Complete necessary assessments before administering medications. Check the patient's allergy bracelet or ask the patient about allergies. Explain the purpose and action of each medication to the patient.**	Assessment is a prerequisite to administration of medications.
16. Scan the patient's bar code on the identification band, if required (Figure 1).	Provides an additional check to ensure that the medication is given to the right patient.
17. **Based on facility policy, the third check of the label may occur at this point. If so, recheck the labels with the eMAR/MAR before administering the medications to the patient.**	Many facilities require the *third* check to occur at the bedside, after identifying the patient and before administration. If facility policy directs the *third* check at this time, this *third* check ensures accuracy and helps to prevent errors.
18. Put on gloves.	Gloves protect the nurse from potential contact with mucous membranes and body fluids.
19. Offer tissue to patient.	Solution and tears may spill from the eye during the procedure.

ACTION

20. Cleanse the eyelids and eyelashes of any drainage with a washcloth, cotton balls, or gauze squares moistened with water or normal saline solution, as indicated by the patient's condition. Use each area of the cleaning surface once, moving from the inner toward the outer canthus (Figure 2).

FIGURE 1. Scanning bar code on patient's identification bracelet.

21. Tilt the patient's head back slightly if sitting, or place the patient's head over a pillow if lying down. **Tilting the patient's head should be avoided if the patient has a cervical spine injury or other condition resulting in limited range-of-notion.** The head may be turned slightly to the affected side to prevent solution or tears from flowing toward the opposite eye (Figure 3).

22. Remove the cap from the medication bottle, being careful not to touch the inner side of the cap or the tip of the container. (See the accompanying Skill Variation for administering ointment.)

23. Invert the monodrip plastic container that is commonly used to instill eye drops. Have the patient look up and focus on something on the ceiling.

24. Place thumb or two fingers near margin of lower eyelid immediately below eyelashes, and apply pressure downward over bony cheek prominence. The lower conjunctival sac is exposed as the lower lid is pulled down (Figure 4).

FIGURE 3. Turning head slightly to affected side.

RATIONALE

Debris can be carried into the eye when the conjunctival sac is exposed. Using each area of the gauze once and moving from the inner canthus to the outer canthus prevents carrying debris to the lacrimal ducts.

FIGURE 2. Cleaning eyelids and eyelashes from the inner toward the outer canthus.

Tilting the patient's head back slightly makes it easier to reach the conjunctival sac. Turning the head to the affected side helps to prevent solution or tears from flowing toward the opposite eye.

Touching the inner side of the cap or tip of container may contaminate the bottle of medication.

By having the patient look up and focus on something else, the procedure is less traumatic and keeps the eye still.

The eye drop should be placed in the conjunctival sac, not directly on the eyeball.

FIGURE 4. Applying pressure downward to expose lower conjunctival sac.

(continued)

Skill 5-15 ▶ Administering Eye Drops *(continued)*

ACTION	RATIONALE
25. Rest the lateral side of your hand on the patient's forehead, just above the eyebrow. **Hold the dropper close to the eye, but avoid touching eyelids or lashes.** Squeeze container and allow prescribed number of drops to fall in lower conjunctival sac (Figure 5).	Stabilizing hand on forehead prevents accidental contamination of the bottle tip and injury to the eye. Touching the eye, eyelids, or lashes can contaminate the medication in the bottle; startle the patient, causing blinking; or injure the eye. Do not allow medication to fall onto the cornea. This may injure the cornea or cause the patient to have an unpleasant sensation.
26. Release lower lid after eye drops are instilled. Ask patient to close eyes gently.	This allows the medication to be distributed over the entire eye.
27. Apply gentle pressure over inner canthus to prevent eye drops from flowing into tear duct (Figure 6).	This minimizes the risk of systemic effects from the medication.

FIGURE 5. Squeezing container to administering drops into conjunctival sac.

FIGURE 6. Applying gentle pressure over inner canthus.

ACTION	RATIONALE
28. Instruct patient not to rub affected eye. Replace the cover on the medication bottle.	This prevents injury and irritation to the eye. Cover prevents contamination.
29. Remove gloves. Assist the patient to a comfortable position.	This ensures patient comfort.
30. Remove additional PPE, if used. Perform hand hygiene.	Proper removal of PPE reduces the risk for infection transmission and contamination of other items. Hand hygiene prevents the spread of microorganisms.
31. Document the administration of the medication immediately after administration. See Documentation section below.	Timely documentation helps to ensure patient safety.
32. Evaluate the patient's response to the medication within an appropriate time frame.	The patient needs to be evaluated for therapeutic and adverse effects from the medication.

EVALUATION   The expected outcomes have been met when the medication is delivered successfully into the eye; the patient experiences the intended effect of the medication; the patient experiences no allergy response; the patient does not exhibit systemic effects of the medication; the patient's eye remains free from injury; and patient understands the rationale for medication administration.

DOCUMENTATION

Guidelines

Document the administration of the medication immediately after administration, including date, time, dose, route of administration, and site of administration, specifically right, left, or both eyes, on the eMAR/MAR or record using the required format. If using a bar-code system, medication administration is automatically recorded when the bar code is scanned. PRN medications require documentation of the reason for administration. Prompt recording avoids the possibility of accidentally repeating the administration of the drug. If the drug was refused or omitted, record this in the appropriate area on the medication record and notify the primary care provider. This verifies the reason medication was omitted and ensures that that health care personnel providing care for the patient are aware of the occurrence.

UNEXPECTED SITUATIONS AND ASSOCIATED INTERVENTIONS

- *Drop is placed on eyelid or outer margin of eyelid due to patient blinking or moving:* Do not count this drop in total number of drops administered. Allow the patient to regain composure and proceed with application of medication. Consider approaching the patient from below the line of sight.
- *You cannot open eyelids due to dried crust and matting of eyelids:* Place a warm, wet washcloth over the eye and allow it to remain there for approximately 3 minutes. Cleanse eye as described previously. You may need to repeat this procedure if there is a large amount of matting.
- *Bottle or tube of medication comes in contact with the eyeball when applying medication:* Bottle is contaminated; discard appropriately. Notify pharmacy or retrieve a new bottle.

SPECIAL CONSIDERATIONS

General Considerations

- Ongoing assessment is an important part of nursing care to evaluate patient response to administered medications and early detection of adverse drug reactions. If an adverse effect is suspected, withhold further medication doses and notify the patient's primary care provider. Additional intervention is based on type of reaction and patient assessment.

Infant and Child Considerations

- To apply eye drops in a small child, two or more people may be needed to restrain the child. Make sure the child does not reach up to the eye, causing the nurse to jab the medication bottle into the eye.

Skill Variation ▶ Administering Eye Ointment

Prepare medication as outlined in steps 1–21 above (Skill 5-15).

1. Have the patient look up and focus on something on the ceiling.
2. Place thumb or two fingers near margin of lower eyelid immediately below eyelashes and exert pressure downward over bony cheek prominence. Lower conjunctival sac is exposed as lower lid is pulled down.
3. Hold the ointment tube close to eye, but avoid touching eyelids or lashes. Squeeze container and apply about 0.5 in of ointment from the tube along the exposed sac. Apply the medication, moving from the inner canthus to the outer canthus. Twist tube to break off ribbon of ointment. **Do not touch the tip to the eye.**
4. Release lower lid after ointment is instilled. Ask the patient to close eyes gently.

5. The patient's body warmth helps to liquefy the ointment. Instruct the patient to keep the eye closed and move the eye in the socket to help to spread the ointment under the lids and over the surface of the eyeball. The patient may then open eye.
6. Assist the patient to a comfortable position. Explain that the ointment may temporarily blur vision; encourage the patient not to rub the eye.

7. Remove gloves and additional PPE, if used. Perform hand hygiene.

8. Document administration of the medication on the eMAR/MAR immediately after administering the medication.
9. Evaluate the patient's response to the medication within an appropriate time frame.

Skill 5-16 ▶ Administering an Eye Irrigation

Eye irrigation is performed to remove secretions or foreign bodies or to cleanse and soothe the eye. In an emergency, eye irrigation can be used to remove chemicals that may burn the eye. When irrigating one eye, take care that the overflowing irrigation fluid does not contaminate the other eye.

DELEGATION CONSIDERATIONS	The administration of an eye irrigation is not delegated to nursing assistive personnel (NAP) or to unlicensed assistive personnel (UAP). Depending on the state's nurse practice act and the organization's policies and procedures, the administration of an eye irrigation may be delegated to licensed practical/vocational nurses (LPN/LVNs). The decision to delegate must be based on careful analysis of the patient's needs and circumstances, as well as the qualifications of the person to whom the task is being delegated. Refer to the Delegation Guidelines in Appendix A.

EQUIPMENT

- Sterile irrigation solution (warmed to 98.6°F [37°C])
- Sterile irrigation set (sterile container and irrigating or bulb syringe)
- Emesis basin or irrigation basin
- Washcloth
- Waterproof pad
- Towel
- Gloves
- Face shield and splash guard
- Additional PPE, as indicated

ASSESSMENT	Assess the appropriateness of the drug for the patient. Review medical history, allergy, assessment, and laboratory data that may influence drug administration. Assess the patient's eyes for redness, erythema, edema, drainage, or tenderness. Assess the patient's knowledge of the procedure. If the patient has a knowledge deficit about the procedure, this may be an appropriate time to begin patient education. Assess the patient's ability to cooperate with the procedure. Verify patient name, dose, route, and time of administration.

NURSING DIAGNOSIS

Determine related factors for the nursing diagnoses based on the patient's current status. Appropriate nursing diagnoses may include:

- Deficient knowledge
- Risk for injury
- Acute pain

OUTCOME IDENTIFICATION AND PLANNING	The expected outcome to achieve is that the eye is cleansed successfully. Other outcomes that may be appropriate include the following: the patient understands the rationale for the procedure and is able to participate; and the patient's eye remains free from additional injury.

IMPLEMENTATION

ACTION	RATIONALE
1. Gather equipment. Check the original order in the patient's health record for the irrigation, according to facility policy. Clarify any inconsistencies. Check the patient's health record for allergies.	This comparison helps to identify errors that may have occurred when orders were transcribed. The primary care provider's order or prescription is the legal record of medication orders for each facility.
2. Know the actions, special nursing considerations, purpose of administration, and potential adverse effects of the medications to be administered. Consider the appropriateness of the medication for this patient.	This knowledge aids the nurse in evaluating the therapeutic effect of the medication in relation to the patient's disorder and can also be used to educate the patient about the medication.
3. Perform hand hygiene and put on PPE, if indicated.	Hand hygiene and PPE prevent the spread of microorganisms. PPE is required based on transmission precautions.

ACTION	RATIONALE
4. Move the medication supply system to the outside of the patient's room or prepare for administration at the medication supply system in the medication area. Alternatively, access the medication administration supply system at or inside the patient's room.	Organization facilitates error-free administration and saves time.
5. Unlock the medication supply system or drawer. Enter pass code into the computer and scan employee identification, if required.	Locking the medication supply system or drawer safeguards each patient's medication supply. Facility accrediting organizations require medication supply systems to be locked when not in use. Entering pass code and scanning ID allows only authorized users into the computer system and identifies the user for documentation by the computer.
6. **Prepare medications for one patient at a time.**	This prevents errors in administration.
7. Read the eMAR/MAR and select the proper irrigation solution from the medication supply system or patient's medication drawer.	This is the *first* check of the medication label.
8. Compare the medication label with the eMAR/MAR. Check expiration dates and perform calculations, if necessary. Scan the bar code on the package, if required.	This is the *second* check of the label. Verify calculations with another nurse to ensure safety, if necessary.
9. **Depending on facility policy, the third check of the label may occur at this point. If so, when all medications for one patient have been prepared, recheck the labels with the eMAR/MAR before taking the medications to the patient. However, many facilities require the third check to occur at the bedside, after identifying the patient.**	This *third* check ensures accuracy and helps to prevent errors. *Note:* Many facilities require the third check to occur at the bedside, after identifying the patient and before administration.
10. **Lock the medication supply system before leaving it.**	Locking the medication supply system or drawer safeguards the patient's medication supply. Facility accrediting organizations require medication supply systems to be locked when not in use.
11. **Ensure that the patient receives the medications at the correct time.**	Check facility policy, which may allow for administration within a period of 30 minutes before or 30 minutes after the designated time.
12. Perform hand hygiene and put on PPE, if indicated.	Hand hygiene and PPE prevent the spread of microorganisms. PPE is required based on transmission precautions.
13. **Identify the patient. Compare the information with the eMAR/MAR. The patient should be identified using at least two of the following methods (The Joint Commission, 2018):**	Identifying the patient ensures the right patient receives the medications and helps prevent errors. The patient's room number or physical location is not used as an identifier (The Joint Commission, 2018). Replace the identification band if it is missing or inaccurate in any way.
a. Check the name on the patient's identification band.	This requires a response from the patient, but illness and strange surroundings often cause patients to be confused.
b. Check the identification number on the patient's identification band.	
c. Check the birth date on the patient's identification band.	
d. Ask the patient to state his or her name and birth date, based on facility policy.	
14. **Complete necessary assessments before administering medications. Check the patient's allergy bracelet or ask the patient about allergies. Explain the purpose and action of each medication to the patient.**	Assessment is a prerequisite to administration of medications. Explanation facilitates cooperation and reassures the patient.

(continued)

Skill 5-16 ▶ Administering an Eye Irrigation *(continued)*

ACTION	RATIONALE
15. Scan the patient's bar code on the identification band, if required.	Provides an additional check to ensure that the medication is given to the right patient.
16. Assemble equipment at the patient's bedside.	This provides for an organized approach to the task.
17. **Based on facility policy, the third check of the medication label may occur at this point. If so, recheck the label with the eMAR/MAR before administering the medications to the patient.**	Many facilities require the *third* check to occur at the bedside, after identifying the patient and before administration. If facility policy directs the *third* check at this time, this *third* check ensures accuracy and helps prevent errors.
18. Have the patient sit or lie with head tilted toward side of affected eye (Figure 1). Protect the patient and bed with a waterproof pad.	Gravity aids flow of the solution away from the unaffected eye and from the inner canthus of the affected eye toward the outer canthus.
19. Put on gloves. Clean lids and lashes with washcloth moistened with water or normal saline or the solution ordered for the irrigation, as indicated by the patient's condition. Wipe from inner canthus toward outer canthus (Figure 2). Use a different corner of washcloth with each wipe.	Gloves protect the nurse from contact with mucous membranes, body fluids, and contaminants. Materials lodged on lids or in lashes may be washed into the eye. Wiping from the inner to outer canthus protects the nasolacrimal duct and the other eye. Use of a different part of the washcloth prevents transmission of bacteria.

FIGURE 1. Tilting head toward affected eye.

FIGURE 2. Cleaning eyelids and eyelashes from inner canthus to outer canthus.

20. Put on face shield/splash guard. Place curved basin at cheek on the side of the affected eye to receive irrigating solution (Figure 3). If patient is able, ask him/her to support the basin.	Face shield/splash guard protects the nurse from contact with splashed body fluids and contaminants. Gravity aids flow of solution.

FIGURE 3. Placing basin to catch irrigating fluid.

ACTION

21. Place thumb near margin of lower eyelid immediately below eyelashes and two fingers above eye. Apply pressure downward over bony cheek prominence to expose the lower conjunctival sac as the lower lid is pulled down. Hold upper lid open with your fingers (Figure 4).

22. Fill the irrigation syringe with the prescribed fluid. **Hold irrigation syringe about 2.5 cm (1 in) from eye (Figure 5). Direct flow of solution from inner to outer canthus along the conjunctival sac.**

RATIONALE

Solution is directed only into lower conjunctival sac because the cornea is sensitive and easily injured. This also prevents reflex blinking.

This minimizes the risk for injury to the cornea. Directing solution toward the outer canthus helps to prevent the spread of contamination from the eye to the lacrimal sac, the lacrimal duct, and the nose.

FIGURE 4. Exposing lower conjunctival sac and holding upper lid open.

FIGURE 5. Holding irrigation syringe about 1 inch from eye.

23. Irrigate until the solution is clear or all the solution has been used. **Use only enough force to remove secretions gently from the conjunctiva. Avoid touching any part of the eye with the irrigating tip.**

24. Pause the irrigation and have the patient close the eye periodically during the procedure.

25. Dry the periorbital area after irrigation with gauze sponge. Offer a towel to the patient if face and neck are wet.

26. Remove gloves. Assist the patient to a comfortable position.

 27. Remove face shield and splash guard and additional PPE, if used. Perform hand hygiene.

28. Evaluate the patient's response to the medication within an appropriate time frame.

Directing solutions with force may cause injury to the tissues of the eye as well as to the conjunctiva. Touching the eye is uncomfortable for the patient and may cause damage to the cornea.

Movement of the eye when the lids are closed helps to move secretions from the upper to the lower conjunctival sac.

Leaving the skin moist after irrigation is uncomfortable for the patient.

This ensures patient comfort.

Proper removal of PPE reduces the risk for infection transmission and contamination of other items. Hand hygiene prevents the spread of microorganisms.

The patient needs to be evaluated for therapeutic and adverse effects from the medication.

EVALUATION

The expected outcomes have been met when the eye was irrigated successfully; the patient understood the rationale for the procedure; and the eye was not injured.

DOCUMENTATION

Guidelines

Document the procedure, site, the type of solution and volume used, length of time irrigation performed, pre- and post-procedure assessments, characteristics of any drainage, and the patient's response to the treatment on the eMAR/MAR or record using the required format. If using a barcode system, medication administration is automatically recorded when the bar code is scanned.

(continued)

Skill 5-16 ▶ Administering an Eye Irrigation *(continued)*

PRN medications require documentation of the reason for administration. Prompt recording avoids the possibility of accidentally repeating the administration of the drug. If the drug was refused or omitted, record this in the appropriate area on the medication record and notify the primary care provider. This verifies the reason medication was omitted and ensures that that health care personnel providing care for the patient are aware of the occurrence.

Sample Documentation

> <u>8/26/20</u> 1820 Sclera of left eye reddened, with periorbital edema and erythema. Thick, yellow liquid draining from left eye. Irrigation of left eye performed using 500 mL of sterile saline. Patient's sclera remains reddened, with slight periorbital edema and erythema. No drainage noted from left eye after irrigation. Patient tolerated procedure with minimal discomfort. Denies need for pain medication at this time. Patient rates pain at present as 1/10.
>
> —B. Clapp, RN

UNEXPECTED SITUATIONS AND ASSOCIATED INTERVENTIONS

- *Patient complains of significant pain during the procedure:* Stop the procedure and notify the primary care provider. Primary care provider may need to check for any foreign objects, such as glass, before proceeding with irrigation.
- *Patient cannot keep the eye open during the procedure:* You may need assistance to help the patient keep the eye open.

SPECIAL CONSIDERATIONS

- Ongoing assessment is an important part of nursing care to evaluate patient response to administered treatments and early detection of adverse drug reactions. If an adverse effect is suspected, notify the patient's primary care provider. Provide additional intervention based on type of reaction and patient assessment.

Skill 5-17 ▶ Administering Ear Drops

Drugs are instilled into the auditory canal for their local effect. They are used to soften wax, relieve pain, apply local anesthesia, and treat infections. If the tympanic membrane is ruptured or has been opened by surgical intervention, the middle ear and the inner ear have a direct passage to the external ear. When this occurs, perform instillations with the greatest of care to prevent forcing materials from the outer ear into the middle ear and the inner ear. Use sterile technique to prevent infection.

DELEGATION CONSIDERATIONS

The administration of medication via drops in the ear is not delegated to nursing assistive personnel (NAP) or to unlicensed assistive personnel (UAP). Depending on the state's nurse practice act and the organization's policies and procedures, the administration of ear drop may be delegated to licensed practical/vocational nurses (LPN/LVNs). The decision to delegate must be based on careful analysis of the patient's needs and circumstances, as well as the qualifications of the person to whom the task is being delegated. Refer to the Delegation Guidelines in Appendix A.

EQUIPMENT

- Ear drop medication (warmed to 98.6°F [37°C])
- Tissue
- Cotton balls (optional)
- Gloves
- Additional PPE, as indicated
- Disposable washcloth or washcloth (optional)
- Normal saline solution or warm water
- Electronic Medication Administration Record (eMAR) or Medication Administration Record (MAR)

ASSESSMENT	Assess the appropriateness of the drug for the patient. Review medical history, allergy, assessment, and laboratory data that may influence drug administration. Assess the affected ear for redness, erythema, edema, drainage, or tenderness. Assess the patient's knowledge of medication and procedure. If the patient has a knowledge deficit about the medication, this may be an appropriate time to begin education about the medication. Assess the patient's ability to cooperate with the procedure. Verify patient name, dose, route, and time of administration.
NURSING DIAGNOSIS	Determine related factors for the nursing diagnoses based on the patient's current status. Appropriate nursing diagnoses may include: • Deficient knowledge • Risk for injury • Acute pain
OUTCOME IDENTIFICATION AND PLANNING	The expected outcome to achieve is that drops are administered successfully and the patient experiences the intended effect of the medication. Other outcomes that may be appropriate include the following: the patient understands the rationale for the ear drop instillation; and the patient does not experience injury.

IMPLEMENTATION

ACTION	**RATIONALE**
1. Gather equipment. Check medication order against the original order in the health record, according to facility policy. Clarify any inconsistencies. Check the patient's health record for allergies.	This comparison helps to identify errors that may have occurred when orders were transcribed. The primary care provider's order or prescription is the legal record of medication orders for each facility.
2. Know the actions, special nursing considerations, safe dose ranges, purpose of administration, and adverse effects of the medication to be administered. Consider the appropriateness of the medication for this patient.	This knowledge aids the nurse in evaluating the therapeutic effect of the medication in relation to the patient's disorder and can also be used to educate the patient about the medication.
3. Perform hand hygiene.	Hand hygiene prevents the spread of microorganisms.
4. Move the medication supply system to the outside of the patient's room or prepare for administration at the medication supply system in the medication area. Alternatively, access the medication administration supply system at or inside the patient's room.	Organization facilitates error-free administration and saves time.
5. Unlock the medication supply system or drawer. Enter pass code and scan employee identification, if required.	Locking the medication supply system or drawer safeguards each patient's medication supply. Facility accrediting organizations require medication supply systems to be locked when not in use. Entering pass code and scanning ID allows only authorized users into the system and identifies the user for documentation by the computer.
6. **Prepare medications for one patient at a time.**	This prevents errors in medication administration.
7. Read the eMAR/MAR and select the proper medication from the patient's medication drawer or medication supply system.	This is the *first* check of the label.
8. Compare the label with the eMAR/MAR. Check expiration dates and perform calculations, if necessary. Scan the bar code on the package, if required.	This is the *second* check of the label. Verify calculations with another nurse to ensure safety, if necessary.

(continued)

Skill 5-17 ▶ Administering Ear Drops *(continued)*

ACTION	RATIONALE
9. Depending on facility policy, the third check of the label may occur at this point. If so, when all medications for one patient have been prepared, recheck the labels with the eMAR/MAR before taking the medications to the patient. However, many facilities require the third check to occur at the bedside, after identifying the patient.	This *third* check ensures accuracy and helps to prevent errors. *Note:* Many facilities require the *third* check to occur at the bedside, after identifying the patient and before administration.
10. Lock the medication supply system before leaving it.	Locking the medication supply system or drawer safeguards the patient's medication supply. Facility accrediting organizations require medication supply systems to be locked when not in use.
11. Transport medications to the patient's bedside carefully, and keep the medications in sight at all times.	Careful handling and close observation prevent accidental or deliberate disarrangement of medications.
12. Ensure that the patient receives the medications at the correct time.	Check facility policy, which may allow for administration within a period of 30 minutes before or 30 minutes after the designated time.
13. Perform hand hygiene and put on PPE, if indicated.	Hand hygiene and PPE prevent the spread of microorganisms. PPE is required based on transmission precautions.
14. Identify the patient. Compare the information with the eMAR/MAR. The patient should be identified using at least two of the following methods (The Joint Commission, 2018):	Identifying the patient ensures the right patient receives the medications and helps prevent errors. The patient's room number or physical location is not used as an identifier (The Joint Commission, 2018). Replace the identification band if it is missing or inaccurate in any way.
a. Check the name on the patient's identification band.	This requires a response from the patient, but illness and strange surroundings often cause patients to be confused.
b. Check the identification number on the patient's identification band.	
c. Check the birth date on the patient's identification band.	
d. Ask the patient to state his or her name and birth date, based on facility policy.	
15. Complete necessary assessments before administering medications. Check the patient's allergy bracelet or ask the patient about allergies. Explain the purpose and action of each medication to the patient.	Assessment is a prerequisite to administration of medications.
16. Scan the patient's bar code on the identification band, if required.	Provides an additional check to ensure that the medication is given to the right patient.
17. Based on facility policy, the third check of the label may occur at this point. If so, recheck the labels with the eMAR/MAR before administering the medications to the patient.	Many facilities require the *third* check to occur at the bedside, after identifying the patient and before administration. If facility policy directs the *third* check at this time, this *third* check ensures accuracy and helps to prevent errors.
18. Put on gloves.	Gloves protect the nurse from potential contact with mucous membranes and body fluids.
19. Cleanse external ear of any drainage with cotton ball or washcloth moistened with normal saline or water (Figure 1).	Debris and drainage may prevent some of the medication from entering the ear canal.
20. Place patient on his or her unaffected side in bed, or, if ambulatory, have patient sit with head well tilted to the side so that the affected ear is uppermost (Figure 2).	This positioning prevents the drops from escaping from the ear.

ACTION	RATIONALE

FIGURE 1. Cleaning external ear.

FIGURE 2. Positioning patient on unaffected side.

21. Remove the cap from the medication bottle, being careful not to touch the inner side of the cap or the tip of the container (Figure 3).

Touching the inner side of the cap or tip of container may contaminate the bottle of medication.

22. Straighten auditory canal by pulling cartilaginous portion of pinna up and back for an adult. (See Infant and Child Considerations for correct positioning for this age group.)

Pulling on the pinna as described helps to straighten the canal properly for ear drop instillation.

23. Invert and hold medication bottle in the ear with its tip above the auditory canal (Figure 4). Do not touch the dropper to the ear.

By holding the medication bottle in the ear, the medication will enter the ear canal. Touching the bottle to the ear contaminates the bottle and medication. The hard tip of the medication bottle can damage the tympanic membrane if it is jabbed into the ear.

FIGURE 3. Removing the cap from the medication bottle.

FIGURE 4. Pulling the pinna up and back and placing dropper tip above auditory canal.

24. **Squeeze container and allow drops to fall on the side of the canal. Avoid instilling in the middle of the canal, to avoid instilling directly onto the tympanic membrane.**

It is uncomfortable for the patient if the drops fall directly onto the tympanic membrane.

25. Release pinna after instilling drops, and have patient maintain the head position to prevent escape of medication.

Medication should remain in ear canal for at least 5 minutes.

(continued)

Skill 5-17 ➤ Administering Ear Drops *(continued)*

ACTION	RATIONALE
26. Gently press on the tragus a few times (Figure 5).	Pressing on the tragus causes medication from the canal to move toward the tympanic membrane.
27. If ordered, loosely insert a cotton ball into the ear canal (Figure 6).	A cotton ball can help prevent medication from leaking out of the ear canal.

FIGURE 5. Applying pressure to tragus.

FIGURE 6. Inserting cotton ball into ear canal.

ACTION	RATIONALE
28. Instruct patient to remain lying down with the affected ear upward for 5 minutes.	This ensures medication remains in ear canal.
29. Replace cap on medication bottle. Remove gloves and additional PPE, if used. Perform hand hygiene.	Replacing cap prevents contamination of tip of bottle. Proper removal of PPE reduces the risk for infection transmission and contamination of other items. Hand hygiene prevents the spread of microorganisms.
30. Document the administration of the medication immediately after administration. See Documentation section below.	Timely documentation helps to ensure patient safety.
31. Evaluate the patient's response to medication within an appropriate time frame.	The patient needs to be evaluated for therapeutic and adverse effects from the medication.

EVALUATION

The expected outcomes have been met when the ear drops have been administered successfully; the patient experiences the intended effect of the medication; the patient understands the rationale for the ear drop instillation; and the patient did not experience injury.

DOCUMENTATION

Guidelines

Document the administration of the medication immediately after administration, including date, time, dose, route of administration, and site of administration, specifically right, left, or both ears, on the eMAR/MAR or record using the required format. If using a bar-code system, medication administration is automatically recorded when the bar code is scanned. PRN medications require documentation of the reason for administration. Prompt recording avoids the possibility of accidentally repeating the administration of the drug. Document pre- and post-administration assessments, characteristics of any drainage, and the patient's response to the treatment, if appropriate. If the drug was refused or omitted, record this in the appropriate area on the medication record and notify the primary care provider. This verifies the reason medication was omitted and ensures that health care personnel providing care for the patient are aware of the occurrence.

UNEXPECTED SITUATIONS AND ASSOCIATED INTERVENTIONS

- *Medication runs from ear into eye:* Notify primary care provider and check with the pharmacy. Eye irrigation may need to be performed.
- *Patient complains of extreme pain when you press on the tragus:* Allow patient to press on tragus. If pressure causes too much pain, this part may be deferred.

SPECIAL CONSIDERATIONS

General Considerations

- If both ears are to be treated, wait 5 minutes before instilling drops into the second ear.
- Ongoing assessment is an important part of nursing care to evaluate patient response to administered treatments and early detection of adverse drug reactions. If an adverse effect is suspected, notify the patient's primary care provider. Additional intervention is based on type of reaction and patient assessment.

Infant and Child Considerations

- Pull pinna up and back for a child older than 3 years (Figure 7) and down and back for an infant or a child younger than 3 years (Figure 8) (Kee et al., 2015; Kyle & Carman, 2017).
- Distraction techniques, such as TV or a quiet toy, may be helpful when attempting to keep a child quiet for 5 minutes. Reading to the child may not be appropriate because the child's hearing may be compromised during medication administration.

FIGURE 7. Pulling pinna up and back for a child older than 3 years.

FIGURE 8. Pulling pinna down and back for an infant or child younger than 3 years.

Skill 5-18 ▶ Administering an Ear Irrigation

Irrigations of the external auditory canal are ordinarily performed for cleaning purposes or for applying heat to the area. Typically, a normal saline solution is used, although an antiseptic solution may be indicated for local action. To prevent pain, make sure the irrigation solution is warmed to body temperature (American Academy of Otolaryngology-Head and Neck Surgery, n.d.). Usually, an irrigation syringe is used. However, a mechanical jet irrigator may also be used (Hayter, 2016). The following skill outlines use of an irrigation syringe.

DELEGATION CONSIDERATIONS

The administration of an irrigation of the ear is not delegated to nursing assistive personnel (NAP) or to unlicensed assistive personnel (UAP). Depending on the state's nurse practice act and the organization's policies and procedures, the irrigation of the ear may be delegated to licensed practical/vocational nurses (LPN/LVNs). The decision to delegate must be based on careful analysis of the patient's needs and circumstances, as well as the qualifications of the person to whom the task is being delegated. Refer to the Delegation Guidelines in Appendix A.

(continued)

Skill 5-18 ▶ Administering an Ear Irrigation *(continued)*

EQUIPMENT

- Prescribed irrigating solution (warmed to 98.6°F to 104.9°F [37°C to 40.5°C])
- Irrigation set (container and irrigating or bulb syringe)
- Waterproof pad
- Emesis basin
- Gloves
- Additional PPE, as indicated
- Cotton balls, disposable washcloth, or washcloth
- Normal saline or water
- Electronic Medication Administration Record (eMAR) or Medication Administration Record (MAR)

ASSESSMENT

Assess the appropriateness of the drug/procedure for the patient. Review medical history, allergy, assessment, and laboratory data that may influence drug administration. Assess for the presence of conditions that indicate irrigation is contraindicated, such as complications from a previous ear irrigation; ear surgery; suspected or actual tympanic puncture or perforation; cleft palate (Harkin, 2015; Hayter, 2016). Assess for the presence of conditions that indicate the need for increased caution when performing an ear irrigation, including patients with anticoagulant use, diabetes, immunocompromised, dizziness and tinnitus or patients who had radiation therapy to the ear (Harkin, 2015; Hayter, 2016). Assess the affected ear for redness, erythema, edema, drainage, or tenderness. Assess the patient's ability to hear. Assess the patient's knowledge of medication and procedure. If the patient has a knowledge deficit about the medication, this may be an appropriate time to begin education about the medication. Assess the patient's ability to cooperate with the procedure. Verify patient name, dose, route, and time of administration.

NURSING DIAGNOSIS

Determine related factors for the nursing diagnoses based on the patient's current status. Appropriate nursing diagnoses may include:

- Acute pain
- Risk for injury
- Deficient knowledge

OUTCOME IDENTIFICATION AND PLANNING

The expected outcome to achieve is that the irrigation is administered successfully and the patient experiences the intended effect of the medication. Other outcomes that may be appropriate include the following: the patient remains free from injury; and the patient understands the rationale for the procedure.

IMPLEMENTATION

ACTION	RATIONALE
1. Gather equipment. Check medication order against the original order in the health record, according to facility policy. Clarify any inconsistencies. Check the patient's health record for allergies.	This comparison helps to identify errors that may have occurred when orders were transcribed. The primary care provider's order or prescription is the legal record of medication orders for each facility.
2. Know the actions, special nursing considerations, safe dose ranges, purpose of administration, and adverse effects of the medication to be administered. Consider the appropriateness of the medication for this patient.	This knowledge aids the nurse in evaluating the therapeutic effect of the medication in relation to the patient's disorder and can also be used to educate the patient about the medication.
3. Perform hand hygiene.	Hand hygiene prevents the spread of microorganisms.
4. Move the medication supply system to the outside of the patient's room or prepare for administration at the medication supply system in the medication area. Alternatively, access the medication administration supply system at or inside the patient's room.	Organization facilitates error-free administration and saves time.

ACTION	**RATIONALE**
5. Unlock the medication supply system or drawer. Enter pass code and scan employee identification, if required.	Locking the medication supply system or drawer safeguards each patient's medication supply. Facility accrediting organizations require medication supply systems to be locked when not in use. Entering pass code and scanning ID allows only authorized users into the computer system and identifies the user for documentation by the computer.
6. **Prepare medications for one patient at a time.**	This prevents errors in medication administration.
7. Read the eMAR/MAR and select the proper medication from medication supply system or the patient's medication drawer.	This is the *first* check of the label.
8. Compare the label with the eMAR/MAR. Check expiration dates and perform calculations, if necessary. Scan the bar code on the package, if required.	This is the *second* check of the label. Verify calculations with another nurse to ensure safety, if necessary.
9. **Depending on facility policy, the third check of the label may occur at this point. If so, when all medications for one patient have been prepared, recheck the labels with the eMAR/MAR before taking the medications to the patient. However, many facilities require the third check to occur at the bedside, after identifying the patient.**	This *third* check ensures accuracy and helps to prevent errors. *Note:* Many facilities require the *third* check to occur at the bedside, after identifying the patient and before administration.
10. **Lock the medication supply system before leaving it.**	Locking the medication supply system or drawer safeguards the patient's medication supply. Facility accrediting organizations require medication supply systems to be locked when not in use.
11. Transport medications to the patient's bedside carefully, and keep the medications in sight at all times.	Careful handling and close observation prevent accidental or deliberate disarrangement of medications.
12. **Ensure that the patient receives the medications at the correct time.**	Check facility policy, which may allow for administration within a period of 30 minutes before or 30 minutes after the designated time.
13. Perform hand hygiene and put on PPE, if indicated.	Hand hygiene and PPE prevent the spread of microorganisms. PPE is required based on transmission precautions.
14. **Identify the patient. Compare the information with the eMAR/MAR. The patient should be identified using at least two of the following methods (The Joint Commission, 2018):**	Identifying the patient ensures the right patient receives the medications and helps prevent errors. The patient's room number or physical location is not used as an identifier (The Joint Commission, 2018). Replace the identification band if it is missing or inaccurate in any way.
a. Check the name on the patient's identification band.	This requires a response from the patient, but illness and strange surroundings often cause patients to be confused.
b. Check the identification number on the patient's identification band.	
c. Check the birth date on the patient's identification band.	
d. Ask the patient to state his or her name and birth date, based on facility policy.	
15. Explain the procedure to the patient.	Explanation facilitates cooperation and reassures the patient.
16. Scan the patient's bar code on the identification band, if required.	Provides an additional check to ensure that the medication is given to the right patient.
17. Assemble equipment at patient's bedside.	This provides for an organized approach to the task.
18. Put on gloves.	Gloves protect the nurse from potential contact with contaminants and body fluids.

(continued)

Skill 5-18 ▶ Administering an Ear Irrigation *(continued)*

ACTION	RATIONALE
19. Have the patient sit up or lie with head tilted slightly toward side of the affected ear. Protect the patient and bed with a waterproof pad. Have the patient support the basin under the ear to receive the irrigating solution (Figure 1).	Gravity causes the irrigating solution to flow from the ear to the basin.
20. Cleanse external ear of any drainage with cotton ball or washcloth moistened with normal saline or water.	Debris and drainage on the external ear may be washed into the ear and/or may prevent some of the medication from entering the ear canal.
21. Pretreat the ear with 2 to 4 drops of warm water or irrigating solution (refer to Skill 5-17) and wait 15 minutes.	Pretreating softens the cerumen and enhances the effectiveness of the ear irrigation (Hayter, 2016).
22. Fill irrigating or bulb syringe with warmed solution. If an irrigating container is used, prime the tubing.	Priming the tubing allows air to escape from the tubing. Air forced into the ear canal is noisy and therefore unpleasant for the patient.
23. Straighten the auditory canal by pulling the cartilaginous portion of pinna up and back for an adult (Figure 2). (See Infant and Child Considerations for correct positioning for this age group.)	Straightening the ear canal allows solution to reach all areas of the canal easily.

FIGURE 1. Positioning for ear irrigation.

FIGURE 2. Pulling pinna up and back to straighten the ear canal.

ACTION	RATIONALE
24. Point the syringe tip superiorly and posteriorly toward the upper back to the ear canal wall. Use a gentle squirting motion to **direct a steady, slow stream of solution against the roof of the auditory canal, using only enough force to remove secretions (Figure 3). Do not occlude the auditory canal with the irrigating nozzle.** Allow solution to flow out unimpeded.	Use of a gentle squirting motion and directing the solution at the roof of the canal help prevent tympanic membrane injury or perforation (Hayter, 2016). Continuous in-and-out flow of the irrigating solution helps to prevent pressure in the canal.
25. When irrigation is complete, place a cotton ball loosely in the auditory meatus (Figure 4) and have the patient lie on side of affected ear on a towel or absorbent pad.	The cotton ball absorbs excess fluid, and gravity allows the remaining solution in the canal to escape from the ear.
26. Remove gloves and any additional PPE, if used. Perform hand hygiene.	Proper removal of PPE reduces the risk for infection transmission and contamination of other items. Hand hygiene prevents the spread of microorganisms.
27. Document the administration of the medication immediately after administration. See Documentation section below.	Timely documentation helps to ensure patient safety.

ACTION

FIGURE 3. Instilling irrigation fluid.

28. Evaluate the patient's response to the procedure. Return in 10 to 15 minutes and remove cotton ball and assess drainage. Evaluate the patient's response to the medication within an appropriate time frame.

RATIONALE

FIGURE 4. Placing cotton ball in ear.

The patient needs to be evaluated for any adverse effects from the procedure. Drainage or pain may indicate injury to the tympanic membrane. The patient needs to be evaluated for therapeutic and adverse effects from the medication.

EVALUATION

The expected outcomes have been met when the irrigation has been administered successfully; the patient experiences the intended effect of the medication; the patient remains free from injury; and the patient understands the rationale for the procedure.

DOCUMENTATION

Guidelines

Document the procedure, site, the type of solution and volume used, length of time irrigation performed, pre- and post-procedure assessments, characteristics of any drainage, and the patient's response to the treatment.

Document the procedure, site, the type of solution and volume used, length of time irrigation performed, characteristics of any drainage, and the patient's response to the treatment on the eMAR/MAR or record using the required format. If using a bar-code system, medication administration is automatically recorded when the bar code is scanned. PRN medications require documentation of the reason for administration. Prompt recording avoids the possibility of accidentally repeating the administration of the drug. Document pre- and post-administration assessments, characteristics of any drainage, and the patient's response to the treatment, if appropriate. If the procedure was refused or omitted, record this in the appropriate area on the medication record and notify the primary care provider. This verifies the reason medication was omitted and ensures that health care personnel providing care for the patient are aware of the occurrence.

Sample Documentation

7/6/20 1830 Right ear noted to be without external edema and redness. No drainage noted. Patient reports slightly decreased hearing in right ear. Slight tenderness noted on palpation. Irrigation of right ear performed using 100 mL of warmed normal saline. Clear return with particles of cerumen noted. Patient tolerated procedure with minimal discomfort. Patient reports no change in hearing in right ear. Denies need for pain medication at this time. Patient rates pain at present as 1/10.

—B. Clapp, RN

UNEXPECTED SITUATIONS AND ASSOCIATED INTERVENTIONS

• *Patient complains of significant pain during irrigation:* Stop the irrigation. Check the temperature of the solution. If the solution has cooled, rewarm it and try again. If the patient still complains of pain, stop the irrigation and notify the primary care provider.

(continued)

Skill 5-18 ▶ Administering an Ear Irrigation   *(continued)*

SPECIAL CONSIDERATIONS

General Considerations

- Ongoing assessment is an important part of nursing care to evaluate patient response to administered medications and early detection of adverse drug reactions. If an adverse effect is suspected, withhold further medication doses and notify the patient's primary care provider. Additional intervention is based on type of reaction and patient assessment.

Infant and Child Considerations

- Pull pinna up and back for a child older than 3 years (Figure 5) and down and back for an infant or a child younger than 3 years (Figure 6) (Kee et al., 2015; Kyle & Carman, 2017).

FIGURE 5. Pulling pinna up and back for child older than 3 years.

FIGURE 6. Pulling pinna down and back for an infant or child younger than 3 years.

Skill 5-19 ▶ Administering a Nasal Spray

Nasal instillations are used to treat allergies, sinus infections, and nasal congestion. Medications with a systemic effect, such as vasopressin, may also be prepared as a nasal instillation. The nose is normally not a sterile cavity, but because of its connection with the sinuses, it is important to observe medical asepsis carefully when using nasal instillations.

The following skill describes the steps to administer a nasal spray. Refer to the accompanying Skill Variation for guidelines to administer medication via nasal drops.

DELEGATION CONSIDERATIONS

The administration of medication using a nasal spray is not delegated to nursing assistive personnel (NAP) or to unlicensed assistive personnel (UAP). Depending on the state's nurse practice act and the organization's policies and procedures, administration of a nasal spray may be delegated to licensed practical/vocational nurses (LPN/LVNs). The decision to delegate must be based on careful analysis of the patient's needs and circumstances, as well as the qualifications of the person to whom the task is being delegated. Refer to the Delegation Guidelines in Appendix A.

EQUIPMENT

- Medication in nasal spray bottle
- Gloves
- Additional PPE, as indicated
- Tissue
- Electronic Medication Administration Record (eMAR) or Medication Administration Record (MAR)

ASSESSMENT	Assess the appropriateness of the drug for the patient. Review medical history, allergy, assessment, and laboratory data that may influence drug administration. Assess the nares for redness, erythema, edema, drainage, or tenderness. Assess the patient's knowledge of medication and the procedure. If the patient has a knowledge deficit about the medication, this may be an appropriate time to begin education about the procedure. Assess the patient's ability to cooperate with the procedure. Verify patient name, dose, route, and time of administration.
NURSING DIAGNOSIS	Determine related factors for the nursing diagnoses based on the patient's current status. Appropriate nursing diagnoses may include: • Deficient knowledge • Risk for allergy reaction
OUTCOME IDENTIFICATION AND PLANNING	The expected outcome to achieve is that the medication is administered successfully into the nose and the patient experiences the intended effect of the medication. Other outcomes that may be appropriate include the following: the patient understands the rationale for the nose spray; the patient experiences no allergy response; and the patient experiences minimal discomfort.

IMPLEMENTATION

ACTION	RATIONALE
1. Gather equipment. Check medication order against the original order in the health record, according to facility policy. Clarify any inconsistencies. Check the patient's health record for allergies.	This comparison helps to identify errors that may have occurred when orders were transcribed. The primary care provider's order or prescription is the legal record of medication orders for each facility.
2. Know the actions, special nursing considerations, safe dose ranges, purpose of administration, and adverse effects of the medication to be administered. Consider the appropriateness of the medication for this patient.	This knowledge aids the nurse in evaluating the therapeutic effect of the medication in relation to the patient's disorder and can also be used to educate the patient about the medication.
3. Perform hand hygiene.	Hand hygiene prevents the spread of microorganisms.
4. Move the medication supply system to the outside of the patient's room or prepare for administration at the medication supply system in the medication area. Alternatively, access the medication administration supply system at or inside the patient's room.	Organization facilitates error-free administration and saves time.
5. Unlock the medication supply system or drawer. Enter pass code and scan employee identification, if required.	Locking the medication supply system or drawer safeguards each patient's medication supply. Facility accrediting organizations require medication supply systems to be locked when not in use. Entering pass code and scanning ID allows only authorized users into the system and identifies the user for documentation by the computer.
6. Prepare medications for one patient at a time.	This prevents errors in medication administration.
7. Read the eMAR/MAR and select the proper medication from the patient's medication drawer or medication supply system.	This is the *first* check of the label.
8. Compare the label with the eMAR/MAR. Check expiration dates and perform calculations, if necessary. Scan the bar code on the package, if required.	This is the *second* check of the label. Verify calculations with another nurse to ensure safety, if necessary.
9. Depending on facility policy, the third check of the label may occur at this point. If so, when all medications for one patient have been prepared, recheck the labels with the eMAR/MAR before taking the medications to the patient. However, many facilities require the third check to occur at the bedside, after identifying the patient.	This *third* check ensures accuracy and helps to prevent errors. *Note:* Many facilities require the *third* check to occur at the bedside, after identifying the patient and before administration.

(continued)

Skill 5-19 ▶ Administering a Nasal Spray *(continued)*

ACTION	RATIONALE

10. Lock the medication supply system before leaving it.

Locking the medication supply system or drawer safeguards the patient's medication supply. Facility accrediting organizations require medication supply systems to be locked when not in use.

11. Transport medications to the patient's bedside carefully, and keep the medications in sight at all times.

Careful handling and close observation prevent accidental or deliberate disarrangement of medications.

12. **Ensure that the patient receives the medications at the correct time.**

Check facility policy, which may allow for administration within a period of 30 minutes before or 30 minutes after the designated time.

13. Perform hand hygiene and put on PPE, if indicated.

Hand hygiene and PPE prevent the spread of microorganisms. PPE is required based on transmission precautions.

14. **Identify the patient. Compare the information with the eMAR/MAR. The patient should be identified using at least two of the following methods (The Joint Commission, 2018):**

Identifying the patient ensures the right patient receives the medications and helps prevent errors. The patient's room number or physical location is not used as an identifier (The Joint Commission, 2018). Replace the identification band if it is missing or inaccurate in any way.

a. Check the name on the patient's identification band.

b. Check the identification number on the patient's identification band.

c. Check the birth date on the patient's identification band.

d. Ask the patient to state his or her name and birth date, based on facility policy.

This requires a response from the patient, but illness and strange surroundings often cause patients to be confused.

15. **Complete necessary assessments before administering medications. Check the patient's allergy bracelet or ask the patient about allergies. Explain the purpose and action of each medication to the patient.**

Assessment is a prerequisite to administration of medications.

16. Scan the patient's bar code on the identification band, if required (Figure 1).

Provides an additional check to ensure that the medication is given to the right patient.

FIGURE 1. Scanning bar code on the patient's identification bracelet.

17. **Based on facility policy, the third check of the label may occur at this point. If so, recheck the labels with the eMAR/MAR before administering the medications to the patient.**

Many facilities require the *third* check to occur at the bedside, after identifying the patient and before administration. If facility policy directs the *third* check at this time, this *third* check ensures accuracy and helps to prevent errors.

18. Put on gloves.

Gloves protect the nurse from potential contact with contaminants and body fluids.

ACTION

19. Provide patient with paper tissues and ask the patient to blow his or her nose.

20. Have the patient sit up with head tilted back. **Tilting the patient's head should be avoided if the patient has a cervical spine injury or other condition resulting in limited range of notion.**

21. Instruct the patient that it is necessary to inhale gently through the nose as the spray is being administered or not to inhale gently as the spray is being administered. Your instruction to the patient will depend on the medication being administered. Consult the manufacturer's instructions for each medication.

22. Agitate the bottle gently, if required for specific medication. Insert the tip of the nosepiece of the bottle into one nostril (Figure 2). Close the opposite nostril with a finger. Instruct the patient to breathe in gently through the nostril, if required. Compress or activate the bottle to release one spray at the same time the patient breathes in.

RATIONALE

Blowing the nose clears the nasal mucosa prior to medication administration.

Allows the spray to flow into the nares. Tilting the head is contraindicated with cervical spine injury.

Inhalation helps to distribute the spray in the nares. Inhalation during administration is not recommended for some medications.

Mixes medication thoroughly to ensure a consistent dose of medication.

FIGURE 2. Inserting tip of bottle into one nostril.

23. Keep the medication container compressed and remove it from the nostril. Release the container from the compressed state. Do not allow the container to return to its original position until it is removed from the patient's nose.

24. Have the patient hold his or her breath for a few seconds, and then breathe out slowly through the mouth. Repeat in the other nostril, as prescribed or indicated.

25. Wipe the outside of the bottle nose piece with a clean, dry tissue or cloth and replace the cap. Instruct the patient to avoid blowing his or her nose for 5 to 10 minutes, depending on the medication.

26. Remove gloves. Assist the patient to a comfortable position.

    27. Remove additional PPE, if used. Perform hand hygiene.

Prevents contamination of the contents of the container.

Allows medication to remain in contact with mucous membranes of nose.

Keeps the end of the bottle clean. Keeps the medication in contact with the mucous membranes of the nose.

This ensures patient comfort.

Proper removal of PPE reduces the risk for infection transmission and contamination of other items. Hand hygiene prevents the spread of microorganisms.

(continued)

Skill 5-19 ▶ Administering a Nasal Spray *(continued)*

ACTION	RATIONALE
28. Document the administration of the medication immediately after administration. See Documentation section below.	Timely documentation helps to ensure patient safety.
29. Evaluate the patient's response to the procedure and medication within an appropriate time frame.	The patient needs to be evaluated for therapeutic and adverse effects from the medication.

EVALUATION

The expected outcomes have been met when the medication has been administered successfully into the nose; the patient experiences the intended effect of the medication; the patient understands the rationale for the nose spray; the patient experiences no allergy response; and the patient experienced minimal discomfort.

DOCUMENTATION

Guidelines

Document the administration of the medication, including date, time, dose, route of administration, and site of administration, specifically right, left, or both nares, on the eMAR/MAR or record using the required format. If using a bar-code system, medication administration is automatically recorded when the bar code is scanned. PRN medications require documentation of the reason for administration. Prompt recording avoids the possibility of accidentally repeating the administration of the drug. Document pre- and post-administration assessments, characteristics of any drainage, and the patient's response to the treatment, if appropriate. If the drug was refused or omitted, record this in the appropriate area on the medication record and notify the primary care provider. This verifies the reason medication was omitted and ensures that health care personnel providing care for the patient are aware of the occurrence.

UNEXPECTED SITUATIONS AND ASSOCIATED INTERVENTIONS

• *Patient sneezes immediately after receiving nose spray:* Do not repeat the dosage, because you cannot determine how much medication was actually absorbed.

SPECIAL CONSIDERATIONS

• Ongoing assessment is an important part of nursing care to evaluate patient response to administered medications and early detection of adverse drug reactions. If an adverse effect is suspected, withhold further medication doses and notify the patient's primary care provider. Additional intervention is based on type of reaction and patient assessment.

Skill Variation ▶ Administering Medication via Nasal Drops

Prepare medication as outlined in steps 1–17 above (Skill 5-19).

1. Put on gloves. Assist the patient to an upright position with the head tilted back.
2. Draw sufficient solution into the dropper for both nares. Do not return excess solution to the bottle to avoid contamination.
3. Have the patient breathe through the mouth. Hold tip of nose up and place dropper just above naris, about 1/3 in. Instill the prescribed number of drops in one naris and then into the other. Avoid touching naris with dropper.

4. Have patient remain in position with head tilted back for 5 minutes to prevent the escape of the medication.

5. Remove gloves and any additional PPE, if used. Perform hand hygiene.

6. Document administration of the medication on the eMAR/MAR immediately after administering the medication. Document the site, if only one nostril is used.

7. Evaluate the patient's response to the medication within an appropriate time frame.

Skill 5-20 ▶ Administering a Vaginal Cream

Creams, foams, and tablets can be applied intravaginally using a narrow, tubular applicator with an attached plunger. Suppositories that melt when exposed to body heat are also administered by vaginal insertion (see the accompanying Skill Variation on page 295). Refrigerate suppositories for storage. Time the administration of vaginal medications to allow the patient to lie down afterward to retain the medication.

DELEGATION CONSIDERATIONS	The administration of medication as a vaginal cream is not delegated to nursing assistive personnel (NAP) or to unlicensed assistive personnel (UAP). Depending on the state's nurse practice act and the organization's policies and procedures, administration of a vaginal cream may be delegated to licensed practical/vocational nurses (LPN/LVNs). The decision to delegate must be based on careful analysis of the patient's needs and circumstances, as well as the qualifications of the person to whom the task is being delegated. Refer to the Delegation Guidelines in Appendix A.
EQUIPMENT	• Medication with applicator, if appropriate • Water-soluble lubricant • Perineal pad • Disposable washcloth or washcloth, skin cleanser, and warm water • Gloves • Additional PPE, as indicated • Electronic Medication Administration Record (eMAR) or Medication Administration Record (MAR)
ASSESSMENT	Assess the appropriateness of the drug for the patient. Review medical history, allergy, assessment, and laboratory data that may influence drug administration. Assess the external genitalia and vaginal canal for redness, erythema, edema, drainage, or tenderness. Assess the patient's knowledge of medication and procedure. If the patient has a knowledge deficit about the medication, this may be an appropriate time to begin education about the medication. Assess the patient's ability to cooperate with the procedure. Verify patient name, dose, route, and time of administration.
NURSING DIAGNOSIS	Determine related factors for the nursing diagnoses based on the patient's current status. Appropriate nursing diagnoses may include: • Deficient knowledge • Risk for injury • Risk for allergy reaction
OUTCOME IDENTIFICATION AND PLANNING	The expected outcome to achieve is that the medication is administered successfully into the vagina and the patient experiences the intended effect of the medication. Other outcomes that may be appropriate include the following: the patient understands the rationale for the vaginal instillation; the patient experiences no allergy response; and the patient experiences minimal discomfort.

IMPLEMENTATION

ACTION	RATIONALE
1. Gather equipment. Check medication order against the original order in the health record, according to facility policy. Clarify any inconsistencies. Check the patient's health record for allergies.	This comparison helps to identify errors that may have occurred when orders were transcribed. The primary care provider's order or prescription is the legal record of medication orders for each facility.
2. Know the actions, special nursing considerations, safe dose ranges, purpose of administration, and adverse effects of the medication to be administered. Consider the appropriateness of the medication for this patient.	This knowledge aids the nurse in evaluating the therapeutic effect of the medication in relation to the patient's disorder and can also be used to educate the patient about the medication.
3. Perform hand hygiene.	Hand hygiene prevents the spread of microorganisms.

(continued)

Skill 5-20 ▶ Administering a Vaginal Cream *(continued)*

ACTION	RATIONALE
4. Move the medication supply system to the outside of the patient's room or prepare for administration at the medication supply system in the medication area. Alternatively, access the medication administration supply system at or inside the patient's room.	Organization facilitates error-free administration and saves time.
5. Unlock the medication supply system or drawer. Enter pass code and scan employee identification, if required.	Locking of the medication supply system or drawer safeguards each patient's medication supply. Facility accrediting organizations require medication supply systems to be locked when not in use. Entering pass code and scanning ID allows only authorized users into the system and identifies the user for documentation by the computer.
6. Prepare medications for one patient at a time.	This prevents errors in medication administration.
7. Read the eMAR/MAR and select the proper medication from medication supply system or the patient's medication drawer.	This is the *first* check of the label.
8. Compare the label with the eMAR/MAR. Check expiration dates and perform calculations, if necessary. Scan the bar code on the package, if required.	This is the *second* check of the label. Verify calculations with another nurse to ensure safety, if necessary.
9. Depending on facility policy, the third check of the label may occur at this point. If so, when all medications for one patient have been prepared, recheck the labels with the eMAR/MAR before taking the medications to the patient. However, many facilities require the third check to occur at the bedside, after identifying the patient.	This *third* check ensures accuracy and helps to prevent errors. *Note:* Many facilities require the *third* check to occur at the bedside, after identifying the patient and before administration.
10. Lock the medication supply system before leaving it.	Locking the medication supply system or drawer safeguards the patient's medication supply. Facility accrediting organizations require medication supply systems to be locked when not in use.
11. Transport medications to the patient's bedside carefully, and keep the medications in sight at all times.	Careful handling and close observation prevent accidental or deliberate disarrangement of medications.
12. Ensure that the patient receives the medications at the correct time.	Check facility policy, which may allow for administration within a period of 30 minutes before or 30 minutes after the designated time.
13. Perform hand hygiene and put on PPE, if indicated.	Hand hygiene and PPE prevent the spread of microorganisms. PPE is required based on transmission precautions.
14. Identify the patient. Compare the information with the eMAR/MAR. The patient should be identified using at least two of the following methods (The Joint Commission, 2018):	Identifying the patient ensures the right patient receives the medications and helps prevent errors. The patient's room number or physical location is not used as an identifier (The Joint Commission, 2018). Replace the identification band if it is missing or inaccurate in any way.
a. Check the name on the patient's identification band.	This requires a response from the patient, but illness and strange surroundings often cause patients to be confused.
b. Check the identification number on the patient's identification band.	
c. Check the birth date on the patient's identification band.	
d. Ask the patient to state his or her name and birth date, based on facility policy.	
15. Complete necessary assessments before administering medications. Check the patient's allergy bracelet or ask the patient about allergies. Explain the purpose and action of each medication to the patient.	Assessment is a prerequisite to administration of medications.

ACTION

16. Scan the patient's bar code on the identification band, if required (Figure 1).

17. **Based on facility policy, the third check of the label may occur at this point. If so, recheck the labels with the eMAR/MAR before administering the medications to the patient.**

18. Ask the patient to void before inserting the medication.

19. Put on gloves.

20. Position the patient so that she is lying on her back with the knees flexed. Maintain privacy with draping. Provide adequate light to visualize the vaginal opening.

21. Perform perineal care. Spread labia with fingers, and cleanse area at vaginal orifice with disposable washcloth or washcloth and warm water, using a different corner of the washcloth with each stroke. Wipe from above the vaginal orifice downward toward the sacrum (front to back) (Figure 2).

22. Remove gloves and put on new gloves.

23. Fill vaginal applicator with prescribed amount of cream (Figure 3). (See the accompanying Skill Variation for administering a vaginal **suppository**.)

RATIONALE

Provides an additional check to ensure that the medication is given to the right patient.

FIGURE 1. Scanning bar code on patient's identification bracelet. (*Photo by B. Proud.*)

Many facilities require the *third* check to occur at the bedside, after identifying the patient and before administration. If facility policy directs the *third* check at this time, this *third* check ensures accuracy and helps to prevent errors.

Empties the bladder and helps to minimize pressure and discomfort during administration.

Gloves protect the nurse from potential contact with contaminants and body fluids.

Position provides access to vaginal canal and helps to retain medication in the canal. Draping limits exposure of the patient and promotes warmth and privacy. Adequate light facilitates ease of administration.

These techniques prevent contamination of the vaginal orifice with debris surrounding the anus.

Prevents spread of microorganisms.

This ensures the correct dosage of medication will be administered.

FIGURE 2. Performing perineal care.

FIGURE 3. Filling vaginal applicator with cream.

(*continued*)

Skill 5-20 ▶ Administering a Vaginal Cream *(continued)*

ACTION	**RATIONALE**
24. Lubricate applicator with the lubricant, as necessary.	Ordinarily, lubrication is unnecessary, but it may be used to reduce friction while inserting the applicator.
25. Spread the labia with your nondominant hand and gently introduce the applicator with your dominant hand, in a rolling manner, while directing it downward and backward.	This follows the normal contour of the vagina for its full length.
26. After the applicator is properly positioned (Figure 4), labia may be allowed to fall in place if necessary to free the hand for manipulating the plunger. Push the plunger to its full length and then gently remove applicator with plunger depressed.	Pushing the plunger will gently deploy the cream into the vaginal orifice.

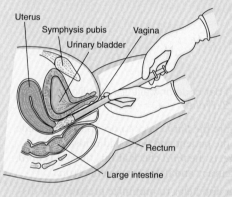

FIGURE 4. Positioning applicator in vagina for administration of medication.

27. **Ask the patient to remain in the supine position for a minimum of 5 to 10 minutes after insertion. Some medications are administered prior to lying down to go to bed.** Offer the patient a perineal pad to collect drainage.	This gives the medication time to be absorbed in the vaginal cavity. As medication heats up, some medication may leak from the vaginal orifice.
28. Dispose of the applicator in an appropriate receptacle or clean the nondisposable applicator according to manufacturer's directions.	Disposal prevents transmission of microorganisms. Cleaning prepares the applicator for future use by same patient for continuing treatment.
29. Remove gloves and additional PPE, if used. Perform hand hygiene.	Proper removal of PPE reduces the risk for infection transmission and contamination of other items. Hand hygiene prevents the spread of microorganisms.
30. Document the administration of the medication immediately after administration. See Documentation section below.	Timely documentation helps to ensure patient safety.
31. Evaluate the patient's response to the medication within an appropriate time frame.	The patient needs to be evaluated for therapeutic and adverse effects from the medication.

EVALUATION

The expected outcomes have been met when the medication is administered successfully into the vagina; the patient experiences the intended effect of the medication; the patient understands the rationale for the vaginal instillation; the patient experiences no allergy response; and the patient experiences minimal discomfort.

DOCUMENTATION

Guidelines

Document the administration of the medication immediately after administration, including date, time, dose, and route of administration on the eMAR/MAR or record using the required format. Prompt recording avoids the possibility of accidentally repeating the administration of the drug. If using a bar-code system, medication administration is automatically recorded when the bar code is scanned. PRN medications require documentation of the reason for administration. Document assessment, characteristics of any drainage, and the patient's response to the treatment, if appropriate. If the drug was refused or omitted, record this in the appropriate area on the medication record and notify the primary care provider. This verifies the reason medication was omitted and ensures that health care personnel providing care for the patient are aware of the occurrence.

Sample Documentation

> <u>7/23/20</u> 2300 Monistat vaginal cream administered as ordered. Small amount of curd-like, white discharge noted from vagina. Perineal skin remains erythematous. Patient states, "It doesn't itch as much as it has been."
>
> —K. Sanders, RN

SPECIAL CONSIDERATIONS

- Ongoing assessment is an important part of nursing care to evaluate patient response to administered medications and early detection of adverse reactions. If an adverse effect is suspected, withhold further medication doses and notify the patient's primary care provider. Additional intervention is based on type of reaction and patient assessment.
- Instruct patients to avoid using tampons, as a tampon will absorb the medication.
- Explain to the patient that she may want to use a sanitary pad to protect clothing from stains from the medication.

Skill Variation ▷ Administering a Vaginal Suppository

Prepare medication as outlined in steps 1–19 above (Skill 5-20).

1. Position the patient so that she is lying on her back with the knees flexed. Maintain privacy with draping. Adequate light should be available to visualize the vaginal opening.
2. Spread labia with fingers, and clean area at vaginal orifice with washcloth and warm water, using a different corner of the washcloth with each stroke. Wipe from above orifice downward toward sacrum (front to back).
3. Remove gloves and put on new gloves.
4. Remove the suppository from its wrapper and lubricate the round end with the water-soluble lubricant (Figure A). Lubricate your gloved index finger on your dominant hand.

FIGURE B. Inserting suppository into vagina.

FIGURE A. Lubricating suppository.

5. Spread the labia with your nondominant hand.
6. Insert the rounded end of the suppository along the posterior wall of the canal (Figure B). Insert to the length of your finger.
7. Remove gloves.

8. **Ask the patient to remain in a supine position for minimum of 5 to 10 minutes after insertion. Some medications are administered prior to lying down to go to bed.**
9. Offer the patient a perineal pad to collect drainage.
10. Remove additional PPE, if used. Perform hand hygiene.
11. Document administration of the medication on the eMAR/MAR immediately after administering the medication.
12. Evaluate the patient's response to the medication within an appropriate time frame.
13. Assist the patient to a comfortable position after the required 5 to 10 minutes in the supine position.

Unexpected Situations and Associated Interventions

- *Upon assessing the patient after administering a vaginal suppository, you note the suppository is not in the vagina but instead is between the labia:* Put on gloves and reinsert the suppository, ensuring that it is inserted fully.

Skill 5-21 ▶ Administering a Rectal Suppository

Rectal suppositories are used primarily for their local action, such as laxatives and fecal softeners. Systemic effects are also achieved with rectal suppositories, such as antiemetic or antipyretic effect. Suppositories may be used when it is difficult or not possible for a patient to take medications orally. It is important to ensure the suppository is placed past the internal anal sphincter and against the rectal mucosa.

DELEGATION CONSIDERATIONS	The administration of medication as a rectal suppository is not delegated to nursing assistive personnel (NAP) or to unlicensed assistive personnel (UAP). Depending on the state's nurse practice act and the organization's policies and procedures, administration of a vaginal cream may be delegated to licensed practical/vocational nurses (LPN/LVNs). The decision to delegate must be based on careful analysis of the patient's needs and circumstances, as well as the qualifications of the person to whom the task is being delegated. Refer to the Delegation Guidelines in Appendix A.
EQUIPMENT	• Suppository (rectal) • Water-soluble lubricant • Nonlatex, disposable gloves • Toilet tissue • Electronic Medication Administration Record (eMAR) or Medication Administration Record (MAR) • Additional PPE, as indicated
ASSESSMENT	Assess the appropriateness of the drug for the patient. Review medical history, allergy, assessment, and laboratory data that may influence drug administration, particularly the patient's white blood cell and platelet counts. Patients who are thrombocytopenic or neutropenic should not receive rectal suppositories. Do not administer rectal suppositories to patients at risk for cardiac arrhythmias. Do not administer suppositories to patients who have had recent rectal or prostate surgery. Assess relevant body systems for the particular medication being administered. Assess the rectal area for any alterations in integrity. Assess the patient's knowledge of the medication and procedure. If the patient has a knowledge deficit about the medication, this may be an appropriate time to begin education about the medication. Assess the patient's ability to cooperate with the procedure. Verify patient name, dose, route, and time of administration.
NURSING DIAGNOSIS	Determine the related factors for the nursing diagnoses based on the patient's current status. Possible nursing diagnoses may include: • Deficient knowledge • Constipation • Risk for injury
OUTCOME IDENTIFICATION AND PLANNING	The expected outcome to achieve is that the medication is administered successfully into the rectum and the patient experiences the intended effect of the medication. Other outcomes that may be appropriate include the following: the patient understands the rationale for the rectal instillation; and the patient experienced minimal discomfort.

IMPLEMENTATION

ACTION	RATIONALE
1. Gather equipment. Check medication order against the original order in the health record, according to facility policy. Clarify any inconsistencies. Check the patient's health record for allergies.	This comparison helps to identify errors that may have occurred when orders were transcribed. The primary care provider's order or prescription is the legal record of medication orders for each facility.
2. Know the actions, special nursing considerations, safe dose ranges, purpose of administration, and adverse effects of the medication to be administered. Consider the appropriateness of the medication for this patient.	This knowledge aids the nurse in evaluating the therapeutic effect of the medication in relation to the patient's mucosa and disorder and can also be used to educate the patient about the medication.
3. Perform hand hygiene.	Hand hygiene prevents the spread of microorganisms.

ACTION	**RATIONALE**
4. Move the medication supply system to the outside of the patient's room or prepare for administration at the medication supply system in the medication area. Alternatively, access the medication administration supply system at or inside the patient's room.	Organization facilitates error-free administration and saves time.
5. Unlock the medication supply system or drawer. Enter pass code and scan employee identification, if required.	Locking the medication supply system or drawer safeguards each patient's medication supply. Facility accrediting organizations require medication supply systems to be locked when not in use. Entering pass code and scanning ID allows only authorized users into the system and identifies the user for documentation by the computer.
6. **Prepare medications for one patient at a time.**	This prevents errors in medication administration.
7. Read the eMAR/MAR and select the proper medication from medication supply system or the patient's medication drawer.	This is the *first* check of the label.
8. Compare the label with the eMAR/MAR. Check expiration dates and perform calculations, if necessary. Scan the bar code on the package, if required.	This is the *second* check of the label. Verify calculations with another nurse to ensure safety, if necessary.
9. **Depending on facility policy, the third check of the label may occur at this point. If so, when all medications for one patient have been prepared, recheck the labels with the eMAR/MAR before taking the medications to the patient. However, many facilities require the third check to occur at the bedside, after identifying the patient.**	This *third* check ensures accuracy and helps to prevent errors. *Note:* Many facilities require the *third* check to occur at the bedside, after identifying the patient and before administration.
10. **Lock the medication supply system before leaving it.**	Locking the medication supply system or drawer safeguards the patient's medication supply. Facility accrediting organizations require medication supply systems to be locked when not in use.
11. Transport medications to the patient's bedside carefully, and keep the medications in sight at all times.	Careful handling and close observation prevent accidental or deliberate disarrangement of medications.
12. **Ensure that the patient receives the medications at the correct time.**	Check facility policy, which may allow for administration within a period of 30 minutes before or 30 minutes after the designated time.
13. Perform hand hygiene and put on PPE, if indicated.	Hand hygiene and PPE prevent the spread of microorganisms. PPE is required based on transmission precautions.
14. **Identify the patient. Compare the information with the eMAR/MAR. The patient should be identified using at least two of the following methods (The Joint Commission, 2018):**	Identifying the patient ensures the right patient receives the medications and helps prevent errors. The patient's room number or physical location is not used as an identifier (The Joint Commission, 2018). Replace the identification band if it is missing or inaccurate in any way.
a. Check the name on the patient's identification band.	This requires a response from the patient, but illness and strange surroundings often cause patients to be confused.
b. Check the identification number on the patient's identification band.	
c. Check the birth date on the patient's identification band.	
d. Ask the patient to state his or her name and birth date, based on facility policy.	
15. **Complete necessary assessments before administering medications. Check the patient's allergy bracelet or ask the patient about allergies. Explain the purpose and action of each medication to the patient.**	Assessment is a prerequisite to administration of medications.

(continued)

Skill 5-21 ► Administering a Rectal Suppository *(continued)*

ACTION	RATIONALE
16. Scan the patient's bar code on the identification band, if required (Figure 1).	Provides an additional check to ensure that the medication is given to the right patient.
17. **Based on facility policy, the third check of the label may occur at this point. If so, recheck the labels with the eMAR/MAR before administering the medications to the patient.**	Many facilities require the *third* check to occur at the bedside, after identifying the patient and before administration. If facility policy directs the *third* check at this time, this *third* check ensures accuracy and helps to prevent errors.
18. Put on gloves.	Gloves protect the nurse from potential contact with contaminants and body fluids.
19. Assist the patient to his or her left side in a Sims' position. Drape accordingly to expose only the buttocks.	Sims' positioning allows for easy access to the anal area. Left side decreases chance of expulsion of the suppository. Proper draping maintains privacy.
20. Remove the suppository from its wrapper. Apply lubricant to the rounded end (Figure 2). Lubricate the index finger of your dominant hand.	Lubricant reduces friction on administration and increases patient comfort.

FIGURE 1. Scanning bar code on patient's identification bracelet. (*Photo by B. Proud.*)

FIGURE 2. Applying lubricant to rounded end of suppository.

21. Separate the buttocks with your nondominant hand and instruct the patient to breathe slowly and deeply through his or her mouth while the suppository is being inserted.	Slow, deep breaths help to relax the anal sphincter and reduce discomfort.
22. Using your index finger, insert the suppository, round end first, **along the rectal wall.** Insert about 3 to 4 in (Figure 3).	Suppository must make contact with the rectal mucosa for absorption to occur. If inserted into stool, it will be ineffective (Peate, 2015).

Anal-rectal ridge

Anal sphincter

Suppository

Rectum

FIGURE 3. Inserting suppository round end first along rectal wall.

ACTION	**RATIONALE**
23. Use toilet tissue to clean any stool or lubricant from around the anus. Release the buttocks. Encourage the patient to remain on his or her side for at least 5 minutes and retain the suppository for the appropriate amount of time for the specific medication.	Prevents skin irritation. Prevents accidental expulsion of suppository and ensures absorption of the medication.
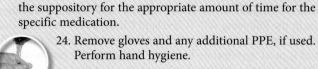 24. Remove gloves and any additional PPE, if used. Perform hand hygiene.	Proper removal of PPE reduces the risk for infection transmission and contamination of other items. Hand hygiene prevents the spread of microorganisms.
25. Document the administration of the medication immediately after administration. See Documentation section below.	Timely documentation helps to ensure patient safety.
26. Evaluate the patient's response to the medication within an appropriate time frame.	The patient needs to be evaluated for therapeutic and adverse effects from the medication.

EVALUATION

The expected outcomes have been met when the medication was administered into the rectum; the patient experiences the intended effect of the medication; the patient understands the rationale for the rectal instillation; and the patient experienced minimal discomfort.

DOCUMENTATION

Guidelines

Document the administration of the medication immediately after administration, including date, time, dose, and route of administration on the eMAR/MAR or record using the required format. If using a bar-code system, medication administration is automatically recorded when the bar code is scanned. PRN medications require documentation of the reason for administration. Prompt recording avoids the possibility of accidentally repeating the administration of the drug. Document your assessments, and the patient's response to the treatment, if appropriate. If the drug was refused or omitted, record this in the appropriate area on the medication record and notify the primary care provider. This verifies the reason medication was omitted and ensures that health care personnel providing care for the patient are aware of the occurrence.

UNEXPECTED SITUATIONS AND ASSOCIATED INTERVENTIONS

- *Patient expels the suppository before it is absorbed:* Put on gloves and apply additional lubricant to the suppository. Reinsert past the internal sphincter. If the suppository has warmed and become too soft, discard the suppository and notify the primary care provider. An additional dose may be ordered.

SPECIAL CONSIDERATIONS

General Considerations

- If the suppository is for laxative purposes, it must remain in position for 35 to 45 minutes, or until the patient feels the urge to defecate.
- Ongoing assessment is an important part of nursing care to evaluate patient response to administered medications and early detection of adverse reactions. If an adverse effect is suspected, withhold further medication doses and notify the patient's primary care provider. Additional intervention is based on type of reaction and patient assessment.

Infant and Child Considerations

- For an infant or child younger than the age of 3 years, use the fifth finger for insertion. For an older child, use the index finger (Kyle & Carmen, 2017).
- It may be necessary to hold the buttocks together for a few minutes to relieve pressure on the anal sphincter and expulsion of the suppository.

Older Adult Considerations

- Older adults may have difficulty retaining rectal suppositories because of decreased muscle tone and loss of sphincter control.

Skill 5-22 ▶ Administering Medication via a Metered-Dose Inhaler (MDI)

Drugs for **inhalation** may be administered via a **metered-dose inhaler** (MDI). An MDI is a handheld inhaler that uses an aerosol spray or mist to deliver a controlled dose of medication with each compression of the canister that is then breathed in by the patient. The medication is then absorbed rapidly through the lung tissue, resulting in local and systemic effects. There are two methods for using an MDI; the preferred method is with a device called a valved holding chamber or spacer, and is outlined in the steps in the following skill (Cleveland Clinic, 2014). An MDI can also be used without a chamber. Refer to the accompanying Skill Variation at the end of this skill. Patients should discuss which method is most appropriate for use with their health care provider. There are a number of different medication inhaler devices. It is imperative that nurses understand the administration technique for the specific type of inhaler in use in order to administer the prescribed medication effectively and to provide appropriate patient education (Alismail et al., 2016).

DELEGATION CONSIDERATIONS

The administration of medication via a metered-dose inhaler is not delegated to nursing assistive personnel (NAP) or to unlicensed assistive personnel (UAP). Depending on the state's nurse practice act and the organization's policies and procedures, administration of a metered-dose inhaler may be delegated to licensed practical/vocational nurses (LPN/LVNs). The decision to delegate must be based on careful analysis of the patient's needs and circumstances, as well as the qualifications of the person to whom the task is being delegated. Refer to the Delegation Guidelines in Appendix A.

EQUIPMENT

- Stethoscope
- Medication in an MDI
- Spacer or holding chamber
- Electronic Medication Administration Record (eMAR) or Medication Administration Record (MAR)
- PPE, as indicated

ASSESSMENT

Assess the appropriateness of the drug for the patient. Review medical history, allergy, assessment, and laboratory data that may influence drug administration. Assess respiratory rate, rhythm, and depth to establish a baseline. Assess lung sounds before and after use to establish a baseline and determine the effectiveness of the medication. If appropriate and/or ordered, assess oxygen saturation level before medication administration. The oxygenation level usually increases after the medication is administered. Assess the patient's ability to manage an MDI; young and older adults may have dexterity problems. Assess the patient's knowledge and understanding of the medication's purpose and action. Verify patient name, dose, route, and time of administration.

NURSING DIAGNOSIS

Determine related factors for the nursing diagnoses based on the patient's current status. Appropriate nursing diagnoses may include:

- Risk for activity intolerance
- Impaired gas exchange
- Deficient knowledge

OUTCOME IDENTIFICATION AND PLANNING

The expected outcome to achieve when using an MDI is that the medication is administered and breathed in by the patient and the patient experiences the intended effect of the medication. Other outcomes that may be appropriate include the following: the patient understands the rationale for the inhaled medication; and the patient demonstrates correct use of an MDI.

IMPLEMENTATION

ACTION	RATIONALE
1. Gather equipment. Check each medication order against the original order in the health record, according to facility policy. Clarify any inconsistencies. Check the patient's health record for allergies.	This comparison helps to identify errors that may have occurred when orders were transcribed. The primary care provider's order or prescription is the legal record of medication orders for each facility.
2. Know the actions, special nursing considerations, safe dose ranges, purpose of administration, and adverse effects of the medications to be administered. Consider the appropriateness of the medication for this patient.	This knowledge aids the nurse in evaluating the therapeutic effect of the medication in relation to the patient's disorder and can also be used to educate the patient about the medication.

ACTION	**RATIONALE**

3. Perform hand hygiene.

Hand hygiene prevents the spread of microorganisms.

4. Move the medication supply system to the outside of the patient's room or prepare for administration at the medication supply system in the medication area. Alternatively, access the medication administration supply system at or inside the patient's room.

Organization facilitates error-free administration and saves time.

5. Unlock the medication supply system or drawer. Enter pass code and scan employee identification, if required.

Locking the medication supply system or drawer safeguards each patient's medication supply. Facility accrediting organizations require medication supply systems to be locked when not in use. Entering pass code and scanning ID allows only authorized users into the computer system and identifies the user for documentation by the computer.

6. **Prepare medications for one patient at a time.**

This prevents errors in medication administration.

7. Read the eMAR/MAR and select the proper medication from the patient's medication drawer or medication supply system.

This is the *first* check of the label.

8. Compare the label with the eMAR/MAR. Check expiration dates and perform calculations, if necessary. Scan the bar code on the package, if required.

This is the *second* check of the label. Verify calculations with another nurse to ensure safety, if necessary.

9. **Depending on facility policy, the third check of the label may occur at this point. If so, when all medications for one patient have been prepared, recheck the labels with the eMAR/MAR before taking the medications to the patient. However, many facilities require the third check to occur at the bedside, after identifying the patient.**

This *third* check ensures accuracy and helps to prevent errors. *Note:* Many facilities require the *third* check to occur at the bedside, after identifying the patient and before administration.

10. **Lock the medication supply system before leaving it.**

Locking the medication supply system or drawer safeguards the patient's medication supply. Facility accrediting organizations require medication supply systems to be locked when not in use.

11. Transport medications to the patient's bedside carefully, and keep the medications in sight at all times.

Careful handling and close observation prevent accidental or deliberate disarrangement of medications.

12. **Ensure that the patient receives the medications at the correct time.**

Check facility policy, which may allow for administration within a period of 30 minutes before or 30 minutes after the designated time.

13. Perform hand hygiene and put on PPE, if indicated.

Hand hygiene and PPE prevent the spread of microorganisms. PPE is required based on transmission precautions.

14. **Identify the patient. Compare the information with the eMAR/MAR. The patient should be identified using at least two of the following methods (The Joint Commission, 2018):**

Identifying the patient ensures the right patient receives the medications and helps prevent errors. The patient's room number or physical location is not used as an identifier (The Joint Commission, 2018). Replace the identification band if it is missing or inaccurate in any way.

a. Check the name on the patient's identification band.

b. Check the identification number on the patient's identification band.

c. Check the birth date on the patient's identification band.

d. Ask the patient to state his or her name and birth date, based on facility policy.

This requires a response from the patient, but illness and strange surroundings often cause patients to be confused.

(continued)

Skill 5-22 ▶ Administering Medication via a Metered-Dose Inhaler (MDI) *(continued)*

ACTION	RATIONALE
15. Complete necessary assessments before administering medications. Check the patient's allergy bracelet or ask the patient about allergies. Explain what you are going to do and the reason for doing it to the patient.	Assessment is a prerequisite to administration of medications. Explanation relieves anxiety and facilitates cooperation.
16. Scan the patient's bar code on the identification band, if required (Figure 1).	Provides an additional check to ensure that the medication is given to the right patient.
17. Based on facility policy, the third check of the label may occur at this point. If so, recheck the labels with the eMAR/MAR before administering the medications to the patient.	Many facilities require the *third* check to occur at the bedside, after identifying the patient and before administration. If facility policy directs the *third* check at this time, this *third* check ensures accuracy and helps to prevent errors.
18. Shake the inhaler well.	The medication and propellant may separate when the canister is not in use. Shaking well ensures that the patient is receiving the correct dosage of medication.
19. Remove the mouthpiece cover from the MDI and the spacer. Attach the MDI to the spacer by inserting in the open end of the spacer, opposite the mouthpiece. (Refer to the accompanying Skill Variation for using an MDI without a spacer.)	The use of a spacer or valved holding chamber is preferred because it traps the medication and aids in delivery of the correct dose.
20. Have patient place the spacer's mouthpiece into mouth, grasping securely with teeth and sealing the lips tightly around the mouthpiece (Figure 2). Have patient breathe normally through the spacer.	Medication should not leak out around the mouthpiece.

FIGURE 1. Scanning bar code on patient's identification bracelet.

FIGURE 2. Placing spacer with MDI into mouth.

ACTION	RATIONALE
21. The patient should breathe out completely, then depress the canister once, releasing one puff into the spacer, then inhale slowly and deeply through the mouth.	The spacer will hold the medication in suspension for a short period so that the patient can receive more of the prescribed medication than if it had been projected into the air. Breathing slowly and deeply distributes the medication deep into the airways.
22. Instruct patient to hold his or her breath for 5 to 10 seconds, or as long as possible, and then to exhale slowly through pursed lips.	This allows better distribution of the medication to the airways and longer absorption time for the medication.
23. Wait 1 to 5 minutes, as prescribed, before administering the next puff, as prescribed.	This ensures that both puffs are absorbed as much as possible. Bronchodilation after the first puff allows for deeper penetration by subsequent puffs.
24. After the prescribed number of puffs has been administered, have the patient remove the MDI from the spacer and replace the caps on both MDI and spacer.	By replacing the caps, the patient is preventing any dust or dirt from entering and being propelled into the bronchioles with later doses.
25. Have the patient gargle and rinse with tap water after using an MDI, as necessary. Clean the MDI according to the manufacturer's directions.	Rinsing removes medication residue from the mouth. Rinsing is necessary when using inhaled steroids because oral fungal infections can occur. The buildup of medication in the device can attract bacteria and affect how the medication is delivered.

ACTION	**RATIONALE**
26. Remove PPE, if used. Perform hand hygiene.	Proper removal of PPE reduces the risk for infection transmission and contamination of other items. Hand hygiene prevents the spread of microorganisms.
27. Document the administration of the medication immediately after administration. See Documentation section below.	Timely documentation helps to ensure patient safety.
28. Evaluate the patient's response to the medication within an appropriate time frame. Reassess lung sounds, oxygen saturation level, and respirations, as indicated.	The patient needs to be evaluated for therapeutic and adverse effects from the medication.

EVALUATION

The expected outcomes have been met when the medication is administered and breathed in by the patient; the patient experiences the intended effect of the medication; the patient understands the rationale for the inhaled medication; and the patient demonstrated correct use of the MDI.

DOCUMENTATION

Guidelines

Document the administration of the medication immediately after administration, including date, time, dose, route of administration and any teaching done with the patient on the eMAR/MAR or record using the required format. If using a bar-code system, medication administration is recorded automatically when the bar code is scanned. PRN medications require documentation of the reason for administration. Prompt recording avoids the possibility of accidentally repeating the administration of the drug. Document respiratory rate, oxygen saturation, if applicable, lung assessment, and the patient's response to the treatment, if appropriate. If the drug was refused or omitted, record this in the appropriate area on the medication record and notify the primary care provider. This verifies the reason medication was omitted and ensures that health care personnel providing care for the patient are aware of the occurrence.

Sample Documentation

> 9/29/20 0820 Wheezes noted in all lobes of lungs before albuterol MDI, O_2 saturation 92%, respiratory rate 24 breaths per minute. After albuterol treatment, lung sounds are clear and equal in all lobes, O_2 saturation 97%, respiratory rate 18 breaths per minute. Patient able to demonstrate accurately the use of an MDI and spacer and verbalizes understanding of medication purpose and action.
>
> —C. Bausler, RN

UNEXPECTED SITUATIONS AND ASSOCIATED INTERVENTIONS

- *Patient uses MDI, but symptoms are not relieved:* Check to make sure that the inhaler still contains medication. The patient may have received only propellant, without medication.
- *Patient is unable to use MDI:* Many companies have adaptive devices that allow patients to use MDIs.
- *Patient reports that relief of symptoms has decreased, even with increased number of puffs:* Have patient demonstrate the technique that he or she is using. Many patients lack an understanding of correct use of an MDI and/or develop poor habits over time (Levy, Hardwell, McKnight, & Holmes., 2013). Poor administration technique can lead to a decrease in effectiveness and a need for an increased dosage of medication.

SPECIAL CONSIDERATIONS

General Considerations

- The plastic holder and provided with the inhaler should be cleaned at least weekly. Remove the medication canister and clean with warm running water. Shake the holder and allow to air dry.
- Some medication canisters cannot be removed from the plastic holder. Wipe the mouthpiece with a cloth or dry cotton swab and/or refer to the manufacturer's directions for cleaning (Cleveland Clinic, 2014).

(continued)

Skill 5-22

Administering Medication via a Metered-Dose Inhaler (MDI) *(continued)*

- Clean the spacer (valved holding chamber) once a week by soaking in warm water with a mild detergent. Rinse well and shake off excess water. Allow to air dry (Cleveland Clinic, 2014).
- Do not store spacer (valved holding chamber) in a plastic bag to prevent moisture retention and possible resulting microorganism growth.
- If the medication being administered is a steroid, the patient should rinse the mouth with water after administration to prevent irritation and secondary infection to the oral mucosa (Cleveland Clinic, 2014).
- Ongoing assessment is an important part of nursing care to evaluate patient response to administered medications and early detection of adverse reactions. If an adverse effect is suspected, withhold further medication doses and notify the patient's primary care provider. Additional intervention is based on type of reaction and patient assessment.

Infant and Child Considerations

- Young children usually require a spacer to use an MDI. Spacers with masks are available for young children; consider using these for children under 5 years of age to aid in the delivery of the medication. The mask must fit securely over both the nose and the mouth to ensure a good seal and prevent medication from escaping.
- Children must be able to seal their lips around the mouthpiece in order to use a spacer without a mask.
- Many medications can also be administered as a nebulizer (see Skill 5-24).

Home Care Considerations

- It is important for patients to know how to tell when medication levels are getting low. The most reliable method is to look on the canister and see how many puffs the canister contains. Divide this number by the number of puffs used daily to ascertain how many days the MDI will last. For instance, if the MDI contains 200 puffs and the patient takes 6 puffs per day, the MDI should last for 33 days. Keep a diary or record of inhaler use and discard the inhaler on reaching the labeled number of doses. This method may be cumbersome and impractical for some patients, but it is a reliable way to determine how much medication remains in an MDI. Another accurate way to know when the canister is depleted is to use a dose counter, which counts down each time the canister is activated (Cleveland Clinic, 2014). **Floating the canister in water is not reliable and is contraindicated. Immersion in water can cause valve obstruction and threatens product integrity** (MedlinePlus, 2016b; Rubin, 2010).

Skill Variation > Using an MDI Without a Spacer

Prepare medication as outlined in steps 1–17 above (Skill 5-22).

1. Remove the cap from the MDI. Shake the inhaler well.
2. Have the patient take a deep breath and exhale.
3. Have the patient hold the inhaler 1 to 2 in away from the mouth (about the width of 2 fingers [MedlinePlus, 2016b]) (Figure A). Have the patient begin to inhale slowly and deeply, depress the medication canister, and continue to inhale for a full breath.
4. **Instruct the patient to hold the breath for 5 to 10 seconds, or as long as possible, and then to exhale slowly through pursed lips.**
5. **Wait 1 to 5 minutes, as prescribed, before administering the next puff.**
6. After the prescribed number of puffs has been administered, have the patient replace the cap on the MDI.
7. Remove additional PPE, if used. Perform hand hygiene.
8. Document administration of the medication on the eMAR/MAR immediately after administering the medication.
9. Evaluate the patient's response to the medication within an appropriate time frame. Reassess lung sounds, oxygen saturation level, if ordered, and respirations.

FIGURE A. Holding the MDI 1 to 2 in from the mouth.

EVIDENCE FOR PRACTICE ▶

INHALED MEDICATIONS

Correct use of a metered-dose inhaler is critical to ensure accurate dosing of medication. Patients who are prescribed medications delivered with an MDI must have accurate knowledge and demonstrate appropriate technique regarding use to ensure accurate medication delivery. Nurses play a key role in patient education and must have adequate knowledge to provide appropriate educational intervention.

Related Research

De Tratto, K., Gomez, C., Ryan, C. J., Bracken, N., Steffen, A., & Corbridge, S. J. (2014). Nurses' knowledge of inhaler technique in the inpatient hospital setting. *Clinical Nurse Specialist: The Journal for Advanced Nursing Practice, 28* (3), 156–160.

The purpose of this study was to examine inpatient staff nurses' self-perceptions of their inhaler technique knowledge, frequency of providing patient education and responsibility for providing education. The study also assessed the nurses demonstrated inhaler technique using both a metered-dose inhaler (MDI) and diskus (a dry powder inhaler). A total of 100 nurses at a large urban academic medical center working on inpatient medical units agreed to participate. Participants completed a Likert-scale written survey to measure self-perceptions of inhaler technique and frequency and responsibility of patient education regarding MDI and diskus inhaler discharge teaching. Participating nurses then demonstrated inhaler-use technique to a data collector who utilized a detailed, validated checklist outlining the steps for use of both types of inhalers to evaluate the nurses' performance. Misuse of both MDI and diskus technique was defined for the study as having less than 75% of the steps correct (<9 of 12 steps for MDI and <8 steps for diskus). Overall misuse rates for both MDI (82%) and diskus (92%) devices were high, with poor correlation between perceived ability and investigator-measured level of performance of inhaler technique. Key steps missed in use of the devices included breathing out fully prior to inhaling with both devices. Ninety percent of participants missed keeping the device horizontal and 78% did not breathe in quickly during use of the diskus. Frequency of teaching for the diskus device by nurses was correlated with higher scores on the validated checklist, but this was not the case with the MDI. The researchers concluded that although nurses are a key component of patient education, nursing staff lack adequate knowledge of inhaler technique.

Relevance to Nursing Practice

Nurses play a large role in patient education and in designing interventions to positively impact patient outcomes. Accurate dosing of inhaled medications, and therefore control of symptoms and disease treatment, depends on correct use of the delivery device. Providing patient education related to self-administration of medications, leading to accurate medication dosing, is a very important nursing intervention. Nurses must take responsibility for acquiring and maintaining accurate knowledge with regard to use of these devices in order to provide accurate patient teaching. Nurses may advocate for education regarding inhaler technique as part of facility-wide professional development interventions.

Refer to thePoint® for additional research on related nursing topics.

Skill 5-23 ▶ Administering Medication via a Dry Powder Inhaler

Drugs for inhalation may be administered via a dry powder inhaler (DPI). A DPI is a handheld inhaler (diskus) that uses a dry powder form of medication, either in a small capsule or disk inserted into the DPI, or in a compartment inside the DPI. DPIs are breath activated. A quick breath by the patient activates the flow of medication, eliminating the need to coordinate activating the inhaler (spraying the medicine) while inhaling the medicine. However, the drug output and size distribution of the aerosol from a DPI is more or less dependent on the flow rate through the device, so the patient must be able to take a powerful, deep inspiration (Alismail et al., 2016). The medication is then absorbed rapidly through the lung tissue, resulting in local and systemic effects.

Many types of DPIs are available, with distinctive operating instructions. Some have to be loaded with a dose of medication each time they are used and some hold a number of preloaded doses. It is important to understand the particular instructions both for the medication and for the particular delivery device being used.

DELEGATION CONSIDERATIONS

The administration of medication via a dry powder inhaler is not delegated to nursing assistive personnel (NAP) or to unlicensed assistive personnel (UAP). Depending on the state's nurse practice act and the organization's policies and procedures, administration of medication using a dry powder inhaler may be delegated to licensed practical/vocational nurses (LPN/LVNs). The decision to delegate must be based on careful analysis of the patient's needs and circumstances, as well as the qualifications of the person to whom the task is being delegated. Refer to the Delegation Guidelines in Appendix A.

EQUIPMENT

- Stethoscope
- DPI and appropriate medication
- Electronic Medication Administration Record (eMAR) or Medication Administration Record (MAR)
- PPE, as indicated

ASSESSMENT

Assess the appropriateness of the drug for the patient. Review medical history, allergy, assessment, and laboratory data that may influence drug administration. Assess respiratory rate, rhythm, and depth to establish a baseline. Assess lung sounds before and after use to establish a baseline and determine the effectiveness of the medication. If appropriate and/or ordered, assess oxygen saturation level before medication administration. The oxygenation level usually increases after the medication is administered. Assess the patient's ability to manage a DPI. Assess the patient's knowledge and understanding of the medication's purpose and action. Verify patient name, dose, route, and time of administration.

NURSING DIAGNOSIS

Determine related factors for the nursing diagnoses based on the patient's current status. Appropriate nursing diagnoses may include:

- Deficient knowledge
- Risk for activity intolerance
- Impaired gas exchange

OUTCOME IDENTIFICATION AND PLANNING

The expected outcome to achieve is that the medication is administered and breathed in by the patient and the patient experiences the intended effect of the medication. Other outcomes that may be appropriate include the following: the patient understands the rationale for the inhaled medication; and the patient demonstrates correct use of the DPI.

IMPLEMENTATION

ACTION	RATIONALE
1. Gather equipment. Check each medication order against the original order in the health record, according to facility policy. Clarify any inconsistencies. Check the patient's health record for allergies.	This comparison helps to identify errors that may have occurred when orders were transcribed. The primary care provider's order or prescription is the legal record of medication orders for each facility.
2. Know the actions, special nursing considerations, safe dose ranges, purpose of administration, and adverse effects of the medications to be administered. Consider the appropriateness of the medication for this patient.	This knowledge aids the nurse in evaluating the therapeutic effect of the medication in relation to the patient's disorder and can also be used to educate the patient about the medication.
3. Perform hand hygiene.	Hand hygiene prevents the spread of microorganisms.
4. Move the medication supply system to the outside of the patient's room or prepare for administration at the medication supply system in the medication area. Alternatively, access the medication administration supply system at or inside the patient's room.	Organization facilitates error-free administration and saves time.
5. Unlock the medication supply system or drawer. Enter pass code and scan employee identification, if required.	Locking the medication supply system or drawer safeguards each patient's medication supply. Facility accrediting organizations require medication supply systems to be locked when not in use. Entering pass code and scanning ID allows only authorized users into the system and identifies the user for documentation by the computer.
6. Prepare medications for one patient at a time.	This prevents errors in medication administration.
7. Read the eMAR/MAR and select the proper medication from the patient's medication drawer or medication supply system.	This is the *first* check of the label.
8. Compare the label with the eMAR/MAR. Check expiration dates and perform calculations, if necessary. Scan the bar code on the package, if required.	This is the *second* check of the label. Verify calculations with another nurse to ensure safety, if necessary.
9. Depending on facility policy, the third check of the label may occur at this point. If so, when all medications for one patient have been prepared, recheck the labels with the eMAR/MAR before taking the medications to the patient. However, many facilities require the third check to occur at the bedside, after identifying the patient.	This *third* check ensures accuracy and helps to prevent errors. *Note:* Many facilities require the *third* check to occur at the bedside, after identifying the patient and before administration.
10. Lock the medication supply system before leaving it.	Locking the medication supply system or drawer safeguards the patient's medication supply. Facility accrediting organizations require medication supply systems to be locked when not in use.
11. Transport medications to the patient's bedside carefully, and keep the medications in sight at all times.	Careful handling and close observation prevent accidental or deliberate disarrangement of medications.
12. Ensure that the patient receives the medications at the correct time.	Check facility policy, which may allow for administration within a period of 30 minutes before or 30 minutes after the designated time.
13. Perform hand hygiene and put on PPE, if indicated.	Hand hygiene and PPE prevent the spread of microorganisms. PPE is required based on transmission precautions.

(continued)

Skill 5-23 ▶ Administering Medication via a Dry Powder Inhaler *(continued)*

ACTION	RATIONALE

 14. Identify the patient. Compare the information with the eMAR/MAR. The patient should be identified using at least two of the following methods (The Joint Commission, 2018):

a. Check the name on the patient's identification band.

b. Check the identification number on the patient's identification band.

c. Check the birth date on the patient's identification band.

d. Ask the patient to state his or her name and birth date, based on facility policy.

Identifying the patient ensures the right patient receives the medications and helps prevent errors. The patient's room number or physical location is not used as an identifier (The Joint Commission, 2018). Replace the identification band if it is missing or inaccurate in any way.

This requires a response from the patient, but illness and strange surroundings often cause patients to be confused.

15. Complete necessary assessments before administering medications. Check the patient's allergy bracelet or ask the patient about allergies. Explain what you are going to do, and the reason for doing it, to the patient.

Assessment is a prerequisite to administration of medications.

16. Scan the patient's bar code on the identification band, if required (Figure 1).

Provides an additional check to ensure that the medication is given to the right patient.

17. **Based on facility policy, the third check of the label may occur at this point. If so, recheck the labels with the eMAR/MAR before administering the medications to the patient.**

Many facilities require the *third* check to occur at the bedside, after identifying the patient and before administration. If facility policy directs the *third* check at this time, this *third* check ensures accuracy and helps to prevent errors.

18. Remove the mouthpiece cover or remove the device from storage container. Load a dose into the device as directed by the manufacturer, if necessary. Alternatively, activate the inhaler, if necessary, according to manufacturer's directions.

This is necessary to deliver the medication.

19. Have the patient breathe out slowly and completely, without breathing into the DPI.

This allows for deeper inhalation with the medication dose. Moisture from the patient's breath can clog the inhaler.

20. Instruct the patient to place teeth over, and seal lips around, the mouthpiece. **It is important to not block the opening with the tongue or teeth (Figure 2).**

Prevents medication from escaping and allows for a tight seal, ensuring maximal dosing of medication. Blocking of opening interferes with medication delivery.

FIGURE 1. Scanning bar code on patient's identification bracelet. (*Photo by B. Proud.*)

FIGURE 2. Patient with teeth over and lips sealed around mouthpiece.

ACTION	**RATIONALE**
21. Instruct patient to breathe in strong, steady and deeply through the mouth, for longer than 2 to 3 seconds.	Activates the flow of medication. Deep inhalation allows for maximal distribution of medication to lung tissue.
22. Remove inhaler from mouth. Instruct patient to hold the breath for 5 to 10 seconds, or as long as possible, and then to exhale slowly through pursed lips.	This allows better distribution and longer absorption time for the medication.
23. Wait 1 to 5 minutes, as prescribed, before administering the next puff.	This ensures that both puffs are absorbed as much as possible. Bronchodilation after the first puff allows for deeper penetration by subsequent puffs.
24. After the prescribed number of puffs has been administered, have the patient replace the cap or storage container.	By replacing the cap, the patient is preventing any dust or dirt from entering the inhaler and being propelled into the bronchioles with later doses or from clogging the inhaler.
25. Have the patient gargle and rinse with tap water after using DPI, as necessary. Clean the DPI according to the manufacturer's directions.	Rinsing is necessary when using inhaled steroids, because oral fungal infections can occur. Rinsing removes medication residue from the mouth. Medication buildup in the device can affect how the medication is delivered, as well as attract bacteria.
26. Remove gloves and additional PPE, if used. Perform hand hygiene.	Proper removal of PPE reduces the risk for infection transmission and contamination of other items. Hand hygiene prevents the spread of microorganisms.
27. Document the administration of the medication immediately after administration. See Documentation section below.	Timely documentation helps to ensure patient safety.
28. Evaluate patient's response to the medication within an appropriate time frame. Reassess lung sounds, oxygen saturation level, and respirations, as indicated.	The patient needs to be evaluated for therapeutic and adverse effects from the medication. Lung sounds and oxygen saturation level may improve after DPI use. Respirations may decrease after DPI use.

EVALUATION

The expected outcomes have been achieved when the medication has been administered and breathed in by the patient; the patient experiences the intended effect of the medication; the patient understands the rationale for the inhaled medication; and the patient demonstrated correct use of the DPI.

DOCUMENTATION

Guidelines

Document the administration of the medication immediately after administration, including date, time, dose, and route of administration on the eMAR/MAR or record using the required format. If using a bar-code system, medication administration is automatically recorded when the bar code is scanned. PRN medications require documentation of the reason for administration. Prompt recording avoids the possibility of accidentally repeating the administration of the drug. Document respiratory rate, oxygen saturation, if applicable, lung assessment, and the patient's response to the treatment, if appropriate. If the drug was refused or omitted, record this in the appropriate area on the medication record and notify the primary care provider. This verifies the reason medication was omitted and ensures that health care personnel providing care for the patient are aware of the occurrence.

(continued)

Skill 5-23 ▶ Administering Medication via a Dry Powder Inhaler *(continued)*

Sample Documentation

12/22/20 1715 Breath sounds slightly decreased in bases of lung pretreatment, respirations 18 breaths per minute and regular. After DPI, lung sounds remain diminished bilaterally in bases, O_2 saturation 97%, respiratory rate 16 breaths per minute. Patient able to demonstrate accurately the use of a DPI and verbalizes understanding of medication purpose and action.

—C. Bausler, RN

UNEXPECTED SITUATIONS AND ASSOCIATED INTERVENTIONS

- *Patient reports that relief of symptoms has decreased:* Have patient demonstrate technique that he or she is using. Many patients develop poor habits over time (O'Conor et al., 2015). Poor administration technique can lead to a decrease in effectiveness of medication.

SPECIAL CONSIDERATIONS

General Considerations

- Instruct the patient never to exhale into the mouthpiece or shake the inhaler.
- If mist can be seen from the mouth or nose, the DPI is being used incorrectly.
- Follow the manufacturer's directions to clean the DPI.
- Store inhaler, capsules, and disks away from moisture at room temperature.
- Explain to the patient that there may not be any taste, smell, or feel associated with inhalation of the medication, which may be different from what they have experienced with another inhaler. As long as the directions for use of the DPI are followed, the patient will receive the full dose of medication (Cleveland Clinic, 2015).
- If the medication being administered is a steroid, the patient should rinse the mouth with water after administration to prevent irritation and secondary infection to the oral mucosa (Cleveland Clinic, 2015).
- Ongoing assessment is an important part of nursing care to evaluate patient response to administered medications and early detection of adverse drug reactions. If an adverse effect is suspected, withhold further medication doses and notify the patient's primary care provider. Additional intervention is based on type of reaction and patient assessment.

Home Care Considerations

- Many DPIs have dosage counters to keep track of remaining doses.
- If a particular DPI does not have a dose counter, teach patients how to tell when medication levels are getting low. The most reliable method is to look on the package and see how many doses the DPI contains. Divide this number by the number of doses used daily to ascertain how many days the DPI will last. Keep a diary or record of DPI use and discard the DPI on reaching the labeled number of doses.

EVIDENCE FOR PRACTICE ▶

INHALED MEDICATIONS

Correct use of a dry powder inhaler (DPI; diskus) is critical to ensure accurate dosing of medication. Patients who are prescribed medications delivered with a DPI must have accurate knowledge and demonstrate appropriate technique regarding use to ensure accurate medication delivery. Nurses play a key role in patient education and must have adequate knowledge to provide appropriate educational intervention.

Related Research

De Tratto, K., Gomez, C., Ryan, C. J., Bracken, N., Steffen, A., & Corbridge, S. J. (2014). Nurses' knowledge of inhaler technique in the inpatient hospital setting. *Clinical Nurse Specialist: The Journal for Advanced Nursing Practice, 28* (3), 156–160.

Refer to details in Skill 5-22, Evidence for Practice, and refer to thePoint® for additional research on related nursing topics.

Skill 5-24 ▶ Administering Medication via a Small-Volume Nebulizer

Many medications prescribed for respiratory problems may be delivered via the respiratory system using a small-volume **nebulizer**. Nebulizers utilize the force of an oxygen stream or compressed air through a fluid medication to disperse fine particles of liquid medication into the deeper passages of the respiratory tract, where absorption occurs. The nebulizer medication treatment continues until all the medication in the nebulizer cup has been inhaled.

DELEGATION CONSIDERATIONS

The administration of medication via a nebulizer is not delegated to nursing assistive personnel (NAP) or to unlicensed assistive personnel (UAP). Depending on the state's nurse practice act and the organization's policies and procedures, administration of medication using a nebulizer may be delegated to licensed practical/vocational nurses (LPN/LVNs). The decision to delegate must be based on careful analysis of the patient's needs and circumstances, as well as the qualifications of the person to whom the task is being delegated. Refer to the Delegation Guidelines in Appendix A.

EQUIPMENT

- Stethoscope
- Medication
- Nebulizer tubing and chamber
- Air compressor or oxygen hookup
- Sterile saline (if medication is not premeasured)
- Electronic Medication Administration Record (eMAR) or Medication Administration Record (MAR)
- PPE, as indicated

ASSESSMENT

Assess the appropriateness of the drug for the patient. Review medical history, allergy, assessment, and laboratory data that may influence drug administration. Assess respiratory rate, rhythm, and depth to establish a baseline. Assess lung sounds before and after use to establish a baseline and determine the effectiveness of the medication. Often, patients have wheezes or coarse lung sounds before medication administration. If ordered, assess patient's oxygen saturation level before medication administration. The oxygen saturation level may increase after the medication has been administered. Assess the patient's knowledge of the medication. If the patient has a knowledge deficit about the medication, this may be the appropriate time to begin education about the medication. If the medication may affect the patient's vital signs, assess them before administration. Verify patient name, dose, route, and time of administration.

NURSING DIAGNOSIS

Determine related factors for the nursing diagnoses based on the patient's current status. Appropriate nursing diagnoses may include:

- Ineffective airway clearance
- Impaired gas exchange
- Ineffective breathing pattern

OUTCOME IDENTIFICATION AND PLANNING

The expected outcome to achieve is that the medication is administered and breathed in by the patient and the patient experiences the intended effect of the medication. Other outcomes that may be appropriate include the following: the patient understands the rationale for the inhaled medication; and the patient demonstrates correct use of the nebulizer.

IMPLEMENTATION

ACTION	RATIONALE
1. Gather equipment. Check each medication order against the original order in the health record, according to facility policy. Clarify any inconsistencies. Check the patient's health record for allergies.	This comparison helps to identify errors that may have occurred when orders were transcribed. The primary care provider's order or prescription/prescription is the legal record of medication orders for each facility.

(continued)

Skill 5-24 ▶ Administering Medication via a Small-Volume Nebulizer *(continued)*

ACTION	**RATIONALE**
2. Know the actions, special nursing considerations, safe dose ranges, purpose of administration, and adverse effects of the medications to be administered. Consider the appropriateness of the medication for this patient.	This knowledge aids the nurse in evaluating the therapeutic effect of the medication in relation to the patient's disorder and can also be used to educate the patient about the medication.
3. Perform hand hygiene.	Hand hygiene prevents the spread of microorganisms.
4. Move the medication supply system to the outside of the patient's room or prepare for administration at the medication supply system in the medication area. Alternatively, access the medication administration supply system at or inside the patient's room.	Organization facilitates error-free administration and saves time.
5. Unlock the medication supply system or drawer. Enter pass code and scan employee identification, if required.	Locking the medication supply system or drawer safeguards each patient's medication supply. Facility accrediting organizations require medication supply systems to be locked when not in use. Entering pass code and scanning ID allows only authorized users into the system and identifies the user for documentation by the computer.
6. **Prepare medications for one patient at a time.**	This prevents errors in medication administration.
7. Read the eMAR/MAR and select the proper medication from medication supply system or the patient's medication drawer.	This is the *first* check of the label.
8. Compare the label with the eMAR/MAR. Check expiration dates and perform calculations, if necessary. Scan the bar code on the package, if required.	This is the *second* check of the label. Verify calculations with another nurse to ensure safety, if necessary.
9. **Depending on facility policy, the third check of the label may occur at this point. If so, when all medications for one patient have been prepared, recheck the labels with the eMAR/MAR before taking the medications to the patient. However, many facilities require the third check to occur at the bedside, after identifying the patient.**	This *third* check ensures accuracy and helps to prevent errors. *Note:* Many facilities require the *third* check to occur at the bedside, after identifying the patient and before administration.
10. **Lock the medication supply system before leaving it.**	Locking the medication supply system or drawer safeguards the patient's medication supply. Facility accrediting organizations require medication supply systems to be locked when not in use.
11. Transport medications to the patient's bedside carefully, and keep the medications in sight at all times.	Careful handling and close observation prevent accidental or deliberate disarrangement of medications.
12. **Ensure that the patient receives the medications at the correct time.**	Check facility policy, which may allow for administration within a period of 30 minutes before or 30 minutes after the designated time.
13. Perform hand hygiene and put on PPE, if indicated.	Hand hygiene and PPE prevent the spread of microorganisms. PPE is required based on transmission precautions.

(continued)

ACTION	RATIONALE

 14. Identify the patient. Compare the information with the eMAR/MAR. The patient should be identified using at least two of the following methods (The Joint Commission, 2018):

Identifying the patient ensures the right patient receives the medications and helps prevent errors. The patient's room number or physical location is not used as an identifier (The Joint Commission, 2018). Replace the identification band if it is missing or inaccurate in any way.

a. Check the name on the patient's identification band.

b. Check the identification number on the patient's identification band.

c. Check the birth date on the patient's identification band.

d. Ask the patient to state his or her name and birth date, based on facility policy.

This requires a response from the patient, but illness and strange surroundings often cause patients to be confused.

15. Complete necessary assessments before administering medications. Check the patient's allergy bracelet or ask the patient about allergies. Explain what you are going to do, and the reason for doing it, to the patient.

Assessment is a prerequisite to administration of medications. Explanation relieves anxiety and facilitates cooperation.

16. Scan the patient's bar code on the identification band, if required.

Scanning provides an additional check to ensure that the medication is given to the right patient.

17. Based on facility policy, the third check of the label may occur at this point. If so, recheck the labels with the eMAR/MAR before administering the medications to the patient.

Many facilities require the *third* check to occur at the bedside, after identifying the patient and before administration. If facility policy directs the *third* check at this time, this *third* check ensures accuracy and helps to prevent errors.

18. Remove the nebulizer cup from the device and open it. Place premeasured unit-dose medication in the bottom section of the cup or use a dropper to place a concentrated dose of medication in the cup (Figure 1). Add prescribed diluent (usually saline), if required.

To get enough volume to make a fine mist, normal saline may need to be added to the concentrated medication.

FIGURE 1. Putting medication into nebulizer.

19. Screw the top portion of the nebulizer cup back in place and attach the cup to the nebulizer. Attach one end of tubing to the stem on the bottom of the nebulizer cuff and the other end to the air compressor or oxygen source.

Air or oxygen must be forced through the nebulizer to form a fine mist.

20. Turn on the air compressor or oxygen. Check that a fine medication mist is produced by opening the valve. Have the patient place the mouthpiece into the mouth and grasp securely with teeth and lips.

If there is no fine mist, make sure that medication has been added to the cup and that the tubing is connected to the air compressor or oxygen outlet. Adjust flow meter if necessary.

Skill 5-24 ▶ Administering Medication via a Small-Volume Nebulizer *(continued)*

ACTION	RATIONALE

21. **Instruct the patient to inhale slowly and deeply through the mouth (Figure 2). A nose clip may be necessary if the patient is also breathing through the nose. Hold each breath for a slight pause, before exhaling.**

While the patient inhales and holds the breath, the medication comes in contact with the respiratory tissue and is absorbed. The longer the breath is held, the more medication can be absorbed.

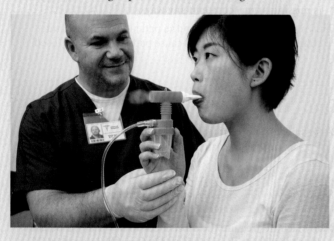

FIGURE 2. Inhaling slowly and deeply through the mouth.

22. Continue this inhalation technique until all medication in the nebulizer cup has been aerosolized (usually about 15 minutes). Once the fine mist decreases in amount, gently flick the sides of the nebulizer cup.

Once the fine mist stops, the medication is no longer being aerosolized. By gently flicking the cup sides, any medication that is stuck to the sides is knocked into the bottom of the cup, where it can become aerosolized.

23. When the medication in the nebulizer cup has been completely aerosolized, the cup will be empty. Have the patient remove the nebulizer from the mouth and gargle and rinse with tap water, as indicated. Clean and store the nebulizer and equipment according to the manufacturer's directions and facility policy.

Rinsing is necessary when using inhaled steroids, because oral fungal infections can occur. Rinsing removes medication residue from the mouth. The buildup of medication in the device can affect how the medication is delivered, as well as attract bacteria.

24. Remove gloves and additional PPE, if used. Perform hand hygiene.

Proper removal of PPE reduces the risk for infection transmission and contamination of other items. Hand hygiene prevents the spread of microorganisms.

25. Document the administration of the medication immediately after administration. See Documentation section below.

Timely documentation helps to ensure patient safety.

26. Evaluate patient's response to the medication within an appropriate time frame. Reassess lung sounds, oxygen saturation level, and respirations, as indicated.

The patient needs to be evaluated for therapeutic and adverse effects from the medication. Lung sounds and oxygen saturation level may improve after nebulizer use. Respirations may decrease after nebulizer use.

EVALUATION

The expected outcomes have been met when the medication has been administered and breathed in by the patient; the patient experiences the intended effect of the medication; the patient understands the rationale for the inhaled medication; and the patient demonstrated correct use of the nebulizer.

DOCUMENTATION

Guidelines

Document the administration of the medication immediately after administration, including date, time, dose, and route of administration on the eMAR/MAR or record using the required format. If using a bar-code system, medication administration is automatically recorded when the bar code is scanned. PRN medications require documentation of the reason for administration. Prompt recording avoids the possibility of accidentally repeating the administration of the drug. Document respiratory rate, oxygen saturation, if applicable, lung assessment, and the patient's response to the treatment, if appropriate. If the drug was refused or omitted, record this in the appropriate area on the medication record and notify the primary care provider. This verifies the reason medication was omitted and ensures that health care personnel providing care for the patient are aware of the occurrence.

Sample Documentation

> <u>9/29/20</u> 2300 Wheezes noted in all lobes of lungs before albuterol nebulizer, O$_2$ saturation 92%, respiratory rate 24 breaths per minute, patient reports "feeling like I can't get my breath." Patient reassessed 20 minutes after albuterol nebulizer treatment; lung sounds are clear and equal in all lobes, O$_2$ saturation 97%, respiratory rate 18 breaths per minute unlabored. Patient verbalizes relief of shortness of breath and an understanding of medication purpose and action.
>
> —C. Bausler, RN

UNEXPECTED SITUATIONS AND ASSOCIATED INTERVENTIONS

- *Patient is unable to hold nebulizer in mouth and/or is unable to keep lips closed around device:* A plain oxygen mask can be attached to the nebulizer device and used to deliver the nebulized medication, eliminating the need to hold the device in the mouth.

SPECIAL CONSIDERATIONS

General Considerations

- Ongoing assessment is an important part of nursing care to evaluate patient response to administered medications and early detection of adverse drug reactions. If an adverse effect is suspected, withhold further medication doses and notify the patient's primary care provider. Additional intervention is based on type of reaction and patient assessment.

Infant and Child Considerations

- A small child may use a mask instead of a mouthpiece. Mask must fit securely over both the nose and the mouth to ensure a good seal and prevent medication escaping.
- Children must be able to seal their lips around the mouthpiece to use a nebulizer without a mask.

Home Care Considerations

- Medicine cup and mouthpiece should be washed with water and air dried (MedlinePlus, 2016d).

Enhance Your Understanding

Focusing on Patient Care: Developing Clinical Reasoning

Consider the case scenarios at the beginning of the chapter as you answer the following questions to enhance your understanding and apply what you have learned.

QUESTIONS

1. When entering Cooper Jackson's room with the antibiotic, Cooper becomes visibly upset and runs to his mother. What is the best technique to administer liquid medication to an uncooperative 2 year old? Thirty minutes after receiving an oral medication, Cooper vomits. Should the nurse re-administer the medication?

2. What are some ways that the nurse can make Erika Jenkins feel more relaxed about receiving her injection?

3. What are some priority points that the nurse needs to discuss with Jonah Dinerman, the patient with type 1 diabetes, if the education needs to be completed in a short time?

You can find suggested answers after the Bibliography at the end of this chapter.

Enhance Your Understanding (Continued)

Integrated Case Study Connection

The case studies in the back of the book focus on integrating concepts. Refer to the following case studies to enhance your understanding of the concepts and skills in this chapter.

- Basic Case Studies: Naomi Bell, page 1103; Claudia Tran, page 1106; Tula Stillwater, page 1111.
- Intermediate Case Studies: Tula Stillwater, page 1117; Jason Brown, page 1119; Kent Clark, page 1121.
- Advanced Case Studies: Damian Wallace, page 1130; Robert Espinoza, page 1132.

Taylor Suite Resources

Explore these additional resources to enhance learning for this chapter:

- NCLEX-Style Questions and other resources on thePoint®, http://thePoint.lww.com/Lynn5e
- Skill Checklists for *Taylor's Clinical Nursing Skills*, 5e
- Taylor's Video Guide to *Clinical Nursing Skills: Oral and Topical Medications, Injectable Medications*, and *Intravenous Medications*
- *Fundamentals of Nursing:* Chapter 29, Medications
- *Lippincott DocuCare* Fundamentals cases

Bibliography

Adams, M., Holland, N., & Urban, C. (2017). *Pharmacology for nurses. A pathophysiologic approach* (5th ed.). Boston, MA: Pearson.

Adhikari, R., Tocher, J., Smith, P., Corcoran, J., & MacArthur, J. (2014). A multi-disciplinary approach to medication safety and the implication for nursing education and practice. *Nurse Education Today, 34*(2), 185–190.

Ağaç, E., & Günes, Ü. Y. (2010). Effect on pain of changing the needle prior to administering medicine intramuscularly: A randomized controlled trial. *Journal of Advanced Nursing, 67*(3), 563–568.

Alismail, A., Song, C. A., Terry, M. H., Daher, N., Almutairi, W. A., & Lo, T. (2016). Diverse inhaler devices: A big challenge for health-care professionals. *Respiratory Care, 61*(5), 593–599.

Allen, S. M. (2015). As a flushing agent for enteral nutrition, does sterile water compared to tap water affect the associated risk of infection in critically ill patients? *The Alabama Nurse, 42*(1), 5–6.

American Academy of Otolaryngology-Head and Neck Surgery. (n.d.). Earwax and care. Retrieved http://www.entnet.org/content/earwax-and-care

American Association of Diabetes Educators. (2014). AADE White Paper. Continuous subcutaneous insulin infusion (CSII). Retrieved https://www.diabeteseducator.org/docs/default-source/legacy-docs/_resources/pdf/publications/csii_pentulimate.pdf?sfvrsn=2

American Diabetes Association (ADA). (2015). Insulin routines. Site rotation. Retrieved http://www.diabetes.org/living-with-diabetes/treatment-and-care/medication/insulin/insulin-routines.html

American Society of Health-System Pharmacists (ASHP). (2009). ASHP statement on bar-code-enabled medication administration technology. *American Journal of Health-System Pharmacy, 66*(6), 588–590. Retrieved https://www.ashp.org/DocLibrary/BestPractices/AutoITStBCMA.aspx

Annersten, M., & Willman, A. (2005). Performing subcutaneous injections: A literature review. *Worldviews on Evidence-Based Nursing, 2*(3), 122–130.

Ball, A., & Smith, K. (2008). Optimizing transdermal drug therapy. *American Journal of Health-System Pharmacy, 65*(14), 1337–1346.

Bankhead, R., Boullata, J., Brantley, S., et al; The American Society for Parenteral and Enteral Nutrition (A.S.P.E.N.) Board of Directors. (2009). Enteral nutrition practice recommendations. *Journal of Parenteral and Enteral Nutrition, 33*(2), 122–167.

Becton, Dickinson and Company. (2016a). How to inject with a pen. Retrieved https://www.bd.com/en-us/company/video-gallery?video=4592430149001

Becton, Dickinson and Company. (2016b). Safety needles. Retrieved http://www.bd.com/hypodermic/products/autoshield/duo

Best, C., & Wilson, N. (2011). Advice on safe administration of medications via enteral feeding tubes. *Nutrition*, Supplement, S6–S8.

Bolton, D. (2015). Clinically indicated replacement of peripheral cannulas. *British Journal of Nursing, 24*(Therapy supplement), S4–S12.

Bravo, K., Cochran, G., & Barrett, R. (2016). Nursing strategies to increase medication safety in inpatient settings. *Journal of Nursing Care Quality, 31*(4), 335–341.

Centers for Disease Control and Prevention (CDC). (2011). Injection safety. Safe injection practices to prevent transmission of infections to patients. Retrieved www.cdc.gov/injectionsafety/IP07_standardPrecaution.html

Centers for Disease Control and Prevention (CDC). (n.d.a). One and only campaign. Retrieved http://www.oneandonlycampaign.org

Centers for Disease Control and Prevention (CDC). (n.d.b). Safe injection practices. Retrieved http://www.oneandonlycampaign.org/safe_injection_practices

Centers for Disease Control and Prevention (CDC). (2013). CDC grand rounds: Preventing unsafe injection practices in the U.S. health-care system. *MMWR: Morbidity and Mortality Weekly Report, 62*(21), 423–425.

Centers for Disease Control and Prevention (CDC). (2015a). Chapter 6. Vaccine administration. *The pink book*. Retrieved https://www.cdc.gov/vaccines/pubs/pinkbook/vac-admin.html

Centers for Disease Control and Prevention (CDC). (2015b). In J. Hamborsky, A. Kroger, & S. Wolfe (Eds.). *Epidemiology and prevention of vaccine-preventable diseases* (13th ed.). Washington, DC: Public Health Foundation. Retrieved http://www.cdc.gov/vaccines/pubs/pinkbook/index.html

Chung, J. W., Ng, W. M., & Wong, T. K. (2002). An experimental study on the use of manual pressure to reduce pain in intramuscular injections. *Journal of Clinical Nursing, 11*(4), 457–461.

Cleveland Clinic. (2014). Inhalers. Retrieved http://my.clevelandclinic.org/health/articles/how-to-use-a-metered-dose-inhaler

Cleveland Clinic. (2015). How to use your diskus dry powder inhaler (DPI). Retrieved http://my.clevelandclinic.org/health/articles/how-to-use-your-diskus-dry-powder-inhaler-dpi

Cocoman, A., & Murray, J. (2010). Recognizing the evidence and changing practice on injection sites. *British Journal of Nursing, 19*(18), 1170–1174.

Cohen, B. J., & Taylor, J. J. (2013). *Memmler's structure and function of the human body* (10th ed.). Philadelphia, PA: Wolters Kluwer Health.

Connor, J. A., Ahern, J. P., Cuccovia, B., Arnold, A., & Hickey, P. A. (2016). Implementing a distraction-free practice with the red zone medication safety initiative. *Dimensions of Critical Care Nursing, 35*(3), 116–124.

Crawford, C. L., & Johnson, J. A. (2012). To aspirate or not: An integrative review of the evidence. *Nursing, 42*(3), 20–25.

Dajkovich, G., & Barkley Jr., T. W. (2015). Understanding insulin pump therapy. *Journal of Community Health Nursing, 32*(3), 131–140.

Davidson, K. M., & Rourke, L. (2013). Teaching best-evidence: Deltoid intramuscular injection technique. *Journal of Nursing Education and Practice, 3*(7), 120–128.

De Tratto, K., Gomez, C., Ryan, C. J., Bracken, N., Steffen, A., & Corbridge, S. J. (2014). Nurses' knowledge of inhaler technique in the inpatient hospital setting. *Clinical Nurse Specialist: The Journal for Advanced Nursing Practice, 28*(3), 156–160.

Diggle, J. (2014). How to help patients achieve correct self-injection technique. *Practice Nursing, 25*(9), 451–454.

Doenges, M. E., Moorhouse, M. F., & Murr, A. C. (2016). *Nursing diagnoses manual. Planning, individualizing, and documenting client care* (5th ed.). Philadelphia, PA: F.A. Davis.

Dolan, S.A., Meehan Arias, K., Felizardo, G., et al. (2016). APIC position paper: Safe injection, infusion, and medication vial practices in health care. *American Journal of Infection Control, 44*(7), 750–757.

Dudek, S. (2017). *Nutrition essentials for nursing practice* (8th ed.). Philadelphia, PA: Wolters Kluwer.

Dulan, A., Sheridan, D., & Laucher, M. A. (2016). Using transdermal drug patches for older adults. *Nursing, 46*(11), 69.

Durand, C., Alhammad, A., & Willett, K. C. (2012). Practical considerations for optimal transdermal drug delivery. *American Journal of Health-System Pharmacy, 69*(2), 116–124.

Eliopoulos, C. (2014). *Gerontological nursing* (8th ed.). Philadelphia, PA: Wolters Kluwer Health.

Fischbach, F. T., & Dunning III, M.B. (2015). *A manual of laboratory and diagnostic tests* (9th ed.). Philadelphia, PA: Wolters Kluwer Health.

Frandsen, G., & Pennington, S. S. (2014). *Abrams' clinical drug therapy: Rationales for nursing practice* (10th ed.). Philadelphia, PA: Wolters Kluwer Health.

Frimpong, A., Caguioa, J., & Octavo, G. (2015). Promoting safe IV management in practice using H.A.N.D.S. *British Journal of Nursing (IV Therapy Supplement), 24*(2), S18, S20–S23.

Gelder, C. (2014). Best practice injection technique for children and young people with diabetes. *Nursing Children and Young People, 26*(7), 32–36.

Grissinger, M. (2014). Ingestion or aspiration of foreign objects or toxic substances is not just a safety concern with children. *Pharmacy and Therapeutics, 39*(7), 462–519.

Grossman, S., & Porth, C. M. (2014). *Porth's pathophysiology: Concepts of altered health states* (9th ed.). Philadelphia, PA: Wolters Kluwer.

Haines, S. T., Miklich, M. A., & Rochester-Eyeguokan, C. (2016). Best practices for safe use of insulin pen devices in hospitals: Recommendations from an expert panel Delphi consensus process. *American Journal of Health-System Pharmacy, Supplement, 73*, S4–S16.

Harding, A. D. (2013). Intravenous smart pumps. *Journal of Infusion Nursing, 36*(3), 191–194.

Harkin, H. (2015). Ear care and irrigation with water: An update. *Practice Nurse, 45*(7), 24–26.

Harper, D. (2014). I.V. Rounds. Infusion therapy: Much more than a simple task. *Nursing, 44*(7), 66–67.

Harrison, D., Sampson, M., Reszel, J., et al. (2014). Too many crying babies: A systematic review of pain management practices during immunizations on You-Tube. *BMC Pediatrics, 14*(1), 134.

Hayter, K. L. (2016). Listen up for safe ear irrigation. *Nursing, 46*(6), 62–65.

Helton, J., Hines, A., & Best, J. (2016). Peripheral IV site rotation based on clinical assessment vs. length of time since insertion. *MEDSURG Nursing, 25*(1), 44–49.

Hess, D. R., MacIntyre, N. R., Galvin, W. F., & Mishoe, S. C. (2016). *Respiratory care. Principles and practice* (3rd ed.). Sudbury, MA: Jones & Bartlett Learning.

Hinkle, J. L., & Cheever, K. H. (2018). *Brunner & Suddarth's textbook of medical-surgical nursing* (14th ed.). Philadelphia, PA: Wolters Kluwer.

Hunt, C. W. (2008). Clinical queries. Which site is best for an I.M. injection? *Nursing, 38*(11), 62.

Infusion Nurses Society (INS). (2016a). *Policies and procedures for infusion therapy* (5th ed.). Norwood, MA: Author.

Infusion Nurses Society (INS). (2016b). Infusion therapy. Standards of practice. *Journal of Infusion Nursing, 39*(Suppl 1), S1–S159.

Institute for Safe Medication Practices (ISMP). (2007). *The five rights: A destination without a map.* Retrieved http://www.ismp.org/newsletters/acutecare/articles/20070125.asp

Institute for Safe Medication Practices (ISMP). (2012a). *ISMP and FDA campaign to eliminate use of error-prone abbreviations.* Retrieved www.ismp.org/tools/abbreviations

Institute for Safe Medication Practices (ISMP). (2012b). *ISMP medication safety alert. Preventing tragedies caused by syringe tip caps.* Retrieved http://www.ismp.org/Newsletters/acutecare/articles/19990310.asp

Institute for Safe Medication Practices (ISMP). (2015). *ISMP safe practice guidelines for adult IV push medications.* Horsham, PA: Author. Retrieved http://www.ismp.org/Tools/guidelines/ivsummitpush/ivpushmedguidelines.pdf

Janssen Pharmaceuticals, Inc. (2009). Instructions for use. Duragesic®. Fentanyl transdermal system. Retrieved http://www.duragesic.com/assets/pdf/duragesic_patient_instructions_0.pdf

Janssen Pharmaceuticals, Inc. (2015). Welcome. What is Duragesic®? Retrieved http://www.duragesic.com

Jarvis, C. (2016). *Physical examination & health assessment.* (7th ed.). St. Louis, MO: Elsevier.

Jenkins, E. J., Knott, J., & Brooks, A. (2016). Insulin pump users require recurrent education for the management of pump failure. *Journal of Diabetes Nursing, 20*(10), 364–369.

Jensen, S. (2015). *Nursing Health Assessment: A best practice approach* (2nd ed.). Philadelphia, PA: Wolters Kluwer.

The Joint Commission. (2018). National patient safety goals. Retrieved https://www.jointcommission.org/standards_information/npsgs.aspx

Karch, A. M. (2017). *Focus on nursing pharmacology* (7th ed.). Philadelphia, PA: Wolters Kluwer.

Katsma, D. L., & Katsma, R. P. (2000). The myth of the 90°-angle intramuscular injection. *Nurse Educator, 25*(1), 34–37.

Kee, J. L., Hayes, E. R., & McCuistion, L. E. (2015). *Pharmacology. A patient-centered nursing process approach* (8th ed.). St. Louis, MO: Elsevier Saunders.

Kyle, T., & Carman, S. (2017). *Essentials of pediatric nursing* (3rd ed.). Philadelphia, PA: Wolters Kluwer.

LeMone, P., Burke, K. M., Bauldoff, G., & Gubrud, P. (2015). *Medical-surgical nursing. Clinical reasoning in patient care* (6th ed.). New York: Pearson.

Levy, M. L., Hardwell, A., McKnight, E., & Holmes, J. (2013). Asthma patients' inability to use a pressurized metered-dose inhaler (pMDI). Correctly correlates with poor asthma control as defined by the Global Initiative for Asthma (GINA) strategy: A retrospective analysis. *Primary Care Respiratory Journal, 22*(4), 406–411.

Loveday, H. P., Wilson, J. A., Pratt, R. J., et al. (2014). Epic3: National evidence-based guidelines for preventing healthcare-associated infections in NHS hospitals in England. *Journal of Hospital Infection, 86*(S1), S1–S70.

Lowry, M. (2016). Rectal drug administration in adults: How, when, why. *Nursing Times, 112*(8), 12–14.

Lutz, M. F., Haines, S. T., Lesch, C. A., & Szumita, P. M. (2016). Facilitating the safe use of insulin pens in hospitals through a mentored quality-improvement program. *American Journal of Health-System Pharmacy, 73*(19), Supplement 5, S17–S31.

The Medicines Company. (2016). Ionsys. Instructions for use and disposal. Retrieved http://www.ionsys.com/use-and-disposal.html

MedlinePlus. (2016a). Miconazole. Retrieved https://medlineplus.gov/druginfo/meds/a688022.html

MedlinePlus. (2016b). How to use an inhaler–no spacer. Retrieved https://medlineplus.gov/ency/patientinstructions/000041.htm

MedlinePlus. (2016c). How to use an inhaler–with spacer. Retrieved https://medlineplus.gov/ency/patientinstructions/000042.htm

MedlinePlus. (2016d). How to use a nebulizer. Retrieved https://medlineplus.gov/ency/patientinstructions/000006.htm

Metheny, N. (2008). Residual volume measurement should be retained in enteral feeding protocols. *American Journal of Critical Care, 17*(1), 62–64.

Mudd, S. S., Leu, K., Sloand, E. D., & Ngo, T. L. (2015). Pediatric asthma and the use of metered dose inhalers with valve holding chambers: Barriers to the implementation of evidence-based practice. *Journal of Emergency Nursing, 41*(1), 13–18.

NANDA International, Inc.: Nursing Diagnoses - Definitions and Classification 2018–2020 © 2017 NANDA International, ISBN 978-1-62623-929-6. Used by arrangement with the Thieme Group, Stuttgart/New York.

National Institutes of Health. Clinical Center. (2008). Patient education. How to put in your eye drops. Retrieved https://www.cc.nih.gov/ccc/patient_education/pepubs/eyedrops.pdf

Nicoll, L., & Hesby, A. (2002). Intramuscular injection: An integrative research review and guideline for evidence-based practice. *Applied Nursing Research, 16*(2), 149–162.

Niemann, D., Bertsche, A., Meyrath, D., et al. (2015). A prospective three-step intervention study to prevent medication errors in drug handling in paediatric care. *Journal of Clinical Nursing, 24*(1/2), 101–114.

O'Conor, R., Wolf, M.S., Smith, S.G., et al. (2015). Health literacy, cognitive function, proper use, and adherence to inhaled asthma controller medications among older adults with asthma. *Chest, 147*(5), 1307–1315.

Paparella, S. F., & Mandrack, M. M. (2016). IV push medication administration Making safe choices; choosing best practice. *Journal of Emergency Nursing, 42*(1), 64–67.

Peate, I. (2015). How to administer suppositories. *Nursing Standard, 30*(1), 34–36.

Pedersen, C. A., Schneider, P. J., & Scheckelhoff, D. J. (2013). ASHP national survey of pharmacy practice in hospital settings: Monitoring and patient education–2012. *American Journal of Health- System Pharmacy, 70*(9), 787–803.

Perry, S. E., Hockenberry, M. J., Lowdermilk, D. L., & Wilson, D. (2014). *Maternal child nursing care* (5th ed.). St. Louis, MO: Elsevier Mosby.

Phillips, A. (2016). Advances in infusion sets and insulin pumps in diabetes care. *British Journal of Community Nursing, 21*(3), 124–127.

Press, V. G., Arora, V. M., Trela, K. C., et al. (2016). Effectiveness of interventions to teach metered-dose and diskus inhaler techniques. *Annals of the American Thoracic Society, 13*(6), 816–824.

Purnell, L. D. (2013). *Transcultural health care. A culturally competent approach* (4th ed.). Philadelphia, PA: F.A. Davis Company.

Rishovd, A. (2014). Pediatric intramuscular injections. Guidelines for best practice. *The American Journal of Maternal Child Nursing, 39*(2), 107–114.

Rubin, B. K. (2010). Air and soul: The science and application of aerosol therapy. *Respiratory Care, 55*(7), 911–921.

Sanofi Aventis. (2013). Lovenox®. Prescribing information. Administration. Retrieved http://products.sanofi.us/lovenox/lovenox.html#section-5.4

Sanofi Aventis. (2016). Know Lovenox®. How to self-inject Lovenox®. Retrieved http://www.lovenox.com/default.aspx

Sanofi Pasteur. (2016). Fluzone® intradermal quadrivalent influenza vaccine. Retrieved http://www.fluzone.com/fluzone-intradermal-quadrivalent-vaccine.cfm

Scheiner, G. (2016, March). Product guide: Insulin pumps. *Diabetes Forecast.* American Diabetes Association. Retrieved http://www.diabetesforecast.org/2016/mar-apr/product-guide-insulin-pumps.html

Sexson, K., Lindauer, A., & Harvath, T. A. (2016). Administration of subcutaneous injections. *American Journal of Nursing, 116*(12), 49–52.

Sisson, H. (2015). Aspirating during the intramuscular injection procedure: A systematic literature review. *Journal of Clinical Nursing, 24*(17-18), 2368–2375.

Smeulers, M., Verweij, L., Maaskant, J. M., et al. (2015). Quality indicators for safe medication preparation and administration: A systematic review. *PLoS ONE, 10*(4), 1–14.

Stango, C., Runyan, D., Stern, J., Macri, I., & Vacca, M. (2014). A successful approach to reducing bloodstream infections based on a disinfection device for intravenous needleless connector hubs. *Journal of Infusion Nursing, 37*(6), 462–465.

Taddio, A., Appleton, M., Bortolussi, R., et al. (2010). Reducing the pain of childhood vaccination: An evidence-based clinical practice guideline. *Canadian Medical Association Journal, 182*(18), E843–E855.

Taylor, C., Lynn, P., & Bartlett, J. (2019). *Fundamentals of nursing: The art and science of person-centered care* (9th ed.). Philadelphia, PA: Wolters Kluwer.

Thomas, C. M., Mraz, M., & Rajcan, L. (2015). Blood aspiration during IM injection. *Clinical Nursing Research, 25*(5), 546–559.

Tucker, M. E. (2015). Pens and needles. These devices make insulin dosing more convenient and portable. *Diabetes Forecast, 68*(2), 67–69.

Tuffaha, H. S., Rickard, C. M., Weber, J., et al. (2014). Cost-effectiveness analysis of clinically indicated versus routine replacement of peripheral intravenous catheters. *Applied Health Economics and Health Policy, 12*(1), 51–58.

University of Maryland Medical Center. (2016). Patient information. How to use eardrops. Ear medications. Retrieved http://umm.edu/programs/hearing/patients/eardrops

U.S. Food and Drug Administration (FDA). (2016a). Drug information for consumers. Retrieved http://www.fda.gov/Drugs/ResourcesForYou/Consumers/default.htm

U.S. Food and Drug Administration (FDA). (2016b). Medication errors related to drugs. Retrieved http://www.fda.gov/Drugs/DrugSafety/MedicationErrors/default.htm#abbreviations

U.S. Food and Drug Administration (FDA). (2017). MedWatch: The FDA safety information and adverse event reporting program. Retrieved http://www.fda.gov/Safety/MedWatch/default.htm

VHA Center for Engineering & Occupational Safety and Health (CEOSH). (2016). Safe patient handling and mobility guidebook. St. Louis, MO: Author. Retrieved http://www.tampavaref.org/safe-patient-handling.htm

Williams, N, T. (2008). Medication administration through enteral feeding tubes. *American Journal of Health-System Pharmacy, 65*(24), 2347–2357.

Williams, T., King, M. W., Thompson, J. A., & Champagne, M. T. (2014). Implementing evidence-based medication safety interventions on a progressive care unit. *American Journal of Nursing, 114*(11), 53–62.

Wilmot, E. G., Choudhary, P., Grant, P., & Hammond, P. (2014). Insulin pump therapy: A practical guide to optimising glycaemic control. *Practical Diabetes, 31*(3), 121–125.

World Health Organization (WHO). (2016). Immunization in practice: A practical guide for health staff– Module 3 Ensuring safe injections. Retrieved http://www.who.int/immunization/documents/training/en

Zhu, L. L., & Zhou, Q. (2013). Therapeutic concerns when oral medications are administered nasogastrically. *Journal of Clinical Pharmacy and Therapeutics, 38*(4), 272–276.

Zimmerman, P. G. (2010). Revisiting IM injections. *American Journal of Nursing, 110*(2), 60–61.

SUGGESTED ANSWERS FOR FOCUSING ON PATIENT CARE: DEVELOPING CLINICAL REASONING

1. Discuss routines and rituals typically used at home with Cooper's mother. Incorporating these routines and rituals if they are safe and positive can provide a positive way to administer medication. Offer simple choices to Cooper, such as allowing him the choice of having the nurse or his mother administer the medication. A toddler may enjoy using an oral syringe to squirt the medicine into his own mouth. The nurse could also allow Cooper to act out medication administration with a favorite toy, pretending to administer liquid medication to the toy.

2. Explore Erika's feelings related to injections and assess her knowledge of the procedure. Allow patients who are fearful of injections to talk about his or her fears. Answer the patient's questions truthfully, and explain the nature and purpose of the injection. Taking the time to offer support often allays fears and decreases discomfort. Explain to Erika how the injection will be given. Discuss possible injection sites and allow Erika to have a say in the location used for the injection, if possible. It is very important that the nurse selects the appropriate needle length and gauge for the medication and patient criteria, including site location, patient's body size, and age. The nurse must use the correct technique to administer the injection and minimize pain. The nurse should consider use of the Z-track technique to reduce pain and discomfort related to the injection.

3. Diabetes is a chronic illness that requires life-long self-management behaviors. However, it is important that, initially, Jonah learns the "survival skills." "Survival skills" are basic information that patients must know to survive. Jonah should have a basic understanding of the definition of diabetes, normal blood glucose ranges and target levels; the effect of insulin and exercise; the effect of food and stress; basic treatment approaches; administration of prescribed medications, including subcutaneous insulin and oral antidiabetes medications; and meal planning. Jonah must also have an understanding of how to recognize, treat, and prevent hypoglycemia and hyperglycemia before discharge. The nurse should include information related to the importance of continued diabetes education, once the basic skills are mastered and information understood. Patient knowledge and compliance with treatment are crucial to preventing complications related to diabetes.

Perioperative Nursing

Learning Objectives

After completing the chapter, you will be able to accomplish the following:

1. Provide patient teaching regarding deep-breathing exercises, coughing, and splinting of an incision.
2. Provide patient teaching regarding leg exercises.
3. Provide safe and effective care for the preoperative patient.
4. Provide safe and effective care for the postoperative patient.
5. Apply a forced-air warming device.

Key Terms

anesthetic: medication that produces such states as loss of consciousness, analgesia, relaxation, and loss of reflexes

atelectasis: incomplete expansion or collapse of a part of the lungs

deep vein thrombosis (DVT): the presence of a blood clot (thrombus) in one or more of the deep veins in the body, most commonly in the lower legs

elective surgery: surgery that is recommended, but can be omitted or delayed without a negative effect

hemorrhage: excessive blood loss due to the escape of blood from blood vessels

hypothermia: core body temperature below 36°C (96°F) (AORN, 2017); complications of poor wound healing, hemodynamic stress, cardiac disturbances, coagulopathy, delayed emergence from anesthesia, and shivering and its associated discomfort.

perioperative nursing: wide variety of nursing activities carried out before, during, and after surgery

perioperative phase: time frame consisting of the preoperative phase (starts with decision that surgery is necessary and lasting until the patient is transferred to the operating room [OR] or procedural bed); the intraoperative phase (starts from the arrival in the OR until transfer to the postanesthesia care unit [PACU]); and the postoperative phase (begins with admission to the PACU or other recovery area and lasts until complete recovery from surgery and last follow-up physician visit)

postanesthesia care unit (PACU): an area often adjacent to the surgical suite designed to provide care for patients recovering from anesthesia or moderate sedation/analgesia.

thrombophlebitis: inflammation in a vein associated with thrombus formation

A wide range of illnesses and injuries may require treatment that includes some type of surgical intervention. Surgical procedures may be inpatient, performed in a hospital; or ambulatory or outpatient, performed in a hospital-based surgical center, a freestanding surgical center, or a physician's office. In an ambulatory or outpatient center, the patient goes to the surgical area the day of surgery and returns home on the same day.

Nursing care provided for the patient before, during, and after surgery is called **perioperative nursing**. Perioperative nursing involves providing care for the patient during the **perioperative phase**; before (*preoperative*), during (*intraoperative*), and after surgery (*postoperative*). The nursing process is used during each phase to meet physical and psychosocial needs and to facilitate the patient's return to health.

Whether the surgery is performed in the inpatient or outpatient setting, one of the most significant roles of the perioperative nurse is that of collaborator—the nurse working directly and indirectly with people from surgery, anesthesia, pharmacy, respiratory therapy, laboratory and radiology, rehabilitation, and other specialties (Riddle & Stannard, 2014). Evidence-based practice that considers patient and family preferences, clinical expertise of the health care provider, and the best evidence available informs decision-making at all stages of the perioperative process. The ultimate, shared goal is to provide safe, quality care for the vulnerable perioperative patient (Riddle & Stannard, 2014).

The nurse follows specific criteria and guidelines while conducting the preadmission assessment, preparation, and patient education. This preoperative care can be provided through a telephone call or a face-to-face interview with the patient. A preoperative teaching plan should include preoperative instructions and patient preparation. This teaching should include both the patient and the patient's family members or guardian/significant others. For certain types of **elective surgery**, such as joint replacements, patients may participate in a group patient teaching session before their admission to the hospital. Refer to Fundamentals Review 6-1, 6-2, and 6-3.

The postoperative care of the patient begins immediately after the surgical procedure is completed. This involves a short stay in the **postanesthesia care unit (PACU)** or other recovery area for about 1 to 2 hours, depending on the type of surgery and the patient's condition. After this time period and when the patient's condition is stabilized, the patient may be transferred either to the intensive care unit (ICU), to the surgical unit in the hospital, or, if the surgery was ambulatory, the patient will be discharged to home. Nursing care throughout the postoperative period includes ongoing assessments, monitoring for complications, implementing specific nursing interventions, and patient and family teaching, as needed. Before discharge from either the hospital or the ambulatory care unit, all patients will receive both oral and written discharge instructions. In addition, to ensure early identification of complications and address any patient concerns, the patient may receive a follow-up telephone call the next day after discharge.

With an increasing trend toward short-stay or same-day surgical treatment, the nursing interventions in each phase of perioperative nursing care may vary somewhat, but they remain basically the same. While caring for the surgical patient, the nurse should keep in mind that a surgical procedure of any extent is a stressor that requires physical and psychosocial adaptations for both the patient and the family (Fundamentals Review 6-4).

This chapter will cover the skills the nurse needs to provide safe perioperative nursing care in the pre- and postoperative phases.

Fundamentals Review 6-1

NURSING ASSESSMENT AND INTERVENTION BEFORE SURGERY

The nurse assesses for the following during preadmission or upon admission:

- Baseline physical status
- Baseline mental status
- Allergies and sensitivities
- Signs of abuse or neglect
- Cultural, emotional, and socioeconomic factors
- Pain (comprehensive assessment)
- Medication history, including nonprescription medications and supplements
- Previous surgeries, complications, and implants
- Anesthetic history
- Results of radiologic examinations and other preoperative testing

- Referrals
- Physical alterations that require additional equipment or supplies

The nurse also:

- Provides preoperative patient teaching
- Determines informed consent and/or knowledge of planned procedure
- Asks about advance directives
- Develops a plan of care
- Documents and communicates all information per facility policy

Source: From Taylor, C., Lynn, P., & Bartlett, J. (2019). *Fundamentals of nursing: The art and science of person-centered care* (9th ed.). Philadelphia, PA: Wolters Kluwer. Association of periOperative Registered Nurses (AORN). (2017). *Guidelines for perioperative practice.* Denver, CO: AORN, Inc.

Fundamentals Review 6-2

PREOPERATIVE INFORMATION FOR OUTPATIENT/SAME DAY SURGERY

Provide verbal and written instructions, in simple language the patient can understand, for patients having ambulatory surgery.

Ask the patient to:

- List all medications routinely taken, and ask the health care provider which medicines should be taken or omitted the morning of surgery.
- Notify the surgeon's office if a cold or infection develops before surgery.
- List all allergies, and be sure the operating staff is aware of these.

- Follow all instructions from your health care provider regarding bathing or showering with a special soap solution.
- Remove nail polish and do not wear makeup on the day of the procedure.
- Leave all jewelry and valuables at home.
- Have someone available for transportation home after recovery from anesthesia.

Inform patient of:

- Limitations on eating or drinking before surgery, with a specific time to begin the limitations.
- When and where to arrive for the procedure, as well as the estimated time when the procedure will be performed.

Fundamentals Review 6-3

SAMPLE PREOPERATIVE TEACHING: ACTIVITIES AND EVENTS FOR IN-PATIENT SURGERY PREOPERATIVE PHASE

- Exercises and physical activities:
  - Deep-breathing exercises
  - Coughing
  - Incentive spirometry
  - Turning
  - Leg exercises
  - Early mobility
  - Pneumatic/graduated compression stockings
- Pain management:
  - Meaning of PRN orders for medications
  - Patient-controlled analgesia (PCA), as appropriate

- Timing for best effect of medications
- Splinting incision
- Nonpharmacologic pain management options
- Visit by anesthesiologist
- Physical preparation:
  - Nothing by mouth (NPO)
  - Medications the night before and day of surgery
  - Preoperative checklist (review items)
- Visitors and waiting room
- Transport to operating room by stretcher

(continued)

Fundamentals Review 6-3 continued

SAMPLE PREOPERATIVE TEACHING: ACTIVITIES AND EVENTS FOR IN-PATIENT SURGERY PREOPERATIVE PHASE

INTRAOPERATIVE PHASE

- Holding area:
  - Skin preparation
  - Intravenous lines and fluids
  - Medications
- Operating room:
  - Operating room bed
  - Lights and common equipment (e.g., cardiac monitor, pulse oximeter, warming device)
  - Safety belt
  - Sensations
  - Staff

POSTOPERATIVE PHASE

- Postanesthesia care unit:
  - Frequent vital signs, assessments (e.g., orientation, movement of extremities, strength of grasp)
  - Dressings, drains, tubes, catheters
  - Intravenous lines
  - Pain medications, comfort measures
  - Family notification
  - Sensations
  - Airway, oxygen therapy, pulse oximetry
  - Staff
- Transfer to unit (on stretcher):
  - Frequent vital signs
  - Sensations
  - Pain medications, nonpharmacologic strategies
  - NPO, diet progression
  - Exercises
  - Early ambulation
  - Family visits

Fundamentals Review 6-4

NURSING INTERVENTIONS TO MEET PSYCHOSOCIAL NEEDS OF PATIENTS HAVING SURGERY

- Establish and maintain a therapeutic relationship, allowing the patient to verbalize fears and concerns.
- Use active listening skills to identify and validate verbal and nonverbal messages revealing anxiety and fear.
- Use touch, as appropriate, to demonstrate genuine empathy and caring.
- Be prepared to respond to common patient questions about surgery:
  - Will I lose control of my body functions while I'm having surgery?
- How long will I be in the operating room and PACU?
- Where will my family be?
- Will I have pain when I wake up?
- Will the anesthetic make me sick?
- Will I need a blood transfusion?
- How long will it be before I can eat?
- What kind of scar will I have?
- When will I be able to be sexually active?
- When can I go back to work?

Skill 6-1 ▶ Teaching Deep-Breathing Exercises, Coughing, and Splinting

During surgery, the cough reflex is suppressed, mucus accumulates in the tracheobronchial passages, and the lungs do not ventilate fully. After surgery, respirations are often less effective as a result of anesthesia, pain medication, and pain from the incision, particularly thoracic and high abdominal incisions. Alveoli do not inflate and may collapse. Along with retained secretions, this increases the risk for **atelectasis** and respiratory infection.

Deep-breathing exercises hyperventilate the alveoli and prevent them from collapsing again, improve lung expansion and volume, help to expel **anesthetic** gases and mucus, and facilitate tissue oxygenation. Coughing, which helps to remove mucus from the respiratory tract, usually is taught in conjunction with deep breathing. Because coughing is often painful for the patient with a thoracic or abdominal incision, it is important to teach the patient how to splint the

Box 6-1   The I COUGH Multidisciplinary Program

The focus of this program is to reduce postoperative respiratory complications.

I COUGH stands for

I   *Incentive Spirometry*: Deep-breathing exercises will help keep your lungs healthy and prevent lung problems. This breathing exercise needs to be done 10 times each hour.

C   *Cough and Deep Breathe*: After surgery taking deep breaths and coughing helps to clear your lungs. This helps the lungs do the vital job of delivering oxygen to the tissues in your body.

O   *Oral Care*: Brushing your teeth and using mouthwash twice a day keeps your mouth clean from germs.

U   *Understanding Patient Education*: Is important for you and your family to take an active part in your recovery. We want your pain to be controlled so you can take deep breaths, cough, get out of bed for a walk and be sitting up at mealtime.

G   *Get out of Bed*: Walking will help clear secretions from your lungs, help your circulation and help to regain your strength.

H   *Head of Bed Elevated*: It is important to keep the head of the bed elevated between 30 and 45 degrees. Being in an upright position after your operation will help with your breathing.

Source: From Boston Medical Center and Boston University School of Medicine. (n.d.). *I COUGH*. Retrieved http://www.bumc.bu.edu/surgery/quality-safety/i-cough. Used with permission.

incision when coughing. This technique provides support to the incision and helps reduce pain during coughing and movement. Some facilities have implemented the I COUGH program to reduce respiratory complications after surgery (Boston Medical Center and Boston University School of Medicine, n.d.; Cassidy, Rosenkranz, McCabe, Rosen, & McAneny, 2013). This multidisciplinary pulmonary care program is outlined in Box 6-1.

DELEGATION CONSIDERATIONS	Preoperative assessment and teaching is not delegated to nursing assistive personnel (NAP) or to unlicensed assistive personnel (UAP). Depending on the state's nurse practice act and the organization's policies and procedures, preoperative teaching may be delegated to licensed practical/vocational nurses (LPN/LVNs) after an assessment of education needs by the registered nurse. The decision to delegate must be based on careful analysis of the patient's needs and circumstances, as well as the qualifications of the person to whom the task is being delegated. Refer to the Delegation Guidelines in Appendix A.
EQUIPMENT	• Small pillow or folded bath blanket • PPE, as indicated
ASSESSMENT	It is important for the nurse to identify patients who are considered at greater risk for respiratory complications after surgery, such as the very young and very old; obese or malnourished patients; patients with fluid and electrolyte imbalances; patients with chronic disease; patients who have underlying lung or cardiac disease; patients who have decreased mobility; and patients who are at risk for decreased compliance with postoperative activities, such as those with alterations in cognitive function. Depending on the particular at-risk patient, specific assessments and interventions may be warranted. Assess the patient's current level of knowledge regarding deep breathing, coughing, and splinting.
NURSING DIAGNOSIS	Determine related factors for the nursing diagnoses based on the patient's current status. Appropriate nursing diagnoses may include: • Deficient knowledge • Ineffective breathing pattern • Impaired physical mobility
OUTCOME IDENTIFICATION AND PLANNING	The expected outcome to achieve when teaching deep breathing, coughing, and splinting of an incision is that the patient and/or significant other verbalizes an understanding of the instructions and is able to demonstrate the activities.

(continued)

Skill 6-1 ▶ Teaching Deep-Breathing Exercises, Coughing, and Splinting *(continued)*

IMPLEMENTATION

ACTION	RATIONALE
1. Check the patient's health record for the type of surgery and review the prescribed orders. Gather the necessary supplies.	This check ensures that the care will be provided for the right patient and any specific teaching based on the type of surgery will be addressed. Preparation promotes efficient time management and an organized approach to the task.
2. Perform hand hygiene and put on PPE, if indicated.	Hand hygiene and PPE prevent the spread of microorganisms. PPE is required based on transmission precautions.
3. Identify the patient.	Identifying the patient ensures the right patient receives the intervention and helps prevent errors.
4. Close curtains around the bed and close the door to the room, if possible. Explain what you are going to do and why you are going to do it to the patient. Place necessary supplies on the bedside stand, overbed table, or other surface within easy reach.	Closing the curtain and door ensures the patient's privacy. Explanation relieves anxiety and facilitates cooperation. Bringing everything to the bedside conserves time and energy. Arranging items nearby is convenient, saves time, and avoids unnecessary stretching and twisting of muscles on the part of the nurse.
5. Identify the patient's learning needs and the patient's level of knowledge regarding deep-breathing exercises, coughing, and splinting of the incision. If the patient has had surgery before, ask about this experience.	Identification of baseline knowledge contributes to individualized teaching. Previous surgical experience may impact preoperative/postoperative care positively or negatively, depending on this experience.
6. Explain the rationale for performing deep-breathing exercises, coughing, and splinting of the incision.	Explanation facilitates patient cooperation. An understanding of the rationale may contribute to increased compliance.
7. Teach the patient how to perform deep-breathing exercises and explain their importance.	Deep-breathing exercises improve lung expansion and volume, help expel anesthetic gases and mucus from the airway, and facilitate the oxygenation of body tissues.
a. Assist or ask the patient to sit up (semi- or high-Fowler's position) (Figure 1), with the neck and shoulders supported. Ask the patient to place the palms of both hands along the lower anterior rib cage.	The upright position promotes chest expansion and lessens exertion of the abdominal muscles. Positioning the hands on the rib cage allows the patient to feel the chest rise and the lungs expand as the diaphragm descends.
b. Ask the patient to exhale gently and completely.	
c. Instruct the patient to breathe in through the nose as deeply as possible and hold breath for 3 to 5 seconds.	Deep inhalation promotes lung expansion.
d. Instruct the patient to exhale through the mouth, pursing the lips like when whistling.	

FIGURE 1. Assisting patient to semi- or high-Fowler's position.

ACTION

e. Have the patient practice the breathing exercise three times. Instruct the patient that this exercise should be performed every 1 to 2 hours for the first 24 hours after surgery, and as necessary thereafter, depending on risk factors and pulmonary status.

8. Provide teaching regarding coughing and splinting.

a. Ask the patient to sit up (semi-Fowler's position), leaning forward. Apply a folded bath blanket or small pillow against the part of the body where the incision will be (e.g., abdomen or chest) (Figure 2).

b. Ask the patient to inhale and exhale deeply and slowly through the nose three times.

c. Ask the patient to take a deep breath and hold it for 3 seconds (Figure 3) and then cough out three short times (Figure 4).

d. Ask the patient to take a quick breath through the mouth and strongly and deeply cough again one or two times.

e. Ask the patient to take another deep breath, then relax and breathe normally.

f. Instruct the patient that he or she should perform these actions every 2 hours when awake after surgery.

RATIONALE

Return demonstration ensures that the patient is able to perform the exercises properly. Practice promotes effectiveness and compliance.

Coughing helps remove retained mucus from the respiratory tract. Splinting minimizes pain while coughing or moving.

These interventions aim to decrease discomfort while coughing.

FIGURE 2. Having patient splint chest or abdominal incision by holding a folded bath blanket or small pillow against the incision.

FIGURE 3. Telling patient to take a deep breath and hold for 3 seconds.

FIGURE 4. Encouraging patient to cough out three short times after holding breath.

(continued)

Skill 6-1 ▶ Teaching Deep-Breathing Exercises, Coughing, and Splinting (continued)

ACTION	RATIONALE
9. Validate the patient's understanding of the information. Ask the patient to give a return demonstration. Ask the patient if he or she has any questions. Encourage the patient to practice the activities and ask questions, if necessary.	Validation facilitates patient's understanding of information and performance of activities.
10. Remove PPE, if used. Perform hand hygiene.	Proper removal of PPE reduces the risk for infection transmission and contamination of other items. Hand hygiene prevents the spread of microorganisms.

EVALUATION

The expected outcomes have been met when the patient and/or significant other verbalizes an understanding of the instructions related to deep breathing, coughing, and splinting and provides an accurate demonstration of the activities.

DOCUMENTATION

Guidelines

Document the components of teaching related to deep-breathing exercises, coughing, and splinting that were reviewed with the patient and family, if present. Record the patient's ability to demonstrate deep-breathing exercises, coughing, and splinting and his or her response to the teaching; note if any follow-up instruction needs to be performed.

Sample Documentation

> 4/2/20 1030 Perioperative teaching points related to deep breathing, coughing, and splinting reviewed with patient and his wife, including the rationale for each of these points. Patient verbalized an understanding of the rationale for the activities. Patient demonstrated proper technique for deep breathing, coughing, and splinting. Patient stated that he was anxious about the surgery because this will be his first time to the OR. Emotional support and reassurance were provided.
>
> —J. Lance, RN

UNEXPECTED SITUATIONS AND ASSOCIATED INTERVENTIONS

• *The patient verbalizes concern about being able to remember steps for deep breathing and coughing:* Discuss with the patient why he or she feels this way. Offer encouragement and support. Reinforce that nurses will assist the patient with postoperative activities and reinforce the required actions. Provide written instructions as necessary to reinforce material.

SPECIAL CONSIDERATIONS

General Considerations

• Respiratory disorders, such as pneumonia, bronchitis, asthma, and chronic obstructive pulmonary diseases increase the risk for respiratory depression from anesthesia as well as postoperative pneumonia and atelectasis.

Infant and Child Considerations

• Deep breathing and coughing can be accomplished through play such as blowing bubbles or a whistle to enhance a child's participation (Kyle & Carman, 2017).

EVIDENCE FOR PRACTICE ▶

REDUCING POSTOPERATIVE PULMONARY COMPLICATIONS

A wide variety of factors increase the risk of postoperative complications. Potential respiratory complications include pulmonary embolus, atelectasis, and pneumonia. It is important to implement ongoing postoperative interventions to decrease the risk for postoperative complications.

Related Research

Cassidy, M. R., Rosenkranz, P., McCabe, K., Rosen, J. E., & McAneny, D. (2013). I COUGH. Reducing postoperative pulmonary complications with a multidisciplinary patient care program. *JAMA Surgery, 148*(8), 740–745.

This quality improvement project was initiated to design, implement, and determine the efficacy of a group of interventions to reduce postoperative pulmonary complications. A multidisciplinary team developed a strategy based on comprehensive patient and family education and a set of standardized electronic physician orders to specify early postoperative mobilization and pulmonary care. The I COUGH program emphasizes **I**ncentive spirometry, **C**oughing and deep breathing, **O**ral care (brushing teeth and using mouthwash twice a day), **U**nderstanding (patient and family education), **G**etting out of bed (at least 3 times a day), and **H**ead-of-bed elevation. An audit of preintervention nursing practice was completed, noting patient activity, availability of incentive spirometry, and head-of-bed elevation were documented at three different time periods over the course of 3 days. The I COUGH program was implemented for all patients undergoing general or vascular surgery. Information regarding incidence of postoperative pneumonia and unplanned intubation were obtained for 1 year prior to and 1 year after implementation of the program. Post I COUGH audits of nursing practice revealed a significant increase in the number of patients out of bed and the availability of an incentive spirometer and appropriate frequency of use significantly increased. The incidence of postoperative pneumonia and unplanned intubation fell. The team concluded use of the I COUGH multidisciplinary postoperative program was effective in reducing postoperative pulmonary complications and had positive effect on patient outcomes.

Relevance for Nursing Practice

Implementation of recommended postoperative interventions to prevent pulmonary complications is an important part of patient care. Basic postoperative patient care can favorably affect patient outcomes (Cassidy et al., 2013). Nurses must include preventative nursing interventions and patient education as part of the plan of care for patients undergoing surgical procedures.

Refer to the**Point** for additional research on related nursing topics.

Skill 6-2 ▶ Teaching Leg Exercises

During surgery, venous blood return from the legs slows. In addition, some patient positions used during surgery decrease venous return. **Thrombophlebitis, deep vein thrombosis (DVT)**, and the risk for emboli are potential complications from circulatory stasis in the legs. Leg exercises increase venous return through flexion and contraction of the quadriceps and gastrocnemius muscles. It is important to individualize leg exercises to patient needs, physical condition, health care provider preference, and facility protocol.

DELEGATION CONSIDERATIONS	Preoperative assessment and teaching is not delegated to nursing assistive personnel (NAP) or to unlicensed assistive personnel (UAP). Depending on the state's nurse practice act and the organization's policies and procedures, preoperative teaching may be delegated to licensed practical/vocational nurses (LPN/LVNs) after an assessment of education needs by the registered nurse. The decision to delegate must be based on careful analysis of the patient's needs and circumstances, as well as the qualifications of the person to whom the task is being delegated. Refer to the Delegation Guidelines in Appendix A.
EQUIPMENT	• PPE, as indicated

(*continued*)

Skill 6-2 ▶ Teaching Leg Exercises *(continued)*

ASSESSMENT	It is important to identify patients who are considered at greater risk, such as those with chronic disease; patients who are obese or who have underlying cardiovascular disease; patients who have decreased mobility; older adults; and patients who are at risk for decreased compliance with post-operative activities, such as those with alterations in cognitive function. Depending on the particular at-risk patient, specific assessments and interventions may be warranted. Assess the patient's current level of knowledge regarding leg exercises.
OUTCOME IDENTIFICATION AND PLANNING	The expected outcome to achieve when teaching leg exercises is that the patient and/or significant other verbalizes an understanding of the instructions and is able to demonstrate the activity.
NURSING DIAGNOSIS	Determine related factors for the nursing diagnoses based on the patient's current status. Appropriate nursing diagnoses may include: • Deficient knowledge • Anxiety • Impaired physical mobility

IMPLEMENTATION

ACTION	RATIONALE
1. Check the patient's health record for the type of surgery and review the prescribed orders. Gather the necessary supplies.	This check ensures that the care will be provided for the right patient and any specific teaching based on the type of surgery will be addressed. Preparation promotes efficient time management and an organized approach to the task.
2. Perform hand hygiene and put on PPE, if indicated.	Hand hygiene and PPE prevent the spread of microorganisms. PPE is required based on transmission precautions.
3. Identify the patient.	Identifying the patient ensures the right patient receives the intervention and helps prevent errors.
4. Close the curtains around the bed and close the door to the room, if possible. Explain what you are going to do and why you are going to do it to the patient. Place necessary supplies on the bedside stand, overbed table, or other surface within easy reach.	Closing the curtain and door ensures the patient's privacy. Explanation relieves anxiety and facilitates cooperation. Bringing everything to the bedside conserves time and energy. Arranging items nearby is convenient, saves time, and avoids unnecessary stretching and twisting of muscles on the part of the nurse.
5. Identify the patient's learning needs. Identify the patient's level of knowledge regarding leg exercises. If the patient has had surgery before, ask about this experience.	Identification of baseline knowledge contributes to individualized teaching. Previous surgical experience may impact preoperative/postoperative care positively or negatively, depending on this experience.
6. Explain the rationale for performing leg exercises.	Explanation facilitates patient cooperation. An understanding of rationale may contribute to increased compliance.
7. Teach leg exercises and explain their purpose.	Leg exercises assist in preventing muscle weakness, promote venous return, and decrease complications related to venous stasis.
a. Assist or ask the patient to sit up (semi-Fowler's position) (Figure 1) and explain to the patient that you will first demonstrate, and then coach him or her to exercise one leg at a time.	

ACTION

b. Bend the patient's knee, raise the foot (Figure 2), and keep it elevated for a few seconds. Then, extend the lower leg, and hold this position for a few seconds (Figure 3). Lower the entire leg (Figure 4). Practice this exercise with the other leg.

FIGURE 1. Assisting patient to semi-Fowler's position.

FIGURE 3. Extending lower portion of the leg and holding for a few seconds.

c. Assist or ask the patient to point the toes of both legs toward the foot of the bed, then relax them (Figure 5). Next, flex or pull the toes toward the chin (Figure 6).

FIGURE 5. Pointing toes of both feet toward foot of bed.

RATIONALE

FIGURE 2. Raising patient's foot with knee straight.

FIGURE 4. Lowering entire leg to bed.

FIGURE 6. Pulling toes toward chin.

(*continued*)

Skill 6-2 ▶ Teaching Leg Exercises *(continued)*

ACTION	**RATIONALE**

d. Assist or ask the patient to keep legs extended and to make circles with both ankles, first circling to the left and then to the right (Figure 7). Instruct the patient to repeat these exercises three to five times with each leg. Instruct the patient to perform leg exercises every 2 to 4 hours when awake after surgery.

FIGURE 7. Having patient make circles with both ankles, first one way and then the other.

8. Validate the patient's understanding of the information. Ask the patient for a return demonstration. Ask the patient if he or she has any questions. Encourage the patient to practice the activities and ask questions, if necessary.

Validation facilitates the patient's understanding of information and performance of activities.

9. Remove PPE, if used. Perform hand hygiene.

Proper removal of PPE reduces the risk for infection transmission and contamination of other items. Hand hygiene prevents the spread of microorganisms.

EVALUATION

The expected outcomes have been met when the patient and/or significant other verbalizes an understanding of the instructions related to leg exercises and provides an accurate demonstration of the activities.

DOCUMENTATION

Guidelines

Document the components of teaching related to leg exercises that were reviewed with the patient and family, if present. Record the patient's ability to demonstrate the leg exercises and response to the teaching; note if any follow-up instruction needs to be performed.

Sample Documentation

> 11/2/20 2230 Perioperative teaching points related to leg exercises reviewed with patient and her husband, including the rationale for each of these points. Patient verbalized an understanding of the rationale for the activities. Patient demonstrated proper technique for leg exercises and asked appropriate questions. Patient stated that she was anxious about the surgery because this will be her first surgical experience. Emotional support and reassurance were provided.
>
> —J. Lynn, RN

UNEXPECTED SITUATIONS AND ASSOCIATED INTERVENTIONS

- *Patient unable to complete full range of motion of lower extremities due to pain from arthritis or other health issue:* Modify exercises based on patient's abilities. Encourage patient to perform to the best of his or her abilities. Document patient's range of motion and limitations related to exercises.

SPECIAL CONSIDERATIONS	• Cardiovascular disorders, such as thrombocytopenia, hemophilia, recent myocardial infarction or cardiac surgery, heart failure, and dysrhythmias, increase the risk for venous stasis, thrombophlebitis, and thromboembolism. • Certain types of surgeries are associated with a higher risk of deep vein thrombosis and pulmonary embolism, including orthopedic, thoracic, abdominal and genitourinary surgery (LeMone, Burke, Bauldoff, & Gubrud, 2015).

Skill 6-3 ▶ Providing Preoperative Patient Care

The preoperative phase consists of the time from when it is decided that surgery is needed until the patient is transferred to the operating room (OR). Preoperative nursing care is focused on addressing key aspects of care involving (Turunen, Miettinen, Setälä, & Vehviläinen-Julkunen, 2017):

- Holistic preoperative screening—complete medical, physical, social, psychological, and personal assessments
- Coordination—collaborate with the entire interprofessional team
- Communication—promote open, clear communication
- Patient and family education—provide specific pre- and postoperative instructions
- Individual patient- and family-centered care—promote empowerment and emotional support/comfort
- Preoperative contact—engage with the patient prior to surgery for screening and patient preparation, providing last-minute instruction as needed
- Scheduling—prioritize and communicate surgical scheduling plans

Preoperative nursing care is affected by the length of the preoperative phase. Refer to Fundamentals Review 6-1, 6-2, and 6-3. There may not be enough time for comprehensive assessments and teaching for patients who enter the hospital through the emergency department needing immediate surgery and those who have outpatient/same-day surgery. In such cases, the nurse uses standardized preoperative plans and individualizes the plan for the particular patient and family, utilizing nursing interventions that are designed to meet the priority needs of individual patients and situations.

DELEGATION CONSIDERATIONS	Preoperative assessment and teaching are not delegated to nursing assistive personnel (NAP) or to unlicensed assistive personnel (UAP). Depending on the state's nurse practice act and the organization's policies and procedures, preoperative teaching may be delegated to licensed practical/vocational nurses (LPN/LVNs) after an assessment of education needs by the registered nurse. The decision to delegate must be based on careful analysis of the patient's needs and circumstances, as well as the qualifications of the person to whom the task is being delegated. Refer to the Delegation Guidelines in Appendix A.

EQUIPMENT (Varies, Depending on the Type of Surgery and Surgical Setting)	• Blood pressure cuff • Electronic blood pressure monitor/sphygmomanometer • Pulse oximeter • IV infusion device • Graduated compression stockings	• Pneumatic compression device • Tubes, drains, vascular access tubing • Incentive spirometer • Small pillow • PPE, as indicated

ASSESSMENT	The preoperative nursing assessment, which includes a complete baseline health assessment, is completed upon admission to the surgical facility. This assessment may begin in various settings, such as the surgeon's office, in the patient's home or by phone, or an inpatient unit, and is often conducted several days before surgery as part of preoperative laboratory screening and teaching.

(continued)

Skill 6-3 ▶ Providing Preoperative Patient Care *(continued)*

Interview the patient to determine the health history; identify risk factors for surgical adverse events and allergies; and determine any emotional, socioeconomic, cultural, and spiritual factors that may influence the patient's care. Ask about and review all medications the patient is taking, including nonprescription drugs, herbs, and supplements, as well as illicit drugs. Determine the teaching and psychosocial needs of the patient and family. If the patient has a preferred speaking language other than English, it is essential to note this in the patient's record.

Perform physical assessments of skin, respiratory, cardiovascular, abdominal, neurologic, and musculoskeletal function. Take the patient's vital signs. Communicate any assessment abnormalities or areas of concern to the health care provider. It is important for the nurse to identify patients who are considered at greater risk, such as the very young and very old; obese or malnourished patients; patients with fluid and electrolyte imbalances; patients with chronic disease; patients taking certain medications (e.g., anticoagulants or analgesics); and patients who are extremely anxious. Depending on the particular at-risk patient, additional specific assessments and interventions may be warranted.

NURSING DIAGNOSIS   Determine related factors for the nursing diagnoses based on the patient's current status. Appropriate nursing diagnoses may include:

- Anxiety
- Risk for imbalanced fluid volume
- Deficient knowledge

OUTCOME IDENTIFICATION AND PLANNING   The expected outcome to achieve when providing preoperative patient care is that the patient will proceed to surgery. Other outcomes that may be appropriate include the following: the patient verbalizes physical- and emotional-readiness for surgery; and the patient verbalizes an understanding of measures to minimize the postoperative risks associated with surgery.

IMPLEMENTATION

ACTION	RATIONALE
1. Check the patient's health record for the type of surgery and review the prescribed orders. Review the nursing database, history, and physical examination. Check that the baseline data are recorded; report those that are abnormal.	These checks ensure that the care will be provided for the right patient and any specific teaching based on the type of surgery will be addressed. Also, this review helps to identify patients who are at increased surgical risk.
2. **Check that all diagnostic testing has been completed and results are available; identify and report abnormal results.** Gather the necessary supplies.	This check may influence the type of surgery performed and anesthetic used, as well as the timing of surgery or the need for additional consultation. Preparation promotes efficient time management and an organized approach to the task.
3. Perform hand hygiene and put on PPE, if indicated.	Hand hygiene and PPE prevent the spread of microorganisms. PPE is required based on transmission precautions.
4. Identify the patient.	Identifying the patient ensures the right patient receives the intervention and helps prevent errors.
5. Close the curtains around the bed and close the door to the room, if possible. Explain what you are going to do and why you are going to do it to the patient and significant other. Place necessary supplies on the bedside stand, overbed table, or other surface within easy reach.	Closing the curtains and door ensures the patient's privacy. Explanation relieves anxiety and facilitates cooperation. Bringing everything to the bedside conserves time and energy. Arranging items nearby is convenient, saves time, and avoids unnecessary stretching and twisting of muscles on the part of the nurse.

ACTION	RATIONALE

ACTION

6. Explore the psychological needs of the patient and family related to the surgery.

   a. Establish a therapeutic relationship, encouraging the patient to verbalize concerns or fears.

   b. Use active listening skills, answering questions and clarifying any misinformation.

   c. Use touch, as appropriate, to convey genuine empathy.

   d. Offer to contact spiritual counselor (e.g., priest, minister, rabbi) to meet spiritual needs.

7. **Identify learning needs of patient and family.** Ensure that the informed consent of the patient for the surgery has been signed, timed, dated, and witnessed. Inquire if the patient has any questions regarding the surgical procedure (Figure 1). Check the patient's record to determine if an advance directive has been completed. If an advance directive has not been completed, discuss with the patient the possibility of completing it, as appropriate. If patient has had surgery before, ask about this experience.

RATIONALE

Meeting the psychological needs of the patient and family before surgery can have a beneficial effect on the postoperative course.

Spiritual beliefs for some patients and family can provide a source of support over the perioperative course.

Patient education enhances surgical recovery and allays anxiety by preparing the patient for postoperative convalescence, discharge plans, and self-care. The surgeon is responsible for explaining the details of the surgical procedure and potential risks and complications. The nurse is responsible for clarifying what the surgeon has explained to the patient and contacting the surgeon if the patient does not understand or has further questions. An advance directive provides written communication of the patient's wishes to the health care team related to the patient's desire for extraordinary life-sustaining treatments if the patient's condition is deemed unsalvageable. Previous surgical experience may impact preoperative care positively or negatively, depending on the patient's experience.

FIGURE 1. Identifying needs of patient and answering questions.

8. Teach deep-breathing exercises. Refer to Skill 6-1.

   Deep-breathing exercises improve lung expansion and volume, help expel anesthetic gases and mucus from the airway, and facilitate the oxygenation of body tissues.

9. Teach coughing and splinting. Refer to Skill 6-1.

   Coughing helps remove retained mucus from the respiratory tract. Splinting minimizes pain while coughing or moving.

10. Teach use of incentive spirometer, as prescribed or indicated. (Refer to Skill 14-2 in Chapter 14, for specific information.)

   Incentive spirometry improves lung expansion, helps expel anesthetic gases and mucus from the airway, and facilitates oxygenation of body tissues. Use of incentive spirometry may be based on patient risk factors and/or health care provider preference; evidence of effectiveness in prevention of postoperative pulmonary complications is controversial (Branson, 2013; Strickland et al., 2013).

(*continued*)

Skill 6-3 ▶ Providing Preoperative Patient Care *(continued)*

ACTION	RATIONALE
11. Teach leg exercises, as appropriate. Refer to Skill 6-2.	Physical activity reduces the risk of postoperative complications. Leg exercises assist in preventing muscle weakness, promote venous return, and decrease complications related to venous stasis. Leg exercises may be contraindicated for patients with certain conditions, such as lower extremity fractures.
12. Teach about early ambulation, as appropriate.	Physical activity reduces the risk of postoperative complications. Early ambulation has positive effects on the respiratory, cardiovascular, integumentary, musculoskeletal, gastrointestinal, and renal systems. Discussing the benefits during the preoperative period help patients fully engage in this activity (as appropriate) despite expected pain and discomfort postoperatively.
13. Assist the patient in putting on graduated compression stockings. Refer to Skill 9-11 in Chapter 9 for specific information. Demonstrate how the pneumatic compression device operates. Refer to Skill 9-12 in Chapter 9 for specific information.	Graduated compression stockings and pneumatic compression devices are used postoperatively for patients who are at risk for a deep vein thrombosis (DVT) and pulmonary embolism.
14. Teach about turning in the bed.	Turning and repositioning of the patient is important to prevent postoperative complications and to minimize pain.

a. Instruct the patient to use a pillow or bath blanket to splint where the incision will be. Ask the patient to raise his or her left knee and reach across to grasp the right side rail of the bed. If the patient is turning to the left side, he or she will bend the right knee and grasp the left side rail.

b. When turning the patient onto the right side, ask the patient to push with bent left leg and pull on the right side rail (Figure 2). Explain to the patient that you will place a pillow behind his/her back to provide support, and that the call bell will be placed within easy reach.

c. Explain to the patient that position change is recommended every 2 hours.

FIGURE 2. Helping patient to roll over to her right side while she pushes with left bent leg and pulls on the side rail.

ACTION	RATIONALE
15. Provide individualized, developmentally appropriate teaching about pain management options, plans and goals.	Individualized use of pharmacologic and nonpharmacologic methods of pain management is an important part of pain management guidelines related to surgery (Chou et al., 2016). Adequate pain control is important; continuing or unresolved pain can increase the patient's length of recovery and delay discharge.
a. Discuss past experiences with pain and interventions that the patient has used to reduce pain.	Past experiences with pain can impact the patient's ability to manage surgical pain. Pain is a subjective experience and the interventions effective in reducing pain vary from patient to patient.
b. Discuss the availability of analgesic medication postoperatively.	Depending on the prescribed order, the patient may need to request analgesic medication, as needed, or a patient-controlled analgesia (PCA) or epidural analgesia may be ordered, for which the patient will need specific instruction on how to use. (See Chapter 10 for more information.)
c. Discuss the use of PCA, as appropriate. Refer to Skill 10-4 in Chapter 10.	Patient understanding of the use of PCA is crucial for effective, safe administration.
d. Explore the use of other alternative and nonpharmacologic methods to reduce pain, such as position change, massage, relaxation/diversion, guided imagery, and meditation. Refer to Skills 10-1 and 10-2 in Chapter 10.	These measures may reduce anxiety and may decrease the amount of pain medication that is needed. Analgesic therapy should involve a multimodal approach influenced by age, weight, and comorbidity.
16. Review equipment that may be used after surgery.	
a. Show the patient various equipment, such as IV infusion devices, electronic blood pressure cuff, tubes, urinary catheters, and surgical drains.	Knowledge can reduce anxiety about equipment. The patient may need an indwelling urinary catheter during and after surgery to keep the bladder empty and to monitor urinary output. Drains are frequently used to remove excess fluid around the surgical incision.
17. Provide skin preparation.	
a. **Ask the patient to bathe or shower with the antibacterial soap or solution. Remind the patient to clean the surgical site.**	An antiseptic shower, bath, or cleansing with antimicrobial-impregnated wipes may be ordered the evening before surgery and repeated the morning of surgery to begin the process of preparing the skin before surgery and to prevent infection. The skin is cleaned at the operative site with an antibacterial soap or solution to remove bacteria. The patient can do this while taking a bath or shower. The specific choice of soap or antiseptic product depends on the patient, the procedure, and the manufacturer recommendations (AORN, 2017; Cowperthwaite & Holm, 2015). This skin antiseptic eliminates skin microorganisms and leaves an antimicrobial film on their skin.
	Evidence-based practice advises against hair removal at the surgical site due to increased potential for infection. If hair removal is necessary, it should be accomplished using hair clippers and be performed immediately before the surgery, using disposable supplies and aseptic technique (AORN, 2017). Follow facility policy regarding skin preparation of the surgical patient. In addition, immediately before the surgical procedure, the skin of the patient's operative site will be cleansed with a product that is compatible with the antiseptic used for showering.

(continued)

Skill 6-3 ▶ Providing Preoperative Patient Care (continued)

ACTION	RATIONALE
18. Provide teaching about and follow dietary/fluid restrictions. **Explain to the patient that both food and fluid will be restricted before surgery to ensure that the stomach contains a minimal amount of gastric secretions. This restriction is important to reduce the risk of aspiration. Emphasize to the patient the importance of avoiding food and fluids during the prescribed time period, because failure to adhere may necessitate cancellation of the surgery.**	Ensure that fluid and dietary restrictions (NPO), as ordered by the health care provider or as per facility protocol, have been followed. These restrictions assist in preventing regurgitation and aspiration.
19. Provide intestinal preparation, as appropriate. In certain situations, such as surgery of the lower gastrointestinal tract, the bowel will need to be prepared by administering enemas or laxatives.	A prescribed bowel prep and cleansing enema may be ordered if the patient is scheduled for surgery of the lower gastrointestinal tract to evacuate the bowel and to reduce the intestinal bacteria to help prevent contamination of the surgical area during surgery. Peristalsis does not return for 24 to 48 hours after the bowel is handled, so preoperative cleansing also helps to decrease postoperative constipation.
a. As needed, explain the purpose of enemas or laxatives before surgery. If the patient will be administered an enema, clarify the steps as needed. Refer to Skills 13-1 and 13-2 in Chapter 13.	Enemas can be stressful, especially when repeated enemas are required to obtain a clear fluid return. Repeated enemas may cause fluid and electrolyte imbalance, orthostatic hypotension, and weakness.
20. **Check administration of regularly scheduled medications.** Review with the patient routine medications, over-the-counter medications, and herbal supplements that are taken regularly. Check the medical orders and review with the patient which medications he or she will be permitted to take the day of surgery.	Many patients take medications for a variety of chronic medical conditions. Adjustments in taking these medications may be needed before surgery. Certain medications, such as aspirin, are stopped days before surgery due to their anticoagulant effect. Certain cardiac and respiratory drugs may be taken the day of surgery per health care provider order. If the patient has diabetes, oral hypoglycemic agent and/or insulin dosages may be reduced.
21. Provide information to the patient and family regarding timing of surgical events and potential sensations that may be experienced. Explain to patients and their families how long the surgery and postanesthesia care will last, as well as what will be done before, during, and after surgery (e.g., procedures, medications, equipment). Explain to patients that they may not drive themselves home or take public transportation alone if they have had any anesthesia or sedation.	Patients and their families require this information to plan activities accordingly. Explanation and knowledge relieve anxiety and facilitates cooperation.
22. Remove PPE, if used. Perform hand hygiene.	Proper removal of PPE reduces the risk for infection transmission and contamination of other items. Hand hygiene prevents the spread of microorganisms.

EVALUATION

The expected outcomes have been when the patient proceeds to surgery; the patient and/or family verbalizes physical- and emotional-readiness for surgery; and the patient and/or family verbalizes an understanding of measures to minimize the postoperative risks associated with surgery.

DOCUMENTATION

Guidelines

Document that the patient's health records were reviewed, including the history, physical assessment, and any laboratory values and diagnostic studies. Record that the surgeon was notified of any abnormal values. Document the components of perioperative teaching that were reviewed with the patient and family, if present, such as use of the incentive spirometer, deep-breathing exercises, splinting, leg exercises, graduated compression stockings, and pneumatic compression devices.

Record the patient's ability to demonstrate the skills and response to the teaching, and note if any follow-up instruction needs to be performed. Document other preoperative teaching, including pain management, intestinal preparation, medications, and preoperative skin preparation. Record any patient concerns about the surgery and whether the surgeon was contacted to provide any further explanations. Document the emotional support that was offered to the patient and if a spiritual counselor was notified per request of patient.

Sample Documentation

4/2/20 1030 Patient's health records were reviewed and no abnormal results were identified. Perioperative teaching points reviewed with patient and his wife, including the rationale for each of these points. Patient demonstrated proper deep breathing, splinting while coughing, and leg exercises. Reviewed pain management, intestinal preparation, medications, and preoperative skin preparation. Patient stated that he was anxious about the surgery because this will be his first time to the OR. Emotional support and reassurance were provided.

—J. Grabes, RN

UNEXPECTED SITUATIONS AND ASSOCIATED INTERVENTIONS

- *Patient's laboratory results are noted to be abnormal:* Notify health care provider. Some abnormalities, such as an elevated international normalized ratio (INR) or abnormalities in the complete blood count (CBC), may postpone the surgery.
- *A patient says to you, "I'm not sure I really want this surgery":* Ask the patient to elaborate on his or her concerns. Discuss with the patient why he or she feels this way. Notify the health care provider. Patients should not undergo surgery until any questions or doubts are resolved and they are sure that surgery is what they want.

SPECIAL CONSIDERATIONS

General Considerations

- Patients who are obese are at increased risk for respiratory, cardiovascular, positional injury, DVT, and gastrointestinal problems. In taking the history of these patients, be alert for other medical conditions, such as diabetes, gastroesophageal reflux disease (GERD), hypertension, and sleep apnea, which also increase the risk of operative complications.
- Current recommendations caution against routine opioid prescription postoperatively, focusing on oral opioid administration with acetaminophen and/or nonsteroidal anti-inflammatory drugs (NSAIDs) as needed, or the use of patient-controlled analgesia (PCA) when the parenteral route is necessary (Chou et al., 2016).

Infant and Child Considerations

- Children have special needs related to their overall health, age, and size. Easing preoperative anxiety of the child is crucial and includes using simple and concrete terms when providing information.
- The nurse needs to be sensitive to the anxiety level of the parent and provide support, explanations, and patient teaching, as needed.
- Accurate weights are essential for correct medication dosages.
- Developmentally appropriate pain assessment and management needs to be initiated to ensure adequate pain management.

Older Adult Considerations

- Age-related changes and pre-existing chronic conditions can affect the postoperative course of the older adult patient.
- It is important to present preoperative teaching information slowly with reinforcement, because processing of information can be slower.
- Management of postoperative pain in older adults may be complicated by a number of factors, including a higher risk of age- and disease-related changes in physiology and disease–drug and drug–drug interactions (Falzone, Hoffmann, & Keita, 2013, p. 81).
- Physiologic changes related to aging need to be carefully considered because aging is individualized and progressive. Assessment of pain management needs to include renal, liver, and cardiac functions (Falzone et al., 2013, p. 81).

(continued)

Skill 6-3 ▶ Providing Preoperative Patient Care   *(continued)*

EVIDENCE FOR PRACTICE ▶	**POSTOPERATIVE INTERVENTIONS TO PREVENT PULMONARY COMPLICATIONS**

Strickland, S. L., Rubin, B. K., Drescher, G. S., et al. (2013). AARC clinical practice guideline: Effectiveness of nonpharmacologic airway clearance therapies in hospitalized patients. *Respiratory Care, 58*(12), 2187–2193.

This clinical practice guideline is the result of a consensus of the committee, informed by a systematic review of the literature and clinical experience. Based on this review, it is recommended that early mobility and ambulation is used to reduce postoperative complications and promote airway clearance. In addition, the use of incentive spirometry is not recommended for routine, prophylactic use in postoperative adult and pediatric patients.

Refer to thePoint° for additional research on related nursing topics.

Skill 6-4 ▶ Providing Preoperative Patient Care: Day of Surgery

Due to the variety of outpatient and inpatient settings where elective surgery is performed, the day before surgery may be spent at home or in the hospital. If the patient will be arriving the morning of surgery to the surgical setting, he or she will receive a phone call the day before from a health care professional reminding the patient of the scheduled surgery, and key points, such as showering with an antiseptic cleansing agent, NPO restrictions, and any other pertinent information related to the particular procedure. Additionally, the nurse will clarify any questions that the patient may have. If the patient is a hospitalized patient, the nurse will review the same information, clarify any concerns, and reinforce any perioperative instructions, as needed. A preoperative checklist is often used to outline the nurse's responsibilities on the day of surgery; some of the activities outlined in Skill 6-3 are part of this checklist and are completed and documented before the patient is transported to surgery. Refer as well to Fundamentals Review 6-1, 6-2, and 6-3.

DELEGATION CONSIDERATIONS

Preoperative measurement of vital signs may be delegated to nursing assistive personnel (NAP) or to unlicensed assistive personnel (UAP), as well as to licensed practical/vocational nurses (LPN/LVNs). Preoperative assessment and teaching is not delegated to NAP or to UAP. Depending on the state's nurse practice act and the organization's policies and procedures, preoperative teaching may be delegated to LPN/LVNs after an assessment of education needs by the registered nurse. The decision to delegate must be based on careful analysis of the patient's needs and circumstances, as well as the qualifications of the person to whom the task is being delegated. Refer to the Delegation Guidelines in Appendix A.

EQUIPMENT

- Blood pressure cuff
- Electronic blood pressure monitor/sphygmomanometer
- Thermometer
- Pulse oximeter
- IV infusion device, IV solution, vascular access tubing

- Graduated compression stockings (as ordered/indicated)
- Pneumatic compression device (as ordered/indicated)
- Incentive spirometer (as ordered/indicated)
- PPE, as indicated

ASSESSMENT

Immediately prior to the surgery, assess the patient's vital signs and report any abnormalities in vital signs, as well as any abnormalities in laboratory and diagnostic results to the surgeon. Also, review and complete the preoperative checklist (see below) and inquire if the patient or family members have any questions. Provide clarification as needed.

NURSING DIAGNOSIS

Determine related factors for the nursing diagnoses based on the patient's current status. Appropriate nursing diagnoses may include:

- Anxiety
- Deficient knowledge
- Risk for aspiration

OUTCOME IDENTIFICATION AND PLANNING

The expected outcome to achieve when providing preoperative patient care on the day of surgery is that the patient will proceed to surgery. Other outcomes that may be appropriate include the following: the patient and/or family verbalize physical- and emotional-readiness for surgery; the patient and/or family verbalize an understanding of measures to minimize the postoperative risks associated with surgery and of what to expect over the remainder of the pre- and postoperative course.

IMPLEMENTATION

ACTION	RATIONALE
1. Check the patient's health record for the type of surgery and review the prescribed orders. Review the nursing database, history, and physical examination. Check that the baseline data are recorded; report those that are abnormal. Gather the necessary supplies.	A review of the health record ensures that the care will be provided for the right patient and any specific teaching based on the type of surgery will be addressed. Also, review identifies patients who are at surgical risks. Preparation promotes efficient time management and an organized approach to the task.
2. Perform hand hygiene and put on PPE, if indicated.	Hand hygiene and PPE prevent the spread of microorganisms. PPE is required based on transmission precautions.
3. Identify the patient.	Identifying the patient ensures the right patient receives the intervention and helps prevent errors.
4. Close the curtains around the bed and close the door to the room, if possible. Explain what you are going to do and why you are going to do it to the patient and significant other. Place necessary supplies on the bedside stand or overbed table, within easy reach.	Closing the curtains and door ensures the patient's privacy. Explanation relieves anxiety and facilitates cooperation. Bringing everything to the bedside conserves time and energy. Arranging items nearby is convenient, saves time, and avoids unnecessary stretching and twisting of muscles on the part of the nurse.
5. Check that preoperative consent forms are signed, witnessed, and correct; that advance directives are in the health record (as applicable); and that the patient's health record is in order.	These steps fulfill legal requirements related to informed consent and educate the patient regarding advance directives.

(continued)

Skill 6-4 ▸ Providing Preoperative Patient Care: Day of Surgery (continued)

ACTION	RATIONALE
6. Measure vital signs (Figure 1). Notify the primary care provider and surgeon of any pertinent changes (e.g., rise or drop in blood pressure, elevated temperature, cough, symptoms of infection).	Vital signs taken now provide baseline data for comparison. Significant findings may require interventions and/or result in postponement of surgery.

FIGURE 1. Obtaining preoperative vital signs.

ACTION	RATIONALE
7. Provide hygiene and oral care. Assess for loose teeth and caps. Remind the patient of food and fluid restrictions before surgery.	These steps promote comfort and prevent intraoperative complications during anesthesia induction.
8. Instruct the patient to remove all personal clothing, including underwear, and to put on a hospital gown.	Having the patient wear only a gown permits access to the operative area and ease of assessment during the operative period.
9. Ask the patient to remove cosmetics, jewelry including body-piercing, nail polish, and prostheses (e.g., contact lenses, false eyelashes, dentures, and so forth). Some facilities allow a wedding band to be left in place depending on the type of surgery, provided it is secured to the finger with tape.	These items interfere with assessment during surgery. Some hospital policies advise having the patient wear eyeglasses and leave hearing aids in place, if needed. Notify the postanesthesia care unit (PACU) nurse if the patient wears hearing aids.
10. If possible, give valuables to a family member or place them in an appropriate area, such as the hospital safe, if this is not possible. They should not be placed in the narcotics drawer.	This ensures safety of valuables and personal possessions. Document where valuables have been secured.
11. Have patient empty bladder and bowel before surgery.	An empty bladder and bowel minimizes risk for injury or complications during and after surgery.
12. Attend to any special preoperative orders, such as starting an IV line.	This prepares the patient for the operative procedure.
13. Complete preoperative checklist and record of patient's preoperative preparation.	This step ensures accurate documentation and communication with the perioperative nurse caring for patient.
14. Question patient regarding the location of the operative site. Document the location in the health record according to facility policy. The actual site will be marked on the patient when the patient arrives in the preoperative holding area by the licensed independent practitioner who will be directly involved in the procedure (The Joint Commission, n.d., 2017).	The Universal Protocol (National Patient Safety Goals) requires marking and documentation to validate the intended site for the procedure. The site will be marked before the patient is moved into the surgical location by a licensed independent practitioner who will be involved directly in the procedure and will be present at the time the procedure is performed (The Joint Commission, n.d., 2017).

ACTION	RATIONALE
15. Administer preoperative medication as prescribed.	Medication reduces anxiety, provides sedation, and diminishes salivary and bronchial secretions. Preoperative medications, including antibiotics, may be given "on call" (when the OR nurse calls to tell the nurse to give the medication) or at a scheduled time. Certain patients undergoing specific surgical procedures also may be given antibiotic prophylaxis before surgery; depending on facility policy and procedure and the specific medication, prophylactic antibiotics may be administered sent to the OR with the patient for administration immediately prior to the surgery.
16. Raise side rails of bed, based on facility policy; place bed in lowest position. Instruct the patient to remain in bed or on stretcher. If necessary, use a safety belt.	These actions ensure the patient's safety once the preoperative medication has been given.
17. Help move the patient from the bed to the transport stretcher, if necessary. Reconfirm patient identification and ensure that all preoperative events and measures are documented.	Helping the patient move prevents injury. Reconfirming the patient identity helps to ensure that the correct patient is being transported to surgery.
18. Tell the patient's family where the patient will be taken after surgery and the location of the waiting area where the surgeon will come to explain the outcome of the surgery. If possible, take the family to the waiting area.	Informing the family members of what to expect helps allay anxiety and avoid confusion.
19. After the patient leaves for the OR, prepare the room for patients returning to a room on a hospital patient care unit and make a postoperative bed for the patient (Figure 2). Anticipate any necessary equipment based on the type of surgery and the patient's history.	Preparing for the patient's return helps to promote efficient care in the postoperative period.

FIGURE 2. Postoperative bed, ready for patient's return.

ACTION	RATIONALE
20. Remove PPE, if used. Perform hand hygiene.	Proper removal of PPE reduces the risk for infection transmission and contamination of other items. Hand hygiene prevents transmission of microorganisms.

EVALUATION

The expected outcomes have been met when the patient proceeds to surgery; the patient and/or family verbalizes physical- and emotional-readiness for surgery; the patient and/or family verbalizes an understanding of measures to minimize the postoperative risks associated with surgery and of what to expect over the remainder of the pre- and postoperative course.

(continued)

Skill 6-4 ▶ Providing Preoperative Patient Care: Day of Surgery *(continued)*

DOCUMENTATION

Guidelines

Document that the preoperative checklist was completed, time of patient's last void, preoperative medications administered, intended procedure site, and any special interventions that were ordered before sending the patient to the OR. Record if there were any abnormal results that were communicated to the surgeon or OR nurse. Note if the patient's valuables were given to a family member. Document that the patient was safely transferred onto the stretcher and escorted to the OR without incident. Record that the patient's family members were instructed as to where to wait to meet the surgeon after the surgery is performed.

Sample Documentation

> 4/3/20 1045 Preoperative checklist completed with no abnormalities noted, patient voided, and operative permit signed. Patient states surgical site is left knee. Maintained NPO status throughout night. IV started into right forearm, #18-gauge needle inserted without difficulty. IV solution of 1,000 mL of D5.45 sodium chloride at 80/mL/hr initiated. No preoperative medications ordered. Patient verbalized that he will be glad when the surgery is over. Patient assisted onto stretcher for transfer to OR without difficulty. Family also accompanied and instructed to wait in surgical waiting lounge.
>
> —A. Lynn, RN

UNEXPECTED SITUATIONS AND ASSOCIATED INTERVENTIONS

- *A patient admits he ate "just a little bit" this morning upon waking from sleep:* Notify the surgeon. The patient's surgery may have to be postponed for a few hours to prevent aspiration during surgery.
- *Identification band is not in place:* Ensure identity of patient and obtain new identification band. Patient cannot proceed to surgery without an identification band. Two patient identifiers are required to meet current patient safety goals.
- *Consent form is not signed:* Notify the surgeon. It is the responsibility of the provider performing the procedure to obtain consent for surgery and anesthesia. Preoperative medications cannot be given until the consent form is signed. The patient should not proceed to surgery without a signed consent form (unless it is an emergency).
- *Patient refuses to take preoperative medication:* Notify surgeon and anesthesiologist before patient goes to the OR. Many medications are necessary to protect the patient pre- or postoperatively.

SPECIAL CONSIDERATIONS

General Considerations

- Preoperative practice guidelines allow patients to drink clear liquids up to 2 hours before surgery with the order of the provider. If clear liquids are allowed, they should be carefully defined for the patient, and include water, fruit juices without pulp, carbonated beverages, clear tea, and black coffee. These liquids do not include any alcohol. Light meals such as tea and toast may be consumed up to 6 hours before surgery; regular meals should be finished 8 hours before surgery (American Society of Anesthesiologists, 2011).
- Bariatric equipment, such as blood pressure cuffs, wide stretchers, and lift devices, need to be available for patients who are obese.

Infant and Child Considerations

- In many institutions, the parents are allowed to enter the preoperative area with the child. This has been shown to decrease the child's and the parents' anxiety.
- Infants may receive breast milk 4 hours before surgery, and may receive infant formula 6 hours before surgery (American Society of Anesthesiologists, 2011). Breast milk is easier for the stomach to digest, so the clearance time is shorter than for formula.

Older Adult Considerations

- Due to the prevalence of hearing and vision loss in this age group, the necessity of wearing eyeglasses and hearing aids is essential for processing preoperative teaching and throughout the postoperative course. The patient who requires glasses and hearing aids to understand and/or read instructions should be sent to the preoperative area with the glasses and/or hearing aid in place and then remove them before entering the OR.

Skill 6-5 ▸ Providing Postoperative Care

Postoperative care facilitates recovery from surgery and supports the patient in coping with physical changes or alterations. Nursing assessments and interventions are consistent with those in the preoperative and intraoperative phases and are carried out to maintain function, promote recovery, and facilitate coping with alterations in structure or function.

After surgery, patients spend time on the postanesthesia care unit (PACU). After this time period and when the patient's condition is stabilized, the patient may be transferred either to the intensive care unit (ICU) if more in-depth monitoring and nursing care is required, or to the surgical unit in the hospital. If the surgery was ambulatory, the patient will be discharged to home.

Nursing care throughout the postoperative period includes ongoing assessments, monitoring for complications, implementing specific nursing interventions, and patient and family teaching, as needed. Before discharge from either the hospital or the ambulatory care unit, all patients will receive both oral and written discharge instructions and information regarding appropriate follow-up appointments, usually with the surgeon at a minimum. Discharge teaching focuses on patient teaching to support and encourage continuation of interventions to prevent postoperative complications. In addition, to ensure early identification of complications and address any patient concerns, the patient may receive a follow-up telephone call the next day after discharge.

Ongoing assessments are crucial for early identification of postoperative complications.

DELEGATION CONSIDERATIONS	Postoperative measurement of vital signs may be delegated to nursing assistive personnel (NAP) or to unlicensed assistive personnel (UAP), as well as to licensed practical/vocational nurses (LPN/LVNs). Postoperative assessment and teaching is not delegated to NAP or to UAP. Depending on the state's nurse practice act and the organization's policies and procedures, postoperative teaching may be delegated to LPN/LVNs after an assessment of education needs by the registered nurse. The decision to delegate must be based on careful analysis of the patient's needs and circumstances, as well as the qualifications of the person to whom the task is being delegated. Refer to the Delegation Guidelines in Appendix A.

EQUIPMENT (Varies, Depending on the Surgery)

- Electronic blood pressure monitor/sphygmomanometer
- Blood pressure cuff
- Electronic thermometer
- Pulse oximeter
- Stethoscope
- IV infusion device, IV solutions
- Graduated compression stockings (as ordered/indicated)
- Pneumatic compression devices (as ordered/indicated)
- Tubes, drains, vascular access tubing
- Incentive spirometer (as ordered/indicated)
- PPE, as indicated
- Blankets and/or forced-air warming device, as needed

ASSESSMENT	Assess the patient's mental status, positioning, and vital signs. Assess the patient's oxygen saturation level, skin color, respiratory status, and cardiovascular status. Assess the patient's neurovascular status, depending on the type of surgery. Assess the operative site, drains/tubes, and IV site(s). Perform a pain assessment. A wide variety of factors increase the risk for postoperative complications. Ongoing postoperative assessments and interventions are used to decrease the risk for postoperative complications. Assessment of the patient's and family's learning needs is also important.

NURSING DIAGNOSIS

Determine the related factors for the nursing diagnoses based on the patient's current status. Appropriate nursing diagnoses may include the following:

- Acute pain
- Impaired gas exchange
- Risk for imbalanced fluid volume

(continued)

Skill 6-5 ▶ Providing Postoperative Care *(continued)*

OUTCOME IDENTIFICATION AND PLANNING

The expected outcome to achieve when providing postoperative care to a patient is that the patient will recover from the surgery. Other outcomes that may be appropriate include the following: patient's temperature remains between 36.5°C and 37.5°C (97.7°F and 99.5°F); patient's vital signs remain stable; patient will remain free from infection; patient will not experience any skin breakdown; patient will regain mobility; patient will have pain managed appropriately; and patient is comfortable with body image. Specific expected outcomes are individualized based on risk factors, the surgical procedure, and the patient's unique needs.

IMPLEMENTATION

ACTION	RATIONALE

Immediate Care

1. When patient returns from the PACU, participate in hand-off report from the PACU nurse and review the OR and PACU data. Gather the necessary supplies.

Obtaining a hand-off report ensures accurate communication and promotes continuity of care. Preparation promotes efficient time management and an organized approach to the task.

2. Perform hand hygiene and put on PPE, if indicated.

Hand hygiene and PPE prevent the spread of microorganisms. PPE is required based on transmission precautions.

3. Identify the patient.

Identifying the patient ensures the right patient receives the intervention and helps prevent errors.

4. Close the curtains around the bed and close the door to the room, if possible. Explain what you are going to do and why you are going to do it to the patient or significant other. Place necessary supplies on the bedside stand, over-bed table, or other surface within easy reach.

Closing the curtains and door ensures the patient's privacy. Explanation relieves anxiety and facilitates cooperation. Bringing everything to the bedside conserves time and energy. Arranging items nearby is convenient, saves time, and avoids unnecessary stretching and twisting of muscles on the part of the nurse.

5. **Place patient in safe position (semi- or high-Fowler's or side-lying). Note level of consciousness.**

A sitting position (head of bed [HOB] elevated) facilitates deep breathing; the side-lying position with neck slightly extended prevents aspiration and airway obstruction. Alternate positions may be appropriate based on the type of surgery.

6. **Obtain vital signs. Monitor and record vital signs frequently.** Assessment order may vary, but usual frequency includes taking vital signs every 15 minutes the first hour, every 30 minutes the next 2 hours, every hour for 4 hours, and finally every 4 hours.

Comparison with baseline preoperative vital signs may indicate impending shock or hemorrhage. Although protocols are used as guidelines in the immediate postoperative period, the nurse is responsible for adjusting the frequency and priorities of assessment to the specific needs of each patient.

7. Assess the patient's respiratory status. (Refer to Skill 3-5 in Chapter 3.) Measure the patient's oxygen saturation level (Figure 1). If oxygen is ordered, ensure accurate delivery device and flow rate.

Comparison with baseline preoperative respiratory assessment may indicate impending respiratory complications.

8. Assess the patient's cardiovascular status. (Refer to Skills 3-6 and 3-10 in Chapter 3.)

Comparison with baseline preoperative cardiovascular assessment may indicate impending cardiovascular complications.

9. Assess the patient's neurovascular status, based on the type of surgery performed. (Refer to Skill 3-10 in Chapter 3.)

Comparison with baseline preoperative neurovascular assessment may indicate impending neurovascular complications.

10. Provide for warmth, using heated or extra blankets, or forced-air warming device as necessary. Refer to Skill 6-6. Assess skin color and condition.

The OR is a cold environment. **Hypothermia** is uncomfortable and may lead to cardiac arrhythmias and impaired wound healing.

ACTION

11. Put on gloves. Assess the surgical site. Check dressings for color, odor, presence of drains, and amount of drainage (Figure 2). Mark the drainage on the dressing by circling the amount, and include the time. Assess dependent areas, such as turning the patient to assess visually under the patient, for bleeding from the surgical site.

RATIONALE

Hemorrhage and shock are life-threatening complications of surgery and early recognition is essential.

FIGURE 1. Obtaining postoperative oxygen saturation level.

FIGURE 2. Checking dressings for color, odor, and amount of drainage.

12. Verify that all tubes and drains are patent and the equipment is working; note the amount of drainage in collection device. If an indwelling urinary catheter is in place, note urinary output.

This ensures function of drainage devices.

13. Verify and maintain IV infusion at prescribed rate.

This replaces fluid loss and prevents dehydration and electrolyte imbalances.

14. Assess for pain. Check health record to verify if analgesic medication was administered in the PACU. Administer analgesics as indicated, prescribed/ordered and appropriate. If the patient has been instructed in the use of PCA for pain management, review its use. Institute nonpharmacologic pain management interventions as appropriate and indicated.

Use a facility-approved pain scale. Observe for nonverbal behavior that may indicate pain, such as grimacing, crying, and restlessness. Analgesics and other nonpharmacologic pain strategies are used for relief of postoperative pain.

15. Assess for nausea and vomiting. Administer antiemetic medication as indicated, prescribed/ordered, and appropriate.

General anesthesia can cause postoperative nausea and vomiting. Vomiting can lead to serious complications, including pulmonary aspiration, dehydration, and dysrhythmias secondary to electrolyte imbalances (Tinsley & Barone, 2013).

16. Provide for a safe environment. Keep bed in low position with side rails up, based on facility policy. Have call bell within patient's reach.

This adjustment to the bed prevents accidental injury. Easy access to call bell permits patient to call for nurse when necessary.

17. Remove PPE, if used. Perform hand hygiene.

Proper removal of PPE reduces the risk for infection transmission and contamination of other items. Hand hygiene prevents transmission of microorganisms.

(continued)

Skill 6-5 ▶ Providing Postoperative Care *(continued)*

ACTION	**RATIONALE**

Ongoing Care

18. Promote optimal respiratory function.

    a. Assess respiratory rate, depth, quality, color, and capillary refill. Ask if the patient is experiencing any difficulty breathing.

    b. Assist with coughing and deep-breathing exercises. (Refer to Skill 6-1.)

    c. Assist with incentive spirometry, as indicated/ordered. (Refer to Skill 14-2 in Chapter 14.)

    d. Assist with early ambulation.

    e. Provide frequent position changes.

    f. Administer oxygen, as ordered.

    g. Monitor pulse oximetry. (Refer to Skill 14-1 in Chapter 14.)

Patient is at risk for respiratory complications postoperatively. Interventions can be implemented to prevent respiratory complications.

Postoperative analgesic medication can reduce the rate and quality of the respiratory effort.

19. Promote optimal cardiovascular function:

    a. Assess apical rate, rhythm, and quality and compare with peripheral pulses, color, and blood pressure. Ask if the patient has any chest pains or shortness of breath.

    b. Provide frequent position changes.

    c. Assist with early ambulation.

    d. Apply graduated compression stockings or pneumatic compression devices, if ordered and not in place. If in place, assess for integrity.

    e. Provide leg and range-of-motion exercises if not contraindicated. (Refer to Skill 6-2.)

Patient is at risk for cardiovascular complications postoperatively. Interventions can be implemented to prevent cardiovascular complications.

20. Promote optimal neurologic function:

    a. Assess level of consciousness, movement, and sensation.

    b. Determine the level of orientation to person, place, and time.

    c. Test motor ability by asking the patient to move each extremity.

    d. Evaluate sensation by asking the patient if he or she can feel your touch on an extremity.

Anesthetic and pain management agents can alter neurologic function.

Anesthesia alters motor and sensory function.

21. Promote optimal renal and urinary function and fluid and electrolyte status. Assess intake and output, evaluate for urinary retention and monitor serum electrolyte levels.

    a. Promote voiding by offering bedpan/bedside commode, or assistance to bathroom at regular intervals, noting the frequency, amount, and if any burning or urgency symptoms.

    b. Monitor urinary catheter drainage if present.

    c. Measure intake and output.

Anesthetic agents and surgical manipulation in the area may temporarily depress bladder tone and response causing urinary retention.

Frequency, burning, or urgency may indicate possible urinary tract abnormality.

The primary care provider needs to be notified if the urinary output is less than 30 mL/hr or 240 mL/8-hr period.

Intake and output are good indicators of fluid balance.

ACTION	RATIONALE
22. Promote optimal gastrointestinal function and meet nutritional needs:	Anesthetic agents and narcotics depress peristalsis and normal functioning of the gastrointestinal tract. Flatus indicates return of peristalsis.
a. Assess abdomen for distention and firmness. Ask if patient feels nauseated, any vomiting, and if passing flatus.	
b. Auscultate for bowel sounds.	Presence of bowel sounds indicates return of peristalsis.
c. Assist with diet progression; encourage fluid intake; monitor intake.	Patients may experience nausea after surgery and are encouraged to resume diet slowly, starting with clear liquids and advancing as tolerated.
d. Medicate for nausea and vomiting, as ordered.	Antiemetics are frequently ordered to alleviate postoperative nausea.
23. Promote optimal wound healing.	Alterations in nutritional, circulatory, and metabolic status may predispose the patient to infection and delayed healing.
a. Assess condition of wound for presence of drains and any drainage.	
b. Use surgical asepsis for dressing changes and drain care. Refer to Skills 8-2 and 8-6 to 8-10 in Chapter 8.	Surgical asepsis reduces the risk of infection.
c. Inspect all skin surfaces for beginning signs of pressure injury and use pressure-relieving supports to minimize potential skin breakdown.	Lying on the OR table in the same position can predispose some patients to pressure injury formation, especially in patients who have undergone lengthy procedures.
24. Promote optimal comfort and relief from pain.	This shortens recovery period and facilitates return to normal function.
a. Assess for pain (location and intensity using pain scale).	Control of postoperative pain promotes patient comfort and recovery.
b. Provide for rest and comfort; provide extra blankets, as needed, for warmth.	Patients may experience chills in the postoperative period.
c. Administer analgesics, as needed, and/or initiate non-pharmacologic methods, as appropriate.	Multimodal analgesia, combining analgesic drugs from different classes, is recommended to reduce the risk of adverse drug effects (Polomano et al., 2017).
25. Promote optimal meeting of psychosocial needs:	This facilitates individualized care, anxiety reduction, and patient's return to normal health.
a. Provide emotional support to patient and family, as needed.	
b. Explain procedures and offer explanations regarding postoperative recovery, as needed, to both patient and family members.	

EVALUATION   The expected outcomes have been met when the patient has recovered from surgery; patient's temperature remains between 36.5°C and 37.5°C (97.7°F and 99.5°F); patient's vital signs remain stable; patient remains free from infection; patient does not experience skin breakdown; patient regains mobility; patient experiences adequate pain control; and patient is comfortable with body image. Specific expected outcomes are individualized based on risk factors, the surgical procedure, and the patient's unique needs.

DOCUMENTATION

Guidelines   Document the time that the patient returns from PACU to the surgical unit. Record the patient's level of consciousness, vital signs, all assessments, and condition of dressing. If patient has oxygen running, an IV, or any other equipment, record this information. Document pain assessment, interventions that were instituted to alleviate pain, and the patient's response to the interventions. Document any patient teaching that is reviewed with the patient, such as use of incentive spirometer.

(continued)

Skill 6-5 ▷ Providing Postoperative Care *(continued)*

Sample Documentation

4/10/20 1330 Patient returned to room at 1315, drowsy but easily aroused; answers to name. Patient's temperature 98.8°F, pulse 78, BP 122/84, O₂ sat 96% on O₂ 2 L/min. Right lower abdominal dressing dry and intact. Rates pain at a "4" on a scale of 1 to 10, was medicated in PACU with 4-mg morphine sulfate IV at 1030. Incentive spirometry completed × 10 cycles, 750 mL each. Patient deep breathing and coughing without production and turned to right side with HOB elevated. See EHR for additional system assessments.

—J. Grabbs, RN

UNEXPECTED SITUATIONS AND ASSOCIATED INTERVENTIONS

- *Vital signs are progressively increasing or decreasing from baseline:* Notify health care provider. A continued decrease in blood pressure or an increase in heart rate could indicate internal bleeding or **hemorrhage**.
- *Dressing was clean before but now has large amount of fresh blood:* Do not remove dressing. Reinforce dressing with more bandages. Removing the bandage could dislodge any clot that is forming and lead to further blood loss. Notify health care provider.
- *Patient reports pain that is not relieved by ordered medication:* After fully assessing pain (location, description, alleviating factors, and aggravating factors), notify health care provider. Pain can be a clue to other problems, such as hemorrhage.
- *Patient is febrile within 12 hours of surgery:* Assist patient with coughing and deep breathing. If ordered, encourage incentive spirometry. Continue to monitor vital signs and laboratory values such as complete blood count (CBC).
- *Adult patient has a urine output of less than 30 mL/hr:* Unless this is expected, notify health care provider. Urine output is a good indicator of tissue perfusion. Patient may need more fluid or may need medication to increase blood pressure if it is low.

SPECIAL CONSIDERATIONS

General Considerations

- Be aware of baseline sensory deficits. Ensure appropriate aids are in place, such as glasses or hearing aids. Lack of appropriate aids may impact postoperative assessments, such as level of consciousness.
- For patients undergoing throat surgery, such as a tonsillectomy, evaluate swallowing pattern. A patient who has had throat surgery and swallows frequently may be bleeding from the incision site.
- Multimodal analgesia, which combines analgesic drugs from different classes and employs analgesic techniques that target different mechanisms of pain, is recommended in the treatment of acute postoperative pain. The synergistic effects maximize pain relief at lower analgesic doses, reducing the risk of adverse drug effects (Polomano et al., 2017, p. S12).
- In patients who are obese, medications may not perform as expected related to the lack of serum proteins that are needed to bind with the drugs to support their effectiveness. In addition, due to the larger kidney mass of the patient who is obese, renal elimination rates of certain drugs are increased, reducing the effectiveness of these drugs.
- Consider need for bariatric mattress or bariatric bed for a patient who is obese because this patient is at greater risk for skin breakdown due to the poor vascular supply of adipose tissue.
- Ensure that written postoperative instructions specific to the patient and follow-up appointments with the surgeon or other health care professionals are provided to each patient upon discharge from the hospital or outpatient center. Information, such as signs and symptoms to report to the health care provider, as well as restrictions in activity and diet, are addressed. In addition, patients discharged the same day as their surgery are required to have a responsible person accompany them home, and a contact telephone number is to be provided in case of emergency. The patient should be alert and oriented, or mental status should be at the patient's baseline. The vital signs of the patient should be stable. Have the patient "teach back" important information/instructions in their own words.

Infant and Child Considerations

- Postoperative complications are often related to the respiratory system in this age group. After receiving general anesthesia, premature infants are at greater risk for apnea.
- Infants and children are at great risk for temperature-related complications because their body temperature can change rapidly. It is essential to have warmed blankets and other warming equipment available to avoid this complication.

Older Adult Considerations

- Older adults may take longer to return to normothermia and their level of orientation before surgery. Drugs and anesthetics will delay this return.

EVIDENCE FOR PRACTICE ▶

PREVENTION OF DEEP VEIN THROMBOSIS

American Association of Critical Care Nurses. (2016). AACN practice alert: Preventing venous thromboembolism in adults. *Critical Care Nurse, 36*(5), e20–e23.

This Practice Alert outlines expected nursing practice related to the prevention of venous thromboembolism (VTE) in adults. Depending on the individual patient's level of risk for VTE, appropriate interventions include anticoagulant therapy, mechanical prophylaxis including graduated compression stockings and intermittent pneumatic compression devices, as well as daily interprofessional rounds to review each patient's VTE risk factors, current status, and response to treatment.

Refer to thePoint® for additional research on related nursing topics.

EVIDENCE FOR PRACTICE ▶

PAIN MANAGEMENT IN THE POSTOPERATIVE PERIOD

Chou, R. Gordon, D. B., de Leon-Casasola, O. A., et al. (2016). Management of postoperative pain: A clinical practice guideline from the American Pain Society, the American Society of Regional Anesthesia and Pain Medicine, and the American Society of Anesthesiologists' Committee on Regional Anesthesia, Executive Committee, and Administrative Council. *The Journal of Pain, 17*(2), 131–157.

This clinical practice guideline is based on a systematic review of the evidence on postoperative pain management. This document provides recommendations developed by a multidisciplinary expert panel. Safe and effective postoperative pain management should be on the basis of a plan of care tailored to the person and the surgical procedure involved, and multimodal regimens are recommended in many situations. These recommendations are intended to facilitate the safety and effectiveness of acute pain management in the postoperative period and reduce the risk of adverse outcomes related to pain management.

Refer to thePoint® for additional research on related nursing topics.

Skill 6-6 ▶ Applying a Forced-Air Warming Device

Patients are at risk for altered body temperature related to the surgical procedure, length of the procedure, anesthetic agents, a cool surgical environment, age, and use of cool irrigating or infusion fluids. Inadvertent hypothermia (temperature below 36°C [96°F]) can lead to complications of poor wound healing, hemodynamic stress, cardiac disturbances, coagulopathy, delayed emergence from anesthesia, and shivering and its associated discomfort (AORN, 2017). Warming methods intra- and postoperatively are tailored to the individual patient and may include a combination of modalities (John, Ford, & Harper, 2014). Warmed blankets and forced-air warming devices are used for rewarming postoperatively. Forced-air warming devices are placed over the patient and circulate warm air around the patient. Covering the patient with the device acts to reduce heat loss from the skin (through convective and radiant loss) and in combination with the transfer of heat to the patient's body from the forced-air acts to raise the patient's body temperature and/or prevent hypothermia (John et al., 2014). It is important to monitor the patient's body temperature and circulatory status during use of these devices. Follow the manufacturer's directions and facility policies for use.

(continued)

Skill 6-6 ▶ Applying a Forced-Air Warming Device *(continued)*

DELEGATION CONSIDERATIONS	Application of a forced-air warming device is not delegated to nursing assistive personnel (NAP) or to unlicensed assistive personnel (UAP). Application of a forced-warm air device may be delegated to licensed practical/vocational nurses (LPN/LVNs). The decision to delegate must be based on careful analysis of the patient's needs and circumstances, as well as the qualifications of the person to whom the task is being delegated. Refer to the Delegation Guidelines in Appendix A.
EQUIPMENT	• Forced-air warming device • Electronic thermometer • Forced-air blanket • PPE, as indicated
ASSESSMENT	Assess patient's temperature and skin color and perfusion. Patients who are hypothermic are generally pale to dusky and cool to the touch and have decreased peripheral perfusion. Inspect nail beds and mucous membranes of patients with darker skin tones for signs of decreased perfusion. Measure the patient's body temperature and assess the patient's vital signs.
NURSING DIAGNOSIS	Determine the related factors for the nursing diagnoses based on the patient's current status. Appropriate nursing diagnoses may include the following: • Risk for ineffective thermoregulation • Risk for perioperative hypothermia • Risk for injury
OUTCOME IDENTIFICATION AND PLANNING	The expected outcome to achieve when applying a forced-air warming device is that the patient will return to and maintain a temperature of 97.7° to 99.5°F (36.5° to 37.5°C). Other outcomes that may be appropriate include the following: skin will become warm; capillary refill will be less than 2 to 3 seconds; and the patient will not experience shivering.

IMPLEMENTATION

ACTION	RATIONALE
1. Check the patient's health record for the order for the use of a forced-air warming device. Gather the necessary supplies.	Reviewing the order validates the correct patient and correct procedure. Organization facilitates performance of the task. Preparation promotes efficient time management and an organized approach to the task.
2. Perform hand hygiene and put on PPE, if indicated.	Hand hygiene and PPE prevent the spread of microorganisms. PPE is required based on transmission precautions.
3. Identify the patient.	Identifying the patient ensures the right patient receives the intervention and helps prevent errors.
4. Close the curtains around the bed and close the door to the room, if possible. Explain what you are going to do and why you are going to do it to the patient or significant other. Place necessary supplies on the bedside stand, over-bed table, or other surface within easy reach.	Closing the curtains and door ensures the patient's privacy. Explanation relieves anxiety and facilitates cooperation. Bringing everything to the bedside conserves time and energy. Arranging items nearby is convenient, saves time, and avoids unnecessary stretching and twisting of muscles on the part of the nurse.
5. Assess the patient's temperature.	Baseline temperature validates the need for use of the device and provides baseline information for future comparison.

ACTION	RATIONALE
6. Plug forced-air warming device into electrical outlet. Place forced-air blanket over patient, with plastic side up (Figure 1). Keep air-hose inlet at foot of bed.	Blanket should always be used with the device. To avoid causing burns, *do not* place air hose under lightweight blankets with airflow blanket.

FIGURE 1. Forced-air blanket on patient, plastic side up, with air hose inlet at foot of bed. (The photograph is reproduced herein with permission. © 3M 2014. All rights reserved.)

ACTION	RATIONALE
7. Securely insert air hose into inlet. Place a lightweight fabric blanket over the forced-air blanket, according to manufacturer's instructions. Turn the machine on and adjust temperature of air to desired effect.	Air hose must be properly inserted to ensure that it will not fall out. Blanket will help keep warmed air near the patient. Adjust air temperature, depending on desired patient temperature. If blanket is being used to maintain an already stable temperature, it may be turned down lower than if needed to raise patient's temperature.
8. Remove PPE, if used. Perform hand hygiene.	Proper removal of PPE reduces the risk for infection transmission and contamination of other items. Hand hygiene prevents transmission of microorganisms.
9. Monitor the patient's temperature at least every 30 minutes while using the forced-air device. If rewarming a patient with hypothermia, do not raise the temperature more than 1°C/hr to prevent a rapid vasodilation effect.	Monitoring the patient's temperature ensures that the patient does not experience too rapid a rise in body temperature, resulting in vasodilation.
10. Discontinue use of the forced-air device once patient's temperature is adequate and the patient can maintain the temperature without assistance.	Forced-air device is not needed once the patient is warm and stable enough to maintain temperature.
11. Remove device and clean according to facility policy and manufacturer's instructions.	Proper care of equipment helps to maintain function of the device.

EVALUATION

The expected outcomes have been met when the patient's temperature has returned to the normal range of 97.7°F to 99.5°F (36.5°C to 37.5°C); the patient is able to maintain this temperature; the patient's skin is warm; and patient is free from shivering.

DOCUMENTATION

Guidelines

Document the patient's temperature and the route used for measurement. Record that the forced-air warming device was applied to the patient. Document appearance of the skin and that the patient did not experience any adverse effects from the warming device. Record that the patient's temperature was monitored every 30 minutes, as well as the actual temperature measurements.

(continued)

Skill 6-6 ▶ Applying a Forced-Air Warming Device *(continued)*

Sample Documentation

<u>4/23/20</u> 1440 Patient's temperature 35.9°C tympanically. Forced-air warming device applied to patient due to decreased temperature. Device temperature set on medium. Patient's temperature after first 30 minutes 36.4°C tympanically. Device temperature setting decreased to low and continued. Will recheck temperature in 30 minutes.

—J. Grabbs, RN

UNEXPECTED SITUATIONS AND ASSOCIATED INTERVENTIONS

- *Patient's temperature is increasing more than 1°C/hr:* Decrease temperature of air-warming device. If air is down to lowest setting, turn device off. If patient's temperature increases too rapidly, it can lead to a vasodilation effect that will cause the patient to become hypotensive.

SPECIAL CONSIDERATIONS

- Use of forced-air warming devices has been associated with thermal injuries, although the occurrence is rare (John et al., 2014). Monitor for correct assembly of warmer hose to the blanket and accidental disconnection to avoid hot air being blown directly on the patients skin for prolong periods of time (John et al., 2014).
- It is important to ensure the correct use of microbial filters and clean forced-air warming systems according to manufacturer's instructions to prevent increased risk of surgical site infections (John et al., 2014; Kellam, Dieckmannm, & Austin, 2013).

Enhance Your Understanding

Focusing on Patient Care: Developing Clinical Reasoning

Consider the case scenarios at the beginning of the chapter as you answer the following questions to enhance your understanding and apply what you have learned.

QUESTIONS

1. In Josie's health record there is an order for a prophylactic antibiotic to be given "on call to the OR," which means the nurse is to administer the prescribed medication after receiving the phone call to send Josie to the OR. However, the phone call comes during a busy period, and the nurse realizes that Josie has been transported down to the preoperative holding area without receiving her dose of prophylactic antibiotics. What should the nurse do?

2. After her surgery, Ms. Kelly rates her pain as 8 of 10. The nurse administers the ordered pain medication.

Fifteen minutes later, Ms. Kelly is now rating her pain as 9 of 10 and is beginning to writhe with pain. She has no more ordered pain medication for another hour. What should the nurse do?

3. Dorothy Gibbs returns from surgery with a core temperature of 95.4°F (35.2°C), blood pressure of 128/72 mm Hg, and pulse of 60 beats per minute. Her skin is pale and cool to the touch. A forced-air warming device is placed on Ms. Gibbs, and the nurse turns the warmer to the highest heat setting. An hour later, the nurse takes Ms. Gibbs' vital signs. Her tympanic temperature is 37.8°C (100.0°F), her blood pressure is 82/48 mm Hg, and her pulse is 100 beats per minute. What should the nurse do?

You can find suggested answers after the Bibliography at the end of this chapter.

UNIT II

Promoting Healthy Physiologic Responses

Hygiene

7

Focusing on Patient Care

This chapter will help you develop some of the skills related to hygiene that may be necessary to care for the following patients:

Denasia Kerr, age 6, who lives in a pediatric long-term care facility, has limited mobility, and needs her hair washed.

Cindy Vortex, age 34, who is in a coma after a car accident and needs her contact lenses removed.

Carl Sheen, age 76, who needs help cleaning his dentures.

Refer to Focusing on Patient Care: Developing Clinical Reasoning at the end of the chapter to apply what you learn.

Learning Objectives

After completing the chapter, you will be able to accomplish the following:

1. Assist with a shower or tub bath.
2. Provide a bed bath.
3. Assist with oral care.
4. Provide oral care for a dependent patient.
5. Provide denture care.
6. Remove contact lenses.
7. Shampoo a patient's hair in bed.
8. Assist with shaving.
9. Provide nail care.
10. Make an unoccupied bed.
11. Make an occupied bed.

Key Terms

caries: cavities of the teeth

dysphagia: inability to swallow or difficulty in swallowing

gingivitis: inflammation of the gingivae (gums)

halitosis: offensive breath

pediculosis: infestation with lice

plaque: transparent, adhesive coating on teeth consisting of mucin, carbohydrate, and bacteria

tartar: hard deposit on the teeth near the gum line formed by plaque buildup and dead bacteria

Personal hygiene involves measures for maintaining a minimal level of personal cleanliness and grooming that promotes physical and psychological well-being. Personal hygiene practices vary widely among people. The time of day one bathes, how often a person shampoos his or her hair, and how often a person changes his or her bed linens are very individualized choices.

People who are well ordinarily are responsible for their own hygiene. In some cases, the nurse may provide teaching to assist a well person to develop personal hygiene habits he or she may lack. Acute and chronic illness, hospitalization, and institutionalization may make it necessary to modify hygiene practices. In these situations, the nurse helps the patient to continue sound hygiene practices and can teach the patient and family members, when necessary, about hygiene. When assisting with basic hygiene, it is important to respect individual patient preferences and give only the care those patients cannot, or should not, provide for themselves. Patient care flow sheets are documentation tools used to record routine aspects of nursing care, and are often used to document hygiene-related interventions. Figure 7-1 shows an example of a patient care flow sheet that is part of an electronic health record.

This chapter covers skills that the nurse needs to promote hygiene, including bathing, skin care, oral care, removing dentures and contact lenses, shampooing hair, shaving, and changing bed linens. Fundamentals Review 7-1 outlines general skin care principles.

FIGURE 7-1. Patient Care Flow Sheet as part of an electronic health record.

Fundamentals Review 7-1

GENERAL SKIN CARE PRINCIPLES

- Assess the patient's skin at least daily and after every episode of incontinence.
- Cleanse the skin, when indicated, such as when soiled, using a no-rinse, pH-balanced cleanser.
- Avoid using soap and hot water; avoid excessive friction and scrubbing.

- Minimize skin exposure to moisture (incontinence, wound leakage); use a skin barrier product as necessary.
- Use skin emollients after bathing and as needed.

Source: Adapted from Bardsley, A. (2015). Principles of skin cleansing in continence management. *British Journal of Nursing (Urology Supplement)*, 24(18), S36-S38; Lichterfeld, A., Hauss, A., Surber, C., Peters, T., Blume-Peytavi, U., & Lottner, J. (2015). Evidence-based skin care: A systematic literature review and the development of a basic skin care algorithm. *Journal of Wound, Ostomy and Continence Nursing, 42*(5), 501–524.

Skill 7-1 — Assisting With a Shower or Tub Bath

A shower may be the preferred method of bathing for patients who are ambulatory and able to tolerate the activity. Tub baths may be an option, particularly in long-term care or other community-based settings, depending on facility policy. Make any necessary adaptations for individual patients. For example, if the patient is confused and becomes agitated as a result of overstimulation when bathing, reduce the stimuli. Turn down the lights and play soft music and/or warm the room before taking the patient into it (Johnson, 2011; Konno, Kang, & Makimoto, 2014). Box 7-1 outlines possible measures to implement to meet the bathing needs of patients with dementia.

Bathing is performed in a matter-of-fact and dignified manner. If this approach is followed, patients generally do not find care provided by a person who does not share the patient's sex or gender to be offensive or embarrassing.

Box 7-1 — Meeting the Bathing Needs of Patients With Dementia

- Shift the focus of the interaction from the "task of bathing" to the needs and abilities of the patient. Focus on comfort, safety, autonomy, and self-esteem, in addition to cleanliness.
- Individualize patient care. Consult the patient, the patient's record, family members, and other caregivers to determine patient preferences.
- Consider what can be learned from the behaviors associated with dementia about the needs and preferences of the patient. A patient's behavior may be an expression of unmet needs; unwillingness to participate may be a response to uncomfortable water temperatures or levels of sound or light in the room.
- Ensure privacy and warmth.
- Consider the use of music to sooth anxiety and agitation.
- Consider other methods for bathing. Showers and tub baths are not the only options in bathing. Towel baths,

washing under clothes, and bathing "body sections" one day at a time are other possible options.
- Maintain a relaxed demeanor. Use calming language. Use one-step commands. Try to determine phrases and terms the patient understands in relation to bathing and make use of them. Offer frequent reassurance.
- Encourage independence. Using hand-over-hand or a guided hand technique to cue the person regarding the purpose of the interaction can allow patients to perform some activities for themselves.
- Explore the need for routine analgesia before bathing. Move limbs carefully and be aware of signs of discomfort during bathing.
- Wash the face and hair at the end of the bath or at a separate time. Water dripping in the face and having a wet head are often the most upsetting parts of the bathing process for people with dementia.

Source: Adapted from Gallagher, M., & Hall, G. R. (2014). Bathing persons with Alzheimer's disease and related dementias. *Journal of Gerontological nursing, 40*(2), 14–20; Gozalo, P., Prakash, S., Qato, D. M., Sloane, P. D., & Mor, V. (2014). Effect of the bathing without a battle training intervention on bathing-associated physical and verbal outcomes in nursing home residents with dementia: A randomized crossover diffusion study. *Journal of the American Geriatrics Society, 62*(5), 797–804; Konno, R., Kang, H. S., & Makimoto, K. (2014). A best-evidence review of intervention studies for minimizing resistance-to-care behaviours for older adults with dementia in nursing homes. *Journal of Advanced Nursing, 70*(10), 2167–2180; and Ray, K. D., & Fitzsimmons, S. (2014). Music-assisted bathing: Making shower time easier for people with dementia. *Journal of Gerontological Nursing, 40*(2), 9–13.

(continued)

Skill 7-1 ▶ Assisting With a Shower or Tub Bath *(continued)*

DELEGATION CONSIDERATIONS	The implementation of a shower or tub bath may be delegated to nursing assistive personnel (NAP) or unlicensed assistive personnel (UAP), as well as to licensed practical/vocational nurses (LPN/LVNs). The decision to delegate must be based on careful analysis of the patient's needs and circumstances, as well as the qualifications of the person to whom the task is being delegated. Refer to the Delegation Guidelines in Appendix A.

EQUIPMENT

- Personal hygiene supplies (deodorant, lotion, and others)
- Skin-cleaning agent
- Emollient and skin barrier, as indicated
- Towels and washcloths
- Robe (as indicated) and slippers or nonskid socks
- Gown or pajamas, or clothing (as indicated)
- Laundry bag
- Shower or tub chair, as needed
- Nonsterile gloves, as indicated
- Additional PPE, as indicated

ASSESSMENT

Assess the patient's knowledge of hygiene practices and bathing preferences: frequency, time of day, and type of hygiene products. Assess for any physical-activity limitations. Assess the patient's ability to perform and participate with bathing activities. Assess the patient's skin for dryness, redness, or areas of breakdown, and gather any other appropriate supplies that may be needed as a result of the assessment.

NURSING DIAGNOSIS

Determine the related factors for the nursing diagnoses based on the patient's current status. Appropriate nursing diagnoses may include:

- Bathing self-care deficit
- Risk for impaired skin integrity
- Readiness for enhanced self-care

OUTCOME IDENTIFICATION AND PLANNING

The expected outcome to achieve when assisting with a shower or tub bath is that the patient will be clean and fresh, and without injury. Other outcomes that may be appropriate include the following: patient regains feelings of control by assisting with the bath; patient verbalizes positive body image; and patient demonstrates understanding about the need for hygiene measures.

IMPLEMENTATION

ACTION	**RATIONALE**
1. Review the patient's health record for any limitations in physical activity. Check presence of medical order for clearing the patient to shower, if required by facility policy.	Identifying limitations prevents patient discomfort and injury. In some settings, a medical order is required for showering.
2. Check to see that the bathroom is available, clean, and safe. Make sure showers and tubs have mats or nonskid strips to prevent patients from falling. Place a mat or towel on the floor in front of the shower or tub. Put a shower or tub chair in place, as appropriate. Place "occupied" sign on door of room, as appropriate for setting.	A clean bathroom prevents transmission of microorganisms. Mats and nonskid materials prevent patients from slipping and falling. Having a place for a weak or physically disabled patient to sit in a shower prevents falls; warm water could cause vasodilation and pooling of blood in lower extremities, contributing to lightheadedness or dizziness. Use of sign allows others to be aware of use of the room and ensures patient privacy.
3. Gather necessary hygienic and toiletry items, and linens. Place within easy reach of shower or tub.	Bringing everything to the bathing location conserves time and energy. Arranging items nearby is convenient, saves time, and avoids unnecessary reaching and possible falls.
4. Perform hand hygiene.	Hand hygiene prevents the spread of microorganisms.

ACTION

5. Identify the patient. Discuss the procedure with the patient and assess the patient's ability to assist in the bathing process, as well as personal hygiene preferences.

6. Assist the patient to bathroom to void or defecate, if appropriate.

7. Assist the patient to put on a robe and slippers or nonskid socks. Cover IV access site(s) according to facility policy.

8. Assist the patient to the shower or tub.

9. Close the curtains around the shower or tub, as appropriate, and close the door to the bathroom. Adjust the room temperature, if necessary.

Shower: Turn shower on. Check to see that the water temperature is safe and comfortable.
Tub: Fill tub halfway with water. Check to see that the water temperature is safe and comfortable.
Adjust water temperature, if appropriate, based on patient preference (Figure 1). **Water temperature should be adjusted to 100°F to less than 120° to 125°F, with the lower temperature limit suggested for children and older adults (Burn Foundation, 2016).**

RATIONALE

Identifying the patient ensures the right patient receives the intervention and helps prevent errors. Discussion promotes reassurance and provides knowledge about the procedure. Dialogue encourages patient participation and allows for individualized nursing care.

Voiding or defecating before the bath lessens the likelihood that the bath will be interrupted, because warm bath water may stimulate the urge to void.

This ensures the patient's privacy, prevents chilling, and decreases the risk for slipping and fallings. Coverage of IV site prevents loosening of dressings from exposure to moisture, and maintains integrity of IV access.

This prevents accidental falls.

This ensures the patient's privacy and lessens the risk for loss of body heat during the bath. Warm water is relaxing, stimulates circulation, and provides for more effective cleansing. Adjusting the water temperature to 100°F to less than 120° to 125°F decreases risk of burns and drying of the skin. The lower temperature is recommended for children and adults over 65 years of age (Burn Foundation, 2016).

FIGURE 1. Adjusting water temperature, based on patient preference.

10. Explain the use of the call device and ensure that it is within the reach of the shower or tub.

11. Put on gloves, as indicated. Help the patient get in and out of the shower or tub, as necessary. Use safety bars. For a tub: Have the patient grasp the handrails at the side of the tub, or place a chair at the side of the tub. The patient sits on the chair and eases to the edge of the tub. After putting both feet into the tub, have the patient reach to the opposite side and ease down into the tub. The patient may kneel first in the tub and then sit in it.

Use of the call device allows the patient to call for help if necessary.

Gloves are required if contact with blood or body fluids is anticipated. Gloves prevent the transmission of microorganisms.
This prevents slipping and falling.

(continued)

Skill 7-1 ▶ Assisting With a Shower or Tub Bath *(continued)*

ACTION	**RATIONALE**
12. If necessary, use a hydraulic lift, when available, to lower patients who are unable to maneuver safely or completely bear their own weight. Some community-based settings have walk-in tubs available.	This prevents slipping and falling and prevents strain and injury to patients and nurses.
13. Keep room door unlocked. Remain in room with the patient to offer assistance, as appropriate. If assistance is needed with bathing, put on gloves. Otherwise, check on the patient every 5 minutes. **Never leave young children or confused patients alone in the bathroom.**	These actions promote safety. Health personnel should be able to enter with ease if the patient needs help. Gloves are required if contact with blood or body fluids is anticipated. Gloves prevent the transmission of microorganisms.
14. Assist the patient out of the shower or tub when bathing is complete. Obtain the assistance of additional personnel, as appropriate. Use safety bars. For a tub: Drain the water from the tub. Have the patient grasp the handrails at the side of the tub. Assist the patient to the edge of the tub. Have the patient ease to a chair placed at the side of the tub, then remove feet out of tub. The patient may kneel first in the tub and then move to the side of the tub.	This prevents slipping and falling. Use of additional personnel prevents strain and injury to patients and nurses.
15. If necessary, use a hydraulic lift, when available, to raise patients who are unable to maneuver safely or completely bear their own weight.	This prevents slipping and falling and prevents strain and injury to patients and nurses.
16. Put on gloves, as indicated. Assist the patient with drying, application of emollients, and dressing, as appropriate or necessary. Remove cover from IV access site.	Gloves are required if contact with blood or body fluids is anticipated. Gloves prevent the transmission of microorganisms. Prevents chilling and promotes patient comfort. Use of emollients is recommended to restore and maintain skin integrity (Andriessen, 2013; Lichterfeld et al., 2015; Voegeli, 2010).
17. Remove gloves, if used. Assist the patient to the room (Figure 2) and into a position of comfort.	Removing gloves properly reduces risk for infection transmission and contamination of other items. Promotes patient comfort and safety.

FIGURE 2. Assisting patient to room.

18. Clean shower or tub according to facility policy. Dispose of soiled linens according to facility policy. Remove "occupied" sign from door of bathroom.	Reduces risk for infection transmission and contamination of other items. Allows others to make use of room.
19. Perform hand hygiene.	Hand hygiene prevents the spread of microorganisms.

EVALUATION	The expected outcomes have been met when the patient is clean; demonstrates some feeling of control in his or her care; verbalizes an improved body image; and verbalizes understanding of the need for hygiene measures.

DOCUMENTATION

Guidelines

Record any significant observations and communication. Document the condition of the patient's skin. Record the procedure, amount of assistance given, and patient participation. Document the application of skin care products, such as an emollient.

Sample Documentation

<u>7/14/20</u> 1030 Shower provided with minimal assistance. Skin intact. Patient states improved sense of cleanliness and increased comfort.

—*C. Stone, RN*

UNEXPECTED SITUATIONS AND ASSOCIATED INTERVENTIONS

- *The patient becomes chilled during bath:* If the room temperature is adjustable, increase temperature. Provide additional assistance to dry and dress quickly, to decrease chilling.
- *The patient becomes excessively fatigued during the bath process:* Allow for rest period sitting down after walking to bathing room and/or completion of bath, before returning to room. Assist the patient to and from bath in wheelchair, to conserve energy. Schedule bath after rest period or nap.

SPECIAL CONSIDERATIONS

General Considerations

- Patients with bariatric needs are at increased risk of skin breakdown (Cowdell & Radley, 2014). Assess the skin of bariatric inpatients twice a day, lifting and separating folds of skin to assess the area, utilizing extra help as necessary (Black & Hotaling, 2015). Nonsoap cleansers should be used and the skin should be dried to prevent retained moisture (Black & Hotaling).
- Incontinent patients require special attention to perineal care. Patients with urinary or fecal incontinence are at risk for perineal skin damage. This damage is related to moisture, changes in the pH of the skin, overgrowth of bacteria and infection of the skin, and erosion of perineal skin from friction on moist skin. Skin care for these patients should include measures to reduce over-hydration (excess exposure to moisture), reduce contact with ammonia and bacteria, and reduce friction. Remove soil and irritants from the skin during routine hygiene, and clean the area when the skin becomes exposed to irritants. Avoid using soap and excessive force for cleaning. The use of perineal skin cleansers, moisturizers, and moisture barriers is recommended for skin care for the incontinent patient. These products help promote healing and prevent further skin damage.
- Basic wound care used for body piercings is usually called "aftercare." Aftercare techniques are used for the new piercing and whenever the piercing fistula has become disrupted through injury or exhibits signs of infection or inflammation (Halliday, 2005; Mayo Foundation for Medical Education and Research [MFMER], 2015a;). Clean the jewelry and the piercing site of all crust and debris. Rinse the site with warm water and use a cotton swab to gently remove any crusting. Rinse well.

Infant and Child Considerations

- When bathing an infant or young child, have supplies within easy reach, and support or hold the child securely at all times to ensure safety.
- Never leave the child alone.

Older Adult Considerations

- Check the temperature of the water carefully before bathing an older adult, because their sensitivity to temperature may be impaired.
- An older, continent adult may not require a bath every day. If dry skin is a problem, water and skin lotion or bath oil may be used on alternate days. Do not use bath oil in tub water, as it can cause tub surfaces to become slippery.

Home Care Considerations

- Evaluate the safety of the bathing area in the home. Tub mats, adhesive strips, grab bars, and shower stools can help prevent falls.
- Instruct patients to apply emollients, lotions, or oils after leaving tub or shower to prevent slipping and falling.

Skill 7-2 ▶ Providing a Bed Bath

Some patients must remain in bed as a part of their therapeutic regimen, but can still bathe themselves. Other patients are not on bed rest, but require total or partial assistance with bathing in bed due to physical limitations, such as fatigue or limited range of motion. A bed bath may be considered a partial bed bath if the patient is well enough to perform most of the bath, and the nurse needs to assist with washing areas that the patient cannot reach easily. A partial bath may also refer to bathing only those body parts that absolutely have to be cleaned, such as the perineal area, and any soiled body parts. Many of the bedside skin-cleaning products available today do not require rinsing. After cleaning the body part, dry it thoroughly. See Table 7-1 for a summary of common bedside cleaning and skincare products. Perform bathing in a matter-of-fact and dignified manner. If this approach is followed, patients generally do not find care provided by a person who does not share the patient's sex or gender to be offensive or embarrassing. This skill reviews providing a bed bath using water, skin cleanser, and a minimal number of wash cloths. An alternative approach is to use multiple cloth washcloths, using a new washcloth for each body area. The Skill Variation at the end of the skill offers guidelines to provide a bath using a disposable bathing system.

Table 7-1 Bedside Cleaning and Skin Care Products

PRODUCT	DESCRIPTION
Bathing cloths	Premoistened, pH-balanced, microwaveable, disposable cloths for rinse-free skin cleaning and moisturizing. Each package provides one complete bath using 8–10 cloths.
Bathing wipes	Packaged dry cloths. Adding water to the cloths causes them to foam, providing rinse-free skin pH-balanced cleaning. Cloths are in a resealable package for multiple uses.
No-rinse body wash and shampoo	No-rinse, concentrated skin cleanser and moisturizer. Mix with water, apply with a cloth, lather, and dry.
Body foam	Foam cleanser and moisturizer to be used as a body wash, no-rinse shampoo, and perineal cleanser. Pump bottle dispenses foam to be applied with a cloth.
Chlorhexidine gluconate	Reduces colonization of skin with pathogens. Bathing with chlorhexidine may be used to reduce the incidence of hospital-acquired infections, such as central line–associated bloodstream infections and surgical site infections, as well as to reduce the acquisition of or decolonization with multidrug-resistant organisms (Cassir et al., 2015; Hines et al., 2015; Petlin et al., 2014; Pyrek, 2015; Shah, Schwartz, & Cullen, 2016; Viray et al., 2014). Chlorhexidine can be added to bath water, but is also available, and easier to use, in prepackaged impregnated cloths.

Make any necessary adaptations for individual patients. For example, if the patient is confused and becomes agitated as a result of overstimulation when bathing, reduce the stimuli. Turn down the lights and play soft music and/or warm the room before giving the patient a bath (Johnson, 2011; Konno et al., 2014). Box 7-1 in Skill 7-1 outlines possible measures to implement to meet the bathing needs of patients with dementia.

DELEGATION CONSIDERATIONS

The implementation of a bed bath may be delegated to nursing assistive personnel (NAP) or to unlicensed assistive personnel (UAP), as well as to licensed practical/vocational nurses (LPN/LVNs). The decision to delegate must be based on careful analysis of the patient's needs and circumstances, as well as the qualifications of the person to whom the task is being delegated. Refer to the Delegation Guidelines in Appendix A.

EQUIPMENT	• Washbasin and warm water • Personal hygiene supplies (deodorant, lotion, and others) • Skin-cleaning agent • Emollient and skin barrier, as indicated • Towels (2)	• Washcloths (2) • Bath blanket • Gown, pajamas, or appropriate clothing • Bedpan or urinal • Laundry bag • Nonsterile gloves; other PPE, as indicated

ASSESSMENT

Assess the patient's knowledge of hygiene practices and bathing preferences: frequency, time of day, and type of hygiene products. Assess for any physical-activity limitations. Assess the patient's ability to bathe him or herself. Allow the patient to do any part of the bath that he or she can do. For example, the patient may be able to wash the face, while the nurse does the rest. Assess the patient's skin for dryness, redness, or areas of breakdown, and gather any other appropriate supplies that may be needed as a result of the assessment.

NURSING DIAGNOSIS

Determine the related factors for the nursing diagnoses based on the patient's current status. Appropriate nursing diagnoses may include:

• Bathing self-care deficit
• Impaired skin integrity
• Risk for impaired skin integrity

OUTCOME IDENTIFICATION AND PLANNING

The expected outcome to achieve when giving a bed bath is that the patient will be clean and fresh. Other outcomes that may be appropriate include the following: patient regains feelings of control by assisting with the bath; patient verbalizes positive body image; and patient demonstrates understanding about the need for hygiene measures.

IMPLEMENTATION

ACTION	RATIONALE
1. Review the patient's health record for any limitations in physical activity.	Identifying limitations prevents patient discomfort and injury.
2. Perform hand hygiene and put on gloves and/or other PPE, if indicated.	Hand hygiene and PPE prevent the spread of microorganisms. PPE is required based on transmission precautions.
3. Identify the patient. Discuss the procedure with the patient and assess the patient's ability to assist in the bathing process, as well as personal hygiene preferences.	Identifying the patient ensures the right patient receives the intervention and helps prevent errors. Discussion promotes reassurance and provides knowledge about the procedure. Dialogue encourages patient participation and allows for individualized nursing care.
4. Assemble equipment on the overbed table or other surface within reach.	Organization facilitates performance of the task.
5. Close the curtains around the bed and close the door to the room, if possible. Adjust the room temperature, if necessary.	This ensures the patient's privacy and lessens the risk for loss of body heat during the bath.
6. Adjust the bed to a comfortable working height; usually elbow height of the caregiver (VHACEOSH, 2016).	Having the bed at the proper height prevents back and muscle strain.
7. Remove sequential compression devices and antiembolism stockings from lower extremities according to facility protocol.	Most manufacturers and facilities recommend removal of these devices before the bath to allow for assessment.
8. Put on gloves. Offer the patient a bedpan or urinal.	Gloves are necessary for potential contact with blood or body fluids. Voiding or defecating before the bath lessens the likelihood that the bath will be interrupted, because warm bath water may stimulate the urge to void.

(continued)

Skill 7-2 ▶ Providing a Bed Bath *(continued)*

ACTION	**RATIONALE**

 9. Remove gloves and perform hand hygiene.

Hand hygiene deters the spread of microorganisms.

10. Put on a clean pair of gloves. Lower the side rail nearest to you and assist the patient to the side of bed where you will work. Have the patient lie on his or her back.

Gloves prevent transmission of microorganisms. Having the patient positioned near the nurse and lowering the side rail prevent unnecessary stretching and twisting of muscles on the part of the nurse.

11. Loosen top covers and remove all except the top sheet. Place a bath blanket over the patient and then remove the top sheet while the patient holds the bath blanket in place. If linen is to be reused, fold it over a chair. Place soiled linen in laundry bag. Take care to prevent linen from coming in contact with your clothing.

The patient is not exposed unnecessarily, and warmth is maintained. If a bath blanket is unavailable, the top sheet may be used in its place.

12. Remove the patient's gown or clothing and keep the bath blanket in place. If the patient has an IV line and is not wearing a gown with snap sleeves, remove gown from other arm first. Lower the IV container and pass the gown over the tubing and the container. **Rehang the container and check the drip rate.**

This provides uncluttered access during the bath and maintains warmth of the patient. IV fluids must be maintained at the prescribed rate.

13. **Raise side rails.** Fill basin with a sufficient amount of comfortably warm water (100°F to less than 120° to 125°F). Add the skin cleanser, if appropriate, according to manufacturer's directions. Change, as necessary, throughout the bath. Lower the side rail nearest to you when you return to the bedside to begin the bath.

Side rails maintain patient safety. Adjusting the water temperature to 100°F to less than 120° to 125°F decreases risk of burns and drying of the skin. The lower temperature is recommended for children and adults over 65 years of age (Burn Foundation, 2016). Warm water is comfortable and relaxing for the patient. It also stimulates circulation and provides for more effective cleansing.

14. Put on gloves, if indicated. Lay a towel across the patient's chest and on top of bath blanket.

Gloves are necessary if there is potential contact with blood or body fluids. The towel prevents chilling and keeps the bath blanket dry.

15. With no cleanser on the washcloth, wipe one eye from the inner part of the eye, near the nose, to the outer part (Figure 1). Rinse or turn the cloth before washing the other eye.

Soap is irritating to the eyes. Moving from the inner to the outer aspect of the eye prevents carrying debris toward the nasolacrimal duct. Rinsing or turning the washcloth prevents spreading organisms from one eye to the other.

FIGURE 1. Washing from the inner corner of the eye outward.

16. Bathe the patient's face, neck, and ears. Apply appropriate emollient.

Use of emollients is recommended to restore and maintain skin integrity (Andriessen, 2013; Lichterfeld et al., 2015; Voegeli, 2010).

ACTION

17. Expose the patient's far arm and place towel lengthwise under it. Using firm strokes, wash hand, arm, and axilla, lifting the arm as necessary to access axillary region (Figure 2). Rinse, if necessary, and dry. Apply appropriate emollient. Cover the area with the bath blanket.

18. Repeat Action 17 for the arm nearest you. Another option might be to bathe one side of the patient first and then move to the other side of the bed to complete the bath.

19. Spread a towel across the patient's chest. Lower the bath blanket to the patient's umbilical area. Wash, rinse, if necessary, and dry chest. Keep chest covered with towel between the wash and rinse. Pay special attention to the folds of skin under the breasts. Apply appropriate emollient.

20. Lower the bath blanket to the perineal area. Place a towel over the patient's chest.

21. Wash, rinse, if necessary, and dry abdomen (Figure 3). Carefully inspect and clean umbilical area and any abdominal folds or creases. Apply appropriate emollient.

FIGURE 2. Exposing the far arm and washing it.

22. Return bath blanket to original position and expose far leg. Place towel under far leg. Using firm strokes, wash, rinse, if necessary, and dry leg from ankle to knee and knee to groin (Figure 4). Apply appropriate emollient.

RATIONALE

The towel helps to keep the bed dry. Washing the far side first eliminates contaminating a clean area once it is washed. Gentle friction stimulates circulation and muscles and helps remove dirt, oil, and organisms. Long, firm strokes are relaxing and more comfortable than short, uneven strokes. Rinsing is necessary when using some cleansing products. Use of emollients is recommended to restore and maintain skin integrity (Andriessen, 2013; Lichterfeld et al., 2015; Voegeli, 2010). Re-covering the body maintains warmth.

Exposing, washing, rinsing, and drying one part of the body at a time avoids unnecessary exposure and chilling. Areas of skin folds may be sources of odor and skin breakdown if not cleaned and dried properly. Use of emollients is recommended to restore and maintain skin integrity (Andriessen, 2013; Lichterfeld et al., 2015; Voegeli, 2010).

Keeping the bath blanket and towel in place avoids exposure and chilling.

Skin-fold areas may be sources of odor and skin breakdown if not cleaned and dried properly. Use of emollients is recommended to restore and maintain skin integrity (Andriessen, 2013; Lichterfeld et al., 2015; Voegeli, 2010).

FIGURE 3. Washing the abdomen, with perineal and chest areas covered.

The towel protects linens and prevents the patient from feeling uncomfortable from a damp or wet bed. Washing from ankle to groin with firm strokes promotes venous return. Use of emollients is recommended to restore and maintain skin integrity (Andriessen, 2013; Lichterfeld et al., 2015; Voegeli, 2010).

FIGURE 4. Washing and drying far leg, keeping the other leg covered.

(*continued*)

Skill 7-2 ▶ Providing a Bed Bath *(continued)*

ACTION	**RATIONALE**
23. Wash, rinse if necessary, and dry the foot. Pay particular attention to the areas between toes. Apply appropriate emollient.	Drying of the feet is important to prevent irritation, possible skin breakdown, and infections (National Institute on Aging, 2015). Use of emollients is recommended to restore and maintain skin integrity (Andriessen, 2013; Lichterfeld et al., 2015; Voegeli, 2010).
24. Repeat Actions 22 and 23 for the other leg and foot.	
25. Make sure the patient is covered with bath blanket. Change water and washcloth at this point or earlier, if necessary.	The bath blanket maintains warmth and privacy. Clean, warm water prevents chilling and maintains patient comfort.
26. Assist the patient to a prone or side-lying position. Put on gloves, if not applied earlier. Position bath blanket and towel to expose only the back and buttocks.	Positioning the towel and bath blanket protects the patient's privacy and provides warmth. Gloves prevent contact with body fluids.
27. Wash, rinse, if necessary, and dry back and buttocks area (Figure 5). **Pay particular attention to cleansing between gluteal folds, and observe for any redness or skin breakdown in the sacral area.**	Fecal material near the anus may be a source of microorganisms. Prolonged pressure on the sacral area or other bony prominences may compromise circulation and lead to development of decubitus ulcer.

FIGURE 5. Washing the back.

28. If not contraindicated, give the patient a backrub, as described in Skill 10-2, Chapter 10. Alternatively, back massage may be given after perineal care. Apply appropriate emollient and/or skin barrier product.	A backrub improves circulation to the tissues and is an aid to relaxation. A backrub may be contraindicated in patients with cardiovascular disease or musculoskeletal injuries. Use of emollients is recommended to restore and maintain skin integrity (Andriessen, 2013; Lichterfeld et al., 2015; Voegeli, 2010). Skin barriers protect the skin from damage caused by excessive exposure to water and irritants, such as urine and feces.
29. Raise the side rail. Refill basin with clean water. Discard washcloth and towel. Remove gloves and put on clean gloves.	The washcloth, towel, and water are contaminated after washing the patient's gluteal area. Changing to clean supplies decreases the spread of organisms from the anal area to the genitals.
30. Clean perineal area or set the patient up so that he or she can complete perineal self-care. If the patient is unable to do so, lower the side rail and complete perineal care. Follow the guidelines in the accompanying Skill Variation at the end of the skill. Apply skin barrier, as indicated. Raise the side rail, remove gloves, and perform hand hygiene.	Providing perineal self-care may decrease embarrassment for the patient. Effective perineal care reduces odor and decreases the risk for infection through contamination. Skin barriers protect the skin from damage caused by excessive exposure to water and irritants, such as urine and feces.
31. Help the patient put on a clean gown or clothing and assist with the use of other personal toiletries, such as deodorant or cosmetics.	This provides for the patient's warmth and comfort.
32. Protect pillow with towel, and groom the patient's hair.	

ACTION	**RATIONALE**
33. When finished, make sure the patient is comfortable, with the side rails up and the bed in the lowest position.	Proper positioning with raised side rails and proper bed height provides for patient comfort and safety.
34. Change bed linens, as described in Skills 7-10 and 7-11. Dispose of soiled linens according to facility policy. Clean bath basin according to facility policy before returning to storage at bedside. Remove gloves and any other PPE, if used. Perform hand hygiene.	Proper disposal of linens and cleaning of bath basin reduce the risk for transmission of microorganisms. Proper removal of PPE reduces the risk for infection transmission and contamination of other items. Hand hygiene prevents the spread of microorganisms.

EVALUATION

The expected outcomes have been met when the patient is clean; demonstrates some feeling of control in his or her care; verbalizes an improved body image; and verbalizes the importance of cleanliness.

DOCUMENTATION

Guidelines

Record any significant observations and communication. Document the condition of the patient's skin. Record the procedure, amount of assistance given, and patient participation. Document the application of skin care products, such as a skin barrier.

Sample Documentation

> 7/14/20 2130 Bath provided with complete assistance; reddened area (3 cm × 3 cm) noted on patient's sacral area; skin-care team consultation made.
>
> —C. Stone, RN

UNEXPECTED SITUATIONS AND ASSOCIATED INTERVENTIONS

- *The patient becomes chilled during bath:* If the room temperature is adjustable, increase it. Another bath blanket may be needed.
- *The patient becomes unstable during the bath:* Critically ill patients often need to be bathed in stages. For instance, the right arm is bathed, and then the patient is allowed to rest for a short period before the left arm is bathed. The amount of rest time needed depends on how unstable the patient is and which parameter is being monitored. The nurse may watch the blood pressure while bathing an unstable patient and stop when it begins to decrease. Once the blood pressure returns to the previous level, the nurse can begin to bathe the patient again.

SPECIAL CONSIDERATIONS

General Considerations

- To remove the gown from a patient with an IV line, take the gown off the uninvolved arm first and then thread the IV tubing and bottle or bag through the arm of the gown. To replace the gown, place the clean gown on the unaffected arm first and thread the IV tubing and bottle or bag from inside the arm of the gown on the involved side. Never disconnect IV tubing to change a gown, because this causes a break in a sterile system and could introduce infection.
- Patients with bariatric needs are at increased risk of skin breakdown (Cowdell & Radley, 2014). Assess the skin of bariatric inpatients twice a day, lifting and separating the folds of skin to assess the area, utilizing extra help as necessary (Black & Hotaling, 2015). Nonsoap cleansers should be used and the skin should be dried to prevent retained moisture (Black & Hotaling).
- Lying flat in bed during the bed bath may be contraindicated for certain patients. The position may have to be modified to accommodate their needs.
- Incontinent patients require special attention to perineal care. Patients with urinary or fecal incontinence are at risk for perineal skin damage. This damage is related to moisture, changes in skin pH, overgrowth of bacteria and skin infection, and erosion of perineal skin from friction on moist skin. Skin care for these patients should include measures to reduce overhydration (excess exposure to moisture), reduce contact with ammonia and bacteria, and reduce friction.

(continued)

Skill 7-2 ▶ Providing a Bed Bath *(continued)*

Remove soil and irritants from the skin during routine hygiene, as well as cleansing when the skin becomes exposed to irritants. Avoid using soap and excessive force for cleaning. The use of perineal skin cleansers, moisturizers, and moisture barriers is recommended for skin care for the incontinent patient. These products help promote healing and prevent further skin damage.

- If the patient has an indwelling catheter, use mild soap and water or a perineal cleanser to clean the perineal area; rinse the area well. Do not use powders and lotions after cleaning. Do not use antibiotic or other antimicrobial cleaners or betadine at the urethral meatus (Herter & Kazer, 2010; SUNA, 2010). Facility policy may recommend use of an antiseptic cleaning agent or plain cleanser and water to clean the actual catheter. Put on clean gloves before cleaning the catheter. Clean 4 to 6 in of the catheter, moving from the meatus downward. Be careful not to pull or tug on the catheter during the cleaning motion (Underwood, 2015). Inspect the meatus for drainage and note the characteristics of the urine.
- The use of chlorhexidine gluconate (CHG) for bathing has been shown to reduce colonization of skin with pathogens and is an important measure utilized by institutions in an attempt to decrease health care–associated infections (HAIs) (Hines et al., 2015). Some facilities' policies include the use of CHG for all inpatient bathing, expect for patients with a history of CHG allergy or intolerance or those less than 2 months of age (Hines et al.). Chlorhexidine can be added to bath water, but is also available, and easier to use, in prepackaged impregnated cloths.
- If applying lotion, warm the lotion in your hands before applying it to the patient to prevent chilling.
- Soaking the patient's hands in a basin of water is an additional comfort measure for the patient. It facilitates thorough washing of the hands and between the fingers and aids in removing debris from under the nails. If appropriate and as indicated, place a folded towel on the bed next to the patient's hand and put the basin of water on it. Wash, rinse if necessary, and dry hand. Apply appropriate emollient. Use of emollients is recommended to restore and maintain skin integrity (Andriessen, 2013; Lichterfeld et al., 2015; Voegeli, 2010).
- Basic wound care used for body piercings is usually called "aftercare." Aftercare techniques are used for the new piercing and whenever the piercing fistula has become disrupted through injury or exhibits signs of infection or inflammation (Halliday, 2005; MFMER, 2015a). Clean the jewelry and the piercing site of all crust and debris. Rinse the site with warm water and use a cotton swab to gently remove any crusting. Rinse well.

Infant and Child Considerations

- When bathing an infant or young child, have supplies within easy reach, and support or hold the child securely at all times to ensure safety.
- Never leave the child alone.
- Consider bathing a newborn using a reverse-order procedure, from "trunk to head," wetting the infant's head last to reduce the amount of time the infant's head is wet. The method supports a more rapid recovery of body temperature and decreased heat loss from evaporation during bathing (So et al., 2014).

Older Adult Considerations

- Check the temperature of the water carefully before bathing an older adult, because sensitivity to temperature may be impaired in older adults.
- An older, continent patient may not require a full bed bath with soap and water every day. If dry skin is a problem, water and skin lotion or bath oil may be used on alternate days.

Home Care Considerations

- Use plastic trash bags or a plastic shower-curtain liner to protect the mattress when bathing or shampooing a patient in bed. Disposable washcloths may also be an option to consider. A large plastic container or baby bathtub can effectively serve as a shampoo basin.
- If linens are soiled with blood or body fluids, instruct family members to wear gloves when handling them. They should be rinsed first in cold water and then washed separately from other household wash, using hot water, laundry detergent, and bleach.
- Teach a family member or caregiver how to perform comfort measures, such as a backrub.
- If patients are home with an indwelling catheter, instruct them or their caregivers to wash the urinary meatus and perineal area twice daily with mild soap and water or a perineal cleanser.
- Teach patients to clean the anal area after each bowel movement. Careful handwashing is imperative.

Skill Variation > Performing Perineal Cleansing

Perineal cleaning should be performed in a matter-of-fact and dignified manner. If this approach is followed, patients generally do not find care provided by a person who does not share the patient's sex or gender to be offensive or embarrassing. When performing perineal care, follow these guidelines:

1. Perform hand hygiene and put on PPE, if indicated.

2. Identify the patient.

3. Explain what you are going to do and the reason for doing it to the patient.
4. Assemble necessary equipment on the bedside stand or overbed table.

5. Close curtains around the bed and close the door to the room, if possible.
6. Put on gloves. Cover the patient with a bath blanket and remove top linens to expose only the perineal area. Wash and rinse the groin area (both male and female patients):
   - **For a female patient**, spread the labia and move the washcloth from the pubic area toward the anal area to prevent carrying organisms from the anal area back over the genital area (Figure A). Always proceed from the least contaminated area to the most contaminated area. Use a clean portion of the washcloth for each stroke. Rinse the washed areas well with plain water.
   - **For a male patient**, clean the tip of the penis first, moving the washcloth in a circular motion from the meatus outward. Wash the shaft of the penis using downward strokes toward the pubic area (Figure B). Always proceed from the least contaminated area to the most

FIGURE A. Performing female perineal care.

FIGURE B. Performing male perineal care.

(continued)

Skill 7-2 ▶ Providing a Bed Bath *(continued)*

Skill Variation ▶ Performing Perineal Cleansing *(continued)*

contaminated area. Rinse the washed areas well with plain water. In an *uncircumcised male patient* (teenage or older), retract the foreskin (prepuce) while washing the penis. **It is not recommended to retract the foreskin for cleaning during infancy and childhood, because injury and scarring could occur** (MedlinePlus, 2015).

- Pull the *uncircumcised male patient's* (teenage or older) foreskin back into place over the glans penis to prevent constriction of the penis, which may result in edema and tissue injury. Wash and rinse the male patient's scrotum. Handle the scrotum, which houses the testicles, with care because the area is sensitive.

7. Dry the cleaned areas and apply an emollient, as indicated. Apply skin barrier (protectant) to area, as indicated. Avoid the use of powder. Powder may become a medium for bacteria growth.

8. Turn the patient on his or her side and continue cleansing the anal area. Continue in the direction of least contaminated to most contaminated area. In the female, cleanse from the vagina toward the anus. In both female and male patients, change the washcloth with each stroke until the area is clean. Rinse and dry the area. Apply skin barrier (protectant) to area, as indicated.

 9. Remove gloves and perform hand hygiene. Continue with additional care as necessary.

Skill Variation ▶ Giving a Bath Using a Disposable Self-Contained Bathing System

A disposable bathing system is packaged with eight to ten premoistened disposable washcloths. If more than eight cloths are available in the package, use a separate cloth for hands and feet. When giving a bath with a disposable system, follow these guidelines:

1. Warm the unopened package in the microwave, according to manufacturer's directions or remove package from storage warmer (Figure A).

 2. Perform hand hygiene and put on PPE, if indicated.

3. Identify the patient.

4. Explain what you are going to do and the reason for doing it to the patient.

5. Assemble necessary equipment on the bedside stand or overbed table.

6. Close the curtains around the bed and close the door to the room, if possible.

7. Put on gloves. Cover the patient with a bath blanket and remove top linens. Remove the patient's gown and keep the bath blanket in place.

8. Remove first cloth from the package. Wipe one eye from the inner part of the eye, near the nose, to the outer part. Use a different part of the cloth for the other eye.

9. Bathe the face, neck, and ears. Allow the skin to air dry for approximately 30 seconds, according to manufacturer's

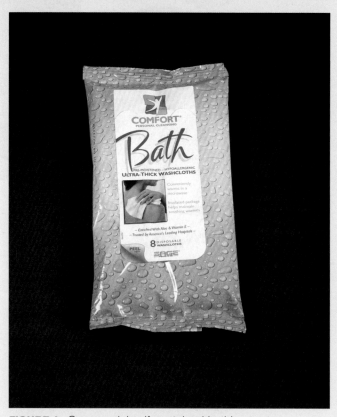

FIGURE A. Commercial self-contained bathing system. (*Photo by B. Proud.*)

directions. Air drying allows the emollient ingredient of the cleanser to remain on the skin. Alternately, dry the skin with a towel, based on the product used. Apply appropriate emollient. Dispose of cloth in trash receptacle.

10. Expose the patient's far arm. Remove another cloth. Using firm strokes, wash hand, arm, and axilla. Allow the skin to air dry for approximately 30 seconds, according to manufacturer's directions. Air drying allows the emollient ingredient of the cleanser to remain on the skin. Alternately, dry the skin with a towel, based on the product used. Apply appropriate emollient. Dispose of cloth in trash receptacle. Cover arm with blanket.

11. Repeat for nearer arm with a new cloth. Cover arm with blanket.

12. Expose the patient's chest. Remove new cloth and cleanse chest. Allow the skin to air dry for approximately 30 seconds, according to manufacturer's directions. Cover chest with a towel. Expose the patient's abdomen. Cleanse abdomen. Allow the skin to air dry for approximately 30 seconds, according to manufacturer's directions. Air drying allows the emollient ingredient of the cleanser to remain on the skin. Alternately, dry the skin with a towel, based on the product used. Apply appropriate emollient. Dispose of cloth in trash receptacle. Cover the patient's body with blanket.

13. Expose far leg. Remove new cloth and cleanse leg and foot. Allow the skin to air dry for approximately 30 seconds, according to manufacturer's directions. Air drying allows the emollient ingredient of the cleanser to remain on the skin. Alternately, dry the skin with a towel, based

on the product used. Apply appropriate emollient. Dispose of cloth in trash receptacle. Cover the patient's leg with blanket.

14. Repeat for nearer leg with a new cloth. Cover leg with blanket.

15. Assist the patient to prone or side-lying position. Put on gloves, if not applied earlier. Position blanket to expose back and buttocks. Remove a new cloth and cleanse back and buttocks area. Allow the skin to air dry for approximately 30 seconds, according to manufacturer's directions. Air drying allows the emollient ingredient of the cleanser to remain on the skin. Alternately, dry the skin with a towel, based on the product used. Apply appropriate emollient. Dispose of cloth in trash receptacle. If not contraindicated, give the patient a back massage. Apply skin barrier, as indicated. Cover the patient with blanket.

16. Remove gloves and put on clean gloves. Remove last cloth and cleanse the perineal area. Refer to the guidelines in the previous Skill Variation. Dispose of cloth in trash receptacle. Apply skin barrier, as indicated.

17. Remove gloves. Assist the patient to put on a clean gown or appropriate clothing. Perform hand hygiene. Assist with the use of other personal toiletries.

18. Change bed linens as described in Skills 7-10 and 7-11. Dispose of soiled linens according to facility policy.

19. Remove gloves and additional PPE, if used. Perform hand hygiene.

EVIDENCE FOR PRACTICE ▶

NO-RINSE DISPOSABLE WASH GLOVES

The use of disposable bath products is an alternative to traditional use of skin cleanser and water. Use of these products has increased and often does not require rinsing. Disposable wash gloves are one alternative that may be implemented to provide personal hygiene.

Related Research

Schoonhoven, L., van Gaal, B. G. I., Teerenstra, S., Adang, E., van der Vleuten, C., & van Achterberg, T. (2015). Cost-consequence analysis of "washing without water" for nursing home residents: A cluster randomized trial. *International Journal of Nursing Studies, 52*(1), 112–120.

   This study examined the use of prepackaged disposable wash gloves versus the traditional bed bath using skin cleanser and water and a bath basin. The study took place over a 19-month period, in 22 nursing homes, and used a cluster randomized design involving 500 adult care-dependent residents. The study compared the use of each type of bathing procedure in relation to effects on skin integrity, resistance on the part of the participants during bathing, and costs. The study also examined satisfaction in residents and nurses in the group using the wash gloves. The bed bath regimens were continued for 6 weeks for each cluster of participants. The disposable wash gloves were impregnated with a no-rinse, quickly vaporizing skin cleaning and caring lotion. Each glove package contained eight disposable gloves and were heated in a microwave before use. The traditional bed bath consisted of a wash basin, towels, tap water, and skin cleanser. Patients who received bathing with the wash gloves experienced slightly decreased skin abnormalities and lesions. There was no statistically significant difference in cost for preparing

(continued)

Skill 7-2 ► Providing a Bed Bath *(continued)*

and performing the baths between the bathing procedures. Cognitively intact residents who received bathing with wash gloves indicated that washing without water was effective in cleaning the skin. They reported feeling refreshed, with skin that felt moister, and indicated that they would replace traditional bathing for washing without water. The majority of nurses indicated sufficient satisfaction with the wash glove product. The authors concluded that washing without water mildly protects the skin without additional costs when compared with traditional bathing, and can be considered the more efficient alternative.

Relevance for Nursing Practice

This study suggests that implementing bathing procedures utilizing alternatives to traditional cleanser and water are effective in providing personal hygiene. Nurses and nursing staff are the primary providers of bathing activities in many health care settings, and should consider implementing efficient interventions, such as wash gloves, to enhance patient experiences related to personal hygiene and improve skin health.

Refer to thePoint® for additional research on related nursing topics.

Skill 7-3 ► Assisting the Patient With Oral Care

Adequate oral hygiene care is imperative to promote the patient's sense of well-being and prevent deterioration of the oral cavity. Poor oral hygiene is reported to lead to the colonization of the oropharyngeal secretions by respiratory pathogens. Diligent oral hygiene care can improve oral health and limit the growth of pathogens in the oropharyngeal secretions, decreasing the incidence of aspiration pneumonia, community-acquired pneumonia, hospital-acquired nonventilator-associated pneumonia, and ventilator-associated pneumonia (AACN, 2010; Coker, Ploeg, Kaasalainen, & Fisher, 2013; Hillier, Wilson, Chamberlain, King, 2013; Quinn & Baker, 2015).

The mouth requires care particularly during illness, but sometimes care must be modified to meet a patient's needs. If the patient can assist with mouth care, provide the necessary materials. Oral care is important not only to prevent dental **gingivitis** and **caries**, but also to improve the patient's self-image. Teeth should be brushed and flossed twice a day; the mouth should be rinsed after meals. If the patient is unable to perform oral hygiene, make certain that the mouth receives care as often as necessary to keep it clean and moist, as often as every 1 or 2 hours if necessary. This is especially important for patients who cannot drink or are not permitted fluids by mouth. Refer to Box 7-2 for suggestions to meet the oral hygiene needs for patients with cognitive impairments.

Box 7-2 Meeting the Oral Hygiene Needs of Patients With Cognitive Impairments

- Choose a time of day when the patient is most calm and accepting of care.
- Enlist the aid of a family member or significant other.
- Break the task into small steps.
- Provide distraction, such as playing favorite music, while providing care.
- Allow the patient to participate. The nurse can put a hand over the patient's hand to guide the activity.

- The nurse can start the activity, show the patient what to do, then let the patient take over.
- If the patient strongly refuses care, withdraw and re-approach later.
- Effective and ineffective interventions should be documented to provide appropriate information for staff to give consistent, person-centered care.

Source: Adapted from Alzheimer's Association. (2016). Dental care. Retrieved https://www.alz.org/care/alzheimers-dementia-dental.asp; Eliopoulos, C. (2014). *Gerontological Nursing* (8th ed.). Philadelphia, PA: Wolters Kluwer Health; and Konno, R., Kang, H. S., & Makimoto, K. (2014). A best-evidence review of intervention studies for minimizing resistance-to-care behaviours for older adults with dementia in nursing homes. *Journal of Advanced Nursing, 70*(10), 2167–2180.

DELEGATION CONSIDERATIONS	The implementation of oral care may be delegated to nursing assistive personnel (NAP) or to unlicensed assistive personnel (UAP), as well as to licensed practical/vocational nurses (LPN/LVNs). The decision to delegate must be based on careful analysis of the patient's needs and circumstances, as well as the qualifications of the person to whom the task is being delegated. Refer to the Delegation Guidelines in Appendix A.

EQUIPMENT

- Toothbrush
- Toothpaste
- Emesis basin
- Glass with cool water
- Disposable gloves
- Additional PPE, as indicated

- Towel
- Mouth rinse
- Washcloth or paper towel
- Lip lubricant (optional)
- Dental floss or other interdental cleaner
- Oral assessment tool, as indicated (Figure 1)

ASSESSMENT

Assess the patient's oral hygiene preferences: frequency, time of day, and type of hygiene products. Assess for any physical activity limitations. An oral assessment tool can assist with assessment of the status of the oral cavity, as well as help to determine the frequency and procedure for oral care (Figure 1 on next page). Assess the patient's oral cavity and dentition. Look for any inflammation or bleeding of the gums. Look for ulcers, lesions, and yellow or white patches. The yellow or white patches may indicate a fungal infection called thrush. Assess for signs of dehydration (dry mucosa) and dental decay. Look at the lips for dryness or cracking. Ask the patient if he or she is having pain, dryness, soreness, or difficulty chewing or swallowing. Assess the patient's ability to perform own care.

NURSING DIAGNOSIS

Determine the related factors for the nursing diagnoses based on the patient's current status. Appropriate nursing diagnoses may include:

- Risk for aspiration
- Impaired oral mucous membrane integrity
- Impaired dentition

OUTCOME IDENTIFICATION AND PLANNING

The expected outcome to achieve is that the patient's mouth and teeth will be clean; the patient will exhibit a positive body image; and the patient will verbalize the importance of oral care.

IMPLEMENTATION

ACTION	RATIONALE
1. Perform hand hygiene and put on gloves if assisting with oral care, and/or other PPE, if indicated.	Hand hygiene and PPE prevent the spread of microorganisms. PPE is required based on transmission precautions.
2. Identify the patient. Explain the procedure to the patient.	Identifying the patient ensures the right patient receives the intervention and helps prevent errors. Explanation facilitates cooperation.
3. Assemble equipment on overbed table or other surface within the patient's reach.	Organization facilitates performance of the task.
4. Close the room door or curtains. Place the bed at an appropriate and comfortable working height; usually elbow height of the caregiver (VHACEOSH, 2016).	Closing the door or curtains provides privacy. Proper bed height helps reduce back strain while performing the procedure.
5. Lower the side rail and assist the patient to a sitting position, if permitted, or turn the patient onto side. Place towel across the patient's chest.	The sitting or side-lying position prevents aspiration of fluids into the lungs. The towel protects the patient from dampness.

(continued)

Skill 7-3 ▶ Assisting the Patient With Oral Care *(continued)*

Oral Health Assessment Tool (OHAT) - Modified
Mouth Care Without a Battle©

Person Assessed:_____ Assessed by:_____ Date:_____

*For each category, circle the one best description. Then, in the column marked score, write the points for the assessment. Add the points in the bottom row. Problems __underlined and in bold__ are indications for immediate referral to a dentist, as they may represent a serious condition. For nursing home residents, problems in **bold** may require documentation on the MDS 3.0 and may trigger the Dental Care CAA, regardless of the total score.*

Category	0 = Healthy	1 = Minor Problems	2 = Major Problems	Score*
Lips	Smooth, pink, moist	Dry, chapped, or red at corners	**New or growing lump, ulcer, or lesion; white, red, and/or ulcerated patch; bleeding and/or ulcer at corners**	
Gums, palate, and insides of cheeks	Pink, moist, smooth, no bleeding	Dry, shiny, rough, red, and/or swollen area; **one small ulcer, lesion, and/or sore spot under dentures**	__Swollen, tender area around a tooth or tooth root (suspected abscess);__ **swollen and/or bleeding ulcer; white, red and/or ulcerated patch; small pimple-like area with pus; widespread redness under dentures**	
Natural teeth	No decay or broken or worn down teeth	1-3 decayed or broken and/or very worn down teeth	__One or more very loose teeth;__ **4 or more decayed or broken or very worn down teeth; fewer than 4 teeth**	
Dentures	No broken areas; teeth, dentures are regularly worn, and dentures are labeled with name	**1 broken area or tooth; denture loose, but adhesive not needed; denture uncleanable; denture not labeled with name;** dentures only worn for 1-2 hrs daily	**More than 1 broken area or tooth; denture so loose adhesive needed;** denture missing or not worn	
Quality of tooth hygiene	Clean and no food particles or tartar in mouth or on dentures	Food particles, tartar, and/or plaque in 1-2 areas of the mouth or on small area of dentures; bad breath (halitosis)	Food particles, tartar, and/or plaque in most areas of the mouth or on most of dentures; severe bad breath (halitosis)	
Tooth pain	No behavioral, verbal, or physical signs of dental pain	**Nonspecific verbal and/or behavioral signs of pain such as pulling at face, chewing lips, or not eating; unexplained aggression**	**Physical signs of pain (swelling of cheek or gum, broken teeth, ulcers); verbal and/or behavioral signs of pain specific to the mouth**	
Saliva / dry mouth	Moist tissues, watery and free flowing saliva	Dry, sticky tissues, little saliva present; person complains of dry mouth	Tissues parched and red; very little/no saliva present; saliva is thick	
Tongue	Normal, moist, roughness, pink	Patchy, fissured, red, coated	Patch that is red and/or white, ulcerated, and/or swollen	
			Total Score	

FIGURE 1. Oral Health Assessment Tool (OHAT). (Mouth Care Without a Battle, UNC Cecil G. Sheps Center for Health Services Research. Used by Permission. Modified from Kayser-Jones et al., *Gerontologist* 35:814–24, 1995, and Chalmers et al., *Journal of Gerontological Nursing*, 30[11]:5–12, 2004.)

ACTION

6. Encourage the patient to brush own teeth according to the following guidelines. Assist, if necessary.

   a. Moisten toothbrush and apply toothpaste to bristles.

   b. Place brush at a 45-degree angle to gum line (Figure 2) and brush from gum line to crown of each tooth (Figure 3). Brush outer and inner surfaces. Brush back and forth across biting surface of each tooth.

FIGURE 2. Placing brush at a 45-degree angle to gum line.

   c. Brush tongue gently with toothbrush (Figure 4).

   d. Have the patient rinse vigorously with water and spit into emesis basin (Figure 5). Repeat until clear. Suction may be used as an alternative for removal of fluid and secretions from the mouth.

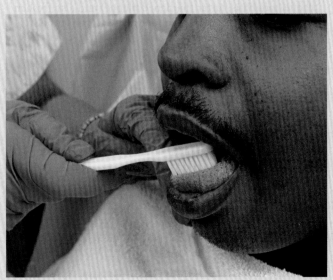

FIGURE 4. Brushing tongue.

RATIONALE

Water softens the bristles.

Facilitates removal of **plaque** and **tartar**. The 45-degree angle of brushing permits cleansing of all tooth surface areas.

FIGURE 3. Brushing from gum line to the crown of each tooth.

Removes coating on the tongue. Gentle motion does not stimulate gag reflex.

The vigorous swishing motion helps to remove debris. Suction is appropriate if the patient is unable to expectorate well.

FIGURE 5. Holding emesis basin for patient to rinse and spit.

(*continued*)

Skill 7-3 ▶ Assisting the Patient With Oral Care (continued)

ACTION	RATIONALE
7. Assist patient to floss teeth, if appropriate:	Flossing aids in removal of plaque and promotes healthy gum tissue.
a. Remove approximately 18 in of dental floss from container or use a plastic floss holder. Wrap most of the floss around one of the middle fingers. Wind the remaining floss around the same finger of the opposite hand, keeping about 1 to 1.5 in of floss taut between the fingers.	The floss must be held taut to get between the teeth.
b. Insert floss gently between teeth, moving it back and forth downward to the gums.	Trauma to the gums can occur if floss is forced between teeth.
c. Move the floss up and down, first on one side of a tooth and then on the side of the other tooth, until the surfaces are clean (Figure 6). Repeat in the spaces between all teeth and the backside of the last teeth.	This ensures that the sides of both teeth are cleaned.
d. Instruct the patient to rinse mouth well with water after flossing.	Vigorous rinsing helps to remove food particles and plaque that have been loosened by flossing.

FIGURE 6. Flossing teeth.

ACTION	RATIONALE
8. Offer a mouth rinse if the patient prefers or if use has been recommended.	Use of a mouth rinse can reduce bacteria and can help reduce plaque, gingivitis, tartar (hardened plaque) and also freshen breath. Anticavity rinses with fluoride help protect tooth enamel to help prevent or control tooth decay (American Dental Association [ADA], n.d.a).
9. Offer lip balm or petroleum jelly.	Lip balm lubricates lips and prevents drying.
10. Remove equipment. Remove gloves and discard. Raise the side rail and lower the bed. Assist the patient to a position of comfort.	Removing gloves properly reduces the risk for infection transmission and contamination of other items. These actions promote patient comfort and safety.
11. Remove any other PPE, if used. Perform hand hygiene.	Proper removal of PPE reduces the risk for infection transmission and contamination of other items. Hand hygiene prevents the spread of microorganisms.

EVALUATION

The expected outcomes have been met when the patient receives oral care, experiences little to no discomfort, states mouth feels refreshed, and demonstrates understanding the reasons for proper oral care.

DOCUMENTATION

Guidelines

Record oral assessment, significant observations, and unusual findings, such as bleeding or inflammation. Document any teaching done. Document procedure and patient response.

Sample Documentation

> <u>10/2020</u> 0930 Patient performed oral care with minimal assistance. Oral cavity mucosa pink and moist. No evidence of bleeding or ulceration. Lips slightly dry; lip moisturizer applied. Reinforcement provided related to importance of flossing teeth every day. Patient demonstrates appropriate flossing technique.
>
> —*L. Schneider, RN*

UNEXPECTED SITUATIONS AND ASSOCIATED INTERVENTIONS

- *While cleaning the teeth, you notice a large amount of bleeding from the gum line:* Stop brushing. Allow the patient to gently rinse mouth with water and spit into emesis basin. Before brushing again, check the patient's most recent platelet level. Consider the use of a softer toothbrush to provide oral hygiene.
- *The patient has braces on teeth:* Braces collect food particles. Brush extra thoroughly. Reinforce the importance of using an appropriate interdental cleaner.

SPECIAL CONSIDERATIONS

General Considerations

- Use a soft-bristled toothbrush with a small head even when the patient has no or few teeth. It is the only effective way to remove plaque and debris from the teeth, gums, and tongue.
- A patient receiving chemotherapy medication may have bleeding gums and extremely sensitive mucous membranes. Use an extra-soft toothbrush after every meal and at bedtime, and rinse the mouth several times a day with a solution of ¼ teaspoon of salt or 1 teaspoon of baking soda in 8 oz of warm water, followed by a plain water rinse (NIH, 2014). If brushing hurts, bristles can be softened in warm water (NIH, 2014).
- Automatic toothbrushes, electric or battery operated, are simple to use and are as good as manual brushes for removing debris and plaque. These devices are very useful for patients with arthritis or other conditions that make it difficult to brush effectively (MFMER, 2016).
- The use of chlorhexidine gluconate (CHG) as part of oral hygiene has been integrated into oral hygiene regimens and is available in an oral spray and dental gel (Ames et al., 2011; Kelly, Timmis, & Twelvetree, 2010; Nicolosi, del Carmen Rubio, Martinez, Gonzáles, Cruz, 2014). The use of CHG as part of protocols for systematic oral care for critically ill patients has been shown to reduce the incidence of health care–associated pneumonia (Nicolosi et al.).

Infant and Child Considerations

- Begin brushing children's teeth as soon as they begin to come into the mouth and begin flossing when the child has two teeth that touch (ADA, 2016a).
- Clean an infant's gums by wiping with a clean, damp cloth.
- Young children should be supervised by an adult until around age six (Jablonski, Mertz, Featherstone, Fulmer, 2014).
- Use smaller amounts of fluoride toothpaste on the toothbrush for children: a smear (size of a grain of rice) for children younger than 3 years of age and a pea-sized amount for children 3 to 6 years of age (ADA, 2016a).

EVIDENCE FOR PRACTICE ▶

ORAL HYGIENE AND OLDER ADULTS

Poor oral hygiene contributes to alterations in oral health, and is associated with increased risk for aspiration pneumonia, community-acquired pneumonia, and other health concerns (Coker et al., 2013; Hillier et al., 2013; Quinn & Baker, 2015). Poor oral health in older adults compounds dental problems associated with aging. Adequate oral hygiene is essential to promote a sense of well-being and prevent deterioration of the oral cavity.

(continued)

Skill 7-3 ▶ Assisting the Patient With Oral Care *(continued)*

Related Research

Jennings, A. (2015). Assessing oral hygiene in hospitalized older veterans. *MEDSURG Nursing*, 24(6), 420–424.

This pilot study surveyed 50 veterans aged 60 and older from two medical units at a veteran's medical center for a period of 3 months. Participants completed a questionnaire designed to assist health care providers in monitoring older adults' oral hygiene regimes. Questions addressed current oral status, denture use, self-care ability, brushing aid and frequency, flossing, denture care, mouth rinses, saliva stimulant, and difficulties with daily oral care. Twenty percent of study participants did not brush their teeth on a regular basis. Eighty percent of participants reported not flossing their teeth, only 18% used denture cleaner, and 16% reported using mouthwash. Participants' responses highlighted several oral cavity issues, including bleeding gums (20%), bleeding with flossing (10%), forgetting to brush teeth (16%), and neglecting regular checkups with a dentist (10%). The authors concluded that oral hygiene care and habits among older veterans need improvement and suggest that further exploration is warranted to identify possible contributing factors as well as barriers that prevent nurses from encouraging and participating in oral care with older adults.

Relevance for Nursing Practice

Poor oral hygiene can contribute to poor oral health and oral diseases, as well as other systemic health problems. By performing oral assessments, providing oral hygiene education, and promoting tooth brushing, flossing, and use of other dental services, nurses can be instrumental in supporting optimal oral health outcomes and prevention of oral diseases in older adults.

EVIDENCE FOR PRACTICE ▶

CLINICAL PRACTICE GUIDELINE
Oral Hygiene Care for Functionally Dependent and Cognitively Impaired Older Adults

Johnson, V. B., & Chalmers, J. (2011). Oral hygiene care for functionally dependent and cognitively impaired older adults. Iowa City, IA: University of Iowa College of Nursing. National Guideline Clearinghouse. Retrieved https://www.guideline.gov/content.aspx?id=34447.

This evidence-based guideline provides practical information for health care providers and caregivers in the provision and documentation of oral hygiene care for functionally dependent and cognitively impaired older adults.

Refer to thePoint® for additional research on related nursing topics.

Skill 7-4 ▶ Providing Oral Care for the Dependent Patient

Physical limitations, such as those associated with aging, often lead to less than adequate oral hygiene. The dexterity required for adequate brushing and flossing may decrease with age or illness. Older adults may be dependent on caregivers for oral hygiene. Patients with cognitive impairment, such as dementia and mental illness, are also at risk for inadequate oral hygiene (Brennan & Strauss, 2014; Kadia, Bawas, Shah, Narang, Lippmann, 2014; Lee et al., 2013). Refer to Box 7-2 in Skill 7-3 for suggestions to meet the oral hygiene needs for patients with cognitive impairments.

Teeth should be brushed and flossed twice a day; the mouth should be rinsed after meals. If the patient is unable to perform oral hygiene, make certain that the mouth receives care as often as necessary to keep it clean and moist, as often as every 1 or 2 hours, if necessary. This is especially important for patients who cannot drink or are not permitted fluids by mouth. Moisten the mouth with water, if allowed, and lubricate the lips often enough to keep the membranes well moistened.

DELEGATION CONSIDERATIONS

The implementation of oral care for a dependent patient may be delegated to nursing assistive personnel (NAP) or to unlicensed assistive personnel (UAP) after assessment by the registered nurse, as well as to licensed practical/vocational nurses (LPN/LVNs). The decision to delegate must be based on careful analysis of the patient's needs and circumstances, as well as the qualifications of the person to whom the task is being delegated. Refer to the Delegation Guidelines in Appendix A.

EQUIPMENT

- Suction toothbrush (Figure 4) or soft toothbrush
- Suction swab
- Suction catheter with suction apparatus
- Toothpaste or other oral cleanser
- Emesis basin
- Glass with cool water
- Disposable gloves
- Additional PPE, as indicated
- Towel
- Mouth rinse (optional)

- Dental floss in holder or other interdental cleaner
- Mouth-prop or second toothbrush (Figure 1)
- Denture-cleaning equipment (if necessary)
  - Denture cup
  - Denture cleaner
  - 4 × 4 gauze
  - Washcloth or paper towel
- Lip lubricant (optional)
- Oral health assessment tool (Figure 1 in Skill 7-3)
- Additional care giver, as indicated

ASSESSMENT

Assess the patient's oral hygiene preferences: frequency, time of day, and type of hygiene products. Assess for any physical activity limitations. Assess the patient's level of consciousness and overall ability to assist with oral care and respond to directions. Assess the patient's risk for oral hygiene problems. Alterations in cognitive function and/or consciousness increase the risk for alterations in oral tissue and structure integrity. Assess the patient's gag reflex. Decreased or absent gag reflex increases the risk for aspiration. An oral assessment tool can assist with assessment of the status of the oral cavity, as well as help to determine the frequency and procedure for oral care (Figure 1 in Skill 7-3). Assess the patient's oral cavity and dentition. Look for any inflammation or bleeding of the gums. Look for ulcers, lesions, and yellow or white patches. The yellow or white patches may indicate a fungal infection called thrush. Assess for signs of dehydration (dry mucosa) and dental decay. Look at the lips for dryness or cracking. If the patient is conscious and/or cognitively able to respond, ask the patient if he or she is having pain, dryness, soreness, or difficulty chewing or swallowing.

NURSING DIAGNOSIS

Determine the related factors for the nursing diagnoses based on the patient's current status. Appropriate nursing diagnoses may include:

- Impaired oral mucous membrane integrity
- Chronic confusion
- Risk for aspiration

OUTCOME IDENTIFICATION AND PLANNING

The expected outcome to achieve when performing oral care is that the patient's mouth and teeth are clean; the patient does not experience impaired oral mucous membranes; and the patient verbalizes, if able, an understanding about the importance of oral care.

IMPLEMENTATION

ACTION	RATIONALE
1. Perform hand hygiene and put on PPE, if indicated.	Hand hygiene and PPE prevent the spread of microorganisms. PPE is required based on transmission precautions.
2. Identify the patient. Explain the procedure to the patient.	Identifying the patient ensures the right patient receives the intervention and helps prevent errors. Explanation facilitates cooperation.

(continued)

Skill 7-4   Providing Oral Care for the Dependent Patient *(continued)*

ACTION	RATIONALE
3. Assemble equipment on overbed table or other surface within reach.	Organization facilitates performance of task.
4. Close the room door or curtains. Place the bed at an appropriate and comfortable working height, usually elbow height of the caregiver (VHACEOSH, 2016). Lower one side rail and position the patient on the side, with head tilted forward. Place towel across the patient's chest and emesis basin in position under chin. Depending on equipment in use, connect the suction toothbrush or suction catheter to suction tubing and turn on suction. Put on gloves.	Cleaning another person's mouth is invasive and may be embarrassing (Holman, Roberts, Nicol, 2005). Closing the door or curtains provides privacy. Proper bed height helps reduce back strain while performing the procedure. The side-lying position with head forward prevents aspiration of fluid into lungs. Towel and emesis basin protect the patient from dampness. Suction provides means to remove oral hygiene products and saliva from oral cavity (Johnson & Chalmers, 2011). Gloves prevent the spread of microorganisms.
5. Gently open the patient's mouth by applying pressure to the lower jaw at the front of the mouth. Do not use fingers to hold the patient's mouth open. Use another toothbrush or mouth prop (Figure 1) to keep the mouth open (Johnson & Chalmers, 2011). Remove dentures, if present. (Refer to Skill 7-5.)	Patients with altered cognition may inadvertently bite fingers inserted into the mouth. Removal of dentures allows for cleaning of dentures and oral cavity.

FIGURE 1. Example of a mouth prop. (Used with permission from Neo-Health Services, Inc. ©2011 OrofacialMyology.com. All rights reserved.)

ACTION	RATIONALE
6. If using a regular toothbrush and suction catheter, one care giver provides oral cleaning and the other removes secretions with the suction catheter.	Allows for efficient care to reduce the risk of aspiration.
7. Brush the teeth and gums carefully with toothbrush and paste or other oral cleanser (Figure 2). Lightly brush the tongue.	Toothbrush provides friction necessary to clean areas where plaque and tartar accumulate.
8. Moisten toothbrush with water to rinse the oral cavity. **Position the patient's head to allow for return of water. If using regular toothbrush, use suction catheter to remove the water and cleanser from oral cavity (Figure 3).**	Rinsing helps clean debris from the mouth. Suction toothbrush removes fluids and cleansers.

FIGURE 2. Carefully brushing patient's teeth.

FIGURE 3. Using suction to remove excess fluid.

ACTION	RATIONALE
9. Using the suction swab, apply a therapeutic antiseptic mouth rinse as indicated. Apply oral moisturizer as indicated.	Therapeutic and antiseptic mouth rinses reduce bacteria and reduce plaque, gingivitis, tartar, and reduce the incidence of health care–associated pneumonia (ADA, n.d.a; Lev, Aied, & Arshed, 2015; Nicolosi et al., 2014). Oral moisturizers provide moisture to the mucosa.
10. Clean the dentures before replacing. (See Skill 7-5.)	Cleaning maintains dentures and oral hygiene. Plaque can accumulate on dentures and promote oropharyngeal colonization of pathogens.
11. Apply lubricant to the patient's lips.	This prevents drying and cracking of lips.
12. Remove equipment and return the patient to a position of comfort. Remove gloves. Raise the side rail and lower the bed.	Promotes patient comfort and safety. Removing gloves properly reduces the risk for infection transmission and contamination of other items.
13. Remove additional PPE, if used. Perform hand hygiene.	Proper removal of PPE reduces the risk for infection transmission and contamination of other items. Hand hygiene prevents the spread of microorganisms.

EVALUATION	The expected outcomes have been met when the patient's oral cavity is clean and free from complications, and, the patient, if able, verbalizes a basic understanding of the need for oral care.
DOCUMENTATION	
Guidelines	Record oral assessment, significant observations, and unusual findings, such as bleeding or inflammation. Document any teaching done. Document care provided and patient response.
Sample Documentation	7/10/20 0945 Oral care performed. Oral cavity mucosa pink and moist. Small amount of bleeding noted from gums after using soft-bristled toothbrush. Resolved spontaneously when brushing completed. No evidence of ulceration. Lips slightly dry; lip moisturizer applied. —C. Stone, RN
UNEXPECTED SITUATIONS AND ASSOCIATED INTERVENTIONS	• *The patient begins to bite the toothbrush:* Do not jerk the toothbrush out. Wait for the patient to relax mouth before removing the toothbrush and continuing with care. Use distraction, gentle touch or massage to divert the patient (Johnson & Chalmers, 2011). • *Mouth is extremely dry with crusts that remain after oral care provided:* Increase frequency of oral hygiene. Apply mouth moisturizer to oral mucosa. Monitor fluid intake and output to ensure adequate intake of fluid.
SPECIAL CONSIDERATIONS	• Suction toothbrushes may be used with patients with **dysphagia** (Figure 4). • A patient receiving chemotherapy medication may have bleeding gums and extremely sensitive mucous membranes. Use an extra-soft toothbrush after every meal and at bedtime, and rinse the mouth several times a day with a solution of ¼ teaspoon of salt or 1 teaspoon of baking soda in 8 oz of warm water, followed by a plain water rinse (NIH, 2014). If brushing hurts, bristles can be softened in warm water (NIH, 2014). • Use a soft bristled toothbrush with a small head even when the patient has no or few teeth. It is the only effective way to remove plaque and debris from the teeth, gums, and tongue.

FIGURE 4. Example of a suction toothbrush. (Permission granted by Sage Products LLC.)

Skill 7-5 ▶ Providing Denture Care

Adequate oral hygiene care is imperative to promote the patient's sense of well-being and prevent deterioration of the oral cavity. Poor oral hygiene is reported to lead to the colonization of the oropharyngeal secretions by respiratory pathogens. Plaque, which can accumulate on dentures, can promote oropharyngeal colonization of pathogens. Diligent oral hygiene care can improve oral health and limit the growth of pathogens in the oropharyngeal secretions, decreasing the incidence of aspiration pneumonia, community-acquired pneumonia, hospital-acquired nonventilator-associated pneumonia, and ventilator-associated pneumonia (AACN, 2010; Coker et al., 2013; Hillier et al., 2013; Quinn & Baker, 2015). It is important to clean dentures daily and to remove and rinse dentures and mouth after meals. Dentures may be cleaned more often, based on need and the patient's personal preference. To reduce or minimize denture stomatitis (irritation of the oral tissues), it is recommended that dentures not be worn continuously (24 hours per day); dentures are often removed at night (ADA, 2016b; Felton et al., 2011). Handle dentures with care to prevent breakage. Refer to Box 7-2 in Skill 7-3 for suggestions to meet the oral hygiene needs for patients with cognitive impairments.

DELEGATION CONSIDERATIONS	The implementation of denture care may be delegated to nursing assistive personnel (NAP) or to unlicensed assistive personnel (UAP), as well as to licensed practical/vocational nurses (LPN/LVNs). The decision to delegate must be based on careful analysis of the patient's needs and circumstances, as well as the qualifications of the person to whom the task is being delegated. Refer to the Delegation Guidelines in Appendix A.

EQUIPMENT

- Soft toothbrush or denture brush
- Denture paste
- Denture cleaner for soaking (optional)
- Denture adhesive (optional)
- Glass of cool water
- Emesis basin
- Denture cup (optional)

- Nonsterile gloves
- Additional PPE, as indicated
- Towel
- Oral hygiene supplies
- Washcloth or paper towel
- Lip lubricant
- Gauze

ASSESSMENT

Assess the patient's oral hygiene preferences: frequency, time of day, and type of hygiene products. Assess for any physical activity limitations. Assess for difficulty chewing, pain, tenderness, and discomfort. An oral assessment tool can assist with assessment of the status of the oral cavity, as well as help to determine the frequency and procedure for oral care. Assess the patient's oral cavity. Look for inflammation, edema, lesions, bleeding, or yellow/white patches. The patches may indicate a fungal infection called thrush. Assess the patient's ability to perform own care.

NURSING DIAGNOSIS

Determine the related factors for the nursing diagnoses based on the patient's current status. Appropriate nursing diagnoses may include:

- Ineffective health management
- Impaired oral mucous membrane integrity

- Disturbed body image

OUTCOME IDENTIFICATION AND PLANNING

The expected outcome to achieve is that the patient's mouth and dentures will be clean; the patient will exhibit a positive body image; and the patient will verbalize the importance of oral care.

IMPLEMENTATION

ACTION	RATIONALE
1. Perform hand hygiene and put on PPE, if indicated.	Hand hygiene and PPE prevent the spread of microorganisms. PPE is required based on transmission precautions.

ACTION

2. Identify the patient. Explain the procedure to the patient.

3. Assemble equipment on overbed table or other surface within reach.

4. Provide privacy for the patient.

5. Lower the side rail and assist the patient to a sitting position, if permitted, or turn the patient onto the side. Place a towel across the patient's chest. Raise the bed to a comfortable working position, usually elbow height of the caregiver (VHACEOSH, 2016). Put on gloves.

6. Apply gentle pressure with 4 × 4 gauze to grasp lower denture plate and remove it. If necessary, use a slight rocking motion to remove plate. Place it immediately in denture cup. Grasp upper denture with gauze and remove it (Figure 1). Place in denture cup.

7. Place paper towels or washcloth in sink while brushing. Using the toothbrush and denture paste, brush all denture surfaces gently but thoroughly (Figure 2). Be sure to completely remove any denture adhesive remaining on the denture (Felton et al., 2011). If the patient prefers, add denture cleaner to cup with water and follow directions on preparation. After denture soaks, brush denture as previously described.

RATIONALE

Identifying the patient ensures the right patient receives the intervention and helps prevent errors. Explanation facilitates cooperation.

Organization facilitates performance of task.

Cleaning another person's mouth is invasive and may be embarrassing (Holman, et al., 2005). The patient may be embarrassed by removal of dentures.

The sitting or side-lying position prevents aspiration of fluids into the lungs. The towel protects the patient from dampness. Proper bed height helps reduce back strain while performing the procedure. Gloves prevent the spread of microorganisms.

Remove bottom denture first, as it is easier to remove and minimizes bite risk (Jablonski, 2012). Rocking motion breaks suction between denture and gum. Using 4 × 4 gauze prevents slippage and discourages spread of microorganisms.

Putting paper towels or a washcloth in the sink protects against breakage. Dentures collect food and microorganisms and require daily cleaning. Removal of any residual denture adhesive prevents buildup, plaque buildup, and potential problems with the fit of the denture.

FIGURE 1. Removing dentures with a gauze sponge.

FIGURE 2. Brushing denture surfaces.

8. Rinse thoroughly with water. Apply denture adhesive, if appropriate, following product directions.

Water aids in removal of debris and acts as a cleaning agent. Denture adhesives, when properly used, can improve the retention and stability of dentures and help seal out the accumulation of food particles beneath the dentures (Felton et al., 2011)

(continued)

Skill 7-5 ▶ Providing Denture Care *(continued)*

ACTION	**RATIONALE**
9. Use a toothbrush and toothpaste to gently clean gums, mucous membranes, and tongue. Offer water and/or mouth rinse so the patient can rinse mouth before replacing dentures. Refer to Skill 7-3 for additional details related to oral hygiene care.	Cleaning removes food particles and plaque, permitting proper fit and preventing infection. Therapeutic and antiseptic mouth rinses reduce bacteria and gingivitis (ADA, n.d.a).
10. Insert upper denture in mouth and press firmly. Insert lower denture. If adhesive is used, ask the patient to bite firmly. Check that the dentures are securely in place and comfortable.	This ensures patient comfort. Biting firmly after insertion spreads the adhesive to the entire tissue-contacting surface (Felton et al., 2011).
11. If the patient desires, dentures can be stored in the denture cup in cold water, instead of returning to the mouth. Label the cup and place it on the patient's bedside table.	Storing in water prevents warping of dentures. Proper storage prevents loss and damage.
12. Remove equipment and return the patient to a position of comfort. Remove your gloves. Raise the side rail and lower the bed.	Promotes patient comfort and safety. Removing gloves properly reduces the risk for infection transmission and contamination of other items.
13. Remove additional PPE, if used. Perform hand hygiene.	Proper removal of PPE reduces the risk for infection transmission and contamination of other items. Hand hygiene prevents transmission of microorganisms.

EVALUATION   The expected outcomes have been met when the patient's oral cavity and dentures are clean, free from complications, and the patient verbalizes or demonstrates improved body image. In addition, the patient verbalizes a basic understanding of the need for oral care.

DOCUMENTATION

Guidelines   Record oral assessment, significant observations and unusual findings, such as bleeding or inflammation. Document any teaching done. Document care provided and patient response.

Sample Documentation

> 7/10/20 0945 Oral care performed. Oral cavity mucosa pink and moist. Denture and oral care given. No evidence of bleeding, ulceration, or inflammation.
>
> —C. Stone, RN

UNEXPECTED SITUATIONS AND ASSOCIATED INTERVENTIONS

- *Food or other material does not come off denture with brushing:* Place denture in a cup with cool water and soak. After soaking, use a toothbrush and denture paste to clean again. If necessary, use commercial denture cleaner added to water in the cup to soak, then brush clean.

SPECIAL CONSIDERATIONS

- Encourage the patient to wear his or her dentures, if not contraindicated. Dentures enhance appearance, assist in eating, facilitate speech, and maintain the gum line. Denture fit may be altered with long periods of nonuse.
- Encourage the patient to refrain from wrapping the denture in paper towels or napkins because they could be mistaken for trash.
- Encourage the patient to refrain from placing the dentures in the bedclothes because they can be lost in the laundry.
- Store dentures in cold water when not in the patient's mouth. Leaving dentures dry can cause warping, leading to discomfort when worn (Felton et al., 2011).

EVIDENCE FOR PRACTICE ▶

CLINICAL PRACTICE GUIDELINE
Care and Maintenance of Complete Dentures
Felton, D., Cooper, L., Duqum, I., et al. (2011). Evidence-based guidelines for the care and maintenance of complete dentures. *The Journal of the American Dental Association, 142* (2 suppl), 1S–20S. Retrieved http://jada.ada.org/article/S0002-8177(14)63742-9/fulltext.
This evidence-based guideline provides information to guide the care and maintenance of removable complete denture prostheses.

Skill 7-6 ▶ Removing Contact Lenses

If a patient wears contact lenses but cannot remove them, the nurse may be responsible for removing them. This may occur, for example, when the nurse is caring for an unconscious patient. Whenever an unconscious patient is admitted without any family present, always assess the patient to determine whether he or she wears contact lenses. Leaving contact lenses in place for long periods could result in permanent eye damage. However, if an eye injury is present, do not try to remove lenses because of the danger of causing an additional injury. Lenses should be cleaned and stored as prescribed. Different types of lenses require special care and certain types of products. Sleeping in any contact lens is not recommended as the incidence of serious eye infections is greatly increased (Cleveland Clinic, 2015b).

DELEGATION CONSIDERATIONS

The removal of contact lenses may be delegated to nursing assistive personnel (NAP) or to unlicensed assistive personnel (UAP), as well as to licensed practical/vocational nurses (LPN/LVNs). The decision to delegate must be based on careful analysis of the patient's needs and circumstances, as well as the qualifications of the person to whom the task is being delegated. Refer to the Delegation Guidelines in Appendix A.

EQUIPMENT

- Disposable gloves
- Additional PPE, if indicated
- Container for contact lenses (if unavailable, two small sterile containers marked "L" and "R" will suffice)
- Sterile normal saline solution and/or appropriate contact disinfecting solution, based on particular contact lenses
- Rubber pincer, if available (for removal of soft lenses)
- Suction-cup remover, if available (for removal of rigid lenses)

ASSESSMENT

Assess both eyes for contact lenses; some people wear them in only one eye. Assess eyes for any redness or drainage, which may indicate an eye infection or an allergic response. Assess for any eye injury. If an injury is present, notify the primary care provider about the presence of the contact lens. Do not try to remove the contact lens in this situation due to the risk for additional eye injury.

NURSING DIAGNOSIS

Determine the related factors for the nursing diagnoses based on the patient's current status. Appropriate nursing diagnoses may include:

- Risk for injury
- Deficient knowledge

OUTCOME IDENTIFICATION AND PLANNING

The expected outcome to achieve when removing contact lenses is that the lenses are removed without trauma to the eye and are stored safely.

(continued)

Skill 7-6 ▶ Removing Contact Lenses *(continued)*

IMPLEMENTATION

ACTION	RATIONALE

 1. Perform hand hygiene and put on PPE, if indicated.

Hand hygiene and PPE prevent the spread of microorganisms. PPE is required based on transmission precautions.

 2. Identify the patient. Explain the procedure to the patient.

Patient identification validates the correct patient and correct procedure. Discussion and explanation help allay anxiety and prepare the patient for what to expect.

3. Assemble equipment on overbed table or other surface within reach.

Organization facilitates performance of task.

4. Close the curtains around the bed and close the door to the room, if possible.

This ensures the patient's privacy.

5. Assist the patient to a supine position. Raise the bed to a comfortable working position, usually elbow height of the caregiver (VHACEOSH, 2016). Lower the side rail closest to you.

Supine position with the bed raised and the side rail down is the least stressful position for removing a contact lens. Proper bed height helps reduce back strain while performing the procedure.

6. If containers are not already labeled, do so now. Place 5 mL of normal saline or appropriate contact disinfecting solution in each container.

Many patients have different prescription strengths for each eye. The saline will prevent the contact from drying out.

7. Put on gloves. Remove soft contact lens:

Gloves prevent the spread of microorganisms.

a. Have the patient look forward. Retract the lower lid with one hand. Using the pad of the index finger of the other hand, move the lens down to the sclera (Figure 1).

b. Using the pads of the thumb and index finger, grasp the lens with a gentle pinching motion and remove it (Figure 2).

FIGURE 1. Retracting lower lid with one hand and using pad of index finger of other hand to move lens down to the sclera.

FIGURE 2. Using the pads of thumb and index finger to grasp lens with a gentle pinching motion to remove it.

See the accompanying Skill Variation figures for other techniques for removing both rigid and soft lenses.

8. Place the first lens in its designated cup in the storage case before removing the second lens (Figure 3).

Lenses may be different for each eye. Avoids mixing them up.

FIGURE 3. Storage cases are marked L and R, designating left and right lenses. Placing first lens in its designated cup before removing second lens avoids mixing them up.

ACTION	RATIONALE

9. Repeat actions to remove other contact lens.

10. If the patient is awake and has glasses at bedside, offer the patient glasses.

Not being able to see clearly creates anxiety.

11. Remove equipment and return the patient to a position of comfort. Remove your gloves. Raise the side rail and lower the bed.

Promotes patient comfort and safety. Removing gloves properly reduces the risk for infection transmission and contamination of other items.

12. Remove additional PPE, if used. Perform hand hygiene.

Proper removal of PPE reduces the risk for infection transmission and contamination of other items. Hand hygiene prevents transmission of microorganisms.

EVALUATION

The expected outcomes have been met when the patient remains free of injury as the contact lenses are removed; eyes exhibit no signs and symptoms of trauma, irritation, or redness; and contacts are stored safely.

DOCUMENTATION

Guidelines

Record your assessment, significant observations, and unusual findings, such as drainage or pain. Document any teaching done. Document the removal of the contact lenses, their storage, and patient response.

Sample Documentation

> 7/15/20 1045 Soft contacts removed from eyes without trauma. Stored in patient's lens case in contact solution. Sclera white with no drainage from eye. Glasses placed at bedside.
>
> —C. Stone, RN

UNEXPECTED SITUATIONS AND ASSOCIATED INTERVENTIONS

- *The contact lens cannot be removed:* Use a tool to remove the lens. For hard lenses, the tool has a small suction cup that is placed over the contact lens. For soft lenses, the tool is a small pair of rubber grippers that can be placed over the contact lens to aid in removal.
- *Hard contact is not over the cornea:* Place a cotton-tipped applicator over the upper eyelid and grasp the lid, inverting the lid over the applicator. Examine the eye for the lens. If the lens is not in the upper portion, place a finger below the eye and gently pull down on the lid while having the patient look up. When the lens is found, gently slide it over the cornea. Soft contacts may be removed from other areas of the eye.

Skill Variation | Removing Different Types of Contact Lens

1. Perform hand hygiene and put on PPE, if indicated.

2. Identify the patient.

3. Explain to the patient what you are going to do and why you are doing it

4. Assemble necessary equipment on the bedside stand or overbed table or other surface within reach.

5. Close the curtains around the bed and close the door to the room, if possible.

6. Assist the patient to a supine position. Raise bed to a comfortable working position, usually elbow height of the caregiver (VHACEOSH, 2016). Lower the side rail closest to you.

7. If containers are not already labeled, do so now. Place 5 mL of normal saline in each container.

8. Put on clean gloves.

(continued)

Skill 7-6 ▶ Removing Contact Lenses *(continued)*

Skill Variation ▶ Removing Different Types of Contact Lens *(continued)*

To Remove Hard Contact Lenses—Patient is Able to Blink

a. If the lens is not centered over the cornea, apply gentle pressure on the lower eyelid to center the lens (Figure A).

b. Gently pull the outer corner of the eye toward the ear (Figure B).

c. Position the other hand below the lens to catch it and ask the patient to blink (Figure C).

To Remove Hard Contact Lenses—Patient is Unable to Blink

a. Gently spread the eyelids beyond the top and bottom edges of the lens (Figure D).

b. Gently press the lower eyelid up against the bottom of the lens (Figure E).

c. After the lens is tipped slightly, move the eyelids toward one another to cause the lens to slide out between the eyelids (Figure F).

To Remove Hard Contact Lenses with a Suction Cup—Patient is Unable to Blink

a. Ensure that contact lens is centered on the cornea. Place a drop of sterile saline on the suction cup.

b. Place the suction cup in the center of the contact lens and gently pull the contact lens off the eye.

c. To remove the suction cup from the lens, slide the lens off sideways.

To Remove Soft Contact Lenses with a Rubber Pincer

a. Locate the contact lens and place the rubber pincers in the center of the lens.

b. Gently squeeze the pincers and remove the lens from the eye.

9. Place the first lens in its designated cup in the storage case before removing the second lens.

10. Repeat actions to remove other contact lens. Remove gloves.

11. If the patient is awake and has glasses at bedside, offer the patient glasses. Lower the bed. Assist the patient to a comfortable position.

12. Remove additional PPE, if used. Perform hand hygiene.

FIGURE A. Centering lens.

FIGURE B. Gently pulling outer corner of eye toward ear.

FIGURE C. Receiving lens as patient blinks.

FIGURE D. Spreading eyelids.

FIGURE E. Pressing lower lid up against bottom of lens.

FIGURE F. Sliding lens out between lids.

Skill 7-7 ▶ Shampooing a Patient's Hair in Bed

The easiest way to wash a patient's hair is to assist him or her in the shower, but not all patients can take showers. If the patient's hair needs to be washed but the patient is unable or not allowed to get out of bed, a bed shampoo can be performed. Shampoo caps are available, and are being used with increasing frequency. These commercially prepared, disposable caps contain a rinseless shampoo product. Refer to the accompanying Skill Variation at the end of the skill.

DELEGATION CONSIDERATIONS	The shampooing of a patient's hair may be delegated to nursing assistive personnel (NAP) or to unlicensed assistive personnel (UAP), as well as to licensed practical/vocational nurses (LPN/LVNs). The decision to delegate must be based on careful analysis of the patient's needs and circumstances, as well as the qualifications of the person to whom the task is being delegated. Refer to the Delegation Guidelines in Appendix A.

EQUIPMENT

- Water pitcher
- Warm water
- Shampoo
- Conditioner (optional)
- Disposable gloves
- Additional PPE, as indicated
- Protective pad for bed

- Shampoo board or tray
- Bucket
- Towels
- Gown
- Comb or brush
- Blow dryer (optional)

ASSESSMENT	Assess the patient's hygiene preferences: frequency, time of day, and type of hygiene products. Assess for any physical activity limitations. Assess the patient's ability to get out of bed to have his or her hair washed. If the medical orders allow it and the patient is physically able to wash his or her hair in the shower, the patient may prefer to do so. If the patient cannot tolerate being out of bed or is not allowed to do so, perform a bed shampoo. Assess for any activity or positioning limitations. Inspect the patient's scalp for any cuts, lesions, or bumps. Note any flaking, drying, or excessive oiliness, or evidence of problems, such as **pediculosis**.

NURSING DIAGNOSIS	Determine the related factors for the nursing diagnoses based on the patient's current status. Appropriate nursing diagnoses may include:

- Bathing self-care deficit
- Fatigue

- Impaired transfer ability

OUTCOME IDENTIFICATION AND PLANNING	The expected outcome to achieve is that the patient's hair will be clean. Other outcomes that may be appropriate include the following: the patient will tolerate the shampoo with little to no difficulty, the patient will demonstrate an improved body image, and the patient will verbalize an increase in comfort.

IMPLEMENTATION

ACTION

1. Review the health record for any limitations in physical activity, or contraindications to the procedure. Confirm the presence of a medical order for shampooing the patient's hair, if required by facility policy.

2. Perform hand hygiene. Put on PPE, as indicated.

3. Identify the patient. Explain the procedure to the patient.

RATIONALE

Identifying limitations prevents patient discomfort and injury. In some settings, a medical order is required for shampooing a patient's hair.

Hand hygiene and PPE prevent the spread of microorganisms. PPE is required based on transmission precautions.

Patient identification validates the correct patient and correct procedure. Discussion and explanation help allay anxiety and prepare the patient for what to expect.

(continued)

Skill 7-7 ▶ Shampooing a Patient's Hair in Bed *(continued)*

ACTION	**RATIONALE**
4. Assemble equipment on overbed table or other surface within reach.	Organization facilitates performance of task.
5. Close the curtains around the bed and close the door to the room, if possible.	Provides for patient privacy.
6. Lower the head of the bed. Raise the bed to a comfortable working position, usually the elbow height of the caregiver (VHACEOSH, 2016). Lower the side rail. Remove the pillow and place a protective pad under the patient's head and shoulders (Figure 1).	Proper bed height helps reduce back strain while performing the procedure. A protective pad keeps the sheets from getting wet.
7. **Fill the pitcher with comfortably warm water (100°F to less than 120° to 125°F).** Position the patient at the top of the bed, in a supine position. Have the patient lift his or her head and place the shampoo board underneath the patient's head (Figure 2). If necessary, pad the edge of the board with a small towel.	Warm water is comfortable and relaxing for the patient. It also stimulates circulation and provides for more effective cleaning. Adjusting the water temperature to 100°F to less than 120° to 125°F decreases risk of burns and drying of the skin. The lower temperature is recommended for children and adults over 65 years of age (Burn Foundation, 2016). Padding the edge of the shampoo board may help increase patient comfort.
8. Place a drain container underneath the drain of the shampoo board (Figure 3).	The container will catch the runoff water, preventing a mess on the floor.

FIGURE 1. Placing protective pad under patient's head.

FIGURE 2. Placing patient's head on shampoo board.

FIGURE 3. Positioning drain container for shampoo board.

ACTION

9. Put on gloves. If the patient is able, have him or her hold a folded washcloth at the forehead. Pour a pitcher of warm water slowly over the patient's head, making sure that all hair is saturated (Figure 4). Refill pitcher, if needed.

10. Apply a small amount of shampoo to the patient's hair. Lather shampoo. Massage deep into the scalp, avoiding any cuts, lesions, or sore spots.

11. Rinse with comfortably warm water until all shampoo is out of hair (Figure 5). Repeat shampoo, if necessary.

12. If the patient has thick hair or requests it, apply a small amount of conditioner to the hair and massage throughout. Avoid any cuts, lesions, or sore spots.

13. If drain container is small, empty before rinsing hair. Rinse with comfortably warm water until all conditioner is out of hair.

14. Remove shampoo board. Place towel around the patient's hair.

15. Pat hair dry, avoiding any cuts, lesions, or sore spots (Figure 6). Remove protective padding, but keep one dry protective pad under the patient's hair.

RATIONALE

Gloves prevent the spread of microorganisms. A washcloth prevents water from running into the patient's eyes. By pouring slowly, more hair will become wet, and it is more soothing for the patient.

Shampoo will help to remove dirt or oil.

Shampoo left in hair may cause pruritus. If hair is still dirty, another shampoo treatment may be needed.

Conditioner eases tangles and moisturizes hair and scalp.

Container may overflow if not emptied. Conditioner left in hair may cause pruritus.

This prevents the patient from getting cold.

Patting dry removes any excess water without damaging hair or scalp.

FIGURE 4. Pouring warm water over patient's head.

FIGURE 5. Rinsing shampoo from patient's head.

FIGURE 6. Patting patient's hair dry.

(*continued*)

Skill 7-7 ▶ Shampooing a Patient's Hair in Bed   *(continued)*

ACTION	RATIONALE
16. Gently brush hair, removing tangles, as needed.	Removing tangles helps hair to dry faster. Brushing hair improves the patient's self-image.
17. Blow-dry hair on a cool setting, if allowed and if the patient wishes. If not, consider covering the patient's head with a dry towel, until hair is dry.	Blow-drying hair helps hair to dry faster and prevents the patient from becoming chilled. Keeping the head covered prevents chilling while hair is drying.
18. Change the patient's gown and remove protective pad. Replace pillow.	If the patient's gown is damp, the patient will become chilled. Protective pad is no longer needed once hair is dry.
19. Remove the equipment and return the patient to a position of comfort. Remove your gloves. Raise the side rail and lower the bed.	Promotes patient comfort and safety. Removing gloves properly reduces the risk for infection transmission and contamination of other items.
20. Remove additional PPE, if used. Perform hand hygiene.	Proper removal of PPE reduces the risk for infection transmission and contamination of other items. Hand hygiene deters spread of microorganisms.

EVALUATION

The expected outcomes have been met when the patient's hair is clean, the patient verbalizes a positive body image, and the patient reports an increase in comfort level.

DOCUMENTATION

Guidelines

Record your assessment, significant observations, and unusual findings, such as bleeding or inflammation. Document any teaching done. Document care provided and patient response.

Sample Documentation

> 7/4/20 1130 Hair washed. Moderate amount of dried blood in hair noted. A 3-cm laceration noted over left parietal area. Edges well approximated, slight redness of wound, surrounding skin consistent with rest of skin tone, sutures intact, and no drainage noted.
>
> —C. Stone, RN

UNEXPECTED SITUATIONS AND ASSOCIATED INTERVENTIONS

- *Glass is found in hair:* Carefully comb through hair before washing to remove as much glass as possible. Discard glass in appropriate container. When massaging the scalp, be alert to signs of pain from the patient; glass could be cutting the patient's head.

SPECIAL CONSIDERATIONS

- If the patient has a spinal cord or neck injury, use of the shampoo board may be contraindicated. In this case, a makeshift protection area can be created to wash the patient's hair without using the board. Place a protective pad underneath the patient's head and shoulders. Roll a towel into the bottom of the protective pad and direct the roll into one area so that water will drain into the container.

Skill Variation ▶ Shampooing a Patient's Hair With a Shampoo Cap

Shampoo caps are available and are being used with increasing frequency. These commercially prepared, disposable caps contain a rinseless shampoo product. The cap is warmed in the microwave or stored in a warmer until use. The cap is placed on the patient's head and the hair and scalp are massaged through the cap, to lather the shampoo. After shampooing for the manufacturer's suggested length of time, the cap is removed and discarded. The patient's hair is towel dried and styled.

1. Review chart for any limitations in physical activity, or contraindications to the procedure. Confirm presence of medical order for shampooing the patient's hair, if required by facility policy.

2. Warm the cap in the microwave, according to the manufacturer's directions, or remove it from the storage warmer.

3. Perform hand hygiene and put on PPE, if indicated.

4. Identify the patient.

5. Explain what you are going to do and the reason for doing it to the patient.

6. Assemble necessary equipment on the bedside stand, overbed table, or other surface within reach.

7. Close the curtains around the bed and close the door to the room, if possible.

8. Put on gloves. Raise bed to a comfortable working position, usually elbow height of the caregiver (VHACEOSH, 2016). Place a towel across the patient's chest. Place the shampoo cap on the patient's head (Figure A).

9. Massage the scalp and hair through the cap to lather the shampoo. Continue to massage according to the time frame specified by the manufacturer's directions (Figure B).

10. Remove and discard the shampoo cap.

11. Dry the patient's hair with a towel.

12. Remove the towel from the patient's chest.

13. Comb and style the hair.

14. Remove gloves. Lower the bed. Assist the patient to a comfortable position.

15. Remove additional PPE, if used. Perform hand hygiene.

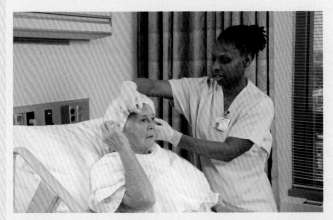

FIGURE A. Placing warmed shampoo cap on the patient's head.

FIGURE B. Massaging the hair and scalp.

Skill 7-8 Assisting the Patient to Shave

For many patients shaving is a daily hygiene ritual. They may feel disheveled and unclean without shaving. Some patients may need help with shaving when using a regular blade or may require that the nurse perform the shaving procedure for them completely. Patients with beards or mustaches may require nursing assistance to keep the beard and mustache clean. However, never trim or shave a patient's beard or mustache without the patient's consent. Female patients may require assistance with shaving underarm and leg hair, depending on the patient's personal preference and abilities. If available and permitted by the facility, electric shavers are usually recommended when the patient is receiving anticoagulant therapy or has a bleeding disorder. Electric shavers are especially convenient for ill and bedridden patients. This skill outlines one technique for shaving with a safety razor.

(continued)

Skill 7-8 ▶ Assisting the Patient to Shave *(continued)*

DELEGATION CONSIDERATIONS

The shaving of a patient's hair may be delegated to nursing assistive personnel (NAP) or to unlicensed assistive personnel (UAP) after assessment by the registered nurse, as well as to licensed practical/vocational nurses (LPN/LVNs). The decision to delegate must be based on careful analysis of the patient's needs and circumstances, as well as the qualifications of the person to whom the task is being delegated. Refer to the Delegation Guidelines Appendix A.

EQUIPMENT

- Shaving cream or gel
- Safety razor
- Towel
- Washcloth
- Bath basin

- Disposable gloves
- Additional PPE, as indicated
- Waterproof pad
- Aftershave or lotion (optional)

ASSESSMENT

Assess the patient's shaving preferences: frequency, time of day, and type of shaving products. Assess for any physical activity limitations. Assess the patient for any bleeding problems. If the patient is receiving any anticoagulant, such as heparin or warfarin (Coumadin), has received an antithrombolytic agent, or has a low platelet count, consider using an electric razor. Inspect the area to be shaved for any lesions or areas of altered skin integrity. Assess the patient's ability to shave independently or for the need of assistance with the procedure.

NURSING DIAGNOSIS

Determine related factors for the nursing diagnoses based on the patient's current status. Appropriate nursing diagnoses may include:

- Risk for injury
- Bathing self-care deficit
- Fatigue

OUTCOME IDENTIFICATION AND PLANNING

The expected outcome to achieve when assisting the patient with shaving is that the patient will be clean, without evidence of hair growth or trauma to the skin. Other outcomes that may be appropriate include the following: the patient tolerates shaving with minimal to no difficulty and the patient verbalizes feelings of improved self-esteem.

IMPLEMENTATION

ACTION	RATIONALE
1. Review the health record for any limitations in physical activity, or contraindications to the procedure. Confirm the presence of a medical order for shaving the patient, if required by facility policy.	Identifying limitations prevents patient discomfort and injury. In some settings, a medical order is required for shaving a patient with certain health problems or taking medications that affect coagulation.
2. Perform hand hygiene. Put on PPE, as indicated.	Hand hygiene and PPE prevent the spread of microorganisms. PPE is required based on transmission precautions.
3. Identify the patient. Explain the procedure to the patient.	Identifying the patient ensures the right patient receives the intervention and helps prevent errors. Explanation facilitates cooperation.
4. Assemble equipment on overbed table or other surface within reach.	Organization facilitates performance of task.
5. Close the curtains around the bed and close the door to the room, if possible.	Provides for patient privacy.

ACTION

6. Raise the bed to a comfortable working position, usually elbow height of the caregiver (VHACEOSH, 2016). Lower the side rail. Cover the patient's chest with a towel or water-proof pad. Fill bath basin with comfortably warm (100°F to less than 120° to 125°F) water. Put on gloves. Wet a wash-cloth in the basin of water. Press the warm washcloth on the area to be shaved.

7. Dispense shaving cream or gel into the palm of the hand. Apply cream to the area to be shaved in a layer about 0.5 in thick (Figure 1). Allow to remain on the skin for a few minutes.

8. With one hand, hold the skin steady at the area to be shaved. Using a smooth stroke, begin shaving. If shaving the face, shave with the direction of hair growth in short strokes (Figure 2). If shaving a leg, shave against the hair in upward, short strokes. If shaving an underarm, hold skin steady and use short, upward strokes.

RATIONALE

Proper bed height helps reduce back strain while performing the procedure. Adjusting the water temperature to 100°F to less than 120° to 125°F decreases risk of burns and dry-ing of the skin. The lower temperature is recommended for children and adults over 65 years of age (Burn Founda-tion, 2016). Warm water is comfortable and relaxing for the patient. Moistens skin and softens hair. Gloves prevent the spread of microorganisms. Warm water softens the hair, making the process easier.

Using shaving cream or gel helps to prevent skin irritation and prevents hair from pulling. Applying cream or gel a few min-utes before shaving softens the hair (MFMER, 2015b).

Holding the skin steady prevents the razor from pulling on the skin. Do not pull the skin taut while shaving to reduce the risk for ingrown hairs (MFMER, 2015b). The skin on the face is more sensitive and needs to be shaved with the direc-tion of hair growth to prevent discomfort.

FIGURE 1. Applying shaving cream to face.

FIGURE 2. Shaving face.

9. Remove residual shaving cream with wet washcloth (Figure 3).

Shaving cream can lead to irritation if left on the skin.

FIGURE 3. Using a wet washcloth to remove remaining shaving cream.

10. If the patient requests, apply aftershave or lotion to the area shaved.

Aftershave and lotion can reduce skin irritation.

(continued)

Skill 7-8 ▶ Assisting the Patient to Shave *(continued)*

ACTION	RATIONALE
11. Remove equipment and return the patient to a position of comfort. Remove your gloves. Raise the side rail and lower the bed.	Promotes patient comfort and safety. Removing gloves properly reduces the risk for infection transmission and contamination of other items.
12. Remove additional PPE, if used. Perform hand hygiene.	Proper removal of PPE reduces the risk for infection transmission and contamination of other items. Hand hygiene deters spread of microorganisms.

EVALUATION

The expected outcome has been met when the patient is clean-shaven without evidence of trauma, irritation, or redness. In addition, the patient verbalizes feeling refreshed and demonstrates improved self-esteem.

DOCUMENTATION

Shaving a patient does not usually require documentation. However, if your skin assessment reveals any unusual findings, document your assessment and the procedure. If the patient or nurse breaks the skin while shaving, document the occurrence and your assessment of the patient.

UNEXPECTED SITUATIONS AND ASSOCIATED INTERVENTIONS

- *The patient is cut and bleeds during shave:* Apply pressure with gauze or towel to injured area. Do not release pressure for 2 to 3 minutes. After bleeding has stopped, resume shaving. The water basin may need to be rewarmed before washing off the shaving cream. Document the occurrence and assessment of area after the shave.
- *The patient has a large amount of hair to be shaved:* If the hair is longer, it may need to be trimmed with scissors before shaving to prevent pulling of hair when shaving.

SPECIAL CONSIDERATIONS

- *The patient is wearing a beard:* Do not shave the patient's beard without consent unless it is an emergency situation, such as insertion of an endotracheal tube. For this procedure, shave only the area needed and leave the rest of the beard.

Skill 7-9 ▶ Providing Nail Care

Care of the nails is important to prevent pain and infection. Long, roughened nails that have not been trimmed or filed may increase the occurrence of traumatic nail injury, such as damage to the nail that may result in the nail plate being torn from the nail bed (Malkin & Berridge, 2009). Poor toenail care may lead to poor mobility. The nurse should document and report to the patient's primary care provider any changes to nail color, such as discoloration of the entire nail or a dark streak under the nail; changes in nail shape, such as curled nails; thinning or thickening of the nails; separation of the nail from the surrounding skin; bleeding around the nails; and redness, swelling, or pain around the nails (MFMER, 2014c).

DELEGATION CONSIDERATIONS

Depending on the organization's policies and procedures, the care of a patient's nails may be delegated to nursing assistive personnel (NAP) or to unlicensed assistive personnel (UAP) after assessment by the registered nurse. The care of a patient's nails may be delegated to licensed practical/vocational nurses (LPN/LVNs). The decision to delegate must be based on careful analysis of the patient's needs and circumstances, as well as the qualifications of the person to whom the task is being delegated. Refer to the Delegation Guidelines in Appendix A.

| EQUIPMENT | • Nail file
• Nail clipper
• Cuticle scissors
• Orangewood stick or cuticle stick
• Emollient
• Disposable waterproof pad | • Towel
• Wash basin and skin cleanser, or commercially prepared bathing system
• Disposable gloves
• Additional PPE, if indicated |

ASSESSMENT

Assess the patient's nail care preferences: frequency, time of day, and type of products. Assess for any physical activity limitations. Assess for conditions that may put the patient at high risk for nail problems, such as diabetes and peripheral vascular disease. Assess the color and temperature of fingers and toes. Assess adequacy of pulses to area and capillary refill. Assess the skin of fingers and toes for dryness, cracking, or inflammation. Assess the nails and surrounding skin for changes in nail color, changes in nail shape, thinning or thickening of the nails, separation of the nail from the surrounding skin, bleeding around the nails, and redness, swelling, or pain around the nails. Nails should appear intact, smooth, firmly attached to nail bed, pink in color, with a white crescent visible at the base. Dark streaks running lengthwise in nails are a normal variation for patients with darker skin tones. Assess the patient's ability for self-care of nails or assist with the procedure.

NURSING DIAGNOSIS

Determine related factors for the nursing diagnoses based on the patient's current status. Appropriate nursing diagnoses may include:

• Risk for injury
• Bathing self-care deficit
• Readiness for enhanced self-care

OUTCOME IDENTIFICATION AND PLANNING

The expected outcome to achieve when assisting the patient with care of the nails is nails are trimmed and clean with smooth edges and intact cuticles, without evidence of trauma to nails or surrounding skin. Other outcomes that may be appropriate include the patient verbalizing feelings of improved self-esteem.

IMPLEMENTATION

ACTION	RATIONALE
1. Review health record for any limitations in physical activity, or contraindications to the procedure. Confirm presence of medical order for nail care, if required by facility policy.	Identifying limitations prevents patient discomfort and injury. In some settings, a medical order is required for nail care, particularly for a patient with certain health problems.
2. Perform hand hygiene. Put on PPE, as indicated.	Hand hygiene and PPE prevent the spread of microorganisms. PPE is required based on transmission precautions.
3. Identify the patient. Explain the procedure to the patient.	Identifying the patient ensures the right patient receives the intervention and helps prevent errors. Explanation facilitates cooperation.
4. Assemble equipment on overbed table or other surface within reach.	Organization facilitates performance of task.
5. Close the curtains around the bed and close the door to the room, if possible.	Provides for patient privacy.
6. Raise bed to a comfortable working position, usually elbow height of the caregiver (VHACEOSH, 2016). Lower the side rail. Place a towel or waterproof pad under the patient's hand or foot.	Proper bed height helps reduce back strain while performing the procedure. Waterproof pad protects bed linens and surrounding surfaces.

(continued)

Skill 7-9 ▶ Providing Nail Care *(continued)*

ACTION	RATIONALE
7. Put on gloves. Wash the patient's hands or feet, depending on the care to be given.	Gloves prevent the spread of microorganisms. Washing removes surface dirt and softens nails and skin, making it easier to trim and care for cuticles (MFMER, 2014c).
8. Gently clean under the nails using the cuticle or orangewood stick (Figure 1). Wash hand or foot.	Washing removes debris and dirt dislodged from under nails.
9. Clip nails, if necessary. Avoid cutting the whole nail in one attempt. Use the tip of the nail clipper and take small cuts. Cut the nail straight across (Figure 2). Do not trim so far down on the sides that the skin and cuticle are injured. **Only file, do not cut, the nails of patients with diabetes or circulatory problems.**	Cutting the entire nail in one attempt may lead to splitting the nail (Malkin & Berridge, 2009). Cutting straight across prevents injury to nail, cuticle, and finger or toe and reduces risk for in-growing nails (MFMER, 2014a, 2014c; Malkin & Berridge, 2009).

FIGURE 1. Gently cleaning under nails.

FIGURE 2. Trimming straight across nails with clipper.

10. File the nail straight across, then round the tips in a gentle curve, to shape the nail. Do not trim so far down on the sides that the skin and cuticle are injured. **Only file, do not cut, the nails of patients with diabetes or circulatory problems.**	Smoothens the nail. Prevents injury to nail, cuticle, and finger or toe and reduces risk for ingrowing nails (Malkin & Berridge, 2009; MFMER, 2011c, 2014a).
11. Remove hangnails, which are broken pieces of cuticle, by carefully trimming them off with cuticle scissors. **Do not pull or rip off hangnails.** Avoid injury to tissue with the cuticle scissors.	Removes dead cuticle. Reduces hangnail formation. Tearing of hangnail can cause injury to live tissue.
12. Gently push cuticles back off the nail using the orangewood or cuticle stick or towel (Figure 3).	Keeps cuticles and nails neat and prevents cracking and drying of cuticles.
13. Dry hand or foot thoroughly, taking care to be sure to dry between fingers or toes (Figure 4). Apply an emollient to the hand or foot, rubbing it into the nails and cuticles. **Do not moisturize between the toes of patients with peripheral artery disease.**	Thorough drying reduces risk of maceration, damage from overly and consistently wet skin. Maceration increases risk for injury from rubbing or friction, and risk for fungal and bacterial infections. Moisturizing between the toes of patients with peripheral artery disease can encourage fungal growth (MFMER, n.d.).
14. Repeat Steps 7-13 for other extremity or extremities.	
15. Remove equipment and return the patient to a position of comfort. Remove your gloves. Raise the side rail and lower the bed.	Promotes patient comfort and safety. Removing gloves properly reduces the risk for infection transmission and contamination of other items.
16. Remove additional PPE, if used. Perform hand hygiene.	Proper removal of PPE reduces the risk for infection transmission and contamination of other items. Hand hygiene deters spread of microorganisms.

ACTION	RATIONALE

FIGURE 3. Gently pushing cuticles back off nail.

FIGURE 4. Drying hand thoroughly.

EVALUATION

The expected outcome has been met when the patient's nails are trimmed and clean with smooth edges and intact cuticles, and are without evidence of trauma to nails or surrounding skin. In addition, the patient verbalizes feeling refreshed and demonstrates improved self-esteem.

DOCUMENTATION

Guidelines

Record your assessment, significant observations, and unusual findings, such as broken nails or inflammation. Document any teaching done. Document care provided and patient response. Nail care is often recorded on routine flow sheet.

Sample Documentation

> <u>7/17/120</u> 2030 Nail care performed for fingernails. Nails intact, supple, nailbed pink in color, with white crescent visible at the base. Significant amount of old food removed from under nails. Skin on fingers and hands dry and cracked; emollient applied.
> —*J. Lyman, RN*

UNEXPECTED SITUATIONS AND ASSOCIATED INTERVENTIONS

- *The patient is cut and bleeds during nail care:* Apply pressure with gauze or towel to the injured area. Do not release pressure for 2 to 3 minutes. Assess the area. Document the occurrence and assessment of area; notify primary care provider according to facility policy. Continue to monitor area for bleeding and inflammation.
- *Cuticles, fingers, or toes are inflamed and tender:* Assess area. Document findings. Notify primary care provider. Resume care as appropriate after consultation with primary care provider and based on facility policy.
- *Calluses, corns, or bunions are present:* Assess area and document findings. Do not cut or file. Consult primary care provider and/or podiatrist for treatment.

SPECIAL CONSIDERATIONS

General Considerations

- Advise the patient to avoid using fingernails as tools to pick, poke, or pry things to prevent nail damage.
- Discourage biting of nails or picking at cuticles. These habits can damage the nail bed. Even a minor cut alongside a fingernail can allow bacteria or fungi to enter and cause an infection (MFMER, 2014c).
- Advise patients to avoid pulling off hangnails. This can cause injury to live tissue that is pulled off along with the hangnail. Instead, carefully clip off hangnails.
- Advise patients to wear appropriate footwear. Break in new shoes gradually. Improperly fitting shoes can lead to corns, calluses, bunions, and blisters.

(continued)

Skill 7-9 ▶ Providing Nail Care *(continued)*

Infant and Child Considerations	• A newborn's nail beds may be cyanotic (blue) for the first few hours of life, and then turn pink. • Infants' nails should be carefully trimmed on a regular basis to prevent scratching.
Older Adult Considerations	• Nails may have lengthwise ridges, due to decreased nail growth rate and injury to the nail bed. • Nails may be brittle or peeling. Toenails may be thickened.
Home Care Considerations	• Advise patients with diabetes or peripheral vascular disease to inspect feet daily for blisters, cuts, cracks, sores, redness, tenderness, or swelling. Encourage patients to report problems to primary care provider for early intervention. • Encourage patients with diabetes or peripheral vascular disease to schedule regular foot checkups with their primary care provider or podiatrist. Schedule foot exams at least once a year or more often if recommended by primary care provider. • Instruct patients with diabetes and/or peripheral vascular disease to trim nails carefully and if necessary, ask for assistance from a caregiver as necessary. • Encourage patients with diabetes and peripheral vascular disease to see a podiatrist for treatment related to bunions, corns, or calluses (MFMER, n.d., 2014a).

Skill 7-10 ▶ Making an Unoccupied Bed

Usually bed linens are changed after the bath, but some facilities change linens only when soiled. If the patient can get out of bed, the nurse should make the bed while it is unoccupied to decrease stress on the patient and the nurse. The following procedure explains how to make the bed using a fitted bottom sheet. Some facilities do not provide fitted bottom sheets, or sometimes a fitted bottom sheet may not be available. If this is the case, refer to the Skill Variation at the end of this skill for using a flat bottom sheet, instead of a fitted sheet.

DELEGATION CONSIDERATIONS	The making of an unoccupied bed may be delegated to nursing assistive personnel (NAP) or to unlicensed assistive personnel (UAP), as well as to licensed practical/vocational nurses (LPN/LVNs). The decision to delegate must be based on careful analysis of the patient's needs and circumstances, as well as the qualifications of the person to whom the task is being delegated. Refer to the Delegation Guidelines in Appendix A.
EQUIPMENT	• One large flat sheet • One fitted sheet • Drawsheet (optional) • Blankets • Bedspread • Pillowcases • Linen hamper or bag • Bedside chair • Waterproof protective pad (optional) • Disposable gloves • Additional PPE, as indicated
ASSESSMENT	Assess facility policies and patient preferences regarding linen changes. Assess for any physical activity limitations. Check for any patient belongings that may have accidentally been placed in the bed linens, such as eyeglasses or prayer cloths.
NURSING DIAGNOSIS	Determine related factors for the nursing diagnoses based on the patient's current status. Appropriate nursing diagnoses may include: • Risk for impaired skin integrity • Risk for activity intolerance • Impaired bed mobility

| **OUTCOME IDENTIFICATION AND PLANNING** | The expected outcome to achieve when making an unoccupied bed is that the bed linens will be changed without injury to the patient or nurse. |

IMPLEMENTATION

ACTION	**RATIONALE**
1. Perform hand hygiene. Put on PPE, as indicated.	Hand hygiene and PPE prevent the spread of microorganisms. PPE is required based on transmission precautions.
2. Explain to the patient what you are going to do and the reason for doing it, if the patient is present in the room.	Explanation facilitates cooperation.
3. Assemble necessary equipment on the bedside stand, over-bed table, or other surface within reach.	Arranging items nearby is convenient, saves time, and avoids unnecessary stretching and twisting of muscles on the part of the nurse.
4. Adjust the bed to a comfortable working height, usually elbow height of the caregiver (VHACEOSH, 2016). Drop the side rails.	Having the bed at the proper height prevents back and muscle strain. Having the side rails down reduces strain on the nurse while working.
5. Disconnect call bell or any tubes from bed linens.	Disconnecting devices prevents damage to the devices.
6. Put on gloves. Loosen all linen as you move around the bed, from the head of the bed on the far side to the head of the bed on the near side.	Gloves prevent the spread of microorganisms. Loosening the linen helps prevent tugging and tearing on linen. Loosening the linen and moving around the bed systematically reduce strain caused by reaching across the bed.
7. Fold reusable linens, such as sheets, blankets, or spread, in place on the bed in fourths and hang them over a clean chair.	Folding saves time and energy when reusable linen is replaced on the bed. Folding linens while they are on the bed reduces strain on the nurse's arms. Some facilities change linens only when soiled.
8. Snugly roll all the soiled linen inside the bottom sheet. Hold linen away from your body and place directly into the laundry hamper (Figure 1). **Do not place on floor or furniture. Do not hold soiled linens against your clothing.**	Rolling soiled linens snugly and placing them directly into the hamper helps prevent the spread of microorganisms. The floor is heavily contaminated; soiled linen will further contaminate furniture. Soiled linen contaminates the nurse's clothing, and this may spread organisms to another patient.

FIGURE 1. Bundling soiled linens in bottom sheet and holding them away from clothing.

| 9. If possible, shift mattress up to head of bed. If mattress is soiled, clean and dry according to facility policy before applying new sheets. | This allows more foot room for the patient. |

(continued)

Skill 7-10 ▶ Making an Unoccupied Bed *(continued)*

ACTION	**RATIONALE**
10. Remove your gloves, unless indicated for transmission-based precautions. Place the bottom sheet on the mattress and secure the bottom sheet over the corners at the head and foot of the mattress.	Gloves are not necessary to handle clean linen. Opening linens on the bed reduces strain on the nurse's arms and diminishes the spread of microorganisms.
11. Push the sheet open to the center of the mattress, pulling the sheet taut from the secured corners (Figure 2). (See the Skill Variation at the end of this skill for using a flat bottom sheet, instead of a fitted sheet.)	Making the bed on one side and then completing the bed-making on the other side saves time. Pulling the sheet taut keeps it in place on the mattress. Having bottom linens free of wrinkles reduces patient discomfort.
12. If using, place the drawsheet with its centerfold in the center of the bed and positioned so it will be located under the patient's midsection. Open the drawsheet and fan-fold to the center of the mattress (Figure 3). If a protective pad is used, place it over the drawsheet in the proper area and open to the centerfold. Not all facilities use drawsheets routinely. The nurse may decide to use one. In some institutions, the protective pad doubles as a drawsheet. Tuck the drawsheet securely under the mattress.	If the patient soils the bed, drawsheet and pad can be changed without the bottom and top linens on the bed. Having all bottom linens in place before tucking them under the mattress avoids unnecessary moving about the bed. A drawsheet can aid moving the patient in bed.

FIGURE 2. Pushing the bottom sheet open to the center of the mattress.

FIGURE 3. Placing drawsheet on bed.

13. Move to the other side of the bed to secure bottom linens. Pull the bottom sheet tightly and secure over the corners at the head and foot of the mattress. Pull the drawsheet tightly and tuck it securely under the mattress.	This removes wrinkles from the bottom linens, which can cause patient discomfort and promote skin breakdown.
14. Place the top sheet on the bed with its centerfold in the center of the bed and with the hem even with the head of the mattress. Unfold the top sheet. Follow same procedure with top blanket or spread, placing the upper edge about 6 in below the top of the sheet.	Opening linens by shaking them spreads organisms into the air. Holding linens overhead to open causes strain on the nurse's arms.
15. Tuck the top sheet and blanket under the foot of the bed on the near side. Miter the corners (Figure 4). (See the Skill Variation at the end of this skill for information to miter a corner.)	This saves time and energy and keeps the top linen in place.
16. Fold the upper 6 in of the top sheet down over the spread and make a cuff.	This makes it easier for the patient to get into bed and pull up the covers.

ACTION	**RATIONALE**
17. Move to the other side of the bed and follow the same procedure for securing top sheets under the foot of the bed and making a cuff (Figure 5).	Working on one side of the bed at a time saves energy and is more efficient.

FIGURE 4. Mitering corner of top sheet and blanket.

FIGURE 5. Cuffing top linens.

ACTION	**RATIONALE**
18. Place the pillows on the bed. Open each pillowcase in the same manner as you opened other linens. Gather the pillowcase over one hand toward the closed end. Grasp the pillow with the hand inside the pillowcase. Keep a firm hold on the top of the pillow and pull the cover onto the pillow. Place the pillow at the head of the bed.	Opening linens by shaking causes organisms to be carried on air currents. Covering the pillow while it rests on the bed reduces strain on the nurse's arms and back.
19. Fan-fold or pie-fold the top linens.	Having linens opened makes it more convenient for the patient to get into bed.
20. Secure the signal device on the bed, according to facility policy.	The patient will be able to call for assistance as necessary. Promotes patient comfort and safety.
21. Raise the side rail and lower the bed.	Promotes patient comfort and safety.
22. Dispose of soiled linen according to facility policy.	Deters the spread of microorganisms.
23. Remove any other PPE, if used. Perform hand hygiene.	Proper removal of PPE reduces the risk for infection transmission and contamination of other items. Hand hygiene prevents the spread of microorganisms.

EVALUATION	The expected outcome is met when the bed linens are changed without any injury to the patient or nurse.
DOCUMENTATION	Changing of bed linens does not require documentation. The use of a specialty bed or bed equipment should be documented.
UNEXPECTED SITUATIONS AND ASSOCIATED INTERVENTIONS	• *Drawsheet is not available:* A flat sheet can be folded in half to substitute for a drawsheet, but extra care must be taken to avoid wrinkles in the bed. • *The patient is frequently incontinent of stool or urine:* More than one protective pad can be placed under the patient to protect the bed, but take care to ensure that the patient is not lying on wrinkles from linens.

(continued)

Skill 7-10 ▶ Making an Unoccupied Bed *(continued)*

- Many different types of specialty beds are available for use as part of treatment and prevention of many health issues, such as treatment of pressure injuries. Refer to manufacturer's recommendations and instructions on use of specialty lines and products with this equipment.

Skill Variation ▶ Making a Bed With a Flat Bottom Sheet

1. Perform hand hygiene and put on PPE, if indicated.

2. If the patient is present in the room, explain to the patient what you are going to do why you are doing it.

3. Assemble necessary equipment on the bedside stand, overbed table or other surface within reach. Two large flat sheets are needed.

4. Raise bed to a comfortable working position, usually elbow height of the caregiver (VHACEOSH, 2016). Disconnect call bell or any other equipment from bed linens.

5. Put on gloves. Loosen all linen as you move around the bed, from the head of the bed on the far side to the head of the bed on the near side.

6. Fold reusable linens, such as sheets, blankets, or spread, in place on the bed in fourths and hang them over a clean chair.

7. Snugly roll all the soiled linen inside the bottom sheet and place directly into the laundry hamper. Do not place on floor or furniture. Do not hold soiled linens against your clothing.

8. If possible, shift mattress up to head of bed.

9. Remove your gloves. Place the bottom sheet with its centerfold in the center of the bed and high enough to be able to tuck it under the head of the mattress. Open the sheet and fan-fold to the center.

10. If using, place the drawsheet with its centerfold in the center of the bed and positioned so it will be located under the patient's midsection. Open the drawsheet and fan-fold it to the center of the mattress. If a protective pad is used, place it over the drawsheet in the proper area and open it to the centerfold.

11. Tuck the bottom sheet securely under the head of the mattress on one side of the bed, making a corner. Corners are usually mitered. Grasp the side edge of the sheet about 18 in down from the mattress top (Figure A). Lay the sheet on top of the mattress to form a triangular, flat fold (Figure B). Tuck under the mattress the portion of the sheet that is hanging loose below the mattress without pulling on the triangular fold (Figure C). Pick the top of the triangle fold and place it over the side of the mattress (Figure D). Tuck this loose portion of the sheet under the mattress. Continue tucking the remaining bottom sheet and drawsheet securely under the mattress (Figure E). Move to the other side of the bed to secure bottom linens. Pull the sheets across the mattress from the centerfold. Secure the bottom of the sheet under the head of the bed and miter the corner. Pull the remainder of the sheet and the drawsheet tightly and tuck under the mattress, starting at the head of the bed and moving toward the foot (Figure F).

12. Place the top sheet on the bed with its centerfold in the center of the bed and with the hem even with the head of the mattress. Unfold the top sheet. Follow the same procedure with the top blanket or spread, placing the upper edge about 6 in below the top of the sheet.

13. Tuck the top sheet and blanket under the foot of the bed on the near side. Miter the corners.

FIGURE A. Grasping side edge of sheet and lifting up to form a triangle.

FIGURE B. Laying sheet on top of bed to make triangular, flat fold.

FIGURE C. Tucking sheet under mattress.

FIGURE D. Placing top of triangular fold over mattress side.

FIGURE E. Tucking end of triangular linen fold under mattress to complete mitered corner.

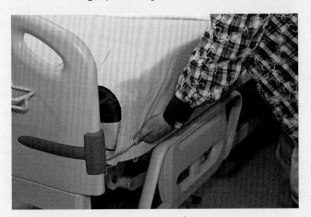

FIGURE F. Tucking sheet snugly under mattress.

14. Fold the upper 6 in of the top sheet down over the spread and make a cuff.
15. Move to the other side of the bed and follow the same procedure for securing top sheet under the foot of the bed and making a cuff.
16. Place the pillows on the bed. Open each pillowcase in the same manner as you opened other linens. Gather the pillowcase over one hand toward the closed end. Grasp the pillow with the hand inside the pillowcase. Keep a firm hold on the top of the pillow and pull the cover onto the pillow. Place the pillow at the head of the bed.

17. Fan-fold or pie-fold the top linens. Remove gloves.
18. Secure the signal device on the bed according to facility policy.
19. Adjust bed to low position. Raise rail.

20. Dispose of soiled linen according to facility policy. Perform hand hygiene.

Skill 7-11 ▶ Making an Occupied Bed

If the patient cannot get out of bed, the linens may need to be changed with the patient still in the bed. This is termed an "occupied" bed. In some instances, creativity and flexibility are necessary when changing linens because of the patient's condition, orthopedic appliances or other equipment in use, or treatments that may be in progress. The following procedure explains how to make the bed using a fitted bottom sheet. Some facilities do not provide fitted bottom sheets, or sometimes a fitted bottom sheet may not be available. If this is the case, refer to the Skill Variation for using a flat bottom sheet instead of a fitted sheet, located at the end of Skill 7-10.

(continued)

Skill 7-11 ▶ Making an Occupied Bed *(continued)*

DELEGATION CONSIDERATIONS	The making of an occupied bed may be delegated to nursing assistive personnel (NAP) or to unlicensed assistive personnel (UAP), as well as to licensed practical/vocational nurses (LPN/LVNs). The decision to delegate must be based on careful analysis of the patient's needs and circumstances, as well as the qualifications of the person to whom the task is being delegated. Refer to the Delegation Guidelines in Appendix A.

EQUIPMENT	• One large flat sheet • Linen hamper or bag • One fitted sheet • Bedside chair • Drawsheet (optional) • Protective pad (optional) • Blankets • Disposable gloves • Bedspread • Additional PPE, as indicated • Pillowcases

ASSESSMENT	Assess the facility policies and patient's preferences regarding linen changes. Assess for any precautions or activity restrictions for the patient. Check the bed for any patient belongings that may have accidentally been placed or fallen there, such as eyeglasses or prayer cloths. Note the presence and position of any tubes or drains that the patient may have.

NURSING DIAGNOSIS	Determine related factors for the nursing diagnoses based on the patient's current status. Appropriate nursing diagnoses may include: • Risk for impaired skin integrity • Impaired bed mobility • Impaired comfort

OUTCOME IDENTIFICATION AND PLANNING	The expected outcome to achieve when making an occupied bed is that the bed linens are applied without injury to the patient or nurse. Other possible outcomes may include the patient participating in moving from side to side, and patient verbalizes feelings of increased comfort.

IMPLEMENTATION

ACTION	RATIONALE
1. Check health care record for limitations on the patient's physical activity.	This facilitates patient cooperation, determines level of activity, and promotes patient safety.
2. Perform hand hygiene. Put on PPE, as indicated.	Hand hygiene and PPE prevent the spread of microorganisms. PPE is required based on transmission precautions.
3. Identify the patient. Explain what you are going to do.	Patient identification validates the correct patient and correct procedure. Discussion and explanation allay anxiety and prepare the patient for what to expect.
4. Assemble equipment on overbed table or other surface within reach.	Organization facilitates performance of task.
5. Close the curtains around the bed and close the door to the room, if possible.	This ensures the patient's privacy.
6. Adjust the bed to a comfortable working height, usually elbow height of the caregiver (VHACEOSH, 2016).	Having the bed at the proper height prevents back and muscle strain.
7. Lower the side rail nearest you, leaving the opposite side rail up. Place the bed in a flat position unless contraindicated.	Having the mattress flat makes it easier to prepare a wrinkle-free bed.
8. Put on gloves. Check bed linens for the patient's personal items. **Disconnect the call bell or any tubes/drains from bed linens.**	Gloves prevent the spread of microorganisms. It is costly and inconvenient when personal items are lost. Disconnecting tubes from linens prevents discomfort and accidental dislodging of the tubes.

ACTION

9. Place a bath blanket over the patient. Have the patient hold on to the bath blanket while you reach under it and remove the top linens (Figure 1). Leave the top sheet in place if a bath blanket is not used. Fold linen that is to be reused over the back of a chair. Discard soiled linen in a laundry bag or hamper. **Do not place on floor or furniture. Do not hold soiled linens against your clothing.**

10. If possible, and another person is available to assist, grasp mattress securely and shift it up to head of bed.

11. Assist the patient to turn toward the opposite side of the bed, and reposition pillow under the patient's head.

12. Loosen all bottom linens from head, foot, and side of bed.

13. Fan-fold or roll soiled linens as close to the patient as possible (Figure 2).

RATIONALE

The blanket provides warmth and privacy. Placing linens directly into the hamper helps prevent the spread of microorganisms. The floor is heavily contaminated; soiled linen will further contaminate furniture. Soiled linen contaminates the nurse's clothing, and this may spread organisms to another patient.

This allows more foot room for the patient.

This allows the bed to be made on the vacant side.

This facilitates removal of linens.

This makes it easier to remove linens when the patient turns to the other side.

FIGURE 1. Removing top linens from under bath blanket.

FIGURE 2. Moving soiled linen as close to patient as possible.

14. Use clean linen and make the near side of the bed. Place the bottom sheet in the center of the bed. Open the sheet and pull the bottom sheet over the corners at the head and foot of the mattress (Figure 3). Push the sheet toward the center of the bed, pulling it taut and positioning it under the old linens (Figure 4). (See the Skill Variation at the end of Skill 7-10 for information on using a flat bottom sheet, instead of a fitted sheet.)

Opening linens on the bed reduces strain on the nurse's arms and diminishes the spread of microorganisms. Centering the sheet ensures sufficient coverage for both sides of the mattress. Positioning under the old linens makes it easier to remove linens.

FIGURE 3. Pulling the bottom sheet over the corners at the head and foot of the mattress.

FIGURE 4. Pushing the bottom sheet toward the center of the bed, positioning it under old linens.

(continued)

Skill 7-11 ▶ Making an Occupied Bed *(continued)*

ACTION	RATIONALE

ACTION

15. If using, place the drawsheet with its centerfold in the center of the bed and positioned so it will be located under the patient's midsection. Open the drawsheet and fan-fold it to the center of the mattress. Tuck the drawsheet securely under the mattress (Figure 5). If a protective pad is used, place it over the drawsheet in the proper area and open to the centerfold. Not all facilities use drawsheets routinely. The nurse may decide to use one.

16. Raise the side rail. Assist the patient to roll over the folded linen in the middle of the bed toward you. Reposition pillow and bath blanket or top sheet. Move to other side of the bed and lower the side rail.

17. Loosen and remove all bottom linen (Figure 6). Discard soiled linen in laundry bag or hamper. **Do not place on floor or furniture. Do not hold soiled linens against your clothing.**

RATIONALE

If the patient soils the bed, drawsheet and pad can be changed without the bottom and top linens on the bed. A drawsheet can aid in moving the patient in bed.

This ensures patient safety. The movement allows the bed to be made on the other side. The bath blanket provides warmth and privacy.

Placing linens directly into the hamper helps prevent the spread of microorganisms. The floor is heavily contaminated; soiled linen will further contaminate the furniture. Soiled linen contaminates the nurse's clothing, and this may spread organisms to another patient.

FIGURE 5. Tucking drawsheet tightly.

FIGURE 6. Removing soiled bottom linens from other side of bed.

18. Ease clean linen from under the patient. Pull the bottom sheet taut and secure at the corners at the head and foot of the mattress. Pull the drawsheet tight and smooth. Tuck the drawsheet securely under the mattress. (See the Skill Variation at the end of Skill 7-10 for information on using a flat bottom sheet, instead of a fitted sheet.)

This removes wrinkles and creases in the linens, which are uncomfortable to lie on.

19. Assist the patient to turn back to the center of bed. Remove pillow and change pillowcase. Open each pillowcase in the same manner as you opened other linens. Gather the pillowcase over one hand toward the closed end. Grasp the pillow with the hand inside the pillowcase. Keep a firm hold on the top of the pillow and pull the cover onto the pillow. Place the pillow under the patient's head.

Opening linens by shaking causes organisms to be carried on air currents.

ACTION	RATIONALE
20. Apply top linen, sheet, and blanket, if desired, so that it is centered. Fold the top linens over at the patient's shoulders to make a cuff. Have the patient hold on to top linen and remove the bath blanket from underneath (Figure 7).	This allows bottom hems to be tucked securely under the mattress and provides for privacy.

FIGURE 7. Removing bath blanket from under top linens.

ACTION	RATIONALE
21. Secure top linens under foot of mattress and miter corners. (Refer to the Skill Variation in Skill 7-10 for information to miter a corner.) Loosen top linens over the patient's feet by grasping them in the area of the feet and pulling gently toward the foot of bed.	This provides for a neat appearance. Loosening linens over the patient's feet gives more room for movement.
22. Return the patient to a position of comfort. Remove your gloves. Raise the side rail and lower the bed. Reattach call bell.	Promotes patient comfort and safety. Removing gloves properly reduces the risk for infection transmission and contamination of other items.
23. Dispose of soiled linens according to facility policy.	Deters the spread of microorganisms.
24. Remove any other PPE, if used. Perform hand hygiene.	Proper removal of PPE reduces the risk for infection transmission and contamination of other items. Hand hygiene prevents the spread of microorganisms.

EVALUATION	The expected outcomes have been met when the bed linens are changed, and the patient and nurse remain free of injury. In addition, the patient assists in moving from side to side and states feelings of increased comfort after the bed is changed.
DOCUMENTATION	Changing of bed linens does not require documentation. The use of a specialty bed or bed equipment should be documented. Document any significant observations and communication.
UNEXPECTED SITUATIONS AND ASSOCIATED INTERVENTIONS	• *Dirty linens are grossly contaminated with urinary or fecal drainage:* Obtain an extra towel or protective pad. Place the pad under and over the soiled linens so that new linens will not be in contact with soiled linens. Clean and dry the mattress according to facility policy before applying new sheets.
SPECIAL CONSIDERATIONS	
Older Adult Considerations	• Using a soft bath blanket or a flannelette blanket as a bottom sheet may solve the problem of "coldness" for older adult patients with vascular problems or arthritis.

Enhance Your Understanding

Focusing on Patient Care: Developing Clinical Reasoning

Consider the case scenarios at the beginning of the chapter as you answer the following questions to enhance your understanding and apply what you have learned.

QUESTIONS

1. Denasia Kerr, the 6-year-old with limited mobility, needs her hair shampooed. How would you accomplish this task?

2. Cindy Vortex, the 34-year-old woman who is now in a coma after a car accident, is wearing contact lenses.

What information would be important to gather before attempting to remove the contact lenses?

3. Carl Sheen, 76 years of age, asks, "How can I clean my dentures with my right hand all tied up with this IV?" How best could you help Mr. Sheen with this hygiene activity while still fostering his independence?

You can find suggested answers after the Bibliography at the end of this chapter.

Integrated Case Study Connection

The case studies in the back of the book focus on integrating concepts. Refer to the following case studies to enhance your understanding of the concepts and skills in this chapter.

- Basic Case Studies: Joe LeRoy, page 1108.
- Intermediate Case Studies: Victoria Holly, page 1115.

Taylor Suite Resources

Explore these additional resources to enhance learning for this chapter:

- NCLEX-Style Questions and other resources on thePoint®, http://thePoint.lww.com/Lynn5e
- Skill Checklists for Taylor's Clinical Nursing Skills, 5e
- Taylor's Video Guide to *Clinical Nursing Skills: Hygiene*
- *Fundamentals of Nursing: Chapter 31, Hygiene*

Bibliography

Alzheimer's Association. (2016). Dental care. Retrieved https://www.alz.org/care/alzheimers-dementia-dental.asp

American Association of Critical-Care Nurses (AACN). (2010). *Practice Alert: Oral care in the critically ill*. Retrieved http://www.aacn.org/wd/practice/content/oral-care-practice-alert.pcms?menu=practice

American Dental Association (ADA). (n.d.a). Mouthrinses. Retrievedhttp://www.ada.org/en/science-research/ada-seal-of-acceptance/product-category-information/mouthrinses

American Dental Association (ADA). (n.d.b). Removable partial dentures. Retrievedhttp://www.mouthhealthy.org/en/az-topics/d/dentures-partial

American Dental Association (ADA). (2016a). MouthHealthy. Babies and kids. Retrievedhttp://www.mouthhealthy.org/en/babies-and-kids

American Dental Association (ADA). (2016b). MouthHealthy. Flossing. Retrievedhttp://www.mouthhealthy.org/en/az-topics/f/flossing

American Dental Association (ADA). (2016c). MouthHealthy. Dentures. Retrievedhttp://www.mouthhealthy.org/en/az-topics/d/dentures

Ames, N. J., Sulima, P., Yates, J. M., et al. (2011). Effects of systematic oral care in critically ill patients: A multicenter study. *American Journal of Critical Care, 20*(5), e103–e113. Available http://ajcc.aacnjournals.org/content/20/5/e103.full.pdf+html

Andriessen, A. (2013). Prevention, recognition and treatment of dry skin conditions. *British Journal of Nursing, 22*(1), 26–30.

Bardsley, A. (2015). Principles of skin cleansing in continence management. *British Journal of Nursing (Urology Supplement), 24*(18), S36–S38.

Bathing bedbound patients. (2015). *Homecare Direction, 23*(5), 11.

Berry, A. M., Davidson, P. M., Masters, J., & Rolls, K. (2007). Systematic literature review of oral hygiene practices for intensive care patients receiving mechanical ventilation. *American Journal of Critical Care, 16*(6), 552–562.

Black, J., & Hotaling, T. (2015). Ten top tips: Bariatric skin care. *Wounds International, 6*(3), 17–21.

Bloomfield, J., & Pegram, A. (2012). Physical healthcare needs: Oral hygiene in the mental health setting. *Mental Health Practice, 15*(6), 32–38.

Bloomfield, J., Pegram, A., & Jones, A. (2008). Recommended procedure for bedmaking in hospital. *Nursing Standard, 22*(23), 41–44.

Brennan, L. J., & Strauss, J. (2014). Cognitive impairment in older adults and oral health considerations: Treatment and management. *Dental Clinics of North America, 58*(4), 815–828.

Burn Foundation. (2016). Burn prevention. Safety facts on scald burns. Retrievedhttp://www.burnfoundation.org/programs/resource.cfm?c=1&a=3

Cassir, N., Thomas, G., Hraiech, S., et al. (2015). Chlorhexidine daily bathing: Impact on health care-associated infections caused by gram-negative bacteria. *American Journal of Infection Control, 43*(6), 640–643.

Chalmers, J. M., King, P. L., Spencer, A. J., Wright, F. A., & Carter, K. D. (2005). The oral health assessment tool – validity and reliability. *Australian Dental Journal, 50*(3), 191–199.

Chen, W., Cao, Q, Li, S., Li, H., & Zhang, W. (2015). Impact of daily bathing with chlorhexidine gluconate on ventilator associated pneumonia in intensive care units: a meta-analysis. *Journal of Thoracic Disease, 7*(4), 746–753.

Cleveland Clinic. (2015a). Contact lenses. Retrievedhttp://my.clevelandclinic.org/health/drugs_devices_supplements/hic_Contact_Lenses

Cleveland Clinic. (2015b). Contact lens care. Retrieved http://my.clevelandclinic.org/health/drugs_devices_supplements/hic_Contact_Lenses/hic_Contact_Lens_Care

Coke, L., Otten, K., Staffileno, B., Minarich, L., & Nowiszewski, C. (2015). The impact of an oral hygiene education module on patient practices and nursing documentation. *Clinical Journal of Oncology Nursing, 19*(1), 75–80.

Coker, E., Ploeg, J., Kaasalainen, S., & Fisher, A. (2013). A concept analysis of oral hygiene care in dependent older adults. *Journal of Advanced Nursing, 69*(10), 2360–2371.

Cowdell, F., & Radley, K. (2014). What do we know about skin-hygiene care for patients with bariatric needs? Implications for nursing practice. *Journal of Advanced Nursing, 70*(3), 543–552.

Davis, C. (2014). Caring for…patients with tattoos and body piercings. *Nursing Made Incredibly Easy, 12*(6), 48–51.

Doenges, M. E., Moorhouse, M. F., & Murr, A. C. (2016). *Nursing diagnoses manual. Planning, individualizing, and documenting client care* (5th ed.). Philadelphia, PA: F.A. Davis.

Eliopoulos, C. (2014). *Gerontological nursing* (8th ed.). Philadelphia, PA: Wolters Kluwer Health.

Felton, D., Cooper, L., Duqum, I., et al. (2011). Evidence-based guidelines for the care and maintenance of complete dentures. *The Journal of the American Dental Association, 142*(2 suppl), 1S–20S.

Gallagher, M., & Hall, G. R. (2014). Bathing persons with Alzheimer's disease and related dementias. *Journal of Gerontological nursing, 40*(2), 14–20.

Gozalo, P., Prakash, S., Qato, D. M., Sloane, P. D., & Mor, V. (2014). Effect of the bathing without a battle training intervention on bathing-associated physical and verbal outcomes in nursing home residents with dementia: A randomized crossover diffusion study. *Journal of the American Geriatrics Society, 62*(5), 797–804.

Hall, G. R., Gallagher, M., & Hoffmann-Snyder, C. (2013). Bathing persons with dementia. Iowa City, IA: University of Iowa College of Nursing, John A. Hartford Foundation Center of Geriatric Nursing Excellence. Retrieved https://www.guideline.gov/content.aspx?id=4 4984&search=hall+bathing

Halliday, K. (2005). Body piercing: Issues and challenges for nurses. *Journal of Forensic Nursing, 1*(2), 47–56.

Herter, R., & Kazer, M. W. (2010). Best practices in urinary catheter. *Home Healthcare Nurse, 28*(6), 342–349.

Hillier, B., Wilson, C., Chamberlain, D. & King, L. (2013). Preventing ventilator-associated pneumonia through oral care, product selection, and application method. *AACN Advanced Critical Care, 24*(1), 38–58.

Hines, A. G., Nuss, S., Rupp, M. E., Lyden, E., Tyner, K., & Hewlett, A. (2015). Chlorhexidine bathing of hospitalized patients: Beliefs and practices of nurses and patient care technicians, and potential barriers to compliance. *Infection Control & Hospital Epidemiology, 36*(8), 993–994.

Hinkle, J. L., & Cheever, K. H. (2018). *Brunner & Suddarth's textbook of medical–surgical nursing* (14th ed.). Philadelphia: Wolters Kluwer.

Holman, C., Roberts, S., & Nicol, M. (2005). Practice update: Clinical skills with older people. Promoting oral hygiene. *Nursing Older People, 16*(10), 37–38.

Jablonski, R. A. (2012). Oral health and hygiene content in nursing fundamentals textbooks. *Nursing Research and Practice.* Article ID 372617. Retrieved http://www.hindawi.com/journals/nrp/2012/372617

Jablonski, R., Mertz, E., Featherstone, J. D., & Fulmer, T. (2014). Maintaining oral health across the life span. *Nurse Practitioner, 39*(6), 39–48.

Jablonski, R. A., Therrien, B., & Kolanowski, A. (2011). No more fighting and biting during mouth care: Applying the theoretical constructs of threat perception to clinical practice. *Research and Theory for Nursing Practice: An International Journal, 25*(3), 163–175.

Jarvis, C. (2016). *Physical Examination & Health Assessment* (7th ed.). St. Louis, MO: Elsevier.

Jennings, A. (2015). Assessing oral hygiene in hospitalized older veterans. *MEDSURG Nursing, 24*(6), 420–424.

Jensen, S. (2015). *Nursing health assessment: A best practice approach* (2nd ed.). Philadelphia, PA: Wolters Kluwer Health.

Johnson, R. H. (2011). Practical care: Creative strategies for bathing. *Nursing & Residential Care, 13*(8), 392–394.

Johnson, V. B. (2012). Evidence-based practice guideline. Oral hygiene care for functionally dependent and cognitively impaired older adults. *Journal of Gerontological Nursing, 38*(11), 11–19.

Johnson, V. B., & Chalmers, J. (2011). *Oral hygiene care for functionally dependent and cognitively impaired older adults.* Iowa City, IA: University of Iowa College of Nursing. National Guideline Clearinghouse. Retrieved http://www.iowanursingguidelines.com

Johnson, R., & Quinn, B. (2013). Supporting the older person with oral hygiene. *Nursing & Residential Care, 15*(4), 201–204.

Kadia, S., Bawas, R., Shah, H., Narang, P., & Lippmann, S. (2014). Poor oral hygiene in the mentally ill: Be aware of the problem, and intervene. *Current Psychiatry, 13*(7), 47–48.

Kelly, T., Timmis, S., & Twelvetree, T. (2010). Review of the evidence to support oral hygiene in stroke patients. *Nursing Standard, 24*(37), 35–38.

Konno, R., Kang, H. S., & Makimoto, K. (2014). A best-evidence review of intervention studies for minimizing resistance-to-care behaviours for older adults

with dementia in nursing homes. *Journal of Advanced Nursing, 70*(10), 2167–2180.

Kyle, T., & Carman, S. (2017). *Essentials of pediatric nursing* (3rd ed.). Philadelphia, PA: Wolters Kluwer Health.

Lee, K. H., Wu, B., & Plassman, B. L. (2013). Cognitive function and oral health-related quality of life in older adults. *Journal of the American Geriatrics Society, 61*(9), 1602–1607.

Lev, A., Aied, A. S., & Arshed, S. (2015). The effect of different oral hygiene treatments on the occurrence of ventilator associated pneumonia (VAP) in ventilated patients. *Journal of Infection Prevention, 16*(2), 76–81.

Lichterfeld, A., Hauss, A., Surber, C., Peters, T., Blume-Peytavi, U., & Lottner, J. (2015). Evidence-based skin care: A systematic literature review and the development of a basic skin care algorithm. *Journal of Wound, Ostomy and Continence Nursing, 42*(5), 501–524.

Malkin, B., & Berridge, P. (2009). Guidance on maintaining personal hygiene in nail care. *Nursing Standard, 23*(41), 35–38.

Mayo Foundation for Medical Education and Research (MFMER). (n.d.). Peripheral Artery Disease (PAD). Lifestyle and Home Remedies. Retrieved http://www.mayoclinic.org/diseases-conditions/peripheral-artery-disease/manage/ptc-20167503

Mayo Foundation for Medical Education and Research (MFMER). (2014a). Amputation and diabetes: How to Protect Your Feet. Retrieved http://www.mayoclinic.org/diseases-conditions/diabetes/in-depth/amputation-and-diabetes/art-20048262

Mayo Foundation for Medical Education and Research (MFMER). (2014b). Denture care: How do I clean dentures? Retrieved http://www.mayoclinic.org/denture-care/expert-answers/faq-20058375

Mayo Foundation for Medical Education and Research (MFMER). (2014c). Fingernails: Do's and Don'ts for Healthy Nails. Retrieved http://www.mayoclinic.org/healthy-lifestyle/adult-health/in-depth/nails/art-20044954

Mayo Foundation for Medical Education and Research (MFMER). (2014d). Skin Care: 5 Tips for Healthy Skin. Retrievedhttp://www.mayoclinic.org/healthy-lifestyle/adult-health/in-depth/skin-care/art-20048237

Mayo Foundation for Medical Education and Research (MFMER). (2015a). Piercings: How to Prevent Complications. Retrieved http://www.mayoclinic.org/healthy-lifestyle/adult-health/in-depth/piercings/art-20047317

Mayo Foundation for Medical Education and Research (MFMER). (2015b). Ingrown Hair. Prevention. Retrieved http://www.mayoclinic.org/diseases-conditions/ingrown-hair/basics/prevention/con-20034717

Mayo Foundation for Medical Education and Research (MFMER). (2016). Oral Health: Brush Up on Dental Care Basics. Retrieved http://www.mayoclinic.org/healthy-lifestyle/adult-health/in-depth/dental/art-20045536

MedlinePlus. (2015). *Penis Care (uncircumcised).* Retrieved http://www.nlm.nih.gov/medlineplus/ency/article/001917.htm

NANDA International, Inc.: Nursing Diagnoses - Definitions and Classification 2018–2020 © 2017 NANDA International, ISBN 978-1-62623-929-6. Used by arrangement with the Thieme Group, Stuttgart/New York.

National Institute on Aging (NIA). (2015). *Age Page. Foot Care.* Retrieved https://www.nia.nih.gov/health/publication/foot-care

National Institute of Health (NIH). National Institute of Dental and Craniofacial Research. (2014). Oral Health. Chemotherapy and Your Mouth. Retrieved http://www.nidcr.nih.gov/oralhealth/Top-

ics/CancerTreatment/ChemotherapyYourMouth. htm#WhatCan

National Institute of Health (NIH). (2015). Keep your mouth healthy. Oral care for older adults. Retrieved https://newsinhealth.nih.gov/issue/oct2015/feature2

Nicolosi, L. N., del Carmen Rubio, M., Martinez, C. D., Gonzáles, N. N., & Cruz, M. E. (2014). Effect of oral hygiene and 0.12% chlorhexidine gluconate oral rinse in preventing ventilator-associated pneumonia after cardiovascular surgery. *Respiratory Care, 59*(4), 504–509.

Perry, S. E., Hockenberry, M. J., Lowdermilk, D. L., & Wilson, D. (2014). *Maternal child nursing care* (5th ed.). St. Louis, MO: Elsevier Mosby.

Petlin, A., Schallom, M., Prentice, D., et al. (2014). Chlorhexidine gluconate bathing to reduce methicillin-resistant *staphylococcus aureus* acquisition. *Critical Care Nurse, 34*(5), 17–26.

Purnell, L. D. (2013). *Transcultural health care. A culturally competent approach* (4th ed.). Philadelphia, PA: F.A. Davis Company.

Pyrek, K. M. (2015). Experts address the promise and challenges of CHG bathing interventions. *Infection Control Today, 19*(1), 32–36.

Quinn, B., & Baker, D. L. (2015). Comprehensive oral care helps prevent hospital-acquired nonventilator pneumonia. *American Nurse Today, 10*(3), 18–22.

Schoonhoven, L., van Gaal, B. G, Teerenstra, S., et al. (2015). Cost-consequence analysis of "washing without water" for nursing home residents: A cluster randomized trial. *International Journal of Nursing Studies, 52*(1), 112–120.

Shah, H. N., Schwartz, J. L., & Cullen, D. L. (2016). Bathing with 2% chlorhexidine gluconate. Evidence and costs associated with central line-associated blood stream infections. *Critical Care Nursing Quarterly, 39*(1), 42–50.

So, H. S., You, M. A., Mun, J. Y., et al. (2014). Effect of trunk to head bathing on physiological responses in newborns. *Journal of Obstetric, Gynecological, & Neonatal Nursing, 43*(6), 742–751.

Society of Urologic Nurses and Associates (SUNA). (2010). *Clinical practice guidelines. Prevention & control of catheter-associated urinary tract infection (CAUTI). [Brochure].* Pitman, NJ: Author.

Taylor, C., Lynn, P., & Bartlett, J. (2019). *Fundamentals of nursing: The art and science of person-centered care* (9th ed.). Philadelphia, PA: Wolters Kluwer.

Underwood, L. (2015). The effect of implementing a comprehensive unit-based safety program on urinary catheter use. *Urologic Nursing, 35*(6), 271–279.

U.S. Food and Drug Administration (FDA). (2014). *A guide to bed safety. Bed rails in hospitals, nursing homes and home health care: The facts.* Retreived http://www.fda.gov/MedicalDevices/ProductsandMedicalProcedures/GeneralHospitalDevicesandSupplies/HospitalBeds/ucm123676.htm

VHA Center for Engineering & Occupational Safety and Health (CEOSH). (2016). *Safe patient handling and mobility guidebook.* St. Louis, MO: Author. Retrieved http://www.tampavaref.org/safe-patient-handling.htm

Viray, M. A., Morley, J., Coopersmith, C. M., Kollef, M. H., Fraser, V. J., & Warren, D. K. (2014). Daily bathing with chlorhexidine-based soap and the prevention of *staphylococcus aureus* transmission and infection. *Infection Control and Hospital Epidemiology, 35*(3), 243–250.

Voegeli, D. (2010). Care or harm: Exploring essential components in skin care regimens. *British Journal of Nursing, 19*(13), 812–819.

Voegeli, D. (2013). Moisture-associated skin damage: An overview for community nurses.*British Journal of Community Nursing, 18*(1), 6–12.

Wolf, Z. R., & Czekanski, K. E. (2015). Bathing disability and bathing persons with dementia. *MEDSURG Nursing, 24*(1), 9–22.

SUGGESTED ANSWERS FOR FOCUSING ON PATIENT CARE: DEVELOPING CLINICAL REASONING

1. Before Denasia's hair is washed, assess the situation. Assess the patient's hygiene preferences: frequency, time of day, and type of shampoo products. Assess for any physical activity limitations. Assess the patient's ability to get out of bed to have her hair washed. If the medical orders allow it and the patient is physically able to wash her hair in the shower, the patient may prefer to do so. Otherwise, the shampoo could take place at the sink, if available. If the patient cannot tolerate being out of bed or is not allowed to do so, or a sink is not available, perform a bed shampoo. Assess for any activity or positioning limitations. Inspect the patient's scalp for any cuts, lesions, or bumps. Note any flaking, drying, or excessive oiliness. Find out if Denasia would prefer a family member to shampoo her hair. If shampooing in bed, a shampoo cap can be used. Otherwise, use a shampoo board or tray, shampoo and water.

2. Before removing Ms. Vortex's contacts assess the following: Assess both eyes for contact lenses, because some people wear them in only one eye. Determine the type of contact lenses worn. Assess eyes for any redness or drainage, which may indicate an eye infection or an allergic response. Assess for any eye injury. If an injury is present, notify the primary care provider about the presence of the contact lens. Do not try to remove the contact lens in this situation due to the risk for additional eye injury.

3. Assess the patient's oral hygiene preferences: frequency, time of day, and type of hygiene products. Assess for any physical activity limitations. Assess the patient's ability to perform own care. Determine if the IV site can be covered with water-protecting material, such as a glove or plastic wrap, to allow Mr. Sheen the ability to care for his dentures. Explore the possibility of discontinuing the IV infusion for a short period of time to keep the IV tubing from interfering with oral hygiene. If this is a possibility, review facility policy and determine the need for medical clearance to implement this option. Encourage Mr. Sheen to do as much as he can; offer assistance, as needed. Patients are often afraid they will damage the IV or hurt themselves. Reinforce the fact that normal range of motion and activity are acceptable and should not interfere with the IV infusion.

8

Skin Integrity and Wound Care

Focusing on Patient Care

This chapter will help you develop some of the skills related to skin integrity and wound care necessary to care for the following patients:

Lori Downs, a patient with diabetes mellitus, is being treated in the outpatient wound center for a chronic wound on her left foot.

Tran Nguyen, diagnosed with breast cancer, has had a modified radical mastectomy and is 3 days post-op.

Arthur Lowes, has an appointment with his surgeon today for a follow-up examination and removal of surgical staples following a colon resection.

Refer to Focusing on Patient Care: Developing Clinical Reasoning at the end of the chapter to apply what you learn.

Learning Objectives

After completing the chapter, you will be able to accomplish the following:

1. Provide interventions to prevent pressure injury.
2. Clean a wound and apply a dry, sterile dressing.
3. Perform wound irrigation.
4. Collect a wound culture.
5. Apply Montgomery straps.
6. Provide care to a Penrose drain.
7. Provide care to a T-tube drain.
8. Provide care to a Jackson–Pratt drain.
9. Provide care to a Hemovac drain.
10. Apply negative pressure wound therapy.
11. Remove sutures.
12. Remove surgical staples.
13. Apply an external heating pad.
14. Apply a warm compress.
15. Assist with a sitz bath.
16. Apply cold therapy.

Key Terms

approximated (wound edges): edges of a wound that are lightly pulled together; epithelialization of wound margins; edges touch, wound is closed

debridement: removal of devitalized tissue and foreign material from a wound

dehiscence: accidental separation of wound edges, especially a surgical wound

ecchymosis: discoloration of an area resulting from infiltration of blood into the subcutaneous tissue

edema: accumulation of fluid in the interstitial tissues

epithelialization: stage of wound healing in which epithelial cells move across the surface of a wound margin (approximation); tissue color ranges from the color of "ground glass" to pink

erythema: redness or inflammation of an area as a result of dilation and congestion of capillaries

eschar: a thick, leathery scab or dry crust composed of dead cells and dried plasma

exudate: fluid that accumulates in a wound; may contain serum, cellular debris, bacteria, and white blood cells

granulation tissue: new tissue that is deep pink/red composed of fibroblasts and small blood vessels that fill an open wound when it starts to heal; characterized by irregular surface-like raspberries

health care–associated infections: infections caused by a wide variety of common and unusual bacteria, fungi, and viruses during the course of receiving medical care (CDC, 2016)

ischemia: insufficient blood supply to a body part due to obstruction of circulation

jaundice: condition characterized by yellowness of the skin, whites of eyes, mucous membranes, and body fluids as a result of deposition of bile pigment resulting from excess bilirubin in the blood

maceration: softening of tissue due to excessive moisture

necrosis: localized tissue death

nonsterile (clean) technique: strategies used in patient care to reduce overall number of microorganisms or to prevent or reduce the risk of transmission of microorganisms from one person to another or from one place to another. Involves meticulous handwashing, maintaining a clean environment by preparing a clean field, using clean gloves and sterile instruments, and preventing direct contamination of materials and supplies (WOCN, 2012)

pathogens: microorganisms that can harm humans

pressure injury: localized damage to the skin and underlying tissue that usually occurs over a bony prominence or is related to the use of a (medical or other) device, resulting from intense and/or prolonged pressure or pressure in combination with shear (NPUAP, 2016c).

sinus tract: cavity or channel underneath a wound that has the potential for infection

sterile technique: strategies used in patient care to reduce exposure to microorganisms and maintain objects and areas as free from microorganisms as possible. Involves meticulous handwashing, use of a sterile field, use of sterile gloves for application of a sterile dressing, and use of sterile instruments (WOCN, 2012)

surgical staples: stainless-steel wire (shaped like a staple) used to close a surgical wound

surgical sutures: thread or wire used to hold tissue and skin together

tunneling: passageway or opening that may be visible at skin level, but with most of the tunnel under the surface of the skin

undermining: areas of tissue destruction underneath intact skin along the margins of a wound

vasoconstriction: narrowing of the lumen of a blood vessel

vasodilation: an increase in the diameter of a blood vessel

The skin is the body's first line of defense, protecting the underlying structures, tissues, and organs. Alteration in skin integrity, disruption in the normal integrity and function of the skin and underlying tissues, is a potentially dangerous and possibly life-threatening situation. Disruptions in skin and tissue integrity are called wounds; wounds resulting from compression of skin and underlying tissues for a prolonged period or pressure in combination with shear are termed pressure injuries (Hess, 2013; NPUAP,

2016c; NPUAP, EPUAP, & PPPIA, 2014b). The term **pressure injury** has replaced the term *pressure ulcer* to more accurately describe pressure injuries to both intact and ulcerated skin (NPUAP, 2016a).

Wounds and pressure injuries often require physical and emotional adaptation and are potential and actual source of stress for a patient, impacting a person's quality of life. Stressors may include pain, anxiety, fear, alterations in activities of daily living, and changes in body image. Patients with a wound and/or pressure injury are at risk for complications such as infection, hemorrhage, **dehiscence**, evisceration, and delayed wound healing.

The nurse plays a major role in maintaining the patient's skin integrity, identifying risk factors that predispose a patient to a break in integrity, intervening to prevent or reduce a patient's risk for impaired skin integrity, and providing specific wound care when breaks in integrity occur. Nursing responsibilities related to skin integrity and wound care involve assessment of the patient and the wound and staging of pressure injuries (Fundamentals Review 8-1, 8-2, and 8-3), followed by the development of the nursing care plan, including the identification of appropriate outcomes, nursing interventions, and evaluation of the nursing care. Depending upon the patient's individualized care plan, specific wound care skills may be needed. Refer to Chapter 3 for additional information related to assessment of the skin and integumentary system.

It is extremely important to use appropriate aseptic technique when caring for wounds and pressure injuries to prevent introduction of microorganisms. Hand hygiene before and after dressing changes is imperative; follow *Standard Precautions* and, if needed, *Transmission-Based Precautions* in providing wound care. Carelessness in adherence to aseptic technique and wound care practice recommendations is a cause of **health care–associated infections** (Ding et al., 2017). Pressure injuries (ulcers) and chronic wounds may be treated using clean technique **(nonsterile technique)** (Baranoski & Ayello, 2016; NPUAP, EPUAP, & PPPIA, 2014b; WOCN, 2012). Fundamentals Review 8-4 identifies basic principles related to the use of clean technique and wound care. Refer to Chapter 1 for a discussion of infection control precautions and additional information related to **sterile technique,** medical asepsis, and clean technique.

Ongoing assessment for possible skin or wound complications is required. An ideal dressing/product maintains a moist environment to promote healing, is absorbent, provides thermal insulation, acts as a barrier to microorganisms, reduces or eliminates pain, and allows for pain-free removal (Baranoski & Ayello, 2016; Doughty & McNichol, 2016; Leaper, et al., 2012; Ousey et al., 2016; Sood et al., 2014). There are hundreds of products available for use, each with distinctive actions, as well as indications, contraindications, advantages, and disadvantages (see Fundamentals Review 8-5). As a result, inclusion of skills related to the use of each type of product is not possible. It is extremely important for the nurse to be familiar with the indications for and correct application of each type of dressing and wound care product in use. Fundamentals Review 8-5 outlines the characteristics, purposes, and the use of some of these wound dressing products. In the past, wet-to-dry gauze (saline-moistened) dressings have been used to debride wounds, but is no longer considered good practice. This type of dressing damages healthy wound bed tissue, disrupts angiogenesis, and can be painful and is not included here (Baranoski & Ayello, 2016; Joanna Briggs Institute, 2013).

Nurses must also be skilled in assessing the patient for pain and employing strategies to minimize the patient's pain experience. Some patients may experience both physiologic and psychological pain related to dressing changes and wound care. Perform a pain assessment at each dressing change; measure and document the level of pain before, during, and after a procedure. Even if pain is never verbalized or expressed, always assume that pain is a definite possibility, and focus on comfort needs (NPUAP, EPUAP, & PPPIA, 2014b). Ask the patient about pain from the wound and determine if the pain is a one-time episode, occurs with dressing changes, or constant pain (Baranoski & Ayello, 2016). If the patient experiences increased or constant pain from the wound, perform further assessments. Increasing pain, especially when accompanied by an increased or purulent flow of drainage, may indicate delayed healing or an infection (NPUAP, EPUAP, & PPPIA, 2014b). Surgical incisional pain is usually most severe for the first 2 to 3 days and then progressively diminishes. Refer to Chapter 10 for additional information related to patient comfort and pain management.

It is often appropriate and necessary to consult with a wound care specialist, often a wound certified nurse specialist, to plan and coordinate the most effective care for a patient.

This chapter covers skills to assist the nurse in providing care related to skin integrity and wounds.

Fundamentals Review 8-1

GENERAL WOUND ASSESSMENT

Wounds are assessed for appearance, size, drainage, pain, presence of sutures, drains, and tubes, and the evidence of complications. Refer to Chapter 3 for additional information related to assessment of the skin and integumentary system.

PERFORMING GENERAL WOUND ASSESSMENT

- Assess the wound's appearance by inspecting and palpating. Look for the approximation of the edges and the color of the wound and surrounding area. The edges should be clean and well **approximated**. Edges may be reddened and slightly swollen for about a week, then closer to normal in appearance. Skin around the wound may be bruised initially.
- Observe for signs of infection: redness, **erythema**, warmth, pain, **edema**/swelling, presence of purulent drainage (WOCN, 2016).
- Observe for these additional signs of infection in chronic wounds, as the classic symptoms of infection may be diminished or altered: serous drainage with concurrent inflammation, delayed healing, discolored and/or friable **granulation tissue**, pocketing at the base of the wound, foul odor, wound breakdown (WOCN, 2016).

- Note the presence of any sutures, drains, and tubes. These areas are assessed in the same manner as the incision. Make sure they are intact and functioning.
- Assess the amount, color, odor, and consistency of any wound drainage.
- Assess the patient's pain, using an objective scale. Incisional pain is usually most severe for the first 2 to 3 days, after which it progressively diminishes. Increased or constant pain, especially an acute change in pain, requires further assessment. It can be a sign of delayed healing, infection, or other complication.
- Assess the patient's general condition for signs and symptoms of infection and hemorrhage.
- Consider use of photography to document the appearance of the wound, based on access and facility policy (Baranoski & Ayello, 2016).
- Consider use of a tool to monitor and document patient symptoms and wound healing, such as the Pressure Ulcer Scale for Healing (PUSH), the Bates-Jensen Wound Assessment Tool (BWAT), and the Toronto Symptom Assessment System for Wounds (TSAS-W) (Baranoski & Ayello, 2016; Doughty & McNichol, 2016; Harris et al., 2010; Maida et al., 2009; NPUAP, 2016e).

Fundamentals Review 8-2

MEASURING WOUNDS AND PRESSURE INJURIES

Wounds are assessed for appearance, size, drainage, pain, presence of sutures, drains, and tubes, and the evidence of complications. Refer to Chapter 3 for additional information related to assessment of the skin and integumentary system.

SIZE OF THE WOUND

- Draw the shape and describe it.
- Measure the length, width, and diameter (if circular).

DEPTH OF THE WOUND

- Perform hand hygiene. Put on gloves.
- Moisten a sterile, flexible applicator with saline and insert it gently into the wound at a 90-degree angle, with the tip down (Figure A).

FIGURE A.

- Mark the point on the swab that is even with the surrounding skin surface, or grasp the applicator with the thumb and forefinger at the point corresponding to the wound's margin (Figure B).

FIGURE B.

- Remove the swab and measure the depth with a ruler (Figure C).

FIGURE C.

Fundamentals Review 8-2 continued

MEASURING WOUNDS AND PRESSURE INJURIES

WOUND TUNNELING

- Perform hand hygiene. Put on gloves.
- Determine direction: Moisten a sterile, flexible applicator with saline and gently insert a sterile applicator into the site where **tunneling** occurs. View the direction of the applicator as if it were the hand of a clock (Figure D). The direction of the patient's head represents 12 o'clock. Moving in a clockwise direction, document the deepest sites where the wound tunnels.
- Determine the depth: While the applicator is inserted into the tunneling, mark the point on the swab that is even with the wound's edge, or grasp the applicator with the thumb and forefinger at the point corresponding to the wound's margin. Remove the swab and measure the depth with a ruler (see Figure C).
- Document both the direction and depth of tunneling.

FIGURE D.

Source: Adapted from Hess, C. (2013). *Clinical guide to skin & wound care* (7th ed.). Philadelphia, PA: Wolters Kluwer.

Fundamentals Review 8-3

PRESSURE INJURY STAGES

PRESSURE INJURY

A pressure injury is localized damage to the skin and underlying soft tissue usually over a bony prominence or related to a medical or other device. The injury can present as intact skin or an open ulcer and may be painful. The injury occurs as a result of intense and/or prolonged pressure or pressure in combination with shear. The tolerance of soft tissue for pressure and shear may also be affected by microclimate, nutrition, perfusion, co-morbidities and condition of the soft tissue.

Healthy skin, lightly pigmented.[a]

Healthy skin, darkly pigmented.[a]

STAGE 1 PRESSURE INJURY: NONBLANCHABLE ERYTHEMA OF INTACT SKIN

Intact skin with a localized area of nonblanchable erythema, which may appear differently in darkly pigmented skin. Presence of blanchable erythema or changes in sensation, temperature, or firmness may precede visual changes. Color changes do not include purple or maroon discoloration; these may indicate deep tissue pressure injury.

Stage 1 pressure injury, lightly pigmented.[a]

Stage 1 pressure injury, darkly pigmented.[a]

(continued)

Fundamentals Review 8-3 continued

PRESSURE INJURY STAGES

STAGE 2 PRESSURE INJURY: PARTIAL-THICKNESS SKIN LOSS WITH EXPOSED DERMIS

Partial-thickness loss of skin with exposed dermis. The wound bed is viable, pink or red, moist, and may also present as an intact or ruptured serum-filled blister. Adipose (fat) is not visible and deeper tissues are not visible. Granulation tissue, slough, and **eschar** are not present. These injuries commonly result from adverse microclimate and shear in the skin over the pelvis and shear in the heel. This stage should not be used to describe moisture-associated skin damage (MASD) including incontinence-associated dermatitis (IAD), intertriginous dermatitis (ITD), medical adhesive–related skin injury (MARSI), or traumatic wounds (skin tears, burns, abrasions).

Stage 2 pressure injury.[a]

STAGE 3 PRESSURE INJURY: FULL-THICKNESS SKIN LOSS

Full-thickness loss of skin, in which adipose (fat) is visible in the ulcer and granulation tissue and epibole (rolled wound edges) are often present. Slough and/or eschar may be visible. The depth of tissue damage varies by anatomical location; areas of significant adiposity can develop deep wounds. **Undermining** and tunneling may occur. Fascia, muscle, tendon, ligament, cartilage, and/or bone are not exposed. If slough or eschar obscures the extent of tissue loss, this is an Unstageable Pressure Injury.

Stage 3 pressure injury.[a]

STAGE 4 PRESSURE INJURY: FULL-THICKNESS SKIN AND TISSUE LOSS

Full-thickness skin and tissue loss with exposed or directly palpable fascia, muscle, tendon, ligament, cartilage or bone in the ulcer. Slough and/or eschar may be visible. Epibole (rolled edges), undermining, and/or tunneling often occur. Depth varies by anatomical location. If slough or eschar obscures the extent of tissue loss, this is an Unstageable Pressure Injury.

Stage 4 pressure injury.[a]

Fundamentals Review 8-3   continued

PRESSURE INJURY STAGES

UNSTAGEABLE PRESSURE INJURY: OBSCURED FULL-THICKNESS SKIN AND TISSUE LOSS

Full-thickness skin and tissue loss in which the extent of tissue damage within the ulcer cannot be confirmed because it is obscured by slough or eschar. If slough or eschar is removed, a stage 3 or stage 4 pressure injury will be revealed. Stable eschar (i.e., dry, adherent, intact without erythema or fluctuance) on the heel or ischemic limb should not be softened or removed.

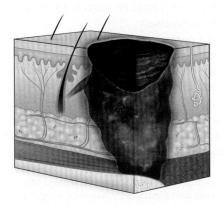

Unstageable pressure injury, dark eschar.[a]

Unstageable pressure injury, slough and eschar.[a]

DEEP TISSUE PRESSURE INJURY: PERSISTENT NONBLANCHABLE DEEP RED, MAROON, OR PURPLE DISCOLORATION

Intact or nonintact skin with localized area of persistent nonblanchable deep red, maroon, or purple discoloration or epidermal separation revealing a dark wound bed or blood-filled blister. Pain and temperature change often precede skin color changes. Discoloration may appear differently in darkly pigmented skin. This injury results from intense and/ or prolonged pressure and shear forces at the bone–muscle interface. The wound may evolve rapidly to reveal the actual extent of tissue injury, or may resolve without tissue loss. If necrotic tissue, subcutaneous tissue, granulation tissue, fascia, muscle, or other underlying structures are visible, this indicates a full-thickness pressure injury (unstageable, stage 3, or stage 4). Do not use DTPI to describe vascular, traumatic, neuropathic, or dermatologic conditions.

Deep tissue pressure injury.[a]

Source: Reprinted with permission from National Pressure Ulcer Advisory Panel (NPUAP). (2016b). *NPUAP Pressure injury stages.* Retrieved http://www.npuap.org/resources/educational-and-clinical-resources/npuap-pressure-injury-stages.
[a]Illustrations redrawn from National Pressure Ulcer Advisory Panel (NPUAP) (2016c). Pressure injury staging illustrations. Retrieved http://www.npuap.org/resources/educational-and-clinical-resources/pressure-injury-staging-illustrations.

Fundamentals Review 8-4

CLEAN (NONSTERILE) TECHNIQUE AND WOUND CARE

Clean technique involves strategies to reduce the overall number of microorganisms or to prevent or reduce the risk of transmission of microorganisms from one person to another or from one place to another (WOCN, 2012, p. S30). The aim of the use of clean technique in wound care is to ensure that contamination of the wound, any supplies and the environment is minimized (Heale, 2014, para 14).

Clean technique in wound care involves:

- Consideration of patient and wound factors, care environment, and likelihood of exposure to microorganisms
- Meticulous hand hygiene before initiating care and before/after glove changes
- Use of clean gloves
- Use of sterile instruments, solutions, supplies, and dressings that are maintained as clean

- Preventing direct contamination of materials and supplies
- Avoiding direct touching of the wound or any surface that might come in contact with the wound
- Sterile gloves should be worn if direct contact with the wound is necessary
- Use of a nonporous material to protect the surface under the wound
- Change gloves after removal of old dressing and after cleaning of the wound
- Cutting dressing materials with sterile scissors and storing dry and uncontaminated cut dressing materials in the original package, sealed and labeled in a clean, plastic storage bag

Source: Adapted from Heale, M. (2014). How 'clean' is your clean dressing technique? Wound Source. Retrieved http://www.wound-source.com/blog/how-clean-your-clean-dressing-technique; and Wound, Ostomy and Continence Nurses Society (WOCN). (2012). Clean vs. sterile dressing techniques for management of chronic wounds. A fact sheet. *Journal of Wound, Ostomy, and Continence Nursing, 39*(Suppl2), S30–S34.

Fundamentals Review 8-5

EXAMPLES OF WOUND DRESSINGS/PRODUCTS

Type	Purposes	Use
Transparent films, such as: • 3M Medipore • 3M Tegaderm • BIOCLUSIVE • ClearSite • DermaView • OPSITE • Suresite	• Allow exchange of oxygen between wound and environment • Are self-adhesive • Protect against contamination; waterproof • Prevent loss of wound fluid • Maintain a moist wound environment • Facilitate autolytic **debridement** • No absorption of drainage • Allow visualization of wound • May remain in place for 4 to 7 days, resulting in less interference with healing	• Wounds that are small; partial thickness • Stage 1 pressure injuries • Wounds with minimal drainage • Cover dressings for gels, foams, and gauze • Secure intravenous catheters, nasal cannulas, chest tube dressing, central venous access devices
Hydrocolloid dressings, such as: • Comfeel • DuoDERM • Exuderm • PrimaCol • Ultec	• Are occlusive or semi-occlusive, limiting exchange of oxygen between wound and environment • Inner layer is self-adherent, gel-forming, and composed of colloid particles • Outer layer seals and protects the wound from contamination • Minimal to moderate absorption of drainage • Maintain a moist wound environment • Thermal insulation • Provide cushioning • Facilitate autolytic debridement • May remain in place for 3 to 7 days, depending on **exudate**	• Partial- and full-thickness wounds • Stage 2 and stage 3 pressure injuries • Prevention at high-risk friction areas • Wounds with light to moderate drainage • Wounds with **necrosis** or slough • First- and second-degree burns • Not for use with wounds that are infected

Fundamentals Review 8-5   continued

EXAMPLES OF WOUND DRESSINGS/PRODUCTS

Type	Purposes	Use
Hydrogels, such as: • Aquasorb • DermaGauze • FlexiGel • Hypergel • INTRASITE Gel	• Polymer gels comprised of an 80% to 99% water base • Available in many sizes and forms (gels, sheets, gauze, strips) • Maintain a moist wound environment • Minimal absorption of drainage • Facilitate autolytic debridement • Thermal insulation • Do not adhere to wound • Less effective barrier than occlusive dressings • Reduce pain • Most require a secondary dressing to secure • May remain in place for 24 to 72 hours, depending on the gel form	• Partial- and full-thickness wounds • Stages 2–4 pressure injuries • Necrotic wounds • First- and second-degree burns • Dry wounds • Wounds with minimal exudate • Infected wounds • Radiation tissue damage
Alginates, such as: • ALGICELL • AQUACEL • Curasorb • KALGINATE • Kaltostat • Melgisorb • Sorbsan	• Contain alginic acid from brown seaweed; covered in calcium–sodium salts • Absorb exudate • Maintain a moist wound environment • Facilitate autolytic debridement • Require secondary dressing to secure • May remain in place for 1 to 3 days	• Partial- and full-thickness wounds • Stage 3 and stage 4 pressure injuries • Infected and noninfected wounds • Wounds with moderate to heavy exudate • Tunneling wounds; undermining • Moist red and yellow wounds • Not for use with wounds with minimal drainage or dry eschar
Foams, such as: • Lyofoam • Mepilex • Optifoam • Polyderm • XuSorb	• Foam covered by hydrophilic polyurethane or gel • Maintain a moist wound environment • Do not adhere to wound • Insulate wound • Highly absorbent • May require a secondary dressing to secure • May remain in place 3 to 5 days (7 days for foams with silver), depending on exudate	• Partial- and full-thickness wounds • Stages 2–4 pressure injuries • Surgical wounds • Absorb light to heavy amounts of drainage • Use around tubes and drains • Not for use with wounds with dry eschar
Antimicrobials, such as: • IODOSORB/IODOFLEX • Kerlix AMD	• Antimicrobial or antibacterial action (reduce and/or prevent infection) • Do not adhere to wound • Can be highly absorbent • May require a secondary dressing to secure • Antimicrobial action may last 7 days	• Partial- and full-thickness wounds • Stages 2–4 pressure injuries • Burns • Primary dressing over skin graft(s) and donor sites • Draining, exuding, and nonhealing wounds of any kind (pressure injury, venous/arterial, diabetic, surgical) • Acute and chronic wounds

(continued)

Fundamentals Review 8-5 continued

EXAMPLES OF WOUND DRESSINGS/PRODUCTS

Type	Purposes	Use
Collagens, such as: • BIOSTEP • Stimulin • PROMOGRAN Matrix	• Protein (collagen derived from bovine, porcine, or avian sources) stimulates cellular migration and fosters new tissue development • Highly absorbent • Maintain a moist wound environment • Do not adhere to wound • Compatible with topical agents • Conform well to the wound surface • Require secondary dressing to secure • May remain in place 3 to 5 days (7 days for foams with silver), depending on exudate	• Partial- or full-thickness wounds • Stage 3 pressure injuries • Infected and noninfected wounds • Primary dressing over skin graft(s) and donor sites • Tunneling wounds • Moist red and yellow wounds
Contact layers, such as: • ACTICOAT • ADAPTIC TOUCH • Profore WCL • Silverlon	• Placed in contact with base of wound, protecting base from trauma during dressing change • Allow exudate to pass to a secondary dressing • Not intended to be changed with every dressing change • May be used with topical medication, wound filler, or gauze dressings • Require secondary dressing to secure	• Partial- and full-thickness wounds • Shallow, dehydrated wounds • Wounds with eschar • Wounds with viscous exudate
Composites, such as: • 3M Medipore • CombiDERM • Stratasorb	• Combine two or more physically distinct products in a single dressing with several functions • Allow exchange of oxygen between wound and environment • May facilitate autolytic debridement • Provide physical bacterial barrier and absorptive layer • Semi-adherent or nonadherent • Primary or secondary dressing	• Partial- and full-thickness wounds • Stages 1–4 pressure injuries • Wounds with minimal to heavy exudate • Necrotic tissue • Mixed (granulation and necrotic tissue) wounds • Infected wounds

Source: Adapted from Baranoski, S., & Ayello, E. A. (2016). Wound care essentials. *Practice principles* (4th ed.). Philadelphia, PA: Wolters Kluwer; Hess, C. (2013). *Clinical guide to skin & wound care* (7th ed.). Philadelphia, PA: Wolters Kluwer; and Sood, A., Granick, M. S., & Tomaselli, N. L. (2014). Wound dressings and comparative effectiveness data. *Advances in Wound Care*, 3(8), 511–529.

Skill 8-1 ▶ Preventing Pressure Injury

"A pressure injury is defined as localized damage to the skin and underlying soft tissue usually over a bony prominence or related to the use of a medical or other device," as a result of intense and/or prolonged pressure or pressure in combination with shear (NPUAP, 2016c, para. 4). The National Pressure Ulcer Advisory Panel (NPUAP, 2016a) recently updated staging definitions and the term *pressure ulcer* was replaced by *pressure injury* to better-represent the early stages of pressure injury where there is not an actual ulcer or break in the skin. A pressure injury may be acute or chronic. Most pressure injuries develop when soft tissue is compressed between a bony prominence and an external surface for a prolonged period of time, or when soft tissue undergoes pressure in combination with shear and/or friction (Hess, 2013; NPUAP, 2016c; NPUAP, EPUAP, & PPPIA, 2014b). The terms *decubitus ulcer, pressure sore,* and *bedsore* are also sometimes still used to refer to this type of wound.

Factors contributing to development of pressure injuries are identified in Box 8-1. A risk assessment tool may be used as part of the assessment of risk; although no one risk assessment tool is universally recommended, these tools are part of an assessment that must be structured, comprehensive, and based on clinical judgment (NPUAP, EPUAP, & PPPIA, 2014a). Several different scales are available to assess risk, such as the Norton scale, Waterlow scale, and the Braden scale (Braden, 2005; Doughty & McNichol, 2016; Waterlow, 1985). Patients may have additional risk factors and/or other health problems not measured by the chosen assessment scale. Therefore, good nursing judgment may reveal the need for a higher intensity of preventive intervention than what may be identified by the scale alone (Braden, 2012).

These risk factors are incorporated into pressure injury prevention plans, which are based on knowledge and assessment data related to the patient's clinical condition, current skin condition overall pressure injury risk status and specific risk factors, and resource availability (Doughty & McNichol, 2016; Taylor et al., 2019). The following skill identifies potential interventions related to prevention of pressure injuries. The interventions are listed sequentially for teaching purposes; after completion of appropriate assessments, the order in which the interventions are completed is not sequential and should be adjusted based on the individual patient assessment, health status and situation, as well as nursing judgment and facility policies. Not every intervention discussed will be appropriate for every patient. Additional interventions related to prevention of pressure injuries are discussed in other chapters. Refer to Chapter 5 for nursing skills related to administering medications for pain relief. Chapter 7 provides skills addressing hygiene and skin care. Interventions related to mobility and repositioning are discussed in Chapter 9.

Box 8-1 ▍ Factors Contributing to Development of Pressure Injuries

Mobility and activity limitations are required conditions in the formation of pressure injury development. In the absence of mobility issues, the risk factors listed below should not result in the formation of a pressure injury. Note that the development of a pressure injury may be unavoidable, even with preventative measures, such as in situations with hemodynamic instability, inadequate nutrition/hydration, and immobility (Alvarez et al., 2016). Inadequate nutrition and dehydration, skin moisture, altered mental status, and advanced age are factors in the development of pressure injuries. In addition, patients compromised by the following conditions are at risk for pressure injury development:

- Advanced age (>65 years of age)
- Poor skin hygiene

- Diabetes mellitus
- Diminished sensory perception (pain awareness)
- Fractures
- History of corticosteroid therapy
- Immunosuppression
- Altered mental status
- Microvascular dysfunction
- Excess exposure to moisture (diaphoresis, incontinence)
- Multiorgan dysfunction syndrome (MODS)
- Altered nutritional and/or hydration status
- Previous pressure injuries
- Significant obesity or thinness
- Spinal cord injury
- Increased body temperature
- Terminal illness/end-of-life/dying process

Source: Adapted from Alvarez, O. M., Brindle, C. T., Langemo, D., et al. (2016). The VCU Pressure Ulcer Summit: The search for a clearer understanding and more precise clinical definition of the unavoidable pressure injury. *Journal of Wound, Ostomy, and Continence Nursing, 43*(5), 455–463; Doughty, D. B., & McNichol, L. L. (2016). *Wound, Ostomy and Continence Nurses Society™ Core Curriculum. Wound Management.* Philadelphia, PA: Wolters Kluwer; Hess, C. (2013). *Clinical guide to skin & wound care* (7th ed.). Philadelphia, PA: Wolters Kluwer; and National Pressure Ulcer Advisory Panel [NPUAP], European Pressure Ulcer Advisory Panel [EPUAP], & Pan Pacific Pressure Injury Alliance [PPPIA]. (2014b). *Prevention and treatment of pressure ulcers: Clinical practice guideline.* In E. Haesler (Ed.). Cambridge Media: Osborne Park, Australia.

(continued)

Skill 8-1 ▶ Preventing Pressure Injury *(continued)*

DELEGATION CONSIDERATIONS

The assessment of a patient's skin is not delegated to nursing assistive personnel (NAP) or to unlicensed assistive personnel (UAP). The assessment of a patient's skin may be delegated to licensed practical/vocational nurses (LPN/LVNs). The use of interventions related to prevention of pressure injuries may be delegated to NAP or to UAP, as well as to LPN/LVNs. The decision to delegate must be based on careful analysis of the patient's needs and circumstances, as well as the qualifications of the person to whom the task is being delegated. Refer to the Delegation Guidelines in Appendix A.

EQUIPMENT

- Pressure injury assessment form and/or risk assessment tool
- Functional assessment tool, as indicated
- Support surfaces, such as integrated bed systems, specialized and/or low-pressure mattresses and overlays, seating surfaces and cushions, heel elevation devices, and foam positioning wedges, as indicated
- Safe patient handling and movement devices, as indicated
- Protective dressings, such as polyurethane foam dressing, as indicated
- Low-friction patient care textiles, such as bed linens and patient gowns
- Personal hygiene and skin barrier products, as indicated
- PPE, as indicated

ASSESSMENT

Review the patient's health record and care plan for information about the patient's status and contraindications to any of the potential interventions. Assess the patient's skin at least daily, paying special attention to the skin over bony prominences and the skin in contact with medical devices (Doughty & McNichol, 2016; NPUAP, EPUAT, PPPIA, 2014a). Assess the patient's risk for pressure injury and nutritional status. Assess the patient's response to a particular intervention to evaluate effectiveness and presence of adverse effects.

NURSING DIAGNOSIS

Determine the related factors for the nursing diagnoses based on the patient's current status. Nursing diagnoses that may be appropriate include:

- Risk for impaired skin integrity
- Deficient knowledge
- Risk for disturbed body image

OUTCOME IDENTIFICATION AND PLANNING

The expected outcome to achieve is that the patient does not experience pressure injury and/or alterations in skin integrity. Other outcomes that may be appropriate include the patient and/or caregivers are able to participate in prevention activities and the patient and caregivers verbalize an understanding of the pressure injury prevention plan.

IMPLEMENTATION

ACTION	RATIONALE
1. Perform hand hygiene and put on PPE, if indicated.	Hand hygiene and PPE prevent the spread of microorganisms. PPE is required based on transmission precautions.
2. Identify the patient.	Identifying the patient ensures the right patient receives the intervention and helps prevent errors.
3. Discuss pressure injury prevention with the patient and/or patient caregivers. Explain what pressure injury is, the causes of pressure injuries, and the importance of a pressure injury prevention plan (WOCN, 2016).	These measures promote a collaborative relationship in which the patient is treated with respect. Explanation encourages patient understanding and cooperation and reduces apprehension. Patient and caregiver education assist patients to implement behaviors to meet goals for care (Doughty & McNichol, 2016).

ACTION

4. Assess the patient's skin at least daily, paying special attention to the skin over bony prominences and the skin in contact with medical devices (Doughty & McNichol, 2016; NPUAP, EPUAT, PPPIA, 2014a). Refer to Chapter 3 for additional skin assessment information.

5. Assess the patient's risk for pressure injury upon entry to a health care setting and on a regularly scheduled basis or when there is a significant change in the patient's condition, incorporating appropriate assessment tools and scales, based on facility policy (WOCN, 2016). Refer to Box 8-1.

6. Utilize appropriate support surfaces to redistribute tissue loads, based on facility policy and availability. Appropriate support surfaces may include, but are not limited to, integrated bed systems, specialized and/or low-pressure mattresses and overlays, seating surfaces and cushions, heel elevation devices, and foam positioning wedges.

   Note: Pressure redistribution devices should serve as adjuncts and not replacements for repositioning of patients (WOCN, 2016). **Do not use foam rings, foam cut-outs or donut-type devices.**

   The Wound, Ostomy and Continence Nurses Society (WOCN, 2016) has developed a content-validated algorithm for support surface selection. Refer to the General Considerations below.

7. Routinely reposition the patient; at least every 2 hours for bedridden patients and every hour for patients in a chair or wheelchair (Doughty & McNichol, 2016). Consider the pressure redistribution support surface in the use as well as the individual patient's status when determining the frequency of repositioning; the use of some types of support surfaces may extend the frequency (Doughty & McNichol; NPUAP, EPUAP, PPPIA, 2014a). Refer to Chapter 9 for additional information related to the repositioning of patients.

   Note: Regular repositioning may not be possible due to the patient's medical condition and alternative strategies such as a "high-specification bed" may be required (NPUAP, EPUAP, PPPIA, 2014a; WOCN, 2016).

8. Use a 30-degree side-lying position (lateral tilt position) when positioning patients at risk for pressure injury in side-lying positions (WOCN, 2016).

9. Encourage and provide early mobilization. Develop a schedule for progressive sitting and ambulation as rapidly as tolerated by the individual patient. Collaborate with the physical and occupational therapists to develop an individualized intervention plan.

10. Maintain the head-of-bed elevation at or below 30 degrees, or at the lowest degree of elevation appropriate for the patient's medical condition.

RATIONALE

Skin assessment provides information related to the patient's current status and detects impending or actual alterations in skin integrity (Doughty & McNichol, 2016). Skin assessment provides information needed to develop an appropriate care plan (Taylor et al., 2019). For patients at risk for pressure injury, the skin should be inspected daily with special attention to the skin over bony prominences (NPUAP, EPUAT, PPPIA, 2014a).

Risk for pressure injury development should be determined on admission and at regular intervals thereafter (NPUAP, EPUAP, PPPIA, 2014a). Identification of people at risk for developing pressure injury is a critical component of prevention (Baranoski & Ayello, 2016).

Support surfaces help prevent pressure injury by cushioning vulnerable parts of the body and redistribute body weight, minimizing interface pressures between the body and the lying or seating surface (Doughty & McNichol, 2016). Foam rings, foam cut-outs or donut-type devices concentrate pressure on the surrounding tissue and should be avoided (WOCN, 2016).

Repositioning reduces or relieves pressure and limits the amount of time tissues are exposed to pressure and contribute to the patient's functional abilities (Doughty & McNichol, 2016; NPUAP, EPUAP, PPPIA, 2014a; WOCN, 2016).

The 30-degree lateral tilt position avoids pressure on the patient's trochanters (Doughty & McNichol, 2016).

Mobilization relieves pressure and contributes to the patient's functional abilities (Taylor et al., 2019). "Ambulation schedules may help offset the clinical deterioration often seen in individuals subjected to prolonged bedrest" (NPUAP, EPUAP, PPPIA, 2014a, p. 26). Physical and occupational therapists are important resources for maximizing patient mobility (Baranoski & Ayello, 2016).

Head-of-bed elevation at or below 30 degrees prevents shear-related injury (WOCN, 2016).

(continued)

Skill 8-1 ▶ Preventing Pressure Injury *(continued)*

ACTION	RATIONALE
11. Consider the use of a prophylactic dressing, such as a polyurethane foam dressing, on bony prominences, such as heels and the sacrum. Replace prophylactic dressings that are damaged, displaced, loosened, or excessively moist (NPUAP, EPUAP, PPPIA, 2014a).	Prophylactic dressings on anatomical areas frequently subjected to friction and shear are an emerging therapy for prevention of pressure injury (Byrne et al., 2016; Cornish, 2017; NPUAP, EPUAP, PPPIA, 2014a, p. 18; WOCN, 2016).
12. Consider the use of low-friction patient care textiles, such as bed linens and patient gowns, and the use of silk-like fabrics instead of cotton or cotton-blend fabrics.	Low-friction textiles reduce frictional forces and wick moisture away from the skin to reduce pressure injury risk (Doughty & McNichol, 2016). These types of fabrics reduce shear and friction (NPUAP, EPUAP, PPPIA, 2014a, p. 18; WOCN, 2016).
13. Utilize proper lifting, positioning, and repositioning techniques (safe patient handling and movement techniques); for example, use lift/repositioning sheets and sufficient caregivers when moving a patient. Collaborate with the physical and occupational therapists to develop an individualized intervention plan. Refer to Chapter 9 for additional information related to safe patient handling and the use of patient handling and mobility devices.	Proper lifting, positioning, and repositioning techniques are critical to prevent injury from shearing forces (Doughty & McNichol, 2016). Physical and occupational therapists are important resources for maximizing patient mobility (Baranoski & Ayello, 2016).
14. Utilize interventions to protect the skin from excessive exposure to moisture from wound exudate, perspiration, mucous, saliva, fistula or stoma effluent, and urinary and fecal incontinence. Refer to Chapters 7, 12, and 13 for additional information related to these interventions.	Exposure to excessive moisture contributes to skin damage and pressure injury development due to decreased tissue tolerance and increases susceptibility to friction, pressure, and shear (Baranoski & Ayello, 2016; Doughty & McNichol, 2016; NPUAP, EPUAP, PPPIA, 2014a; WOCN, 2016).
15. Provide appropriate interventions to support the patient's nutritional status and ensure adequate intake. Interventions may include strategies to enhance oral intake, nutritional supplements, fortified foods, and/or enteral or parenteral feeding (Baranoski & Ayello, 2016). Collaborate with the registered dietician and dietary staff to develop an individualized nutrition intervention plan (NPUAP, EPUAP, PPPIA, 2014a).	Adequate calories, protein, fluids, vitamins, and minerals are required for health and tissue maintenance (Doughty & McNichol, 2016). Nutritional management is an important aspect of a comprehensive care plan for pressure injury prevention (Doughty & McNichol; NPUAP, EPUAP, PPPIA, 2014a; WOCN, 2016).
16. Implement interventions to prevent pressure injury related to the use of medical devices, based on the individual patient's situation.	Interventions are necessary to prevent pressure injury related to the use of medical devices (NPUAP, EPUAP, PPPIA, 2014a; WOCN, 2016).
a. Ensure correct for patient size and application of devices in use.	Correct size and accurate application minimizes pressure and shear.
b. Use cushioning dressings under the device, as appropriate to the individual patient and clinical use (NPUAP, EPUAP, PPPIA, 2014a).	Appropriate use of prophylactic dressing manages moisture and provides cushioning to reduce pressure (NPUAP, EPUAP, PPPIA, 2014a).
c. Inspect the skin under the devices and observe for edema under the devices at least twice daily or more often, as indicated.	Presence of edema increases risk for alterations in skin integrity (Doughty & McNichol, 2016).
d. Remove device as soon as medically feasible. Reposition or rotate any medical device daily when possible.	Removal prevents pressure injury. Repositioning or rotating redistributes pressure and decreases shear (NPUAP, EPUAP, PPPIA, 2014a).
e. Keep the skin clean and dry under medical devices.	Moisture underneath medical device increases risk of alterations in skin integrity (NPUAP, EPUAP, PPPIA, 2014a).
17. Provide education to the patient and caregiver(s) about the prevention plan and ways to minimize the risk of pressure injury.	These measures promote a collaborative relationship in which the patient is treated with respect. Explanation encourages patient understanding and cooperation and reduces apprehension. Patient and caregiver education assist patients to implement behaviors to meet goals for care (Doughty & McNichol, 2016; NPUAP, EPUAP, PPPIA, 2014a; Taylor et al., 2019; WOCN, 2016).

ACTION	**RATIONALE**

 18. Remove gloves and additional PPE, if used. Perform hand hygiene.

Removing gloves and PPE properly reduces the risk for infection transmission and contamination of other items. Hand hygiene prevents the transmission of microorganisms.

19. Evaluate the patient's response to interventions. Reassess and alter care plan as indicated by facility policies and procedures, as appropriate.

Evaluation allows for individualization of care plan and promotes optimal patient comfort.

EVALUATION

The expected outcomes have been met when the patient did not experience pressure injury and/or alterations in skin integrity; the patient and/or caregivers participated in prevention activities; and the patient and caregivers verbalized and demonstrated an understanding of the pressure injury prevention plan and interventions.

DOCUMENTATION

Guidelines

Document assessments, as indicated in the individualized patient care plan. Document interventions provided and patient responses. Record alternative treatments to consider, if appropriate. Document reassessment after interventions, at an appropriate interval, based on specific interventions used. Documentation related to pressure injury prevention is often completed on checklists or other tools on the patient's health record. Include any pertinent patient and family education provided.

UNEXPECTED SITUATIONS AND ASSOCIATED INTERVENTIONS

- *Patient develops a pressure injury:* Reassess the patient's condition. Perform assessment to differentiate pressure injuries from wounds and/or injuries due to other causes (WOCN, 2016). Consult with the patient's health care provider to report the injury and collaborate on a revised care plan. Review and revise the current nursing care plan to reflect the change in the patient's status and ensure implementation of appropriate interventions. Implement appropriate wound care as prescribed and indicated in facility policy. Continue vigilant preventive interventions to avoid further pressure injury.

SPECIAL CONSIDERATIONS

General Considerations

- Preventive interventions related to pressure injury prevention should be based on nursing clinical judgment, the use of a reliable risk assessment tool, and assessment of individual patient extrinsic and intrinsic risk factors (WOCN, 2016).
- Nurses must participate in continued pressure injury prevention and treatment education to ensure provision of evidence-based nursing care, achieve desired outcomes and provide patients the best possible care (Doughty & McNichol, 2016; NPUAP, EPUAP, PPPIA, 2014a).
- Numerous risk assessment tools have been validated for use in assessing pressure injury risk, including those for general use and others for specific populations, such as critical care/intensive care units, pediatrics, older adults, and palliative care (Fletcher, 2017; NPUAP, EPUAP, PPPIA, 2014a; Taylor et al., 2019).
- WOCN (2016) has developed a content-validated algorithm for support surface selection. This evidence- and consensus-based algorithm for support surface selection had a Content Validity Index (CVI) of 0.95 with an overall mean score of 3.72, indicating strong content validity and steps that are appropriate to the purpose of the algorithm (McNichol et al., 2015). Refer to thePoint° to access literature describing the Support Surface Algorithm, including the algorithm (McNichol et al.). Visit the WOCN website at http://www.WOCN.org and search the site for the Support Surface Algorithm to access the interactive algorithm tool.

Infant and Child Considerations

- An age-appropriate risk assessment for pediatric and neonate populations considers risk factors of specific concern, including activity and mobility levels; body mass index and/or birth weight; skin maturity; ambient temperature and humidity; nutritional indicators; perfusion and oxygenation; presence of an external device; and duration of hospitalization (NPUAP, EPUAP, PPPIA, 2014a, p. 61).

(continued)

Skill 8-1 ▶ Preventing Pressure Injury *(continued)*

Home Care Considerations
- Pressure injury prevention in home settings can be challenging and may be compromised by access to resources and devices. Assessment of the patient and individual risk factors, as well as implementation of pressure injury prevention interventions in the home are critical in meeting patients' needs (Ellis, 2017).
- Education of the patient, family, and caregivers is critical to ensure successful implementation of the pressure injury prevention care plan (Payne, 2016).

EVIDENCE FOR PRACTICE ▶

PRESSURE INJURY PREVENTION AND THE USE OF SUPPORT SURFACES

McNichol, L., Watts, C., Mackey, D., Beitz, J. M., & Gray, M. (2015). Identifying the right surface for the right patient at the right time: Generation and content validation of an algorithm for support surface selection. *Journal of Wound, Ostomy, and Continence Nursing, 42*(1), 19–37.

The Wound, Ostomy, and Continence Nurses Society (WOCN) is an international nursing society of health care professionals who are experts in the care of patients with wound, ostomy, and incontinence and is recognized for the promotion of safe and effective wound, ostomy, and continence care (WOCN, 2017). The WOCN has developed an evidence- and consensus-based algorithm for support surface use in the prevention and treatment of pressure injuries. This algorithm has undergone content validation and provides clinical guidance for selecting support surfaces to match individual patient needs (McNichol et al., 2015).

Refer to thePoint° for a link to this article and to the Support Surface Algorithm and additional research on related nursing topics.

Skill 8-2 ▶ Cleaning a Wound and Applying a Dressing (General Guidelines)

The goal of wound care is to promote tissue repair and regeneration to restore skin integrity. Often, wound care includes cleaning of the wound and the use of a dressing as a protective covering and to maintain an environment to promote healing (Baranoski & Ayello, 2016). Wound cleansing is performed to remove debris, contaminants, and excess exudate. Normal saline (0.9% sodium chloride) is the preferred cleansing solution (Taylor et al., 2019). Commercially prepared cleansing solutions are also available, including antiseptics or surfactants, and may be used in wounds with debris, confirmed infection, or high levels of bacterial colonization (Baranoski & Ayello, 2016; NPUAP, EPUAP, & PPPIA, 2014a). Sterile equipment and solutions are required for irrigating an open wound, even in the presence of an existing infection (Taylor et al., 2019). Nonsterile solutions are generally used to clean the skin surface if the wound edges are approximated (Taylor et al., 2019).

There is no standard frequency for how often dressings should be changed. It depends on the amount of drainage, the primary health care provider's preference, the nature of the wound, and the particular wound care product being used. It is customary for the surgeon or other advanced practice provider to perform the first dressing change on a surgical wound, usually within 24 to 48 hours after surgery.

There are many commercially prepared wound care products; cleaning of a wound and application of many of these products are applied in a similar manner using the same underlying principles. It is very important for the nurse to be aware of the products available in a particular facility and be knowledgeable of the indications for and correct use of each type of dressing and wound care product in use. Refer to Fundamentals Review 8-4 and 8-5 for additional information.

This skill provides general guidelines and focuses on application of a dry, sterile dressing; specifics may change based on the particular dressing and/or wound care product in use.

DELEGATION CONSIDERATIONS	Wound care and procedures requiring the use of a sterile field and other sterile items are not delegated to nursing assistive personnel (NAP) or unlicensed assistive personnel (UAP). Depending on the state's nurse practice act and the organization's policies and procedures, these procedures may be delegated to licensed practical/vocational nurses (LPN/LVNs). The decision to delegate must be based on careful analysis of the patient's needs and circumstances, as well as the qualifications of the person to whom the task is being delegated. Refer to the Delegation Guidelines in Appendix A.

EQUIPMENT

- Sterile gloves, as indicated
- Clean, disposable gloves
- Additional PPE, as indicated
- Gauze dressings
- Surgical or abdominal pads
- Sterile dressing set or suture set (for the sterile scissors and forceps)
- Sterile cleaning solution as ordered (commonly 0.9% normal saline solution, or a commercially prepared wound cleanser)
- Skin protectant/barrier wipes

- Sterile basin (may be optional)
- Sterile drape (may be optional)
- Plastic bag or other appropriate waste container for soiled dressings
- Waterproof pad and bath blanket
- Tape or ties
- Bath blanket or other linens for draping patient
- Additional dressings and supplies needed or required based on the wound dressing/care prescribed for the patient

ASSESSMENT

Assess the situation to determine the need for wound cleaning and a dressing change. Confirm any prescribed orders relevant to wound care and any wound care included in the nursing care plan. Assess the patient's level of comfort and the need for analgesics before wound care. Assess if the patient experienced any pain related to prior dressing changes and the effectiveness of interventions employed to minimize the patient's pain. Assess the current dressing to determine if it is intact. Assess for excess drainage, bleeding, or saturation of the dressing. Inspect the wound and the surrounding tissue. Assess the appearance of the wound for the approximation of wound edges, the color of the wound and surrounding area, and signs of dehiscence. Assess for the presence of sutures, staples, or adhesive closure strips. Note the stage of the healing process and characteristics of any drainage. Also assess the surrounding skin for color, temperature, and edema, **ecchymosis**, or **maceration**.

NURSING DIAGNOSIS

Determine the related factors for the nursing diagnoses based on the patient's current status. Appropriate nursing diagnoses may include:

- Risk for infection
- Impaired skin integrity

- Delayed surgical recovery

OUTCOME IDENTIFICATION AND PLANNING

The expected outcome to achieve when cleaning a wound and applying a dry, sterile dressing is that the wound is cleaned and dressed without contaminating the wound area, causing trauma to the wound, and/or causing the patient to experience pain or discomfort. Other outcomes that are appropriate include the following: the wound continues to show signs of progression of healing, and the patient demonstrates an understanding of the wound care and dressing.

IMPLEMENTATION

ACTION	RATIONALE
1. Review the patient's health record for prescribed wound care or the nursing care plan related to wound care. Gather necessary supplies.	Reviewing the health record and care plan validates the correct patient and correct procedure. Preparation promotes efficient time management and an organized approach to the task.
2. Perform hand hygiene and put on PPE, if indicated.	Hand hygiene and PPE prevent the spread of microorganisms. PPE is required based on transmission precautions.

(continued)

Skill 8-2 ▶ Cleaning a Wound and Applying a Dressing (General Guidelines) *(continued)*

<table>
<tr><td>ACTION</td><td>RATIONALE</td></tr>
<tr>
<td> 3. Identify the patient.</td>
<td>Identifying the patient ensures the right patient receives the intervention and helps prevent errors.</td>
</tr>
<tr>
<td>4. Assemble equipment on the overbed table or other surface within reach.</td>
<td>Organization facilitates performance of the task.</td>
</tr>
<tr>
<td>5. Close the curtains around the bed and close the door to the room, if possible. Explain to the patient what you are going to do and why you are going to do it.</td>
<td>This ensures the patient's privacy. Explanation relieves anxiety and facilitates cooperation.</td>
</tr>
<tr>
<td>6. Assess the patient for the possible need for nonpharmacologic pain-reducing interventions or analgesic medication before wound care dressing change. Administer appropriate prescribed analgesic. Allow enough time for the analgesic to achieve its effectiveness.</td>
<td>Pain is a subjective experience influenced by past experience. Wound care and dressing changes may cause pain for some patients.</td>
</tr>
<tr>
<td>7. Place a waste receptacle or bag at a convenient location for use during the procedure.</td>
<td>Having a waste container handy means the soiled dressing may be discarded easily, without the spread of microorganisms.</td>
</tr>
<tr>
<td>8. Adjust the bed to a comfortable working height, usually elbow height of the caregiver (VHA Center for Engineering & Occupational Safety and Health [CEOSH], 2016).</td>
<td>Having the bed at the proper height prevents back and muscle strain.</td>
</tr>
<tr>
<td>9. Assist the patient to a comfortable position that provides easy access to the wound area. Use the bath blanket to cover any exposed area other than the wound. Place a waterproof pad under the wound site.</td>
<td>Patient positioning and the use of a bath blanket provide for comfort and warmth. Waterproof pad protects underlying surfaces.</td>
</tr>
<tr>
<td>10. Check the position of drains, tubes, or other adjuncts before removing the dressing. Put on clean, disposable gloves and loosen the tape or adhesive edge on the old dressings by removing in the direction of hair growth and the use of a push–pull method (Figure 1). Push–pull method: lift a corner of the dressing away from the skin, and then gently push the skin away from the dressing/adhesive. Continue moving fingers of the opposite hand to support the skin as the product is removed (McNichol, Lund, Rose, & Gray, 2013). Carefully lift the adhesive barrier from the surrounding skin to prevent medical adhesive–related skin injury (MARSI). Remove the sides/edges first, then the center. If there is resistance, use an adhesive remover (McNichol et al., 2013).</td>
<td>Checking ensures that a drain is not removed accidentally if one is present. Gloves protect the nurse from contaminated dressings and prevent the spread of microorganisms. Removal of the tape in the direction of hair growth minimizes trauma to the skin (Taylor et al., 2019). The use of adhesive remover allows for the easy, rapid, and painless removal without the associated problems of skin stripping and helps reduce patient discomfort (McNichol et al., 2013).</td>
</tr>
</table>

FIGURE 1. Loosening dressing tape or adhesive edge.

ACTION	RATIONALE
11. Carefully remove the soiled dressings. If any part of the dressing sticks to the underlying skin, use small amounts of sterile saline to help loosen and remove it.	Cautious removal of the dressing is more comfortable for the patient and ensures that any drain present is not removed. Sterile saline moistens the dressing for easier removal and minimizes damage and pain.
12. After removing the dressing, note the presence, amount, type, color, and odor of any drainage on the dressings (Figure 2). Place soiled dressings in the appropriate waste receptacle. Remove your gloves and dispose of them in an appropriate waste receptacle.	The presence of drainage should be documented. Proper disposal of soiled dressings and used gloves prevents the spread of microorganisms.

FIGURE 2. Noting characteristics of drainage on dressing that has been removed.

ACTION	RATIONALE
13. Perform hand hygiene.	Hand hygiene prevents the transmission of microorganisms.
14. Inspect the wound site for size, appearance, and drainage (Refer to Fundamentals Review 8-2). Assess if any pain is present. Check the status of sutures, adhesive closure strips, staples, and drains or tubes, if present. Note any problems to include in your documentation.	Wound healing or the presence of irritation or infection should be documented.
15. **Using sterile technique, prepare a sterile work area and open the needed supplies.**	Supplies are within easy reach and sterility is maintained.
16. Open the sterile cleaning solution. Depending on the amount of cleaning needed, the solution might be poured directly over gauze sponges over a container for small cleaning jobs, or into a basin for more complex or larger cleaning.	Sterility of dressings and solution is maintained.
17. Put on sterile gloves. Alternatively, clean gloves (clean technique) may be used when cleaning a chronic wound or pressure injury.	The use of sterile gloves maintains surgical asepsis and sterile technique and reduces the risk for spreading microorganisms. Clean technique is appropriate for cleaning chronic wounds or pressure injuries (Baranoski & Ayello, 2016; NPUAP, EPUAP, & PPPIA, 2014b; Taylor et al., 2019).
18. Clean the wound. **Clean from top to bottom and/or from the center to the outside.** Refer to Box 8-2. Use new gauze for each wipe, placing the used gauze in the waste receptacle (Figure 3). Alternatively, spray the wound from top to bottom with a commercially prepared wound cleanser; wound irrigation is often used to clean open wounds and may also be used for other types of wounds. Refer to Skill 8-3.	Cleaning from top to bottom and center to outside ensures that cleaning occurs from the least to most contaminated area and a previously cleaned area is not contaminated again. Using a single gauze for each wipe ensures that the previously cleaned area is not contaminated again.

(continued)

Skill 8-2 ▶ Cleaning a Wound and Applying a Dressing (General Guidelines) *(continued)*

Box 8-2 | Cleaning a Wound

Cleaning a Wound with Approximated Edges

- Use standard precautions; use appropriate transmission-based precautions when indicated.
- Moisten a sterile gauze pad or swab with the prescribed cleansing agent.
- Use a new swab or gauze for each downward stroke.
- Clean from top to bottom.
- Work outward from the incision in lines parallel to it (Figure A).
- Wipe from the clean area toward the less clean area.

Cleaning a Wound with Unapproximated Edges

- Use standard precautions; use appropriate transmission-based precautions when indicated.
- Moisten a sterile gauze pad or swab with the prescribed cleansing agent and squeeze out excess solution.
- Use a new swab or gauze for each circle.
- Clean the wound in full or half circles, beginning in the center and working toward the outside (Figure B).
- Clean to at least 1 in beyond the end of the new dressing.
- If a dressing is not being applied, clean to at least 2 in beyond the wound margins.

FIGURE A.

FIGURE B.

Source: Hess, C. (2013). *Clinical guide to skin & wound care* (7th ed.). Philadelphia, PA: Wolters Kluwer; Taylor, C., Lynn, P., & Bartlett, J. (2019). *Fundamentals of nursing: The art and science of person-centered care* (9th ed.). Philadelphia, PA: Wolters Kluwer.

FIGURE 3. Cleaning the wound.

ACTION	RATIONALE
19. Once the wound is cleaned, dry the area using a gauze sponge in the same manner.	Moisture provides a medium for the growth of microorganisms.
20. If a drain is in use at the wound location, clean around the drain. Refer to Skills 8-6, 8-7, 8-8, and 8-9.	Cleaning the insertion site helps prevent infection.
21. Remove gloves and place in the waste receptacle. Perform hand hygiene.	Proper disposal of used gloves and hand hygiene prevent the spread of microorganisms.
22. Put on sterile gloves. Alternately, clean gloves (clean technique) may be used when cleaning a chronic wound or pressure injury. Apply a skin protectant or barrier to the healthy skin around the wound where the dressing adhesive or tape will be placed and where wound drainage may come in contact with the skin (Figure 4).	The use of sterile gloves maintains surgical asepsis and sterile technique and reduces the risk for spreading microorganisms. Clean technique is appropriate for cleaning chronic wounds or pressure injuries (Baranoski & Ayello, 2016; NPUAP, EPUAP, & PPPIA, 2014b; Taylor et al., 2019). Skin barrier/protectant prevents skin irritation and excoriation from tape, adhesives, and wound drainage (McNichol et al., 2013).
23. Apply any topical medications, foams, gels, and/or gauze to the wound as prescribed; ensure products stay confined to the wound and do not impact on intact surrounding tissue/skin (Figure 5).	The growth of microorganisms may be inhibited and the healing process improved with the use of prescribed medications, foams, gels and/or other wound care product.

FIGURE 4. Applying skin protectant to skin surrounding wound.

FIGURE 5. Applying prescribed wound care product.

24. Gently place a layer of dry, sterile dressing, or other prescribed cover dressing at the wound center and extend it at least 1 in beyond the wound in all directions. Alternately, follow the manufacturer's directions for application (Figure 6). Forceps may be used to apply the dressing.

Extending the dressing at least 1 in past the wound edges ensures the dressing covers and protects the wound. The use of forceps helps ensure that sterile technique is maintained.

FIGURE 6. Applying cover dressing to site.

(*continued*)

Skill 8-2 ▶ Cleaning a Wound and Applying a Dressing (General Guidelines) *(continued)*

ACTION	**RATIONALE**
25. As necessary, apply a surgical or abdominal pad (ABD) over the gauze at the site of the outermost layer of the dressing, with the side of the dressing with the blue line facing away from the patient. Alternately, note the side of the dressing that contains the moisture barrier and place away from the patient, based on the dressing material in use. Note: May not be necessary or appropriate, based on the cover dressing used in step 22.	The dressing acts as additional protection for the wound against microorganisms in the environment and increased absorption of drainage. The blue line on the dressing indicates the side of the dressing with a moisture barrier and should not be placed against the wound. The moisture barrier prevents leaking of fluid.
26. Apply tape, Montgomery straps, or roller gauze to secure the dressings. Alternately, many commercial wound products are self-adhesive and do not require additional tape. Remove and discard gloves.	Tape or other securing products keep the dressing in place. Proper disposal of gloves prevents the spread of microorganisms.
27. After securing the dressing, label it with date and time. Remove all remaining equipment; place the patient in a comfortable position, with side rails up as indicated and bed in the lowest position.	Recording date and time provides communication and demonstrates adherence to care plan. Proper patient and bed positioning promotes safety and comfort.
28. Remove PPE, if used. Perform hand hygiene.	Proper removal of PPE reduces the risk for infection transmission and contamination of other items. Hand hygiene prevents the spread of microorganisms.
29. Check all wound dressings at least every shift. More frequent checks may be needed if the wound is more complex or dressings become saturated quickly.	Checking dressings ensures the assessment of changes in patient condition and timely intervention to prevent complications.

EVALUATION

The expected outcomes have been met when the wound was cleaned and dressed without contaminating the wound area or causing trauma to the wound; the patient did not experience pain or discomfort; the wound continued to show signs of progression of healing; and the patient demonstrated an understanding of the wound care and dressing.

DOCUMENTATION

Guidelines

Document the location of the wound and that the dressing was removed. Record your assessment of the wound, including approximation of wound edges; presence of sutures, staples, or adhesive closure strips; and the condition of the surrounding skin. Note if redness, edema, or drainage is observed and document characteristics if present. Document cleansing of wound and application of topical medications, foams, gels, and/or gauze to the wound as prescribed. Record the type of dressing that was reapplied. Note pertinent patient and family education and any patient reaction to the procedure, including patient's pain level and effectiveness of nonpharmacologic interventions or analgesia if administered.

Sample Documentation

DocuCare Practice documenting wound care in *Lippincott DocuCare.*

<u>9/8/20</u> 0600 Dressing removed from left lateral calf incision. Scant purulent secretions noted on dressing. Incision edges approximately 1 mm apart, red, with ecchymosis and edema present. Small amount of purulent drainage from wound noted. Area cleansed with normal saline, dried, antibiotic ointment applied per order. Surrounding tissue red and ecchymotic. Redressed with nonadhering dressing, gauze, and wrapped with stretch gauze. Patient reports adequate pain control after preprocedure analgesic; states pain is dull ache, 1/10 on pain scale.

—*N. Joiner, RN*

UNEXPECTED SITUATIONS AND ASSOCIATED INTERVENTIONS	

UNEXPECTED SITUATIONS AND ASSOCIATED INTERVENTIONS

- *The previous wound assessment states that the incision was clean and dry and the wound edges were approximated, with the staples and surgical drain intact. The surrounding tissue was without inflammation, edema, or erythema. After the dressing is removed, the nurse notes the incision edges are not approximated at the distal end, multiple staples are evident in the old dressing, the surrounding skin tissue is red and swollen, and purulent drainage is on the dressing and leaking from the wound:* Assess the patient for any other signs and symptoms, such as pain, malaise, fever, and paresthesias. Place a dry sterile dressing over the wound site. Report the findings to the primary health care provider and document the event in the patient's record. Be prepared to obtain a wound culture and implement any changes in wound care as ordered.
- *After the nurse has put on sterile gloves, the patient moves too close to the edge of the bed and the nurse must support her with his hands to prevent the patient from falling:* If nothing else in the sterile field was touched, remove the contaminated gloves and put on new sterile gloves. If you did not bring a second pair, use the call bell to summon a coworker to provide a new pair of gloves.
- *The nurse has set up dressing supplies, removed the old dressing, and put on sterile gloves to clean the wound. The nurse then realizes that a necessary piece of dressing material has been forgotten:* Ask the patient to press the call bell to summon a coworker to provide the missing supplies.
- *When removing a patient's dressing, the assessment reveals eschar in the wound:* Notify the primary health care provider or wound care specialist, as a different treatment modality and/or debridement may be necessary. Note: The presence of eschar in a pressure injury wound precludes staging the wound. The eschar must be removed for adequate pressure injury staging to be done. However, stable (dry, adherent, intact, without erythema or movement) eschar on pressure injuries on the heels serves as "the body's natural (biologic) cover" and should not be removed (NPUAP, 2014a).

SPECIAL CONSIDERATIONS

General Considerations

- Instruct the patient, if appropriate, and other members of the health care team to observe for excessive drainage that may overwhelm the dressing. They should also report when dressings become soiled or loosened from the skin.
- There are many dressing types and manufacturers—the nurse needs to collaborate with the provider to ensure the correct dressing type is chosen, ongoing assessment occurs, and updates to the treatment plan (dressing choice) are made as the wound evolves (Taylor et al., 2019).
- Products designed to assist with dressing removal can reduce pain, avoid damaging the peri-wound skin and resulting skin stripping and MARSI and result in time savings (Reevell, Anders, & Morgan, 2016).
- When using adherent dressings, such as a hydrocolloid dressing, cut the dressing to size, allowing at least a 1-in margin of healthy skin around the wound to be covered with the dressing. Apply the dressing to the wound without stretching the dressing.
- Appropriate nutritional support is critical in achieving successful wound healing and may be overlooked (Quain & Khardori, 2015). Collaborate with the registered dietician and dietary staff to develop an individualized nutrition intervention plan for the patient (NPUAP, EPUAP, PPPIA, 2014a).

Infant and Child Considerations

- The skin of neonates is more fragile as a result of incomplete epidermal-to-dermal cohesion; use paper tape or nonadherent dressings to prevent tearing of the skin (Baranoski, LeBlanc, & Gloeckner, 2016).

Older Adult Considerations

- The skin of older adults is less elastic and more fragile as a result of age-related changes; use paper tape, nonadherent dressings, or roller gauze (on extremities) to prevent tearing of the skin (Baranoski, LeBlanc, & Gloeckner, 2016).

(continued)

Skill 8-3 ▶ Performing Irrigation of a Wound

Irrigation is a directed flow of solution over tissues. Wound irrigations are ordered to clean the area of **pathogens** and other debris and to promote wound healing. Irrigation procedures may also be ordered to apply heat or antiseptics locally. If the wound edges are approximated, nonsterile solutions and clean technique may be used; if the wound edges are not approximated, sterile equipment and solutions are used for irrigation (Taylor et al., 2019). Normal saline (0.9% sodium chloride) is often the solution of choice when irrigating wounds, but sterile water, commercially prepared wound cleansers, potable tap water, or antiseptics may be used (Taylor et al.; WOCN, 2016).

DELEGATION CONSIDERATIONS	Irrigation of a wound and procedures requiring the use of a sterile field and other sterile items are not delegated to nursing assistive personnel (NAP) or to unlicensed assistive personnel (UAP). Depending on the state's nurse practice act and the organization's policies and procedures, these procedures may be delegated to licensed practical/vocational nurses (LPN/LVNs). The decision to delegate must be based on careful analysis of the patient's needs and circumstances, as well as the qualifications of the person to whom the task is being delegated. Refer to the Delegation Guidelines in Appendix A.

EQUIPMENT	• A sterile irrigation set, including a basin, irrigant container, and irrigation syringe
	  • A bulb syringe may be used to provide gentle flushing to cleanse a clean wound (in the proliferative phase of repair) (WOCN, 2016)
	  • A 35-mL syringe and a 19-gauge catheter or a commercial cleanser packaged in a pressurized container may be used to provide low pressure irrigation to cleanse a necrotic or infected wound (WOCN, 2016)
	• Sterile irrigation solution as prescribed, warmed to body temperature, commonly 0.9% normal saline solution or other solution as prescribed
	• Alternately, irrigation solution may be packaged in individual, single-use syringe
	• Plastic bag or other waste container to dispose of soiled dressings
	• Sterile gloves
	• Sterile drape (may be optional)
	• Clean, disposable gloves
	• Moisture-proof gown; mask, and eye protection or face shield
	• Additional PPE, as indicated
	• Sterile dressing set or suture set (for the sterile scissors and forceps)
	• Waterproof pad and bath blanket, as needed
	• Sterile gauze dressings
	• Sterile packing gauze, as needed
	• Tape or ties
	• Skin protectant/barrier wipes
	• Additional dressings and supplies needed or required based on the wound dressing/care prescribed for the patient

ASSESSMENT	Assess the situation to determine the need for wound irrigation. Confirm any prescribed orders relevant to wound care and any wound care included in the nursing care plan. Assess the current dressing to determine if it is intact. Assess the patient's level of comfort and the need for analgesics before wound care. Assess if the patient experienced any pain related to previous dressing changes and the effectiveness of interventions employed to minimize the patient's pain. Assess for excess drainage or bleeding or saturation of the dressing. Inspect the wound and the surrounding tissue. Assess the location, appearance of the wound, stage (if appropriate), drainage, and types of tissue present in the wound. Measure the wound. Note the stage of the healing process and characteristics of any drainage. Also assess the surrounding skin for color, temperature, and edema, ecchymosis, or maceration.

| NURSING DIAGNOSIS | Determine the related factors for the nursing diagnoses based on the patient's current health status. Appropriate nursing diagnoses may include: |

- Acute pain
- Impaired skin integrity
- Impaired tissue integrity

| OUTCOME IDENTIFICATION AND PLANNING | The expected outcome to achieve when irrigating a wound is that the wound is cleaned without contamination or trauma; without damaging proliferative cells and newly formed tissues; and without causing the patient to experience pain or discomfort. Other outcomes that might be appropriate include the following: the wound continues to show signs of progression of healing, and the patient demonstrates an understanding of the wound care and dressing. |

IMPLEMENTATION

ACTION

1. Review the patient's health record for prescribed wound care or the nursing care plan related to wound care. Gather necessary supplies.

2. Perform hand hygiene and put on PPE, if indicated.

3. Identify the patient.

4. Assemble equipment on the overbed table or other surface within reach.

5. Close the curtains around the bed and close the door to the room if possible. Explain what you are going to do and why you are going to do it to the patient.

6. Assess the patient for possible need for nonpharmacologic pain-reducing interventions or analgesic medication before wound care and/or dressing change. Administer appropriate prescribed analgesic. Allow enough time for the analgesic to achieve its effectiveness before beginning the procedure.

7. Place a waste receptacle or bag at a convenient location for use during the procedure.

8. Adjust the bed to a comfortable working height, usually elbow height of the caregiver (VHACEOSH, 2016).

9. Assist the patient to a comfortable position that provides easy access to the wound area. Position the patient so the irrigation solution will flow from the clean end of the wound toward the dirtier end or top to bottom. Use the bath blanket to cover any exposed area other than the wound. Place a waterproof pad under the wound site.

10. Put on a gown, mask, and eye protection or face shield.

RATIONALE

Reviewing the health record and care plan validates the correct patient and correct procedure. Preparation promotes efficient time management and an organized approach to the task.

Hand hygiene and PPE prevent the spread of microorganisms. PPE is required based on transmission precautions.

Identifying the patient ensures the right patient receives the intervention and helps prevent errors.

Organization facilitates performance of the task.

This ensures the patient's privacy. Explanation relieves anxiety and facilitates cooperation.

Pain is a subjective experience influenced by past experience. Wound care and dressing changes may cause pain for some patients.

Having a waste container handy means the soiled dressing may be discarded easily, without the spread of microorganisms.

Having the bed at the proper height prevents back and muscle strain.

Patient positioning and the use of a bath blanket provide for comfort and warmth. Gravity directs the flow of liquid from the least contaminated to the most contaminated area. Waterproof pad protects underlying surfaces.

Using PPE, such as gowns, masks, and eye protection, is part of *Standard Precautions*. A gown protects clothes from contamination should splashing occur. Appropriate personal protective equipment, including a mask and eye protection or face shield is essential when irrigating a wound with any degree of pressure (WOCN, 2016).

(continued)

Skill 8-3 ▶ Performing Irrigation of a Wound *(continued)*

ACTION	RATIONALE
11. Check the position of drains, tubes, or other adjuncts before removing the dressing. Put on clean, disposable gloves and loosen the tape on the old dressings by removing in the direction of hair growth and the use of a push–pull method (see Figure 1, Skill 8-2). Push–pull method: lift a corner of the dressing away from the skin, then gently push the skin away from the dressing/adhesive. Continue moving fingers of the opposite hand to support the skin as the product is removed (McNichol et al., 2013). Carefully lift the adhesive barrier from the surrounding skin to prevent medical adhesive–related skin injury (MARSI). Remove the sides/edges first, then the center. If there is resistance, use an adhesive remover (McNichol et al., 2013).	Checking ensures that a drain is not removed accidentally if one is present. Gloves protect the nurse from contaminated dressings and prevent the spread of microorganisms. Removal of the tape in the direction of hair growth minimizes trauma to the skin (Taylor et al., 2019). The use of adhesive remover allows for the easy, rapid, and painless removal without the associated problems of skin stripping and helps reduce patient discomfort (McNichol et al., 2013).

FIGURE 1. Drawing up sterile solution from sterile container into irrigation syringe.

ACTION	RATIONALE
12. Carefully remove the soiled dressings. If any part of the dressing sticks to the underlying skin, use small amounts of sterile saline to help loosen and remove it.	Cautious removal of the dressing is more comfortable for the patient and ensures that any drain present is not removed. Sterile saline moistens the dressing for easier removal and minimizes damage and pain.
13. After removing the dressing, note the presence, amount, type, color, and odor of any drainage on the dressings. Place soiled dressings in the appropriate waste receptacle.	The presence of drainage should be documented. Proper disposal of soiled dressings and used gloves prevents the spread of microorganisms.
14. Assess the wound for appearance, stage, presence of eschar, granulation tissue, **epithelialization**, undermining, tunneling, necrosis, **sinus tract**, and drainage. Assess the appearance of the surrounding tissue. Measure the wound. Refer to Fundamentals Review 8-2.	This information provides evidence about the wound healing process and/or the presence of infection.

 15. Remove your gloves and put them in the receptacle. Perform hand hygiene.

Discarding gloves prevents the spread of microorganisms. Hand hygiene prevents the spread of microorganisms.

ACTION	RATIONALE
16. Set up a sterile field, if indicated, and wound cleaning and irrigation supplies. Pour warmed sterile irrigating solution into the sterile container. Put on the sterile gloves. Alternately, clean gloves (clean technique) may be used when cleaning a chronic wound or pressure injury.	Using warmed solution prevents chilling the patient and may minimize patient discomfort. Sterile technique and gloves maintain surgical asepsis. Clean technique is appropriate for irrigating chronic wounds or pressure injuries (Baranoski & Ayello, 2016; NPUAP, EPUAP, & PPPIA, 2014b; Taylor et al., 2019).

ACTION

17. Position the sterile basin below the wound to collect the irrigation fluid.

18. Fill the irrigation syringe with solution (Figure 1). **Alternately, irrigation solution may be packaged in individual, single-use syringe; remove cap on syringe. Using your nondominant hand, gently apply pressure to the basin against the skin below the wound to form a seal with the skin (Figure 2).**

19. **Direct a stream of solution into the wound (Figure 3). Keep the tip of the syringe at least 1 in above the upper edge of the wound. Flush all wound areas.**

RATIONALE

Patient and bed linens are protected from contaminated fluid.

The solution will collect in the basin and prevent the irrigant from running down the skin. Patient and bed linens are protected from contaminated fluid.

Debris and contaminated solution flow from the least contaminated to most contaminated area. High-pressure irrigation flow may cause patient discomfort as well as damage granulation tissue.

FIGURE 2. Applying pressure to basin to form seal.

FIGURE 3. Irrigating wound with a stream of solution. Solution drains into collection container.

20. Watch for the solution to flow smoothly and evenly. When the solution from the wound flows out clear, discontinue irrigation.

21. Once the wound is cleaned, dry the surrounding skin using a gauze sponge (Figure 4).

Irrigation removes exudate and debris.

Moisture provides a medium for the growth of microorganisms.

FIGURE 4. Drying around wound, not in wound, with gauze pad.

(*continued*)

Skill 8-3 ▶ Performing Irrigation of a Wound (continued)

ACTION	**RATIONALE**
22. If a drain is in use at the wound location, clean around the drain. Refer to Skills 8-6, 8-7, 8-8, and 8-9.	Cleaning the insertion site helps prevent infection.
23. Remove gloves and place in a waste receptacle. Perform hand hygiene.	Proper disposal of used gloves and hand hygiene prevent the spread of microorganisms.
24. Put on sterile gloves. Alternately, clean gloves (clean technique) may be used when cleaning a chronic wound or pressure injury. Apply a skin protectant or barrier to the healthy skin around the wound where the dressing adhesive or tape will be placed and where wound drainage may come in contact with skin.	The use of sterile gloves maintains surgical asepsis and sterile technique and reduces the risk for spreading microorganisms. Clean technique is appropriate for cleaning chronic wounds or pressure injuries (Baranoski & Ayello, 2016; NPUAP, EPUAP, & PPPIA, 2014b; Taylor et al., 2019). Skin barrier/protectant prevents skin irritation and excoriation from tape, adhesives, and wound drainage (McNichol et al., 2013).
25. Apply any topical medications, foams, gels, and/or gauze to the wound as prescribed; ensure products stay confined to the wound and do not impact on intact surrounding tissue/skin (Figure 5).	The growth of microorganisms may be inhibited and the healing process improved with the use of prescribed medications, foams, gels and/or other wound care product.

FIGURE 5. Applying wound contact material.

26. Gently place a layer of dry, sterile dressing or other prescribed cover dressing at the wound center and extend it at least 1 in beyond the wound in all directions. Alternately, follow the manufacturer's directions for application. Forceps may be used to apply the dressing.	Extending the dressing at least 1 in past the wound edges ensures the dressing covers and protects the wound. The use of forceps helps ensure that sterile technique is maintained.
27. Apply tape, Montgomery straps, or roller gauze to secure the dressings, if needed. Alternately, many commercial wound products are self-adhesive and do not require additional tape. Remove and discard gloves.	Tape or other securing products keep the dressing in place. Proper disposal of gloves prevents the spread of microorganisms.
28. After securing the dressing, label it with date and time. Remove all remaining equipment; place the patient in a comfortable position, with side rails up as indicated and bed in the lowest position.	Recording date and time provides communication and demonstrates adherence to care plan. Proper patient and bed positioning promotes safety and comfort.
29. Remove PPE, if used. Perform hand hygiene.	Proper removal of PPE reduces the risk for infection transmission and contamination of other items. Hand hygiene prevents the spread of microorganisms.
30. Check all wound dressings at least every shift. More frequent checks may be needed if the wound is more complex or dressings become saturated quickly.	Checking dressings ensures the assessment of changes in patient condition and timely intervention to prevent complications.

EVALUATION

The expected outcomes have been met when the wound was cleaned without contamination or trauma, without damaging proliferative cells and newly formed tissues, and without causing the patient to experience pain or discomfort; the wound continued to show signs of progression of healing; and the patient demonstrated an understanding of the wound care and dressing.

DOCUMENTATION

Guidelines

Document the location of the wound and that the dressing was removed. Record your assessment of the wound, including evidence of granulation tissue, presence of necrotic tissue, stage (if pressure injury), and characteristics of drainage. Include the appearance of the surrounding skin. Document the irrigation of the wound and solution used. Record the type of dressing that was applied. Note pertinent patient and family education and any patient reaction to this procedure, including patient's pain level and effectiveness of nonpharmacologic interventions or analgesia if administered.

Sample Documentation

> <u>3/5/20</u> 1700 Dressing removed from left outer heel area. Minimal serosanguineous drainage noted on dressings. Wound 4 cm × 5 cm × 2 cm, pink, with granulation tissue evident. Surrounding skin tone consistent with patient's skin, no edema or redness noted. Irrigated with normal saline and hydrogel dressing applied.
>
> —*J. Lark, RN*

UNEXPECTED SITUATIONS AND ASSOCIATED INTERVENTIONS

- *The patient experiences pain when the wound irrigation is begun:* Stop the procedure and administer an analgesic, as prescribed. Obtain new sterile supplies and begin the procedure after an appropriate amount of time has elapsed to allow the analgesic to begin working. Note the patient's pain on the nursing care plan so that pain medication can be given before future wound treatments.
- *During the wound irrigation, the nurse notes bleeding from the wound. This has not been documented as happening with previous irrigations:* Stop the procedure. Assess the patient for other symptoms. Obtain vital signs. Report the findings to the primary health care provider and document the event in the patient's record.

General Considerations

- Antiseptic solutions can potentially damage viable wound disuse and use should be a short-term intervention (WOCN, 2016). Once the bacterial loads have been controlled and the volume of necrotic tissue has been reduced to <40% of the wound bed, the use of an antiseptic should be discontinued (WOCN, p. 133).
- Appropriate nutritional support is critical in achieving successful wound healing and may be overlooked (Quain & Khardori, 2015). Collaborate with the registered dietician and dietary staff to develop an individualized nutrition intervention plan for the patient (NPUAP, EPUAP, PPPIA, 2014a).

Skill 8-4 ▶ Collecting a Wound Culture

A wound culture may be ordered to identify the causative organism(s) of an infected wound. Identifying the invading microorganism will provide useful information for selecting the most appropriate therapy. A wound culture involves collecting a specimen of exudate, drainage or tissue by swab, aspiration, or tissue removal. Nurses generally perform collection of a culture by swab; wound cultures collected by aspiration and tissue removal are performed by advanced practice professionals and physicians. The collection of a wound culture by swab is addressed in the following skill.

Maintaining strict asepsis is crucial so that only the pathogen present in the wound is isolated. It is essential to use optimal technique and the correct collection device based on the tests ordered for the collection of a specimen to isolate aerobic and/or anaerobic organisms (WOCN, 2016).

(*continued*)

Skill 8-4 ▶ Collecting a Wound Culture *(continued)*

DELEGATION CONSIDERATIONS	The collection of a wound culture is not delegated to nursing assistive personnel (NAP) or to unlicensed assistive personnel (UAP). Depending on the state's nurse practice act and the organization's policies and procedures, the collection of a wound culture may be delegated to licensed practical/vocational nurses (LPN/LVNs). The decision to delegate must be based on careful analysis of the patient's needs and circumstances, as well as the qualifications of the person to whom the task is being delegated. Refer to the Delegation Guidelines in Appendix A.

EQUIPMENT

- A sterile Culturette kit (aerobic and/or anaerobic) with swab, or a culture tube with individual sterile swabs
- Sterile gloves
- Clean, disposable gloves
- Additional PPE, as indicated
- Plastic bag or appropriate waste receptacle
- Patient label for the sample tube
- Biohazard specimen bag
- Bath blanket (if necessary to drape the patient)
- Supplies to clean the wound and reapply a sterile dressing after obtaining the culture. (Refer to Skills 8-2 and 8-3.)

ASSESSMENT	Assess the situation to determine the need for wound culture. Confirm any prescribed orders relevant to obtaining a wound culture, as well as wound care, and/or any wound care included in the nursing care plan. Assess the patient's level of comfort and the need for analgesics before obtaining the wound culture. Inspect the wound and the surrounding tissue. Assess the location, appearance of the wound, stage (if appropriate), drainage, and types of tissue present in the wound. Measure the wound. Note the stage of the healing process and characteristics of any drainage. Also assess the surrounding skin for color, temperature, and edema, ecchymosis, or maceration.

NURSING DIAGNOSIS	Determine the related factors for the nursing diagnoses based on the patient's current health status. Appropriate nursing diagnoses may include: - Impaired skin integrity - Impaired tissue integrity - Risk for infection

OUTCOME IDENTIFICATION AND PLANNING	The expected outcome to achieve when collecting a wound culture is that the culture is obtained without contamination, exposing the patient to additional pathogens, or causing discomfort for the patient, and the patient demonstrates an understanding of the reason for the wound culture.

IMPLEMENTATION

ACTION	RATIONALE
1. Review the patient's health record for prescribed orders for obtaining a wound culture. Gather necessary supplies. If possible, obtain the wound culture prior to the start of antimicrobial therapy.	Reviewing the health record and care plan validates the correct patient and correct procedure. Preparation promotes efficient time management and an organized approach to the task. Antimicrobial therapy interferes with microorganism growth, so it is important to obtain the wound culture prior to the start of antimicrobial therapy (Huddleston Cross, 2014; Van Leeuwen & Bladh, 2017).
2. Perform hand hygiene and put on PPE, if indicated.	Hand hygiene and PPE prevent the spread of microorganisms. PPE is required based on transmission precautions.
3. Identify the patient.	Identifying the patient ensures the right patient receives the intervention and helps prevent errors.

ACTION	**RATIONALE**
4. Assemble equipment on the overbed table or other surface within reach.	Organization facilitates performance of the task.
5. Close the curtains around the bed and close the door to the room, if possible. Explain to the patient what you are going to do and why you are going to do it.	This ensures the patient's privacy. Explanation relieves anxiety and facilitates cooperation.
6. Assess the patient for possible need for nonpharmacologic pain-reducing interventions or analgesic medication before obtaining the wound culture. Administer appropriate pre-scribed analgesic. Allow enough time for the analgesic to achieve its effectiveness before beginning the procedure.	Pain is a subjective experience influenced by past experience. Wound care and dressing changes may cause pain for some patients.
7. Place an appropriate waste receptacle within easy reach for use during the procedure.	Having the waste container handy means that soiled mate-rials may be discarded easily, without the spread of microorganisms.
8. Adjust the bed to a comfortable working height, usually elbow height of the caregiver (VHACEOSH, 2016).	Having the bed at the proper height prevents back and muscle strain.
9. Assist the patient to a comfortable position that provides easy access to the wound. If necessary, drape the patient with the bath blanket to expose only the wound area. Place a waterproof pad under the wound site. Check the culture label against the patient's identification bracelet (Figure 1).	Patient positioning and the use of a bath blanket provide for com-fort and warmth. Checking the culture label with the patient's identification ensures the correct patient and the correct procedure.

FIGURE 1. Checking culture label with the patient's identification band.

10. If there is a dressing in place on the wound, put on clean gloves and carefully remove the dressing. Refer to Skill 8-2. Note the presence, amount, type, color, and odor of any drainage on the dressings. Place soiled dressings in the appropriate waste receptacle.	Gloves protect the nurse from handling contaminated dress-ings. The dressing must be removed to allow access to the wound.
11. Remove gloves and perform hand hygiene.	Hand hygiene prevents the transmission of microorganisms.
12. Assess and clean the wound, **using a nonantimicrobial cleanser,** as outlined in Skills 8-2 and 8-3. Refer also to Fundamentals Review 8-1, 8-2, 8-3, and 8-4.	This information provides evidence about the wound heal-ing process and/or the presence of infection. Cleaning the wound removes previous drainage and wound debris, which could introduce extraneous organisms into the collected specimen, resulting in inaccurate results.
13. Dry the surrounding skin with gauze dressings. Put on clean gloves.	Excess moisture can contribute to skin irritation and breakdown. The use of a culture swab does not require immediate contact with the skin or wound, so clean gloves are appropriate to pro-tect the nurse from contact with blood and/or body fluids.

(continued)

Skill 8-4 ▶ Collecting a Wound Culture *(continued)*

ACTION	RATIONALE

ACTION

14. Twist the cap to loosen the swab on the Culturette tube, or open the separate swab(s) and remove the cap from the culture tube. **Keep the swab and inside of the culture tube(s) sterile (Figure 2).**

FIGURE 2. Removing cap from culture tube.

15. If contact with the wound is necessary to separate wound margins to permit insertion of the swab deep into the wound, put a sterile glove on one hand to manipulate the wound margins. Clean gloves may be appropriate for contact with pressure injuries and chronic wounds.

16. **Identify a 1 cm area of the wound that is free from necrotic tissue.** Carefully insert the swab into this area of clean viable tissue. **Press the swab to apply sufficient pressure to express fluid from the wound tissue and rotate the swab several times. Avoid touching the swab to intact skin at the wound edges (Figure 3).**

17. Place the swab back in the culture tube (Figure 4). **Do not touch the outside of the tube with the swab.** Secure the cap. Some swab containers have an ampule of medium at the bottom of the tube. It might be necessary to crush this ampule to activate. Follow the manufacturer's instructions for use.

RATIONALE

Supplies are ready to use and within easy reach, and aseptic technique is maintained.

If contact with the wound is necessary to collect the specimen, a sterile glove is necessary to prevent contamination of the wound. Clean technique may be appropriate for cleaning chronic wounds or pressure injuries (Baranoski & Ayello, 2016; NPUAP, EPUAP, & PPPIA, 2014b; Taylor et al., 2019).

Cotton tip absorbs wound drainage. This technique (Levine technique) is considered to provide more accurate results and current best practice (Huddleston Cross, 2014; WOCN, 2016). Contact with skin could introduce extraneous organisms into the collected specimen, resulting in inaccurate results.

The outside of the container is protected from contamination with microorganisms, and the sample is not contaminated with organisms not in the wound. Surrounding the swab with culture medium is necessary for accurate culture results.

FIGURE 3. Rotating swab several times over wound surface.

FIGURE 4. Placing swab in culture tube.

ACTION

RATIONALE

18. Use another swab if collecting a specimen from another area of the wound or site and repeat the procedure.

Using another swab at a different site prevents cross-contamination of the wound.

 19. Remove gloves and discard them accordingly. Perform hand hygiene.

Removing gloves properly reduces the risk for infection transmission and contamination of other items. Hand hygiene prevents the transmission of microorganisms.

 20. Put on gloves. Place a dressing on the wound, as appropriate, based on prescribed orders and/or the nursing care plan. Refer to Skill 8-2. Remove gloves. Perform hand hygiene.

Wound dressings protect, absorb drainage, provide a moist environment, and promote wound healing. Removing gloves properly reduces the risk for infection transmission and contamination of other items.

21. After securing the dressing, label dressing with date and time. Remove all remaining equipment; place the patient in a comfortable position, with side rails up as indicated and bed in the lowest position.

Recording date and time provides communication and demonstrates adherence to care plan. Proper patient and bed positioning promotes safety and comfort.

22. Label the specimen according to your institution's guidelines. Information included may include wound site, time the specimen was collected, any antimicrobials the patient is receiving, and the identity of the person who obtained the specimen (Huddleston Cross, 2014). Send or transport specimen to the laboratory in a biohazard bag immediately or within the optimal time from for transport as indicated by facility policy and guidelines (Figure 5).

Proper labeling ensures proper identification of the specimen. Specimens must be sent to the laboratory immediately or within the optimal time from for transport as indicated by facility policy and guidelines to ensure accurate results (Huddleston Cross, 2014; Van Leeuwen & Bladh, 2017; WOCN, 2016).

FIGURE 5. Labeled culture container in biohazard bag.

 23. Remove PPE, if used. Perform hand hygiene.

Proper removal of PPE reduces the risk for infection transmission and contamination of other items. Hand hygiene prevents the spread of microorganisms.

EVALUATION

The expected outcomes have been met when the culture was obtained without contamination; the patient was not exposed to additional pathogens; the patient did not experience discomfort; and the patient demonstrated an understanding of the reason for the wound culture.

Skill 8-4 ▶ Collecting a Wound Culture *(continued)*

DOCUMENTATION

Guidelines

Document the location of the wound, the assessment of the wound, including the type of tissue present, presence of necrotic tissue, stage (if appropriate), and characteristics of drainage. Include the appearance of the surrounding skin. Document cleansing of the wound and the obtained culture. Record any skin care and/or dressing applied. Note pertinent patient and family education and any patient reaction to this procedure, including patient's pain level and effectiveness of nonpharmacologic interventions or analgesia, if administered.

Sample Documentation

> 6/22/20 2100 Wound noted on patient's hand; 2 cm × 3 cm × 1 cm, red, tender, with purulent drainage present. Edges macerated, without erythema and tenderness. Wound cleaned with normal saline, culture obtained. Skin protectant/barrier applied to surrounding area, wound redressed with alginate, cover dressing, and roller gauze. Hand elevated. Culture labeled and sent to lab.
>
> —J. Wentz, RN

UNEXPECTED SITUATIONS AND ASSOCIATED INTERVENTIONS

- *The nurse has inserted the culture swab into the patient's wound to obtain the specimen and realizes that the wound was not cleaned:* Discard this swab. Obtain the additional supplies needed to clean the wound according to facility policy and a new culture swab. Cleaning the wound prior to obtaining a specimen for culture removes previous drainage and wound debris, which could introduce extraneous organisms into the collected specimen, resulting in inaccurate results. Clean the wound using a nonantimicrobial cleanser and then proceed to obtain the culture specimen.
- *As the nurse prepares to insert the culture swab into the wound, the nurse inadvertently touches the swab to the patient's bedclothes or other surface:* Discard this swab, obtain a new culture swab, and collect the specimen.

GENERAL CONSIDERATIONS

- Tissue biopsy is considered the "gold standard" of wound cultures; however it and the aspiration technique are invasive and are performed by physicians and advanced practice professionals (WOCN, 2016). Swab specimens are more commonly used because they are most easily collected, readily available, and may be collected by nurses in general practice (Wounds International, 2012, as cited in Huddleston Cross, 2014).
- Final culture results may take 24 to 72 hours depending on the method used and organism suspected; antimicrobial therapy based on the pathogens most commonly involved in a particular type of wound may be started immediately and changed if indicated when culture and sensitivity results are available (Van Leeuwen & Bladh, 2017; WOCN, 2016).

Skill 8-5 ▶ Applying Montgomery Straps

Montgomery straps are prepared strips of nonallergenic tape with ties inserted through holes at one end. One set of straps is placed on either side of a wound, and the straps are tied like shoelaces to secure the dressings. When it is time to change the dressing, the straps are untied, the wound is cared for, and then the straps are retied to hold the new dressing. A skin protectant/barrier or hydrocolloid dressing is applied to the skin before the straps are placed to protect the skin. The straps or ties need to be changed only if they become loose or soiled.

Montgomery straps may be appropriate to secure dressings on wounds that require frequent dressing changes, such as wounds with increased drainage. These straps allow the nurse to perform wound care without the need to remove adhesive strips, such as tape, with each dressing change, thus decreasing the risk of skin irritation and medical adhesive–related skin injury (MARSI).

DELEGATION CONSIDERATIONS	Application of Montgomery Straps is not delegated to nursing assistive personnel (NAP) or to unlicensed assistive personnel (UAP). Depending on the state's nurse practice act and the organization's policies and procedures, this procedure may be delegated to licensed practical/vocational nurses (LPN/LVNs). The decision to delegate must be based on careful analysis of the patient's needs and circumstances, as well as the qualifications of the person to whom the task is being delegated. Refer to the Delegation Guidelines in Appendix A.

EQUIPMENT

- Clean, disposable gloves
- Additional PPE, as indicated
- Dressings for wound care, as indicated and prescribed for the patient
- Montgomery straps
- Supplies to clean the wound, based on the wound care prescribed for the patient
- Normal saline solution
- Skin protectant/barrier wipes
- Skin-barrier sheet (hydrocolloidal or nonhydrocolloidal)
- Disposable scissors, if available, or scissors
- Antimicrobial wipes

ASSESSMENT

Assess the situation to determine the need for wound cleaning and a dressing change. Assess the integrity of any straps currently in use. Replace loose or soiled straps or ties. Confirm any prescribed orders relevant to wound care and any wound care included in the nursing care plan. Assess the patient's level of comfort and the need for analgesics before wound care. Assess if the patient experienced any pain related to prior dressing changes and the effectiveness of interventions employed to minimize the patient's pain. Assess the current dressing to determine if it is intact. Assess for excess drainage or bleeding or saturation of the dressing. Inspect the wound and the surrounding tissue. Assess the appearance of the wound for the approximation of wound edges, the color of the wound and surrounding area, and signs of dehiscence. Assess for the presence of sutures, staples, or adhesive closure strips. Note the stage of the healing process and characteristics of any drainage. Also assess the surrounding skin for color, temperature, and edema, ecchymosis, or maceration.

NURSING DIAGNOSIS

Determine the related factors for the nursing diagnoses based on the patient's current health status. Appropriate nursing diagnoses may include:

- Impaired skin integrity
- Acute pain
- Delayed surgical recovery

OUTCOME IDENTIFICATION AND PLANNING

The expected outcome to achieve when applying Montgomery straps is that the Montgomery straps are applied and the patient's skin is free from irritation and injury. Other outcomes that may be appropriate include that the care is accomplished without contaminating the wound area, causing trauma to the wound, and/or causing the patient to experience pain or discomfort.

IMPLEMENTATION

ACTION	**RATIONALE**
1. Review the patient's health record for prescribed wound care or the nursing care plan related to wound care. Gather necessary supplies.	Reviewing the health record and care plan validates the correct patient and correct procedure. Preparation promotes efficient time management and an organized approach to the task.
2. Perform hand hygiene and put on PPE, if indicated.	Hand hygiene and PPE prevent the spread of microorganisms. PPE is required based on transmission precautions.
3. Identify the patient.	Identifying the patient ensures the right patient receives the intervention and helps prevent errors.

(continued)

Skill 8-5 ▶ Applying Montgomery Straps *(continued)*

ACTION	RATIONALE
4. Assemble equipment on the overbed table or other surface within reach.	Organization facilitates performance of the task.
5. Close the curtains around the bed and close the door to the room, if possible. Explain what you are going to do and why you are going to do it to the patient.	This ensures the patient's privacy. Explanation relieves anxiety and facilitates cooperation.
6. Assess the patient for possible need for nonpharmacologic pain-reducing interventions or analgesic medication before wound care dressing change. Administer appropriate prescribed analgesic. Allow enough time for the analgesic to achieve its effectiveness before beginning the procedure.	Pain is a subjective experience influenced by past experience. Wound care and dressing changes may cause pain for some patients.
7. Place a waste receptacle at a convenient location for use during the procedure.	Having a waste container handy means that the soiled dressing may be discarded easily, without the spread of microorganisms.
8. Adjust the bed to a comfortable working height, usually elbow height of the caregiver (VHACEOSH, 2016).	Having the bed at the proper height prevents back and muscle strain.
9. Assist the patient to a comfortable position that provides easy access to the wound area. Use a bath blanket to cover any exposed area other than the wound. Place a waterproof pad under the wound site.	Patient positioning and the use of a bath blanket provide for comfort and warmth. Waterproof pad protects underlying surfaces.
10. Perform wound care and a dressing change as ordered and outlined in Skills 8-2 and 8-3.	Wound care aids in healing and protects the wound.
11. Put on clean gloves. Clean the skin on either side of the wound with the gauze, moistened with normal saline. Dry the skin.	Gloves prevent the spread of microorganisms. Cleaning and drying the skin prevents irritation and injury.
12. **Apply a skin protectant/barrier to the skin where the straps will be placed.**	Skin barrier/protectant prevents skin irritation and excoriation from tape, adhesives, and wound drainage (McNichol et al., 2013).
13. Cut the Montgomery strap to size, based on the size of the wound. Write the date and time of application on strap.	Strap should be large enough to hold the dressing in place.
14. Cut the hydrocolloidal or nonhydrocolloidal skin barrier sheet to the size of the strap and apply to the patient's skin, near the dressing. Apply the sticky side of each strap to the skin barrier sheet, so the openings for the strings are at the edge of the dressing (Figure 1). Repeat for the other side.	Skin protectant/barrier and skin barrier sheet prevent skin irritation and medical adhesive–related skin injury (MARSI). Recording date and time provides a baseline for changing straps.
15. Tie the opposing ties together, over the dressing, like a shoelace (Figure 2). **Do not secure too tightly.**	Ties hold the dressing in place. Tying too tightly puts additional stress on the surrounding skin.

FIGURE 1. Applying Montgomery straps to skin barrier sheet on patient's abdomen.

FIGURE 2. Tying Montgomery straps.

ACTION	RATIONALE
16. Remove gloves. Perform hand hygiene. Label dressing with date and time. Remove all remaining equipment; place the patient in a comfortable position, with side rails up as indicated and the bed in the lowest position.	Hand hygiene prevents the transmission of microorganisms. Recording date and time provides communication and demonstrates adherence to care plan. Proper patient and bed positioning promotes safety and comfort.
17. If nondisposable scissors were used, put on gloves. Clean scissors with antimicrobial wipe.	Cleaning of scissors prevents the transmission of microorganisms.
18. Remove gloves and additional PPE, if used. Perform hand hygiene.	Proper removal of PPE reduces the risk for infection transmission and contamination of other items. Hand hygiene prevents the spread of microorganisms.
19. Check all wound dressings at least every shift. More frequent checks may be needed if the wound is more complex or dressings become saturated quickly.	Checking dressings ensures the assessment of changes in patient condition and timely intervention to prevent complications.
20. Replace the ties and straps whenever they are soiled, or every 2 to 3 days. Straps can be reapplied onto skin barrier. Skin barrier can remain in place up to 7 days. Use a silicone-based adhesive remover to help remove the skin barrier.	Replacing soiled ties and straps prevents the growth of pathogens. Minimizing removal of skin barrier sheet prevents skin irritation and MARSI. The use of adhesive remover allows for the easy, rapid, and painless removal without the associated problems of skin stripping and helps reduce patient discomfort (McNichol et al., 2013).

EVALUATION

The expected outcomes have been met when the Montgomery straps are applied and the patient's skin is free from irritation and injury; the care was accomplished without contaminating the wound area or causing trauma to the wound; and the patient did not experience pain or discomfort.

DOCUMENTATION

Guidelines

Document the procedure, the patient's response, and your assessment of the area before and after application of Montgomery straps. Record a description of the wound, amount and character of the wound drainage, and an assessment of the surrounding skin. Note the type of dressing that was applied, including the application of skin protectant/barrier and a skin barrier sheet. Document that Montgomery straps were applied to secure the dressings. Record the patient's response to the dressing care and associated pain assessment. Include any pertinent patient and family education.

Sample Documentation

> 10/20/20 1930 Patient's abdominal wound has large amounts of serosanguineous drainage, saturating multiple layers of gauze and ABDs, requiring dressing changes at least q3h. Surrounding skin cleansed, skin protectant/barrier applied, and Montgomery straps applied to secure wound dressings.
>
> —D. Rightner, RN

UNEXPECTED SITUATIONS AND ASSOCIATED INTERVENTIONS

• *A patient has had an abdominal wound for several weeks. Despite careful wound and skin care, the nurse observes signs of redness and irritation where the adhesive for the dressings has been repeatedly placed:* Obtain the supplies listed in this skill. Apply Montgomery straps, being sure to move the skin barrier sheet at least 1 in away from the area of irritation. Consult with the advanced practice wound nurse regarding the care plan.

SPECIAL CONSIDERATIONS

• Wound care is often uncomfortable, and patients may experience significant pain. Assess the patient's comfort level and past experiences with wound care. Offer analgesics, as ordered, and nonpharmacologic comfort/pain interventions to maintain the patient's level of comfort.

Skill 8-6 ▶ Caring for a Penrose Drain

Drains are inserted into or near a wound when it is anticipated that a collection of fluid in a closed area would delay healing. A Penrose drain is a hollow, soft, flexible, open-ended rubber tube. It does not have a collection device and allows fluid to drain passively, with the drainage moving from the area of greater pressure (in the wound) to the area of less pressure (the dressing). Penrose drains are commonly used after a surgical procedure or for drainage of an abscess. After a surgical procedure, the surgeon places one end of the drain in or near the area to be drained. The other end passes through the skin, directly through the incision or through a separate opening referred to as a stab wound. A Penrose drain is not sutured. A large safety pin is usually placed in the part of the drain outside the wound to prevent the drain from slipping back into the incised area. The patency and placement of the drain are included in the wound assessment.

DELEGATION CONSIDERATIONS

Care for a Penrose drain insertion site and wound care is not delegated to nursing assistive personnel (NAP) or to unlicensed assistive personnel (UAP). Depending on the state's nurse practice act and the organization's policies and procedures, these procedures may be delegated to licensed practical/vocational nurses (LPN/LVNs). The decision to delegate must be based on careful analysis of the patient's needs and circumstances, as well as the qualifications of the person to whom the task is being delegated. Refer to the Delegation Guidelines in Appendix A.

EQUIPMENT

- Sterile gloves
- Gauze dressings
- Sterile cotton-tipped applicators, if appropriate
- Sterile drain sponges
- Surgical or abdominal pads
- Sterile dressing set or suture set (for the sterile scissors and forceps)
- Sterile cleaning solution as ordered (commonly 0.9% normal saline solution)
- Sterile container to hold cleaning solution
- Clean safety pin
- Clean, disposable gloves
- Plastic bag or other appropriate waste container for soiled dressings
- Waterproof pad and bath blanket
- Tape or ties
- Skin protectant/barrier wipes
- Additional dressings and supplies needed or as required for ordered wound care

ASSESSMENT

Assess the situation to determine the necessity for wound cleaning and a dressing change. Confirm any prescribed orders relevant to drain care and any drain care included in the nursing care plan. Assess the patient's level of comfort and the need for analgesics before wound care. Assess if the patient experienced any pain related to prior dressing changes and the effectiveness of interventions employed to minimize the patient's pain. Assess the current dressing to determine if it is intact, and assess for the presence of excess drainage, bleeding, or saturation of the dressing. Assess the patency of the Penrose drain.

Inspect the wound and the surrounding tissue. Assess the appearance of the wound for the approximation of wound edges, the color of the wound and surrounding area, and signs of dehiscence. Note the stage of the healing process and the characteristics of any drainage. Assess the surrounding skin for color, temperature, and the presence of edema, ecchymosis, or maceration.

NURSING DIAGNOSIS

Determine the related factors for the nursing diagnoses based on the patient's current health status. Appropriate nursing diagnoses may include:

- Risk for infection
- Disturbed body image
- Deficient knowledge

OUTCOME IDENTIFICATION AND PLANNING

The expected outcome to achieve when performing care for a Penrose drain is that the Penrose drain remains patent and intact; the wound care is accomplished without contaminating the wound area, or causing trauma to the wound, and without causing the patient to experience pain or discomfort. Other outcomes that are appropriate may include the following: the wound shows signs of progressive healing without evidence of complications, and the patient demonstrates an understanding of drain care.

IMPLEMENTATION

ACTION	RATIONALE
1. Review the patient's health record for prescribed wound care or the nursing care plan related to wound/drain care. Gather necessary supplies.	Reviewing the health record and care plan validates the correct patient and correct procedure. Preparation promotes efficient time management and an organized approach to the task.
2. Perform hand hygiene and put on PPE, if indicated.	Hand hygiene and PPE prevent the spread of microorganisms. PPE is required based on transmission precautions.
3. Identify the patient.	Identifying the patient ensures the right patient receives the intervention and helps prevent errors.
4. Assemble equipment on the overbed table or other surface within reach.	Organization facilitates performance of the task.
5. Close the curtains around the bed and close the door to the room, if possible. Explain what you are going to do and why you are going to do it to the patient.	This ensures the patient's privacy. Explanation relieves anxiety and facilitates cooperation.
6. Assess the patient for possible need for nonpharmacologic pain-reducing interventions or analgesic medication before wound care dressing change. Administer appropriate prescribed analgesic. Allow enough time for the analgesic to achieve its effectiveness before beginning the procedure.	Pain is a subjective experience influenced by past experience. Wound care and dressing changes may cause pain for some patients.
7. Place a waste receptacle at a convenient location for use during the procedure.	Having a waste container handy means that the soiled dressing may be discarded easily, without the spread of microorganisms.
8. Adjust the bed to a comfortable working height, usually elbow height of the caregiver (VHACEOSH, 2016).	Having the bed at the proper height prevents back and muscle strain.
9. Assist the patient to a comfortable position that provides easy access to the drain and/or wound area. Use a bath blanket to cover any exposed area other than the wound. Place a waterproof pad under the wound site.	Patient positioning and the use of a bath blanket provide for comfort and warmth. Waterproof pad protects underlying surfaces.
10. Put on clean, disposable gloves. Check the position of the drain or drains before removing the dressing. Loosen the tape on the old dressings by removing in the direction of hair growth and the use of a push–pull method. Push–pull method: lift a corner of the dressing away from the skin, then gently push the skin away from the dressing/adhesive. Continue moving fingers of the opposite hand to support the skin as the product is removed (McNichol et al., 2013). Carefully lift the adhesive from the surrounding skin to prevent medical adhesive–related skin injury (MARSI). Remove the sides/edges first, then the center. If there is resistance, use an adhesive remover (McNichol et al., 2013).	Checking ensures that a drain is not removed accidentally if one is present. Gloves protect the nurse from contaminated dressings and prevent the spread of microorganisms. Removal of the tape in the direction of hair growth minimizes trauma to the skin (Taylor et al., 2019). The use of adhesive remover allows for the easy, rapid, and painless removal without the associated problems of skin stripping and helps reduce patient discomfort (McNichol et al., 2013).
11. Carefully remove the soiled dressings. If any part of the dressing sticks to the underlying skin, use small amounts of sterile saline to help loosen and remove it. Note the presence, amount, type, color, and odor of any drainage on the dressings. Place soiled dressings in the appropriate waste receptacle.	Cautious removal of the dressing is more comfortable for the patient and ensures that any drain present is not removed. Sterile saline moistens the dressing for easier removal and minimizes damage and pain. The presence of drainage should be documented. Discarding dressings appropriately prevents the spread of microorganisms.
12. Inspect the drain site for appearance and drainage. Assess if any pain is present.	The wound healing process and/or the presence of irritation or infection must be documented.

(continued)

Skill 8-6 ▶ Caring for a Penrose Drain *(continued)*

ACTION	RATIONALE

13. Remove gloves and perform hand hygiene.

Removal of gloves and performance of hand hygiene prevent the transmission of microorganisms.

14. Using sterile technique, prepare a sterile work area and open the needed supplies.

Supplies are within easy reach and sterility is maintained.

15. Open the sterile cleaning solution. Pour it into the basin. Add the gauze sponges.

Sterility of dressings and solution is maintained.

16. Put on sterile gloves.

Sterile gloves help to maintain surgical asepsis and sterile technique and prevent the spread of microorganisms.

17. Cleanse the drain site with the cleaning solution. Use the forceps and the moistened gauze or cotton-tipped applicators. **Start at the drain insertion site, moving in a circular motion toward the periphery (Figure 1). Use each gauze sponge or applicator only once.** Discard and use new gauze if additional cleansing is needed.

Using a circular motion ensures that cleaning occurs from the least to most contaminated area and a previously cleaned area is not contaminated again.

18. Dry the skin with a new gauze pad in the same manner. Apply skin protectant/barrier to the skin around the drain; extend out to include the area of skin that will be taped. Place a pre-split drain sponge under and around the drain (Figure 2). Closely observe the safety pin in the drain. If the pin or drain is crusted, replace the pin with a new sterile pin. **Take care not to dislodge the drain.**

Drying prevents skin irritation. Skin barrier/protectant prevents skin irritation and excoriation from tape, adhesives, and wound drainage (McNichol et al., 2013). The gauze absorbs drainage and prevents the drainage from accumulating on the patient's skin.

Microorganisms grow more easily in a soiled environment. The safety pin ensures proper placement because the drain is not sutured in place.

FIGURE 1. Cleaning drain site in circular motion toward periphery.

FIGURE 2. Placing pre-split dressing around Penrose drain.

19. Apply gauze pads over the drain (Figure 3). Apply surgical pad, ABD, or other cover dressing over the gauze.

The gauze absorbs drainage. Pads provide both extra absorption for excess drainage and a moisture barrier.

20. Apply tape, Montgomery straps, or roller gauze to secure the dressings. Remove and discard gloves. Perform hand hygiene.

Tape or other securing products keep the dressing in place. Proper disposal of gloves prevents the spread of microorganisms. Hand hygiene prevents the transmission of microorganisms.

21. After securing the dressing, label dressing with date and time. Remove all remaining equipment; place the patient in a comfortable position, with side rails up as indicated and bed in the lowest position.

Recording date and time provides communication and demonstrates adherence to care plan. Proper patient and bed positioning promotes safety and comfort.

ACTION

FIGURE 3. Applying gauze pads over drain.

RATIONALE

 22. Remove additional PPE, if used. Perform hand hygiene.

Proper removal of PPE reduces the risk for infection transmission and contamination of other items. Hand hygiene prevents the spread of microorganisms.

23. Check all wound dressings at least every shift. More frequent checks may be needed if the wound is more complex or dressings become saturated quickly.

Checking dressings ensures the assessment of changes in patient condition and timely intervention to prevent complications.

EVALUATION

The expected outcomes have been met when the Penrose drain remained patent and intact; the wound care was accomplished without contaminating the wound area or causing trauma to the wound; the patient did not experience pain or discomfort; the wound showed signs of progressive healing without evidence of complications; and the patient demonstrated an understanding of drain care.

DOCUMENTATION

Guidelines

Document the location of the wound and drain, the assessment of the wound and drain site, and patency of the Penrose drain. Document the presence of drainage and characteristics on the old dressing upon removal. Include the appearance of the surrounding skin. Document cleansing of the drain site. Record any skin care and the dressing applied. Note pertinent patient and family education and any patient reaction to this procedure, including patient's pain level and effectiveness of nonpharmacologic interventions or analgesia if administered.

Sample Documentation

3/13/20 1400 Patient medicated with morphine 3 mg IV, as ordered, prior to dressing change. Dressing to right forearm removed. Dressings noted with small amount of serosanguineous drainage. Forearm with gross edema and erythema. Penrose drain intact, with safety pin in place. Incision edges approximated, staples intact. Area cleansed with normal saline, dried, and redressed with nonadherent gauze, ABD pads, and roller gauze. Reinforced the importance of keeping arm elevated on pillows, with patient verbalizing understanding.

—P. Towns, RN

UNEXPECTED SITUATIONS AND ASSOCIATED INTERVENTIONS

- *Assessment of the drain site reveals significantly increased edema, erythema, and drainage from the site, in addition to drainage via the drain:* Cleanse the site, as ordered, or per the nursing care plan. Obtain vital signs, including the patient's temperature. Document care and assessments. Notify the primary health care provider of the findings.

(continued)

Skill 8-6 ▶ Caring for a Penrose Drain *(continued)*

- *Assessment of the drain site reveals that the drain has slipped back into the incision:* Follow facility policy and the prescribed orders related to advancing Penrose drains. Document assessments and interventions. Notify the primary health care provider of the findings and interventions.
- *When preparing to change a dressing on a Penrose drain site, the nurse's assessment reveals that the drain is completely out, lying in the dressing material:* Assess the site and the patient for symptoms of pain, increased edema/erythema/drainage. Provide site care, as ordered. Notify the primary health care provider. Often, depending on the patient's stage of recovery, the drain is left out. Document the findings and interventions.

SPECIAL CONSIDERATIONS	- Evaluate a sudden increase in the amount of drainage or bright red drainage and notify the primary health care provider of these findings. - Wound care is often uncomfortable, and patients may experience significant pain. Assess the patient's comfort level and past experiences with wound care. Offer analgesics, as ordered, and nonpharmacologic comfort/pain interventions to maintain the patient's level of comfort. - Appropriate nutritional support is critical in achieving successful wound healing and may be overlooked (Quain & Khardori, 2015). Collaborate with the registered dietician and dietary staff to develop an individualized nutrition intervention plan for the patient (NPUAP, EPUAP, PPPIA, 2014a).

Skill 8-7 ▶ Caring for a T-Tube Drain

A biliary drain, or T-tube (Figure 1) is sometimes placed in the common bile duct after removal of the gallbladder (cholecystectomy) or a portion of the bile duct (choledochostomy). The tube passively drains bile while the surgical site is healing. A portion of the tube is inserted into the common bile duct and the remaining portion is anchored to the abdominal wall, passed through the skin, and connected to a closed drainage system. Often, a three-way valve is inserted between the drain tube and the drainage system to allow for clamping and flushing of the tube, if necessary. The drainage amount is measured every shift, recorded, and included in output totals.

FIGURE 1. T-tube.

DELEGATION CONSIDERATIONS	Care for a T-tube drain insertion site is not delegated to nursing assistive personnel (NAP) or to unlicensed assistive personnel (UAP). Depending on the organization's policies and procedures, the drain may be emptied and reconstituted by NAP or UAP. Depending on the state's nurse practice act and the organization's policies and procedures, these procedures may be delegated to licensed practical/vocational nurses (LPN/LVNs). The decision to delegate must be based on careful analysis of the patient's needs and circumstances, as well as the qualifications of the person to whom the task is being delegated. Refer to the Delegation Guidelines in Appendix A.

EQUIPMENT	
• Sterile gloves	• Tape or a commercial securement/ stabilization device
• Clean, disposable gloves	• Graduated collection container
• Additional PPE, as indicated	• Waste receptacle
• Sterile gauze pads	• Sterile basin
• Sterile drain sponges	• Sterile forceps
• Cleansing solution, usually sterile normal saline	• Tape
• Sterile cotton-tipped applicators (if appropriate)	• Skin protectant/barrier wipes
• Transparent or other cover dressing, as indicated	• Waterproof pad and bath blanket

ASSESSMENT

Assess the situation to determine the need for wound cleaning, a dressing change, or emptying of the drain. Confirm any prescribed orders relevant to drain care and any drain care included in the nursing care plan. Assess the patient's level of comfort and the need for analgesics before wound care. Assess if the patient experienced any pain related to prior dressing changes and the effectiveness of interventions employed to minimize the patient's pain. Assess the current dressing to determine if it is intact, and assess for evidence of excessive drainage or bleeding or saturation of the dressing. Assess the patency of the T-tube and the drain site. Note the characteristics of the drainage in the collection bag.

Inspect the wound and the surrounding tissue. Assess the appearance of the incision for the approximation of wound edges, the color of the wound and surrounding area, and signs of dehiscence. Note the stage of the healing process and characteristics of any drainage. Assess the surrounding skin for color, temperature, and edema, ecchymosis, or maceration.

NURSING DIAGNOSIS

Determine the related factors for the nursing diagnoses based on the patient's current health status. Appropriate nursing diagnoses may include:

• Risk for infection
• Deficient knowledge
• Disturbed body image

OUTCOME IDENTIFICATION AND PLANNING

The expected outcome to achieve when performing care for a T-tube drain is that the drain remains patent and intact; drain care is accomplished without contaminating the wound area and/or without causing trauma to the wound; and the patient does not experience pain or discomfort. Other outcomes that are appropriate may include the following: the drainage amounts are measured accurately at the frequency required by facility policy and recorded as part of the intake and output record; and the patient demonstrates an understanding of drain care.

IMPLEMENTATION

ACTION	RATIONALE
1. Review the patient's health record for prescribed wound care or the nursing care plan related to wound/drain care. Gather necessary supplies.	Reviewing the health record and care plan validates the correct patient and correct procedure. Preparation promotes efficient time management and an organized approach to the task.
2. Perform hand hygiene and put on PPE, if indicated.	Hand hygiene and PPE prevent the spread of microorganisms. PPE is required based on transmission precautions.
3. Identify the patient.	Identifying the patient ensures the right patient receives the intervention and helps prevent errors.

(continued)

Skill 8-7 ▶ Caring for a T-Tube Drain *(continued)*

ACTION	RATIONALE
4. Assemble equipment on the overbed table or other surface within reach.	Organization facilitates performance of the task.
5. Close the curtains around the bed and close the door to the room, if possible. Explain what you are going to do and why you are going to do it to the patient.	This ensures the patient's privacy. Explanation relieves anxiety and facilitates cooperation.
6. Assess the patient for possible need for nonpharmacologic pain-reducing interventions or analgesic medication before wound care dressing change. Administer appropriate prescribed analgesic. Allow enough time for the analgesic to achieve its effectiveness before beginning the procedure.	Pain is a subjective experience influenced by past experience. Wound care and dressing changes may cause pain for some patients.
7. Place a waste receptacle at a convenient location for use during the procedure.	Having a waste container handy means that the soiled dressing may be discarded easily, without the spread of microorganisms.
8. Adjust the bed to a comfortable working height, usually elbow height of the caregiver (VHACEOSH, 2016).	Having the bed at the proper height prevents back and muscle strain.
9. Assist the patient to a comfortable position that provides easy access to the drain and/or wound area. Use a bath blanket to cover any exposed area other than the drain. Place a waterproof pad under the drain site.	Patient positioning and the use of a bath blanket provide for comfort and warmth. Waterproof pad protects underlying surfaces.

Emptying Drainage

10. Put on clean gloves; put on mask or face shield, as indicated.	Gloves prevent the spread of microorganisms; mask reduces the risk of transmission should splashing occur.
11. Using sterile technique, open a gauze pad, making a sterile field with the outer wrapper.	Using sterile technique deters the spread of microorganisms.
12. Place the graduated collection container under the outlet valve of the drainage bag. **Without touching the outlet, pull off the cap and empty the bag's contents completely into the container (Figure 2). Use the gauze to wipe the outlet, and replace the cap (Figure 3).**	Draining contents into a container allows for accurate measurement of the drainage. Touching the outlet with gloves or other surface contaminates the valve, potentially introducing pathogens. Wiping the outlet with gauze prevents contamination of the valve. Recapping prevents the spread of microorganisms.

FIGURE 2. Emptying bag's contents into collection container.

FIGURE 3. Replacing outlet cap.

13. Carefully measure and note the characteristics of the drainage. Discard the drainage according to facility policy.	Documentation promotes continuity of care and communication. Appropriate disposal of biohazard material reduces the risk for microorganism transmission.
14. Remove gloves and perform hand hygiene.	Proper glove removal and performing hand hygiene prevent the spread of microorganisms.

ACTION	**RATIONALE**

Cleaning the Drain Site

15. Put on clean, disposable gloves. Check the position of the drain before removing the dressing. Loosen the tape on the old dressings by removing in the direction of hair growth and the use of a push–pull method. Push–pull method: lift a corner of the dressing away from the skin, then gently push the skin away from the dressing/adhesive. Continue moving fingers of the opposite hand to support the skin as the product is removed (McNichol et al., 2013). Carefully lift the adhesive from the surrounding skin to prevent medical adhesive–related skin injury (MARSI). Remove the sides/edges first, then the center. If there is resistance, use an adhesive remover (McNichol et al., 2013).

Checking ensures that a drain is not removed accidentally if one is present. Gloves protect the nurse from contaminated dressings and prevent the spread of microorganisms. Removal of the tape in the direction of hair growth minimizes trauma to the skin (Taylor et al., 2019). The use of adhesive remover allows for the easy, rapid, and painless removal without the associated problems of skin stripping and helps reduce patient discomfort (McNichol et al., 2013).

16. Carefully remove the soiled dressings. If any part of the dressing sticks to the underlying skin, use small amounts of sterile saline to help loosen and remove it. Note the presence, amount, type, color, and odor of any drainage on the dressings. Place soiled dressings in the appropriate waste receptacle.

Cautious removal of the dressing is more comfortable for the patient and ensures that any drain present is not removed. Sterile saline moistens the dressing for easier removal and minimizes damage and pain. The presence of drainage should be documented. Discarding dressings appropriately prevents the spread of microorganisms.

17. Inspect the drain site for appearance and drainage. Assess if any pain is present.

Wound healing process and/or the presence of irritation or infection should be documented.

18. Remove gloves and perform hand hygiene.

Removal of gloves and performance of hand hygiene prevent transmission of microorganisms.

19. Using sterile technique, prepare a sterile work area and open the needed supplies.

Preparing a sterile work area ensures that supplies are within easy reach and sterility is maintained.

20. Open the sterile cleaning solution. Pour it into the basin. Add the gauze sponges.

Sterility of dressings and solution is maintained.

21. Put on sterile gloves.

The use of sterile gloves maintains surgical asepsis and sterile technique and reduces the risk of microorganism transmission.

22. Cleanse the drain site with the cleaning solution. Use the forceps and the moistened gauze or cotton-tipped applicators. **Start at the drain insertion site, moving in a circular motion toward the periphery. Use each gauze sponge only once.** Discard and use new gauze if additional cleansing is needed. (Refer to Figure 1 in Skill 8-6.)

Cleaning is done from the least to most contaminated area so that a previously cleaned area is not contaminated again.

23. Dry with new sterile gauze in the same manner. Apply skin protectant/barrier to the skin around the drain; extend out to include the area of skin that will be taped.

Drying prevents skin irritation. Skin barrier/protectant prevents skin irritation and excoriation from tape, adhesives, and wound drainage (McNichol et al., 2013).

24. Place a pre-split drain sponge under the drain. (Refer to Figure 2 in Skill 8-6.) Apply gauze pads or other cover dressing, such as a transparent dressing, as indicated by facility policy, over the drain. Secure the dressings with tape, as needed. Remove and discard gloves. Perform hand hygiene.

The gauze absorbs drainage and prevents the drainage from accumulating on the patient's skin. Proper disposal of gloves prevents the spread of microorganisms. Hand hygiene prevents the transmission of microorganisms.

25. Secure the drain tubing to the patient's skin using a tape or a commercial securement/stabilization device, allowing slack in the tubing to avoid excessive tension. **Be careful not to kink the tubing and ensure the collection bag remains below the drain site.**

Securing the tubing prevents accidental dislodgement or movement and avoids excessive tension on tube. Kinked tubing could block drainage. Maintaining the drain collection bag remains below the drain site facilitates proper drainage.

(continued)

Skill 8-7 ▶ Caring for a T-Tube Drain *(continued)*

ACTION	RATIONALE
26. Label the dressing with date and time. Remove all remaining equipment; place the patient in a comfortable position, with side rails up as indicated and bed in the lowest position.	Recording date and time provides communication and demonstrates adherence to care plan. Proper patient and bed positioning promotes safety and comfort.
27. Remove additional PPE, if used. Perform hand hygiene.	Proper removal of PPE reduces the risk for infection transmission and contamination of other items. Hand hygiene prevents the spread of microorganisms.
28. Check drain status at least every 4 hours. Check all wound dressings every shift. Perform more frequent checks if the wound is more complex or dressings become saturated quickly.	Checking drain ensures proper functioning and early detection of problems. Checking dressings ensures the assessment of changes in patient condition and timely intervention to prevent complications.

EVALUATION

The expected outcomes have been met when the T-tube drain remains patent and intact; drain care was accomplished without contaminating the wound area and/or without causing trauma to the wound; the patient did not experience pain or discomfort; the drainage amounts were measured accurately at the frequency required by facility policy and were recorded as part of the intake and output record; and the patient demonstrated an understanding of drain care.

DOCUMENTATION

Guidelines

Document the location of the drain, the assessment of the drain site, and patency of the drain. Note if sutures are intact. Document the presence and characteristics of drainage on the old dressing upon removal. Include the appearance of the surrounding skin. Document cleansing of the drain site. Record any skin care and the dressing applied. Note pertinent patient and family education and any patient reaction to this procedure, including patient's pain level and effectiveness of nonpharmacologic interventions or analgesia, if administered. Document the amount of bile drainage obtained from the drainage bag on the appropriate intake and output record.

Sample Documentation

> 8/9/20 1500 Dressing removed from T-tube site. No drainage noted on dressings. Drain site without redness, edema, drainage, or ecchymosis. Suture intact. Exit site cleaned with normal saline, dried, skin protectant/barrier applied, and redressed with dry dressing. Patient denies pain. Emptied collection bag of 20 mL bile-colored drainage.
> —*L. Saunders, RN*

UNEXPECTED SITUATIONS AND ASSOCIATED INTERVENTIONS

- *A patient's T-tube has been consistently draining 30 to 50 mL a shift, but now there is no output for the current shift. You check the tubing and site and do not observe kinks or other exterior obstructions:* Assess for signs of obstructed bile flow, including chills, fever, tachycardia, nausea, right upper quadrant fullness and pain, **jaundice**, dark foamy urine, and clay-colored stools. Obtain vital signs. Notify the primary health care provider of the situation and findings and document the event in the patient's record. Flushing of the tube with sterile saline via the three-way valve may be ordered as part of the patient's care.
- *Patient had a T-tube placed after surgery. The surgeon has asked that the tube be clamped for 1 hour before and after meals:* This diverts bile into the duodenum to aid in digestion and is accomplished by turning the three-way access valve so the drain is closed to the drainage bag or occluding the tube with a clamp. Monitor the patient's response to clamping the tube. If the patient reports new symptoms, such as right upper quadrant pain, nausea, or vomiting, unclamp the tube. Assess for other symptoms and obtain vital signs. Report the findings to the surgeon and document the intervention in the patient's record.

SPECIAL CONSIDERATIONS	• When the patient with a drain is ready to ambulate, empty the drain collection bag before activity. Ensure that the collection bag is secured to the patient's gown below the wound, making sure there is no tension on the drainage tubing. This allows for optimal drainage and avoids strain on the drain's suture line and the drain site.
	• Appropriate nutritional support is critical in achieving successful wound healing and may be overlooked (Quain & Khardori, 2015). Collaborate with the registered dietician and dietary staff to develop an individualized nutrition intervention plan for the patient (NPUAP, EPUAP, PPPIA, 2014a).

Skill 8-8 ▶ Caring for a Jackson–Pratt Drain

A Jackson–Pratt (JP) or grenade drain collects wound drainage in a bulblike device that is compressed to create low suction (negative) pressure (Figure 1). It consists of perforated tubing connected to a portable vacuum unit. After a surgical procedure, the surgeon places one end of the drain in or near the area to be drained. The other end passes through the skin via a separate incision. These drains are usually sutured in place. The site may be treated as an additional surgical wound, but often these sites are left open to air 24 hours after surgery. They are typically used with breast and abdominal surgery.

As the drainage accumulates in the bulb, the bulb expands and suction is lost, requiring recompression. Typically, these drains are emptied every 4 to 8 hours, and when they are half full of drainage or air. However, based on nursing assessment and judgment, the drain could be emptied and recompressed more frequently.

FIGURE 1. Jackson-Pratt drain.

DELEGATION CONSIDERATIONS	Care for a JP drain insertion site is not delegated to nursing assistive personnel (NAP) or to unlicensed assistive personnel (UAP). Depending on the organization's policies and procedures, the drain may be emptied and reconstituted by NAP or UAP. Depending on the state's nurse practice act and the organization's policies and procedures, these procedures may be delegated to licensed practical/vocational nurses (LPN/LVNs). The decision to delegate must be based on careful analysis of the patient's needs and circumstances, as well as the qualifications of the person to whom the task is being delegated. Refer to the Delegation Guidelines in Appendix A.

EQUIPMENT	• Graduated container for measuring drainage	• Sterile gauze pads
	• Clean, disposable gloves	• Skin protectant/barrier wipes
	• Additional PPE, as indicated	• Dressing materials for site dressing, if used
	• Cleansing solution, usually sterile normal saline	

(continued)

Skill 8-8 ▶ Caring for a Jackson–Pratt Drain *(continued)*

ASSESSMENT

Assess the situation to determine the need for wound cleaning, a dressing change, or emptying of the drain. Assess the patient's level of comfort and the need for analgesics before wound care. Assess if the patient experienced any pain related to prior dressing changes and the effectiveness of interventions employed to minimize the patient's pain. Assess the current dressing. Assess for the presence of excess drainage or bleeding or saturation of the dressing. Assess the patency of the JP drain and the drain site. Note the characteristics of the drainage in the collection bag.

Inspect the wound and the surrounding tissue. Assess the appearance of the incision for the approximation of wound edges, the color of the wound and surrounding area, and signs of dehiscence. Note the stage of the healing process and characteristics of any drainage. Also assess the surrounding skin for color, temperature, and edema, ecchymosis, or maceration.

NURSING DIAGNOSIS

Determine the related factors for the nursing diagnoses based on the patient's current health status. Appropriate nursing diagnoses may include:

- Risk for infection
- Disturbed body image
- Deficient knowledge

OUTCOME IDENTIFICATION AND PLANNING

The expected outcome to achieve when performing care for a JP drain is that the drain is patent and intact; drain care is accomplished without contaminating the wound area and/or without causing trauma to the wound; and the patient does not experience pain or discomfort. Other outcomes that are appropriate may include the following: the drainage amounts are measured accurately at the frequency required by facility policy and recorded as part of the intake and output record; and the patient demonstrates an understanding of drain care.

IMPLEMENTATION

ACTION	RATIONALE
1. Review the patient's health record for prescribed wound care or the nursing care plan related to wound/drain care. Gather necessary supplies.	Reviewing the health record and care plan validates the correct patient and correct procedure. Preparation promotes efficient time management and organized approach to the task.
2. Perform hand hygiene and put on PPE, if indicated.	Hand hygiene and PPE prevent the spread of microorganisms. PPE is required based on transmission precautions.
3. Identify the patient.	Identifying the patient ensures the right patient receives the intervention and helps prevent errors.
4. Assemble equipment on the overbed table or other surface within reach.	Organization facilitates performance of the task.
5. Close the curtains around the bed and close the door to the room, if possible. Explain what you are going to do and why you are going to do it to the patient.	This ensures the patient's privacy. Explanation relieves anxiety and facilitates cooperation.
6. Assess the patient for possible need for nonpharmacologic pain-reducing interventions or analgesic medication before wound care dressing change. Administer appropriate prescribed analgesic. Allow enough time for the analgesic to achieve its effectiveness before beginning the procedure.	Pain is a subjective experience influenced by past experience. Wound care and dressing changes may cause pain for some patients.
7. Place a waste receptacle at a convenient location for use during the procedure.	Having a waste container handy means that the soiled dressing may be discarded easily, without the spread of microorganisms.
8. Adjust the bed to a comfortable working height, usually elbow height of the caregiver (VHACEOSH, 2016).	Having the bed at the proper height prevents back and muscle strain.

ACTION

9. Assist the patient to a comfortable position that provides easy access to the drain and/or wound area. Use a bath blanket to cover any exposed area other than the drain. Place a waterproof pad under the drain site.

10. Put on clean gloves; put on mask or face shield, as indicated.

11. Using sterile technique, open a gauze pad, making a sterile field with the outer wrapper.

12. Place the graduated collection container under the drain outlet. Without contaminating the outlet valve, pull off the cap. The chamber will expand completely as it draws in air. **Empty the chamber's contents completely into the container (Figure 2). Use the gauze pad to wipe the outlet. Fully compress the chamber with one hand and replace the cap with your other hand (Figure 3).**

RATIONALE

Patient positioning and the use of a bath blanket provide for comfort and warmth. Waterproof pad protects underlying surfaces.

Gloves prevent the spread of microorganisms; mask reduces the risk of transmission should splashing occur.

Using sterile technique deters the spread of microorganisms.

Emptying the drainage allows for accurate measurement. Cleaning the outlet reduces the risk of contamination and helps prevent the spread of microorganisms. Compressing the chamber reestablishes the suction.

FIGURE 2. Emptying contents of Jackson-Pratt drain into collection container.

FIGURE 3. Compressing Jackson-Pratt drain and replacing cap.

13. Check the patency of the equipment. Bulb should remain compressed. **Check that the tubing is free from twists and kinks.**

14. Secure the JP drain to the patient's gown below the wound with a safety pin, **making sure that there is no tension on the tubing.**

 15. Carefully measure and record the character, color, and amount of the drainage. Discard the drainage according to facility policy. Remove gloves. Perform hand hygiene.

16. Put on clean gloves. If the drain site has a dressing, remove the dressing (as outlined in Skill 8-7) and assess the site.

17. Remove gloves and perform hand hygiene.

18. Cleanse the drain site and redress as outlined in Skill 8-7.

Compressed chamber establishes suction. Patent, untwisted, or unkinked tubing promotes appropriate wound drainage.

Securing the drain prevents injury to the patient and accidental removal of the drain.

Documentation promotes continuity of care and communication. Appropriate disposal of biohazard material reduces the risk for microorganism transmission. Hand hygiene prevents the transmission of microorganisms.

Dressing protects the site. Cleaning and drying sutures deters the growth of microorganisms.

Removal of gloves and performance of hand hygiene prevent transmission of microorganisms.

Cleaning of wound removes microorganisms and promotes healing.

(continued)

Skill 8-8 ▶ Caring for a Jackson–Pratt Drain *(continued)*

ACTION	RATIONALE
19. If the drain site is open to air, observe the sutures that secure the drain to the skin. Look for signs of pulling, tearing, swelling, or infection of the surrounding skin. Gently clean the sutures with the gauze pad moistened with normal saline. Dry with a new gauze pad. Apply skin protectant/barrier to the surrounding skin.	Early detection of problems leads to prompt intervention and prevents complications. Gentle cleaning and drying prevent the growth of microorganisms. Skin barrier/protectant prevents skin irritation and excoriation from tape, adhesives, and wound drainage (McNichol et al., 2013).
20. Remove and discard gloves. Perform hand hygiene.	Proper removal of gloves prevents the spread of microorganisms. Hand hygiene prevents the transmission of microorganisms.
21. Remove all remaining equipment; place the patient in a comfortable position, with side rails up as indicated and bed in the lowest position.	Proper patient and bed positioning promotes safety and comfort.
22. Remove additional PPE, if used. Perform hand hygiene.	Proper removal of PPE reduces the risk for infection transmission and contamination of other items. Hand hygiene prevents the spread of microorganisms.
23. Check drain status at least every 4 hours. Empty and reengage suction (compress device) when device is half to two thirds full. Check all wound dressings at least every shift. More frequent checks may be needed if the wound is more complex or dressings become saturated quickly.	Checking drain ensures proper functioning and early detection of problems. Emptying and compression ensure appropriate suction. Checking dressings ensures the assessment of changes in patient condition and timely intervention to prevent complications.

EVALUATION

The expected outcome has been met when the drain remained patent and intact; drain care was accomplished without contaminating the wound area and/or without causing trauma to the wound; the patient did not experience pain or discomfort; the drainage amounts were measured accurately at the frequency required by facility policy and recorded as part of the intake and output record; and the patient demonstrated an understanding of drain care.

DOCUMENTATION

Guidelines

Document the location of the drain, the assessment of the drain site, and patency of the drain. Note if sutures are intact. Document the presence and characteristics of drainage on the old dressing upon removal. Include the appearance of the surrounding skin. Document cleansing the drain site. Record any skin care and the dressing applied. Note that the drain was emptied and recompressed. Note pertinent patient and family education and any patient reaction to this procedure, including patient's pain level and effectiveness of nonpharmacologic interventions or analgesia, if administered. Document the amount and characteristics of drainage obtained on the appropriate intake and output record.

Sample Documentation

> 2/7/20 2400 Right chest incision and drain open to air. Wound edges approximated, slight ecchymosis, no edema, redness, or drainage. Steri-Strips intact. JP drain patent and secured with suture. Exit site without edema, drainage, or redness. Drain emptied and recompressed. 40-mL sanguineous drainage recorded.
>
> —C. White, RN

UNEXPECTED SITUATIONS AND ASSOCIATED INTERVENTIONS

- *A patient has a JP drain in the right lower quadrant following abdominal surgery. The record indicates it has been draining serosanguineous fluid, 40 to 50 mL every shift. While performing your initial assessment, you note that the dressing around the drain site is saturated with serosanguineous secretions and there is minimal drainage in the collection chamber:* Inspect the tubing for kinks or obstruction. Assess the patient for changes in condition. Remove the dressing and assess the site. Often, if the tubing becomes blocked with a blood clot or drainage particles, the wound drainage will leak around the exit site of the drain. Cleanse the area and redress the site. Notify the primary health care provider of the findings and document the event in the patient's record.

- *Your patient calls you to the room and says, "I found this in the bed when I went to get up." He has his JP drain in his hand. It is completely removed from the patient:* Assess the patient for any new and abnormal signs or symptoms, and assess the surgical site and drain site. Apply a sterile dressing with gauze and tape to the drain site. Notify the primary health care provider of the findings and document the event in the patient's record.

SPECIAL CONSIDERATIONS

- Often patients have more than one JP drain. Number or letter the drains for easy identification. Record the drainage from each drain separately, identified by the number or letter, on the intake and output record.
- When the patient with a drain is ready to ambulate, empty and compress the drain before activity. Secure the drain to the patient's gown below the wound, making sure there is no tension on the drainage tubing. This removes excess drainage, maintains maximum suction, and avoids strain on the drain's suture line.
- Appropriate nutritional support is critical in achieving successful wound healing and may be overlooked (Quain & Khardori, 2015). Collaborate with the registered dietician and dietary staff to develop an individualized nutrition intervention plan for the patient (NPUAP, EPUAP, PPPIA, 2014a).

Skill 8-9 ▶ Caring for a Hemovac Drain

A Hemovac drain is placed into a vascular cavity where blood drainage is expected after surgery, such as with abdominal and orthopedic surgery. The drain consists of perforated tubing connected to a portable suction (vacuum) unit (Figure 1). Suction is maintained by compressing a spring-like device in the collection unit. After a surgical procedure, the surgeon places one end of the drain in or near the area to be drained. The other end passes through the skin via a separate incision. These drains are usually sutured in place. The site may be treated as an additional surgical wound, but often these sites are left open to air 24 hours after surgery.

As the drainage accumulates in the collection unit, it expands and suction is lost, requiring recompression. Typically, the drain is emptied every 4 or 8 hours and when it is half full of drainage or air. However, based on the prescribed orders and nursing assessment and judgment, it could be emptied and recompressed more frequently.

FIGURE 1. Hemovac drain.

DELEGATION CONSIDERATIONS

Care for a Hemovac drain insertion site is not delegated to nursing assistive personnel (NAP) or to unlicensed assistive personnel (UAP). Depending on the organization's policies and procedures, the drain may be emptied and reconstituted by NAP or to UAP. Depending on the state's nurse practice act and the organization's policies and procedures, these procedures may be delegated to licensed practical/vocational nurses (LPN/LVNs). The decision to delegate must be based on careful analysis of the patient's needs and circumstances, as well as the qualifications of the person to whom the task is being delegated. Refer to the Delegation Guidelines in Appendix A.

(continued)

Skill 8-9 ▶ Caring for a Hemovac Drain *(continued)*

EQUIPMENT	
• Graduated container for measuring drainage	• Sterile gauze pads
• Clean, disposable gloves	• Skin protectant/barrier wipes
• Additional PPE, as indicated	• Dressing materials for site dressing, if used
• Cleansing solution, usually sterile normal saline	

ASSESSMENT

Assess the situation to determine the need for wound cleaning, a dressing change, or emptying of the drain. Assess the patient's level of comfort and the need for analgesics before wound care. Assess if the patient experienced any pain related to prior dressing changes and the effectiveness of interventions employed to minimize the patient's pain. Assess the current dressing. Assess for the presence of excess drainage or bleeding or saturation of the dressing. Assess the patency of the Hemovac drain and the drain site. Note the characteristics of the drainage in the collection bag.

Inspect the wound and the surrounding tissue. Assess the appearance of the incision for the approximation of wound edges, the color of the wound and surrounding area, and signs of dehiscence. Note the stage of the healing process and characteristics of any drainage. Also assess the surrounding skin for color, temperature, and edema, ecchymosis, or maceration.

NURSING DIAGNOSIS

Determine the related factors for the nursing diagnoses based on the patient's current health status. Appropriate nursing diagnoses may include:

• Risk for infection
• Disturbed body image
• Deficient knowledge

OUTCOME IDENTIFICATION AND PLANNING

The expected outcome to achieve when performing care for a Hemovac drain is that the drain is patent and intact; drain care is accomplished without contaminating the wound area and/or without causing trauma to the wound; and the patient does not experience pain or discomfort. Other outcomes that are appropriate may include the following: the drainage amounts are measured accurately at the frequency required by facility policy and recorded as part of the intake and output record; and the patient demonstrates an understanding of drain care.

IMPLEMENTATION

ACTION	RATIONALE
1. Review the patient's health record for prescribed wound care or the nursing care plan related to wound/drain care. Gather necessary supplies.	Reviewing the health record and care plan validates the correct patient and correct procedure. Preparation promotes efficient time management and an organized approach to the task.
2. Perform hand hygiene and put on PPE, if indicated.	Hand hygiene and PPE prevent the spread of microorganisms. PPE is required based on transmission precautions.
3. Identify the patient.	Identifying the patient ensures the right patient receives the intervention and helps prevent errors.
4. Assemble equipment on the overbed table or other surface within reach.	Organization facilitates performance of the task.
5. Close the curtains around the bed and close the door to the room, if possible. Explain what you are going to do and why you are going to do it to the patient.	This ensures the patient's privacy. Explanation relieves anxiety and facilitates cooperation.

ACTION

6. Assess the patient for possible need for nonpharmacologic pain-reducing interventions or analgesic medication before wound care dressing change. Administer appropriate prescribed analgesic. Allow enough time for analgesic to achieve its effectiveness before beginning the procedure.

7. Place a waste receptacle at a convenient location for use during the procedure.

8. Adjust the bed to a comfortable working height, usually elbow height of the caregiver (VHACEOSH, 2016).

9. Assist the patient to a comfortable position that provides easy access to the drain and/or wound area. Use a bath blanket to cover any exposed area other than the drain. Place a waterproof pad under the drain site.

10. Put on clean gloves; put on mask or face shield, as indicated.

11. Using sterile technique, open a gauze pad, making a sterile field with the outer wrapper.

12. Place the graduated collection container under the drain outlet. **Without contaminating the outlet, pull off the cap. The chamber will expand completely as it draws in air. Empty the chamber's contents completely into the container (Figure 2). Use the gauze pad to wipe the outlet. Fully compress the chamber by pushing the top and bottom together with your hands. Keep the device tightly compressed while you apply the cap (Figure 3).**

RATIONALE

Pain is a subjective experience influenced by past experience. Wound care and dressing changes may cause pain for some patients.

Having a waste container handy means that the soiled dressing may be discarded easily, without the spread of microorganisms.

Having the bed at the proper height prevents back and muscle strain.

Patient positioning and the use of a bath blanket provide for comfort and warmth. Waterproof pad protects underlying surfaces.

Gloves prevent the spread of microorganisms; mask reduces the risk of transmission should splashing occur.

Using sterile technique deters the spread of microorganisms.

Emptying the drainage allows for accurate measurement. Cleaning the outlet reduces the risk of contamination and helps prevent the spread of microorganisms. Compressing the chamber reestablishes the suction.

FIGURE 2. Emptying Hemovac drain into collection container.

FIGURE 3. Compressing Hemovac and securing cap.

13. Device should remain compressed. Check the patency of the equipment. **Make sure the tubing is free from twists and kinks.**

14. Secure the Hemovac drain to the patient's gown below the wound with a safety pin, **making sure that there is no tension on the tubing.**

Compressed device establishes suction. Patent, untwisted, or unkinked tubing promotes appropriate drainage from the wound.

Securing the drain prevents injury to the patient and accidental removal of the drain.

(continued)

Skill 8-9 ▶ Caring for a Hemovac Drain *(continued)*

ACTION	**RATIONALE**

15. Carefully measure and record the character, color, and amount of the drainage. Discard the drainage according to facility policy. Remove gloves. Perform hand hygiene.

Documentation promotes continuity of care and communication. Appropriate disposal of biohazard material reduces the risk for microorganism transmission. Proper disposal of gloves deters transmission of microorganisms. Hand hygiene prevents the transmission of microorganisms.

16. Put on clean gloves. If the drain site has a dressing, remove the dressing, assess and clean the site, and replace the dressing as outlined in Skill 8-7. Include cleaning of the sutures with the gauze pad moistened with normal saline. Dry sutures with gauze before applying new dressing.

Dressing protects the site. Cleaning and drying sutures deters the growth of microorganisms.

17. If the drain site is open to air, observe the sutures that secure the drain to the skin. Look for signs of pulling, tearing, swelling, or infection of the surrounding skin. Gently clean the sutures with the gauze pad moistened with normal saline. Dry with a new gauze pad. Apply skin protectant/barrier to the surrounding skin, if needed.

Early detection of problems leads to prompt intervention and prevents complications. Gentle cleaning and drying prevent the growth of microorganisms. Skin barrier/protectant prevents skin irritation and excoriation from tape, adhesives, and wound drainage (McNichol et al., 2013).

18. Remove and discard gloves. Perform hand hygiene.

Proper removal of gloves prevents the spread of microorganisms. Hand hygiene prevents the transmission of microorganisms.

19. Remove all remaining equipment; place the patient in a comfortable position, with side rails up as indicated and bed in the lowest position.

Proper patient and bed positioning promotes safety and comfort.

20. Remove additional PPE, if used. Perform hand hygiene.

Proper removal of PPE reduces the risk for infection transmission and contamination of other items. Hand hygiene prevents the spread of microorganisms.

21. Check drain status at least every 4 hours. Empty and reengage suction (compress device) when device is half to two thirds full. Check all wound dressings at least every shift. More frequent checks may be needed if the wound is more complex or dressings become saturated quickly.

Checking the drain ensures proper functioning and early detection of problems. Emptying and compression ensure appropriate suction. Checking dressings ensures the assessment of changes in patient condition and timely intervention to prevent complications.

EVALUATION

The expected outcomes have been met when the drain remains patent and intact; drain care was accomplished without contaminating the wound area and/or without causing trauma to the wound; the patient did not experience pain or discomfort; the drainage amounts were measured accurately at the frequency required by facility policy and recorded as part of the intake and output record; and the patient demonstrated an understanding of drain care.

DOCUMENTATION

Guidelines

Document the location of the drain, the assessment of the drain site, and patency of the drain. Note if sutures are intact. Document the presence and characteristics of drainage on the old dressing upon removal. Include the appearance of the surrounding skin. Document cleansing of the drain site. Record any skin care and any dressing applied. Note that the drain was emptied and recompressed. Note pertinent patient and family education and any patient reaction to this procedure, including patient's pain level and effectiveness of nonpharmacologic interventions or analgesia, if administered. Document the amount and characteristics of drainage obtained on the appropriate intake and output record.

Sample Documentation

> <u>1/18/20</u> 1000 Hemovac drain in place at lateral aspect of left knee. Gauze dressing removed, no drainage noted on dressing. Suture intact; exit site slightly pink, without redness, edema, or drainage. Surrounding skin without edema, ecchymosis, or redness. Exit site and suture cleansed with normal saline and redressed with dry gauze dressing. Hemovac emptied of 90-mL sanguineous secretions and recompressed.
>
> —A. Smith, RN

UNEXPECTED SITUATIONS AND ASSOCIATED INTERVENTIONS	• *A patient has a Hemovac drain placed in the left knee following surgery. The record indicates it has been draining serosanguineous secretions, 40 to 50 mL every shift. While performing your initial assessment, you note that the collection chamber is completely expanded. The nurse empties the device and compresses to resume suction. A short time later, the nurse observes that the chamber is completely expanded again:* Inspect the tubing for kinks or obstruction. Inspect the device, looking for breaks in the integrity of the chamber. Make sure the cap is in place and closed. Assess the patient for changes in condition. Remove the dressing and assess the site. Make sure the drainage tubing has not advanced out of the wound, exposing any of the perforations in the tubing. If you are not successful in maintaining the suction, notify the primary health care provider of the findings and interventions and document the event in the patient's record.
SPECIAL CONSIDERATIONS	• When the patient with a drain is ready to ambulate, empty and compress the drain before activity. Secure the drain to the patient's gown below the wound, making sure there is no tension on the drainage tubing. This removes excess drainage, maintains maximum suction, and avoids strain on the drain's suture line. • Appropriate nutritional support is critical in achieving successful wound healing and may be overlooked (Quain & Khardori, 2015). Collaborate with the registered dietician and dietary staff to develop an individualized nutrition intervention plan for the patient (NPUAP, EPUAP, PPPIA, 2014a).

Skill 8-10 ▶ Applying Negative Pressure Wound Therapy

Negative pressure wound therapy (NPWT), also known as topical negative pressure, vacuum therapy, and VAC (vacuum-assisted closure), promotes wound healing and wound closure through the application of controlled, uniform suction (vacuum) to the wound surface (Apelqvist et al., 2017; Hurd et al., 2017; Milne, 2013; Taylor et al., 2019). NPWT results in reduction in bacteria in the wound and the removal of excess wound fluid, while providing a moist wound healing environment. The negative pressure results in mechanical tension on the wound tissues, stimulating cell proliferation, blood flow to wounds, and the growth of new blood vessels. NPWT also acts to pull the wound edges together. Refer to Figure 1 for an illustration of the principles of NPWT.

A wound contact material is applied to fit the contours of the wound. There are various wound contact materials, including open-cell foam dressings or fillers and open weave gauze dressing fillers (Milne, 2015). An airtight adhesive polyurethane drape that is permeable to water vapor, transparent, and bacteria proof is used to seal the wound (Apelqvist et al., 2017). A small hole is made in the drape and a connection pad is applied over the hole, sealing the opening, and is connected to tubing and a vacuum source (Apelqvist et al.). This system prevents air from entering the system from the external environment and provides for the application of the negative pressure. Excess wound fluid, small tissue debris, and infectious materials are removed through tubing into a collection container (Apelqvist et al.; Benbow, 2016). A cycle of continuous, intermittent, or variable pressure (typically between –60 and 125 mm Hg) is achievable, depending on the particular device, the patient's condition, the location and type of wound, type of filler material, and the amount of drainage (Apelqvist et al.; Milne, 2013; Schreiber, 2016). Refer to Figure 2 for examples of components of an NPWT system.

(continued)

Skill 8-10 ▶ Applying Negative Pressure Wound Therapy *(continued)*

A

B

The wound (A) and a foam, cut to fit to the wound geometry, which is placed inside the wound (B).

C

D

The wound is sealed airtight with a thin adhesive drape (C) with the attached "suction pad" (connecting pad) including the drainage tube (D).

E

Suction
0 mmHg

F

Suction
−125 mmHg

The wound is hermetically sealed with a thin adhesive drape and connected to the vacuum source by means of the attached "suction pad" (suction strength 0 mmHg) (E). At suction strength −125 mmHg, the foam has collaped and the exudate collection reservoir is already partly filled (F).

FIGURE 1. Principles of negative pressure wound therapy.

FIGURE 2. Examples of components of an NPWT system. (From Hess, C. [2013]. *Clinical guide to skin & wound care* [7th ed.]. Philadelphia, PA: Wolters Kluwer, p. 482 and 484.)

NPWT is used to treat a variety of acute or chronic wounds, wounds with heavy drainage, wounds failing to heal, or wounds healing slowly. Examples of such wounds include pressure injuries; arterial, venous, and diabetic ulcers; dehisced surgical wounds; infected wounds; skin graft sites; and burns. NPWT is contraindicated for use in the presence of: clotting disorders and acute mild to moderate bleeding in the wound region after injury/debridement; bleeding or risk of bleeding; wounds with exposed blood vessels, organs, or nerves; untreated osteomyelitis; wounds with a necrotic wound bed; nonenteric and unexplored fistulas; anastomotic sites; surgical suction; pleural, mediastinal, or chest tubing drainage; and malignancy in the wound tissue (Apelqvist et al., 2017; Milne, 2013; Milne, 2015).

There are several modifications of conventional NPWT in use as well. Instillation therapy (NPWTi) is a modification of NPWT to treat acute and chronic wound infections after initial surgery (Apelqvist et al., 2017). NPWTi involves retrograde instillation of an antiseptic or antibiotic substance into the sealed wound using a computer-controlled programmable therapy unit (Apelqvist et al.). Closed incision negative pressure therapy (ciNPWT) is another variation of NPWT that involves the use of negative pressure therapy immediately postoperatively over closed incisions to prevent surgical site infections (Apelqvist et al.).

NPWT dressings are changed every 48 to 72 hours, depending on the manufacturer's specifications and prescribed orders. Infected wounds may require dressing changes every 12 to 24 hours. The following Skill outlines one procedure for one example of NPWT. There are many manufacturers of NPWT systems. **The nurse must be familiar with the components of and procedures related to the particular system in use for an individual patient.**

DELEGATION CONSIDERATIONS	The application of negative pressure wound therapy is not delegated to nursing assistive personnel (NAP) or to unlicensed assistive personnel (UAP). Depending on the state's nurse practice act and the organization's policies and procedures, the application of negative pressure wound therapy may be delegated to licensed practical/vocational nurses (LPN/LVNs). The decision to delegate must be based on careful analysis of the patient's needs and circumstances, as well as the qualifications of the person to whom the task is being delegated. Refer to the Delegation Guidelines in Appendix A.
EQUIPMENT	• Negative pressure unit • Evacuation/collection canister • Wound contact material, as indicated by wound care plan and device/materials in use • Transparent adhesive drape • Connection pad/tubing port • Drainage tubing • Skin protectant/barrier wipes • Sterile gauze sponge • Sterile irrigation set, including a basin, irrigant container, and irrigation syringe • Sterile irrigation solution as ordered, warmed to body temperature • Waste receptacle to dispose of contaminated materials • Sterile gloves (two pairs) • Sterile scissors • Clean, disposable gloves • Gown, mask, eye protection • Additional PPE, as indicated • Sterile scissors • Waterproof pad and bath blanket
ASSESSMENT	Confirm the prescribed orders for the application of NPWT. Check the patient's chart and question the patient about current treatments and medications that may make the application contraindicated. Assess the situation to determine the need for a dressing change. Confirm any prescribed orders relevant to wound care and any wound care included in the nursing care plan. Assess the patient's level of comfort and the need for analgesics before wound care. Assess if the patient experienced any pain related to prior dressing changes and the effectiveness of interventions employed to minimize the patient's pain. Assess the current dressing to determine if it is intact. Assess for excess drainage or bleeding or saturation of the dressing. Inspect the wound and the surrounding tissue. Assess the location, appearance of the wound, stage (if appropriate), drainage, and types of tissue present in the wound. Measure the wound. Note the stage of the healing process and characteristics of any drainage. Also assess the surrounding skin for color, temperature, and edema, ecchymosis, or maceration.
NURSING DIAGNOSIS	Determine the related factors for the nursing diagnoses based on the patient's current health status. Appropriate nursing diagnoses may include:

- Impaired skin integrity
- Disturbed body image
- Deficient knowledge

(*continued*)

Skill 8-10 ▶ Applying Negative Pressure Wound Therapy (continued)

OUTCOME IDENTIFICATION AND PLANNING	The expected outcome to achieve when applying NPWT is that the application is accomplished without contaminating the wound area, causing trauma to the wound, causing the patient to experience pain or discomfort and the device functions correctly. Other outcomes that may be appropriate include the following: the appropriate and prescribed pressure is maintained throughout therapy; and the wound exhibits progression in healing.

IMPLEMENTATION

ACTION	RATIONALE
1. Review the patient's health record for prescribed application of NPWT therapy, including the ordered pressure setting for the device. Gather necessary supplies.	Reviewing the health record validates the correct patient and correct procedure. Preparation promotes efficient time management and an organized approach to the task.
2. Perform hand hygiene and put on PPE, if indicated.	Hand hygiene and PPE prevent the spread of microorganisms. PPE is required based on transmission precautions.
3. Identify the patient.	Identifying the patient ensures the right patient receives the intervention and helps prevent errors.
4. Assemble equipment on the overbed table or other surface within reach.	Organization facilitates performance of task.
5. Close the curtains around the bed and close the door to the room, if possible. Explain what you are going to do and why you are going to do it to the patient.	This ensures the patient's privacy. Explanation relieves anxiety and facilitates cooperation.
6. Assess the patient for possible need for nonpharmacologic pain-reducing interventions or analgesic medication before wound care dressing change. Administer appropriate prescribed analgesic. Allow enough time for the analgesic to achieve its effectiveness before beginning the procedure.	Pain is a subjective experience influenced by past experience. Wound care and dressing changes may cause pain for some patients.
7. Adjust the bed to a comfortable working height, usually elbow height of the caregiver (VHACEOSH, 2016).	Having the bed at the proper height prevents back and muscle strain.
8. Assist the patient to a comfortable position that provides easy access to the wound area. Position the patient so the cleaning/irrigation solution will flow from the clean end of the wound toward the dirty end. Expose the area and drape the patient with a bath blanket, if needed. Put a waterproof pad under the wound area.	Patient positioning and draping provide for comfort and warmth. Gravity directs the flow of liquid from the least contaminated to the most contaminated area. Waterproof pad protects the patient and the bed linens.
9. Have the disposal bag or waste receptacle within easy reach for use during the procedure.	Having a waste container handy allows for easy disposal of the soiled dressings and supplies, without the spread of microorganisms.
10. Using sterile technique, prepare a sterile field and add all the sterile supplies needed for the procedure to the field. Pour warmed, sterile irrigating solution into the sterile container, as indicated.	Proper preparation ensures that supplies are within easy reach and sterility is maintained. Warmed solution may result in less discomfort.
11. Put on a gown, mask, and eye protection.	The use of PPE is part of *Standard Precautions*. A gown protects your clothes from contamination if splashing should occur. Goggles protect mucous membranes of your eyes from contact with irrigant fluid.

ACTION

RATIONALE

12. If NPWT is currently in use, turn off the negative pressure unit. Put on clean, disposable gloves. Loosen the tape on the old dressings by removing in the direction of hair growth and the use of a push–pull method. Push–pull method: lift a corner of the dressing away from the skin, then gently push the skin away from the dressing/adhesive (Refer to Skill 8-2). Continue moving fingers of the opposite hand to support the skin as the product is removed (McNichol et al., 2013). Carefully lift the adhesive from the surrounding skin to prevent medical adhesive–related skin injury (MARSI). Remove the sides/edges first, then the center. If there is resistance, use an adhesive remover (McNichol et al., 2013).

Gloves protect the nurse from contaminated dressings and prevent the spread of microorganisms. Removal of the tape in the direction of hair growth minimizes trauma to the skin (Taylor et al., 2019). The use of adhesive remover allows for the easy, rapid, and painless removal without the associated problems of skin stripping and helps reduce patient discomfort (McNichol et al., 2013).

13. Carefully remove the soiled dressings. If any part of the dressing sticks to the underlying skin, use small amounts of sterile saline to help loosen and remove it.

Cautious removal of the dressing is more comfortable for the patient and ensures that any drain present is not removed. Sterile saline moistens the dressing for easier removal and minimizes damage and pain.

14. Note the presence, amount, type, color, and odor of any drainage on the dressings. **Note the number of pieces of wound contact material removed from the wound. Compare with the documented number from the previous dressing change.**

The presence and characteristics of drainage should be documented. Counting the number of pieces of wound contact material assures the removal of all foam that was placed during the previous dressing change (Schreiber, 2016).

15. Discard the dressings in the receptacle. Remove your gloves and put them in the receptacle. Perform hand hygiene.

Proper disposal of dressings and used gloves prevents the spread of microorganisms. Hand hygiene prevents the transmission of microorganisms.

16. Put on sterile gloves. Using sterile technique, clean or irrigate the wound, based on wound care plan and prescribed wound care (see Skill 8-3).

Aseptic technique maintains sterility of items to come in contact with wound. Cleaning and/or irrigation remove exudate and debris.

17. Clean the area around the wound with normal saline or prescribed skin cleanser. Dry the surrounding skin with a sterile gauze sponge.

Cleaning of skin removes debris and aids in adherence of dressing materials. Moisture provides a medium for the growth of microorganisms.

18. Assess the wound for appearance, stage, presence of eschar, granulation tissue, epithelialization, undermining, tunneling, necrosis, sinus tract, and drainage. Assess the appearance of the surrounding tissue. Measure the wound. Refer to Fundamentals Review 8-2 and 8-3.

This information provides evidence about the wound healing process and/or the presence of infection.

19. Remove gloves and perform hand hygiene.

Hand hygiene prevents the transmission of microorganisms.

20. Put on sterile gloves. **Wipe intact skin around the wound with a skin protectant/barrier wipe and allow it to dry.**

Aseptic technique maintains sterility of items to come in contact with wound. Skin barrier/protectant prevents skin irritation and excoriation from adhesive drape (Baranoski & Ayello, 2016; McNichol et al., 2013).

21. If the use of a wound contact layer (impregnated porous gauze or silicone adhesive contact layer) is indicated, use sterile scissors to cut the wound contact layer to fit the wound bed. Apply wound contact layer to the wound bed.

Impregnated porous gauze or silicone adhesive contact layer may be indicated, depending on wound filler material in use, to prevent adherence of wound filler to wound be to protect the wound bed (Doughty & McNichol, 2016).

(continued)

Skill 8-10 ▶ Applying Negative Pressure Wound Therapy *(continued)*

ACTION	**RATIONALE**
22. Fit the wound contact material to the shape of the wound. • If using foam wound contact material, use sterile scissors to cut the foam to the shape and measurement of the wound. **Do not cut foam over the wound.** More than one piece of foam may be necessary if the first piece is cut too small. Carefully place the foam in the wound (Figure 3). **Ensure foam-to-foam contact if more than one piece is required.** • If using gauze wound filler, carefully place in wound to fill cavity. • **Note the number of pieces of wound filler placed in the wound.** • **Do not under- or over-fill.**	Wound contact material should fill the wound, but not cover intact surrounding skin. Foam fragments may fall into the wound if cutting is performed over the wound. Foam-to-foam contact allows for even distribution of negative pressure. Recording the number of pieces of wound contact material aids in assuring the removal of all dressing material with next dressing change (Schreiber, 2016). Appropriate filling of wound is necessary to ensure safe and effective application of NPWT (Apelqvist et al., 2017; Milne, 2013; Schreiber, 2016).
23. Trim and place the transparent adhesive drape to cover the wound contact material and an additional 3 to 5 cm border of intact periwound tissue (Figure 4). **Avoid stretching the transparent adhesive drape tight over the wound.**	The occlusive air-permeable V.A.C. Drape provides a seal, allowing the application of the negative pressure. Tight stretching of transparent adhesive drape during application may cause periwound damage (Schreiber, 2016).

FIGURE 3. Cutting wound contact material (foam) to shape and measurement of wound. (Used with permission. Courtesy of KCI, an Acelity Company.)

FIGURE 4. Placing transparent adhesive drape to cover the wound. (Used with permission. Courtesy of KCI, an Acelity Company.)

24. Choose an appropriate site to apply the connector pad/tubing port. Pinch the transparent adhesive drape and cut a hole through it (Figure 5). Apply the connector pad/tubing port and connective tubing over the hole (Figure 6). Position tubing away from the periwound area and anchor (Schreiber, 2016).	Position the connector pad/tubing port and tubing to avoid placement over pressure areas, bony prominences, or skin creases to avoid excess pressure on the underlying skin and tissues (Schreiber, 2016). A hole in the drape and application of connector pad/tubing port and connective tubing are necessary for the application of negative pressure and removal of fluid and/or exudate. Securing the tubing prevents accidental excessive tension on the dressing (Schreiber).

FIGURE 5. Cutting a hole in the drape.

ACTION	RATIONALE

FIGURE 6. Applying the connecting pad over the hole.

25. Remove the drainage collection canister from the package and insert into the negative pressure unit until it locks into place. Attach the connective tubing to the canister and check that the clamps on the tubing are open, if present.

The tubing and canister provides means for the collection of drainage. Clamps must be open for the device to work properly.

 26. Remove gloves and discard. Perform hand hygiene. Turn on the power to the negative pressure unit. Select the prescribed therapy settings (suction and cycle type) and start the device.

Removal of gloves, proper disposal, and hand hygiene prevent transmission of microorganisms.

27. **Assess the dressing to ensure seal integrity. The dressing should be collapsed, shrinking to the wound contact material and skin (Figure 7). Observe drainage in tubing.**

Shrinkage confirms a good seal, allowing for accurate application of pressure and treatment. Observation of drainage in device tubing ensures proper flow (Schreiber, 2016).

FIGURE 7. Dressing is collapsed, shrinking to wound contact material and skin. (Used with permission. Courtesy of KCI, an Acelity Company.)

28. Label dressing with date and time. Remove all remaining equipment; place the patient in a comfortable position, with side rails up as indicated and bed in the lowest position.

Recording the date and time provides communication and demonstrates adherence to the care plan. Proper patient and bed positioning promotes safety and comfort.

 29. Remove PPE, if used. Perform hand hygiene.

Proper removal of PPE reduces the risk for infection transmission and contamination of other items. Hand hygiene prevents the spread of microorganisms.

30. Check all wound dressings at least every shift. More frequent checks may be needed if the wound is more complex or dressings become saturated quickly. Check negative pressure settings at least every shift. Assess the patient's tolerance of and response to the therapy at least every shift.

Checking dressings, the device, and patient response ensures the assessment of changes in patient condition and timely intervention to prevent complications.

(continued)

Skill 8-10 ▶ Applying Negative Pressure Wound Therapy (continued)

EVALUATION

The expected outcomes have been met when the application of NPWT was accomplished without contaminating the wound area, causing trauma to the wound, and causing the patient to experience pain or discomfort; the device functions correctly; the appropriate and prescribed pressure was maintained throughout therapy; and the wound exhibited progression in healing.

DOCUMENTATION

Guidelines

Record your assessment of the wound, including evidence of granulation tissue, stage (if appropriate), and characteristics of drainage. Include the appearance of the surrounding skin. Document the cleansing or irrigation of the wound and solution used. Document the application of the NPWT, noting the pressure setting, patency, and seal of the dressing. Describe the color and characteristics of the drainage in the collection chamber. Record pertinent patient and family education and any patient reaction to this procedure, including the presence of pain and effectiveness or ineffectiveness of pain interventions.

Sample Documentation

> <u>4/5/20</u> 0800 NPWT dressing intact with good seal maintained, system patent, pressure setting 80 mm Hg. Purulent, sanguineous drainage noted in collection chamber and tubing. Surrounding tissue without edema, redness, ecchymosis, or signs of irritation. Patient verbalizes an understanding of use of the device and movement limitations related to the system.
>
> —B. Clark, RN

UNEXPECTED SITUATIONS AND ASSOCIATED INTERVENTIONS

- *While assessing the patient, the nurse notes that the seal between the transparent adhesive drape and the wound contact material and skin is not tight:* Check the dressing seals, tubing connections, and canister insertion, and ensure the clamps are open. If a leak in the transparent drape is identified, the appropriate pressure is not being applied to the wound. Apply additional transparent dressing to reseal. If this application does not correct the break, change the dressing.
- *The patient complains of acute pain while NPWT is operating:* Assess the patient for other symptoms, obtain vital signs, assess the wound, and assess the vacuum device for proper functioning. Report your findings to the primary health care provider and document the event in the patient's record. Administer analgesics, as ordered. Continue or change the wound therapy, as ordered. Some patients may be unable to tolerate NPWT and may require a change in the type of wound contact material used, addition of a wound contact layer, intermittent therapy cycling, a reduction in suction pressure, or discontinuation of the therapy (Apelqvist et al., 2017; Milne, 2015; Schreiber, 2016; Waldie, 2013).

SPECIAL CONSIDERATIONS

- The wound should be debrided of as much necrotic tissue as possible before using NPWT; it is best to have the wound bed free of necrotic tissue (Baranoski & Ayello, 2016).
- NPWT dressings are typically changed every 48 to 72 hours (Doughty & McNichol, 2016). Time dressing changes to allow for wound assessment by other members of the health care team.
- Monitor infected wounds often; dressings may need to be changed more often than 48 to 72 hours (Hess, 2013).
- Measure and record the amount of drainage each shift as part of the intake and output record.
- Check the fluid level in the canister periodically. Depending on the particular device in use, replace the canister whenever full or nearly full.
- Be alert for audible and visual alarms on the vacuum device to alert you to problems, such as tipping of the device greater than 45 degrees, a full collection canister, an air leak in the dressing, or dislodgment of the canister.
- NPWT should operate for 24 hours a day. It should not be shut off for more than 2 hours in a 24-hour period. Remove the dressing any time therapy cannot be reestablished within the 2-hour time period (Doughty & McNichol, 2016). When suction is lost, there is no mechanism for exudate control and allowing the dressing to remain in place without suction significantly increases the risk of wound infection (Doughty & McNichol, p. 192). When NPWT is restarted, clean/irrigate the wound per prescribed order or facility policy, and apply a new NPWT dressing.

- When maceration of the surrounding skin beneath the occlusive dressing occurs, this may be treated by placing a barrier/wafer dressing beneath the transparent dressing to protect the skin. Verify with facility policy, as needed.
- A weekly reduction in wound area of 10% to 15% or more indicates a positive response to treatment with NPWT (Milne, 2015, p. 14).
- NPWT is discontinued when there is a plateau in response or any deterioration in the wound (Doughty & McNichol, 2016).
- Approaches to NPWT continue to change, including the size of the vacuum pumps, types of wound contact materials and length of time recommended for the use of NPWT (Benbow, 2016).
- Appropriate nutritional support is critical in achieving successful wound healing and may be overlooked (Quain & Khardori, 2015). Collaborate with the registered dietician and dietary staff to develop an individualized nutrition intervention plan for the patient (NPUAP, EPUAP, PPPIA, 2014a).

Home Care Considerations
- Vacuum pumps are available in small sizes and as disposable devices designed for single use, facilitating the use of NPWT in outpatient and community settings (Benbow, 2016; Brandon, 2016; Milne, 2015).
- Patients and caregivers must be educated about NPWT: how NPWT works; the risks and benefits of NPWT; device operation; signs of and actions for possible complications; response to alarms and emergencies; and when to seek and who to contact for assistance (Benbow, 2016; Schreiber, 2016).

EVIDENCE FOR PRACTICE ▶

NEGATIVE PRESSURE WOUND THERAPY AND QUALITY OF LIFE

Because the skin is a sensory organ and plays a major role in communication with others and self-image, wounds and pressure injuries require emotional as well as physical adaptation. Although stress and adaptation vary greatly among people, actual and potential emotional stressors are common in all patients with wounds. Therapies related to wound care are also a source of stress. These stressors impact the quality of life (QoL) of the patient and caregivers and include pain, anxiety, fear, activities of daily living, and changes in body image.

Related Research

Janssen, A. H., Mommers, E. H., Notter, J., de Vries Rellingh, T. S., & Wegdam, J. A. (2016). Negative pressure wound therapy versus standard wound care on quality of life: A systematic review. *Journal of Wound Care, 25*(3), 154–159.

This systematic literature review examined the effect of negative pressure wound therapy (NPWT) versus standard wound care (SWC) on the QoL of patients. A range of databases were searched using the search terms "standard wound care, wound dressing, dressing treatment, OR NPWT, OR vacuum-assisted closure AND QoL, patient satisfaction OR experiences." The methodologic index for nonrandomized studies (MINORS) checklist was used to assess the methodologic quality of the resulting studies. There were 42 studies identified with 5 matching the inclusion criteria. Median MINORS score was 75%, with a range of 58% to 96%. Seven different questionnaires were used to measure QoL or a subsidiary outcome. QoL in the NPWT group was temporarily lower in the first week of treatment along with increased anxiety, compared with SWC. The systematic review established that the QoL improved at the end of the therapy, independent of which therapy was used. The authors concluded that NPWT led to lower QoL during the first week of treatment, possibly as a result of increased anxiety related to treatment with NPWT.

Relevance for Nursing Practice

Using the best treatment for a wound or pressure injury is important. However, the best treatment may not produce the best patient experience, if the patient's emotional needs are not met. Nurses need to be holistic in their approach with patients receiving wound care and be aware of patient experiences related to any prescribed treatments for wounds and pressure injuries. Interventions, including patient education, support, and encouragement, can foster hope and reduce anxiety for patients.

Refer to thePoint® for additional research on related nursing topics.

(continued)

Skill 8-10 ▶ Applying Negative Pressure Wound Therapy (continued)

EVIDENCE FOR PRACTICE ▶

NEGATIVE PRESSURE WOUND THERAPY: OVERVIEW OF PRESENT KNOWLEDGE

Apelqvist, J., Willy, C., Fagerdah, A. M., et al. (2017). European Wound Management Association (EWMA). EWMA document: Negative pressure wound therapy. Overview, challenges and perspectives. *Journal of Wound Care, 26*(Sup 3), S1–S154.

The European Wound Management Association established an interdisciplinary working group to describe the present knowledge with regard to NPWT. The resulting document provides an overview of the implications of NPWT for organization of patient care, documentation, communication, patient safety, and the health economic aspects of NPWT. This comprehensive summary details the principles of NPWT, provides a review of the literature evidence on NPWT and identifies treatment specifics. Discussion related to the patient perspective and patient safety is provided, as well as other aspects of NPWT, including future perspectives.

Refer to thePoint° for additional research on related nursing topics.

Skill 8-11 ▶ Removing Sutures

Skin sutures are used to hold the tissue and skin together. Sutures may be black silk, synthetic material, or fine wire. **Surgical sutures** are removed when enough tensile strength has developed to hold the wound edges together during healing. The time frame varies depending on the patient's age, nutritional status, and wound location. Frequently, after skin sutures are removed, adhesive wound closure strips are applied across the wound to give additional support as it continues to heal. The removal of sutures may be done by the primary health care provider, and advanced practice professional, or by the nurse, as indicated in facility policy.

DELEGATION CONSIDERATIONS

The removal of surgical sutures is not delegated to nursing assistive personnel (NAP) or to unlicensed assistive personnel (UAP). Depending on the state's nurse practice act and the organization's policies and procedures, the removal of surgical sutures may be delegated to licensed practical/vocational nurses (LPN/LVNs). The decision to delegate must be based on careful analysis of the patient's needs and circumstances, as well as the qualifications of the person to whom the task is being delegated. Refer to the Delegation Guidelines in Appendix A.

EQUIPMENT

- Suture removal kit or forceps and scissors
- Gauze
- Wound cleansing agent, according to facility policy
- Clean, disposable gloves
- Additional PPE, as indicated
- Adhesive wound closure strips, as indicated
- Skin protectant/barrier wipes

ASSESSMENT

Inspect the surgical incision and the surrounding tissue. Assess the appearance of the wound for the approximation of wound edges, the color of the wound and surrounding area, presence of wound drainage noting color, volume, and odor, and for signs of dehiscence. Note the stage of the healing process and characteristics of any drainage. Assess the surrounding skin for color, temperature, and the presence of edema, maceration, or ecchymosis.

| NURSING DIAGNOSIS | Determine the related factors for the nursing diagnoses based on the patient's current health status. Appropriate nursing diagnoses may include: |

- Deficient knowledge
- Risk for infection
- Impaired skin integrity

| OUTCOME IDENTIFICATION AND PLANNING | The expected outcome to achieve when removing surgical sutures is that the sutures are removed without contaminating the incisional area, causing trauma to the wound, and/or causing the patient to experience pain or discomfort. In addition, other outcomes that are appropriate include the following: the patient remains free of complications that would delay recovery; and the patient verbalizes an understanding of the procedure. |

IMPLEMENTATION

ACTION	RATIONALE
1. Review the patient's health record for prescribed orders for suture removal. Gather necessary supplies.	Reviewing the health record and care plan validates the correct patient and correct procedure. Preparation promotes efficient time management and an organized approach to the task.
2. Perform hand hygiene and put on PPE, if indicated.	Hand hygiene and PPE prevent the spread of microorganisms. PPE is required based on transmission precautions.
3. Identify the patient.	Identifying the patient ensures the right patient receives the intervention and helps prevent errors.
4. Assemble equipment on the overbed table or other surface within reach.	Organization facilitates performance of task.
5. Close the curtains around the bed and close the door to the room, if possible. Explain what you are going to do and why you are going to do it to the patient. Describe the sensation of suture removal as a pulling or slightly uncomfortable experience.	This ensures the patient's privacy. Explanation relieves anxiety and facilitates cooperation.
6. Assess the patient for possible need for nonpharmacologic pain-reducing interventions or analgesic medication before beginning the procedure. Administer appropriate prescribed analgesic. Allow enough time for the analgesic to achieve its effectiveness before beginning the procedure.	Pain is a subjective experience influenced by past experience. Wound care and dressing changes may cause pain for some patients.
7. Place a waste receptacle at a convenient location for use during the procedure.	Having a waste container handy means that the soiled dressing may be discarded easily, without the spread of microorganisms.
8. Adjust the bed to a comfortable working height, usually elbow height of the caregiver (VHACEOSH, 2016).	Having the bed at the proper height prevents back and muscle strain.
9. Assist the patient to a comfortable position that provides easy access to the incision area. Use a bath blanket to cover any exposed area other than the incision. Place a waterproof pad under the incision site.	Patient positioning and the use of a bath blanket provide for comfort and warmth. Waterproof pad protects underlying surfaces.
10. Put on clean gloves. Carefully and gently remove any dressings that may be in place. Refer to Skill 8-2.	Gloves protect the nurse from handling contaminated dressings. Cautious removal of the dressing is more comfortable for the patient and prevents medical adhesive–related skin injury (MARSI) (McNichol et al., 2013).

(continued)

Skill 8-11 ▶ Removing Sutures *(continued)*

ACTION	**RATIONALE**

11. Clean the incision, according to prescribed wound care or facility policy and procedure. Refer to Skill 8-2. Assess the wound (Refer to Assessment section of skill and Fundamentals Review 8-1) (Figure 1).

Incision cleaning prevents the spread of microorganisms and contamination of the wound. Assessment provides validation of healing related to timing of suture removal.

 12. Perform hand hygiene. Open the suture removal kit. Put on clean disposable gloves.

Hand hygiene prevents the transmission of microorganisms. Gloves prevent contact with blood and body fluids.

13. Using the forceps, grasp the knot of the first suture and gently lift the knot up off the skin.

Raising the suture knot prevents accidental injury to the wound or skin when cutting.

14. Using the scissors, cut one side of the suture below the knot, close to the skin (Figure 2). Grasp the knot with the forceps and pull the cut suture through the skin. **Avoid pulling the visible portion of the suture through the underlying tissue.**

Cutting close to the skin results in minimal exposed suture to pull through skin. Pulling the cut suture through the skin helps reduce the risk for contamination of the incision area and resulting infection.

FIGURE 1. Incision with sutures.

FIGURE 2. Using forceps to pull up on a suture and cutting suture with sterile scissors.

15. Remove every other suture to be sure the wound edges are healed. If the wound edges remain approximated, remove the remaining sutures, as ordered. Dispose of sutures according to facility policy.

Removing every other suture allows for inspection of the wound, while leaving adequate suture in place to promote continued healing if the edges are not totally approximated. Follow *Standard Precautions* in disposing of sutures.

16. If wound closure strips are to be used, apply skin protectant/barrier to skin around incision. **Do not apply to incision.** Apply adhesive closure strips (Figure 3). Take care to handle the strips by the paper backing.

Skin protectant helps adherence of closure strips and prevents skin irritation and excoriation from tape, adhesives, and wound drainage (McNichol et al., 2013). Adhesive wound closure strips provide additional support to the wound as it continues to heal. Handling by the paper backing avoids contamination.

17. Reapply the dressing, based on the prescribed orders and facility policy.

A new dressing protects the wound. Some policies advise leaving the area uncovered.

 18. Remove and discard gloves. Perform hand hygiene.

Proper removal of gloves prevents the spread of microorganisms. Hand hygiene prevents the transmission of microorganisms.

ACTION

RATIONALE

FIGURE 3. Applying adhesive closure strips on incision.

19. Remove all remaining equipment; place the patient in a comfortable position, with side rails up as indicated and bed in the lowest position.

Proper patient and bed positioning promotes safety and comfort.

 20. Remove additional PPE, if used. Perform hand hygiene.

Proper removal of PPE reduces the risk for infection transmission and contamination of other items. Hand hygiene prevents the spread of microorganisms.

21. Assess all wounds every shift. More frequent checks may be needed if the wound is more complex.

Checking wound and dressings ensures the assessment of changes in patient condition and timely intervention to prevent complications.

EVALUATION

The expected outcomes have been met when the sutures were removed without contaminating the incisional area, causing trauma to the wound, and/or causing the patient to experience pain or discomfort; the patient remained free of complications that would delay recovery; and the patient verbalized an understanding of the procedure.

DOCUMENTATION

Guidelines

Document the location of the incision and the assessment of the site. Include the appearance of the surrounding skin. Document cleansing of the site and suture removal. Record any skin care, application of wound closure strips, and the dressing applied, if appropriate. Note pertinent patient and family education and any patient reaction to this procedure, including the patient's pain level and effectiveness of nonpharmacologic interventions or analgesia if administered.

Sample Documentation

> 3/4/20 1800 Right lower lateral leg surgical wound appears healed. Incision edges are approximated, without erythema, edema, ecchymosis, or drainage. Skin warm with consistent tone. Sutures removed without difficulty; skin protectant/barrier applied to skin surrounding incision and adhesive wound closure strips applied. Patient instructed on how to care for wound and expectations regarding wound closure strips; patient and wife verbalized an understanding of information and asked appropriate questions.
>
> —L. Downs, RN

(continued)

Skill 8-11 ▸ Removing Sutures *(continued)*

UNEXPECTED SITUATIONS AND ASSOCIATED INTERVENTIONS	• *Sutures are crusted with dried blood or secretions, making them difficult to remove:* Moisten sterile gauze with sterile saline and gently loosen crusts before removing sutures. • *Resistance is met when attempting to pull suture through the tissue:* Use a gentle, continuous pulling motion to remove the suture. If the suture still does not come out, do not use excessive force. Report findings to the primary health care provider and document the event in the patient's record.
SPECIAL CONSIDERATIONS	• After suture removal, continue to encourage the patient to splint chest and abdominal wounds during activity, such as changing position, ambulating, coughing, and sneezing. This provides increased support for the skin and underlying tissues and can decrease discomfort.

Skill 8-12 ▸ Removing Surgical Staples

Skin staples made of stainless steel are used to hold the tissue and skin together. Staples decrease the risk of infection and allow for faster wound closure. **Surgical staples** are removed when enough tensile strength has developed to hold the wound edges together during healing. The time frame for removal varies depending on the patient's age, nutritional status, and wound location. After skin staples are removed, adhesive wound closure strips are applied across the wound to keep the skin edges approximated as it continues to heal. The removal of sutures may be done by the primary health care provider, and advanced practice professional, or by the nurse, as indicated in facility policy.

DELEGATION CONSIDERATIONS	The removal of surgical staples is not delegated to nursing assistive personnel (NAP) or to unlicensed assistive personnel (UAP). Depending on the state's nurse practice act and the organization's policies and procedures, the removal of surgical staples may be delegated to licensed practical/vocational nurses (LPN/LVNs). The decision to delegate must be based on careful analysis of the patient's needs and circumstances, as well as the qualifications of the person to whom the task is being delegated. Refer to the Delegation Guidelines in Appendix A.
EQUIPMENT	• Staple remover • Gauze • Wound cleansing agent, according to facility policy • Clean, disposable gloves • Additional PPE, as indicated • Adhesive wound closure strips, as indicated • Skin protectant/barrier wipes
ASSESSMENT	Inspect the surgical incision and the surrounding tissue. Assess the appearance of the wound for the approximation of wound edges, the color of the wound and surrounding area, and signs of dehiscence. Note the stage of the healing process and the characteristics of any drainage. Assess the surrounding skin for color, temperature, and the presence of edema or ecchymosis.
NURSING DIAGNOSIS	Determine the related factors for the nursing diagnoses based on the patient's current health status. Appropriate nursing diagnoses may include: • Impaired skin integrity • Acute pain • Delayed surgical recovery
OUTCOME IDENTIFICATION AND PLANNING	The expected outcome to achieve when removing surgical staples is that the staples are removed without contaminating the incisional area, causing trauma to the wound, and/or causing the patient to experience pain or discomfort. In addition, other outcomes that are appropriate include the following: the patient remains free of complications that would delay recovery; and the patient verbalizes an understanding of the procedure.

IMPLEMENTATION

ACTION	RATIONALE
1. Review the patient's health record for prescribed order for staple removal. Gather necessary supplies.	Reviewing the health record and care plan validates the correct patient and correct procedure. Preparation promotes efficient time management and an organized approach to the task.
2. Perform hand hygiene and put on PPE, if indicated.	Hand hygiene and PPE prevent the spread of microorganisms. PPE is required based on transmission precautions.
3. Identify the patient.	Identifying the patient ensures the right patient receives the intervention and helps prevent errors.
4. Assemble equipment on the overbed table or other surface within reach.	Organization facilitates the performance of the task.
5. Close the curtains around the bed and close the door to the room, if possible. Explain what you are going to do and why you are going to do it to the patient. Describe the sensation of staple removal as a pulling experience.	This ensures the patient's privacy. Explanation relieves anxiety and facilitates cooperation.
6. Assess the patient for possible need for nonpharmacologic pain-reducing interventions or analgesic medication before beginning the procedure. Administer the appropriate prescribed analgesic. Allow enough time for the analgesic to achieve its effectiveness before beginning the procedure.	Pain is a subjective experience influenced by past experience. Wound care and dressing changes may cause pain for some patients.
7. Place a waste receptacle at a convenient location for use during the procedure.	Having a waste container handy means that the soiled dressing may be discarded easily, without the spread of microorganisms.
8. Adjust the bed to a comfortable working height, usually elbow height of the caregiver (VHACEOSH, 2016).	Having the bed at the proper height prevents back and muscle strain.
9. Assist the patient to a comfortable position that provides easy access to the incision area. Use a bath blanket to cover any exposed area other than the incision. Place a waterproof pad under the incision site.	Patient positioning and the use of a bath blanket provide for comfort and warmth. Waterproof pad protects underlying surfaces.
10. Put on clean gloves. Carefully remove any dressings that may be in place. Refer to Skill 8-2.	Gloves protect the nurse from handling contaminated dressings. Cautious removal of the dressing is more comfortable for the patient and prevents medical adhesive–related skin injury (MARSI) (McNichol et al., 2013).
11. Clean the incision, according to prescribed wound care or facility policy and procedure. Refer to Skill 8-2. Assess the wound (Figure 1). Refer to assessment section of this skill.	Incision cleaning prevents the spread of microorganisms and contamination of the wound. Assessment provides validation of healing related to timing of suture removal.

FIGURE 1. Incision with surgical staples.

(continued)

Skill 8-12 ▶ Removing Surgical Staples (continued)

ACTION	RATIONALE

 12. Perform hand hygiene. Open the staple remover kit. Put on clean disposable gloves.

Hand hygiene prevents the transmission of microorganisms. Gloves prevent contact with blood and body fluids.

13. Grasp the staple remover (Figure 2). **Position the staple remover under the staple to be removed. Firmly close the staple remover. The staple will bend in the middle and the edges will pull up out of the skin** (Figure 3).

Correct use of the staple remover prevents accidental injury to the wound and contamination of the incision area and resulting infection.

FIGURE 2. Grasping staple remover.

FIGURE 3. Firmly closing the staple remover, bending the staple in the middle, pulling the edges up out of the skin.

14. Remove every other staple to be sure the wound edges are healed. If the wound edges remain approximated, remove the remaining staples, as ordered. Dispose of staples in the sharps container.

Removing every other staple allows for inspection of the wound, while leaving an adequate number of staples in place to promote continued healing if the edges are not totally approximated.

15. If wound closure strips are to be used, apply skin protectant to the skin around the incision. **Do not apply to the incision.** Apply adhesive closure strips. Take care to handle the strips by the paper backing (Refer to Skill 8-11, step 16).

Skin protectant helps adherence of closure strips and prevents skin irritation and excoriation from tape, adhesives, and wound drainage (McNichol et al., 2013). Adhesive wound closure strips provide additional support to the wound as it continues to heal. Handling by the paper backing avoids contamination.

16. Reapply the dressing, based on the prescribed orders and facility policy.

A new dressing protects the wound. Some policies advise leaving the area uncovered.

 17. Remove and discard gloves. Perform hand hygiene.

Proper removal of gloves prevents the spread of microorganisms. Hand hygiene prevents the transmission of microorganisms.

18. Remove all remaining equipment; place the patient in a comfortable position, with side rails up as indicated and bed in the lowest position.

Proper patient and bed positioning promotes safety and comfort.

 19. Remove additional PPE, if used. Perform hand hygiene.

Proper removal of PPE reduces the risk for infection transmission and contamination of other items. Hand hygiene prevents the spread of microorganisms.

20. Assess all wounds every shift. More frequent checks may be needed if the wound is more complex.

Checking wound and dressings ensures the assessment of changes in patient condition and timely intervention to prevent complications.

EVALUATION	The expected outcomes have been met when the staples were removed without contaminating the incisional area, causing trauma to the wound, and/or causing the patient to experience pain or discomfort; the patient remained free of complications that would delay recovery; and the patient verbalized an understanding of the procedure.
DOCUMENTATION *Guidelines*	Document the location of the incision and the assessment of the site. Include the appearance of the surrounding skin. Document cleansing of the site and staple removal. Record any skin care and the dressing applied, if appropriate. Note pertinent patient and family education and any patient reaction to this procedure, including the patient's pain level and effectiveness of nonpharmacologic interventions or analgesia if administered.
Sample Documentation	3/4/20 1800 Left upper lateral leg surgical wound appears healed. Incision edges are approximated, without erythema, edema, ecchymosis, or drainage. Skin warm with consistent tone. Staples removed without difficulty; skin protectant/barrier applied to skin surrounding incision and adhesive wound closure strips applied. Patient instructed in how to care for wound and expectations regarding wound closure strips; patient and wife verbalized an understanding of information and asked appropriate questions. —*S. Hoffman, RN*
UNEXPECTED SITUATIONS AND ASSOCIATED INTERVENTIONS	• *The wound edges appear approximated before staple removal but pull apart afterward:* Report the findings to the primary health care provider and document the event in the patient's record. Apply adhesive wound closure strips and/or further wound care according to facility policy or prescribed order. • *The staples are stuck to the wound because of dried blood or secretions:* Per facility policy or prescribed order, apply moist saline compresses to loosen crusts before attempting to remove the staples.
SPECIAL CONSIDERATIONS	• Encourage the patient to splint chest and abdominal wounds (before and after surgical staple removal) during activity, such as changing position, ambulating, coughing, and sneezing. This provides increased support for the skin and underlying tissues and can help decrease patient discomfort.

Skill 8-13 Applying an External Heating Pad

Heat applications accelerate the inflammatory response, promoting healing. Heat is also used to reduce muscle tension, and to relieve muscle spasm and joint stiffness. Heat also helps relieve pain. It is used to treat infections, surgical wounds, inflammation, arthritis, joint pain, muscle pain, and chronic pain.

Heat may be applied by moist and dry methods. The prescribed order should include the type of application, the body area to be treated, the frequency of application, and the length of time for the applications. Water used for heat applications needs to be at the appropriate temperature to avoid skin damage: set the temperature of the water within a range of 105° to 109°F (40.5° to 43°C), which is considered to be physiologically effective and comfortable for the patient (Taylor et al., 2019). **Water temperature should not exceed 125°F** (Burn Foundation, 2016).

Common types of external heating devices include aquathermia pads (e.g., Aqua-K) and crushable, microwaveable hot packs. Aquathermia pads are used in health care facilities and are safer to use than heating pads. Microwaveable packs are easy and inexpensive to use, but have several disadvantages. They may leak and pose a danger from burns related to improper use. Microwaveable packs are used most often in the home setting.

(continued)

Skill 8-13 ▶ Applying an External Heating Pad *(continued)*

DELEGATION CONSIDERATIONS	The application of an external heating pad may be delegated to nursing assistive personnel (NAP) or to unlicensed assistive personnel (UAP), as well as to licensed practical/vocational nurses (LPN/LVNs). The decision to delegate must be based on careful analysis of the patient's needs and circumstances, as well as the qualifications of the person to whom the task is being delegated. Refer to the Delegation Guidelines in Appendix A.
EQUIPMENT	• Aquathermia heating pad with electronic unit • Distilled water • Cover for the pad, if not part of pad • Gauze bandage or tape to secure the pad • Bath blanket • PPE, as indicated
ASSESSMENT	Assess the situation to determine the appropriateness for the application of heat. Assess the patient's physical and mental status and the condition of the body area to be treated with heat. Assess for circulatory compromise in the area where the heat will be applied, including skin color, pulses distal to the site, evidence of edema, and the presence of sensation. Confirm the prescribed order for heat therapy, including frequency, type of therapy, body area to be treated, and length of time for the application. Check the equipment to be used, including the condition of cords, plugs, and heating elements. Look for fluid leaks. Once the equipment is turned on, make sure there is a consistent distribution of heat and the temperature is within safe limits. Assess the application site frequently during the treatment, as tissue damage can occur.
NURSING DIAGNOSIS	Determine the related factors for the nursing diagnoses based on the patient's current health status. Appropriate nursing diagnoses may include: • Chronic pain • Acute pain • Risk for impaired skin integrity
OUTCOME IDENTIFICATION AND PLANNING	The expected outcome to achieve when applying an external heat source depends on the patient's nursing diagnosis and the rationale for application. Outcomes that may be appropriate include the following: the patient experiences increased comfort; the patient experiences decreased muscle spasms; the patient exhibits improved wound healing; the patient experiences a reduction in inflammation; the patient remains free from injury; and the patient demonstrates knowledge of safe application of the external heat source.

IMPLEMENTATION

ACTION	RATIONALE
1. Review the patient's health record for prescribed order for the application of heat therapy, including frequency, type of therapy, body area to be treated, and length of time for the application. Gather necessary supplies.	Reviewing the health record and care plan validates the correct patient and correct procedure. Preparation promotes efficient time management and an organized approach to the task.
2. Perform hand hygiene and put on PPE, if indicated.	Hand hygiene and PPE prevent the spread of microorganisms. PPE is required based on transmission precautions.
3. Identify the patient.	Identifying the patient ensures the right patient receives the intervention and helps prevent errors.
4. Assemble equipment on the overbed table or other surface within reach.	Organization facilitates performance of task.
5. Close the curtains around the bed and close the door to the room if possible. Explain what you are going to do and why you are going to do it to the patient.	This ensures the patient's privacy. Explanation relieves anxiety and facilitates cooperation.

ACTION

6. Adjust the bed to a comfortable working height, usually elbow height of the caregiver (VHACEOSH, 2016).

7. Assist the patient to a comfortable position that provides easy access to the area where the heat will be applied; use a bath blanket to cover any other exposed area.

8. Assess the condition of the skin where the heat is to be applied.

9. Check that the water in the electronic unit (Figure 1) is at the appropriate level. Fill the unit two thirds full or to the fill mark, with distilled water, if necessary. Check the temperature setting on the unit to ensure it is within the safe range.

FIGURE 1. External heating pad electronic unit.

10. Attach pad tubing to the electronic unit tubing (Figure 2).

11. Plug in the unit and warm the pad before use. Apply the aquathermia pad to the prescribed area (Figure 3). Secure with gauze bandage or tape.

RATIONALE

Having the bed at the proper height prevents back and muscle strain.

Patient positioning and the use of a bath blanket provide for comfort and warmth.

Assessment supplies baseline data for post-treatment comparison and identifies conditions that may contraindicate the application.

Sufficient water in the unit is necessary to ensure proper function of the unit. Tap water leaves mineral deposits in the unit. Checking the temperature setting helps to prevent skin or tissue damage.

Allows flow of warmed water through the heating pad.

Plugging in the pad readies it for use. Heat travels by conduction from one object to another. Gauze bandage or tape holds the pad in position; **do not use pins, as they may puncture and damage the pad.**

FIGURE 2. Attaching pad tubing to electronic unit tubing.

FIGURE 3. Applying heating pad to the prescribed area.

(continued)

Skill 8-13 ▶ Applying an External Heating Pad *(continued)*

ACTION	**RATIONALE**
12. Remove PPE, if used, and perform hand hygiene.	Proper removal of PPE reduces the risk for infection transmission and contamination of other items. Hand hygiene prevents the spread of microorganisms.
13. **Monitor the condition of the skin and the patient's response to the heat at frequent intervals, according to facility policy. Do not exceed the prescribed length of time for the application of heat.**	Maximum **vasodilation** and therapeutic effects from the application of heat occur within 20 to 30 minutes. Using heat for more than this amount of time results in tissue congestion and **vasoconstriction**, known as the rebound phenomenon. Prolonged heat application may also result in an increased risk of burns and tissue damage (Taylor et al., 2019). Assessment of the patient's skin is necessary for early detection of adverse effects, thereby allowing prompt intervention to avoid complications.
14. After the prescribed time for the treatment (up to 30 minutes), remove the aquathermia pad. **Do not exceed the prescribed amount of time.** Reassess the patient and area of application, noting the effect and presence of any adverse effects.	Using heat for more than this amount of time results in tissue congestion and vasoconstriction, known as the rebound phenomenon. Prolonged heat application may also result in an increased risk of burns and tissue damage (Taylor et al., 2019). Assessment provides input as to the effectiveness of the treatment.
15. Remove all remaining equipment; place the patient in a comfortable position, with side rails up as indicated and bed in the lowest position.	Proper patient and bed positioning promotes safety and comfort.
16. Remove additional PPE, if used. Perform hand hygiene.	Proper removal of PPE reduces the risk for infection transmission and contamination of other items. Hand hygiene prevents the spread of microorganisms.

EVALUATION

The expected outcomes have been met when (depending on the patient's nursing diagnosis) the patient experienced increased comfort; the patient experienced decreased muscle spasms; the patient exhibited improved wound healing; the patient experienced a reduction in inflammation; the patient remained free from injury; and the patient demonstrated knowledge of safe application of the external heat source.

DOCUMENTATION

Guidelines

Document the rationale for application of heat therapy. If the patient is receiving heat therapy for pain, document the assessment of pain pre- and postintervention. Specify the type of heat therapy and location where it is applied, as well as the length of time applied. Record the condition of the skin, noting any redness or irritation before the heat application and after the application. Document the patient's reaction to the heat therapy. Record any appropriate patient or family education.

Sample Documentation

> 9/13/20 2300 Patient states he has lower back pain, rating it 5 of 10, constant and aching. Aquathermia pad applied to patient's lower back for 30 minutes; patient now rating pain as 2 of 10 and intermittent. Skin without signs of redness or irritation before and after application.
>
> —M. Martinez, RN

UNEXPECTED SITUATIONS AND ASSOCIATED INTERVENTIONS

- *When performing a periodic assessment of the site during the application of heat, the nurse notes excessive swelling and redness at the site and the patient complains of pain that was not present prior to the application of heat:* Remove the heat source. Assess the patient for other symptoms and obtain vital signs. Report your findings to the primary health care provider and document the interventions in the patient's record.

SPECIAL CONSIDERATIONS

General Considerations

- Direct heat treatment may be contraindicated for patients at risk for bleeding, patients with a sprained limb in the acute stage, or patients with a condition associated with acute inflammation. Use cautiously with children and older adults. Patients with diabetes, stroke, spinal cord injury, and peripheral neuropathy are at risk for thermal injury, as are patients with very thin or damaged skin. Be extremely careful when applying to heat-sensitive areas, such as scar tissue and stomas.
- Instruct the patient not to lean or lie directly on the heating device, as this reduces air space and increases the risk of burns.
- Check the water level in the aquathermia unit periodically. Evaporation may occur. If the unit runs dry, it could become damaged. Refill with distilled water periodically.

Older Adult Considerations

- Older adults are more at risk for skin and tissue damage because of their thin skin, loss of heat sensation, decreased subcutaneous tissue, and changes in the body's ability to regulate temperature. Check these patients more frequently during therapy.

Home Care Considerations

- A hot water bag or commercially prepared hot pack may be used in the home to apply heat. If using a hot water bag, fill with hot tap water to warm the bag, then empty it to detect any leaks. Check the temperature of the water with a thermometer or test on your inner wrist, adjusting the temperature as ordered. (The temperature of the water should be within a range of 105° to 109°F [40.5° to 43°C], which is considered to be physiologically effective and comfortable for the patient [Taylor et al., 2019]. **Water temperature should not exceed 125°F [Burn Foundation, 2016].)** Fill the bag one half to two thirds full. Partial filling keeps the bag lightweight and flexible so that it can be molded to the treatment area. Squeeze the bag until the water reaches the neck; this expels air, which would make the bag inflexible and would reduce heat conduction. Fasten the top and cover the bag with an absorbent cloth. The covering protects the skin from direct contact with the bag. If using a commercially prepared hot pack, follow manufacturer's directions and carefully assess skin before and after heat application.
- Electric heating pads may be used in the home to apply heat. Avoid the use of pins to prevent electric shocks. Use a dry covering over the pad to protect skin. Place a heating pad anteriorly or laterally to, not under, the body part. If the heating pad is between the patient and the mattress, heat dissipation may be inadequate, leading to burning of the patient or the bed linens. Caution the patient to use a heating pad with a selector switch that cannot be turned up beyond a safe temperature. After heat has been applied and a certain amount of adaptation of heat receptors takes place, the patient may be tempted to increase the heat because the pad does not seem sufficiently warm, resulting in burns (Taylor et al., 2019).

Skill 8-14 ▶ Applying a Warm Compress

Warm, moist compresses are used to help promote circulation, encourage healing, decrease edema, promote consolidation of exudate, and decrease pain and discomfort. Moist heat softens crusted material and is less drying to the skin. Moist heat also penetrates tissues more deeply than dry heat.

A heat application needs to be at the appropriate temperature to avoid skin damage: set the temperature of the soak within a range of 105° to 109°F (40.5° to 43°C), which is considered to be physiologically effective and comfortable for the patient (Taylor et al., 2019). **Water temperature should not exceed 125°F** (Burn Foundation, 2016). Many facilities have warming devices to heat the dressing package to an appropriate temperature for the compress. These devices help reduce the risk of burning or skin damage.

The heat of a warm compress dissipates quickly, so the compresses must be changed frequently. If a constant warm temperature is required, a heating device such as an aquathermia pad (refer to Skill 8-13) is applied over the compress. However, **because moisture conducts heat, a low temperature setting is needed on the heating device.**

(continued)

Skill 8-14 ▶ Applying a Warm Compress   *(continued)*

DELEGATION CONSIDERATIONS	The application of a warm compress may be delegated to nursing assistive personnel (NAP) or to unlicensed assistive personnel (UAP), as well as to licensed practical/vocational nurses (LPN/LVNs). The decision to delegate must be based on careful analysis of the patient's needs and circumstances, as well as the qualifications of the person to whom the task is being delegated. Refer to the Delegation Guidelines in Appendix A.

EQUIPMENT

- Prescribed solution to moisten the compress material, warmed to 105° to 109°F (40.5° to 43°C)
- Container for solution
- Gauze dressings or compresses
- Alternately, obtain the appropriate number of commercially packaged, prewarmed dressings from the warming device
- Clean, disposable gloves
- Additional PPE, as indicated
- Waterproof pad and bath blanket
- Dry bath towel
- Tape or ties
- Aquathermia or other external heating device, if ordered or required to maintain the temperature of the compress

ASSESSMENT

Assess the situation to determine the appropriateness for the application of heat. Assess the patient's physical and mental status and the condition of the body area to be treated with heat. Assess for circulatory compromise in the area where the compress will be applied, including skin color, pulses distal to the site, evidence of edema, and the presence of sensation. Confirm the prescribed order for the compresses, including the solution to be used, frequency, body area to be treated, and length of time for the application. Assess the equipment to be used, if necessary, including the condition of cords, plugs, and heating elements. Look for fluid leaks. Once the equipment is turned on, make sure there is a consistent distribution of heat and the temperature is within safe limits. Assess the application site frequently during the treatment, as tissue damage can occur.

NURSING DIAGNOSIS

Determine the related factors for the nursing diagnoses based on the patient's current health status. Appropriate nursing diagnoses may include:

- Deficient knowledge
- Chronic pain
- Risk for impaired skin integrity

OUTCOME IDENTIFICATION AND PLANNING

The expected outcome to achieve when applying a warm compress depends on the patient's nursing diagnosis and the rationale for application. Outcomes that may be appropriate include the following: the patient shows signs such as decreased inflammation, decreased muscle spasms, or decreased pain that indicate problems have been relieved; the patient experiences improved healing; and the patient remains free from injury.

IMPLEMENTATION

ACTION	RATIONALE
1. Review the patient's health record for prescribed order for the application of a moist warm compress, including the frequency and length of time for the application. Gather necessary supplies.	Reviewing the health record and care plan validates the correct patient and correct procedure. Preparation promotes efficient time management and an organized approach to the task.
2. Perform hand hygiene and put on PPE, if indicated.	Hand hygiene and PPE prevent the spread of microorganisms. PPE is required based on transmission precautions.
3. Identify the patient.	Identifying the patient ensures the right patient receives the intervention and helps prevent errors.

ACTION	RATIONALE
4. Assemble equipment on the overbed table or other surface within reach.	Organization facilitates performance of task.
5. Assess the patient for possible need for nonpharmacologic pain-reducing interventions or analgesic medication before beginning the procedure. Administer appropriate analgesic, as ordered, and allow enough time for the analgesic to achieve its effectiveness before beginning the procedure.	Pain is a subjective experience influenced by past experience. Depending on the site of application, manipulation of the area may cause pain for some patients.
6. Close the curtains around the bed and close the door to the room, if possible. Explain what you are going to do and why you are going to do it to the patient.	This ensures the patient's privacy. Explanation relieves anxiety and facilitates cooperation.
7. If using an electronic heating device with the compress, check that the water in the unit is at the appropriate level. Fill the unit two thirds full with distilled water, or to the fill mark, if necessary. Check the temperature setting on the unit to ensure it is within the safe range (refer to Skill 8-13).	Sufficient water in the unit is necessary to ensure proper function of the unit. Tap water leaves mineral deposits in the unit. Checking the temperature setting helps to prevent skin or tissue damage.
8. Assist the patient to a comfortable position that provides easy access to the area. Use a bath blanket to cover any exposed area other than the intended site. Place a waterproof pad under the site.	Patient positioning and the use of a bath blanket provide for comfort and warmth. Waterproof pad protects underlying surfaces.
9. Place a waste receptacle at a convenient location for use during the procedure.	Having a waste container handy means that the used materials may be discarded easily, without the spread of microorganisms.
10. Pour the warmed solution into the container and drop the gauze for the compress into the solution. Alternately, if commercially packaged, prewarmed gauze is used, open packaging.	Prepares compress for application.
11. Put on clean gloves. Assess the application site for inflammation, skin color, and ecchymosis.	Gloves protect the nurse from potential contact with microorganisms. Assessment provides information about the area, the healing process, and the presence of infection, and allows for documentation of the condition of the area before the compress is applied.
12. Retrieve the compress from the warmed solution, squeezing out any excess moisture. Alternately, remove pre-warmed gauze from open package. **Apply the compress by gently and carefully molding it to the intended area (Figure 1). Ask the patient if the application feels too hot.**	Excess moisture may contaminate the surrounding area and is uncomfortable for the patient. Molding the compress to the skin promotes retention of warmth around the site.
13. Cover the site with a clean dry bath towel (Figure 2); secure in place with a tape or roller gauze, if necessary.	Towel provides extra insulation.

FIGURE 1. Applying compress to the intended area.

FIGURE 2. Covering site with clean dry bath towel.

(continued)

Skill 8-14 ▶ Applying a Warm Compress *(continued)*

ACTION	**RATIONALE**
14. Place the aquathermia or heating device, if used, over the towel. Refer to Skill 8-13.	The use of a heating device maintains the temperature of the compress and extends the therapeutic effect.
15. Remove gloves and discard them appropriately. Perform hand hygiene and remove additional PPE, if used.	Hand hygiene prevents the spread of microorganisms. Proper removal of PPE reduces the risk for infection transmission and contamination of other items.
16. **Monitor the time the compress is in place to prevent burns and skin/tissue damage. Monitor the condition of the patient's skin and the patient's response at frequent intervals.**	Extended use of heat results in an increased risk for burns from the heat. Impaired circulation may affect the patient's sensitivity to heat. Assessment of the patient's skin is necessary for early detection of adverse effects, thereby allowing prompt intervention to avoid complications.
17. After the prescribed time for the treatment (up to 30 minutes), remove the external heating device (if used). **Do not exceed the prescribed amount of time.** Put on gloves.	Using heat for more than this amount of time results in tissue congestion and vasoconstriction, known as the rebound phenomenon. Prolonged heat application may also result in an increased risk of burns and tissue damage (Taylor et al., 2019). Gloves protect the nurse from potential contact with microorganisms.
18. Carefully remove the compress while assessing the skin condition around the site and observing the patient's response to the heat application. Note any changes in the application area.	Assessment provides information about the healing process; the presence of irritation or infection should be documented.
19. Remove gloves. Perform hand hygiene.	Proper removal of gloves prevents the spread of microorganisms. Hand hygiene prevents the transmission of microorganisms.
20. Place the patient in a comfortable position. Lower the bed. Dispose of any other supplies appropriately.	Repositioning promotes patient comfort and safety.
21. Remove additional PPE, if used. Perform hand hygiene.	Proper removal of PPE reduces the risk for infection transmission and contamination of other items. Hand hygiene prevents the spread of microorganisms.

EVALUATION

The expected outcomes have been met when the patient experienced decreased inflammation, decreased muscle spasms, or decreased pain that indicate problems have been relieved; the patient experienced improved healing; and the patient remained free from injury.

DOCUMENTATION

Guidelines

Document the procedure, the length of time the compress was applied, including any use of an aquathermia pad. Record the temperature of the aquathermia pad and length of application time. Include a description of the application area, noting any edema, redness, or ecchymosis. Document the patient's reaction to the procedure including pain assessment. Record any patient and family education provided.

Sample Documentation

> <u>7/6/20</u> 0900 Left forearm with positive radial pulse, sensation and movement within normal limits, skin pale with brisk capillary refill. Left medial forearm (IV access infiltration site) positive for redness, edema; no evidence of maceration or drainage. Moist saline compress applied with aquathermia pad set at 100°F for 30 minutes. Site assessed every 10 minutes; no evidence of injury noted. Left arm elevated on pillows.
>
> —S. Tran, RN

UNEXPECTED SITUATIONS AND ASSOCIATED INTERVENTIONS	• *The nurse is monitoring a patient with a warm compress. Procedure requires that the nurse check the area of application every 5 minutes for tissue tolerance. The nurse notes excessive redness and slight maceration of the surrounding skin, and the patient verbalizes increased discomfort:* Stop the heat application. Remove the compress. Assess the patient for other symptoms. Obtain vital signs. Report the findings to the primary health care provider and document the event in the patient's record.
SPECIAL CONSIDERATIONS	• Use warm moist compresses cautiously with children and older adults. • Patients with diabetes, stroke, spinal cord injury, and peripheral neuropathy are at increased risk for thermal injury, as are patients with very thin or damaged skin. • Be extremely careful when applying to heat-sensitive areas, such as scar tissue and stomas.
Older Adult Considerations	• Older adults are more at risk for skin and tissue damage because of their thin skin, loss of heat sensation, decreased subcutaneous tissue, and changes in the body's ability to regulate temperature. Check these patients more frequently during therapy.

Skin 8-15 ▶ Assisting With a Sitz Bath

A sitz bath is a method of applying tepid or warm water to the perineal, pelvic, or rectal areas by sitting in a basin filled with this water. A sitz bath can help relieve pain and discomfort in the perineal area, such as after childbirth or surgery, and can increase circulation to the tissues, promoting healing.

DELEGATION CONSIDERATIONS	Assisting with a sitz bath may be delegated to nursing assistive personnel (NAP) or to unlicensed assistive personnel (UAP), as well as to licensed practical/vocational nurses (LPN/LVNs). The decision to delegate must be based on careful analysis of the patient's needs and circumstances, as well as the qualifications of the person to whom the task is being delegated. Refer to the Delegation Guidelines in Appendix A.
EQUIPMENT	• Clean gloves • Additional PPE, as indicated • Towel • Adjustable IV pole • Disposable sitz bath bowl with water bag
ASSESSMENT	Assess the situation to determine the appropriateness for the application of heat. Assess the patient's physical and mental status and the condition of the body area to be treated with heat. Determine the patient's ability to ambulate to the bathroom and maintain a sitting position for 15 to 20 minutes. Prior to the sitz bath, inspect perineal/rectal area for swelling, drainage, redness, warmth, and tenderness. Assess bladder fullness and encourage the patient to void before sitz bath. Confirm the prescribed order for the sitz bath, including frequency and length of time for the application. Assess the application site frequently during the treatment, as tissue damage can occur.
NURSING DIAGNOSIS	Determine related factors for the nursing diagnoses based on the patient's current status. Possible nursing diagnoses may include: • Acute pain • Risk for infection • Impaired tissue integrity
OUTCOME IDENTIFICATION AND PLANNING	The expected outcome to achieve when administering a sitz bath is that the patient verbalizes an increase in comfort. Other outcomes that may be appropriate include the following: the patient remains free of any signs and symptoms of infection, and exhibits signs and symptoms of healing.

(*continued*)

Skill 8-15 ▶ Assisting With a Sitz Bath *(continued)*

IMPLEMENTATION

| ACTION | RATIONALE |

ACTION

RATIONALE

1. Review the patient's health record for prescribed order for the application of a sitz bath, including the frequency and length of time for the application. Gather necessary supplies.

Reviewing the health record and care plan validates the correct patient and correct procedure. Preparation promotes efficient time management and an organized approach to the task.

2. Perform hand hygiene and put on PPE, if indicated.

Hand hygiene and PPE prevent the spread of microorganisms. PPE is required based on transmission precautions.

3. Identify the patient.

Identifying the patient ensures the right patient receives the intervention and helps prevent errors.

4. Close the curtains around the bed and close the door to the room, if possible.

This ensures the patient's privacy.

5. Put on gloves. Assemble equipment either at the bedside if using a bedside commode or in the bathroom.

Gloves prevent exposure to blood and body fluids. Organization facilitates performance of task.

6. Raise the lid of the toilet or commode. Place the bowl of the sitz bath, with drainage ports to the rear and infusion port in front, in the toilet (Figure 1). Fill the bowl of the sitz bath about halfway full with tepid to warm water (within a range of 105° to 109°F (40.5° to 43°C) (Taylor et al., 2019). **Water temperature should not exceed 125°F (Burn Foundation, 2016).**

Sitz bath will not drain appropriately if placed in the toilet backward. Tepid water can promote relaxation and help with edema; warm water can help with circulation. A range of 105° to 109°F (40.5° to 43°C) in temperature is considered to be physiologically effective and comfortable for the patient (Taylor et al., 2019).

FIGURE 1. Disposable sitz bath in place in toilet.

7. Clamp tubing on the bag. Fill the bag with same temperature water as mentioned above. Hang the bag above the patient's shoulder height on the IV pole.

If the bag is hung lower, the flow rate will not be sufficient and water may cool too quickly.

8. Assist the patient to sit on the toilet or commode. The patient should be able to sit in the basin or tub with the feet flat on the floor without any pressure on the sacrum or thighs. Wrap a blanket around the shoulders and provide extra draping, if needed. Insert tubing into the infusion port of the sitz bath. Slowly unclamp tubing and allow the sitz bath to fill.

Excessive pressure on the sacrum or thighs could cause tissue injury. Blanket and draping protects from chilling and exposure. If tubing is placed into the sitz bath before the patient sits on the toilet, the patient may trip over tubing. Filling the sitz bath ensures that the tissue is submerged in water.

ACTION	**RATIONALE**
9. Clamp tubing once the sitz bath is full. Instruct the patient to open clamp when water in bowl becomes cool. **Ensure that the call bell is within reach. Instruct the patient to call if he or she feels light-headed or dizzy or has any problems. Instruct the patient not to try standing without assistance.**	Cool water may produce hypothermia. The patient may become light-headed due to vasodilation, so call bell should be within reach.
10. Remove gloves and perform hand hygiene.	Hand hygiene deters the spread of microorganisms.
11. When the patient is finished (in about 15 to 20 minutes, or prescribed time), put on clean gloves. Assist the patient to stand and gently pat the perineal area dry. Remove gloves. Perform hand hygiene.	Gloves prevent contact with blood and body fluids. The patient may be light-headed and dizzy due to vasodilation. The patient should not stand alone, and bending over to dry self may cause the patient to fall.
12. Assist the patient to bed or chair. Ensure that the call bell is within reach.	The patient should not stand or walk alone. Having call bell within reach ensures the patient is able to ring for assistance as needed.
13. Put on gloves. Empty and disinfect sitz bath bowl according to facility policy.	Proper equipment cleaning deters the spread of microorganisms.
14. Remove gloves and any additional PPE, if used. Perform hand hygiene.	Proper removal of PPE reduces the risk for infection transmission and contamination of other items. Hand hygiene prevents the spread of microorganisms.

EVALUATION

The expected outcomes have been met when the patient verbalized an increase in comfort; the patient remained free of any signs and symptoms of infection; the patient exhibits signs and symptoms of healing.

DOCUMENTATION

Guidelines

Document administration of the sitz bath, including water temperature and duration. Document patient response, and assessment of perineum, pelvic and/or rectal areas before and after administration.

Sample Documentation

> 7/30/20 1620 Perineum assessed. Episiotomy edges well approximated, no drainage noted. Patient assisted to sitz bath. Patient took warm water sitz bath (temperature 99°F) for 20 minutes. Denies feeling light-headed or dizzy. Assisted back to bed after bath. Patient states pain level has dropped "from a 5 to a 2."
>
> —C. Stone, RN

UNEXPECTED SITUATIONS AND ASSOCIATED INTERVENTIONS

- *Patient complains of feeling light-headed or dizzy during sitz bath:* Stop sitz bath. Do not attempt to ambulate the patient alone. Use the call bell to summon help. Let the patient sit on the toilet until feeling subsides or help has arrived to assist the patient back to bed.
- *Temperature of water is uncomfortable:* The water may be too warm or cold, depending on the patient's preference. If this happens, clamp the tubing, disconnect the water bag, and refill it with water that is comfortable for the patient, but no warmer than 125°F.

Skill 8-16 ▶ Applying Cold Therapy

Cold constricts the peripheral blood vessels, reducing blood flow to the tissues and decreasing the local release of pain-producing substances. Cold reduces the formation of edema and inflammation, reduces muscle spasm, and promotes comfort by slowing the transmission of pain stimuli. The application of cold therapy (hypothermia therapy) reduces bleeding and hematoma formation. The application of cold is appropriate after direct trauma, for dental pain, for muscle spasms, after muscle sprains, and for the treatment of chronic pain. Ice can be used to apply cold therapy, usually in the form of an ice bag or ice collar, or in a glove. Commercially prepared cold packs are also available. For electronically controlled cooling devices, see the accompanying Skill Variation.

DELEGATION CONSIDERATIONS	The application of cold therapy may be delegated to nursing assistive personnel (NAP) or to unlicensed assistive personnel (UAP), as well as to licensed practical/vocational nurses (LPN/LVNs). The decision to delegate must be based on careful analysis of the patient's needs and circumstances, as well as the qualifications of the person to whom the task is being delegated. Refer to the Delegation Guidelines in Appendix A.
EQUIPMENT	• Ice bag, ice collar, glove, and ice • Commercially prepared cold packs • Small towel or washcloth • PPE, as indicated • Disposable waterproof pad • Gauze wrap or tape • Bath blanket
ASSESSMENT	Assess the situation to determine the appropriateness for the application of cold therapy. Assess the patient's physical and mental status and the condition of the body area to be treated with the cold therapy. Assess for circulatory compromise in the area where the compress will be applied, including skin color, pulses distal to the site, evidence of edema, and the presence of sensation. Confirm the prescribed order for the application of cold, including frequency, type of therapy, body area to be treated, and length of time for the application. Assess the equipment to be used to make sure it will function properly. Once the equipment is turned on, make sure there is a consistent distribution of heat and the temperature is within safe limits. Assess the application site frequently during the treatment, as tissue damage can occur.
NURSING DIAGNOSIS	Determine the related factors for the nursing diagnoses based on the patient's current health status. Appropriate nursing diagnoses may include: • Acute pain • Risk for injury • Deficient knowledge
OUTCOME IDENTIFICATION AND PLANNING	The expected outcome to achieve when applying an external cold source depends on the patient's nursing diagnosis. Outcomes that may be appropriate include the following: the patient experiences increased comfort; the patient experiences decreased muscle spasms; the patient experiences decreased inflammation; and the patient does not show signs of bleeding or hematoma at the treatment site.

IMPLEMENTATION

ACTION	RATIONALE
1. Review the patient's health record for prescribed order or nursing care plan for the application of cold therapy, including frequency, type of therapy, body area to be treated, and length of time for the application. Gather necessary supplies.	Reviewing the health record validates the correct patient and correct procedure. Preparation promotes efficient time management and an organized approach to the task.

ACTION	**RATIONALE**

2. Perform hand hygiene and put on PPE, if indicated.

Hand hygiene and PPE prevent the spread of microorganisms. PPE is required based on transmission precautions.

3. Identify the patient. Determine if the patient has had any previous adverse reaction to hypothermia therapy.

Identifying the patient ensures the right patient receives the intervention and helps prevent errors. Individual differences exist in tolerating specific therapies.

4. Assemble equipment on the overbed table or other surface within reach.

Organization facilitates performance of task.

5. Close the curtains around the bed and close the door to the room, if possible. Explain what you are going to do and why you are going to do it to the patient.

This ensures the patient's privacy. Explanation relieves anxiety and facilitates cooperation.

6. Assess the condition of the skin where the cold is to be applied.

Assessment supplies baseline data for post-treatment comparison and identifies any conditions that may contraindicate the application.

7. Assist the patient to a comfortable position that provides easy access to the area to be treated. Expose the area and drape the patient with a bath blanket, if needed. Put the waterproof pad under the wound area, if necessary.

Patient positioning and the use of a bath blanket provide for comfort and warmth. Waterproof pad protects the patient and the bed linens.

8. Prepare device: Fill the bag, collar, or glove about three fourths full with ice (Figure 1). Remove any excess air from the device. Securely fasten the end of the bag or collar; tie the glove closed, checking for holes and leakage of water. Prepare commercially prepared ice pack, according to the manufacturer's directions, if appropriate.

Ice provides a cold surface. Excess air interferes with cold conduction. Fastening the end prevents leaks.

9. **Cover the device with a towel or washcloth; commercially prepared devices may come with a cover (Figure 2). (If the device has a cloth exterior, this is not necessary.)**

The cover protects the skin and absorbs condensation.

FIGURE 1. Filling ice bag with ice.

FIGURE 2. Covering ice bag with cover.

(continued)

Skill 8-16 ▶ Applying Cold Therapy *(continued)*

ACTION	**RATIONALE**
10. Positioning the ice bag on the intended area and lightly secure in place, as needed (Figure 3).	Proper positioning ensures the cold therapy to the specified body area.

FIGURE 3. Positioning ice bag on the intended area and securing in place.

ACTION	**RATIONALE**
11. **Remove the ice and assess the site for redness after 30 seconds. Ask the patient about the presence of burning sensations.**	These actions prevent tissue injury.
12. Replace the device snugly against the site if no problems are evident. Secure it in place with gauze wrap, ties, or tape.	Wrapping or taping stabilizes the device in the proper location.
13. **Monitor the time the compress is in place to prevent burns and skin/tissue damage. Monitor the condition of the patient's skin and the patient's response at frequent intervals.**	Assessment of the patient's skin is necessary for early detection of adverse effects, thereby allowing prompt intervention to avoid complications.
14. After the prescribed time for the treatment (up to 30 minutes), remove the ice and dry the skin. **Do not exceed the prescribed amount of time.**	Limiting the time of application prevents injury due to overexposure to cold. Prolonged application of cold may result in decreased blood flow with resulting tissue **ischemia**. A compensatory vasodilation or rebound phenomenon may also occur as a means to provide warmth to the area.
15. Remove PPE, if used. Perform hand hygiene.	Proper removal of PPE reduces the risk for infection transmission and contamination of other items. Hand hygiene prevents the spread of microorganisms.
16. Place the patient in a comfortable position. Lower the bed. Dispose of any other supplies appropriately.	Repositioning promotes patient comfort and safety.
17. Remove additional PPE, if used. Perform hand hygiene.	Proper removal of PPE reduces the risk for infection transmission and contamination of other items. Hand hygiene prevents the spread of microorganisms.

EVALUATION

The expected outcomes have been met when (depending on the patient's nursing diagnosis) the patient reported relief of pain and increased comfort; patient verbalized a decrease in muscle spasms; the patient exhibited a reduction in inflammation; and the patient remained free from injury.

DOCUMENTATION

Guidelines

Document the location of the application, time of placement, and time of removal of the cold source. Record the assessment of the area where the cold therapy was applied, including the patient's mobility, sensation, color, temperature, and any presence of numbness, tingling, or pain. Document the patient's response, such as any decrease in pain or change in sensation. Include any pertinent patient and family education.

Sample Documentation

> 11/1/20 1430 Swelling noted on right lower extremity from mid-calf to foot. Toes warm, pink, positive sensation and movement, negative for numbness, tingling, and pain. Ice bags wrapped in cloth applied to right ankle and lower calf. Patient instructed to communicate any changes in sensation or pain; verbalizes an understanding of information.
>
> —L. Semet, RN
>
> 11/1/20 1450 Ice removed from right lower extremity; neurovascular assessment unchanged. Right lower extremity elevated on two pillows.
>
> —L. Semet, RN

UNEXPECTED SITUATIONS AND ASSOCIATED INTERVENTIONS

- *When performing a skin assessment during therapy, the nurse notes increased pallor at the treatment site and sluggish capillary refill, and the patient reports alterations in sensation at the application site:* Discontinue therapy, obtain vital signs, assess for other symptoms, notify the primary health care provider, and document the event in the patient's record.

SPECIAL CONSIDERATIONS

General Considerations

- The patient may experience a secondary defense reaction, vasodilation, causing body temperature to rebound, defeating the purpose of the therapy.
- Allow at least 1 hour between episodes of application of cold therapy (Taylor et al., 2019).

Older Adult Considerations

- Older adults are more at risk for skin and tissue damage because of their thin skin, loss of cold sensation, decreased subcutaneous tissue, and changes in the body's ability to regulate the temperature. Check these patients more frequently during therapy.

Home Care Considerations

- A bag of frozen vegetables (such as peas) makes a good substitute for an ice bag (Taylor et al., 2019).

Skill Variation | Applying an Electronically Controlled Cooling Device

Electronically controlled cooling devices are used in situations to deliver a constant cooling effect. After orthopedic surgery, those patients as well as other patients with acute musculoskeletal injuries may benefit from this therapy. A prescription or order is required for the use of this device. Initial assessment of the extremity is involved, as well as ongoing assessment throughout the period of use. As with application of any electronic device, ongoing monitoring for proper functioning and temperature regulation is necessary.

1. Gather equipment and verify the prescribed order.
2. Perform hand hygiene. Put on PPE, as indicated.

(continued)

Skill 8-16 ▶ Applying Cold Therapy *(continued)*

Skill Variation ▶ Applying an Electronically Controlled Cooling Device *(continued)*

3. Identify the patient and explain the procedure.
4. Assess the involved extremity or body part.
5. Set the correct temperature on the device.
6. Assess to ensure that the cooling pads are functioning properly.
7. Wrap the cooling water-flow pad around the involved body part.
8. Wrap an Ace bandage or gauze pads around the water-flow pads.

9. Remove PPE, if used. Perform hand hygiene.
10. Monitor frequently to ensure proper functioning of equipment.
11. Unwrap at intervals to assess skin integrity of the body part.
12. Remove device after the prescribed time for the treatment (up to 30 minutes). **Do not exceed the prescribed amount of time.**

EVIDENCE FOR PRACTICE ▶

COLD APPLICATION AND PAIN RELIEF

Chest tube removal is a painful procedure for many, if not most, patients. Pharmacologic and nonpharmacologic interventions have been used to decrease patients' discomfort during this procedure.

Related Research

Sinha, V. R., Dave, K., Goyal, H., & Mathur, R. G. (2015). Effects of cold application on pain & anxiety during chest tube removal among postoperative cardiac surgery adult patients. *IOSR Journal of Nursing and Health Science, 4*(6), 64–68. Retrieved https://www.scribd.com/document/290932063/Effects-of-cold-application-on-pain-anxiety-during-chest-tube-removal-among-post-operative-cardiac-surgery-adult-patients

The objective of this study was to determine whether the application of cold to the chest wall had an effect on pain and anxiety related to chest tube removal. The study was conducted with 60 postoperative cardiac surgery adult patients, divided evenly between an experimental group and a control group. The control group received usual standard of care during chest tube removal. The experimental group received an application of cold using a gel pack at the chest tube site for 15 minutes prior to chest tube removal. Pain intensity, using a Numerical Pain Intensity Scale, was measured at various points before and after the tube removal process. The mean postintervention pain scores were significantly lower in the experimental group ($p < 0.05$). Anxiety related to chest tube removal was assessed using the State Trait Anxiety inventory (STAI) scale and measured at various points before and after the tube removal process. The mean postintervention anxiety scores were significantly lower in the experimental group ($p < 0.05$). The authors concluded the application of cold was effective in reducing pain and anxiety among postoperative cardiac adult surgery patients related to removal of chest tubes. The authors stated cold application is a simple, inexpensive nonpharmacologic anxiety and pain management strategy to implement related to chest tube removal.

Relevance for Nursing Practice

Nursing interventions related to decreasing pain and increasing patient comfort are an important nursing responsibility. Interventions should include the use of nonpharmacologic interventions, in addition to the administration of analgesics. The application of cold to the chest wall could significantly decrease the pain and discomfort experienced by a patient during removal of a chest tube. Nurses could easily incorporate this simple intervention as part of nursing care for these patients.

Refer to thePoint® for additional research on related nursing topics.

Enhance Your Understanding

Focusing on Patient Care: Developing Clinical Reasoning

Consider the case scenarios at the beginning of the chapter as you answer the following questions to enhance your understanding and apply what you have learned.

QUESTIONS

1. While providing wound care for Lori Downs' foot wound, you note that the drainage, which was scant and yellow 2 days ago, is now green and has saturated the old dressing. Should you continue with the prescribed wound care?

2. Three days ago Tran Nguyen underwent a modified radical mastectomy. She has three Jackson–Pratt drains at her surgical site. She has started asking questions about her surgery and has anticipated discharge home. Until this morning, she has avoided looking at her surgical

site. You are helping her with her bathing and dressing. As you help her remove her gown, she becomes visibly upset and anxious and exclaims, "Oh no! What's wrong? I'm bleeding from the cuts!" You realize she is looking at her drains. How should you respond?

3. Arthur Lowes has come to his surgeon's office today for a follow-up examination after a colon resection. After he sees the health care provider, you, the treatment nurse, will remove the surgical staples from the incision and apply adhesive wound strips. As you prepare to remove the staples, Mr. Lowes comments, "I hope my stomach doesn't pop out now!" What should you tell him?

You can find suggested answers after the Bibliography at the end of this chapter.

Integrated Case Study Connection

The case studies in the back of the book focus on integrating concepts. Refer to the following case studies to enhance your understanding of the concepts and skills in this chapter.

- Basic Case Studies: Tula Stillwater, page 1111.
- Intermediate Case Studies: Tula Stillwater, page 1117.
- Advanced Case Studies: Robert Espinoza, page 1132.

Taylor Suite Resources

Explore these additional resources to enhance learning for this chapter:

- NCLEX-Style Questions and other resources on thePoint®, http://thePoint.lww.com/Lynn5e
- *Skill Checklists for Taylor's Clinical Nursing Skills*, 5e
- *Taylor's Video Guide to Clinical Nursing Skills*: Skin Integrity and Wound Care
- *Fundamentals of Nursing*: Chapter 32, Skin Integrity and Wound Care
- *Lippincott DocuCare* Fundamentals cases

Bibliography

Alvarez, O. M., Brindle, C. T., Langemo, D., et al. (2016). The VCU Pressure Ulcer Summit: The search for a clearer understanding and more precise clinical definition of the unavoidable pressure injury. *Journal of Wound, Ostomy, and Continence Nursing*, 43(5), 455–463.

Apelqvist, J., Willy, C., Fagerdah, A. M., et al. (2017). European Wound Management Association (EWMA). EWMA document: Negative pressure wound therapy. Overview, challenges and perspectives. *Journal of Wound Care*, 26(Suppl3), S1–S154.

Association of Perioperative Registered Nurses (AORN). (2015). *Perioperative standards and recommended practices*. Denver, CO: AORN, Inc.

Baranoski, S., & Ayello, E. A. (2016). *Wound care essentials. Practice principles* (4th ed.). Philadelphia, PA: Wolters Kluwer.

Baranoski, S., LeBlanc, K., & Gloeckner, M. (2016). Preventing, assessing, and managing skin tears: A clinical review. *American Journal of Nursing*, 116(11), 24–30.

Barratt, N. (2014). Nutrition and wound healing. Implications for practice. *Journal of the Dermatology Nurses' Association*, 6(1), 27–32.

Beldon, P. (2013). How to select and choose appropriate wound dressings. *Nurse Prescribing*, 11(10), 487–492.

Benbow, M. (2016). Understanding safe practice in the use of negative pressure wound therapy in the community. *British Journal of Community Nursing*, 21(Suppl12), S32–S34.

Bergstrom, N., Braden, B., Laguzza, A., Holman, V. (1987). The Braden scale for predicting pressure sore risk. *Nursing Research*, 36(4), 205–210.

Blenman, J., & Marks-Maran, D. (2017). Pressure ulcer prevention is everyone's business: The PUPS project. *British Journal of Nursing*, 26(6), S16–S26.

Braden, B. J. (2012). The Braden Scale for predicting pressure sore risk: Reflections after 25 years. *Advances in Skin & Wound Care*, 25(2), 61.

Braden, B., & Maklebust, J. (2005). Preventing pressure ulcers with the Braden scale. *American Journal of Nursing*, 105(6), 70–72.

Brandon, T. (2016). Using a single-use, disposable negative pressure wound therapy system in the management of small wounds. Wounds UK, EWMA Special Issue, 70–73.

Broussard, K. C., & Powers, J. G. (2013). Wound dressings: Selecting the most appropriate type. *American Journal of Clinical Dermatology*, 14(6), 449–459.

Burn Foundation. (2016). Burn prevention. Safety facts on scald burns. Retrieved http://www.burnfoundation.org/programs/resource.cfm?c=1&a=3

Byrne, J., Nichols, P., Sroczynski, M., et al. (2016). Prophylactic sacral dressing for pressure ulcer prevention in high-risk patients. *American Journal of Critical Care*, 25(3), 228–234.

Centers for Disease Control and Prevention (CDC). (2010). Healthcare-associated infections (HAIs). Fre-

quently asked questions about surgical site infections. Retrieved https://www.cdc.gov/HAI/ssi/faq_ssi.html

Centers for Disease Control and Prevention (CDC). (2016). *Healthcare-associated infections (HAIs)*. Retrieved https://www.cdc.gov/hai

Cornish, L. (2017). The use of prophylactic dressings in the prevention of pressure ulcers: A literature review. *British Journal of Community Nursing*, 22(Suppl6), S26–S32.

Cross, H. H. (2014). Obtaining a wound swab culture specimen. *Nursing*, 44(7), 68–69.

Ding, S., Lin, F., Marshall, A. P., & Gillespie, B. M. (2017). Nurses' practice in preventing postoperative wound infections: An observational study. *Journal of Wound Care*, 26(1), 28–37.

Doenges, M. E., Moorhouse, M. F., & Murr, A. C. (2016). *Nursing diagnoses manual. Planning, individualizing, and documenting client care* (5th ed.). Philadelphia, PA: F. A. Davis.

Doughty, D. B., & McNichol, L. L. (2016). *Wound, Ostomy and Continence Nurses Society™ Core Curriculum: Wound Management*. Philadelphia, PA: Wolters Kluwer.

Dudek, S. (2018). *Nutrition essentials for nursing practice* (8th ed.). Philadelphia, PA: Wolters Kluwer.

Eliopoulos, C. (2018). *Gerontological Nursing* (9th ed.). Philadelphia, PA: Wolters Kluwer.

Ellis, M. (2017). Pressure ulcer prevention in care home settings. *Nursing Older People*, 29(3), 29–35.

Fletcher, J. (2017). An overview of pressure ulcer risk assessment tools. *Wounds UK, 13*(1), 18–26.

Gabriel, A. (2015). Wound irrigation. *Medscape*. Retrieved http://emedicine.medscape.com/article/1895071-overview#a1

Grossman, S., & Porth, C. M. (2014). *Porth's pathophysiology: Concepts of altered health states* (9th ed.). Philadelphia, PA: Wolters Kluwer.

Harris, C., Bates-Jensen, B., Parslow, N., Raizman, R., Singh, M., & Ketchen, R. (2010). Bates-Jensen Wound Assessment Tool: Pictorial guide validation project. *Journal of Wound, Ostomy, and Continence Nursing, 37*(3), 253–259.

Heale, M. (2014). How 'clean' is your clean dressing technique? *Wound Source*. Retrieved http://www.woundsource.com/blog/how-clean-your-clean-dressing-technique

Hess, C. (2013). *Clinical guide to skin & wound care* (7th ed.). Philadelphia, PA: Wolters Kluwer.

Hinkle, J. L., & Cheever, K. H. (2018). *Brunner & Suddarth's textbook of medical-surgical nursing* (14th ed.). Philadelphia, PA: Wolters Kluwer.

Hogan-Quigley, B., Palm, M. L., & Bickley, L. (2017). *Bates' nursing guide to physical examination and history taking* (2nd ed.). Philadelphia, PA: Wolters Kluwer.

Hurd, T., Rossington, A., Trueman, P., & Smith, J. (2017). A retrospective comparison of the performance of two negative pressure wound therapy systems in the management of wounds of mixed etiology. *Advances in Wound Care, 6*(1), 33–37.

Janssen, A .H., Mommers, E. H., Notter, J., de Vries Rellingh, T. S., & Wegdam, J. A. (2016). Negative pressure wound therapy versus standard wound care on quality of life: A systematic review. *Journal of Wound Care, 25*(3), 154–159.

Jarvis, C. (2016). *Physical Examination & Health Assessment*. (7th ed.). St. Louis, MO: Elsevier.

Jensen, S. (2015). *Nursing Health Assessment: A best practice approach* (2nd ed.). Philadelphia, PA: Wolters Kluwer.

The Joanna Briggs Institute. (2013, Update) Wound Healing and Management Node Group. Evidence summary. Wound management: Debridement – Wet-to-dry moistened gauze. *Wound Practice and Research, 21*(4), 190–192. Retrieved http://www.woundsaustralia.com.au/journal/2104_08.pdf

Kyle, T., & Carman, S. (2017). *Essentials of pediatric nursing* (3rd ed.). Philadelphia, PA: Wolters Kluwer.

Leaper, D. J., Schultz, G., Carville, K., Fletcher, J., Swanson, T., & Drake, R. (2012). Extending the TIME concept: What have we learned in the past 10 years? *International Wound Journal, 9*(Suppl2), 1–19.

LeMone, P., Burke, K. M., Bauldoff, G., & Gubrud, P. (2015). *Medical-surgical nursing. Clinical reasoning in patient care* (6th ed.). New York: Pearson.

Maida, V., Ennis, M., & Kuziemsky, C. (2009). The Toronto Symptom Assessment System for Wounds: A new clinical and research tool. *Advances in Skin & Wound Care, 22*(10), 468–474.

McNichol, L., Lund, C., Rosen, T., & Gray, M. (2013). Medical adhesives and patient safety: State of the science. Consensus statements for the assessment, prevention and treatment of adhesive-related skin injuries. *Journal of Wound, Ostomy, and Continence Nursing, 40*(4), 365–380.

McNichol, L., Watts, C., Mackey, D., Beitz, J. M., & Gray, M. (2015). Identifying the right surface for the right patient at the right time: Generation and content validation of an Algorithm for Support Surface selection. *Journal of Wound, Ostomy, and Continence Nursing, 42*(1), 19–37.

Milne, J. (2013). Effective use of negative pressure wound therapy. *Practice Nursing, 24*(1), 14–19.

Milne, J. (2015). Using disposable negative pressure wound therapy in the community. *Journal of Community Nursing*, Supplement Oct/Nov, 10–15.

NANDA International, Inc.: *Nursing diagnoses – Definitions and classification 2018–2020* © 2017 NANDA International, ISBN 978-1-62623-929-6. Used by arrangement with the Thieme Group, Stuttgart/New York.

National Pressure Ulcer Advisory Panel (NPUAP). (2016a). National Pressure Ulcer Advisor Panel (NPUAP) announces a change in terminology from pressure ulcer to pressure injury and updates the states of pressure injury. Retrieved http://www.npuap.org/national-pressure-ulcer-advisory-panel-npuap-announces-a-change-in-terminology-from-pressure-ulcer-to-pressure-injury-and-updates-the-stages-of-the-pressure-injury

National Pressure Ulcer Advisory Panel (NPUAP). (2016b). Pressure injury prevention points. Retrieved http://www.npuap.org/wp-content/uploads/2016/04/Pressure-Injury-Prevention-Points-2016.pdf

National Pressure Ulcer Advisory Panel (NPUAP). (2016c). NPUAP Pressure injury stages. Retrieved http://www.npuap.org/resources/educational-and-clinical-resources/npuap-pressure-injury-stages

National Pressure Ulcer Advisory Panel (NPUAP) (2016d). Pressure injury staging illustrations. Retrieved http://www.npuap.org/resources/educational-and-clinical-resources/pressure-injury-staging-illustrations

National Pressure Ulcer Advisory Panel (NPUAP) (2016e). PUSH tool. Retrieved http://www.npuap.org/resources/educational-and-clinical-resources/push-tool

National Pressure Ulcer Advisory Panel [NPUAP], European Pressure Ulcer Advisory Panel [EPUAP], & Pan Pacific Pressure Injury Alliance [PPPIA]. (2014a). Prevention and treatment of pressure ulcers: Quick reference guide. Retrieved http://www.npuap.org/wp-content/uploads/2014/08/Quick-Reference-Guide-DIGITAL-NPUAP-EPUAP-PPPIA.pdf

National Pressure Ulcer Advisory Panel [NPUAP], European Pressure Ulcer Advisory Panel [EPUAP], & Pan Pacific Pressure Injury Alliance [PPPIA]. (2014b). *Prevention and treatment of pressure ulcers: Clinical practice guideline*. In E. Haesler (Ed.). Cambridge Media: Osborne Park, Australia.

Ousey, K., Rogers, A. A., & Rippon, M. G. (2016). Hydro-responsive wound dressings simplify T.I.M.E. wound management framework. *British Journal of Community Nursing, 21*(Suppl12), S39–S49.

Padula, W. V., Mishra, M. K., Makic, M. B., et al. (2015). Increased adoption of quality improvement interventions to implement evidence-based practices for pressure ulcer prevention in U.S. academic medical centers. *Worldviews on Evidence-Based Nursing, 12*(6), 328–336.

Pagnamenta, F. (2017). The provision of therapy mattresses for pressure ulcer prevention. *British Journal of Nursing, 26*(6), S28–S33.

Payne, D. (2016). Strategies to support prevention, identification and management of pressure ulcers in the community. *British Journal of Community Nursing, 21*(Suppl6), S10–S18.

Perry, S. E., Hockenberry, M. J., Lowdermilk, D. L., & Wilson, D. (2014). *Maternal child nursing care* (5th ed.). St. Louis, MO: Elsevier Mosby.

Quain, A. M., & Khardori, N. M. (2015). Nutrition in wound care management: A comprehensive overview. *Wounds, 27*(12), 327–335.

Rabess, C. (2015). Understanding the link between wound care and nutrition. *Journal of Community Nursing, 29*(4), 60–65.

Reevell, G., Anders, T., & Morgan, T. (2016). Improving patients' experience of dressing removal in practice. *Journal of Community Nursing, 30*(5), 44–49.

Schreiber, M. L. (2016). Negative pressure wound therapy. *MedSurg Nursing, 25*(6), 425–428.

Sinha, V. R., Dave, K., Goyal, H., & Mathur, R. G. (2015). Effects of cold application on pain & anxiety during chest tube removal among postoperative cardiac surgery adult patients. *IOSR Journal of Nursing and Health Science, 4*(6), 64–68. Retrieved https://www.scribd.com/document/290932063/Effects-of-cold-application-on-pain-anxiety-during-chest-tube-removal-among-post-operative-cardiac-surgery-adult-patients

Smart, L., & Acton, C. (2016). Wound dressings: Surgical dressings. *Dermatological Nursing, 15*(2), 36–40.

Sood, A., Granick, M. S., & Tomaselli, N. L. (2014). Wound dressings and comparative effectiveness data. *Advances in Wound Care, 3*(8), 511–529.

Steven, M., Struble, L., & Larson, J. L. (2015). Recognizing pressure injury in the darkly pigmented skin type. *Medsurg Nursing, 24*(5), 342–348.

Taylor, C., Lynn, P., & Bartlett, J. (2019). *Fundamentals of nursing: The art and science of person-centered care* (9th ed.). Philadelphia, PA: Wolters Kluwer.

Van Leeuwen, A.M., & Bladh, M.L. (2017). *Davis's comprehensive handbook of laboratory & diagnostic tests with nursing implications* (7th ed.). Philadelphia: F.A. Davis Company.

VHA Center for Engineering & Occupational Safety and Health (CEOSH). (2016). *Safe patient handling and mobility guidebook*. St. Louis, MO: Author. Retrieved http://www.tampavaref.org/safe-patient-handling.htm

Voegeli, D. (2013). Moisture-associated skin damage: An overview for community nurses. *British Journal of Community Nursing, 18*(1), 6–12.

Waldie, K. (2013). Pain associated with negative pressure wound therapy. *British Journal of Nursing, 22*(6), S15–S21.

Waterlow, J. (1985). Pressure sores: A risk assessment card. *Nursing Times, 81*(48), 49–55.

Wilkins, R. G., & Unverdorben, M. (2013). Wound cleaning and wound healing: A concise review. *Advances in Skin & Wound Care, 26*(4), 160–163.

Wound, Ostomy and Continence Nurses Society (WOCN). (2017). About the WOCN Society. Retrieved https://www. WOCN.org/?page = about_us

Wound, Ostomy and Continence Nurses Society (WOCN) Wound Committee; Association for Professionals in Infection Control and Epidemiology, Inc. (APIC) 2000 Guidelines Committee. (2012). Clean vs. sterile dressing techniques for management of chronic wounds. A fact sheet. *Journal of Wound, Ostomy, and Continence Nursing, 39*(Suppl2), S30–S34.

Wound, Ostomy and Continence Nurses Society (WOCN). Wound Guidelines Task Force. (2016). WOCH 2016 guideline for prevention and management of pressure injuries (ulcers). *Journal of Wound Ostomy & Continence Nursing, 44*(3), 241–246.

Yarwook-Ross, L. (2013). Theory of moist wound healing. *Independent Nurse*. Retrieved http://www.independentnurse.co.uk/clinical-article/theory-of-moist-wound-healing/63534

SUGGESTED ANSWERS FOR FOCUSING ON PATIENT CARE: DEVELOPING CLINICAL REASONING

1. This is a significant change in the patient's assessment. Perform a thorough wound assessment and obtain vital signs. Assess the patient for any new symptoms, such as increased pain, chills, or abnormal sensation (e.g., numbness, tingling). Report findings to the primary health care provider; a change in wound care, additional assessments (e.g., diagnostic tests, laboratory tests), or change/addition of medication may be required.

2. Reassure the patient regarding her wound status. Explain what the drains are, how they work, and their intended purpose. Provide information regarding wound care, drain care, and recording of drainage amounts. Discuss anticipated care requirements at home and potential arrangements to ensure required care is performed, either by the patient or significant other.

3. Reassure the patient regarding his wound status. Explain the purpose of the staples, the process of wound healing, and the purpose of adhesive wound strips. Discuss the patient's responsibilities for wound care at this point in his healing.

Activity

Learning Objectives

After completing the chapter, you will be able to accomplish the following:

1. Assist a patient with turning in bed.
2. Move a patient up in bed with the assistance of another caregiver.
3. Transfer a patient from the bed to a stretcher.
4. Transfer a patient from the bed to a chair.
5. Transfer a patient using a full-powered body sling lift.
6. Provide range-of-motion exercises.
7. Assist a patient with ambulation.
8. Assist a patient with ambulation using a walker.
9. Assist a patient with ambulation using crutches.
10. Assist a patient with ambulation using a cane.
11. Apply and remove graduated compression stockings.
12. Apply pneumatic compression devices.
13. Apply a continuous passive motion device.
14. Apply a sling.
15. Apply a figure-eight bandage.
16. Assist with a cast application.
17. Care for a patient with a cast.

18. Apply and care for a patient in skin traction.
19. Care for a patient in skeletal traction.
20. Care for a patient with an external fixation device.

Key Terms

abduction: Lateral movement away from the center or median line of the body

adduction: Lateral movement toward the center or median line of the body

arthroplasty: surgical formation or reformation of a joint

compartment syndrome: occurs when there is increased tissue pressure within a limited space; leads to compromises in the circulation and the function of the involved tissue

contracture: permanent shortening or tightening of a muscle due to spasm or paralysis

contusion: an injury in which the skin is not broken; a bruise

deep vein thrombosis (DVT): the formation or development of a blood clot in a blood vessel originating in the large veins of the legs

extension: the return movement from flexion; the joint angle is increased

flexion: bending of a joint so that the angle of the joint diminishes

fracture: a break in the continuity of a bone

goniometer: an apparatus to measure joint movement and angles

hyperextension: extreme or abnormal extension (angle >180 degrees)

patient care ergonomics: the practice of designing equipment and work tasks to conform to the capability of the worker in relation to patient care. It provides a means for adjusting the work environment and work practices to prevent injuries before they occur and is part of best practices for providing safe patient care (Occupational Safety and Health Administration [OSHA], 2009; VHACEOSH, 2016).

pronation: the act of lying face downward; the act of turning the hand so the palm faces downward or backward

range of motion (ROM): the complete extent of movement of which a joint is normally capable.

rotation: process of turning on an axis; twisting or revolving

shearing force: force created by the interplay of gravity and friction on the skin and underlying tissues; shear causes tissue layers to slide over one another and blood vessels to stretch and twist, and disrupts the microcirculation of the skin and subcutaneous tissue

supination: turning of the palm or foot upward

thrombophlebitis: a blood clot that accompanies vein inflammation

venous stasis: decrease in blood flow in the venous system related to dysfunctional valves or inactivity of the muscles of the affected extremity

The ability to move is closely related to the fulfillment of other basic human needs. Regular exercise contributes to the healthy functioning of each body system. Conversely, lack of exercise and immobility affect each body system negatively. A summary of the effects of immobility on the body is outlined in Fundamentals Review 9-1. An important nursing role is to encourage activity and exercise to promote wellness, prevent illness, and restore health.

Nursing interventions are directed at preventing potential problems and treating actual problems related to a patient's activity and mobility status. Strategies designed to promote correct body alignment, mobility, and fitness are important parts of nursing care. Nurses use knowledge of **patient care ergonomics** and of mobility and safe patient handling techniques along with specific nursing interventions to promote fitness and to resolve mobility problems.

An effective approach to safe patient transfers is thought to include patient assessment criteria; algorithms for patient handling and movement decisions; specialized patient handling equipment; and the use of lift teams (Nelson, Motacki, & Menzel, 2009; VHACEOSH, 2016). The OSHA advocates for "no lift" policies for all health care facilities and recommends the use of patient handling aids and mechanical lifting equipment on patients who are unable to assist in their transfer (OSHA, 2013). Many devices and equipment are available to aid in transferring, repositioning, and lifting patients. It is important to use the right equipment and appropriate device based on patient assessment and desired movement. It is equally important for caregivers to utilize proper body position to minimize peak pulling forces and avoid musculoskeletal injury (Bacharach, Miller, & von Duvillard, 2016).

Always check facility practices and guidelines and available equipment related to safe patient handling and movement. Samples of algorithms to aid decision making to prevent injury to staff and patients during patient movement and handling are provided in the appropriate skills. When using any equipment, check for proper functioning before using with the patient. Fundamentals Review 9-2 presents guidelines for safe patient handling and movement. Fundamentals Review 9-3 discusses examples of equipment and assistive devices that are available to aid with safe patient movement and handling. Fundamentals Review 9-4 provides an example of an assessment tool to aid in patient assessment and decision making regarding safe patient handling and movement.

This chapter covers skills to assist the nurse in providing care related to activity, inactivity, and health care problems related to the musculoskeletal system.

Fundamentals Review 9-1

EFFECTS OF IMMOBILITY ON THE BODY

- Decreased muscle strength and tone, decreased muscle size
- Decreased joint mobility and flexibility
- Limited endurance and activity intolerance
- Bone demineralization
- Lack of coordination and altered gait
- Decreased ventilatory effort and increased respiratory secretions, atelectasis, respiratory congestion
- Increased cardiac workload, orthostatic hypotension, venous thrombosis
- Impaired circulation and skin breakdown
- Decreased appetite, constipation
- Urinary stasis, infection
- Altered sleep patterns, pain, depression, anger, anxiety

Fundamentals Review 9-2

GUIDELINES FOR SAFE PATIENT HANDLING AND MOVEMENT

Keep the patient in good alignment and protect from injury while being moved. Follow these recommended guidelines when moving and lifting patients:

- Assess the patient. Know the patient's medical diagnosis, capabilities, and any movement not allowed. Put in place braces or any device the patient wears before helping the patient from the bed.
- Assess the patient's ability to assist with the planned movement. Encourage the patient to assist in own transfers. Encouraging the patient to perform tasks

that are within his or her capabilities promotes independence. Eliminating or reducing unnecessary tasks by the nurse reduces the risk of injury.

- Assess the patient's ability to understand instructions and cooperate with the staff to achieve the movement (see Box 9-1 in Skill 9-1 for general guidelines related to mobility and safe handling of people with dementia).
- During any patient transferring task, if any caregiver is required to lift more than 35 lb of a patient's weight,

(continued)

Fundamentals Review 9-2   continued

GUIDELINES FOR SAFE PATIENT HANDLING AND MOVEMENT

consider the patient to be fully dependent and use assistive devices for the transfer (Smith et al., 2015).

- Ensure sufficient staff is available and present to move the patient safely.
- Assess the area for clutter, accessibility to the patient, and availability of devices. Remove any obstacles that may make moving and lifting inconvenient.
- Decide which equipment to use. Use handling aids whenever possible to help reduce risk of injury to the nurse and patient.
- Plan carefully what you will do before moving or lifting a patient. Assess the mobility of attached equipment. You may injure the patient or yourself if you have not planned well. If necessary, enlist the support of another nurse. This reduces the strain on everyone involved. Communicate the plan with staff and the patient to ensure coordinated movement.
- Explain to the patient what you plan to do. Then, use what abilities the patient has to assist you. This technique often decreases the effort required and the possibility of injury to you.
- If the patient is in pain, administer the prescribed analgesic sufficiently in advance of the transfer to allow the patient to participate in the move comfortably.
- Elevate the bed, as necessary, so that you are working at a height that is comfortable and safe for you.

- Lock the wheels of the bed, wheelchair, or stretcher so that they do not slide while you are moving the patient.
- Observe the principles of patient care ergonomics to prevent injuring yourself while you work.
- Be sure the patient is in good body alignment while being moved and lifted, to protect the patient from strain and muscle injury.
- Support the patient's body properly. Avoid grabbing and holding an extremity by its muscles.
- Use friction-reducing devices, whenever possible, especially during lateral transfers.
- Move your body and the patient in a smooth, rhythmic motion. Jerky movements tend to put extra strain on muscles and joints and are uncomfortable for the patient.
- Use mechanical devices, such as lifts, slides, transfer chairs, or gait belts, for moving patients. Be sure that you understand how the device operates and that the patient is properly secured and informed of what will occur. If you are not comfortable with the operation of the equipment, obtain assistance from a caregiver who is. Patients who do not understand or are afraid may be unable to cooperate and may cause injury to the staff as well as suffer injury as a result.
- Assure equipment used meets weight requirements. Bariatric patients (body mass index [BMI] greater than 50) require bariatric transfer aids and equipment (VHACEOSH, 2016).

Fundamentals Review 9-3

EQUIPMENT AND ASSISTIVE DEVICES

Many devices and equipment are available to aid in transferring, repositioning, and lifting patients. It is important to use the right equipment and appropriate device based on patient assessment and desired movement.

GAIT BELTS

A gait belt is a belt, often with handles, used for transferring patients and assisting with ambulation. It is placed around the patient's waist and secured. The handles can be placed in a variety of configurations so the caregiver can have better access to, improved grasp, and control of the patient. Some belts are hand-held slings that go around the patient, providing a firm grasp for the caregiver and facilitating the transfer (Smith et al., 2015). Do not use gait belts on patients with abdominal or thoracic incisions. Patients seeking to avoid the social stigma of a gait belt can wear a "Sturdily constructed" fanny pack for the same

purpose (Smith et al., 2015) (see Figure A for an example of a gait belt).

FIGURE A. Using a gait belt.

Fundamentals Review 9-3 continued

EQUIPMENT AND ASSISTIVE DEVICES

STAND-ASSIST AND REPOSITIONING AIDS

Some patients need minimal assistance to stand up. With an appropriate support to grasp, they can lift themselves. Many types of secure devices can help a patient to stand. These devices are freestanding or attach to the bed or wheelchair. One type of stand-assist aid attaches to the bed. Other aids have a pull bar to assist the patient to stand, and then a seat unfolds under the patient. After sitting on the seat, the device can be wheeled to the toilet, chair, shower, or bed. Sliding assists are useful for patients who are cooperative, partially dependent but have some weight-bearing capability, and have upper body mobility and strength sufficient to grip device handles.

LATERAL-ASSIST DEVICES

Lateral-assist devices reduce patient-surface friction during lateral transfers. Roller boards, slide boards, transfer boards, inflatable mattresses, and friction-reducing, lateral-assist devices are examples of these devices that make transfers safer and more comfortable for the patient. An inflatable lateral-assist device is a flexible mattress that is placed under the patient. An attached, portable air supply inflates the mattress, which provides a layer of air under the patient. This air cushion allows nursing staff to perform the move with much less effort, but may place the care providers at an increased risk of injury because of the horizontal reach required, posture adopted during transfer, and lack of handles. Transfer boards are placed under the patient. They provide a slick surface for the patient during transfers, reducing friction and the force required to move the patient. Transfer boards are made of smooth, rigid, low-friction material, such as coated wood or plastic. In order to use a board for transfers to or from a chair, the chair must have retractable or removable arm rests (Smith et al., 2015). Another lateral-sliding aid is made of a special fabric that reduces friction. Some devices have long handles that reduce reaching by staff, to improve safety and make the transfer easier (Figure B).

FIGURE B. Lateral-assist device with long handles to reduce reaching by staff.

FRICTION-REDUCING SHEETS

Friction-reducing sheets can be used under patients to prevent skin shearing when moving a patient in the bed and to assist with lateral transfers. The use of these sheets when moving the patient up in bed, turning, and repositioning reduces friction and the force required to move the patient. They can also be used to assist patients to perform range-of-motion exercises in bed (Smith et al., 2015). However, use of these sheets may require use of excessive force by the caregiver and exceed the recommended hand force of 35 lb, increasing the risk of musculoskeletal injuries (Bartnik & Rice, 2013).

MECHANICAL LATERAL-ASSIST DEVICES

Mechanical lateral-assist devices eliminate the need to slide the patient manually. Some devices are motorized and some use a hand crank (Figure C). A portion of the device moves from the stretcher to the bed, sliding under the patient, bridging the bed and stretcher. The device is then returned to the stretcher, effectively moving the patient without pulling by staff members.

FIGURE C. Mechanical lateral-assist device.

TRANSFER CHAIRS

Chairs that can convert into stretchers are available. These are useful with patients who have no weight-bearing capacity, cannot follow directions, and/or cannot cooperate. The back of the chair bends back and the leg supports elevate to form a stretcher configuration, eliminating the need for lifting the patient. Some of these chairs have built-in mechanical aids to perform the patient transfer, as detailed above.

(continued)

Fundamentals Review 9-3   continued

EQUIPMENT AND ASSISTIVE DEVICES

POWERED STAND-ASSIST AND REPOSITIONING LIFTS

Powered stand-assist and repositioning devices can be used with patients who have weight-bearing ability in at least one leg, who can follow directions, and are cooperative. A simple sling is placed around the patient's back and under the arms (Figure D). The patient's feet rest on the device's footrest and then the patient places his or her hands on the handle. The device mechanically assists the patient to stand, without any lifting by the nurse. Once the patient is standing, the device can be wheeled to a chair, the toilet, or bed. Some devices have removable footrests and can be used as a walker. Some have scales incorporated into the device that can be used to weigh the patient.

FIGURE D. Stand-assist device. © Invacare Corporation. Used with permission.

POWERED FULL-BODY LIFTS

Powered full-body lifts are used with patients who cannot bear any weight to move them out of bed, into and out of a chair, and to a commode or stretcher. A full-body sling is placed under the patient's body, including head and torso, and then the sling is attached to the lift. The device slowly lifts the patient. Some devices can be lowered to the floor to pick up a patient who has fallen. These devices are available on portable bases and ceiling-mounted tracks (see Figure 6 in Skill 9-5). Note: For safe operation, a mobile lifts' wheels must be positioned under the patient, which makes them unsuitable for use with platform beds used typically in psychiatric units (Smith et al., 2015). The duration of time spent in slings should be limited to reduce risks for pressure injuries, especially for vulnerable populations (Peterson et al., 2015).

Fundamentals Review 9-4

ASSESSMENT CRITERIA AND CARE PLAN FOR SAFE PATIENT HANDLING AND MOVEMENT

I. Patient's Level of Assistance:

_____ Independent—Patient performs task safely, with or without staff assistance, with or without assistive devices.

_____ Partial Assist—Patient requires no more help than standby, cueing, or coaxing, or caregiver is required to lift no more than 35 lb of a patient's weight.

_____ Dependent—Patient requires nurse to lift more than 35 lb of the patient's weight, or patient is unpredictable in the amount of assistance offered. In this case, assistive devices should be used.

An assessment should be made prior to each task if the patient has varying levels of ability to assist due to medical reasons, fatigue, medications, etc. When in doubt, assume the patient cannot assist with the transfer/repositioning.

II. Weight-Bearing Capability

_____ Full

_____ Partial

_____ None

III. Bilateral Upper-Extremity Strength

_____ Yes

_____ No

Fundamentals Review 9-4 continued

ASSESSMENT CRITERIA AND CARE PLAN FOR SAFE PATIENT HANDLING AND MOVEMENT

IV. Patient's level of cooperation and comprehension:

_____ Cooperative—May need prompting; able to follow simple commands.

_____ Unpredictable or varies (patient whose behavior changes frequently should be considered as unpredictable), not cooperative, or unable to follow simple commands.

V. Weight: _____ Height: _____

Body Mass Index (BMI) (needed if patient's weight is over 300 lb)[a]:_____
  If BMI exceeds 50, institute Bariatric Algorithms

The presence of the following conditions is likely to affect the transfer/repositioning process and should be considered when identifying equipment and technique needed to move the patient.

VI. Check applicable conditions likely to affect transfer/repositioning techniques.

_____ Hip/Knee/Shoulder Replacements	_____ Respiratory/Cardiac Compromise	_____ Fractures
_____ History of Falls	_____ Wounds Affecting Transfer/Positioning	_____ Splints/Traction
_____ Paralysis/Paresis	_____ Amputation	_____ Severe Osteoporosis
_____ Unstable Spine	_____ Urinary/Fecal Stoma	_____ Severe Pain/Discomfort
_____ Severe Edema	_____ **Contractures**/Spasms	_____ Postural Hypotension
_____ Very Fragile Skin	_____ Tubes (e.g., IV, Chest)	

Comments:_____
_____
_____

VII. Appropriate Lift/Transfer Devices Needed:

Vertical Lift: _____
_____

Horizontal Lift: _____
_____

Other Patient Handling Devices Needed: _____
_____

Sling Type: Seated _____ Seated (Amputee) _____ Standing _____ Supine _____ Ambulation _____ Limb Support _____

Sling Size: _____

Signature: _____ **Date:** _____

[a]If patient's weight is over 300 lb, the BMI is needed.

For Online BMI table and calculator see: http://www.nhlbi.nih.gov/guidelines/obesity/bmi_tbl.htm; (*Source:* VHA Center for Engineering & Occupational Safety and Health (CEOSH). (2016). *Safe patient handling and mobility guidebook.* St. Louis, MO: Author. Retrieved http://www.tampavaref.org/safe-patient-handling.htm.)

Skill 9-1   Assisting a Patient With Turning in Bed

Patients experiencing decreased mobility as a result of illness or injury may be unable to reposition themselves. Knowledge of correct body alignment, principles of patient care ergonomics, safe patient handling and movement techniques, and assistive devices to turn the patient in bed are crucial to achieve patient movement and avoid injury. The Safe Patient Handling Algorithm 3 (Figure 1) can help you make decisions about safe patient handling and movement. Mastering and using these techniques will help you maintain a turn schedule to prevent complications for a patient who is immobile. During any patient handling task, if any caregiver is required to lift more than 35 lb of a patient's weight, consider the patient to be fully dependent and use assistive devices (Smith, Gibbs, Rosen, & Lee, 2015). Refer to Box 9-1 for general guidelines related to mobility and safe handling of people with dementia.

(continued)

Skill 9-1 ► Assisting a Patient With Turning in Bed *(continued)*

Algorithm 3: Reposition in Bed

Notes:
- DO NOT PULL FROM HEAD OF BED. Manual patient repositioning is dangerous.
- Discourage and remove draw sheets from beds and replace them with full body slings for repositioning. Using draw sheets on beds gives conflicting messages and makes the transition to technology use more difficult.
- The repositioning sling should be placed before a dependent patient is transferred to the surface.
- Inflate mattress of low air loss beds to maximum setting to assist in repositioning.
- Although some specialty beds turn and/or rotate the patient, most specialists confirm that bed rotations are not sufficient to off load pressure off patient and recommend that use of a repositioning sling is the best option for full turns. Confirm with Wound Care that off-loading pressure is accomplished appropriately.
- When using bed repositioning option, caregiver must assess skin integrity, support the turn, adjust limbs, and provide pillow supports.
- For patients with delicate skin or pressure ulcers, care must be taken to avoid shearing force.
- Working height should be appropriate for staff safety, at about elbow height.
- For patients that can assist in moving up in bed, to encourage them to help, ask the patient to hold on the side rails above head, to help pull themselves up in bed, then to flex knees and push on the count of three.
- Verify equipment is locked prior to transfer/movement.
- If using seated sling, air assisted lateral transfer device, or friction reducing device, obtain facility direction for leaving under patient.
- The force required to logroll a patient is about 32% of the patient's body weight.
- The force required to pull a dependent patient on a draw sheet is about 72.6% of the patient's body weight.
- Caregivers should avoid push or pull forces greater than 20% of their own weight.

FIGURE 1. Step-by-step procedure or algorithm used to outline safe technique for repositioning a patient in bed. (From VHA Center for Engineering & Occupational Safety and Health [CEOSH]. [2016]. *Safe patient handling and mobility guidebook.* St. Louis, MO: Author. Retrieved http://www.tampavaref.org/safe-patient-handling.htm.)

DELEGATION CONSIDERATIONS

Assisting a patient to turn in bed may be delegated to nursing assistive personnel (NAP) or to unlicensed assistive personnel (UAP), as well as to licensed practical/vocational nurses (LPN/LVNs). The decision to delegate must be based on careful analysis of the patient's needs and circumstances, as well as the qualifications of the person to whom the task is being delegated. Refer to the Delegation Guidelines in Appendix A.

EQUIPMENT

- Friction-reducing sheet or draw sheet
- Bed surface that inflates to aid in turning
- Pillows or other supports to help the patient maintain the desired position after turning and to maintain correct body alignment for the patient
- Additional caregivers and/or safe handling equipment to assist, based on assessment
- Nonsterile gloves, if indicated; other PPE as indicated

Box 9-1 | Safe Handling of Patients With Dementia

- Be aware that communication problems and weakness can make the handling of patients with dementia challenging.
- Face the patient when speaking.
- Use clear, short sentences.
- Call patient by name.
- Use calm, reassuring tone of voice.
- Offer simple, step-by-step instructions.
- Repeat verbal cues and prompts, as necessary. This assists when thought processes are delayed.
- Determine if the patient experiencing dementia has receptive aphasia. This inability to understand what is being said results in noncompliance with verbal instructions.
- Phrase instructions positively. For example, remind the patient to "Stand up" until the chair is correctly positioned, instead of saying "Don't sit down." The patient may not register the "Don't" and will try to sit too early.

Positive instructions are more likely to result in successful maneuvers.
- Ask one question at a time, allow the patient to answer, and repeat the question, if necessary.
- Allow the patient to focus on the task; avoid correcting the process of the action unless it would be dangerous to the patient not to do so.
- Identify the patient's established patterns of behavior, customs, traits, and everyday habits and try to incorporate these habits into desired activities. For instance, a patient with dementia may resist or become frightened when a morning shower is attempted if the patient was accustomed to evening baths. Another person may have difficulty getting out of bed in the morning for the simple reason that he is being asked to get out on what he considers the wrong side of the bed.

Source: Adapted from Jootun, D., & Pryde, A. (2013). Moving and handling of patients with dementia. *Journal of Nursing Education and Practice, 3*(2), 126–131; Miller, C. (2008). Communication difficulties in hospitalized older adults with dementia: Try these techniques to make communicating with patients easier and more effective. *American Journal of Nursing, 108*(3), 58–66; and Varnam, W. (2011). How to mobilise patients with dementia to a standing position. *Nursing Older People, 23*(8), 31–36.

ASSESSMENT	Before moving a patient, check the medical record for any conditions or orders that will limit mobility. Perform a pain assessment before the time for the activity. If the patient reports pain, administer the prescribed medication in sufficient time to allow for the full effect of the analgesic. Use available algorithms to aid in assessment and decision making. Assess the patient's ability to assist with moving, the need for assistive devices, and the need for a second or third person to assist with the activity. Determine the need for bariatric equipment. Assess the patient's skin for signs of irritation, redness, edema, or blanching.
NURSING DIAGNOSIS	Determine the related factors for the nursing diagnoses based on the patient's current status. Appropriate nursing diagnoses may include: • Activity intolerance • Impaired bed mobility • Acute pain
OUTCOME IDENTIFICATION AND PLANNING	The expected outcome to achieve when assisting a patient with turning in bed is that the activity takes place without injury to patient or nurse. An additional outcome is that the patient is comfortable and maintains proper body alignment.

IMPLEMENTATION

ACTION	RATIONALE
1. Review the medical orders and nursing care plan for patient activity. Identify any movement limitations and the ability of the patient to assist with turning. **Consult patient handling algorithm, if available, to plan appropriate approach to moving the patient.**	Checking the medical orders and care plan validates the correct patient and correct procedure. Identification of limitations and ability along with use of an algorithm helps to prevent injury and aids in determining the best plan for patient movement.
2. Gather any positioning aids or supports, if necessary.	Having aids readily available promotes efficient time management.
3. Perform hand hygiene. Put on PPE, as indicated.	Hand hygiene and PPE prevent the spread of microorganisms. PPE is required based on transmission precautions.

(continued)

Skill 9-1 ▶ Assisting a Patient With Turning in Bed *(continued)*

ACTION	**RATIONALE**

 4. Identify the patient. Explain the procedure to the patient.

Patient identification validates the correct patient and correct procedure. Discussion and explanation help allay anxiety and prepare the patient for what to expect.

5. Close the curtains around the bed and close the door to the room, if possible. Position at least one nurse on either side of the bed. Place pillows, wedges, or any other support to be used for positioning within easy reach. Place the bed at an appropriate and comfortable working height, usually elbow height of the caregiver (VHACEOSH, 2016). Lower both side rails.

Closing the door or curtains provides for privacy. Proper bed height helps reduce back strain while performing the procedure. Proper positioning and lowering of the side rails facilitates moving the patient and minimizes strain on the nurses.

6. If not already in place, position a friction-reducing sheet under the patient.

Friction-reducing sheets aid in preventing shearing and in reducing friction and the force required to move the patient.

7. Using the friction-reducing sheet, move the patient to the edge of the bed, opposite the side to which he or she will be turned. Raise the side rails.

With this placement, the patient will be on the center of the bed after turning is accomplished. Raising side rails ensures patient safety.

8. If the patient is able, have the patient grasp the side rail on the side of the bed toward which he or she is turning (Figure 2). Alternately, place the patient's arms across his or her chest and cross his or her far leg over the leg toward which they are turning.

This encourages the patient to assist as much as possible with the movement. This facilitates the turning motion and protects the patient's arms during the turn.

FIGURE 2. Having patient grasp side rail on side of bed toward which he or she is turning. (*Note: Patient's covers have been pulled back in this series of photos to show skill action. Covers should be folded back just enough to work, not to expose patients unnecessarily.*) (*Photo by B. Proud.*)

9. If available, activate the bed-turn mechanism to inflate the side of the bed behind the patient's back.

Activating the turn mechanism inflates the side of the bed for approximately 10 seconds, aiding in propelling the patient to turn, and reducing the work required by the nurse. This helps avoid straining the nurse's lower back.

10. The nurse on the side of the bed toward which the patient is turning should stand opposite the patient's center with his or her feet spread about shoulder width and with one foot ahead of the other (Figure 3). Tighten your gluteal and abdominal muscles and flex your knees. Use your leg muscles to do the pulling. The other nurse should position his or her hands on the patient's shoulder and hip, assisting to roll the patient to the side. Instruct the patient to pull on the bed rail at the same time. Use the friction-reducing sheet to gently pull the patient over on his or her side (Figure 4).

Each nurse is in a stable position with good body alignment and prepared to use large muscle masses to turn the patient. These maneuvers support the patient's body and use the nurses' weight to assist with turning.

11. Use a pillow or other support behind the patient's back. Pull the shoulder blade forward and out from under the patient.

Pillow will provide support and help the patient maintain the desired position. Positioning the shoulder blade removes pressure from the bony prominence.

ACTION	**RATIONALE**

FIGURE 3. Standing opposite patient's center with feet spread about shoulder width and with one foot ahead of the other. (*Photo by B. Proud.*)

FIGURE 4. Using friction-reducing sheet to position the patient over on her side. (*Photo by B. Proud.*)

12. Make the patient comfortable and position in proper alignment, using pillows or other supports under the leg and arm, as needed. Readjust the pillow under the patient's head. Elevate the head of the bed as needed for comfort.

Positioning in proper alignment with supports ensures that the patient will be able to maintain the desired position and will be comfortable.

13. Place the bed in the lowest position, with the side rails up, as indicated. Make sure the call bell and other necessary items are within easy reach.

Adjusting the bed height ensures patient safety. Having the call bell and essential items readily available helps promote safety.

14. Clean transfer aids, per facility policy, if not indicated for single patient use. Remove gloves and other PPE, if used. Perform hand hygiene.

Proper cleaning of equipment between patient use prevents the spread of microorganisms. Proper removal of PPE reduces the risk for infection transmission and contamination of other items. Hand hygiene prevents the spread of microorganisms.

EVALUATION

The expected outcome has been met when the patient is turned and repositioned without injury to patient or nurse; and the patient is comfortable and maintains proper body alignment.

DOCUMENTATION

Guidelines

Many facilities provide areas on the bedside flow sheet to document repositioning. Be sure to document the time the patient's position was changed, use of supports, and any pertinent observations, including skin assessment. Document the patient's tolerance of the position change. Document completed assessment algorithm for patient handling and movement decision and aids used to facilitate movement.

Sample Documentation

> <u>11/10/20</u> 1130 Patient repositioned from right side to left side; alignment maintained with wedge support behind back and pillow between legs. Skin on pressure points on right side without signs of irritation, edema, or redness. Patient reports no pain with movement. Friction-reducing sheet used to facilitate transfer and left in place under patient. Three caregivers required for repositioning.
>
> —B. Clapp, RN

(continued)

Skill 9-1 ▶ Assisting a Patient With Turning in Bed (continued)

UNEXPECTED SITUATIONS AND ASSOCIATED INTERVENTIONS

- *You are turning a patient by yourself, but you realize that the patient cannot help as much as you thought and is heavier than you anticipated:* Use the call bell to summon assistance from a coworker. Alternatively, cover the patient, make sure all rails are up, lower the bed to the lowest position, and get someone to assist you. Consider using an algorithm for patient handling and movement to identify appropriate interventions, a friction-reducing sheet and two to three additional caregivers.

SPECIAL CONSIDERATIONS

- Calculate the body mass index (BMI) for patients weighing over 300 lb. If BMI exceeds 50, institute Bariatric Algorithms.

EVIDENCE FOR PRACTICE ▶

SAFE PATIENT HANDLING

VHA Center for Engineering & Occupational Safety and Health (CEOSH). (2016). *Safe patient handling and mobility guidebook.* St. Louis, MO: Author. Retrieved http://www.tampavaref.org/safe-patient-handling.htm.

   Derived from best practices within and outside health care, this guide outlines a comprehensive program to eradicate job-related musculoskeletal injuries in nursing. The program elements described in this guidebook have been tested within the Veterans Health Administration (VHA). Data from VHA and outside organizations suggest a decrease in the frequency and severity of injuries to caregivers through the use of this approach. In the long run, a decrease in the costs associated with such injuries, reductions in musculoskeletal pain, improved quality of life, and reductions in disability are anticipated.

   Refer to thePoint° for additional research on related nursing topics.

Skill 9-2 ▶ Moving a Patient Up in Bed With the Assistance of Another Caregiver

When a patient needs to be moved up in bed, it is important to avoid injuring yourself and the patient. The patient is at risk for injuries from **shearing forces** while being moved. Evaluate the patient's condition, any activity restrictions, the patient's ability to assist with positioning and to understand directions, and the patient's body weight to decide how much additional assistance is needed. This is not a one-person task. Safe Patient Handling Algorithm 4 (Figure 1 in Skill 9-1) can assist in making decisions about patient handling and movement. It is imperative to use principles of patient care ergonomics in conjunction with assistance, appropriate lifting and repositioning devices, and correct technique to avoid injuries to yourself and the patient. During any patient handling task, if any caregiver is required to lift more than 35 lb of a patient's weight, consider the patient to be fully dependent and use assistive devices (Smith et al., 2015).

Fundamentals Review 9-3 reviews examples of equipment and assistive devices that are available to aid in patient movement and handling. Box 9-1 in Skill 9-1 outlines general guidelines related to mobility and safe handling of people with dementia. The procedure below describes moving a patient using a friction-reducing sheet; the Skill Variation at the end of the skill discusses using a full-body sling to reposition the patient.

DELEGATION CONSIDERATIONS

Moving a patient up in bed may be delegated to nursing assistive personnel (NAP) or to unlicensed assistive personnel (UAP), as well as to licensed practical/vocational nurses (LPN/LVNs). The decision to delegate must be based on careful analysis of the patient's needs and circumstances, as well as the qualifications of the person to whom the task is being delegated. Refer to the Delegation Guidelines in Appendix A.

EQUIPMENT	• Friction-reducing sheet or other friction-reducing device • Nonsterile gloves, if indicated; other PPE, as indicated • Additional caregivers to assist, based on assessment • Full-body sling lift and cover sheet, if necessary, based on assessment

ASSESSMENT	Assess the situation to determine the need to move the patient up in the bed. Review the medical record and nursing care plan for conditions that may influence the patient's ability to move or to be positioned. Assess for tubes, IV lines, incisions, or equipment that may alter the positioning procedure. Assess the patient's level of consciousness, ability to understand and follow directions, and ability to assist with moving. Assess the patient's weight and your strength to determine the number of caregivers required to assist with the activity. Use available algorithms to aid in assessment and decision making. Determine the need for bariatric equipment. Assess the patient's skin for signs of irritation, redness, edema, or blanching.

NURSING DIAGNOSIS	Determine the related factors for the nursing diagnoses based on the patient's current status. Appropriate nursing diagnoses may include: • Activity intolerance • Impaired bed mobility • Risk for injury

OUTCOME IDENTIFICATION AND PLANNING	The expected outcome to achieve when moving a patient up in bed with the assistance of another caregiver is that the patient is repositioned, remains free from injury, and maintains proper body alignment. Additional outcomes may include the following: the patient reports improved comfort; and the patient's skin is clean, dry, and intact, and without any redness, irritation, or breakdown.

IMPLEMENTATION

ACTION	RATIONALE
1. Review the medical record and nursing care plan for conditions that may influence the patient's ability to move or to be positioned. Assess for tubes, IV lines, incisions, or equipment that may alter the positioning procedure. Identify any movement limitations. **Consult patient handling algorithm, if available, to plan appropriate approach to moving the patient.**	Reviewing the order and care plan validates the correct patient and correct procedure. Identification of limitations and ability and use of an algorithm helps to prevent injury and aids in determining best plan for patient movement.
2. Perform hand hygiene and put on PPE, if indicated.	Hand hygiene and PPE prevent the spread of microorganisms. PPE is required based on transmission precautions.
3. Identify the patient. Explain the procedure to the patient.	Patient identification validates the correct patient and correct procedure. Discussion and explanation help allay anxiety and prepare the patient for what to expect.
4. Close the curtains around the bed and close the door to the room, if possible. Place the bed at an appropriate and comfortable working height, usually elbow height of the caregiver (VHACEOSH, 2016). Adjust the head of the bed to a flat position or as low as the patient can tolerate. Place the bed in slight Trendelenburg position, if the patient is able to tolerate it.	Closing the door or curtains provides for privacy. Proper bed height helps reduce back strain while you are performing the procedure. Flat positioning helps to decrease the gravitational pull of the upper body. Placing the bed in slight Trendelenburg position aids movement.
5. Remove all pillows from under the patient. Leave one at the head of the bed, leaning upright against the headboard.	Removing pillows from under the patient facilitates movement; placing a pillow at the head of the bed prevents accidental head injury against the top of the bed.

(continued)

Skill 9-2 ▶ Moving a Patient Up in Bed With the Assistance of Another Caregiver *(continued)*

ACTION	RATIONALE
6. Position at least one nurse on either side of the bed, and lower both side rails.	Proper positioning and lowering the side rails facilitate moving the patient and minimize strain on the nurses.
7. If a friction-reducing sheet (or device) is not in place under the patient, place one under the patient's midsection.	A friction-reducing device supports the patient's weight and reduces friction during the repositioning.
8. Ask the patient (if able) to bend his or her legs and put his or her feet flat on the bed to assist with the movement.	Patient can use major muscle groups to push. Even if the patient is too weak to push on the bed, placing the legs in this fashion will assist with movement and prevent skin shearing on the heels.
9. Have the patient fold the arms across the chest. Have the patient (if able) lift the head with chin on chest.	Positioning in this manner provides assistance, reduces friction, and prevents **hyperextension** of the neck.
10. One nurse should be positioned on each side of the bed, at the patient's midsection, with feet spread shoulder width apart and one foot slightly in front of the other.	Doing so positions each nurse opposite the center of the body mass, lowers the center of gravity, and reduces the risk for injury.
11. If available on bed, engage mechanism to make the bed surface firmer for repositioning.	Decreases friction and effort needed to move the patient.
12. Grasp the friction-reducing sheet securely, close to the patient's body.	Having the sheet close to the body brings the patient's center of gravity closer to each nurse and provides for a secure hold.
13. Flex your knees and hips. Tighten your abdominal and gluteal muscles and keep your back straight.	Using the legs' large muscle groups and tightening muscles during transfer prevent back injury.
14. If possible, the patient can assist with the move by pushing with the legs. Shift your weight back and forth from your back leg to your front leg and count to three (Figure 1). On the count of three, move the patient up in bed (Figure 2). Repeat the process, if necessary, to get the patient to the right position.	If the patient assists, the nurses exert less effort. The rocking motion uses the nurses' weight to counteract the patient's weight. Rocking develops momentum, which provides a smooth lift with minimal exertion by the nurses.

FIGURE 1. Nurses positioned at patient's midsection, shifting weight from back leg to front leg in preparation for move. (*Note: Patient's covers have been pulled back in this series of photos to show skill action. Covers should be folded back just enough to work, not expose patients unnecessarily.*)

FIGURE 2. Patient moved up in bed.

ACTION

15. Assist the patient to a comfortable position and readjust the pillows and supports, as needed. Take bed out of Trendelenburg position and return bed surface to normal setting, if necessary. Raise the side rails. Place the bed in the lowest position (Figure 3). Make sure the call bell and other necessary items are within easy reach.

FIGURE 3. Adjusting bed to a safe and comfortable position.

16. Clean transfer aids, per facility policy, if not indicated for single patient use. Remove gloves or other PPE, if used. Perform hand hygiene.

RATIONALE

Readjusting the bed and adjusting the bed height ensure patient safety and comfort. Having the call bell and essential items readily available helps promote safety.

Proper cleaning of equipment between patient use prevents the spread of microorganisms. Proper removal of PPE reduces the risk for infection transmission and contamination of other items. Hand hygiene prevents the spread of microorganisms.

EVALUATION

The expected outcome has been met when the patient is moved up in bed without injury, maintains proper body alignment, is comfortable, and demonstrates intact skin without evidence of any breakdown.

DOCUMENTATION

Guidelines

Many facilities provide areas on the bedside flow sheet to document repositioning. Document the time the patient's position was changed, use of supports, and any pertinent observations, including skin assessment. Document the completed assessment algorithm for patient handling and movement decision and the patient's tolerance of the position change. Document aids used to facilitate movement.

Sample Documentation

11/10/20 1130 Patient repositioned from right side to left side; alignment maintained with wedge support behind back and pillow between legs. Skin on pressure points on right side without signs of irritation, edema, or redness. Patient reports no pain with movement. Tolerated without adverse effect.

—B. Clapp, RN

(continued)

Skill 9-2 ▶ Moving a Patient Up in Bed With the Assistance of Another Caregiver *(continued)*

UNEXPECTED SITUATIONS AND ASSOCIATED INTERVENTIONS

- *You are attempting to move a patient up in the bed with another nurse. Your first attempt is unsuccessful, and you realize the patient is too heavy for only two people to move:* Obtain the assistance of at least two other coworkers. Make use of available friction-reducing devices. Use full-body lift, if available. Position opposing pairs at the patient's shoulders and buttocks to distribute the weight. If necessary, have a fifth person lift the patient's legs or heels. The movement of a very large patient is aided by putting the bed in a slight Trendelenburg position temporarily, provided the patient can tolerate it.

SPECIAL CONSIDERATIONS

- When moving a patient with a leg or foot problem, such as a cast, wound, or **fracture**, one assistant should be assigned to lift and move that extremity.
- Calculate the BMI for patients weighing over 300 lb. If BMI exceeds 50, institute Bariatric Algorithms.

Skill Variation ▶ Using Full-Body Sling to Reposition Patient

1. Review the medical record and nursing care plan for conditions that may influence the patient's ability to move or to be positioned. Assess for tubes, IV lines, incisions, or equipment that may alter the positioning procedure. Identify any movement limitations. **Consult patient handling algorithm, if available, to plan appropriate approach to moving the patient** (see Figure 1 in Skill 9-1).
2. Check equipment for proper functioning.

3. Perform hand hygiene and put on gloves and/or other PPE, as indicated.

4. Identify the patient. Explain the procedure to the patient.

5. Close the curtains around the bed and close the door to the room, if possible. Place the bed at an appropriate and comfortable working height. Adjust the head of the bed to a flat position or as low as the patient can tolerate.
6. Remove all pillows from under the patient. Leave one at the head of the bed, leaning upright against the headboard.
7. Position at least one nurse on either side of the bed, and lower both side rails.
8. Place cover sheet on sling surface. Place sling under patient.

9. Roll the base of the lift under the side of the bed nearest to the chair. **Center the frame over the patient. Lock the wheels of the lift.**
10. **Using the base-adjustment lever, widen the stance of the base of the device.**
11. Position yourself and the other caregiver at the patient's midsection. If necessary, additional staff can support the patient's legs.
12. Crank or engage the mechanism to raise the sling, with the patient, up off the bed. Raise the patient just high enough to clear the bed surface.
13. Guide the sling and relocate the patient to the appropriate place at the head of the bed.
14. Release the sling slowly or activate the lowering device on the lift and slowly lower the patient to the bed surface.
15. Remove the sling or leave in place for future use, based on facility policy.
16. Assist the patient to a comfortable position and readjust the pillows and supports, as needed.
17. Raise the side rails. Place the bed in the lowest position. Make sure the call bell and other necessary items are within easy reach.

18. Clean transfer aids, per facility policy, if not indicated for single patient use. Remove gloves and any other PPE, if used, and perform hand hygiene.

EVIDENCE FOR PRACTICE ▶

SAFE PATIENT HANDLING
VHA Center for Engineering & Occupational Safety and Health (CEOSH). (2016). *Safe patient handling and mobility guidebook.* St. Louis, MO: Author. Retrieved http://www.tampavaref.org/safe-patient-handling.htm.

Refer to details in Skill 9-1, Evidence for Practice, and refer to thePoint® for additional research on related nursing topics.

Skill 9-3 ▶ Transferring a Patient From the Bed to a Stretcher

Considerable care must be taken when moving someone from one surface to another, such as from a bed to a stretcher or from a stretcher to a bed, to prevent injury to the patient or staff. Refer to Figure 1, Safe Patient Handling Algorithm 2, to help in making decisions about safe patient handling and movement. It is imperative to use principles of patient care ergonomics in conjunction with assistance, appropriate lifting and repositioning devices, and correct technique to avoid injuries to yourself and the patient. During any patient handling task, if any caregiver is required to lift more than 35 lb of a patient's weight, consider the patient to be fully dependent and use assistive devices (Smith et al., 2015). Be familiar with the proper way to use lateral-assist devices, based on the manufacturer's directions. Fundamentals Review 9-3 reviews examples of equipment and assistive devices that are available to aid in patient movement and handling. Box 9-1 in Skill 9-1 outlines general guidelines to consider related to mobility and safe handling of people with dementia.

Algorithm 2: Lateral Transfer to/from Supine Positions: Bed, Stretcher, Trolley, Procedure Table

Notes:
- Confirm destination surfaces (bed, stretcher, exam table, etc.) and patient handling equipment MEET WEIGHT, WIDTH, and HEIGHT REQUIREMENTS of patient.
- If patient needs to be pulled up in bed prior to transfer, see Repositioning in Bed (Algorithm 3).
- High/low beds, adjustable exam tables, and stretchers are ideal for making transfers easier.
- Lock all wheeled equipment before transfer.
- When using air assisted lateral transfer device, ALWAYS move feet first, followed by upper torso and head, to determine if is safe to continue the move and to prevent patient from falling through the space between sending and receiving surfaces.
- Destination surface should be ½-inch lower than sending surface for all lateral patient moves.
- Ensure that at least one caregiver is on the destination side.
- For patients with delicate skin or pressure ulcers, care must be taken to avoid shearing force by dragging patient against surfaces.
- Friction reducing devices vary greatly in design and efficiency. Sometimes a combination of a slide board and another type can reduce forces more than either one alone.
- The force required to logroll a patient is about 32% of the patient's body weight.
- Caregivers should avoid push or pull forces greater than 20% of their own weight.

FIGURE 1. Step-by-step procedure or algorithm used to outline safe technique for transferring a patient from bed to a stretcher. (From VHA Center for Engineering & Occupational Safety and Health [CEOSH]. [2016]. *Safe patient handling and mobility guidebook.* St. Louis, MO: Author. Retrieved http://www.tampavaref.org/safe-patient-handling.htm.)

(continued)

Skill 9-3 ▸ Transferring a Patient From the Bed to a Stretcher (continued)

DELEGATION CONSIDERATIONS

The transfer of a patient from bed to stretcher may be delegated to nursing assistive personnel (NAP) or to unlicensed assistive personnel (UAP), as well as to licensed practical/vocational nurses (LPN/LVNs). The decision to delegate must be based on careful analysis of the patient's needs and circumstances, as well as the qualifications of the person to whom the task is being delegated. Refer to the Delegation Guidelines in Appendix A.

EQUIPMENT

- Transport stretcher
- Friction-reducing sheet
- Lateral-assist device, such as a transfer board, roller board, or mechanical lateral-assist device, if available
- Bath blanket
- Regular blanket
- At least two assistants, depending on the patient's condition
- Nonsterile gloves and/or other PPE, as indicated

ASSESSMENT

Review the medical record and nursing care plan for conditions that may influence the patient's ability to move or to be transferred. Assess for tubes, IV lines, incisions, or equipment that may alter the transfer process. Assess the patient's level of consciousness, ability to understand and follow directions, and ability to assist with the transfer. Assess the patient's weight and your strength to determine if a fourth person (or more) is required to assist with the activity. Use available algorithms to aid in assessment and decision making. Determine a need for bariatric equipment. Assess the patient's comfort level; if needed, medicate, as ordered, with analgesics.

NURSING DIAGNOSIS

Determine the related factors for the nursing diagnoses based on the patient's current status. Appropriate nursing diagnoses may include:

- Activity intolerance
- Risk for injury
- Impaired transfer ability

OUTCOME IDENTIFICATION AND PLANNING

The expected outcome to achieve when transferring a patient from the bed to a stretcher is that the patient is transferred without injury to patient or nurse.

IMPLEMENTATION

ACTION	RATIONALE
1. Review the medical record and nursing care plan for any conditions that may influence the patient's ability to move or to be positioned. Assess for tubes, IV lines, incisions, or equipment that may alter the positioning procedure. Identify any movement limitations. **Consult patient handling algorithm, if available, to plan appropriate approach to moving the patient.**	Reviewing the medical record and care plan validates the correct patient and correct procedure. Checking for interfering equipment helps reduce the risk for injury. Identification of limitations and ability along with use of an algorithm helps to prevent injury and aids in determining the best plan for patient movement.
2. Perform hand hygiene and put on PPE, if indicated.	Hand hygiene and PPE prevent the spread of microorganisms. PPE is required based on transmission precautions.
3. Identify the patient. Explain the procedure to the patient.	Patient identification validates the correct patient and correct procedure. Discussion and explanation help allay anxiety and prepare the patient for what to expect.

ACTION	RATIONALE
4. Close the curtains around the bed and close the door to the room, if possible. Adjust the head of the bed to a flat position or as low as the patient can tolerate. Raise the bed to a height that is even with the transport stretcher (VHA-CEOSH, 2016). Lower the side rails, if in place.	Closing the door or curtains provides for privacy. Proper bed height and lowering side rails make transfer easier and decrease the risk for injury.
5. Place the bath blanket over the patient and remove the top covers from underneath.	Bath blanket provides privacy and warmth.
6. If a friction-reducing transfer sheet is not in place under the patient, place one under the patient's midsection. Have patient fold arms against chest and move chin to chest. Use the friction-reducing sheet to move the patient to the side of the bed where the stretcher will be placed. Alternately, place a lateral-assist device under the patient. Follow manufacturer's directions for use.	A friction-reducing sheet supports the patient's weight, reduces friction during the lift, and provides for a secure hold. Positioning with chin to chest and arms folded provides assistance, reduces friction, and prevents hyperextension of the neck. A transfer board or other lateral-assist device makes it easier to move the patient and minimizes the risk for injury to the patient and nurses.
7. Position the stretcher next (and parallel) to the bed. **Lock the wheels on the stretcher and the bed.**	Positioning equipment makes the transfer easier and decreases the risk for injury. Locking the wheels keeps the bed and stretcher from moving.
8. Two nurses should stand on the stretcher side of the bed. A third nurse should stand on the side of the bed without the stretcher.	Team coordination provides for patient safety during transfer.
9. Use the friction-reducing sheet to roll the patient away from the stretcher (Figure 2). Place the transfer board across the space between the stretcher and the bed, partially under the patient (Figure 3). Roll the patient onto his or her back, so that the patient is partially on the transfer board.	The transfer board or other lateral-assist device reduces friction, easing the workload to move patient.

FIGURE 2. Using sheet to roll patient away from stretcher.

FIGURE 3. Positioning transfer board under patient.

10. The nurse on the side of the bed without the stretcher should grasp the friction-reducing sheet at the head and chest areas of the patient. The nurse on the stretcher side of the bed should grasp the friction-reducing sheet at the head and chest, and the other nurse on that side should grasp the friction-reducing sheet at the chest and leg areas of the patient.

Grasping the friction-reducing sheet at these locations evenly supports the patient.

(continued)

Skill 9-3 ▶ Transferring a Patient From the Bed to a Stretcher *(continued)*

ACTION	RATIONALE
11. At a signal given by one of the nurses, have the nurses standing on the stretcher side of the bed pull the friction-reducing sheet. At the same time, the nurse (or nurses) on the other side push, transferring the patient's weight toward the transfer board, and pushing the patient from the bed to the stretcher (Figure 4).	Working in unison distributes the work of moving the patient and facilitates the transfer.
12. Once the patient is transferred to the stretcher, remove the transfer board, and secure the patient until the side rails are raised (Figure 5). Raise the side rails. To ensure the patient's comfort, cover the patient with blanket and remove the bath blanket from underneath. Leave the friction-reducing sheet in place for the return transfer. Make sure the call bell and other necessary items are within easy reach.	Side rails promote safety. Blanket promotes comfort and warmth. Having the call bell and essential items readily available helps promote safety.

FIGURE 4. Transferring patient onto stretcher.

FIGURE 5. Securing patient on stretcher.

13. Clean transfer aids, per facility policy, if not indicated for single patient use. Remove gloves and any other PPE, if used. Perform hand hygiene.	Proper cleaning of equipment between patient use prevents the spread of microorganisms. Proper removal of PPE reduces the risk for infection transmission and contamination of other items. Hand hygiene prevents the spread of microorganisms.

EVALUATION   The expected outcome has been met when the patient has been transferred to the stretcher without injury to patient or nurse.

DOCUMENTATION

Guidelines   Document the time and method of transport, and patient's destination, according to facility policy. Document the completed assessment algorithm for patient handling and movement decision and the use of transfer aids and number of staff required for transfer.

Sample Documentation

> <u>5/12/20</u> 1005 Patient transferred to stretcher via three-person assistance and lateral-assist transfer sheet. Transported to radiology for chest x-ray.
>
> —*M. Joliet, RN*

UNEXPECTED SITUATIONS AND ASSOCIATED INTERVENTIONS

- *Your patient needs to be transported to another department by stretcher. The patient is very heavy and somewhat confused, so you are concerned about his ability to cooperate with the transfer:* Consult a Bariatric Algorithm. Obtain the assistance of three or more additional coworkers. Use a mechanical lateral-transfer device or air-assisted transfer device to move the patient.

SPECIAL CONSIDERATIONS

- If the patient is fully able to assist in the transfer, allow the patient to complete the movement independently, with supervision for safety. If the patient is partially able or not able to assist at all and weighs less than 200 lb, use a friction-reducing device and/or a lateral-transfer board. If the patient is partially able or not able to assist at all and weighs more than 200 lb, a ceiling lift with supine sling, a mechanical lateral-transfer device or air-assisted device, and three caregivers are required (VHACEOSH, 2016). If the patient is unconscious or weakened, additional nurses are needed to support the extremities and the head. When returning the patient to the bed from the stretcher, the same techniques are used.
- Some mechanical lateral-transfer aids are motorized and others use a hand crank. If a mechanical lateral-assist device is used, follow the manufacturer's directions for safe movement of the patient. Be familiar with weight restrictions for individual pieces of equipment.
- Keep in mind that the transfer of patients is often delegated to unlicensed personnel. Before moving patients, all personnel need to complete instructions about this skill and must be able to provide return demonstrations of transfer skills. When a patient is being transferred, communicate clearly any mobility restrictions or special care needs.
- Calculate the BMI for patients weighing over 300 lb. If BMI exceeds 50, institute Bariatric Algorithms.

EVIDENCE FOR PRACTICE ▶

PATIENT TRANSFER AND ASSISTIVE DEVICES

Patient care providers are at risk for musculoskeletal injuries associated with patient transfer and mobility activities. The use of patient transfer devices is recommended to reduce the risk of low back injuries from patient handling.

Related Research

Bacharach, D. W., Miller, K., & von Duvillard, S. P. (2016). Saving your back: How do horizontal patient transfer devices stack up? *Nursing, 46*(1), 59–64.

This study evaluated the use of a roller tray and compared its use with three other transfer devices: a slide board, a nylon tube, and a roller board. A roller tray is a new transfer device consisting of a sleeve made of synthetic material covered by a disposable absorbent under pad. Transfers were coordinated with several caregivers: one pusher and one or two pullers, as well as a third or fourth caregiver to transfer the subject's legs. The third and fourth caregivers were not included in measurements. Each of the devices was used to transfer three subjects from an exam table to a hospital bed three times each. During these transfers, static and dynamic friction were measured, as was flexor torque (the load on the lower back of the caregivers). Caregivers also ranked each device for functionality and ease of use. Statistical analyses were used to determine differences in static friction, dynamic friction, and peak trunk torque between conditions. Caregivers experienced the greatest L4–5 torque and the greatest low back stress moving patients weighing 70 to 90 kg (approx. 150 to 200 lb). In their ranking of the devices, caregivers favored the new roller tray over the other devices. Use of the new roller tray was associated with minimal effort to move a patient of any size; fastest total transfer time; minimal requirements for rolling and/or repositioning patients after transfer; cleanliness; and improved patient comfort. The nylon tube, roller board, and roller tray were associated with reduced static and dynamic friction and should be used whenever possible. The roller tray was favored due to time, cleanliness, and convenience considerations. The authors also concluded that "middle-weight" patients are often moved using only two instead of three caregivers, whereas three caregivers are often used to transfer heavier patients. The researchers suggested caregivers should use three caregivers (two pullers and one pusher) or a lift team, even when patients are medium weight to reduce pulling force, torque, and low back stress.

(continued)

Skill 9-3 ▶ Transferring a Patient From the Bed to a Stretcher *(continued)*

Relevance for Nursing Practice

Nurses have a responsibility to maintain up-to-date knowledge regarding best practice guidelines in providing nursing care, including the means to accomplish safe patient transfers. Appropriate transfer devices, proper body positioning, and appropriate transfer techniques are critical to reduce and eliminate injuries to nurses and other health care professionals, and contribute to safe patient care.

Refer to thePoint° for additional research on related nursing topics.

EVIDENCE FOR PRACTICE ▶

SAFE PATIENT HANDLING

VHA Center for Engineering & Occupational Safety and Health (CEOSH). (2016). *Safe patient handling and mobility guidebook.* St. Louis, MO: Author. Retrieved http://www.tampavaref.org/safe-patient-handling.htm.

Refer to details in Skill 9-1, Evidence for Practice, and refer to thePoint° for additional research on related nursing topics.

Skill 9-4 ▶ Transferring a Patient From the Bed to a Chair

Moving a patient from the bed to a chair helps him or her begin engaging in physical activity. Also, changing a patient's position will help prevent complications related to immobility. Safety and comfort are key concerns when assisting the patient out of bed. Assessing the patient's response to activity is a major nursing responsibility. Before performing the transfer, identify any restrictions related to the patient's condition and determine how activity levels may be affected. The Safe Patient Handling Algorithm 1 (Figure 1) can assist in making decisions about safe patient handling and movement. It is imperative to use principles of patient care ergonomics in conjunction with assistance, appropriate lifting and repositioning devices, and correct technique to avoid injuries to yourself and the patient. During any patient handling task, if any caregiver is required to lift more than 35 lb of a patient's weight, consider the patient to be fully dependent and use assistive devices (Smith et al., 2015). Fundamentals Review 9-3 reviews examples of equipment and assistive devices that are available to aid in patient movement and handling. Box 9-1 in Skill 9-1 outlines general guidelines to consider related to mobility and safe handling of people with dementia.

DELEGATION CONSIDERATIONS

The transfer of a patient from bed to a chair may be delegated to nursing assistive personnel (NAP) or to unlicensed assistive personnel (UAP), as well as to licensed practical/vocational nurses (LPN/LVNs). The decision to delegate must be based on careful analysis of the patient's needs and circumstances, as well as the qualifications of the person to whom the task is being delegated. Refer to the Delegation Guidelines in Appendix A.

EQUIPMENT

- Chair or wheelchair
- Gait belt
- Stand-assist aid, if available
- Additional staff person to assist
- Blanket to cover the patient in the chair
- Nonsterile gloves and/or other PPE, as indicated

Algorithm 1: Transfer to/from Seated Positions: Bed to Chair, Chair to Chair, Chair to Exam Table

Notes:
- If patient has partial weight-bearing capacity, transfer toward stronger side.
- Ensure all chairs, beds, stretchers, etc. are locked
- To use seated transfer aid, chair arms must recess or be removable.
- High/low beds, adjustable exam tables, and stretchers are ideal for making transfers easier.
- Always transfer toward stronger side.
- NEVER use a gait belt to lift, transfer, or catch a patient.

FIGURE 1. Step-by-step procedure or algorithm used to outline safe techniques for transferring a patient to and from bed to chair. (From VHA Center for Engineering & Occupational Safety and Health [CEOSH]. [2016]. *Safe patient handling and mobility guidebook*. St. Louis, MO: Author. Retrieved http://www.tampavaref.org/safe-patient-handling.htm.)

ASSESSMENT

Assess the situation to determine the need to get the patient out of bed. Review the medical record and nursing care plan for conditions that may influence the patient's ability to move or to be transferred. Check for tubes, IV lines, incisions, or equipment that may require modifying the transfer procedure. Assess the patient's level of consciousness, ability to understand and follow directions, and ability to assist with the transfer. Assess the patient's weight and your strength to determine if additional assistance is needed. Use available algorithms to aid in assessment and decision making. Determine the need for bariatric equipment. Assess the patient's comfort level; if needed, medicate as ordered with analgesics.

(continued)

Skill 9-4 ▶ Transferring a Patient From the Bed to a Chair *(continued)*

NURSING DIAGNOSIS	Determine the related factors for the nursing diagnoses based on the patient's current status. Appropriate nursing diagnoses may include:

- Activity intolerance
- Risk for falls
- Impaired transfer ability

OUTCOME IDENTIFICATION AND PLANNING	The expected outcome to achieve when transferring a patient from the bed to a chair is that the transfer is accomplished without injury to patient or nurse.

IMPLEMENTATION

ACTION	RATIONALE
1. Review the medical record and nursing care plan for conditions that may influence the patient's ability to move or to be positioned. Assess for tubes, IV lines, incisions, or equipment that may alter the positioning procedure. Identify any movement limitations. **Consult patient handling algorithm, if available, to plan appropriate approach to moving the patient.**	Reviewing the medical record and care plan validates the correct patient and correct procedure. Identification of limitations and ability and use of an algorithm help to prevent injury and aid in determining best plan for patient movement.
2. Perform hand hygiene and put on PPE, as indicated.	Hand hygiene and PPE prevent spread of microorganisms. PPE is required based on transmission precautions.
3. Identify the patient. Explain the procedure to the patient.	Patient identification validates the correct patient and correct procedure. Discussion and explanation help allay anxiety and prepare the patient for what to expect.
4. If needed, move equipment to make room for the chair. Close the curtains around the bed and close the door to the room, if possible.	A clear pathway from the bed to the chair facilitates the transfer. Closing the door or curtains provides for privacy.
5. Place the bed in the lowest position. Raise the head of the bed to a sitting position, or as high as the patient can tolerate.	Proper bed height and positioning facilitate the transfer. The amount of energy needed to move from a sitting position or elevated position to a sitting position is decreased.
6. **Make sure the bed brakes are locked. Put the chair next to the bed. If available, lock the brakes of the chair. If the chair does not have brakes, brace the chair against a secure object.**	Locking brakes or bracing the chair prevents movement during transfer and increases stability and patient safety.
7. Encourage the patient to make use of a stand-assist aid, either freestanding or attached to the side of the bed, if available, to move to the side of the bed and to a side-lying position, facing the side of the bed on which the patient will sit.	Encourages independence, reduces strain for staff, and decreases risk for patient injury.
8. Lower the side rail, if necessary, and stand near the patient's hips. Stand with your legs shoulder width apart with one foot near the head of the bed, slightly in front of the other foot.	The nurse's center of gravity is placed near the patient's greatest weight to assist the patient to a sitting position safely.
9. Encourage the patient to make use of the stand-assist device. Assist the patient to sit up on the side of the bed; ask the patient to swing his or her legs over the side of the bed. At the same time, pivot on your back leg to lift the patient's trunk and shoulders. Keep your back straight; avoid twisting.	Gravity lowers the patient's legs over the bed. The nurse transfers weight in the direction of motion and protects his or her back from injury.

ACTION	**RATIONALE**
10. Stand in front of the patient, and assess for any balance problems or complaints of dizziness (Figure 2). Allow the patient's legs to dangle a few minutes before continuing.	Standing in front of the patient prevents falls or injuries from orthostatic hypotension. The sitting position facilitates transfer to the chair and allows the circulatory system to adjust to a change in position.
11. Assist the patient to put on a robe, as necessary and nonskid footwear.	Robe provides warmth and privacy. Nonskid soles reduce the risk for falling.
12. Wrap the gait belt around the patient's waist, based on assessed need and facility policy (Figure 3).	Gait belts improve the caregiver's grasp, reducing the risk of musculoskeletal injuries to staff and the patient. Provides firmer grasp for the caregiver if patient should lose his or her balance.

FIGURE 2. Standing in front of patient and assessing for any balance problems or complaints of dizziness.

FIGURE 3. Wrapping gait belt around patient's waist.

13. Stand facing the patient. Spread your feet about shoulder width apart and flex your hips and knees.	This position provides stability and allows for smooth movement using the legs' large muscle groups.
14. Ask the patient to slide his or her buttocks to the edge of the bed until the feet touch the floor. Position yourself as close as possible to the patient, with your foot positioned on the outside of the patient's foot. If a second staff person is assisting, have him or her assume a similar position. Grasp the gait belt (Figure 4).	Doing so provides balance and support.
15. Encourage the patient to make use of the stand-assist device. If necessary, have second staff person grasp the gait belt on opposite side. Rock back and forth while counting to three. **On the count of three, using the gait belt and your legs (not your back), assist the patient to a standing position (Figure 5).** If indicated, brace your front knee against the patient's weak extremity as he or she stands. Assess the patient's balance and leg strength. If the patient is weak or unsteady, return the patient to bed.	Holding at the gait belt prevents injury to the patient. Bracing your knee against a weak extremity prevents a weak knee from buckling and the patient from falling. Assessing balance and strength helps to identify the need for additional assistance to prevent falling.

FIGURE 4. Standing close to patient and grasping gait belt.

FIGURE 5. Using gait belt and pushing with legs to help raise the patient to a standing position.

(continued)

Skill 9-4 ▶ Transferring a Patient From the Bed to a Chair *(continued)*

ACTION	RATIONALE
16. Pivot on your back foot and assist the patient to turn until the patient feels the chair against his or her legs.	This action ensures proper positioning before sitting.
17. Ask the patient to use his or her arm to steady him- or herself on the arm of the chair while slowly lowering to a sitting position. Continue to brace the patient's knees with your knees and hold the gait belt. Flex your hips and knees when helping the patient sit in the chair (Figure 6).	The patient uses his or her own arm for support and stability. Flexing hips and knees uses major muscle groups to aid in movement and to reduce strain on the nurse's back.

FIGURE 6. Assisting patient to sit.

18. Assess the patient's alignment in the chair. Remove gait belt, if desired. Depending on patient comfort, it could be left in place to use when returning to bed. Cover with a blanket, if needed. Make sure call bell and other essential items are within easy reach.	Assessment promotes comfort; blanket provides warmth and privacy; having the call bell and other essential items readily available helps promote safety.

19. Clean transfer aids, per facility policy, if not indicated for single patient use. Remove gloves and any other PPE, if used. Perform hand hygiene.	Proper cleaning of equipment between patient use prevents the spread of microorganisms. Proper removal of PPE reduces the risk for infection transmission and contamination of other items. Hand hygiene prevents the spread of microorganisms.

EVALUATION

The expected outcome has been met when the patient transfers from the bed to the chair without injury to the patient or nurse.

DOCUMENTATION

Guidelines

Document the activity, including the length of time the patient sat in the chair, any other pertinent observations, and the patient's tolerance of and reaction to the activity. Document the completed assessment algorithm for patient handling and movement decision and the use of transfer aids and number of staff required for transfer.

Sample Documentation

> 5/13/20 1135 Patient dangled at side of bed for 5 minutes without complaints of dizziness or lightheadedness. Patient assisted out of bed to chair with minimal difficulty; gait belt in place. Tolerated sitting in chair for 30 minutes. Assisted back to bed. Resting in semi-Fowler's position. Both upper side rails up.
>
> —J. Minkins, RN

UNEXPECTED SITUATIONS AND ASSOCIATED INTERVENTIONS	• *You are assisting a patient out of bed. The previous times the patient has gotten up, you have not had any difficulty helping him by yourself, so you are working alone at this time. The patient is positioned on the side of the bed. You flex your hips and knees to help him stand. As you move to pivot to the chair, the patient becomes very lightheaded and weak and his knees buckle. The patient is too heavy for you to lift to the chair:* Do not continue the move to the chair. Lower the patient back to the side of the bed. Pivot him back into bed, cover him, and raise the side rails. Check vital signs and assess for any other symptoms. After his symptoms have subsided and you are ready to get him up again, arrange for the assistance of another staff member. Have the patient dangle his legs for a longer period of time before standing. Assess for lightheadedness or dizziness before helping him to stand. Notify the primary care provider if there are any significant findings or if his symptoms persist.
SPECIAL CONSIDERATIONS	• Transfer of a patient to a chair or toilet can be accomplished using a powered stand-assist and repositioning lift, if available. These devices can be used with patients who have weight-bearing ability on at least one leg and who can follow directions and are cooperative. A simple sling is placed around the patient's back and under the arms. The patient rests feet on the device's footrest and places his or her hands on the handle. The device mechanically assists the patient to stand, without any lifting by the nurse (see Fundamentals Review 9-3). Once the patient is standing, the device can be wheeled to a chair, the toilet, or bed. Some devices have removable footrests and can be used as a walker. Some have scales incorporated into the device that can be used to weigh the patient. • Patients who are unable to bear partial weight or full weight or who are uncooperative, as well as bariatric patients, should be transferred using a full-body sling lift (VHACEOSH, 2016) (refer to Skill 9-5). • Calculate the BMI for patients weighing over 300 lb. If BMI exceeds 50, institute Bariatric Algorithms. • The transfer of patients is often delegated to unlicensed personnel. Before moving patients, all personnel need to complete instructions and must be able to provide return demonstrations of transfer skills. Before the transfer, communicate clearly any mobility restrictions or special care needs.

EVIDENCE FOR PRACTICE ▶	**SAFE PATIENT HANDLING** VHA Center for Engineering & Occupational Safety and Health (CEOSH). (2016). *Safe patient handling and mobility guidebook.* St. Louis, MO: Author. Retrieved http://www.tampavaref.org/safe-patient-handling.htm. Refer to details in Skill 9-1, Evidence for Practice, and refer to thePoint for additional research on related nursing topics.

Skill 9-5 ▶ Transferring a Patient Using a Powered Full-Body Sling Lift

When it has been determined through the use of a transfer assessment and/or the patient cannot bear any weight, use a powered full-body sling lift device to move him or her up in or out of bed, into and out of a chair, and to a commode or stretcher (refer to Fundamentals Review 9-3). During any patient handling task, if any caregiver is required to lift more than 35 lb of a patient's weight, consider the patient to be fully dependent and use assistive devices (Smith et al., 2015). A full-body sling is placed under the patient's body, including head and torso, and then the sling is attached to the lift. The device slowly lifts the patient. Some devices can be lowered to the floor to pick up a patient who has fallen. These devices are available on portable bases and ceiling-mounted tracks. Each manufacturer's device is slightly different, so review the instructions for your particular device (see Fundamentals Review 9-3). Box 9-1 in Skill 9-1 outlines general guidelines related to mobility and safe handling of people with dementia.

(continued)

Skill 9-5 ▶ Transferring a Patient Using a Powered Full-Body Sling Lift (continued)

DELEGATION CONSIDERATIONS	The transfer of a patient from bed to a chair may be delegated to nursing assistive personnel (NAP) or to unlicensed assistive personnel (UAP), as well as to licensed practical/vocational nurses (LPN/LVNs). The decision to delegate must be based on careful analysis of the patient's needs and circumstances, as well as the qualifications of the person to whom the task is being delegated. Refer to the Delegation Guidelines in Appendix A.
EQUIPMENT	• Powered full-body sling lift • Sheet or pad to cover the sling, if sling is not dedicated to only one patient • Chair or wheelchair • One or more caregivers for assistance, based on assessment • Nonsterile gloves and/or other PPE, as indicated
ASSESSMENT	Assess the situation to determine the need to use the lift. Review the medical record and nursing care plan for conditions that may influence the patient's ability to move or to be transferred. Use available algorithms to aid in assessment and decision making. Determine the need for bariatric equipment. Assess for tubes, IV lines, incisions, or equipment that may alter the transfer procedure. Assess the patient's level of consciousness and ability to understand and follow directions. Assess the patient's comfort level; if needed, medicate, as ordered, with analgesics. Assess the condition of the equipment to ensure proper functioning before using with the patient.
NURSING DIAGNOSIS	Determine the related factors for the nursing diagnoses based on the patient's current status. Appropriate nursing diagnoses may include: • Risk for injury • Risk for falls • Impaired transfer ability
OUTCOME IDENTIFICATION AND PLANNING	The expected outcome to achieve when transferring a patient using a powered full-body sling lift is that the transfer is accomplished without injury to patient or nurse.

IMPLEMENTATION

ACTION	RATIONALE
1. Review the medical record and nursing care plan for conditions that may influence the patient's ability to move or to be positioned. Assess for tubes, IV lines, incisions, or equipment that may alter the positioning procedure. Identify any movement limitations. **Consult patient handling algorithm, if available, to plan appropriate approach to moving the patient.**	Reviewing the medical record and care plan validates the correct patient and correct procedure. Checking for equipment and limitations reduces the risk for injury during the transfer.
2. Perform hand hygiene and put on PPE, if indicated.	Hand hygiene and PPE prevent the spread of microorganisms. PPE is required based on transmission precautions.
3. Identify the patient. Explain the procedure to the patient.	Patient identification validates the correct patient and correct procedure. Discussion and explanation allay anxiety and prepare the patient for what to expect.
4. If needed, move the equipment to make room for the chair. Close the curtains around the bed and close the door to the room, if possible.	Moving equipment out of the way provides a clear path and facilitates the transfer. Closing the door or curtains provides for privacy.
5. Adjust the bed to a comfortable working height, usually elbow height of the caregiver (VHACEOSH, 2016). **Lock the bed brakes.**	Having the bed at the proper height prevents back and muscle strain. Locking the brakes prevents bed movement and ensures patient safety.

ACTION	**RATIONALE**
6. Lower the side rail, if in use, on the side of the bed you are working. If the sling is for use with more than one patient, place a cover or pad on the sling. Place the sling evenly under the patient. Roll the patient to one side and place half of the sling with the sheet or pad on it under the patient from shoulders to mid-thigh (Figure 1). Raise the rail and move to the other side. Lower the rail, if necessary. Roll the patient to the other side and pull the sling under the patient (Figure 2). Raise the side rail.	Lowering the side rail prevents strain on the nurse's back. Covering the sling prevents transmission of microorganisms. Some facilities, such as long-term care institutions, provide each patient with own transport sling. Rolling the patient positions the patient on the sling with minimal movement. Even distribution of the patient's weight in the sling provides for patient comfort and safety.

FIGURE 1. Rolling patient to one side and placing rolled sling underneath patient.

FIGURE 2. Rolling patient to opposite side and pulling sling under patient.

ACTION	**RATIONALE**
7. Bring the chair to the side of the bed. **Lock the wheels, if present.**	Bringing the chair close to the bed minimizes the distance needed for transfer. Locking the wheels prevents chair movement and ensures patient safety.
8. Lower the side rail on the chair side of the bed. Roll the base of the lift under the side of the bed nearest to the chair. **Center the frame over the patient. Lock the wheels of the lift.**	Lowering the rail allows for ease of transfer. Doing so reduces the distance necessary for transfer. Centering the frame helps maintain the balance of the lift. Locking the lift's wheels prevents the lift from rolling.
9. **Using the base-adjustment lever, widen the stance of the base (Figure 3).**	A wider stance provides greater stability and prevents tipping.
10. Lower the arms close enough to attach the sling to the frame (Figure 4).	Lowering the arms is necessary to allow for the attachment of the sling's hooks.

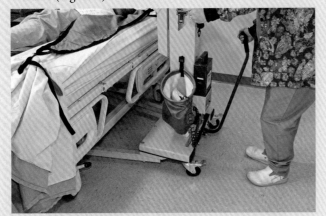

FIGURE 3. Widening stance of lift base.

FIGURE 4. Lowering lift arms.

(continued)

Skill 9-5 ▶ Transferring a Patient Using a Powered Full-Body Sling Lift *(continued)*

ACTION	RATIONALE
11. Attach the straps on the sling to the hooks on the frame (Figure 5). Short straps attach behind the patient's back and long straps attach at the other end of the sling. Check the patient to make sure the straps are not pressing into the skin. Some lifts have straps or chains with hooks that attach to holes in the sling. Check the manufacturer's instructions for each lift.	Connecting the straps or chains permits attachment of the sling to the lift. Checking the patient's skin for pressure from the hooks prevents injury.
12. Check all equipment, lines, and drains attached to the patient so that they are not interfering with the device. Have the patient fold his or her arms across the chest.	Ensuring that equipment and lines are free of the device prevents dislodgement and possible injury.
13. With a person standing on each side of the lift, tell the patient that he or she will be lifted from the bed. Support injured limbs as necessary. Engage the pump to raise the patient about 6 in above the bed (Figure 6).	Having the necessary people available provides for safety. Supporting injured limbs helps maintain stability. Informing the patient about what will occur reassures the patient and reduces fear.

FIGURE 5. Connecting lift straps.

FIGURE 6. Raising patient 6 in above bed.

14. Unlock the wheels of the lift. **Carefully wheel the patient straight back and away from the bed. Support the patient's limbs, as needed.**	Moving in this manner promotes stability and safety.
15. Position the patient over the chair with the base of the lift straddling the chair (Figure 7). Lock the wheels of the lift.	Proper positioning of the patient and device promotes stability and safety.
16. Gently lower the patient to the chair until the hooks or straps are slightly loosened from the sling or frame (Figure 8). Guide the patient into the chair with your hands as the sling lowers.	Gently lowering the patient in this manner places the patient fully in the chair and reduces the risk for injury.

FIGURE 7. Positioning patient in sling over chair.

FIGURE 8. Lowering patient in sling into chair.

ACTION	RATIONALE
17. Disconnect the hooks or strap from the frame. Keep the sling in place under the patient.	Disconnecting the hooks or straps allows the patient to be supported by the chair and promotes comfort. The sling will need to be reattached to the lift to move the patient back to bed.
18. Adjust the patient's position, using pillows, if necessary. Check the patient's alignment in the chair. Cover the patient with a blanket, if necessary. Make sure call bell and other essential items are within easy reach. When it is time for the patient to return to bed, reattach the hooks or straps and reverse the steps.	Pillows and proper alignment provide for patient safety and comfort. Having the call bell and other essential items readily available helps promote safety. Reattaching the hooks or straps allows the lift to support the patient for transfer back to bed.
19. Clean transfer aids, per facility policy, if not indicated for single patient use. Remove gloves and any other PPE, if used. Perform hand hygiene.	Proper cleaning of equipment between patient use prevents the spread of microorganisms. Proper removal of PPE reduces the risk for infection transmission and contamination of other items. Hand hygiene prevents the spread of microorganisms.

EVALUATION

The expected outcome has been met when the transfer has been accomplished without injury to patient or nurse.

DOCUMENTATION

Guidelines

Document the activity, transfer, any other pertinent observations, the patient's tolerance of the procedure, and the length of time in the chair. Document the completed assessment algorithm for patient handling and movement decision and the use of transfer aids and number of staff required for transfer.

Sample Documentation

> 5/13/20 1430 Patient transferred out of bed to chair using powered full-body sling lift. Tolerated sitting in chair for 25 minutes without complaints of dizziness or pain. Assisted back to bed via lift. Patient sitting in semi-Fowler's position with upper two side rails up.
> —P. Jefferson, RN

UNEXPECTED SITUATIONS AND ASSOCIATED INTERVENTIONS

- *You are preparing to move a patient using a powered full-body sling lift. After you apply the sling and attach it to the frame, the patient becomes anxious and tells you she is afraid:* Acknowledge the patient's feelings and explain the procedure again. Reassure the patient about the safety of the device. Obtain an additional person to support the patient during the move by holding her hand or supporting her head. If possible, plan the transfer when a family member or friend is present to offer support.

SPECIAL CONSIDERATIONS

- The duration of time spent in slings should be limited to reduce risk for pressure injuries, especially for vulnerable populations (Peterson, Kahn, Kerrigan, Gutmann, & Harrow, 2015).
- The transfer of patients is often delegated to unlicensed personnel. Before moving patients, all personnel need to complete instructions and must be able to provide return demonstrations of transfer skills. Before the transfer, communicate clearly any mobility restrictions or special care needs.
- Calculate the BMI for patients weighing over 300 lb. If BMI exceeds 50, institute Bariatric Algorithms.

EVIDENCE FOR PRACTICE ▶

SAFE PATIENT HANDLING
VHA Center for Engineering & Occupational Safety and Health (CEOSH). (2016). *Safe patient handling and mobility guidebook.* St. Louis, MO: Author. Retrieved http://www.tampavaref.org/safe-patient-handling.htm.

Refer to details in Skill 9-1, Evidence for Practice, and refer to thePoint® for additional research on related nursing topics.

(continued)

Skill 9-6 ▶ Providing Range-of-Motion Exercises

Range of motion (ROM) is the complete extent of movement of which a joint is normally capable. When a person performs routine activities of daily living (ADLs), he or she is using muscle groups that help to keep many joints in an effective ROM. When all or some of the normal ADLs are impossible due to illness or injury, it is important to give attention to the joints not being used or to those that have limited use. When the patient does the exercise for him- or herself, it is referred to as *active ROM*. Exercises performed by the nurse without participation by the patient are referred to as *passive ROM*. Exercises should be as active as the patient's physical condition permits. Allow the patient to do as much individual activity as his or her condition permits. Initiate ROM exercises as soon as possible because body changes can occur after only 3 days of impaired mobility.

DELEGATION CONSIDERATIONS	Patient teaching regarding ROM exercises cannot be delegated to nursing assistive personnel (NAP) or to unlicensed assistive personnel (UAP). Reinforcement or implementation of ROM exercises may be delegated to NAP or UAP, as well as to licensed practical/vocational nurses (LPN/LVNs). The decision to delegate must be based on careful analysis of the patient's needs and circumstances, as well as the qualifications of the person to whom the task is being delegated. Refer to the Delegation Guidelines in Appendix A.
EQUIPMENT	No special equipment or supplies are necessary to perform ROM exercises. Wear nonsterile gloves and/or other PPE, as appropriate.
ASSESSMENT	Review the medical record and nursing care plan for any conditions or orders that will limit mobility. Perform a pain assessment before the time for the exercises. If the patient reports pain, administer the prescribed medication in sufficient time to allow for the full effect of the analgesic. Assess the patient's ability to perform ROM exercises. Inspect and palpate joints for redness, tenderness, pain, swelling, or deformities.
NURSING DIAGNOSIS	Determine the related factors for the nursing diagnoses based on the patient's current status. Appropriate nursing diagnoses may include: • Risk for disuse syndrome • Deficient knowledge • Fatigue
OUTCOME IDENTIFICATION AND PLANNING	The expected outcome to achieve when performing ROM exercises is that the patient completes the exercises and maintains or improves joint mobility. Other outcomes include improving or maintaining muscle strength, and preventing muscle atrophy and **contractures**.

IMPLEMENTATION

ACTION	**RATIONALE**
1. Review the medical orders and nursing care plan for patient activity. Identify any movement limitations.	Reviewing the order and care plan validates the correct patient and correct procedure. Identification of limitations prevents injury.
2. Perform hand hygiene and put on PPE, if indicated.	Hand hygiene and PPE prevent the spread of microorganisms. PPE is required based on transmission precautions.
3. Identify the patient. Explain the procedure to the patient.	Patient identification validates the correct patient and correct procedure. Discussion and explanation help allay anxiety and prepare the patient for what to expect.
4. Close the curtains around the bed and close the door to the room, if possible. Place the bed at an appropriate and comfortable working height, usually elbow height of the caregiver (VHACEOSH, 2016). Adjust the head of the bed to a flat position or as low as the patient can tolerate.	Closing the door or curtains provides for privacy. Proper bed height helps reduce back strain while performing the procedure.

ACTION

5. Stand on the side of the bed where the joints are to be exercised. Lower side rail on that side, if in place. Uncover only the limb to be used during the exercise.

6. Perform the exercises slowly and gently, providing support by holding the areas proximal and distal to the joint. Repeat each exercise two to five times, moving each joint in a smooth and rhythmic manner. **Stop movement if the patient complains of pain or if you meet resistance.**

7. While performing the exercises, begin at the head and move down one side of the body at a time. **Encourage the patient to do as many of these exercises independently as possible.**

8. Move the chin down to rest on the chest (Figure 1). Return the head to a normal upright position (Figure 2). Tilt the head as far as possible toward each shoulder (Figure 3).

9. Move the head from side to side, bringing the chin toward each shoulder (Figure 4).

RATIONALE

Standing on the side to be exercised and lowering the side rail prevent strain on the nurse's back. Proper draping provides for privacy and warmth.

Slow, gentle movements with support prevent discomfort and muscle spasms resulting from jerky movements. Repeated movement of muscles and joints improves flexibility and increases circulation to the body part. Pain may indicate the exercises are causing damage.

Proceeding from head to toe, one side at a time, promotes efficient time management and an organized approach to the task. Both active and passive exercises improve joint mobility and increase circulation to the affected part, but only active exercise increases muscle mass, tone, and strength and improves cardiac and respiratory functioning.

These movements provide for **flexion**, **extension**, and lateral flexion of the head and neck.

These movements provide for **rotation** of neck.

FIGURE 1. Moving patient's chin down to rest on chest.

FIGURE 2. Holding patient's head upright and centered.

FIGURE 3. Moving patient's head to one shoulder.

FIGURE 4. Moving patient's chin toward one shoulder.

(continued)

Skill 9-6 ▶ Providing Range-of-Motion Exercises *(continued)*

ACTION	RATIONALE

10. Start with the arm at the patient's side (Figure 5) and lift the arm forward to above the head (Figure 6). Return the arm to the starting position at the side of the body.

These movements provide for flexion and extension of the shoulder.

FIGURE 5. Holding patient's arm at side.

FIGURE 6. Lifting patient's arm above patient's head.

11. With the arm back at the patient's side, move the arm laterally to an upright position above the head (Figure 7), and then return it to the original position. Move the arm across the body as far as possible (Figure 8).

These movements provide for **abduction** and **adduction** of the shoulder.

FIGURE 7. Moving patient's arm laterally to an upright position above patient's head.

FIGURE 8. Moving arm across patient's body as far as possible.

12. Raise the arm at the side until the upper arm is in line with the shoulder. Bend the elbow at a 90-degree angle (Figure 9) and move the forearm upward and downward, then return the arm to the side.

These movements provide for internal and external rotation of the shoulder.

13. Bend the elbow and move the lower arm and hand upward toward the shoulder (Figure 10). Return the lower arm and hand to the original position while straightening the elbow.

These movements provide for flexion and extension of the elbow.

FIGURE 9. Raising patient's arm until upper arm is in line with patient's shoulder, with elbow bent.

FIGURE 10. Bending patient's elbow, lower arm, and hand upward toward shoulder.

ACTION

14. Rotate the lower arm and hand so the palm is up (Figure 11). Rotate the lower arm and hand so the palm of the hand is down.

FIGURE 11. Rotating patient's lower arm and hand so palm is up.

15. Move the hand downward toward the inner aspect of the forearm (Figure 12). Return the hand to a neutral position even with the forearm (Figure 13). Then move the dorsal portion of the hand backward as far as possible.

FIGURE 12. Moving patient's hand downward toward inner aspect of forearm.

FIGURE 13. Returning hand to neutral position.

16. Bend the fingers to make a fist (Figure 14), and then straighten them out (Figure 15). Spread the fingers apart (Figure 16) and return them back together. Touch the thumb to each finger on the hand (Figure 17).

FIGURE 14. Bending patient's fingers to make a fist.

FIGURE 15. Straightening out patient's fingers.

RATIONALE

These movements provide for **supination** and **pronation** of the forearm.

These movements provide for flexion, extension, and hyperextension of the wrist.

These movements provide for flexion, extension, abduction, and adduction of the fingers.

(continued)

Skill 9-6 ▶ Providing Range-of-Motion Exercises *(continued)*

ACTION	RATIONALE

FIGURE 16. Spreading patient's fingers apart.

FIGURE 17. Assisting patient to touch thumb to each finger on hand.

17. Extend the leg and lift it upward (Figure 18). Return the leg to the original position beside the other leg.

These movements provide for flexion and extension of the hip.

FIGURE 18. Extending and lifting patient's leg.

18. Lift the leg laterally away from the patient's body (Figure 19). Return the leg back toward the other leg and try to extend it beyond the midline (Figure 20).

These movements provide for abduction and adduction of the hip.

FIGURE 19. Lifting patient's leg laterally away from body (abduction).

FIGURE 20. Returning leg back toward other leg and trying to extend it beyond midline, if possible.

ACTION

RATIONALE

19. Turn the foot and leg toward the opposite leg to rotate it internally (Figure 21). Turn the foot and leg outward away from the opposite leg to rotate it externally (Figure 22).

These movements provide for internal and external rotation of the hip.

FIGURE 21. Turning patient's foot and leg toward opposite leg to rotate it internally.

FIGURE 22. Turning patient's foot and leg outward, away from opposite leg, to rotate it externally.

20. Bend the leg and bring the heel toward the back of the leg (Figure 23). Return the leg to a straight position (Figure 24).

These movements provide for flexion and extension of the knee.

FIGURE 23. Bending patient's leg and bringing heel toward back of leg.

FIGURE 24. Returning leg to a straight position.

21. At the ankle, move the foot up and back until the toes are upright (Figure 25). Move the foot with the toes pointing downward (Figure 26).

These movements provide for dorsiflexion and plantar flexion of the ankle.

FIGURE 25. At the ankle, moving patient's foot up and back until toes are upright.

FIGURE 26. Moving patient's foot with toes pointing down.

(continued)

Skill 9-6 ▶ Providing Range-of-Motion Exercises *(continued)*

ACTION	RATIONALE

22. Turn the sole of the foot toward the midline (Figure 27). Turn the sole of the foot outward (Figure 28).

These movements provide for inversion and eversion of the ankle.

FIGURE 27. Turning sole toward midline.

FIGURE 28. Turning sole outward.

23. Curl the toes downward (Figure 29), and then straighten them out (Figure 30). Spread the toes apart (Figure 31) and bring them together (Figure 32).

These movements provide for flexion, extension, abduction, and adduction of the toes.

FIGURE 29. Curling patient's toes downward.

FIGURE 30. Straightening patient's toes.

FIGURE 31. Spreading patient's toes apart.

FIGURE 32. Bringing patient's toes together.

ACTION	**RATIONALE**
24. Repeat these exercises on the other side of the body. Encourage the patient to do as many of these exercises independently as possible.	Repeating motions on the other side provides exercise for the entire body. Self-esteem, self-care, and independence are encouraged through the patient performing the exercises on his or her own.
25. When finished, make sure the patient is comfortable, with the side rails up and the bed in the lowest position. Place call bell and other essential items within reach.	Proper positioning with raised side rails and proper bed height provide for patient comfort and safety. Having the call bell and other essential items within reach promotes safety.
26. Remove gloves and any other PPE, if used. Perform hand hygiene.	Proper removal of PPE reduces the risk for infection transmission and contamination of other items. Hand hygiene prevents the spread of microorganisms.

EVALUATION

The expected outcome has been met when the patient completes the exercises and maintains or improves joint mobility and muscle strength, and muscle atrophy and contractures are prevented.

DOCUMENTATION

Guidelines

Document the exercises performed, any significant observations, and the patient's reaction to the activities.

Sample Documentation

> <u>5/1/20</u> 0945 Range-of-motion exercises performed to all joints. Patient able to perform active ROM of head, neck, shoulders, and arms. Required moderate assistance with ROM to lower extremities. Denied any complaints of pain during exercises. Patient tolerated exercise session well. Sitting in semi-Fowler's position with two upper side rails up, watching television.
>
> —*J. Chrisp, RN*

UNEXPECTED SITUATIONS AND ASSOCIATED INTERVENTIONS

- *While you are performing ROM exercises, the patient complains of feeling tired:* Stop the activity for that time. Reevaluate the nursing care plan. Space the exercises out at different times of the day. Schedule exercise times for the parts of the day the patient is typically feeling more rested.
- *While exercising your patient's leg, he complains of sudden, sharp pain:* Stop the exercises. Assess the patient for other symptoms. Notify the primary care provider of the event, the patient's uncomfortable reaction, and your assessment findings. Joints should be moved until there is resistance, but not pain. Report uncomfortable reactions and halt exercises. Revise activity plan, if necessary.

SPECIAL CONSIDERATIONS

General Considerations

- Incorporate the exercises when possible into daily activities, such as during bathing.
- Obtain a medical order and specific instructions to perform ROM exercises for patients with acute arthritis, fractures, torn ligaments, joint dislocation, acute myocardial infarction, and bone tumors or metastases.

Older Adult Considerations

- Avoid neck hyperextension and attempts to achieve full ROM in all joints with older adults.

(continued)

Skill 9-6 ▶ Providing Range-of-Motion Exercises *(continued)*

**EVIDENCE
FOR PRACTICE ▶**

EXERCISE AND RESPIRATORY FUNCTION

ROM exercises improve joint mobility; increase circulation, muscle mass, muscle tone, and muscle strength; and improves cardiac and respiratory functioning. Exercises should be as active as the patient's physical condition permits. ROM exercises should be initiated as soon as possible as part of a patient's care plan, because body changes can occur after only a few days of impaired mobility.

Related Research

Cho, S. H., Lee, J. H., & Jang, S. H. (2015). Efficacy of pulmonary rehabilitation using cervical range of motion exercise in stroke patients with tracheostomy tubes. *Journal of Physical Therapy Science, 27*(5), 1329–1331.

This study examined the effect of cervical range-of-motion exercises on pulmonary and coughing function in poststroke patients with tracheostomy tubes who had no history of respiratory disease. Participants were randomly assigned to either an experimental group or a control group. The experimental group performed cervical range-of-motion exercises with a physical therapist five times a week for 8 weeks; the control group did not perform cervical range-of-motion exercises. Measurements of pulmonary function and coughing ability were obtained for both groups at the beginning and at the end of the 8 weeks. When the measurements were compared, the control group did not show any significant changes in pulmonary or coughing function. The experimental group showed a statistically significant increase in pulmonary and coughing function. The researchers concluded that cervical range-of-motion exercises can effectively improve the pulmonary function and coughing ability of stroke patients with tracheostomy tubes.

Relevance for Nursing Practice

An exercise program that includes ROM exercises can generate positive effects in enhancing physical function of stroke survivors. Methods to assist patients in maintaining or increasing physical activity should be a part of routine nursing care. Nurses are in ideal positions to discuss the effects of exercise with patients and include exercise programs in the care plan.

Refer to thePoint® for additional research on related nursing topics.

Skill 9-7 ▶ Assisting a Patient With Ambulation

Walking exercises most of the body's muscles and increases joint flexibility. It improves respiratory and gastrointestinal function. Ambulating also reduces the risk for complications of immobility. However, even a short period of immobility can decrease a person's tolerance for ambulating. If necessary, make use of appropriate equipment and assistive devices to aid in patient movement and handling (refer to Fundamentals Review 9-3 for examples of assistive equipment and devices). Box 9-1 in Skill 9-1 outlines general guidelines related to mobility and safe handling of people with dementia.

**DELEGATION
CONSIDERATIONS**

Assisting a patient with ambulation may be delegated to nursing assistive personnel (NAP) or to unlicensed assistive personnel (UAP), as well as to licensed practical/vocational nurses (LPN/ LVNs). The decision to delegate must be based on careful analysis of the patient's needs and circumstances, as well as the qualifications of the person to whom the task is being delegated. Refer to the Delegation Guidelines in Appendix A.

EQUIPMENT

- Gait belt, as necessary
- Nonskid shoes or slippers
- Nonsterile gloves and/or other PPE, as indicated
- Stand-assist device, as necessary, if available
- Additional staff for assistance, as needed

ASSESSMENT	Assess the patient's ability to walk and the need for assistance (one nurse, two nurses, walker, cane, walking belt, or crutches). Review the patient's record for conditions that may affect ambulation. Perform a pain assessment before the time for the activity. If the patient reports pain, administer the prescribed medication in sufficient time to allow for the full effect of the analgesic. Take vital signs and assess the patient for dizziness or lightheadedness with position changes.
NURSING DIAGNOSIS	Determine the related factors for the nursing diagnoses based on the patient's current status. Appropriate nursing diagnoses may include: • Activity intolerance • Risk for falls • Impaired walking
OUTCOME IDENTIFICATION AND PLANNING	The expected outcome to achieve when assisting a patient with ambulation is that the patient ambulates safely, without falls or injury. Additional appropriate outcomes include the patient demonstrates improved muscle strength and joint mobility; and the patient's level of independence increases.

IMPLEMENTATION

ACTION	RATIONALE
1. Review the medical record and nursing care plan for conditions that may influence the patient's ability to move and ambulate. Assess for tubes, IV lines, incisions, or equipment that may alter the procedure for ambulation. Identify any movement limitations.	Reviewing the medical record and care plan validates the correct patient and correct procedure. Checking for equipment and limitations reduces the risk for patient injury.
2. Perform hand hygiene. Put on PPE, as indicated.	Hand hygiene and PPE prevent the spread of microorganisms. PPE is required based on transmission precautions.
3. Identify the patient. Explain the procedure to the patient. Ask the patient to report any feelings of dizziness, weakness, or shortness of breath while walking. Decide how far to walk.	Patient identification validates the correct patient and correct procedure. Discussion and explanation help allay anxiety and prepare the patient for what to expect.
4. Place the bed in the lowest position.	Proper bed height ensures safety when getting the patient out of bed.
5. Encourage the patient to make use of a stand-assist aid, either freestanding or attached to the side of the bed, if available, to move to the side of the bed. Assist the patient to the side of the bed, if necessary.	Encourages independence, reduces strain for staff, and decreases risk for patient injury.
6. Have the patient sit on the side of the bed for several minutes and assess for dizziness or lightheadedness. Have the patient stay sitting until he or she feels secure.	Having the patient sit at the side of the bed minimizes the risk for blood pressure changes (orthostatic hypotension) that can occur with position change. Allowing the patient to sit until he or she feels secure reduces anxiety and helps prevent injury.
7. Assist the patient to put on footwear and a robe, if desired.	Doing so ensures safety and patient warmth.
8. Wrap the gait belt around the patient's waist, based on assessed need and facility policy.	Gait belts improve the caregiver's grasp, reducing the risk of musculoskeletal injuries to staff and the patient. The belt also provides a firmer grasp for the caregiver if the patient should lose his or her balance.
9. Encourage the patient to make use of the stand-assist device. Assist the patient to stand, using the gait belt, if necessary. Assess the patient's balance and leg strength. If the patient is weak or unsteady, return the patient to the bed or assist to a chair.	Use of gait belt prevents injury to the nurse and to the patient. Assessing balance and strength helps to identify the need for additional assistance to prevent falling.

(continued)

Skill 9-7 ▶ Assisting a Patient With Ambulation *(continued)*

ACTION	**RATIONALE**
10. If you are the only person assisting, position yourself to the side and slightly behind the patient. Support the patient by the waist or transfer belt (Figure 1).	Positioning to the side and slightly behind the patient encourages the patient to stand and walk erect. It also places the nurse in a safe position if the patient should lose his or her balance or begin to fall.

10. If you are the only person assisting, position yourself to the side and slightly behind the patient. Support the patient by the waist or transfer belt (Figure 1).
   - When two caregivers assist, position yourself to the side and slightly behind the patient, supporting the patient by the waist or gait belt. Have the other caregiver carry or manage equipment or provide additional support from the other side.
   - Alternately, when two caregivers assist, stand at the patient's sides (one nurse on each side) with near hands grasping the gait belt and far hands holding the patient's lower arm or hand.

Positioning to the side and slightly behind the patient encourages the patient to stand and walk erect. It also places the nurse in a safe position if the patient should lose his or her balance or begin to fall.

Gait belts improve the caregiver's grasp, reducing the risk of musculoskeletal injuries to staff and the patient, and allow for a firmer grasp for the caregiver if the patient should lose his or her balance.

Gait belts improve the caregiver's grasp, reducing the risk of musculoskeletal injuries to staff and the patient, and allow for a firmer grasp for the caregiver if the patient should lose his or her balance.

FIGURE 1. Nurse positioned to side and slightly behind patient while walking, supporting patient by gait belt or waist.

11. Take several steps forward with the patient. Continue to assess the patient's strength and balance. Remind the patient to stand erect.

Taking several steps with the patient and standing erect promote good balance and stability. Continued assessment helps maintain patient safety.

12. Continue with ambulation for the planned distance and time. Return the patient to the bed or chair based on the patient's tolerance and condition. Remove gait belt.

Ambulation as prescribed promotes activity and prevents fatigue.

13. Ensure the patient is comfortable, with the side rails up and the bed in the lowest position, as necessary. Place call bell and other essential items within reach.

Proper positioning with raised side rails and proper bed height provide for patient comfort and safety. Having the call bell and other essential items within reach promotes safety.

14. Clean transfer aids per facility policy, if not indicated for single patient use. Remove gloves and any other PPE, if used. Perform hand hygiene.

Proper cleaning of equipment between patient use prevents the spread of microorganisms. Proper removal of PPE reduces the risk for infection transmission and contamination of other items. Hand hygiene prevents the spread of microorganisms.

EVALUATION

The expected outcome has been met when the patient ambulates safely for the prescribed distance and time and remains free from falls or injury; and the patient exhibits increasing muscle strength, joint mobility, and independence.

DOCUMENTATION

Guidelines

Document the activity, any other pertinent observations, the patient's tolerance of the procedure, and the distance walked. Document the use of transfer aids and number of staff required for transfer.

Sample Documentation

> 5/14/20 1720 Patient ambulated with assistance in hallway for a distance of approximately 15 ft. Patient tolerated ambulation well; denied any complaints of dizziness, pain, or fatigue. Ambulated back to room and sitting in chair listening to music.
> —J. Minkins, RN

UNEXPECTED SITUATIONS AND ASSOCIATED INTERVENTIONS

- *You are walking with a patient in the hallway. She tells you she feels faint and begins to lean over as if she is going to fall:* Place your feet wide apart, with one foot in front. Rock your pelvis out on the side nearest the patient. This widens and stabilizes the base of support. Grasp the gait belt. This ensures a safe hold on the patient. Support the patient by pulling her weight backward against your body. Gently slide her down your body to the floor, protecting her head. This enables you to support the patient's weight with large muscle groups and protects you from back strain. Stay with the patient. Call for help. If another staff member was assisting you with ambulation, each of you should use one hand to grasp the gait belt and grasp the patient's hand or wrist with your other hand. Slowly lower her to the floor.

SPECIAL CONSIDERATIONS

- Secure all equipment, such as indwelling urinary catheters, drains, or IV infusions, to a pole for ambulation. Do not carry equipment while helping the patient. Your hands should be free to provide support.

EVIDENCE FOR PRACTICE ▶

EARLY AMBULATION AND PREVENTION OF THROMBOSIS
Guyatt, G. H., Akl, E. A., Crowther, M., Gutterman, D. D., Schuünemann, H. J.; American College of Chest Physicians Antithrombotic Therapy and Prevention of Thrombosis Panel. (2012). Executive summary: Antithrombotic therapy and prevention of thrombosis, 9th ed.: American College of Chest Physicians evidence-based clinical practice guidelines. *Chest*, *141*(2 Suppl), 7S–47S.

This evidence-based guideline outlines best practices for the prevention of venous thromboembolism (VTE). The implementation of early ambulation as part of prophylaxis is included in the discussion.

Refer to thePoint® for additional research on related nursing topics.

Skill 9-8 ▶ Assisting a Patient With Ambulation Using a Walker

A walker is a lightweight metal frame with four legs. Walkers provide stability and security for patients with insufficient strength and balance to use other ambulatory aids. There are several kinds of walkers; the choice of which to use is based on the patient's arm strength and balance. Regardless of the type used, the patient stands between the back legs of the walker with arms relaxed at the side; the top of the walker should line up with the crease on the inside of the patient's wrist. When the patient's hands are placed on the grips, elbows should be flexed about 30 degrees (American Academy of Orthopaedic Surgeons [AAOS], 2015b). Usually, the legs of the walker can be adjusted to the appropriate height. Box 9-1 in Skill 9-1 outlines general guidelines related to mobility and safe handling of people with dementia.

(continued)

Skill 9-8 ▶ Assisting a Patient With Ambulation Using a Walker (continued)

DELEGATION CONSIDERATIONS	Patient teaching regarding use of a walker cannot be delegated to nursing assistive personnel (NAP) or to unlicensed assistive personnel (UAP). Reinforcement or implementation of ambulation using a walker may be delegated to NAP or UAP. Assisting a patient with ambulation using a walker may be delegated to licensed practical/vocational nurses (LPN/LVNs). The decision to delegate must be based on careful analysis of the patient's needs and circumstances, as well as the qualifications of the person to whom the task is being delegated. Refer to the Delegation Guidelines in Appendix A.
EQUIPMENT	• Walker, adjusted to the appropriate height • Nonskid shoes or slippers • Nonsterile gloves and/or other PPE, as indicated • Additional staff for assistance, as needed • Stand-assist device, as necessary, if available • Gait belt, based on assessment
ASSESSMENT	Assess the patient's ability to walk and the need for assistance. Review the patient's record for conditions that may affect ambulation. Perform a pain assessment before the time for the activity. If the patient reports pain, administer the prescribed medication in sufficient time to allow for the full effect of the analgesic. Take vital signs and assess the patient for dizziness or lightheadedness with position changes. Assess the patient's knowledge regarding the use of a walker. Ensure that the walker is at the appropriate height for the patient.
NURSING DIAGNOSIS	Determine the related factors for the nursing diagnoses based on the patient's current status. Appropriate nursing diagnoses may include: • Risk for falls • Deficient knowledge • Impaired walking
OUTCOME IDENTIFICATION AND PLANNING	The expected outcome to achieve is that the patient ambulates safely with the walker and is free from falls or injury. Additional appropriate outcomes include the following: the patient demonstrates proper use of the walker and verbalizes an understanding of the rationale for use of the walker; and the patient demonstrates increasing muscle strength, joint mobility, and independence.

IMPLEMENTATION

ACTION	**RATIONALE**
1. Review the medical record and nursing care plan for conditions that may influence the patient's ability to move and ambulate, and for specific instructions for ambulation, such as distance. Assess for tubes, IV lines, incisions, or equipment that may alter the procedure for ambulation. Assess the patient's knowledge and previous experience regarding the use of a walker. Identify any movement limitations.	Reviewing the medical record and care plan validates the correct patient and correct procedure. Checking for equipment and limitations helps minimize the risk for injury.
2. Perform hand hygiene. Put on PPE, if indicated.	Hand hygiene and PPE prevent the spread of microorganisms. PPE is required based on transmission precautions.
3. Identify the patient. Explain the procedure to the patient. Tell the patient to report any feelings of dizziness, weakness, or shortness of breath while walking. Decide how far to walk.	Patient identification validates the correct patient and correct procedure. Discussion and explanation help allay anxiety and prepare the patient for what to expect.

ACTION

4. Place the bed in the lowest position, if the patient is in bed.

5. Encourage the patient to make use of a stand-assist aid, either freestanding or attached to the side of the bed, if available, to move to the side of the bed.

6. Assist the patient to the side of the bed, if necessary. Have the patient sit on the side of the bed. Assess for dizziness or lightheadedness. Have the patient stay seated until he or she feels secure.

7. Assist the patient to put on footwear and a robe, if desired.

8. Wrap the gait belt around the patient's waist, based on assessed need and facility policy.

9. Place the walker directly in front of the patient (Figure 1). Ask the patient to push him- or herself off the bed or chair; make use of the stand-assist device, or assist the patient to stand (Figure 2). Once the patient is standing, have him or her hold the walker's handgrips firmly and equally. Stand slightly behind the patient, on one side.

RATIONALE

Proper bed height ensures safety when getting the patient out of bed.

Use of assistive devices encourages independence, reduces strain for staff, and decreases risk for patient injury.

Having the patient sit on the side of the bed minimizes the risk for blood pressure changes (orthostatic hypotension) that can occur with position change. Assessing patient complaints helps prevent injury.

Doing so ensures safety and warmth.

Gait belts improve the caregiver's grasp, reducing the risk of musculoskeletal injuries to staff and the patient and provide for a firmer grasp if patient should lose his or her balance.

Proper positioning with the walker ensures balance. Standing within the walker and holding the handgrips firmly provide stability when moving the walker and help ensure safety. Positioning to the side and slightly behind the patient encourages the patient to stand and walk erect. It also places the nurse in a safe position if the patient should lose his or her balance or begin to fall.

FIGURE 1. Setting walker in front of a seated patient.

FIGURE 2. Assisting patient to stand.

10. Have the patient move the walker forward 6 to 8 in and set it down, making sure all four feet of the walker stay on the floor. Then, tell the patient to step forward with either foot into the walker, supporting him- or herself on his or her arms. Follow through with the other leg.

Having all four feet of the walker on the floor provides a broad base of support. Moving the walker and stepping forward moves the center of gravity toward the walker, ensuring balance and preventing tipping of the walker.

(continued)

Skill 9-8 ▶ Assisting a Patient With Ambulation Using a Walker (continued)

ACTION	RATIONALE
11. Move the walker forward again, and continue the same pattern. Continue with ambulation for the planned distance and time (Figure 3). Return the patient to the bed or chair based on the patient's tolerance and condition, ensuring that the patient is comfortable. Remove gait belt.	Moving the walker promotes activity. Continuing for the planned distance and time prevents the patient from becoming fatigued.

FIGURE 3. Assisting patient to walk with walker.

ACTION	RATIONALE
12. Ensure the patient is comfortable, with the side rails up and the bed in the lowest position, as necessary. Place call bell and other essential items within reach.	Proper positioning with raised side rails and proper bed height provides for patient comfort and safety. Having the call bell and other essential items within reach promotes safety.
13. Clean transfer aids per facility policy, if not indicated for single patient use. Remove gloves and any other PPE, if used. Perform hand hygiene.	Proper cleaning of equipment between patient use prevents the spread of microorganisms. Proper removal of PPE reduces the risk for infection transmission and contamination of other items. Hand hygiene prevents the spread of microorganisms.

EVALUATION

The expected outcome has been met when the patient uses the walker to ambulate safely and remains free of injury; and the patient exhibits increased muscle strength, joint mobility, and independence.

DOCUMENTATION

Guidelines

Document the activity, any other pertinent observations, the patient's ability to use the walker, the patient's tolerance of the procedure, and the distance walked. Document the use of transfer aids and number of staff required for transfer.

Sample Documentation

5/15/20 0900 Patient ambulated with walker from bed to bathroom for morning care with minimal assistance; demonstrated proper steps in using walker. Able to ambulate back to bed using walker independently.

—P. Collins, RN

UNEXPECTED SITUATIONS AND ASSOCIATED INTERVENTIONS	• *You are assisting a patient ambulating in the hallway using a walker. She becomes extremely tired and says she cannot pick up the walker anymore ("it's too heavy"). However, she cannot walk without the walker:* Call for assistance. Have a coworker obtain a wheelchair to transport the patient back to her room. Assess the patient for other symptoms, if necessary. In the future, plan to ambulate for shorter distances to prevent the patient from becoming fatigued.
SPECIAL CONSIDERATIONS	• Never use a walker on the stairs. • Wear nonskid shoes or slippers. • Some walkers have wheels on the front legs. These walkers are best for patients with a gait that is too fast for a walker without wheels and for patients who have difficulty lifting a walker. This type of walker is rolled forward while the patient walks as normally as possible. Because lifting repeatedly is not required, energy expenditure and stress to the back and upper extremities are less than with a standard walker. • Keep in mind, walkers often prove to be difficult to maneuver through doorways and congested areas. • Advise the patient to check the walker before use for signs of damage, frame deformity, or loose or missing parts. • Teach patients to use the arms of the chair or a stand-assist device for leverage when getting up from a chair. Explain to patients that they should not pull on the walker to get up; the walker could tip over or become unbalanced.

EVIDENCE FOR PRACTICE ▶	**EARLY AMBULATION AND PREVENTION OF THROMBOSIS** Guyatt, G. H., Akl, E. A., Crowther, M., Gutterman, D. D., Schünemann, H. J.; American College of Chest Physicians Antithrombotic Therapy and Prevention of Thrombosis Panel. (2012). Executive summary: Antithrombotic therapy and prevention of thrombosis, 9th ed.: American College of Chest Physicians evidence-based clinical practice guidelines. *Chest, 141*(2 Suppl), 7S–47S. Refer to the details in Skill 9-7, Evidence for Practice, and refer to thePoint® for additional research on related nursing topics.

Skill 9-9 ▶ Assisting a Patient With Ambulation Using Crutches

Crutches enable a patient to walk and remove weight from one or both legs. The patient uses the arms to support the body weight. Crutches can be used for the short or the long term. This section will discuss short-term crutch use. Crutches must be fitted to each person. Have the patient stand up straight with the palm of the hand pressed against the body under the arm. The hand should fit between the top of the crutches and the armpit. When using crutches, the elbow should be slightly bent at about 30 degrees and the hands, not the armpits, should support the patient's weight. Weight on the armpits can cause nerve damage. A physical therapist usually teaches the procedure for crutch walking, but it is important for the nurse to be knowledgeable about the patient's progress and the gait being taught. Be prepared to guide the patient at home or in the hospital after the initial teaching is completed. Remind the patient that the support of body weight should be primarily on the hands and arms while using the crutches. There are a number of different ways to walk using crutches, based on how much weight the patient is allowed to bear on one or both legs.

DELEGATION CONSIDERATIONS	Patient teaching regarding use of crutches cannot be delegated to nursing assistive personnel (NAP) or unlicensed assistive personnel (UAP). Reinforcement or implementation of the use of crutches may be delegated to NAP or UAP. Assisting a patient with ambulation using crutches may be delegated to licensed practical/vocational nurses (LPN/LVNs). The decision to delegate must be based on careful analysis of the patient's needs and circumstances, as well as the qualifications of the person to whom the task is being delegated. Refer to the Delegation Guidelines in Appendix A.

(continued)

Skill 9-9 ▶ Assisting a Patient With Ambulation Using Crutches *(continued)*

EQUIPMENT
- Crutches with axillary pads, handgrips, and rubber suction tips
- Nonskid shoes or slippers
- PPE, as indicated
- Stand-assist device, as necessary, if available
- Gait belt, based on assessment

ASSESSMENT

Review the patient's record and nursing care plan to determine the reason for using crutches and instructions for weight bearing. Check for specific instructions from physical therapy. Perform a pain assessment before the time for the activity. If the patient reports pain, administer the prescribed medication in sufficient time to allow for the full effect of the analgesic. Determine the patient's knowledge regarding the use of crutches and assess the patient's ability to balance on the crutches. Assess for muscle strength in the legs and arms. Determine the appropriate gait for the patient to use.

NURSING DIAGNOSIS

Determine the related factors for the nursing diagnosis based on the patient's current status. Appropriate nursing diagnoses may include:
- Impaired walking
- Deficient knowledge
- Risk for falls

OUTCOME IDENTIFICATION AND PLANNING

The expected outcome to achieve when assisting a patient with ambulation using crutches is that the patient ambulates safely without experiencing falls or injury and the patient demonstrates proper crutch-walking technique.

IMPLEMENTATION

ACTION	RATIONALE
1. Review the medical record and nursing care plan for conditions that may influence the patient's ability to move and ambulate. Assess for tubes, IV lines, incisions, or equipment that may alter the procedure for ambulation. Assess the patient's knowledge and previous experience regarding the use of crutches. Determine that the appropriate size crutch has been obtained.	Reviewing the medical record and care plan validates the correct patient and correct procedure. Assessment helps identify problem areas to minimize the risk for injury.
2. Perform hand hygiene. Put on PPE, if indicated.	Hand hygiene and PPE prevent the spread of microorganisms. PPE is required based on transmission precautions.
3. Identify the patient. Explain the procedure to the patient. Tell the patient to report any feelings of dizziness, weakness, or shortness of breath while walking. Decide how far to walk.	Patient identification validates the correct patient and correct procedure. Discussion and explanation help allay anxiety and prepare the patient for what to expect.
4. Place the bed in the lowest position, if the patient is in bed.	Proper bed height ensures safety when getting the patient out of bed.
5. Encourage the patient to make use of a stand-assist aid, either freestanding or attached to the side of the bed, if available, to move to the side of the bed.	Use of assistive devices encourages independence, reduces strain for staff, and decreases risk for patient injury.
6. Assist the patient to the side of the bed, if necessary. Have the patient sit on the side of the bed. Assess for dizziness or lightheadedness. Have the patient stay seated until he or she feels secure.	Having the patient sit on the side of the bed minimizes the risk for blood pressure changes (orthostatic hypotension) that can occur with position change. Assessing patient complaints helps prevent injury.
7. Assist the patient to put on footwear and a robe, if desired.	Doing so ensures safety and warmth.

ACTION

8. Wrap the gait belt around the patient's waist, based on assessed need and facility policy.

9. Assist the patient to stand erect, face forward in the tripod position (Figure 1). This means the patient holds the crutches 12 in in front of, and 12 in to the side of, each foot.

FIGURE 1. Assisting patient to stand erect facing forward in tripod position.

10. For the four-point gait:
    a. Have the patient move the right crutch forward 12 in and then move the left foot forward to the level of the right crutch.
    b. Then have the patient move the left crutch forward 12 in and then move the right foot forward to the level of the left crutch.

11. For the three-point gait:
    a. Have the patient move the affected leg and both crutches forward about 12 in.
    b. Have the patient move the stronger leg forward to the level of the crutches.

12. For the two-point gait:
    a. Have the patient move the left crutch and the right foot forward about 12 in at the same time.
    b. Have the patient move the right crutch and left leg forward to the level of the left crutch at the same time.

13. For the swing-to gait:
    a. Have the patient move both crutches forward about 12 in.
    b. Have the patient lift the legs and swing them to the crutches, supporting his or her body weight on the crutches.

RATIONALE

Gait belts improve the caregiver's grasp, reducing the risk of musculoskeletal injuries to staff and the patient and provide for a firmer grasp if patient should lose his or her balance.

Positioning the crutches in this manner provides a wide base of support to increase stability and balance.

This movement ensures stability and safety.

Patient bears weight on the stronger leg.

Patient bears partial weight on both feet.

Swing-to gait provides mobility for patients with weakness or paralysis of the hips or legs.

(continued)

Skill 9-9 ▶ Assisting a Patient With Ambulation Using Crutches *(continued)*

ACTION	RATIONALE
14. Continue with ambulation for the planned distance and time. Return the patient to the bed or chair based on the patient's tolerance and condition. Remove gait belt.	Continued ambulation promotes activity. Adhering to the planned distance and time prevents the patient from becoming fatigued.
15. Ensure the patient is comfortable, with the side rails up and the bed in the lowest position, as necessary. Place call bell and other essential items within reach.	Proper positioning with raised side rails and proper bed height provide for patient comfort and safety. Having the call bell and other essential items within reach promotes safety.
16. Clean transfer aids per facility policy, if not indicated for single patient use. Remove gloves and any other PPE, if used. Perform hand hygiene.	Proper cleaning of equipment between patient use prevents the spread of microorganisms. Proper removal of PPE reduces the risk for infection transmission and contamination of other items. Hand hygiene prevents the spread of microorganisms.

EVALUATION

The expected outcome has been met when the patient ambulates safely without experiencing falls or injury and the patient demonstrates proper crutch-walking technique.

DOCUMENTATION

Guidelines

Document the activity, any other pertinent observations, the patient's ability to use the crutches, the patient's tolerance of the procedure, and the distance walked. Document the use of transfer aids and number of staff required for transfer.

Sample Documentation

> <u>5/10/20</u> 1830 Patient instructed in crutch walking using four-point gait. Patient return demonstrated gait, ambulating for approximately 15 ft in hallway, without difficulty.
>
> —H. Pointer, RN

UNEXPECTED SITUATIONS AND ASSOCIATED INTERVENTIONS

- *You are assisting a patient ambulating in the hallway using crutches when the patient reports fatigue. You notice that the patient is bearing weight on the axillary area:* Call for assistance and have a coworker obtain a wheelchair to transport the patient back to the room. Once the patient is back in bed, reinforce instructions about avoiding pressure on the axillary area. In the future, plan to ambulate for a shorter distance to prevent the patient from becoming fatigued. Talk with the multidisciplinary health care team about possible exercises for upper-extremity strengthening.

SPECIAL CONSIDERATIONS

- Crutches can be used when climbing stairs. The patient grasps both crutches as one, on one side of the body and uses the stair railing. Have the patient stand in the tripod position facing the stairs. The patient transfers his or her weight to the crutches and holds the railing. The patient places the unaffected leg on the first stair tread. The patient then transfers his or her weight to the unaffected leg, moving up onto the stair tread. The patient moves the crutches and affected leg up to the stair tread and continues to the top of the stairs. Using this process, the crutches always support the affected leg.
- Long-term use of the swing-to gait can lead to atrophy of the hips and legs. Include appropriate exercises in the patient's care plan to avoid this complication.
- Patients should not lean on the crutches. Prolonged pressure on the axillae can damage the brachial nerves, causing brachial nerve palsy, with resulting loss of sensation and inability to move the upper extremities.
- Patients using crutches should perform arm- and shoulder-strengthening exercises to aid with crutch walking.

Skill 9-10 ▶ Assisting a Patient With Ambulation Using a Cane

Canes are useful for patients who can bear weight, but need support for balance. They are also useful for patients who have decreased strength in one leg. Canes provide an additional point of support during ambulation. Canes are made of wood or metal and often have a rubberized cap on the tip to prevent slipping. Canes come in three variations: single-ended canes with half-circle handles (recommended for patients requiring minimal support and for those who will be using stairs frequently); single-ended canes with straight handles (recommended for patients with hand weakness because the handgrip is easier to hold, but not recommended for patients with poor balance); and canes with three (tripod) or four prongs (quad cane) or legs to provide a wide base of support (recommended for patients with poor balance). The cane should rise from the floor to the crease in the patient's wrist and the elbow should be flexed about 15 degrees when holding the cane. The patient holds the cane in the hand opposite the weak or injured leg. Box 9-1 in Skill 9-1 outlines general guidelines to consider related to mobility and safe handling of people with dementia.

DELEGATION CONSIDERATIONS	Patient teaching regarding use of a cane cannot be delegated to nursing assistive personnel (NAP) or unlicensed assistive personnel (UAP). Reinforcement or implementation of the use of a cane may be delegated to NAP or UAP. Assisting a patient with ambulation using a cane may be delegated to licensed practical/vocational nurses (LPN/LVNs). The decision to delegate must be based on careful analysis of the patient's needs and circumstances, as well as the qualifications of the person to whom the task is being delegated. Refer to the Delegation Guidelines in Appendix A.

EQUIPMENT

- Cane of appropriate size with rubber tip
- Nonskid shoes or slippers
- Nonsterile gloves and/or other PPE, as indicated
- Stand-assist aid, if necessary and available
- Gait belt, based on assessment

ASSESSMENT

Assess the patient's upper body strength, ability to bear weight and to walk, and the need for assistance. Review the patient's record for conditions that may affect ambulation. Perform a pain assessment before the time for the activity. If the patient reports pain, administer the prescribed medication in sufficient time to allow for the full effect of the analgesic. Take vital signs and assess the patient for dizziness or lightheadedness with position changes. Assess the patient's knowledge regarding the use of a cane.

NURSING DIAGNOSIS

Determine the related factors for the nursing diagnoses based on the patient's current status. Appropriate nursing diagnoses may include:

- Risk for falls
- Impaired walking
- Deficient knowledge

OUTCOME IDENTIFICATION AND PLANNING

The expected outcome to achieve when assisting a patient with ambulation using a cane is that the patient ambulates safely without falls or injury. Additional appropriate outcomes include the following: the patient demonstrates proper use of the cane; and the patient demonstrates increased independence.

IMPLEMENTATION

ACTION	RATIONALE
1. Review the medical record and nursing care plan for conditions that may influence the patient's ability to move and ambulate. Assess for tubes, IV lines, incisions, or equipment that may alter the procedure for ambulation.	Review of the medical record and care plan validates the correct patient and correct procedure. Identification of equipment and limitations helps reduce the risk for injury.
2. Perform hand hygiene. Put on PPE, as indicated.	Hand hygiene and PPE prevent the spread of microorganisms. PPE is required based on transmission precautions.

(continued)

Skill 9-10 ▶ Assisting a Patient With Ambulation Using a Cane *(continued)*

ACTION	RATIONALE

3. Identify the patient. Explain the procedure to the patient. Tell the patient to report any feelings of dizziness, weakness, or shortness of breath while walking. Decide how far to walk.

Patient identification validates the correct patient and correct procedure. Discussion and explanation help allay anxiety and prepare the patient for what to expect.

4. Place the bed in the lowest position, if the patient is in bed.

Proper bed height ensures safety when getting the patient out of bed.

5. Encourage the patient to make use of a stand-assist aid, either freestanding or attached to the side of the bed, if available, to move to the side of the bed.

Use of assistive devices encourages independence, reduces strain for staff, and decreases risk for patient injury.

6. Assist the patient to the side of the bed, if necessary. Have the patient sit on the side of the bed. Assess for dizziness or lightheadedness. Have the patient stay seated until he or she feels secure.

Having the patient sit on the side of the bed minimizes the risk for blood pressure changes (orthostatic hypotension) that can occur with position change. Assessing patient complaints helps prevent injury.

7. Assist the patient to put on footwear and a robe, if desired.

Doing so ensures safety and warmth.

8. Wrap the gait belt around the patient's waist, based on assessed need and facility policy.

Gait belts improve the caregiver's grasp, reducing the risk of musculoskeletal injuries to staff and the patient and provide firmer grasp for the caregiver if patient should lose his or her balance.

9. Encourage the patient to make use of the stand-assist device to stand with weight evenly distributed between the feet and the cane.

A stand-assist device reduces strain for caregiver and decreases risk for patient injury. Evenly distributed weight provides a broad base of support and balance.

10. Have the patient hold the cane on his or her stronger side, close to the body, while the nurse stands to the side and slightly behind the patient (Figure 1).

Holding the cane on the stronger side helps to distribute the patient's weight away from the involved side and prevents leaning. Positioning to the side and slightly behind the patient encourages the patient to stand and walk erect. It also places the nurse in a safe position if the patient should lose his or her balance or begin to fall.

FIGURE 1. Nurse stands slightly behind patient. Cane is held on patient's stronger side, close to body.

ACTION	**RATIONALE**
11. Tell the patient to advance the cane 4 to 12 in (10 to 30 cm) and then, while supporting his or her weight on the stronger leg and the cane, advance the weaker foot forward, parallel with the cane.	Moving in this manner provides support and balance.
12. While supporting his or her weight on the weaker leg and the cane, have the patient advance the stronger leg forward to finish the step.	Moving in this manner provides support and balance.
13. Continue with ambulation for the planned distance and time. Return the patient to the bed or chair based on the patient's tolerance and condition. Remove gait belt.	Continued ambulation promotes activity. Adhering to the planned distance and time prevents the patient from becoming fatigued.
14. Ensure the patient is comfortable, with the side rails up and the bed in the lowest position, as necessary. Place call bell and other essential items within reach.	Proper positioning with raised side rails and proper bed height provides for patient comfort and safety. Having the call bell and other essential items within reach promotes safety.
15. Clean transfer aids per facility policy, if not indicated for single patient use. Remove gloves and any other PPE, if used. Perform hand hygiene.	Proper cleaning of equipment between patient use prevents the spread of microorganisms. Proper removal of PPE reduces the risk for infection transmission and contamination of other items. Hand hygiene prevents the spread of microorganisms.

EVALUATION

The expected outcome has been met when the patient uses the cane to ambulate safely without falls or injury; the patient demonstrates proper use of the cane; and the patient demonstrates increased independence.

DOCUMENTATION

Guidelines

Document the activity, any other pertinent observations, the patient's ability to use the cane, the patient's tolerance of the procedure, and the distance walked. Document the use of transfer aids and the number of staff required for transfer.

Sample Documentation

> 5/14/20 1330 Patient instructed in cane use. Patient return demonstrated gait, ambulating approximately 10 ft in room. Patient needed continued reminders about leaning to one side. Requires continued instruction in cane use. Another teaching session planned for early evening.
>
> —J. Phelps, RN

UNEXPECTED SITUATIONS AND ASSOCIATED INTERVENTIONS

- *You are assisting a patient ambulating in the hallway using a cane when the patient says she "can't walk any more":* Call for assistance. Have a coworker obtain a wheelchair to transport the patient back to her room. Assess the patient for possible causes, such as anxiety, fatigue, or a change in her condition. In the future, plan shorter distances to prevent the patient from becoming fatigued. Anticipate the need for referral to physical therapy for muscle strengthening.

SPECIAL CONSIDERATIONS

- Patients with bilateral weakness should not use a cane. Crutches or a walker would be more appropriate.
- To climb stairs, the patient should advance the stronger leg up the stair first, followed by the cane and weaker leg. To descend, reverse the process.
- When less support is required from the cane, the patient can advance the cane and weaker leg forward simultaneously, while the stronger leg supports the patient's weight.
- Teach patients to position their canes within easy reach when they sit down so that they can rise easily.
- While a cane might help with mobility, it can also make it more difficult for people to stabilize themselves during a fall.

(continued)

Skill 9-11 ▶ Applying and Removing Graduated Compression Stockings

Graduated compression stockings are often used for patients at risk for **deep vein thrombosis (DVT)** and pulmonary embolism, and to help prevent phlebitis. Manufactured by several companies, graduated compression stockings are made of elastic material and are available in either knee- or thigh-high length. By applying pressure, graduated compression stockings increase the velocity of blood flow in the superficial and deep veins and improve venous valve function in the legs, promoting venous return to the heart. An order is required from the patient's health care provider for their use.

Be prepared to apply the stockings in the morning before the patient is out of bed and while the patient is supine. If the patient is sitting or has been up and about, have the patient lie down with legs and feet elevated for at least 15 minutes before applying the stockings. Otherwise, the leg vessels are congested with blood, reducing the effectiveness of the stockings.

DELEGATION CONSIDERATIONS

The application and removal of graduated compression stockings may be delegated to nursing assistive personnel (NAP) or to unlicensed assistive personnel (UAP), as well as to licensed practical/vocational nurses (LPN/LVNs). The decision to delegate must be based on careful analysis of the patient's needs and circumstances, as well as the qualifications of the person to whom the task is being delegated. Refer to the Delegation Guidelines in Appendix A.

EQUIPMENT

- Elastic graduated compression stockings in the ordered length and correct size. See Assessment for appropriate measurement procedure.
- Measuring tape
- Talcum powder (optional)
- Skin cleanser, basin, towel
- PPE, as indicated

ASSESSMENT

Assess the skin condition and neurovascular status of the legs. Report any abnormalities before continuing with the application of the stockings. Assess patient's legs for any redness, swelling, warmth, tenderness, or pain that may indicate DVT. If any of these symptoms are noted, notify the health care provider before applying stockings. Measure the patient's legs to obtain the correct size stocking. For knee-high length: Measure around the widest part of the calf and the leg length from the bottom of the heel to the back of the knee, at the bend. For thigh-high length: Measure around the widest part of the calf and the thigh. Measure the length from the bottom of the heel to the gluteal fold. Follow the manufacturer's specifications to select the correct-sized stockings. Each leg should have a correctly fitted stocking; if measurements differ, then two different sizes of stocking need to be ordered to ensure correct fitting on each leg (Muñoz-Figueroa & Ojo, 2015).

NURSING DIAGNOSIS

Determine related factors for the nursing diagnoses based on the patient's current status. Appropriate nursing diagnoses may include:

- Ineffective peripheral tissue perfusion
- Risk for impaired skin integrity
- Deficient knowledge

OUTCOME IDENTIFICATION AND PLANNING

The expected outcome to achieve when applying and removing graduated compression stockings is that the stockings will be applied and removed with minimal discomfort to the patient. Other outcomes that may be appropriate include the following: edema will decrease in the lower extremities; patient will understand the rationale for stocking application; and patient will remain free from deep vein thrombosis.

IMPLEMENTATION

ACTION	RATIONALE
1. Review the medical record and medical orders to determine the need for graduated compression stockings.	Reviewing the medical record and order validates the correct patient and correct procedure.
2. Perform hand hygiene. Put on PPE, as indicated.	Hand hygiene and PPE prevent the spread of microorganisms. PPE is required based on transmission precautions.

ACTION

3. Identify the patient. Explain what you are going to do and the rationale for use of elastic stockings.

4. Close the curtains around the bed and close the door to the room, if possible.

5. Adjust the bed to a comfortable working height, usually elbow height of the caregiver (VHACEOSH, 2016).

6. Assist patient to supine position. If patient has been sitting or walking, have him or her lie down with legs and feet well elevated for at least 15 minutes before applying stockings.

7. Expose legs one at a time. Wash and dry legs, if necessary. Powder the leg lightly unless patient has a respiratory problem, dry skin, or sensitivity to the powder. If the skin is dry, a lotion may be used. Powders and lotions are not recommended by some manufacturers; check the package material for manufacturer specifications.

8. Stand at the foot of the bed. Place hand inside stocking and grasp heel area securely. Turn stocking inside-out to the heel area, leaving the foot inside the stocking leg (Figure 1).

RATIONALE

Patient identification validates the correct patient and correct procedure. Discussion and explanation allay anxiety and prepare the patient for what to expect.

This ensures the patient's privacy.

Having the bed at the proper height prevents back and muscle strain.

Dependent position of legs encourages blood to pool in the veins, reducing the effectiveness of the stockings if they are applied to congested blood vessels.

Helps maintain patient's privacy. Powder and lotion reduce friction and make application of stockings easier.

Inside-out technique provides for easier application; bunched elastic material can compromise extremity circulation.

FIGURE 1. Pulling graduated compression stocking inside-out.

9. With the heel pocket down, ease the stocking foot over the foot and heel (Figure 2). Check that the patient's heel is centered in heel pocket of stocking (Figure 3).

Wrinkles and improper fit interfere with circulation.

FIGURE 2. Putting foot of stocking onto patient.

FIGURE 3. Ensuring heel is centered after stocking is on foot.

(*continued*)

Skill 9-11 ▶ Applying and Removing Graduated Compression Stockings *(continued)*

ACTION	RATIONALE
10. Using your fingers and thumbs, carefully grasp edge of stocking and pull it up smoothly over ankle and calf, toward the knee (Figure 4). Make sure it is distributed evenly.	Easing the stocking carefully into position ensures proper fit of the stocking to the contour of the leg. Even distribution prevents interference with circulation.
11. Pull forward slightly on toe section. If the stocking has a toe window, make sure it is properly positioned. Adjust if necessary to ensure material is smooth.	Ensures toe comfort and prevents interference with circulation.
12. If the stockings are knee-length, make sure each stocking top is 1 to 2 in below the patella. Make sure the stocking does not roll down.	Prevents pressure and interference with circulation. Rolling stockings may have a constricting effect on veins.
13. If applying thigh-length stocking, continue the application. Flex the patient's leg. Stretch the stocking over the knee.	This ensures even distribution.
14. Pull the stocking over the thigh until the top is 1 to 3 in below the gluteal fold (Figure 5). Adjust the stocking, as necessary, to distribute the fabric evenly. Make sure the stocking does not roll down.	Prevents excessive pressure and interference with circulation. Rolling stockings may have a constricting effect on veins.
15. Remove equipment and return patient to a position of comfort. Remove gloves. Raise side rail and lower bed. Place call bell and other essential items within reach.	Promotes patient comfort and safety. Removing gloves properly reduces the risk for infection transmission and contamination of other items. Having the call bell and other essential items within reach promotes safety.

FIGURE 4. Pulling stocking up leg.

FIGURE 5. Pulling stocking up over thigh.

16. Remove any other PPE, if used. Perform hand hygiene.	Proper removal of PPE reduces the risk for infection transmission and contamination of other items. Hand hygiene prevents the spread of microorganisms.

Removing Stockings

17. To remove stocking, grasp top of stocking with your thumb and fingers and smoothly pull stocking off inside-out to heel. Support foot and ease stocking over it.	This preserves the elasticity and contour of the stocking. It allows assessment of circulatory status and condition of skin on lower extremity and for skin care.

EVALUATION   The expected outcome has been met when the stockings are applied and removed, as indicated, with minimal discomfort to the patient; patient exhibits a decrease in peripheral edema in the lower extremities; the patient verbalizes an understanding of the rationale for stocking application; and remains free from deep vein thrombosis.

DOCUMENTATION

Guidelines   Document the patient's leg measurements as a baseline. Document the application of the stockings, size stocking applied, skin and leg assessment, and neurovascular assessment.

Sample Documentation

> 7/22/20 0945 Leg measurements: calf 14½ in, length heel to knee 16 in. Measurements equal bilaterally. Knee-high graduated compression stockings (medium/regular) applied bilaterally. Posterior tibial and dorsalis pedis pulses + 2 bilaterally; capillary refill less than 2 seconds and skin on toes consistent with rest of skin and warm. Skin on lower extremities is intact bilaterally.
>
> —C. Stone, RN

UNEXPECTED SITUATIONS AND ASSOCIATED INTERVENTIONS

- Patient's leg measurements are outside the guidelines for the available sizes: Notify prescriber. Patient may require custom-fitted stockings.
- Patient has a lot of pain with application of stockings: If pain is expected (e.g., if the patient has a leg incision), it may be necessary to premedicate the patient and apply the stockings once the medication has had time to take effect. If the pain is unexpected, notify the primary care provider because the patient may be developing a deep vein thrombosis.
- Patient has an incision on the leg: When applying and removing stockings, be careful not to hit the incision. If the incision is draining, apply a small bandage to the incision so that it does not drain onto the stockings. If the stockings become soiled by drainage, wash and dry according to instructions.
- Patient is to ambulate with stockings: Place skid-resistant socks or slippers on before patient attempts to ambulate.

SPECIAL CONSIDERATIONS

General Considerations

- Each leg should have a correct fitting stocking; if measurements are different, then two different sizes of stocking need to be ordered to ensure correct fitting on each leg (Muñoz-Figueroa & Ojo, 2015). The manufacturer whose stockings are being used provides directions for measuring. Some stockings fit either leg; others are designated right or left. An improperly fitting stocking is uncomfortable and ineffective and possibly even harmful (Muñoz-Figueroa & Ojo).
- Remove stockings daily and inspect legs. Wash and air-dry, as necessary, according to manufacturer's directions.
- Assess the patient's extremities at least every shift for skin color, temperature, sensation, swelling, and the ability to move. If complications are evident, remove the stockings and notify the primary care provider.
- Evaluate stockings to ensure the top or toe opening does not roll with movement. Rolled stocking edges can cause excessive pressure and interfere with circulation.
- Despite the use of elastic stockings, a patient may develop deep vein thrombosis or phlebitis. Unilateral swelling, redness, tenderness, pain, and warmth are possible indicators of these complications. Notify the primary care provider of the presence of any symptoms.

Home Care Considerations

- Make sure that the patient has an extra pair of stockings ordered during hospitalization before discharge (for payment and convenience purposes).
- Generally it is best to take time to wash stockings by hand; stockings may be laundered with other "white" clothing. Avoid excessive bleach. Remove from dryer as soon as "low-heat" cycle is complete to avoid shrinkage. Stockings may also be air-dried; lay on a flat surface to prevent stretching. Check manufacturer's directions.
- Take all jewelry off before putting on stockings as rings and bracelets can snag on the compression hose, causing rips and tears.
- If putting on stockings is difficult, try wearing a pair of latex or rubber gloves, which will make it easier to grip the stockings (Kim & Lee, 2015).

(*continued*)

Skill 9-11 ▶ Applying and Removing Graduated Compression Stockings *(continued)*

EVIDENCE FOR PRACTICE ▶	**VENOUS THROMBOEMBOLISM PREVENTION** American Association of Critical-Care Nurses (AACN). (2010; updated 2016). AACN Practice alert. Preventing venous thromboembolism in adults. Retrieved https://www.aacn.org/clinical-resources/practice-alerts/venous-thromboembolism-prevention. The American Association of Critical-Care Nurses provides Practice Alerts. Practice Alerts, are succinct, dynamic directives that are supported by authoritative evidence to ensure excellence in practice and a safe and humane work environment. Almost all hospitalized patients have at least one risk factor for VTE. VTE, a common complication, contributes to excess length of stay, excess charges, and mortality. This Venous Thromboembolism Prevention Practice Alert supports the use of mechanical methods of prophylaxis, including graduated compression stockings, to reduce the risk of VTE. Nurses must select the correct size of stockings, properly apply them, and ensure that they are removed for only a short time each day. Refer to thePoint° for additional research on related nursing topics.
EVIDENCE FOR PRACTICE ▶	**VENOUS THROMBOEMBOLISM PREVENTION** Guyatt, G. H., Akl, E. A., Crowther, M., Gutterman, D. D., Schuünemann, H. J.; American College of Chest Physicians Antithrombotic Therapy and Prevention of Thrombosis Panel. (2012). Executive summary: Antithrombotic therapy and prevention of thrombosis, 9th ed.: American College of Chest Physicians evidence-based clinical practice guidelines. *Chest, 141*(2 suppl), 7S–47S. This evidence-based guideline outlines best practices for the prevention of venous thromboembolism (VTE). The use of mechanical methods of prophylaxis is included in the discussion. Refer to thePoint° for additional research on related nursing topics.

Skill 9-12 ▶ Applying Pneumatic Compression Devices

Pneumatic compression devices (PCDs) consist of fabric sleeves containing air bladders that apply brief pressure to the legs. Intermittent compression pushes blood from the smaller blood vessels into the deeper vessels and into the femoral veins. This action enhances blood flow and venous return and promotes fibrinolysis, deterring venous thrombosis. The sleeves are attached by tubing to an air pump. The sleeve may cover the entire leg or may extend from the foot to the knee.

PCDs may be used in combination with graduated compression stockings (antiembolism stockings) and anticoagulant therapy to prevent thrombosis formation. They can be used preoperatively and postoperatively with patients at risk for blood clot formation. They are also prescribed for patients with other risk factors for clot formation, including inactivity or immobilization, chronic venous disease, and malignancies.

DELEGATION CONSIDERATIONS	The application and removal of PCDs may be delegated to nursing assistive personnel (NAP) or unlicensed assistive personnel (UAP), as well as to licensed practical/vocational nurses (LPN/LVNs). The decision to delegate must be based on careful analysis of the patient's needs and circumstances, as well as the qualifications of the person to whom the task is being delegated. Refer to the Delegation Guidelines in Appendix A.
EQUIPMENT	• Compression sleeves of appropriate size based on the manufacturer's guidelines • Inflation pump with connection tubing • PPE, as indicated

ASSESSMENT	Assess the patient's history, medical record, and current condition and status to identify risk for development of deep vein thrombosis. Assess lower-extremity skin integrity. Identify any leg conditions that would be exacerbated by the use of the compression device or would contraindicate its use.

NURSING DIAGNOSIS	Determine the related factors for the nursing diagnoses based on the patient's current status. Appropriate nursing diagnoses may include: • Impaired physical mobility • Risk for peripheral neurovascular dysfunction • Delayed surgical recovery

OUTCOME IDENTIFICATION AND PLANNING	The expected outcome to achieve when applying a PCD is that the patient maintains adequate circulation in extremities and is free from symptoms of neurovascular compromise and deep vein thrombosis.

IMPLEMENTATION

ACTION	RATIONALE
1. Review the medical record and nursing care plan to determine the need for a pneumatic compression device (PCD) and for conditions that may contraindicate its use.	Reviewing the medical record and care plan validates the correct patient and correct procedure and minimizes the risk for injury.
2. Perform hand hygiene. Put on PPE, as indicated.	Hand hygiene and PPE prevent the spread of microorganisms. PPE is required based on transmission precautions.
3. Identify the patient. Explain the procedure to the patient.	Patient identification validates the correct patient and correct procedure. Discussion and explanation help allay anxiety and prepare the patient for what to expect.
4. Close the curtains around the bed and close the door to the room, if possible. Place the bed at an appropriate and comfortable working height, usually elbow height of the caregiver (VHACEOSH, 2016).	Closing the door or curtains provides for privacy. Proper bed height helps reduce back strain.
5. Hang the compression pump on the foot of the bed and plug it into an electrical outlet (Figure 1). Attach the connecting tubing to the pump.	Equipment preparation promotes efficient time management and provides an organized approach to the task.

FIGURE 1. PCD machine at foot of bed.

(continued)

Skill 9-12 ▶ Applying Pneumatic Compression Devices *(continued)*

ACTION	RATIONALE
6. Remove the compression sleeves from the package and unfold them. Lay the unfolded sleeves on the bed with the cotton lining facing up. **Note the markings indicating the correct placement for the ankle and popliteal areas.**	Proper placement of the sleeves prevents injury.
7. Apply graduated compression stockings, if ordered. Place a sleeve under the patient's leg with the tubing toward the heel (Figure 2). Each one fits either leg. **For total leg sleeves, place the behind-the-knee opening at the popliteal space to prevent pressure there. For knee-high sleeves, make sure the back of the ankle is over the ankle marking.**	Proper placement prevents injury.
8. Wrap the sleeve snugly around the patient's leg so that two fingers fit between the leg and the sleeve. Secure the sleeve with the Velcro fasteners. Repeat for the second leg, if bilateral therapy is ordered. Connect each sleeve to the tubing, following manufacturer's recommendations (Figure 3).	Correct placement ensures appropriate, but not excessive, compression of the extremity.

FIGURE 2. Placing PCD sleeves under patient's legs with tubing toward heel.

FIGURE 3. PCD sleeves snugly around patient's legs with sleeve tubing connected to device.

ACTION	RATIONALE
9. Set the pump to the prescribed maximal pressure (usually 35 to 55 mm Hg). Make sure the tubing is free from kinks. Check that the patient can move about without interrupting the airflow. Turn on the pump. Initiate cooling setting, if available.	Proper pressure setting ensures patient safety and prevents injury. Some devices have a cooling setting available to increase patient comfort.
10. **Observe the patient and the device during the first cycle. Check the audible alarms. Check the sleeves and pump at least once per shift or per facility policy.**	Observation and frequent checking ensure proper fit and inflation and reduce the risk for injury from the device.
11. Place the bed in the lowest position. Make sure the call bell and other essential items are within easy reach.	Returning the bed to the lowest position and having the call bell and other essential items readily available promote patient safety.
12. Remove PPE, if used. Perform hand hygiene.	Proper removal of PPE reduces the risk for infection transmission and contamination of other items. Hand hygiene prevents the spread of microorganisms.
13. Assess the extremities for peripheral pulses, edema, changes in sensation, and movement. Remove the sleeves and assess for document skin integrity every 8 hours.	Assessment provides for early detection and prompt intervention for possible complications, including skin irritation.

| EVALUATION | The expected outcome is met when the patient exhibits adequate circulation in extremities without symptoms of neurovascular compromise and deep vein thrombosis. |

DOCUMENTATION

Guidelines

Document the time and date of application of the PCD, the patient's response to the therapy, and the patient's understanding of the therapy. Document the status of the alarms and pressure settings. Note the use of the cooling setting, if appropriate. Document your assessment of the extremities.

Sample Documentation

> 4/27/20 1615 Patient instructed regarding reason for PCD therapy; verbalizes understanding of therapy. Knee-high PCD applied to both lower extremities; pressure set at 45 mm Hg, as ordered. Patient denies any complaints of numbness or tingling. Feet and toes warm and pink; quick capillary refill; bilateral pedal pulses present and equal. Alarms and cooling settings as ordered.
>
> —J. Trotter, RN

UNEXPECTED SITUATIONS AND ASSOCIATED INTERVENTIONS

- *Your postoperative patient is wearing PCD on both legs. While you are performing a routine assessment, he tells you that he has started to have pain in his left leg, along with tingling and numbness:* Remove the PCD and assess both lower extremities. Perform skin and neurovascular assessments. Assess the extremities for peripheral pulses, edema, changes in sensation, and movement. Report the patient's symptoms and assessment to the health care provider.

SPECIAL CONSIDERATIONS

- PCDs are contraindicated in patients with suspected or existing DVT. They should not be used for patients with arterial occlusive disease, severe edema, cellulitis, phlebitis, a skin graft, or an infection of the extremity.
- Use the cooling setting, if the unit has one. The skin under the sleeve can become wet with diaphoresis, which can increase the risk for impaired skin integrity.
- Generally, the PCD should be worn continuously. It may be removed for bathing, walking, and physical therapy. Use is usually discontinued when the patient is ambulating consistently.
- The risk for DVT formation and injury is greater if the sleeves are not applied correctly.

EVIDENCE FOR PRACTICE ▶

VENOUS THROMBOEMBOLISM PREVENTION

American Association of Critical-Care Nurses (AACN). (2010; updated 2016). AACN Practice alert. Preventing venous thromboembolism in adults. Retrieved https://www.aacn.org/clinical-resources/practice-alerts/venous-thromboembolism-prevention.

Refer to details in Skill 9-11, Evidence for Practice, and refer to thePoint° for additional research on related nursing topics.

EVIDENCE FOR PRACTICE ▶

VENOUS THROMBOEMBOLISM PREVENTION

Guyatt, G. H., Akl, E. A., Crowther, M., Gutterman, D. D., Schuünemann, H. J.; American College of Chest Physicians Antithrombotic Therapy and Prevention of Thrombosis Panel. (2012). Executive summary: Antithrombotic therapy and prevention of thrombosis, 9th ed.: American College of Chest Physicians evidence-based clinical practice guidelines. *Chest, 141*(2 Suppl), 7S–47S.

This evidence-based guideline outlines best practices for the prevention of venous thromboembolism (VTE). The use of mechanical methods of prophylaxis is included in the discussion.

Refer to thePoint° for additional research on related nursing topics.

Skill 9-13 ▶ Applying a Continuous Passive Motion Device

A continuous passive motion (CPM) device passively moves a joint within a certain ROM (Viswanathan & Kidd, 2010). The impact and benefit of CPM therapy is controversial, with many studies reporting little to no added benefit from use (Chen et al., 2013; Harvey, Brosseau, & Herbert, 2014; Herbold et al., 2014; White, Delitto, Nanal, & Miller, 2015). However, CPM may be prescribed after total knee **arthroplasty** as well as after surgery on other joints, such as shoulders, elbows, or ankles. The degree of flexion and **extension** of the joint and the cycle rate (the number of revolutions per minute) are determined by the prescriber, but nurses place the patient in and out of the device and monitor the patient's response to the therapy.

DELEGATION CONSIDERATIONS	The application and removal of a CPM device is not delegated to nursing assistive personnel (NAP) or to unlicensed assistive personnel (UAP). The application and removal of a CPM device may be delegated to licensed practical/vocational nurses (LPN/LVNs). The decision to delegate must be based on careful analysis of the patient's needs and circumstances, as well as the qualifications of the person to whom the task is being delegated. Refer to the Delegation Guidelines in Appendix A.

EQUIPMENT

- CPM device
- Single patient use soft-goods kit
- Tape measure
- Goniometer
- Nonsterile gloves and/or other PPE, if indicated

ASSESSMENT

Review the medical record and nursing care plan for orders for degrees of flexion and extension. Assess the neurovascular status of the involved extremity. Perform a pain assessment. Administer the prescribed medication in sufficient time to allow for the full effect of the analgesic before starting the device. Assess for proper alignment of the joint in the CPM device. Assess the patient's ability to tolerate the prescribed treatment.

NURSING DIAGNOSIS

Determine the related factors for the nursing diagnoses based on the patient's current status. Appropriate nursing diagnoses may include:

- Impaired bed mobility
- Risk for impaired skin integrity
- Risk for peripheral neurovascular dysfunction

OUTCOME IDENTIFICATION AND PLANNING

The expected outcome to achieve when applying a CPM device is that the patient experiences increased joint mobility and does not exhibit atrophy or contractures.

IMPLEMENTATION

ACTION	RATIONALE
1. Review the medical record and nursing care plan for the appropriate degrees of flexion and extension, the cycle rate, and the length of time the CPM is to be used.	Reviewing the medical record and care plan validates the correct patient and correct procedure and reduces the risk for injury.
2. Obtain equipment. Apply the soft goods to the CPM device.	Equipment preparation promotes efficient time management and provides an organized approach to the task. The soft goods help to prevent friction to the extremity during motion.
3. Perform hand hygiene. Put on PPE, as indicated.	Hand hygiene and PPE prevent the spread of microorganisms. PPE is required based on transmission precautions.
4. Identify the patient. Explain the procedure to the patient.	Patient identification validates the correct patient and correct procedure. Discussion and explanation help allay anxiety and prepare the patient for what to expect.

ACTION

5. Close the curtains around the bed and close the door to the room, if possible. Place the bed at an appropriate and comfortable working height, usually elbow height of the caregiver (VHACEOSH, 2016).

6. Using the tape measure, determine the distance between the gluteal crease and the popliteal space.

7. Measure the leg from the knee to 14 in beyond the bottom of the foot.

8. Position the patient in the middle of the bed. Make sure the affected extremity is in a slightly abducted position.

9. Support the affected extremity and elevate it, placing it in the padded CPM device (Figure 1).

10. **Make sure the knee is at the hinged joint of the CPM device.**

11. **Adjust the footplate to maintain the patient's foot in a neutral position (Figure 2). Assess the patient's position to make sure the leg is not internally or externally rotated.**

RATIONALE

Closing the door or curtains provides for privacy. Proper bed height helps reduce back strain.

The thigh length on the CPM device is adjusted based on this measurement.

The position of the footplate is adjusted based on this measurement.

Proper positioning promotes correct body alignment and prevents pressure on the unaffected extremity.

Support and elevation assist in movement of the affected extremity without injury.

Proper positioning in the device prevents injury.

Adjustment helps ensure proper positioning and prevents injury.

FIGURE 1. Placing patient's leg into CPM machine.

FIGURE 2. Adjusting footplate to maintain patient's foot in a neutral position.

12. Apply the restraining straps under the CPM device and around the leg. **Check that two fingers fit between the strap and the leg (Figure 3).**

Restraining straps maintain the leg in position. Leaving a space between the strap and leg prevents injury from excessive pressure from the strap.

FIGURE 3. Using two fingers to check fit between straps and leg.

(continued)

Skill 9-13 ▶ Applying a Continuous Passive Motion Device *(continued)*

ACTION	RATIONALE
13. Explain the use of the STOP/GO button to the patient. Set the controls to the prescribed levels of flexion and extension and cycles per minute. Turn on the power to the CPM.	Explanation decreases anxiety by allowing the patient to participate in care.
14. Set the device to ON and start the therapy by pressing the GO button. Observe the patient and the device during the first cycle. Determine the angle of flexion when the device reaches its greatest height using the goniometer (Figure 4). Compare with prescribed degree.	Observation ensures that the device is working properly, thereby ensuring patient safety. Measuring with a **goniometer** ensures the device is set to the prescribed parameters.

FIGURE 4. Determining angle of joint flexion using goniometer.

ACTION	RATIONALE
15. Place the bed in the lowest position, with the side rails up. Make sure the call bell and other essential items are within easy reach.	Having the bed at the proper height and having the call bell and other items handy ensure patient safety.
16. Remove PPE, if used. Perform hand hygiene.	Proper removal of PPE reduces the risk for infection transmission and contamination of other items. Hand hygiene prevents the spread of microorganisms.
17. Check the patient's level of comfort and perform skin and neurovascular assessments at least every 4 hours or per facility policy.	Frequent assessments provide for early detection and prompt intervention should problems arise.

EVALUATION

The expected outcome has been met when the patient demonstrates increased joint mobility and does not exhibit atrophy or contractures.

DOCUMENTATION

Guidelines

Document the time and date of application of the CPM, the extension and flexion settings, the speed of the device, the patient's response to the therapy, and your assessment of the extremity.

Sample Documentation

> 5/03/20 1430 Right knee incision clean and dry; dressing intact. Right toes pink and warm, with brisk capillary refill; equal to left. Pedal pulses present and equal bilaterally. CPM device applied with range of motion at 30 degrees of knee flexion, for 5 cycles/min for 30 minutes. Patient complains of slight increase in pain from a rating of 4/10 to 5/10, but states, "I don't want anything for the pain right now." Plan to reassess in 15 minutes and offer analgesic as ordered.
>
> —K. Dugas, RN

| UNEXPECTED SITUATIONS AND ASSOCIATED INTERVENTIONS | • *A patient is prescribed therapy with a CPM device. After you initiate the prescribed flexion and extension of the joint, the patient complains of sudden pain in the joint:* Stop the CPM device. Check the settings to make sure the device is set correctly for the prescribed therapy. Assess the patient for other signs and symptoms and obtain vital signs. Perform a neurovascular assessment of the affected extremity. Notify the primary care provider of the patient's pain and any other findings. When therapy is resumed, evaluate the need for premedication with analgesics. Continue pain intervention with analgesics, as prescribed. |

Skill 9-14 ▶ Applying a Sling

A sling is a bandage that can provide support for an arm or immobilize an injured arm, wrist, or hand. Slings can be used to restrict movement of a fracture or dislocation and to support a muscle sprain. They may also be used to support a splint or secure dressings. Health care facilities usually use commercial slings. The sling should distribute the supported weight over a large area, not the back of the neck, to prevent pressure on the cervical spinal nerves.

DELEGATION CONSIDERATIONS	The application of a sling may not be delegated to nursing assistive personnel (NAP) or to unlicensed assistive personnel (UAP). The application of a sling may be delegated to licensed practical/vocational nurses (LPN/LVNs). The decision to delegate must be based on careful analysis of the patient's needs and circumstances, as well as the qualifications of the person to whom the task is being delegated. Refer to the Delegation Guidelines in Appendix A.
EQUIPMENT	• Commercial arm sling • ABD gauze pad	• Nonsterile gloves and/or other PPE, as indicated
ASSESSMENT	Assess the situation to determine the need for a sling. Assess the affected limb for pain and edema. Perform a neurovascular assessment of the affected extremity. Assess body parts distal to the site for cyanosis, pallor, coolness, numbness, tingling, swelling, and absent or diminished pulses.
NURSING DIAGNOSIS	Determine the related factors for the nursing diagnoses based on the patient's current status. Appropriate nursing diagnoses may include: • Acute pain • Risk for impaired skin integrity • Risk for peripheral neurovascular dysfunction
OUTCOME IDENTIFICATION AND PLANNING	The expected outcome to achieve when applying a sling is that the arm is immobilized in proper alignment. In addition, the patient shows no evidence of contractures, **venous stasis**, thrombus formation, or skin breakdown; and the patient demonstrates proper use of the sling.

IMPLEMENTATION

ACTION	**RATIONALE**
1. Review the medical record and nursing care plan to determine the need for the use of a sling.	Reviewing the medical record and care plan validates the correct patient and correct procedure and prevents injury.
2. Perform hand hygiene. Put on PPE, as indicated.	Hand hygiene and PPE prevent the spread of microorganisms. PPE is required based on transmission precautions.

(continued)

Skill 9-14 ▶ Applying a Sling (continued)

ACTION	**RATIONALE**

 3. Identify the patient. Explain the procedure to the patient.

Patient identification validates the correct patient and correct procedure. Discussion and explanation help allay anxiety and prepare the patient for what to expect.

4. Close the curtains around the bed and close the door to the room, if possible. Place the bed at an appropriate and comfortable working height, usually elbow height of the caregiver (VHACEOSH, 2016).

Closing the door or curtains provides for privacy. Proper bed height helps reduce back strain.

5. Perform a pain assessment. If the patient reports pain, administer the prescribed medication in sufficient time to allow for the full effect of the analgesic.

Injury to the arm requiring the use of a sling may cause discomfort and/or pain. Allowing sufficient time for analgesic to take effect promotes optimal patient comfort.

6. Assist the patient to a sitting position. Place the patient's forearm across the chest with the elbow flexed and the palm against the chest. Measure the sleeve length, if indicated.

Proper positioning facilitates sling application. Measurement ensures proper sizing of the sling and proper placement of the arm.

7. Enclose the arm in the sling, making sure the elbow fits into the corner of the fabric (Figure 1). Run the strap up the patient's back and across the shoulder opposite the injury, then down the chest to the fastener on the end of the sling (Figure 2).

This position ensures adequate support and keeps the arm out of a dependent position, preventing edema.

FIGURE 1. Placing patient's arm into canvas sling with elbow flush in corner of sling.

FIGURE 2. Placing strap around patient's neck.

8. Place the ABD pad under the strap, between the strap and the patient's neck (Figure 3). **Ensure that the sling and forearm are slightly elevated and at a right angle to the body (Figure 4).**

Padding prevents skin irritation and reduces pressure on the neck. Proper positioning ensures alignment, provides support, and prevents edema.

FIGURE 3. Placing padding between strap and patient's neck.

FIGURE 4. Patient with sling in place.

ACTION

9. Place the bed in the lowest position, with the side rails up. Make sure the call bell and other essential items are within easy reach.

 10. Remove PPE, if used. Perform hand hygiene.

11. Check the patient's level of comfort, pain, arm positioning, and neurovascular status of the affected limb every 4 hours or according to facility policy. Assess the axillary and cervical skin frequently for irritation or breakdown.

RATIONALE

Having the bed at proper height and leaving the call bell and other items within reach ensure patient safety.

Proper removal of PPE reduces the risk for infection transmission and contamination of other items. Hand hygiene prevents the spread of microorganisms.

Frequent assessment ensures patient safety, prevents injury, and provides early intervention for skin irritation and other complications.

EVALUATION

The expected outcome has been met when the patient's arm has been immobilized in proper alignment. In addition, the patient shows no evidence of contractures, venous stasis, thrombus formation, or skin breakdown; and the patient demonstrates proper use of the sling.

DOCUMENTATION

Guidelines

Document the time and date the sling was applied. Document the patient's response to the sling and the neurovascular status of the extremity. Document the pain assessment and associated interventions, as well as patient response.

Sample Documentation

5/22/20 2015 Sling applied to left arm, as ordered. Left hand and fingers warm to touch and pink. Brisk capillary refill. Left radial pulse present and equal to right. Patient denies any complaints of numbness, pain, or tingling of left upper extremity.

—P. Peterson, RN

UNEXPECTED SITUATIONS AND ASSOCIATED INTERVENTIONS

- *Your patient needs a sling to support a wrist fracture, but you cannot obtain a commercially prepared sling:* Make a sling using a triangular bandage or cloth. Place the cloth or bandage on the chest with a corner of the cloth at the elbow. Place the affected arm across the chest with the elbow flexed and the palm on the chest. Wrap the end closest to the head around the neck, on the opposite side from the injured arm. Bring the end of the cloth that is farthest from the head up over the injured arm and tie it at the side of the neck. Make sure that the sling and forearm are slightly elevated and at a right angle to the body.

SPECIAL CONSIDERATIONS

- Be sure that the patient's wrist is enclosed in the sling. Do not allow it to hang out and down over the edge. This prevents pressure on nerves and blood vessels and prevents muscle contractures, deformity, and discomfort.
- Assess circulation and comfort at regular intervals.

Skill 9-15 ▶ Applying a Figure-Eight Bandage

Bandages are used to apply pressure over an area, immobilize a body part, prevent or reduce edema, and secure splints and dressings. Bandages can be elasticized or made of gauze, flannel, or muslin. In general, narrow bandages are used to wrap feet, the lower legs, hands, and arms, and wider bandages are used for the thighs and trunk. A roller bandage is a continuous strip of material wound on itself to form a roll. The free end is anchored and the roll is passed or rolled around the body part, maintaining equal tension with all turns. The bandage is unwound gradually and only as needed. The bandage should overlap itself evenly and by one half to two thirds the width of the bandage. The figure-eight turn consists of oblique overlapping turns that ascend and descend alternately. It is used around the knee, elbow, ankle, and wrist.

DELEGATION CONSIDERATIONS

The application of a figure-eight bandage may not be delegated to nursing assistive personnel (NAP) or to unlicensed assistive personnel (UAP). The application of a figure-eight bandage may be delegated to licensed practical/vocational nurses (LPN/LVNs). The decision to delegate must be based on careful analysis of the patient's needs and circumstances, as well as the qualifications of the person to whom the task is being delegated. Refer to the Delegation Guidelines in Appendix A.

EQUIPMENT

- Elastic or other bandage of the appropriate width
- Tape, pins, or self-closures
- Gauze pads
- Nonsterile gloves and/or other PPE, as indicated

ASSESSMENT

Review the medical record and nursing care plan and assess the situation to determine the need for a bandage. Assess the affected limb for pain and edema. Perform a neurovascular assessment of the affected extremity. Assess body parts distal to the site for evidence of cyanosis, pallor, coolness, numbness, tingling, and swelling and absent or diminished pulses. Assess the distal circulation of the extremity after the bandage is in place and at least every 4 hours thereafter.

NURSING DIAGNOSIS

Determine the related factors for the nursing diagnoses based on the patient's current status. Appropriate nursing diagnoses may include:

- Acute pain
- Risk for peripheral neurovascular dysfunction
- Risk for impaired skin integrity

OUTCOME IDENTIFICATION AND PLANNING

The expected outcome to achieve when applying a figure-eight bandage is that the bandage is applied correctly without injury or complications. Other outcomes that may be appropriate include the following: patient maintains circulation to the affected part and remains free of neurovascular complications.

IMPLEMENTATION

ACTION	RATIONALE
1. Review the medical record and nursing care plan to determine the need for a figure-eight bandage.	Reviewing the medical record and care plan validates the correct patient and correct procedure and reduces risk for injury.
2. Perform hand hygiene. Put on PPE, as indicated.	Hand hygiene and PPE prevent the spread of microorganisms. PPE is required based on transmission precautions.
3. Identify the patient. Explain the procedure to the patient.	Patient identification validates the correct patient and correct procedure. Discussion and explanation help allay anxiety and prepare the patient for what to expect.

ACTION

4. Close the curtains around the bed and close the door to the room, if possible. Place the bed at an appropriate and comfortable working height, usually elbow height of the caregiver (VHACEOSH, 2016).

5. Assist the patient to a comfortable position, with the affected body part in a normal-functioning position.

6. Hold the bandage roll with the roll facing upward in one hand, while holding the free end of the roll in the other hand. Make sure to hold the bandage roll so it is close to the affected body part.

7. Wrap the bandage around the limb twice, below the joint, to anchor it (Figure 1).

RATIONALE

Closing the door or curtains provides for privacy. Proper bed height helps reduce back strain.

Keeping the body part in a normal-functioning position promotes circulation and prevents deformity and discomfort.

Proper handling of the bandage allows application of even tension and pressure.

Anchoring the bandage ensures that it will stay in place.

FIGURE 1. Wrapping bandage around patient's limb twice, below joint, to anchor it.

8. Use alternating ascending and descending turns to form a figure eight (Figure 2). Overlap each turn of the bandage by one half to two thirds the width of the strip (Figure 3).

Making alternating ascending and descending turns helps to ensure the bandage will stay in place on a moving body part.

FIGURE 2. Using alternating ascending and descending turns to form a figure eight.

FIGURE 3. Overlapping each turn of bandage by one half to two thirds strip width.

9. Unroll the bandage as you wrap, not before wrapping.

Unrolling the bandage with wrapping prevents uneven pressure, which could interfere with blood circulation.

10. **Wrap firmly, but not tightly. Assess the patient's comfort as you wrap. If the patient reports tingling, itching, numbness, or pain, loosen the bandage.**

Firm wrapping is necessary to provide support and prevent injury, but wrapping too tightly interferes with circulation. Patient complaints are helpful indicators of possible circulatory compromise.

(continued)

Skill 9-15 ▶ Applying a Figure-Eight Bandage *(continued)*

ACTION	RATIONALE
11. After the area is covered, wrap the bandage around the limb twice, above the joint, to anchor it (Figure 4). Secure the end of the bandage with tape, pins, or self-closures. Avoid metal clips.	Anchoring at the end ensures the bandage will stay in place. Metal clips can cause injury.

FIGURE 4. Wrapping bandage around patient's limb twice, above joint, to anchor it.

ACTION	RATIONALE
12. Place the bed in the lowest position, with the side rails up. Make sure the call bell and other necessary items are within easy reach.	Repositioning the bed and having items nearby ensure patient safety.
13. Remove PPE, if used. Perform hand hygiene.	Proper removal of PPE reduces the risk for infection transmission and contamination of other items. Hand hygiene prevents the spread of microorganisms.
14. Elevate the wrapped extremity for 15 to 30 minutes after application of the bandage.	Elevation promotes venous return and reduces edema.
15. Assess the distal circulation after the bandage is in place.	Elastic may tighten as it is wrapped. Frequent assessment of distal circulation ensures patient safety and prevents injury.
16. Lift the distal end of the bandage and assess the skin for color, temperature, and integrity. Assess for pain and perform a neurovascular assessment of the affected extremity after applying the bandage and at least every 4 hours thereafter, or per facility policy.	Assessment aids in prompt detection of compromised circulation and allows for early intervention for skin irritation and other complications.

EVALUATION

The expected outcome has been achieved when the patient exhibits a bandage that is applied correctly, without causing injury or neurovascular compromise.

DOCUMENTATION

Guidelines

Document the time, date, and site that the bandage was applied and the size of the bandage used. Include the skin assessment and care provided before application. Document the patient's response to the bandage and the neurovascular status of the extremity.

Sample Documentation

> 5/27/20 1615 3-in bandage applied to right knee using figure-eight technique. Skin pink, warm, and dry, with quick capillary refill; pedal and dorsalis pedis pulses present and equal bilaterally. Patient denies any complaints of pain, numbness, or tingling. Patient instructed to report any complaints immediately. Right lower extremity resting on two pillows at present.
>
> —J. Wilkins, RN

UNEXPECTED SITUATIONS AND ASSOCIATED INTERVENTIONS	• *After you have applied a figure-eight bandage to a patient's elbow to hold dressings in place, the patient reports tingling, numbness, and pain in his hand during a routine assessment:* Remove the bandage, wait 30 minutes, and reapply the bandage with less tension. Continue to monitor the neurovascular status of the extremity. Symptoms should subside fairly quickly. If symptoms persist, notify the health care provider. • *You remove the bandage on a patient's ankle and note the bandage is limp and less elastic than when it was applied:* Obtain a new bandage and apply it to the ankle. Launder the old bandage to restore its elasticity. Keep two bandages at the bedside: one can be applied while the other is being laundered.
SPECIAL CONSIDERATIONS	• Keep in mind that a figure-eight bandage may be contraindicated if skin breakdown or lesions are present on the area to be wrapped. • When wrapping an extremity, elevate it for 15 to 30 minutes before applying the bandage, if possible. This promotes venous return and prevents edema. Avoid applying the bandage to a dependent extremity. • Place gauze pads or cotton between skin surfaces, such as toes and fingers, to prevent skin irritation. Skin surfaces should not touch after the bandage is applied. • Include the heel when wrapping the foot, but do not wrap the toes or fingers unless necessary. Assess distal body parts to detect impaired circulation. • Avoid leaving gaps in bandage layers or leaving skin exposed, because this may result in uneven pressure on the body part. • Remove and change the bandage at least once a day, or per medical order or facility policy. Cleanse the skin and dry thoroughly before applying a new bandage. Assess the skin for irritation and breakdown.

Skill 9-16 ▶ Assisting With Cast Application

A cast is a rigid external immobilizing device that encases a body part. Casts are used to immobilize a body part in a specific position and to apply uniform pressure on the encased soft tissue. They may be used to treat injuries, correct a deformity, stabilize weakened joints, or promote healing after surgery. Casts generally allow the patient mobility while restricting movement of the affected body part. Casts may be made of plaster or synthetic materials, such as fiberglass. Each material has advantages and disadvantages. Nonplaster casts set in 15 minutes and can sustain weight bearing or pressure in 15 to 30 minutes. Plaster casts can take 24 to 72 hours to dry, and weight bearing or pressure is contraindicated during this period. Patient safety is of utmost importance during the application of a cast. Typically, a physician or other advanced practice professional applies the cast. Nursing responsibilities include preparing the patient and equipment and assisting during the application. The nurse provides skin care to the affected area before, during, and after the cast is applied. In some settings, nurses with special preparation may apply or change casts.

DELEGATION CONSIDERATIONS	Assisting with the application of a cast may not be delegated to nursing assistive personnel (NAP) or to unlicensed assistive personnel (UAP). Depending on the state's nurse practice act and the organization's policies and procedures, assisting with the application of a cast may be delegated to licensed practical/vocational nurses (LPN/LVNs). The decision to delegate must be based on careful analysis of the patient's needs and circumstances, as well as the qualifications of the person to whom the task is being delegated. Refer to the Delegation Guidelines in Appendix A.
EQUIPMENT	• Casting materials, such as plaster rolls or fiberglass, depending on the type of cast being applied • Padding material, such as stockinette or sheet wadding, depending on the type of cast being applied	• Plastic bucket or basin filled with warm water • Disposable, nonsterile gloves and aprons • Scissors • Waterproof, disposable pads • PPE, as indicated

(*continued*)

Skill 9-16 ▶ Assisting With Cast Application *(continued)*

ASSESSMENT	Assess the skin condition in the affected area, noting redness, **contusions**, or open wounds. Assess the neurovascular status of the affected extremity, including distal pulses, color, temperature, presence of edema, capillary refill to fingers or toes, weakness, sensation, and motion. Perform a pain assessment. If the patient reports pain, administer the prescribed analgesic in sufficient time to allow for the full effect of the medication. Assess for muscle spasms and administer the prescribed muscle relaxant in sufficient time to allow for the full effect of the medication. Assess for the presence of disease processes that may contraindicate the use of a cast or interfere with wound healing, including skin diseases, peripheral vascular disease, diabetes mellitus, and open or draining wounds.
NURSING DIAGNOSIS	Determine the related factors for the nursing diagnoses based on the patient's current status. Appropriate nursing diagnoses may include: • Risk for impaired skin integrity • Risk for peripheral neurovascular dysfunction • (Bathing; Dressing; Feeding; Toileting) self-care deficit
OUTCOME IDENTIFICATION AND PLANNING	The expected outcome to achieve when assisting with a cast application is that the cast is applied without interfering with neurovascular function. Other outcomes that may be appropriate include that the patient is free from complications; and the patient experiences increased comfort.

IMPLEMENTATION

ACTION	**RATIONALE**
1. Review the medical record and medical orders to determine the need for the cast.	Reviewing the medical record and order validates the correct patient and correct procedure.
2. Perform hand hygiene. Put on gloves and/or other PPE, as indicated.	Hand hygiene and PPE prevent the spread of microorganisms. PPE is required based on transmission precautions.
3. Identify the patient. Explain the procedure to the patient and verify area to be casted.	Patient identification validates the correct patient and correct procedure. Discussion and explanation help allay anxiety and prepare the patient for what to expect.
4. Perform a pain assessment and assess for muscle spasm. Administer prescribed medications in sufficient time to allow for the full effect of the analgesic and/or muscle relaxant.	Assessment of pain and analgesic administration ensures patient comfort and enhances cooperation.
5. Close the curtains around the bed and close the door to the room, if possible. Place the bed at an appropriate and comfortable working height, usually elbow height of the caregiver (VHACEOSH, 2016).	Closing the door or curtains provides for privacy. Proper bed height helps reduce back strain while you are performing the procedure.
6. Position the patient, as needed, depending on the type of cast being applied and the location of the injury. Support the extremity or body part to be casted. Remove any rings or other jewelry from area to be casted.	Proper positioning minimizes movement, maintains alignment, and increases patient comfort. Rings or other jewelry could produce pressure points and contribute to alterations in circulation and perfusion.
7. Drape the patient with the waterproof pads.	Draping provides warmth and privacy and helps protect other body parts from contact with casting materials.
8. Cleanse and dry the affected body part.	Skin care before cast application helps prevent skin breakdown.

ACTION

9. Position and maintain the affected body part in the position indicated by the physician or advanced practice professional as the stockinette, sheet wadding, and padding are applied (Figure 1). The stockinette should extend beyond the ends of the cast. As the wadding is applied, check for wrinkles.

10. Continue to position and maintain the affected body part in the position indicated by the physician or advanced practice professional as the casting material is applied (Figure 2). Assist with finishing by folding the stockinette or other padding down over the outer edge of the cast.

RATIONALE

Stockinette and other materials protect the skin from casting materials and create a smooth, padded edge, protecting the skin from abrasion. Padding protects the skin, tissues, and nerves from the pressure of the cast.

Smooth edges lessen the risk for skin irritation and abrasion.

FIGURE 1. Stockinette in place.

FIGURE 2. Casting material being applied.

11. **Support the cast during hardening.** Handle hardening plaster casts with the palms of hands, not fingers (Figure 3). Support the cast on a firm, smooth surface. Do not rest it on a hard surface or sharp edges. Avoid placing pressure on the cast.

Proper handling avoids denting of the cast and development of pressure areas.

FIGURE 3. Using palms to handle casted limb.

12. **Elevate the injured limb at heart level with pillow or bath blankets, as ordered, making sure pressure is evenly distributed under the cast.**

Elevation promotes venous return. Evenly distributed pressure prevents molding and denting of the cast and development of pressure areas.

(continued)

Skill 9-16 ▶ Assisting With Cast Application *(continued)*

ACTION	**RATIONALE**
13. Place the bed in the lowest position, with the side rails up. Make sure the call bell and other essential items are within easy reach.	Having the bed at proper height and leaving the call bell and other items within reach ensure patient safety.
14. Remove gloves and any other PPE, if used. Perform hand hygiene.	Proper removal of PPE reduces the risk for infection transmission and contamination of other items. Hand hygiene prevents the spread of microorganisms.
15. Obtain x-rays, as ordered.	X-rays identify that the affected area is positioned properly.
16. Instruct the patient to report pain, odor, drainage, changes in sensation, abnormal sensation, or the inability to move fingers or toes of the affected extremity.	Pressure within a cast may increase with edema and lead to **compartment syndrome**. Patient complaints allow for early detection of, and prompt intervention for, complications such as skin irritation or impaired tissue perfusion.
17. Leave the cast uncovered and exposed to the air. Reposition the patient every 2 hours. Depending on facility policy, a fan may be used to dry the cast.	Keeping the cast uncovered promotes drying. Repositioning prevents development of pressure areas. Using a fan helps increase airflow and speeds drying.

EVALUATION

The expected outcome is achieved when neurovascular function is maintained and healing occurs. In addition, the patient is free from complications, has knowledge of the treatment regimen, and experiences increased comfort.

DOCUMENTATION

Guidelines

Document the time, date, and site that the cast was applied. Include the skin assessment and care provided before application. Document the patient's response to the cast and the neurovascular status of the extremity.

Sample Documentation

> 6/1/20 1245 Fiberglass cast applied to right forearm from mid-upper arm to middle of hand. Cast clean and dry; edges padded. No signs of irritation noted. Patient able to move fingers freely. Fingers pale pink, warm, and dry. Capillary refill less than 2 seconds. Patient denies any numbness, tingling, or pain. Right forearm resting on two pillows. Patient instructed to report any complaints of pain, pressure, numbness, tingling, or decreased ability to move fingers.
>
> —P. Collins, RN

Unexpected Situations and Associated Interventions

- *Your patient, who has a cast on his hand and forearm, has been experiencing pain relief in the extremity with ice application and oral analgesics. He now reports pain unrelieved by the analgesic and a feeling of tightness in his arm. In addition, his fingers are cool, with sluggish capillary refill:* Compartment syndrome may be developing. Adjust the position of the arm so that it is no higher than heart level. This enhances arterial perfusion and controls edema. Notify the primary care provider of the situation immediately. Prepare for bivalving of the cast (cutting of the cast in half longitudinally) to relieve pressure.

SPECIAL CONSIDERATIONS

General Considerations

- Perform frequent, regular assessment of neurovascular status. Early recognition of diminished circulation and nerve function is essential to prevent loss of function. Be alert for the presence of compartment syndrome.
- If a fiberglass cast was applied, remove any fiberglass resin residue on the skin with alcohol or acetone.
- Synthetic casts are lightweight, easy to clean, and somewhat water-resistant. If a Gore-Tex liner is used when the cast is applied, the cast may be immersed in water without affecting the cast integrity.

Infant and Child Considerations

- Synthetic casts come in different colors and with designs, such as cartoons and stripes. These features may make the experience more pleasant for a child.

Skill 9-17 ▸ Caring for a Cast

A cast is a rigid external immobilizing device that encases a body part. Casts, made of plaster or synthetic materials, such as fiberglass, are used to immobilize a body part in a specific position and to apply uniform pressure on the encased soft tissue. They may be used to treat injuries, correct a deformity, stabilize weakened joints, or promote healing after surgery. Casts generally allow the patient mobility while restricting movement of the affected body part. Nursing responsibilities after the cast is in place include maintaining the cast, preventing complications, and providing patient teaching related to cast care.

DELEGATION CONSIDERATIONS	Care of a cast may not be delegated to nursing assistive personnel (NAP) or to unlicensed assistive personnel (UAP). Depending on the state's nurse practice act and the organization's policies and procedures, care of a cast may be delegated to licensed practical/vocational nurses (LPN/LVNs). The decision to delegate must be based on careful analysis of the patient's needs and circumstances, as well as the qualifications of the person to whom the task is being delegated. Refer to the Delegation Guidelines in Appendix A.

EQUIPMENT

- Disposable cleansing wipes or washcloth, towel, skin cleanser, and basin of warm water
- Waterproof pads
- Tape
- Pillows
- PPE, as indicated

ASSESSMENT

Review the patient's medical record and nursing care plan to determine the need for cast care and care of the affected area. Perform a pain assessment and administer the prescribed medication in sufficient time to allow for the full effect of the analgesic before starting care. Assess the neurovascular status of the affected extremity, including distal pulses, color, temperature, presence of edema, capillary refill to fingers or toes, and sensation and motion. Assess the skin distal to the cast. Note any indications of infection, including any foul odor from the cast, pain, fever, edema, and extreme warmth over an area of the cast. Assess for complications of immobility, including alterations in skin integrity, reduced joint movement, decreased peristalsis, constipation, alterations in respiratory function, and signs of **thrombophlebitis**. Inspect the condition of the cast. Be alert for cracks, dents, or the presence of drainage from the cast. Assess the patient's knowledge of cast care.

NURSING DIAGNOSIS

Determine the related factors for the nursing diagnoses based on the patient's current status. Appropriate nursing diagnoses may include:

- Risk for peripheral neurovascular dysfunction
- (Bathing; Dressing; Feeding; Toileting) self-care deficit
- Risk for impaired skin integrity

OUTCOME IDENTIFICATION AND PLANNING

The expected outcome to achieve when caring for a patient with a cast is that the cast remains intact, and the patient does not experience neurovascular compromise. Other outcomes include that the patient is free from infection; the patient experiences only mild pain and slight edema or soreness; the patient experiences only slight limitations of range-of-joint motion; the skin around the cast edges remains intact; the patient participates in ADLs; and the patient demonstrates appropriate cast-care techniques.

IMPLEMENTATION

ACTION	RATIONALE
1. Review the medical record and the nursing care plan to determine the need for cast care and care for the affected body part.	Reviewing the medical record and care plan validates the correct patient and correct procedure.
2. Perform hand hygiene. Put on PPE, as indicated.	Hand hygiene and PPE prevent the spread of microorganisms. PPE is required based on transmission precautions.
3. Identify the patient. Explain the procedure to the patient.	Patient identification validates the correct patient and correct procedure. Discussion and explanation help allay anxiety and prepare the patient for what to expect.

(continued)

Skill 9-17 ▶ Caring for a Cast *(continued)*

ACTION	**RATIONALE**
4. Close the curtains around the bed and close the door to the room, if possible. Place the bed at an appropriate and comfortable working height, usually elbow height of the caregiver (VHACEOSH, 2016).	Closing the door or curtains provides for privacy. Proper bed height helps reduce back strain while you are performing the procedure.
5. If a plaster cast was applied, handle the casted extremity or body area with the palms of your hands for the first 24 to 36 hours, until the cast is fully dry.	Proper handling of a plaster cast prevents dents in the cast, which may create pressure areas on the inside of the cast.
6. If the cast is on an extremity, elevate the affected area on pillows covered with waterproof pads. **Maintain the normal curvatures and angles of the cast (Figure 1).**	Elevation helps reduce edema and enhances venous return. Use of a waterproof pad prevents soiling of linen. Maintaining curvatures and angles maintains proper joint alignment, helps prevent flattened areas on the cast as it dries, and prevents pressure areas.

FIGURE 1. Elevating casted limb, maintaining normal curvatures and angles of the cast.

ACTION	**RATIONALE**
7. Keep cast (plaster) uncovered until fully dry.	Keeping the cast uncovered allows heat and moisture to dissipate and air to circulate to speed drying.
8. Assess the condition of the cast (Figure 2). Be alert for cracks, dents, or the presence of drainage from the cast. Perform skin assessment, particularly around edges of the cast, and neurovascular assessment according to facility policy, as often as every 1 to 2 hours. **Check for pain, edema, inability to move body parts distal to the cast, pallor, pulses, and abnormal sensations. If the cast is on an extremity, compare it with the noncasted extremity (Figure 3).**	Assessment helps detect abnormal neurovascular function or infection and allows for prompt intervention. Assessing the neurovascular status determines the circulation and oxygenation of tissues. Pressure within a cast may increase with edema and lead to compartment syndrome.

FIGURE 2. Assessing condition of cast.

FIGURE 3. Assessing skin and neurovascular function, comparing with noncasted extremity.

ACTION

9. If breakthrough bleeding or drainage is noted on the cast, mark the area on the cast, according to facility policy (Figure 4). Indicate the date and time next to the area. Follow medical orders or facility policy regarding the amount of drainage that needs to be reported to the primary care provider.

10. Assess for signs of infection. Monitor the patient's temperature. Assess for a foul odor from the cast, increased pain, or extreme warmth over an area of the cast.

11. Reposition the patient every 2 hours. Provide back and skin care frequently. Encourage range-of-motion exercise for unaffected joints. Encourage the patient to cough and breathe deeply.

12. Instruct the patient to report pain, odor, drainage, changes in sensation, abnormal sensation, or the inability to move fingers or toes of the affected extremity.

13. Place the bed in the lowest position, with the side rails up. Make sure the call bell and other essential items are within easy reach.

 14. Remove PPE, if used. Perform hand hygiene.

RATIONALE

Marking the area provides a baseline for monitoring the amount of bleeding or drainage.

FIGURE 4. Marking any breakthrough bleeding on cast, indicating date and time.

Infection deters healing. Assessment allows for early detection and prompt intervention.

Repositioning promotes even drying of the cast and reduces the risk for the development of pressure areas under the cast. Frequent skin and back care prevents patient discomfort and skin breakdown. ROM exercises maintain joint function of unaffected areas. Coughing and deep breathing reduce the risk for respiratory complications associated with immobility.

Pressure within a cast may increase with edema and lead to compartment syndrome. The patient's understanding of signs and symptoms allows for early detection and prompt intervention.

Having the bed at proper height and leaving the call bell and other items within reach ensures patient safety.

Proper removal of PPE reduces the risk for infection transmission and contamination of other items. Hand hygiene prevents the spread of microorganisms.

EVALUATION

The expected outcome has been achieved when the patient exhibits a cast that is intact without evidence of neurovascular compromise to the affected body part; the patient remains free from infection; the patient verbalizes only mild pain and slight edema or soreness; the patient maintains range-of-joint motion; the patient demonstrates intact skin at cast edges; the patient is able to perform ADLs; and the patient demonstrates appropriate cast-care techniques.

DOCUMENTATION
Guidelines

Document all assessments and care provided. Document the patient's response to the cast, repositioning, and any teaching.

(*continued*)

Skill 9-17 ▶ Caring for a Cast *(continued)*

Sample Documentation

> 9/1/20 0845 Fiberglass cast in place on right lower extremity from just below knee to toes. Patient repositioned from right side to back. Cast clean and dry; edges padded. No signs of irritation noted. Patient able to move toes freely. Skin tone on right toes somewhat paler tone compared with left toes; toes warm and dry. Capillary refill less than 2 seconds. Patient denies any numbness, tingling, or pain. Right lower extremity elevated on two pillows. Patient instructed to report any complaints of pain, pressure, numbness, tingling, or decreased ability to move toes.
>
> —P. Collins, RN

UNEXPECTED SITUATIONS AND ASSOCIATED INTERVENTIONS

- *Your patient, who has a cast on his hand and forearm, has been experiencing pain relief in the extremity with ice application and oral analgesics. He now reports pain unrelieved by the analgesic and a feeling of tightness in his arm. In addition, his fingers are cool, with sluggish capillary refill:* Compartment syndrome may be developing. Adjust the arm so that it is no higher than heart level. This enhances arterial perfusion and controls edema. Notify the primary care provider of the situation immediately. Prepare for bivalving of the cast (cutting of the cast in half longitudinally) to relieve pressure.

SPECIAL CONSIDERATIONS
General Considerations

- Explain that itching under the cast is normal, but the patient should not stick objects down or in the cast to scratch.
- Begin patient teaching immediately after the cast is applied and continue until the patient or a significant other can provide care.
- If a cast is applied after surgery or trauma, monitor vital signs (the most accurate way to assess for bleeding).
- Synthetic casts are lightweight, easy to clean, and somewhat water-resistant. If a Gore-Tex liner is used when the cast is applied, the cast may be immersed in water without affecting the cast integrity.

Infant and Child Considerations

- Do not allow the child to put anything inside the cast.
- Remove toys, hazardous floor rugs, pets, or other items that might cause the child to stumble.
- Keep in mind that synthetic casts come in different colors and with designs, such as cartoons and stripes. These features may make the experience more pleasant for a child.
- Cover a synthetic cast with a plastic bag for bathing.
- Instruct the parents/guardians of a child with a cast not to alter standard car seats to accommodate a cast. Specially designed car seats and restraints are available for travel in a car.

Older Adult Considerations

- Older adults may experience changes in circulation related to their age. They may have slow or poor capillary refill related to peripheral vascular disease. Obtain baseline information for comparison after the cast is applied. Use more than one neurovascular assessment to assess circulation. Compare extremities or sides of the body for symmetry.

Home Care Considerations

- Instruct patients to rest the extremity, apply ice to the extremity, and elevate the extremity to prevent pain and swelling after the application of the cast (AAOS, 2015a; Satryb, Wilson, & Patterson, 2011).
- To control itching after the cast is dry, teach patients to tap on the outside of the cast with a pen or use a hair dryer on cool setting to blow cool air into the cast. Instruct patients to never insert an object into the cast and immediately to report a wet cast to their health care provider (Satryb et al., 2011).

Skill 9-18 ▶ Applying Skin Traction and Caring for a Patient in Skin Traction

Traction is the application of a pulling force to a part of the body. It is used to reduce fractures, treat dislocations, correct or prevent deformities, improve or correct contractures, or decrease muscle spasms. It must be applied in the correct direction and magnitude to obtain the therapeutic effects desired. The affected body part is immobilized by pulling with equal force on each end of the injured area, mixing traction and countertraction. Weights provide the pulling force or traction. The use of additional weights or positioning of the patient's body weight against the traction pull provides the countertraction. Skin traction is applied directly to the skin, exerting indirect pull on the bone. The force may be applied using adhesive or nonadhesive traction tape or a boot, belt, or halter. Skin traction immobilizes a body part intermittently. See Box 9-2 Principles of Effective Traction.

Types of skin traction for adults include Buck's extension traction (lower leg), a cervical head halter, Russel's traction, Bryant's traction, and the pelvic belt. Nursing care for skin traction includes setting the traction up, applying the traction, monitoring the application and patient response, and preventing complications from the therapy and immobility.

Box 9-2 | Principles of Effective Traction

- Countertraction must be applied for effective traction.
- Traction must be continuous to be effective.
- Skeletal traction is never interrupted.
- Weights are not removed unless intermittent traction is prescribed.

- Patient must maintain good body alignment in the center of the bed.
- Ropes must be unobstructed.
- Weights must hang free.

Source: Adapted from Hinkle, J. L., & Cheever, K. H. (2018). *Brunner & Suddarth's textbook of medical-surgical nursing* (14th ed.). Philadelphia, PA: Wolters Kluwer.

DELEGATION CONSIDERATIONS	The application of, and care for a patient with, skin traction may not be delegated to nursing assistive personnel (NAP) or unlicensed assistive personnel (UAP). Depending on the state's nurse practice act and the organization's policies and procedures, this care may be delegated to licensed practical/vocational nurses (LPN/LVNs). The decision to delegate must be based on careful analysis of the patient's needs and circumstances, as well as the qualifications of the person to whom the task is being delegated. Refer to the Delegation Guidelines in Appendix A.
EQUIPMENT	• Bed with traction frame and trapeze • Weights • Velcro straps or other straps • Rope and pulleys • Boot with footplate • Graduated compression stocking, as appropriate • Nonsterile gloves and/or other PPE, as indicated • Skin-cleansing supplies
ASSESSMENT	Assess the patient's medical record and the nursing care plan to determine the type of traction, traction weight, and line of pull. Assess the traction equipment to ensure proper function, including inspecting the ropes for fraying and proper positioning. Assess the patient's body alignment. Perform skin and neurovascular assessments. Assess for complications of immobility, including alterations in respiratory function, skin integrity, urinary and bowel elimination, and muscle weakness, contractures, thrombophlebitis, pulmonary embolism, and fatigue.
NURSING DIAGNOSIS	Determine the related factors for the nursing diagnoses based on the patient's current status. Appropriate nursing diagnoses may include: • Risk for injury • (Bathing; Dressing; Feeding; Toileting) self-care deficit • Risk for impaired skin integrity

(continued)

Skill 9-18 ▶ Applying Skin Traction and Caring for a Patient in Skin Traction *(continued)*

<table>
<tr>
<td>

OUTCOME IDENTIFICATION AND PLANNING

</td>
<td>

The expected outcome to achieve when applying and caring for a patient in skin traction is that the traction is maintained with the appropriate counterbalance and the patient maintains proper body alignment. Other outcomes that may be appropriate include that the patient reports an increased level of comfort and the patient is free from injury.

</td>
</tr>
</table>

IMPLEMENTATION

ACTION	RATIONALE
1. Review the medical record and the nursing care plan to determine the type of traction being used and care for the affected body part.	Reviewing the medical record and care plan validates the correct patient and correct procedure.
2. Perform hand hygiene. Put on PPE, as indicated.	Hand hygiene and PPE prevent the spread of microorganisms. PPE is required based on transmission precautions.
3. Identify the patient. Explain the procedure to the patient, emphasizing the importance of maintaining counterbalance, alignment, and position.	Patient identification validates the correct patient and correct procedure. Discussion and explanation help allay anxiety and prepare the patient for what to expect.
4. Perform a pain assessment and assess for muscle spasm. Administer prescribed medications in sufficient time to allow for the full effect of the analgesic and/or muscle relaxant.	Assessing pain and administering analgesics promote patient comfort.
5. Close the curtains around the bed and close the door to the room, if possible. Place the bed at an appropriate and comfortable working height, usually elbow height of the caregiver (VHACEOSH, 2016).	Closing the door or curtains provides for privacy. Proper bed height prevents back and muscle strain.

Applying Skin Traction

6. Ensure the traction apparatus is attached securely to the bed. Assess the traction setup.	Assessment of traction setup and weights promotes safety.
7. Check that the ropes move freely through the pulleys. Check that all knots are tight and are positioned away from the pulleys. Pulleys should be free from the linens.	Checking ropes and pulleys ensures that weight is being applied correctly, promoting accurate counterbalance and traction function.
8. Place the patient in a supine position with the foot of the bed elevated slightly. The patient's head should be near the head of the bed and in alignment.	Proper patient positioning maintains proper counterbalance and promotes safety.
9. Cleanse the affected area. Place the compression stocking on the affected limb, as appropriate.	Skin care aids in preventing skin breakdown. Use of graduated compression stockings prevents edema and neurovascular complications.
10. Place the traction boot over the patient's leg (Figure 1). Be sure the patient's heel is in the heel of the boot. Secure the boot with the straps.	The boot provides a means for attaching traction; proper application ensures proper pull.

FIGURE 1. Applying traction boot with a compression stocking in place on leg.

ACTION

11. Attach the traction cord to the boot footplate. Pass the rope over the pulley fastened at the end of the bed. Attach the weight to the hook on the rope, usually 5 to 10 lb for an adult (Figure 2). Gently let go of the weight. **The weight should hang freely, not touching the bed or the floor.**

FIGURE 2. Applying weight for skin traction.

12. Check the patient's alignment with the traction.

13. Check the boot for placement and alignment. Make sure the line of pull is parallel to the bed and not angled downward.

14. Place the bed in the lowest position that still allows the weight to hang freely. Make sure the call bell and other essential items are within easy reach.

 15. Remove PPE, if used. Perform hand hygiene.

Caring for a Patient With Skin Traction

16. Perform a skin-traction assessment per facility policy. This assessment includes checking the traction equipment, examining the affected body part, maintaining proper body alignment, and performing skin and neurovascular assessments.

17. Remove the straps every 4 hours per the health care provider's order or facility policy. Check bony prominences for skin breakdown, abrasions, and pressure areas. Remove the boot, per medical order or facility policy, every 8 hours. Put on gloves and wash, rinse, and thoroughly dry the skin.

RATIONALE

Weight attachment applies the pull for the traction. Gently releasing the weight prevents a quick pull on the extremity and possible injury and pain. Properly hanging weights and correct patient positioning ensure accurate counterbalance and traction function.

Proper alignment is necessary for proper counterbalance and ensures patient safety.

Misalignment causes ineffective traction and may interfere with healing. A properly positioned boot prevents pressure on the heel.

Proper bed positioning ensures effective application of traction without patient injury. Having call bell and other items in easy reach contributes to patient safety.

Proper removal of PPE decreases the risk for infection transmission and contamination of other items. Hand hygiene prevents the spread of microorganisms.

Assessment provides information to determine proper application and alignment, thereby reducing the risk for injury. Misalignment causes ineffective traction and may interfere with healing.

Removing the straps provides assessment information for early detection and prompt intervention of potential complications should they arise. Washing the area enhances circulation to skin; thorough drying prevents skin breakdown. Using gloves prevents transfer of microorganisms.

(*continued*)

Skill 9-18 ▶ Applying Skin Traction and Caring for a Patient in Skin Traction *(continued)*

ACTION	RATIONALE
18. Assess the extremity distal to the traction for edema, and assess peripheral pulses (Figure 3). Assess the temperature, color, and capillary refill (Figure 4), and compare with the unaffected limb. Check for pain, inability to move body parts distal to the traction, pallor, and abnormal sensations. Assess for indicators of deep vein thrombosis, including calf tenderness and swelling.	Doing so helps detect signs of abnormal neurovascular function and allows for prompt intervention. Assessing neurovascular status determines the circulation and oxygenation of tissues. Pressure within the traction boot may increase with edema.

FIGURE 3. Assessing distal pulses.

FIGURE 4. Assessing capillary refill.

19. Replace the traction; remove gloves and dispose of them appropriately.	Replacing traction is necessary to provide immobilization and facilitate healing. Proper disposal of gloves prevents the transmission of microorganisms.
20. Check the boot for placement and alignment. Make sure the line of pull is parallel to the bed and not angled downward.	Misalignment causes ineffective traction and may interfere with healing. A properly positioned boot prevents pressure on the heel.
21. Ensure the patient is positioned in the center of the bed, with the affected leg aligned with the trunk of the patient's body. Check overall alignment of the patient's body.	Misalignment interferes with the effectiveness of traction and may lead to complications.
22. Examine the weights and pulley system. Weights should hang freely, off the floor and bed. Knots should be secure. Ropes should move freely through the pulleys. The pulleys should not be constrained by knots (Figure 5).	Checking the weights and pulley system ensures proper application and reduces the risk for patient injury from traction application.

FIGURE 5. Skin traction in place.

ACTION	**RATIONALE**
23. Keep the bedsheets wrinkle free.	Wrinkles may create areas of increased pressure and contribute to alterations in skin integrity and patient discomfort.
24. Perform range-of-motion exercises on all unaffected joint areas, unless contraindicated. Encourage the patient to cough and deep breathe every 2 hours.	ROM exercises maintain joint function. Coughing and deep breathing help to reduce the risk for respiratory complications related to immobility.
25. Raise the side rails. Place the bed in the lowest position that still allows the weight to hang freely. Make sure the call bell and other essential items are within easy reach.	Raising the side rails promotes patient safety. Proper bed positioning ensures effective application of traction without patient injury. Having call bell and other items in easy reach contributes to patient safety.
26. Remove PPE, if used. Perform hand hygiene.	Proper removal of PPE decreases the risk for infection transmission and contamination of other items. Hand hygiene prevents the spread of microorganisms.

EVALUATION

The expected outcome has been met when traction is maintained with the appropriate counterbalance and the patient maintains proper body alignment; the patient reports an increased level of comfort; and the patient is free from injury.

DOCUMENTATION

Guidelines

Document the time, date, type, amount of weight used, and the site where the traction was applied. Include the skin assessment and care provided before application. Document the patient's response to the traction and the neurovascular status of the extremity.

Sample Documentation

> 6/3/20 1500 Patient complaining of pain in left hip due to fracture, rating it 7/10. Administered oxycodone (2 tablets), as ordered. Pain rated 3/10, 30 minutes later. Buck's extension traction with 5 lb of weight applied to left extremity. Skin intact. Pedal pulses present and equal, feet pale pink, warm, and dry, with brisk capillary refill bilaterally. Patient able to wiggle toes freely. Denies numbness or tingling. Patient lying flat in bed with head of bed elevated approximately 15 degrees. Surgery planned for tomorrow.
>
> —L. James, RN

UNEXPECTED SITUATIONS AND ASSOCIATED INTERVENTIONS

- *Your patient in Buck's traction reports pain in the heel of the affected leg:* Remove traction and perform skin and neurovascular assessments. Reapply the traction and reassess the neurovascular status in 15 to 20 minutes. Notify the primary care provider.

SPECIAL CONSIDERATIONS

General Considerations

- Unless contraindicated, encourage the patient to do active flexion–extension ankle exercise and calf-pumping exercises at regular intervals to decrease venous stasis.
- Be alert for pressure on peripheral nerves with skin traction. Take care with Buck's traction to avoid pressure on the peroneal nerve at the point where it passes around the neck of the fibula just below the knee.
- Assess patients who are in traction for extended periods for the development of helplessness, isolation, confinement, and loss of control. Diversional activities, therapeutic communication, and frequent visits by staff and significant others are an important part of care.

Older Adult Considerations

- Be extra vigilant with older adults in skin traction. Older adults are susceptible to alterations in skin integrity due to a decreased amount of subcutaneous fat and thinner, drier, more fragile skin, as well as constipation due to being confined to bed.

Skill 9-19 ▶ Caring for a Patient in Skeletal Traction

Skeletal traction provides pull to a body part by attaching weight directly to the bone using pins, screws, wires, or tongs. It is used to immobilize a body part for prolonged periods. This method of traction is used to treat fractures of the femur, tibia, and cervical spine. Box 9-2 in Skill 9-18 outlines principles of effective traction. Nursing responsibilities related to skeletal traction include maintaining the traction, maintaining body alignment, monitoring neurovascular status, promoting exercise, preventing complications from the therapy and immobility, and preventing infection by providing pin-site care. A growing evidence base supports effective management of pin sites, but no clear consensus (Cam & Korkmaz, 2013; Ktistakis, Guerado, & Giannoudis, 2015; Lagerquist et al., 2012; Lethaby, Temple, & Santy-Tomlinson, 2013). Pin-site care often varies based on primary care provider and facility policy. Dressings are often applied for the first 48 to 72 hours, and then sites may be left open to air. Pin-site care may be performed frequently in the first 48 to 72 hours after application, when drainage may be heavy; other evidence suggests pin care should begin after the first 48 to 72 hours. Pin-site care may be done daily or weekly (Lagerquist et al., 2012; Timms & Pugh, 2012). Pin-site care is completed using aseptic technique in the immediate postoperative period. Refer to specific patient medical orders and facility guidelines.

DELEGATION CONSIDERATIONS

The care of a patient with skeletal traction may not be delegated to nursing assistive personnel (NAP) or to unlicensed assistive personnel (UAP). Depending on the state's nurse practice act and the organization's policies and procedures, care for these patients may be delegated to licensed practical/vocational nurses (LPN/LVNs). The decision to delegate must be based on careful analysis of the patient's needs and circumstances, as well as the qualifications of the person to whom the task is being delegated. Refer to the Delegation Guidelines in Appendix A.

EQUIPMENT

- Sterile gloves
- Sterile applicators
- Cleansing agent for pin care, usually sterile normal saline, but may be an antimicrobial such as chlorhexidine, per primary care provider order or facility policy
- Sterile container
- Antimicrobial ointment, per primary care provider order or facility policy
- Sterile gauze or dressing, per primary care provider order or facility policy
- Analgesic, as ordered
- Sterile gloves for performing pin care, depending on facility policy
- Additional PPE, as indicated

ASSESSMENT

Review the patient's medical record and nursing care plan to determine the type of traction, traction weight, and line of pull. Assess the traction equipment to ensure proper function, including inspecting the ropes for fraying and proper positioning. Assess the patient's body alignment. Assess the patient's pain and need for analgesia before providing care. Perform skin and neurovascular assessments. Inspect the pin insertion sites for inflammation and infection, including swelling, cloudy or offensive drainage, pain, or redness. Assess for complications of immobility, including alterations in respiratory function, constipation, alterations in skin integrity, alterations in urinary elimination, and muscle weakness, contractures, thrombophlebitis, pulmonary embolism, and fatigue.

NURSING DIAGNOSIS

Determine the related factors for the nursing diagnoses based on the patient's current status. Appropriate nursing diagnoses may include:

- (Bathing; Dressing; Feeding; Toileting) self-care deficit
- Risk for infection
- Disturbed body image

OUTCOME IDENTIFICATION AND PLANNING

The expected outcome to achieve when applying and caring for a patient in skeletal traction is that the traction is maintained appropriately and the patient maintains proper body alignment. Other outcomes that may be appropriate include that the patient reports an increased level of comfort and the patient is free from injury.

IMPLEMENTATION

ACTION	RATIONALE

1. Review the medical record and the nursing care plan to determine the type of traction being used and the prescribed care.

   Reviewing the medical record and care plan validates the correct patient and correct procedure.

2. Perform hand hygiene. Put on PPE, as indicated.

   Hand hygiene and PPE prevent the spread of microorganisms. PPE is required based on transmission precautions.

3. Identify the patient. Explain the procedure to the patient, emphasizing the importance of maintaining counterbalance, alignment, and position.

   Patient identification validates the correct patient and correct procedure. Discussion and explanation help allay anxiety and prepare the patient for what to expect.

4. Perform a pain assessment and assess for muscle spasm. Administer prescribed medications in sufficient time to allow for the full effect of the analgesic and/or muscle relaxant.

   Assessing for pain and administering analgesics promote patient comfort.

5. Close the curtains around the bed and close the door to the room, if possible. Place the bed at an appropriate and comfortable working height, usually elbow height of the caregiver (VHACEOSH, 2016).

   Closing the door or curtains provides for privacy. Proper bed height prevents back and muscle strain.

6. Ensure the traction apparatus is attached securely to the bed. Assess the traction setup, including application of the ordered amount of weight. **Be sure that the weights hang freely, not touching the bed or the floor (Figure 1).**

   Proper traction application reduces the risk of injury by promoting accurate counterbalance and traction function.

FIGURE 1. Skeletal traction in place, weights hanging freely. (From Farrell M. [2017]. *Smeltzer & Bare's Textbook of Medical-Surgical Nursing* [4ᵗʰ Australia/ New Zealand edition]; Lippincott Williams & Wilkins Pty Ltd.)

7. **Check that the ropes move freely through the pulleys. Check that all knots are tight and are positioned away from the pulleys. Pulleys should be free from the linens.**

   Free ropes and pulleys ensure accurate counterbalance and traction function.

8. Check the alignment of the patient's body, as prescribed.

   Proper alignment maintains an effective line of pull and prevents injury.

9. Perform a skin assessment. Pay attention to pressure points, including the ischial tuberosity, popliteal space, Achilles tendon, sacrum, and heel.

   Skin assessment provides early intervention for skin irritation, impaired tissue perfusion, and other complications.

(continued)

Skill 9-19 ► Caring for a Patient in Skeletal Traction *(continued)*

ACTION	RATIONALE
10. Perform a neurovascular assessment. Assess the extremity distal to the traction for edema and peripheral pulses. Assess the temperature and color and compare with the unaffected limb. Check for pain, inability to move body parts distal to the traction, pallor, and abnormal sensations. Assess for indicators of deep vein thrombosis, including calf tenderness, and swelling.	Neurovascular assessment aids in early identification and allows for prompt intervention should compromised circulation and oxygenation of tissues develop.
11. Assess the site at and around the pins for redness, edema, and odor. Assess for skin tenting, prolonged or purulent drainage, elevated body temperature, elevated pin-site temperature, and bowing or bending of the pins.	Pin sites provide a possible entry for microorganisms. Skin inspection allows for early detection and prompt intervention should complications develop.
12. Provide pin-site care.	Performing pin-site care prevents crusting at the site that could lead to fluid buildup, infection, and osteomyelitis.
a. Using sterile technique, open the applicator package and pour the cleansing agent into the sterile container.	Using sterile technique reduces the risk for transmission of microorganisms.
b. Put on the sterile gloves.	Gloves prevent contact with blood and/or body fluids.
c. Place the applicators into the solution.	
d. **Clean the pin site, starting at the insertion area and working outward, away from the pin site (Figure 2).**	Cleaning from the center outward ensures movement from the least to most contaminated area.
e. **Use each applicator once. Use a new applicator for each pin site.** Gently remove crusts or scabs appearing at the pin site if they can be removed easily; leave in place if there is difficulty during removal.	Using an applicator once reduces the risk of transmission of microorganisms. Removal of crusts prevents excessive pressure at site and allows for drainage. Scab formation can lead to infection at the site (Cam & Korkmaz, 2013).

FIGURE 2. Cleaning around pin sites with normal saline on an applicator.

ACTION	RATIONALE
13. Depending on medical order and facility policy, apply the antimicrobial ointment to pin sites and apply a dressing. Remove gloves and dispose of them appropriately.	Antimicrobial ointment helps reduce the risk of infection. A dressing aids in protecting the pin sites from contamination and in containing any drainage. Disposing of gloves reduces the risk of microorganism transmission.
14. Perform ROM exercises on all joint areas, unless contraindicated. Encourage the patient to cough and deep breathe every 2 hours.	Range-of-motion exercises promote joint mobility. Coughing and deep breathing reduce the risk of respiratory complications related to immobility.
15. Place the bed in the lowest position that still allows the weight to hang freely. Make sure the call bell and other essential items are within easy reach.	Proper bed positioning ensures effective application of traction without patient injury. Having call bell and other items in easy reach contributes to patient safety.
16. Remove PPE, if used. Perform hand hygiene.	Proper removal of PPE reduces the risk for infection transmission and contamination of other items. Hand hygiene prevents the spread of microorganisms.

EVALUATION

The expected outcome has been met when the traction is maintained appropriately and the patient maintains proper body alignment; the patient reports an increased level of comfort; and the patient is free from injury.

DOCUMENTATION

Guidelines

Document the time, date, type of traction, and the amount of weight used. Include skin and pin-site assessments, and pin-site care. Document the patient's response to the traction and the neurovascular status of the extremity.

Sample Documentation

6/5/20 1020 Pin-site care performed. Pin sites cleaned with normal saline and open to the air. Sites slightly red with serosanguineous crusting noted. Neurovascular status intact. Balanced suspension skeletal traction maintained as ordered.

—M. Leroux, RN

UNEXPECTED SITUATIONS AND ASSOCIATED INTERVENTIONS

- *While performing a pin-site assessment for your patient with skeletal traction, you note that several of the pins move and slide in the pin tract:* Assess the patient for other symptoms, including signs of infection at the pin sites, pain, and fever. Assess for neurovascular changes. Notify the primary care provider of the findings.

SPECIAL CONSIDERATIONS

- If a pin site becomes unusually painful or tender, or if you notice any fluid discharge, it may be a signal that the pin has loosened or become infected. In the event of unusual pain or irritation, notify the primary care provider. Pin loosening may also be indicated by a "tight" feeling or a "clicking" sound (Lagerquist et al., 2012).
- Assess the patient for chronic conditions, such as diabetes mellitus, peripheral vascular disease, and chronic obstructive pulmonary disease, which can significantly increase a patient's risk for complications when skeletal traction is in use.
- Never remove the weights from skeletal traction unless a life-threatening situation occurs. Removal of the weights interferes with therapy and can result in injury to the patient.
- Jarring movements can disrupt traction. Use smooth, coordinated effort whenever you must reposition the patient.
- Inspect the pin sites for inflammation and evidence of infection at least every 8 hours. Prevention of osteomyelitis is of utmost importance.

EVIDENCE FOR PRACTICE ▶

EXTERNAL FIXATOR PIN SITES—CLINICAL EVIDENCE REVIEW

Lethaby, A., Temple, J., & Santy-Tomlinson, J. (2013). Pin site care for preventing infections associated with external bone fixators and pins (Review). *Cochrane Database of Systematic Reviews, 12,* CD004551. doi: 10.1002/14651858.CD004551.pub3.

This clinical evidence review was conducted by the Cochrane Wounds Group Specialised Trials Register; The Cochrane Central Register of Controlled Trials (CENTRAL) (*The Cochrane Library*); Ovid MEDLINE; Ovid MEDLINE (In-Process & Other Non-Indexed Citations); Ovid EMBASE; and EBSCO CINAHL. The authors evaluated all randomized controlled trials that compared different methods of cleansing or dressing orthopedic percutaneous pin sites, based on associated infection and other complication rates. Eleven trials were reviewed in total. Three trials examined cleansing regimen with no cleansing; three trials compared alternative sterile cleansing solutions; three trials compared methods of cleansing; one trial compared daily site care with no care; and six trials compared different dressings. The authors concluded the evidence was not extensive, was very heterogeneous, and generally of poor quality, so there was no strong evidence that one pin care technique was any better than any other. In addition, the researchers concluded there was insufficient evidence to identify a strategy of pin-site care that minimizes infection rates.

Refer to thePoint® for additional research on related nursing topics.

Skill 9-20 ▶ Caring for a Patient With an External Fixation Device

External fixation devices are used to manage open fractures with soft tissue damage. They consist of one of a variety of frames to hold pins that are drilled into or through bones. External fixators provide stable support for severely crushed or splintered fractures and access to, and treatment for, soft tissue injuries. The use of these devices allows treatment of the fracture and damaged soft tissues while promoting patient comfort, early mobility, and active exercise of adjacent uninvolved joints. Complications related to disuse and immobility are minimized. Nursing responsibilities include reassuring the patient, maintaining the device, monitoring neurovascular status, promoting exercise, preventing complications from the therapy, preventing infection by providing pin-site care, and providing teaching to ensure compliance and self-care.

A growing evidence base supports effective management of pin sites, but no clear consensus (Cam & Korkmaz, 2013; Ktistakis et al., 2015; Lagerquist et al., 2012; Lethaby et al., 2013). Pin-site care often varies based on primary care provider and facility policy. Dressings are often applied for the first 48 to 72 hours, and then sites may be left open to air. Pin-site care may be performed frequently in the first 48 to 72 hours after application, when drainage may be heavy; other evidence suggests pin care should begin after the first 48 to 72 hours. Pin-site care may be done daily or weekly (Lagerquist et al., 2012; Timms & Pugh, 2012). Pin-site care is completed using aseptic technique in the immediate postoperative period. Refer to specific patient medical orders and facility guidelines.

Nurses play a major role in preparing the patient psychologically for the application of an external fixator. The devices appear clumsy and large. In addition, the nurse needs to clarify misconceptions regarding pain and discomfort associated with the device.

DELEGATION CONSIDERATIONS

The care of a patient with an external fixator device may not be delegated to nursing assistive personnel (NAP) or to unlicensed assistive personnel (UAP). Depending on the state's nurse practice act and the organization's policies and procedures, care for these patients may be delegated to licensed practical/vocational nurses (LPN/LVNs). The decision to delegate must be based on careful analysis of the patient's needs and circumstances, as well as the qualifications of the person to whom the task is being delegated. Refer to the Delegation Guidelines in Appendix A.

EQUIPMENT

Equipment varies with the type of fixator and the type and location of the fracture, but may include:

- Sterile applicators
- Cleansing solution, usually sterile normal saline but may be an antimicrobial such as chlorhexidine, per primary care provider order or facility policy
- Ice bag

- Antimicrobial ointment, per primary care provider order or facility policy
- Sterile gauze or dressing, per primary care provider order or facility policy
- Analgesic, as ordered
- Sterile gloves for performing pin care, depending on facility policy
- Additional PPE, as indicated

ASSESSMENT

Review the patient's medical record and the nursing care plan to determine the type of device being used and prescribed care. Assess the patient's pain and need for analgesia before providing care. Assess the external fixator to ensure proper function and position. Perform skin and neurovascular assessments. Inspect the pin-insertion sites for signs of inflammation and infection, including swelling, cloudy or offensive drainage, pain, or redness. Assess the patient's knowledge regarding the device and self-care activities and responsibilities.

NURSING DIAGNOSIS

Determine the related factors for the nursing diagnoses based on the patient's current status. Appropriate nursing diagnoses may include:

- Risk for infection
- Deficient knowledge
- Disturbed body image

OUTCOME IDENTIFICATION AND PLANNING

The expected outcome to achieve when caring for a patient with an external fixator device is that the patient shows no evidence of complication, such as infection, contractures, venous stasis, thrombus formation, or skin breakdown. Additional outcomes that may be appropriate include that the patient shows signs of healing; the patient reports an increased level of comfort; and the patient is free from injury.

IMPLEMENTATION

ACTION	RATIONALE
1. Review the medical record and the nursing care plan to determine the type of device being used and prescribed care.	Reviewing the medical record and care plan validates the correct patient and correct procedure.
2. Perform hand hygiene. Put on PPE, as indicated.	Hand hygiene and PPE prevent the spread of microorganisms. PPE is required based on transmission precautions.
3. Identify the patient. Explain the procedure to the patient. Assure the patient that there will be little pain after the fixation device is in place. Reinforce that the patient will be able to adjust to the device and will be able to move about with the device, allowing him or her to resume normal activities more quickly.	Patient identification validates the correct patient and correct procedure. Discussion and explanation allay anxiety and prepare the patient psychologically for the application of the device.
4. **After the fixation device is in place (Figure 1), apply ice to the surgical site, as ordered or per facility policy. Elevate the affected body part, if appropriate.**	Ice and elevation help reduce swelling, relieve pain, and reduce bleeding.

FIGURE 1. External fixation device in place.

5. Perform a pain assessment and assess for muscle spasm. Administer prescribed medications in sufficient time to allow for the full effect of the analgesic and/or muscle relaxant.	Pain assessment and analgesic administration help promote patient comfort.
6. Administer analgesics, as ordered, before exercising or mobilizing the affected body part.	Administration of analgesics promotes patient comfort and facilitates movement.
7. Perform neurovascular assessments, per facility policy or medical order, usually every 2 to 4 hours for 24 hours, then every 4 to 8 hours. Assess the affected body part for color, motion, sensation, edema, capillary refill, and pulses. If appropriate, compare with the unaffected side. Assess for pain not relieved by analgesics, and for burning, tingling, and numbness.	Assessment promotes early detection and prompt intervention for abnormal neurovascular function, nerve damage, or circulatory impairment. Assessment of neurovascular status determines the circulation and oxygenation of tissues.

(continued)

Skill 9-20 | Caring for a Patient With an External Fixation Device *(continued)*

ACTION	RATIONALE
8. Close the curtains around the bed and close the door to the room, if possible. Place the bed at an appropriate and comfortable working height, usually elbow height of the caregiver (VHACEOSH, 2016).	Closing the door or curtains provides for privacy. Proper bed height prevents back and muscle strain.
9. Assess the pin site for redness, tenting of the skin, prolonged or purulent drainage, swelling, and bowing, bending, or loosening of the pins. Monitor body temperature.	Assessing pin sites aids in early detection of infection and stress on the skin and allows for appropriate intervention.
10. Perform pin-site care.	Performing pin-site care prevents crusting at the site that could lead to fluid buildup, infection, and osteomyelitis.
a. Using sterile technique, open the applicator package and pour the cleansing agent into the sterile container.	Using sterile technique reduces the risk for transmission of microorganisms.
b. Put on the sterile gloves.	Gloves prevent contact with blood and/or body fluids.
c. Place the applicators into the solution.	
d. Clean the pin site starting at the insertion area and working outward, away from the pin site (Figure 2).	Cleaning from the center outward promotes movement from the least to most contaminated area.
e. **Use each applicator once. Use a new applicator for each pin site.** Gently remove crusts or scabs appearing at the pin site if they can be removed easily; leave in place if there is difficulty during removal.	Using an applicator once reduces the risk of transmission of microorganisms. Removal of crusts prevents excessive pressure at site and allows for drainage. Scab formation can lead to infection at the site (Cam & Korkmaz, 2013).

FIGURE 2. Cleaning around pin sites with normal saline on an applicator.

11. Depending on medical order and facility policy, apply the antimicrobial ointment to pin sites and apply a dressing. Remove gloves and dispose of them appropriately.	Antimicrobial ointment helps reduce the risk of infection. A dressing aids in protecting the pin sites from contamination and containing any drainage. Disposing of gloves reduces the risk of microorganism transmission.
12. Perform ROM exercises on all joint areas, unless contraindicated. Encourage the patient to cough and deep breathe every 2 hours.	Range-of-motion exercises promote joint mobility. Coughing and deep breathing reduce the risk of respiratory complications related to immobility.
13. Place the bed in the lowest position that still allows the weight to hang freely, with the side rails up. Make sure the call bell and other essential items are within easy reach.	Proper bed positioning ensures effective application of traction without patient injury. Leaving the call bell and other items within reach ensures patient safety.
14. Remove PPE, if used. Perform hand hygiene.	Proper removal of PPE reduces the risk for infection transmission and contamination of other items. Hand hygiene prevents the spread of microorganisms.

EVALUATION

The expected outcome has been met when the patient exhibits an external fixation device in place with pin sites that are clean, dry, and intact, without evidence of infection; the patient remains free of complications, such as contractures, venous stasis, thrombus formation, or skin breakdown; the patient reports an increased level of comfort; the patient remains free of injury, and the patient demonstrates knowledge of pin-site care.

DOCUMENTATION

Guidelines

Document the time, date, and type of device in place. Include the skin assessment, pin-site assessment, and pin-site care. Document the patient's response to the device and the neurovascular status of the affected area.

Sample Documentation

> 7/6/20 1020 External fixator in place on left forearm. Pin-site care performed. Pin sites cleaned with normal saline and open to the air. Sites slightly red with serosanguineous crusting noted. Neurovascular status intact. Instruction given regarding ROM exercises to left fingers and elbow; patient verbalizes an understanding and is able to demonstrate.
>
> —B. Clapp, RN

SPECIAL CONSIDERATIONS

- Teach the patient and significant others how to provide pin-site care and how to recognize the signs of pin-site infection. External fixator devices are in place for prolonged periods. Clean technique can be used at home instead of sterile technique.
- Teach the patient and significant others to identify early signs of infection, signs of a loose pin, and how to contact the orthopedic team, if necessary.
- Reinforce the importance of keeping the affected body part elevated when sitting or lying down to prevent edema.
- Do not adjust the clamps on the external fixator frame. It is the physician's or advanced practice professional's responsibility to adjust the clamps.
- Fractures often require additional treatment and stabilization with a cast or molded splint after the fixator device is removed.

EVIDENCE FOR PRACTICE ▶

EXTERNAL FIXATOR PIN SITES—CLINICAL EVIDENCE REVIEW

Lethaby, A., Temple, J., & Santy-Tomlinson, J. (2013). Pin site care for preventing infections associated with external bone fixators and pins (Review). *Cochrane Database of Systematic Reviews, 12*, CD004551. doi: 10.1002/14651858.CD004551.pub3.

Refer to details in Skill 9-19, Evidence for Practice, and refer to thePoint® for additional research on related nursing topics.

Enhance Your Understanding

Focusing on Patient Care: Developing Clinical Reasoning

Consider the case scenarios at the beginning of the chapter as you answer the following questions to enhance your understanding and apply what you have learned.

QUESTIONS

1. You are preparing to discharge Bobby Rowden from the emergency room. Discuss the teaching you should include for Bobby and his parents related to his injury and his plaster cast.
2. A pneumatic compression device has been ordered as part of the treatment orders for Esther Levitz. You

bring the pump and sleeves into the room, and she asks, "What is that? It looks like a torture machine!" How will you respond?
3. You are caring for Manuel Esposito the evening before his surgery. Your assessment of his affected extremity reveals skin that is warm to the touch, rapid capillary refill, and positive sensation and movement. What other assessments should you perform as part of your care for Mr. Esposito?

You can find suggested answers after the Bibliography at the end of this chapter.

Integrated Case Study Connection

The case studies in the back of the book focus on integrating concepts. Refer to the following case studies to enhance your understanding of the concepts and skills in this chapter.

- Basic Case Studies: Abigail Cantonelli, page 1099.
- Intermediate Case Studies: Jason Brown, page 1119; Kent Clark, page 1121.

Taylor Suite Resources

Explore these additional resources to enhance learning for this chapter:

- NCLEX-Style Questions and other resources on thePoint®, http://thePoint.lww.com/Lynn5e
- *Skill Checklists for Taylor's Clinical Nursing Skills,* 5e
- *Taylor's Video Guide to Clinical Nursing Skills:* Activity
- *Fundamentals of Nursing:* Chapter 33, Activity

Bibliography

American Academy of Orthopedic Surgeons (AAOS). (2015a). OrthoInfo. Care of casts and splints. Retrieved https://orthoinfo.aaos.org/en/recovery/care-of-casts-and-splints

American Academy of Orthopedic Surgeons (AAOS). (2015b). How to use crutches, canes, and walkers. Retrieved https://orthoinfo.aaos.org/en/recovery/how-to-use-crutches-canes-and-walkers

American Association of Critical-Care Nurses (AACN). (2010; updated 2016). AACN Practice alert. Preventing venous thromboembolism in adults. Retrieved https://www.aacn.org/clinical-resources/practice-alerts/venous-thromboembolism-prevention

American Association of Neuroscience Nurses (AANN). (2014). *Cervical spine surgery. A guide to preoperative and postoperative patient care. AANN Clinical Practice Guideline Series.* Glenview, IL: Author.

American Family Physician. (2009). *Casting and splinting. [Handout].* Retrieved http://www.aafp.org/afp/2009/0101/p23.html

American Geriatrics Society, Health in Aging Foundation. (2016). *Choosing the right cane or walker.* Retrieved http://www.healthinaging.org/files/documents/tipsheets/canes_walkers.pdf

American Nurses Association (ANA). (2016). *Safe patient handling and mobility.* Retrieved http://www.nursingworld.org/MainMenuCategories/Occupationaland Environmental/occupationalhealth/handlewithcare.aspx

Bacharach, D. W., Miller, K., & von Duvillard, S. P. (2016). Saving your back: How do horizontal patient transfer devices stack up? *Nursing, 46*(1), 59–64.

Bartnik, L. M., & Rice, M. S. (2013). Comparison of caregiver forces required for sliding a patient up in bed using an array of slide sheets. *Workplace Health & Safety, 61*(9), 393–400.

Boyd, A. S., Benjamin, H. J., & Asplund, C. (2009). Principles of casting and splinting. *American Family Physician, 79*(1), 16–22.

Boynton, T., Kelly, L., & Perez, A. (2014). Implementing a mobility assessment tool for nurses. *American Nurse Today, 9*(Suppl), 13–16.

Cam, R., & Korkmaz, F. D. (2013). The effect of long-term care and follow-up on complications in patients with external fixators. *International Journal of Nursing Practice, 20*(1), 89–96.

Chen, L. H., Chen, C. H., Lin, S. Y., et al. (2013). Aggressive continuous passive motion exercise does not improve knee range of motion after total knee arthroplasty. *Journal of Clinical Nursing, 22*(3–4), 389–394.

Cho, S. H., Lee, J. H., & Jang, S. H. (2015). Efficacy of pulmonary rehabilitation using cervical range of motion exercise in stroke patients with tracheostomy tubes. *Journal of Physical Therapy Science, 27*(5), 1329–1331.

Clark, M., Phillips, L., & Knibbe, H. J. J. (2015). Lifting and transfer devices: A bridge between safe patient handling and pressure ulcer prevention. *American Journal of Safe Patient Handling & Movement, 5*(4), 154–160.

Cleveland Clinic. (2014). Crutches. Retrieved https://my.clevelandclinic.org/health/articles/15543-crutches

Cohen, B. J., & Taylor, J. J. (2013). *Memmler's structure and function of the human body* (10th ed.). Philadelphia, PA: Wolters Kluwer Health.

Darragh, A. R., Shiyko, M., Margulis, H., & Campo, M. (2014). Effects of a safe patient handling and mobility program on patient self-care outcomes. *The American Journal of Occupational Therapy, 68*(5), 589–596.

Doenges, M. E., Moorhouse, M. F., & Murr, A. C. (2016). *Nursing diagnoses manual. Planning, individualizing, and documenting client care* (5th ed.). Philadelphia, PA: F.A. Davis Company.

Eliopoulos, C. (2014). *Gerontological nursing* (8th ed.). Philadelphia, PA: Wolters Kluwer Health.

Guyatt, G. H., Akl, E. A., Crowther, M., Gutterman, D. D., Schünemann, H. J.; American College of Chest Physicians Antithrombotic Therapy and Prevention of Thrombosis Panel. (2012). Executive summary: Antithrombotic therapy and prevention of thrombosis,

9th ed.: American College of Chest Physicians evidence-based clinical practice guidelines. *Chest, 141*(2 Suppl), 7S–47S.

Harvey, L. A., Brosseau, L., & Herbert, R. D. (2014). Continuous passive motion following total knee arthroplasty in people with arthritis. *Cochrane Database of Systematic Reviews, 2*, CD004260. doi: 10.1002/14651858.CD004260.pub3

Herbold, J. A., Bonistall, K., Blackburn, M., et al. (2014). Randomized controlled trial of the effectiveness of continuous passive motion after total knee replacement. *Archives of Physical Medicine and Rehabilitation, 95*(7), 1240–1245.

Hinkle, J.L., & Cheever, K.H. (2018). *Brunner & Suddarth's textbook of medical–surgical nursing* (14th ed.). Philadelphia, PA: Wolters Kluwer.

Hoogerduijn, J. G., Grobbee, D. E., & Schuurmans, M. J. (2014). Prevention of functional decline in older hospitalized patients: Nurses should play a key role in safe and adequate care. *International Journal of Nursing Practice, 20*(1), 106–113.

Invoflo L. L. C. (2010). Gait belt handle helps during transfers. *Journal of Gerontological Nursing, 36*(12), 8–9.

Jarvis, C. (2016). *Physical examination & health assessment* (7th ed.). St. Louis, MO: Elsevier.

Jensen, S. (2015). *Nursing health assessment: A best practice approach* (2nd ed.). Philadelphia, PA: Wolters Kluwer Health.

Jootun, D., & Pryde, A. (2013). Moving and handling of patients with dementia. *Journal of Nursing Education and Practice, 3*(2), 126–131.

Kim, H., & Lee, E. S. (2015). Major difficulties and information needs recognised by nurses in applying graduated compression stocking and intermittent pneumatic compression for deep vein thrombosis prophylaxis. *Journal of Clinical Nursing, 24*(1–2), 308–311.

Kresevic, D. M. (2015). Reducing functional decline in hospitalized older adults. *American Nurse Today, 10*(5), 8–10.

Ktistakis, I., Guerado, E., & Giannoudis, P. V. (2015). Pin-site care: Can we reduce the incidence of infections? *Injury, 46*(Suppl 3), S35–S39.

Kyle, T., & Carman, S. (2017). *Essentials of pediatric nursing* (3rd ed.). Philadelphia, PA: Wolters Kluwer Health.

Lagerquist, D., Dabrowski, M., Dock, C., et al. (2012). Care of external fixator pin sites. *American Journal of Critical Care, 21*(4), 288–292.

LeMone, P., Burke, K. M., Bauldoff, G., & Gubrud, P. (2015). *Medical-surgical nursing: Clinical reasoning in patient care* (6th ed.). New York: Pearson.

Lethaby, A., Temple, J., & Santy-Tomlinson, J. (2013). Pin site care for preventing infections associated with external bone fixators and pins (Review). *Cochrane Database of Systematic Reviews, 12*, CD004551. doi: 10.1002/14651858.CD004551.pub3.

Mayeda-Letourneau, J. (2014). Safe patient handling and movement: A literature review. *Rehabilitation Nursing, 39*(3), 123–129.

Mayo Clinic. (n.d a.). Healthy lifestyle. Walker tips. Slide show: Tips for choosing and using walkers. Retrieved http://www.mayoclinic.org/healthy-lifestyle/healthy-aging/multimedia/walker/sls-20076469

Mayo Clinic. (n.d b.). Healthy lifestyle. Cane tips. Slide show: Tips for choosing and using canes. Retrieved https://www.mayoclinic.org/healthy-lifestyle/healthy-aging/multimedia/canes/sls-20077060

Mayo Clinic. (2014). *Exercise: 7 benefits of regular physical activity*. Retrieved http://www.mayoclinic.org/healthy-lifestyle/fitness/in-depth/exercise/art-20048389

Mayo Clinic. (2016). *Adult health. Back pain at work: Preventing pain and injury*. Retrieved http://www.mayoclinic.org/healthy-lifestyle/adult-health/in-depth/back-pain/art-20044526

Muñoz-Figueroa, G. P., & Ojo, O. (2015). Venous thromboembolism: Use of graduated compression stockings. *British Journal of Nursing, 24*(13), 680–685.

NANDA International, Inc. Nursing diagnoses: Definitions & classification 2018–2020 © 2017 NANDA International, ISBN 978-1-62623-929-6. Used by arrangement with the Thieme Group, Stuttgart/New York.

National Institute for Occupational Safety and Health (NIOSH). (n.d.). *Step-by-step guide: NIOSH short form. [Booklet]*. Retrieved http://ergo-plus.com/wp-content/uploads/Guide-to-Evaluating-Lifting-Injury-Risk.pdf

Nehan-Babalola, L. (2015). Manual handling considerations for people with dementia. *Equipment Services*, 64–69.

Nelson, A., Motacki, K., & Menzel, N. (2009). *The illustrated guide to safe patient handling and movement*. New York: Springer Publishing Company.

Neville Regan, E., Phillips, F., & Magri, T. (2013). Get a leg (or two) up on total knee. *Nursing, 43*(7), 32–38.

Occupational Safety and Health Administration (OSHA), U.S. Department of Labor. (n.d.a.). *Safe patient handling*. Retrieved https://www.osha.gov/SLTC/healthcarefacilities/safepatienthandling.html

Occupational Safety and Health Administration (OSHA), U.S. Department of Labor. (n.d.b.). *Safe patient handling equipment*. Retrieved https://www.osha.gov/dsg/hospitals/patient_handling_equipment.html

Occupational Safety and Health Administration (OSHA), U.S. Department of Labor. (n.d.c.). *Healthcare wide hazards module–Ergonomics*. Washington, DC:

Author. Retrieved https://www.osha.gov/SLTC/etools/hospital/hazards/ergo/ergo.html

Occupational Safety and Health Administration (OSHA), U.S. Department of Labor. (2009). *Guidelines for nursing homes: Ergonomics for the prevention of musculoskeletal disorders*. Retrieved www.osha.gov/ergonomics/guidelines/nursinghome/final_nh_guidelines.pdf

Occupational Safety and Health Administration (OSHA), U.S. Department of Labor. (2013) *Caring for our caregivers: Facts about hospital worker safety. [Booklet]*. Retrieved https://www.osha.gov/dsg/hospitals/documents/1.2_Factbook_508.pdf

Perry, S. E., Hockenberry, M. J., Lowdermilk, D. L., & Wilson, D. (2014). *Maternal child nursing care* (5th ed.). St. Louis, MO: Elsevier Mosby.

Peterson, M. J., Kahn, J. A., Kerrigan, M. V., Gutmann, J. M., & Harrow, J. J. (2015). Pressure ulcer risk of patient handling sling use. *Journal of Rehabilitation Research & Development, 52*(3), 291–300.

Powell-Cope, G., & Rugs, D. (2015). What elements of the 2013 American Nurses Association Safe Patient Handling and Mobility Standards are reflected in state legislation? *American Journal of Safe Patient Handling & Movement, 5*(1), 13–18.

Purnell, L. D. (2013). *Transcultural health care: A culturally competent approach* (4th ed.). Philadelphia, PA: F.A. Davis Company.

Roman de Mettelinge, T., & Cambier, D. (2015). Understanding the relationship between walking aids and falls in older adults: A prospective cohort study. *Journal of Geriatric Physical Therapy, 38*(4), 155–161.

Sachdeva, A., Dalton, M., Amaragiri, S. V., & Lees, T. (2014). Graduated compression stockings for prevention of deep vein thrombosis. *Cochrane Database of Systematic Reviews, 12*, CD001484.

Sadowski, C., & Jones, A. (2014). Ambulatory assistive devices. How to appropriately measure and use canes, crutches and walkers. *Pharmacy Practice, 1*(10), 24–31.

Santy-Tomlinson, J., Vincent, M., Glossop, N., Jomeen, J., & Pearcey, P. (2011). Calm, irritated or infected? The experience of the inflammatory states and symptoms of pin site infection and irritation during external fixation: A grounded theory study. *Journal of Clinical Nursing, 20*(21–22), 3163–3173.

Satryb, S. A., Wilson, T. J., & Patterson, M. M. (2011). Casting: All wrapped up. *Orthopaedic Nursing, 30*(1), 37–41.

Smith, M. A., & Dahlen, N. R. (2013). Clinical practice guideline surgical site infection prevention. *Orthopaedic Nursing, 32*(5), 242–248.

Smith, S. R., Gibbs, R. L., Rosen, B. S., & Lee, J. T. (2015). The critical lift zone: Recognizing the need for safe patient handling equipment across the broader spectrum of patient weights. *American Journal of Safe Patient Handling & Movement, 5*(3), 108–116.

Stevens, L., Rees, S., Lamb, K., & Dalsing, D. (2013). Creating a culture of safety for safe patient handling. *Orthopaedic Nursing, 32*(3), 155–164.

Sturman-Floyd, M. (2013a). Moving and handling: Assessment of the resident. *Nursing & Residential Care, 15*(3), 150–156.

Sturman-Floyd, M. (2013b). Moving and handling: Supporting bariatric residents. *Nursing & Residential Care, 15*(6), 432–437.

Sturman-Floyd, M. (2013c). Moving and handling: Support for residents with dementia. *Nursing & Residential Care, 15*(5), 276–280.

Taylor, C., Lynn, P., & Bartlett, J. (2019). *Fundamentals of nursing: The art and science of person-centered care* (9th ed.). Philadelphia, PA: Wolters Kluwer.

Timms, A., & Pugh, H. (2012). Pin site care: Guidance and key recommendations. *Nursing Standard, 27*(1), 50–55.

U.S. Department of Health and Human Services (DHHS), Office of Disease Prevention and Health Promotion. (2016). *Physical activity guidelines for Americans*. Retrieved http://health.gov/paguidelines/guidelines

U.S. National Library of Medicine, MedlinePlus (2015). *How to make a sling*. Retrieved http://www.nlm.nih.gov/medlineplus/ency/article/000017.htm

Varnam, W. (2011). How to mobilise patients with dementia to a standing position. *Nursing Older People, 23*(8), 31–36.

VHA Center for Engineering & Occupational Safety and Health (CEOSH). (2016). *Safe patient handling and mobility guidebook*. St. Louis, MO: Author. Retrieved http://www.tampavaref.org/safe-patient-handling.htm

Viswanathan, P., & Kidd, M. (2010). Effect of continuous passive motion following total knee arthroplasty on knee range of motion and function: A systematic review. *New Zealand Journal of Physiotherapy, 38*(1), 14–22.

Walker, J. (2012). Pin site infection in orthopaedic external fixation devices. *British Journal of Nursing, 21*(3), 148–151.

Walker, L., & Lamont, S. (2008). Graduated compression stockings to prevent deep vein thrombosis. *Nursing Standard, 22*(40), 35–38.

Wanless, M., & Wanless, S. (2012). Hoisting a patient: Principles and advice for safer practice. *Nursing & Residential Care, 14*(6), 306–310.

Waters, T. R., Nelson, A., Hughes, N., & Menzel, N.; Department of Health and Human Services (DHHS), Centers for Disease Control and Prevention (CDC), National Institute for Occupational Safety and Health (NIOSH). (2009). *Safe patient handling training for schools of nursing: Curricular materials*. Retrieved http://www.cdc.gov/niosh/docs/2009-127/pdfs/2009-127.pdf

White, N. T., Delitto, A., Nanal, T. J., & Miller, S. (2015). The American Physical Therapy Association's top five choosing wisely recommendations. *Physical Therapy, 95*(1), 9–24.

Williams, J. W., Jr. (2016). Effectiveness of intermittent pneumatic compression devices for venous thromboembolism prophylaxis in high-risk surgical patients: A systematic review. *Journal of Arthroplasty, 31*(2), 524–532.

Winslow, E. H., & Brosz, D. L. (2010). Unraveling the mystery of graduated compression stockings. *OR Nurse, 4*(3), 56.

Yeung, Y. L. (2015). Increase access to healthcare services with safe patient handling and mobility equipment. *American Journal of Safe Patient Handling & Movement, 5*(4), 140–147.

Zisberg, A., Shadmi, E., Gur-Yaish, N., Tonkikh, O., & Sinoff, G. (2015). Hospital-associated functional decline: The role of hospitalization processes beyond individual risk factors. *Journal of the American Geriatrics Society, 63*(1), 55–62.

SUGGESTED ANSWERS FOR FOCUSING ON PATIENT CARE: DEVELOPING CLINICAL REASONING

1. Teaching that should be included for Bobby and his parents related to his injury and his plaster cast includes the following: keeping the extremity elevated on pillows to reduce edema; handling the cast with the palm of the hands for the first 24 to 36 hours; keeping the cast uncovered until fully dry; reporting pain, odor, drainage, changes in sensation, abnormal sensation, or the inability to move his fingers; and avoiding putting anything in the cast.

2. Reassure the patient, Esther Levitz, that the device will not hurt. Explain how the pneumatic compression device works and the rationale for its use. In addition, describe potential adverse symptoms, such as pain or discomfort in the legs and changes in sensation that the patient should report while the pneumatic compression device is in use.

3. Additional assessments that should be performed as part of Mr. Esposito's care include the following: assessing the traction equipment to ensure proper function, including inspecting the ropes for fraying and proper positioning; assessing the patient's body alignment; performing skin and neurovascular assessments; assessing for complications of immobility, including alterations in respiratory function, skin integrity, urinary and bowel elimination, and muscle weakness, contractures, thrombophlebitis, pulmonary embolism, and fatigue.

Comfort and Pain Management

Learning Objectives

After completing the chapter, you will be able to accomplish the following:

1. Promote patient comfort.
2. Give a back massage.
3. Apply and care for a patient using a transcutaneous electrical nerve stimulation (TENS) unit.
4. Care for a patient receiving PCA.
5. Care for a patient receiving epidural analgesia.
6. Care for a patient receiving continuous wound perfusion pain management.

Key Terms

acute pain: pain that is generally rapid in onset and varies in intensity from mild to severe

adjuvant: substances or treatments that enhance the effect of another treatment, especially substances that enhance the effect of drugs

analgesic: agent used to relieve pain

breakthrough pain: a temporary flare-up of moderate to severe pain that occurs even when the patient is taking around-the-clock medication for persistent pain

caregiver-controlled analgesia (CCA): a method of pain control in which a consistently available and competent person is authorized by a prescriber and properly educated to activate the dosing button of an analgesic infusion pump in response to a patient's pain when that patient is unable to do so; the authorized agent is a nonprofessional person (e.g., parent, significant other) (Wuhrman et al., 2007).

chronic pain: pain that may be limited, intermittent, or persistent, but lasts beyond the normal healing period

continuous wound perfusion pain management system: device that delivers a continuous infusion of local analgesia to a surgical wound bed

epidural route: administration of analgesia via an infusion catheter placed in the epidural space

nonpharmacologic interventions: interventions without the use of medicine or drugs; interventions in addition to the use of medicines or drugs

nurse-controlled analgesia (NCA): a method of pain control in which a consistently available and competent person is authorized by a prescriber and properly educated to activate the dosing button of an analgesic infusion pump in response to a patient's pain when that patient is unable to do so; the authorized agent is the nurse responsible for the patient (Wuhrman et al., 2007)

pain tolerance: point beyond which a person is no longer willing to endure pain

perineural route: administration of local anesthetic for pain management via an infusion catheter placed along most or all of the length of a wound

Comfort is an important need and ensuring a patient's comfort is a major nursing responsibility. Providing comfort can be as simple as straightening the patient's bed linens, offering to hold the patient's hand, or assisting with hygiene needs. Often, providing comfort includes providing pain relief. The classic definition of pain that is probably of greatest benefit to nurses and patients is that offered by McCaffery (1968): "Pain is whatever the experiencing person says it is, existing whenever the experiencing person says it does" (p. 95). This definition rests on the belief that the only one who can be a real authority on whether, and how, a person is experiencing pain is that person. The International Association for the Study of Pain (IASP) further defines pain as "an unpleasant sensory and emotional experience associated with actual or potential tissue damage, or described in terms of such damage" (IASP, 2014, p. 3).

Differences in individual pain perception and response to pain, as well as the multiple and diverse causes of pain, require the use of highly specialized abilities to promote comfort and relieve pain. The most important of these are the nurse's belief that the patient's pain is real, a willingness to become involved in the patient's pain experience, and competence in developing effective pain management regimens.

Routine pain assessment is an integral part of providing nursing care. Current emphasis is on individualized pain assessment, treatment, and management. Any indication of pain requires a thorough pain assessment. Fundamentals Review 10-1 outlines factors to include in a pain assessment. Because pain is subjective, self-report is generally considered the most reliable way to assess pain and the nurse should use this method whenever possible. According to Pasero and McCaffery (2011), additional methods to assess a person's pain include the following: identification of pathologic conditions or procedures that may be causing pain; take into account the report of a family member, another person close to the patient, or caregiver who is familiar with the patient; the nonverbal behaviors that may indicate the presence of pain (restlessness, grimacing, crying, clenching fists, protecting the painful area); and physiologic measures (increased blood pressure and pulse), although most research verifies that reliance on vital signs to indicate the presence of pain should be minimized. **The absence of an increase in vital signs does not mean that pain is not present.** Infants, young children, patients who are nonverbal or have difficulty communicating verbally, and cognitively impaired adults, such as those with dementia, are at high risk for underassessment and undertreatment of pain (Booker & Haedtke, 2016; Horgas, Yoon, & Grall, 2012).

Use of a pain scale should be part of the initial and continued assessment of pain and evaluation of pain control measures. Choosing an appropriate tool for patient assessment is necessary to obtain an accurate assessment and valid pain ratings. Fundamentals Review 10-2 is an example of a pain assessment tool. Pain rating scales attempt to confirm and, if possible, quantify the presence of pain in a variety of populations and situations. Alternative approaches to pain assessment for special populations ensure that unacceptable levels of pain are addressed and treated. For example, a nurse caring for a patient in an intensive care unit would use a valid and reliable pain assessment tool that considers the unresponsive and/or noncommunicative nature of the patient. Fundamentals Review 10-3 provides a listing of pain assessment scales that can be used in adults and children who can self-report, as well as scales that can be used to assess pain in adults and children who cannot self-report discomfort and pain. Fundamentals Review 10-4 is an example of a scale that can be used to assess discomfort and pain in patients who are unable to self-report.

This chapter covers skills to assist the nurse in providing for patient comfort, including pain relief. Fundamentals Review 10-5 provides a summary of additional information to assist in understanding the skills related to comfort and pain relief. Refer to *Fundamentals of nursing* textbook for further, in-depth discussions of the physiology, assessment, and treatment of pain.

Fundamentals Review 10-1

GENERAL GUIDELINES FOR PAIN ASSESSMENT

Factors to Assess	Questions and Approaches
Characteristics of the pain Location	*Where is your pain? Is it external or internal?* Asking the patient with **acute pain** to point to the painful area with one finger may help to localize the pain. Patients with chronic pain may have difficulty trying to localize their pain.
Duration	*How long have you been experiencing pain? How long does a pain episode last? How often does a pain episode occur?*
Quantity	Ask the patient to indicate the degree (amount) of pain currently experienced using a scale. One example of a scale appears below. Note that it is important to give patients *zero/no pain* as an option. 0 1 2 3 4 5 6 7 8 9 10 No pain Mild Moderate Severe Pain as bad as it can be It is also helpful to ask how much pain the patient has (on the same scale) when the pain is at its least and at its worst: Least_____ Worst_____
Quality	*What words would you use to describe your pain?*
Chronology	*How does the pain develop and progress? Has the pain changed since it first began? If so, how?* If a pattern can be identified, interventions early in a pain sequence will often be far more effective than those used after the pain is well established.
Aggravating factors	*What makes the pain occur or increase in intensity?*
Alleviating factors	*What makes the pain go away or lessen? What methods of relief have you tried in the past? How long were they used? How effective were they?* Pharmacologic and **nonpharmacologic** methods of relief currently in effect for hospitalized patients should be apparent from the chart. It is important to verify the use of current prescriptions and their effectiveness with the patient. Outpatients may need to be asked to record a medication profile, a thorough and accurate account of all medications they are taking.
Associated phenomena	*Are there any other factors that seem to relate consistently to your pain? Any other symptoms that occur just before the pain begins?*

[a]Increases in vital signs may occur briefly in acute pain and may be absent in chronic pain (Pasero & McCaffery, 2011). Reliance on vital signs to indicate the presence of pain should be minimized. **Absence of an increase in vital signs does not mean that pain is not present** (Pasero & McCaffery).

Fundamentals Review 10-1 continued

GENERAL GUIDELINES FOR PAIN ASSESSMENT

Factors to Assess	Questions and Approaches
Physiologic responses Vital signs (blood pressure, pulse, respirations)[a] Skin color Perspiration Pupil size Nausea	Signs of sympathetic stimulation can occur with acute pain, but need not be present to verify the presence of pain. Signs of parasympathetic stimulation (decreased blood pressure and pulse, rapid and regular respirations, pupil constriction, nausea and vomiting, and warm, dry skin) may occur, especially with prolonged, severe pain, visceral, or deep pain.
Muscle tension	Observe. Ask the patient whether he or she is aware of any tight, tense muscles.
Anxiety	Are signs of anxiety evident? May include decreased attention span or ability to follow directions, frequent asking of questions, shifting topics of conversation, avoiding discussion of feelings, acting out, somatizing.
Behavioral responses Posture, gross motor activities	Does patient rub or support a particular area? Make frequent position changes? Walk, pace, kneel, or assume a rolled-up position? Does patient rest a particular body part? Protect an area from stimulation? Lie quietly? In acute pain, postural and gross motor activities are often altered; in **chronic pain**, the only signs of change may be postures characteristic of withdrawal.
Facial features	Does the patient have a pinched look? Are there facial grimaces? Knotted brow? Overall taut, anxious appearance? A look of fatigue is more characteristic of chronic pain.
Verbal expressions	Does the patient sigh, moan, scream, cry, or repetitively use the same words?
Affective responses Anxiety	*Do you feel anxious? Are you afraid? If so, how bad are these feelings?*
Depression	*Do you feel depressed, down, or low? If so, how bad are these feelings? Are your feelings about yourself mostly good or bad? Do you have feelings of failure? Do you see yourself or your illness as a burden to those you care about?*
Interactions with others	How does the patient act when he or she is in pain in the presence of others? How does the patient respond to others when he or she is not in pain? How do significant others and caregivers respond to the patient when the patient is in pain? When the patient is not in pain?
Degree to which pain interferes with patient's life (use past performance as baseline)	*Does the pain interfere with sleep? If so, to what extent? Is fatigue a major factor in the pain experience? Is the conduct of intimate or peer relationships affected by the pain? Is work function affected? Participation in recreational–diversional activities?* An activity diary is often helpful—sometimes crucial. One to several weeks of hourly activity recorded by the patient may be necessary. Pain level, food intake, and sleep–rest periods are noted along with activities performed. Separate diaries for inpatient and outpatient episodes may be necessary because hospitalization markedly affects the nature and type of activities performed.
Perception of pain and meaning to patient	*Are you worried about your illness? Do you see any connection between your pain and the nature or course of illness? If so, how do you see them as related? Do you find any meaning in your pain? If so, is this beneficial or detrimental to you? Are you struggling to find some meaning for your pain?*
Adaptive mechanisms used to cope with pain	*What do you usually do to relieve stress? How well do these things work? What techniques do you use at home to help cope with the pain? How well have they worked? Do you use these in the hospital? If not, why not?*
Outcomes	*What would you like to be doing right now, this week, this month, if the pain were better controlled? How much would the pain have to decrease (on the 0 to 10 or other scale) for you to begin to accomplish these goals? What is your pain goal (on the 0 to 10 or other scale)?* Keep in mind that a response of "NO pain" may not be an option for some patients. Helping a patient to identify a realistic goal promotes effective pain management.
Factors that affect expression of pain	Patterned attitudes related to cultural, ethnic and/or social group; family, sex, biological sex and age variables; spirituality; religious beliefs; environment and supports; past pain experience

Fundamentals Review 10-2

PAIN ASSESSMENT TOOL

Prescott, Martin	**Gender:** Male	**Diagnosis:** Diverticular disease	**Adm Provider:**
MRN: 22432	**DOB:** 8/29/1971	**Isolation Precaution:** Standard	**Facility:** General Mass
Allergies: None	**Age:** 46 Years	**Adv Directive:** Full Code	**Room:** 2
	Height: 67 in		**Adm On:** 2/21/2018 15:49 [0 day(s)]
	Weight: 175 lb		

Patient Info   Assessment   ADLs   Notes   Nursing Dx   Orders   MAR   I/O   Vital Signs   Diagnostics   OT   Flowsheet

HEENT   Neuro   Cardio   Respiratory   GI   GU   Musculoskeletal   Mental Health   Pain Scale   Integumentary   Vascular Access

Add New Site

Documented By: [▼]

Documented At: [0] days [0] hours [0] minutes [after admission ▼]

Pain Location: [ ]

Onset: [0] days [0] hours [0] minutes [after admission ▼]

Pain Duration: [ ]

Pain Frequency: [▼]

Type Of Pain: [▼]

Pain Goal: [▼]

[Pain Goal Comments]

Aggravating Factors:
☐ Movement
☐ Coughing
☐ Breathing
☐ Eating

[Aggravating Factors Comments]

Alleviating Factors:
☐ Rest
☐ Compression
☐ Medication
☐ Ice
☐ Immobility

[Alleviating Factors Comments]

Pain Scale Used: [ ]

Pain Rating: [▼]

Pain Characteristics:
☐ Aching
☐ Throbbing
☐ Dull
☐ Stabbing
☐ Burning
☐ Piercing
☐ Sore
☐ Crushing
☐ Radiating

Notes: [ ]

Fundamentals Review 10-3

PAIN ASSESSMENT SCALES

Resource	Website	Indications
COMFORT Scale	https://www.verywell.com/pain-scales-assessment-tools-4020329	Infants, children, adults who are unable to use Numerical Rating Pain Scale or Wong-Baker Faces Pain Rating Scale
CRIES Pain Scale	https://www.verywell.com/pain-scales-assessment-tools-4020329	Neonates (0 to 6 months)
FLACC Scale	https://www.verywell.com/pain-scales-assessment-tools-4020329	Infants and children (2 months–7 years) who are unable to validate the presence of or quantify the severity of pain
FPS-R (Faces Pain Scale, Revised)	https://www.iasp-pain.org/Education/Content.aspx?ItemNumber=1519&navItemNumber=577	Young children in parallel with numerical self-rating scales (0 to 10). Patients choose the depiction of a facial expression that best corresponds with their pain
Oucher Pain Scale	http://www.oucher.org/the_scales.html	Young children who can point to a face to indicate their level of pain
PAINAD Scale	https://consultgeri.org/try-this/dementia/issue-d2.pdf	Patients whose dementia is so advanced that they cannot verbally communicate
Payen Behavioral Pain Scale	https://www.mdcalc.com/behavioral-pain-scale-bps-pain-assessment-intubated-patients	Can be used with intubated, critically ill patients; measures bodily indicators of pain and tolerance of intubation
Wong-Baker Faces Pain Rating Scale	https://www.verywell.com/pain-scales-assessment-tools-4020329	Adults and children (>3 years) in all patient care settings
0–10 Numerical Rating Pain Scale	https://www.verywell.com/pain-scales-assessment-tools-4020329	Adults and children (>9 years) in all patient care settings who are able to use numbers to rate the intensity of their pain

Fundamentals Review 10-4

FLACC BEHAVIORAL SCALE

This display presents two ways of demonstrating the FLACC Behavioral Scale.

Categories	Scoring		
	0	1	2
Face	No particular expression or smile	Occasional grimace or frown, withdrawn, disinterested	Frequent to constant frown, clenched jaw, quivering chin
Legs	Normal position or relaxed	Uneasy, restless, tense	Kicking, or legs drawn up
Activity	Lying quietly, normal position, moves easily	Squirming, shifting back and forth, tense	Arched, rigid, or jerking
Cry	No cry (awake or asleep)	Moans or whimpers, occasional complaint	Crying steadily, screams or sobs, frequent complaints
Consolability	Content, relaxed	Reassured by occasional touching, hugging, or being talked to, distractible	Difficult to console or comfort

Each of the five categories (**F**) Face; (**L**) Legs; (**A**) Activity; (**C**) Cry; (**C**) Consolability is scored from 0 to 2, which results in a total score between 0 and 10.

Patients who are awake: Observe for at least 1 to 2 minutes. Observe legs and body uncovered. Reposition the patient or observe activity; assess body for tenseness and tone. Initiate consoling interventions, if needed.

Patients who are asleep: Observe for at least 2 minutes or longer. Observe body and legs uncovered. If possible, reposition the patient. Touch the body and assess for tenseness and tone.

Face

Score 0 points if patient has a relaxed face, eye contact, and interest in surroundings.

Score 1 point if patient has a worried look to face, with eyebrows lowered, eyes partially closed, cheeks raised, mouth pursed.

Score 2 points if patient has deep furrows in forehead, with closed eyes, open mouth, and deep lines around the nose/lips.

Legs

Score 0 points if patient has usual tone and motion to limbs (legs and arms).

Score 1 point if patient has increased tone; rigidity; tense, intermittent flexion/extension of limbs.

Score 2 points if patient has hypertonicity, legs pulled tight, exaggerated flexion/extension of limbs, tremors.

Activity

Score 0 points if patient moves easily and freely, with normal activity/restrictions.

Score 1 point if patient shifts positions, is hesitant to move or is guarding, has tense torso, pressure on body part.

Score 2 points if patient is in fixed position, rocking, has side-to-side head movements, is rubbing body part.

Cry

Score 0 points if patient has no cry/moan (awake or asleep).

Score 1 point if patient has occasional moans, cries, whimpers, sighs.

Score 2 points if patient has frequent/continuous moans, cries, grunts.

Consolability

Score 0 points if patient is calm and does not require consoling.

Score 1 point if patient responds to comfort by touch or talk in 30 seconds to a minute.

Score 2 points if patient requires constant consoling or is unable to be consoled after an extended time.

Whenever feasible, behavioral measurement of pain should be used in conjunction with self-report. When self-report is not possible, interpretation of pain behaviors and decision making regarding treatment of pain requires careful consideration of the context in which pain behaviors were observed.

Each category is scored on the 0 to 2 scale, which results in a total score of 0 to 10.

Assessment of Behavioral Scale

0 = Relaxed and comfortable

1–3 = Mild discomfort

4–6 = Moderate pain

7–10 = Severe discomfort/pain

Source: Printed with permission. © 2002, *The Regents of the University of Michigan.* All rights reserved.

Fundamentals Review 10-5

ADDITIONAL TERMS USED BY PATIENTS TO DESCRIBE PAIN

QUALITY

Sharp	Pain that is sticking in nature and is intense.
Dull	Pain that is not as intense or acute as sharp pain, possibly more annoying than painful. It is usually more diffuse than sharp pain.
Diffuse	Pain that covers a large area. Usually, the patient is unable to point to a specific area without moving the hand over a large surface, such as the entire abdomen.
Shifting	Pain that moves from one area to another, such as from the lower abdomen to the area over the stomach.

Other terms used to describe the quality of pain include sore, stinging, pinching, cramping, gnawing, cutting, throbbing, shooting, and viselike pressure.

SEVERITY

Severe or excruciating Moderate Slight or mild	These terms depend on the patient's interpretation of pain. Behavioral and physiologic signs help assess the severity of pain. On a scale of 1 to 10, slight pain could be described as being between about 1 and 3; moderate pain, between about 4 and 7; and severe pain, between about 8 and 10.

PERIODICITY

Continuous	Pain that does not stop.
Intermittent	Pain that stops and starts again.
Brief or transient	Pain that passes quickly.

Skill 10-1 ▶ Promoting Patient Comfort

The nurse can promote increased comfort and relieve patient discomfort and pain through various interventions and therapies. Interventions can include comfort measures, emotional support, nonpharmacologic interventions, and the administration of analgesics and/or other medications to remove or alter the intensity of painful stimuli. **Nonpharmacologic** methods of comfort and pain management can diminish the emotional components of pain, strengthen coping abilities, give patients a sense of control, contribute to pain relief, decrease fatigue, and promote sleep (LeMone, Burke, Bauldoff, & Gubrud, 2015). Refer to the Evidence for Practice display at the end of this skill. The following skill identifies potential interventions related to discomfort and pain. The interventions are listed sequentially for teaching purposes; the order is not sequential and should be adjusted based on patient assessment and nursing judgment. Not every intervention discussed will be appropriate for every patient. Additional interventions for discomfort and pain are discussed in other chapters. Refer to Chapter 5, for nursing skills related to administering topical medications for pain relief. The application of heat or cold therapy is discussed in Chapter 8.

DELEGATION CONSIDERATIONS

The assessment of a patient's pain is not delegated to nursing assistive personnel (NAP) or to unlicensed assistive personnel (UAP). The assessment of a patient's pain may be delegated to licensed practical/vocational nurses (LPN/LVNs). The use of nonpharmacologic interventions related to patient comfort may be delegated to NAP or to UAP, as well as to LPN/LVNs. The decision to delegate must be based on careful analysis of the patient's needs and circumstances, as well as the qualifications of the person to whom the task is being delegated. Refer to the Delegation Guidelines in Appendix A.

EQUIPMENT

- Pain assessment tool and pain scale
- Oral hygiene supplies
- Nonsterile gloves, if necessary
- Additional PPE, as indicated
- Additional supplies, depending on specific intervention utilized

(continued)

Skill 10-1 ▶ Promoting Patient Comfort *(continued)*

ASSESSMENT	Review the patient's health record and care plan for information about the patient's status and contraindications to any of the potential interventions. Inquire about any allergies. Assess the patient's level of discomfort. Assess the patient's pain using an appropriate assessment tool and pain scale. Assess the characteristics of any pain and for other symptoms that often occur with the pain, such as headache or restlessness. Ask the patient what interventions have and have not been successful in the past to promote comfort and relieve pain. Assess the patient's vital signs. Check the patient's medication administration record for the time an analgesic was last administered. Assess cultural beliefs related to pain. Assess the patient's response to a particular intervention to evaluate effectiveness and presence of adverse effects.
NURSING DIAGNOSIS	Determine the related factors for the nursing diagnoses based on the patient's current status. Nursing diagnoses that may be appropriate include: • Acute pain • Disturbed sleep pattern • Chronic pain
OUTCOME IDENTIFICATION AND PLANNING	The expected outcome to achieve is that the patient experiences relief from discomfort and/or pain without adverse effect. Other outcomes that may be appropriate include the patient experiences decreased anxiety and improved relaxation; is able to participate in activities of daily living (ADLs); and verbalizes an understanding of, and satisfaction with, the comfort and pain management plan.

IMPLEMENTATION

ACTION	**RATIONALE**
1. Perform hand hygiene and put on PPE, if indicated.	Hand hygiene and PPE prevent the spread of microorganisms. PPE is required based on transmission precautions.
2. Identify the patient.	Identifying the patient ensures the right patient receives the intervention and helps prevent errors.
3. Discuss pain with the patient, acknowledging that the patient's pain exists. Explain how pain medications and other pain management therapies work together to provide pain relief. Allow the patient to help choose interventions for pain relief. Discuss the patient's expectations for comfort and pain relief.	These measures promote a collaborative relationship in which the patient is treated with respect. Pain discussion and patient involvement strengthen the nurse–patient relationship and promote pain relief (Taylor, Lynn, & Bartlett, 2019). Explanation encourages patient understanding and cooperation and reduces apprehension.
4. Assess the patient's pain using an appropriate assessment tool and measurement scale (see Fundamentals Review 10-1 through 10-5).	Accurate assessment is necessary to guide treatment/relief interventions and evaluate the effectiveness of pain control measures.
5. Provide pharmacologic interventions, if indicated and ordered.	Analgesics and **adjuvant** drugs reduce perception of pain and alter responses to discomfort.
6. Adjust the patient's environment to promote comfort.	The environment can improve or detract from the patient's sense of well-being and can be a source of stimulation that aggravates pain and reduces comfort.
a. Adjust and maintain the room temperature per the patient's preference.	A too warm or too cool environment can be a source of stimulation that aggravates pain and reduces comfort.
b. Reduce harsh lighting, but provide adequate lighting per the patient's preference.	Harsh lighting can be a source of stimulation that aggravates pain and reduces comfort.
c. Reduce harsh and unnecessary noise. Avoid having conversations immediately outside the patient's room.	Noise, including talking, can be a source of stimuli that aggravates pain and reduces comfort.

ACTION	RATIONALE
d. Close the room door and/or curtain whenever possible.	Closing the door or curtain provides privacy and reduces noise and other extraneous stimuli that may aggravate pain and reduce comfort.
e. Provide good ventilation in the patient's room. Reduce unpleasant odors by promptly emptying bedpans, urinals, and emesis basins after use. Remove trash and laundry promptly.	Odors can be a source of stimuli that aggravate pain and reduce comfort.
7. Prevent unnecessary interruptions and coordinate patient activities to group activities together. Allow for and plan rest periods without disturbance.	Frequent interruptions and disturbances for assessment or treatment can be a source of stimuli that aggravate pain and reduce comfort. Fatigue reduces tolerance for pain and can increase the pain experience.
8. Assist the patient to change position frequently. Assist the patient to a comfortable position, maintaining good alignment and supporting extremities, as needed. Raise the head of the bed, as appropriate (see Chapter 9 for more information on positioning).	Positioning in proper alignment with supports ensures that the patient will be able to maintain the desired position and reduces pressure.
9. Provide oral hygiene as often as necessary (e.g., every 1 to 2 hours) to keep the mouth and mucous membranes clean and moist. This is especially important for patients who cannot drink or are not permitted fluids by mouth (see Chapter 7 for additional information about mouth care).	Moisture helps maintain the integrity of mucous membranes. Dry mucous membranes can be a source of stimuli that aggravate pain and reduce comfort.
10. Ensure the availability of appropriate fluids for drinking, unless contraindicated. Make sure the patient's water pitcher is filled and within reach. Have other fluids of the patient's choice available.	Thirst and dry mucous membranes can be sources of stimuli that reduce comfort and aggravate pain.
11. Remove physical situations that might cause discomfort.	
a. Change soiled and/or wet dressings; replace soiled and/or wet bed linens.	Moisture can cause discomfort and irritation to skin.
b. Smooth wrinkles in bed linens.	Wrinkled bed linens apply pressure to skin and can cause discomfort and irritation to skin.
c. Ensure patient is not lying or sitting on tubes, tubing, wires, or other equipment.	Tubing and equipment apply pressure to skin and can cause discomfort and irritation to skin.
12. Assist the patient, as necessary, with ambulation, and active or passive range-of-motion exercises (ROM), as appropriate (see Chapter 9 for more information about activity).	Activity prevents stiffness and loss of mobility, which can reduce comfort and aggravate pain.
13. Assess the patient's spiritual needs related to the pain experience. Ask the patient if he or she would like a spiritual counselor to visit.	Some people's spiritual beliefs facilitate positive coping with the effects of illness, including pain.
14. Consider the use of distraction. Distraction requires the patient to focus on something other than the pain.	Conscious attention often appears to be necessary to experience pain. Preoccupation with other things has been observed to distract the patient from pain. Distraction is thought to raise the threshold of pain and/or increase **pain tolerance** (Taylor et al., 2019).
a. Have the patient recall a pleasant experience or focus attention on an enjoyable experience.	
b. Offer age or developmentally appropriate games, toys, books, audiobooks, access to television, and/or videos, or other items of interest to the patient.	
c. Encourage the patient to hold or stroke a loved person, pet, or toy.	

(continued)

Skill 10-1 ▶ Promoting Patient Comfort *(continued)*

ACTION	RATIONALE
d. Offer access to music the patient prefers. Turn on the music when pain begins, or before anticipated painful stimuli. The patient can close his or her eyes and concentrate on listening. Raising or lowering the volume as pain increases or decreases can be helpful.	
15. Consider the use of guided imagery.	Guided imagery helps the patient gradually become less aware of the discomfort or pain. Positive emotions evoked by the image help reduce the pain experience.
a. Help the patient to identify a scene or experience that the patient describes as happy, pleasant, or peaceful.	
b. Encourage the patient to begin with several minutes of focused breathing, relaxation, or meditation (refer to specific information in steps 16 and 17).	
c. Help the patient concentrate on the peaceful, pleasant image.	
d. If indicated, read a description of the identified scene or experience, using a soothing, soft voice.	
e. Encourage the patient to concentrate on the details of the image, such as its sight, sounds, smells, tastes, and touch.	
16. Consider the use of relaxation activities, such as deep breathing.	Relaxation techniques reduce skeletal muscle tension and lessen anxiety, both of which can reduce comfort and aggravate pain. Relaxation can also be a distraction, providing help in reducing the pain experience (Taylor et al., 2019; Ward, 2016).
a. Have the patient sit or recline comfortably and place hands on stomach. Close the eyes.	
b. Ask the patient to mentally count to maintain a comfortable rate and rhythm. Have the patient inhale slowly and deeply while letting the abdomen expand as much as possible. Have the patient hold his or her breath for a few seconds.	
c. Tell the patient to exhale slowly through the mouth, blowing through puckered lips. Have the patient continue to count to maintain comfortable rate and rhythm, concentrating on the rise and fall of the abdomen.	
d. When the patient's abdomen feels empty, have the patient begin again with a deep inhalation.	
e. Encourage patient to practice at least twice a day, for 10 minutes, and then use the technique, as needed, to assist with pain management.	
17. Consider the use of relaxation activities, such as progressive muscle relaxation.	Relaxation techniques reduce skeletal muscle tension and lessen anxiety, both of which can reduce comfort and aggravate pain. Relaxation can also be a distraction, providing help in reducing the pain experience (Taylor et al., 2019; Ward, 2016).
a. Assist the patient to a comfortable position.	
b. Direct the patient to focus on a particular muscle group. Start with the muscles of the jaw, then repeat with the muscles of the neck, shoulder, upper and lower arm, hand, abdomen, buttocks, thigh, lower leg, and foot.	

ACTION	RATIONALE

c. Ask the patient to tighten the muscle group and note the sensation that the tightened muscles produce. After 5 to 7 seconds, tell the patient to relax the muscles all at once and concentrate on the sensation of the relaxed state, noting the difference in feeling in the muscles when contracted and relaxed.

d. Have the patient continue to tighten–hold–relax each muscle group until the entire body has been covered.

e. Encourage the patient to practice at least twice a day, for 10 minutes, and then use the technique, as needed, to assist with pain management.

18. Consider the use of cutaneous stimulation, such as the intermittent application of heat or cold, or both (see Chapter 8 for additional information on heat and cold therapy).

Heat helps relieve pain by stimulating specific nerve fibers, closing the gate that allows the transmission of pain stimuli to centers in the brain. Heat accelerates the inflammatory response to promote healing, and reduces muscle tension to promote relaxation and help to relieve muscle spasms and joint stiffness. Cold reduces blood flow to tissues and decreases the local release of pain-producing substances, such as histamine, serotonin, and bradykinin, and reduces the formation of edema and inflammation.

Cold reduces muscle spasm, alters tissue sensitivity (producing numbness), and promotes comfort by slowing the transmission of pain stimuli (Taylor et al., 2019).

19. Consider the use of cutaneous stimulation, such as massage (see Skill 10-2).

Cutaneous stimulation techniques stimulate the skin's surface, closing the gating mechanism in the spinal cord, decreasing the number of pain impulses that reach the brain for perception.

20. Discuss consideration of consultation with a nurse trained in Healing Touch (HT) with the patient.

HT is a complementary health approach that has proved valuable as an adjunct to traditional medicine (Taylor et al., 2019). Studies have indicated that it has been effective in reducing pain and anxiety in hospitalized patients (Weaver, 2017).

21. Discuss the potential for use of cutaneous stimulation, such as TENS, with the patient and health care provider (see Skill 10-3).

Cutaneous stimulation techniques stimulate the skin's surface, closing the gating mechanism in the spinal cord, decreasing the number of pain impulses that reach the brain for perception.

22. Remove equipment and return patient to a position of comfort. Remove gloves, if used. Raise side rail and lower bed.

Equipment removal and repositioning promote patient comfort. Removing gloves properly reduces the risk for infection transmission and contamination of other items. Lowering bed promotes patient safety.

 23. Remove additional PPE, if used. Perform hand hygiene.

Proper removal of PPE reduces the risk for infection transmission and contamination of other items. Hand hygiene prevents transmission of microorganisms.

24. Evaluate the patient's response to interventions. Reassess level of discomfort or pain using original assessment tools. Reassess and alter care plan, as appropriate.

Evaluation allows for individualization of care plan and promotes optimal patient comfort.

(continued)

Skill 10-1 ▶ Promoting Patient Comfort *(continued)*

EVALUATION

The expected outcomes have been met when the patient experienced relief from discomfort and/or pain without adverse effect; experienced decreased anxiety and improved relaxation; was able to participate in activities of daily living (ADLs); and verbalized an understanding of, and satisfaction with, the comfort and pain management plan.

DOCUMENTATION

Guidelines

Document pain assessment and other significant assessments. Document comfort and pain relief therapies used and patient responses. Record alternative treatments to consider, if appropriate. Document reassessment of comfort and pain after interventions, at an appropriate interval, based on specific interventions used.

Sample Documentation

> <u>5/12/20</u> 2030 Patient reports increased pain in lower extremities, rating the pain at 5/10, and described it as burning and constant, consistent with previous pain. Medicated with oxycodone 5 mg PO, as ordered for breakthrough pain. Patient using relaxation and deep-breathing techniques, as well as listening to music. Reviewed instructions for use of relaxation and deep breathing; patient verbalized understanding.
>
> —R. Curry, RN
>
> <u>5/12/20</u> 2145 Patient reports pain reduced to 2/10. OOB to solarium with family.
>
> —R. Curry, RN

UNEXPECTED SITUATIONS AND ASSOCIATED INTERVENTIONS

- *Patient reports, or assessment reveals, ineffective/or lack of pain relief:* Reassess pain and evaluate response to implemented therapies. Implement additional or alternate interventions until desired level of comfort is achieved.
- *Intervention increases patient discomfort or pain:* Immediately stop intervention. Document intervention used and the effect. Communicate changes in the patient's condition to the health care provider, as appropriate. Revise care plan, noting adverse effect of intervention, so other caregivers avoid using same intervention.

SPECIAL CONSIDERATIONS

General Considerations

- The use of alternate and adjunct therapies is often a "try-and-see" process. Many interventions can be tried to achieve the best combination for a particular patient. People respond to pain differently; what works for one person may not help another.

Infant and Child Considerations

- Assessment, measurement, and treatment of discomfort and pain in infants and children frequently involve the use of more than one technique. Communication with parents, guardians, or significant others is vital for accurate pediatric pain assessment and management.
- Nonpharmacologic therapies can be very beneficial in decreasing acute and chronic pain, as well as pain related to procedures in infants and children (Kyle & Carman, 2017; Taylor et al., 2019).

Older Adult Considerations

- In addition to medical problems, poor positioning or posture, inactivity, emotional issues, and adverse drug reactions could be at the root of new or worsened pain. Improving these underlying factors is the first step in pain management (Eliopoulos, 2018, p. 170).
- Pain negatively impacts on the emotional well-being, functional ability, sleep, coping, and resources of older adults. Although pain is not a normal part of aging, pain occurs secondary to many chronic illnesses that are present in older adults (Taylor et al., 2019).
- Assessment of pain in the older adult can be problematic. Vision or hearing impairments may influence the assessment format. Multiple-drug regimens that are common in older people can also affect reliable reporting of pain. Many older adults view pain as a forecast of serious illness or death, thus are reluctant to admit its occurrence or report it (Taylor et al., 2019).

HEALING TOUCH AND PATIENT COMFORT

There is a growing trend toward the use of complementary health approaches (Hausladen Foley, Anderson, Mallea, Morrison, & Downey, 2016). Complementary health approaches are being integrated into patient care plans related to the management of pain. HT is an energy therapy that has proved valuable as an adjunct to traditional medicine in reducing pain (Taylor et al., 2019).

Related Research

Hausladen Foley, M. K., Anderson, J., Mallea, L., Morrison, K., & Downey, M. (2016). Effects of healing touch on postsurgical adult outpatients. *Journal of Holistic Nursing, 34*(3), 271–279.

This prospective pilot study was undertaken to determine the effect of HT on postoperative pain, anxiety, blood pressure and pulse rates in adult postoperative outpatients. Participants were randomly assigned to the control or intervention groups. The control group received traditional nursing care. The intervention group received an HT treatment in addition to traditional nursing care. Pre- and postmeasurements of pain, anxiety, blood pressure, and pulse were collected. Results indicated HT treatment was at least as effective as traditional nursing care for reduction in pain and more effective in reducing anxiety. Participants in the intervention group experienced a significant decrease in anxiety ($p = 0.029$). Neither group showed any difference pre- versus posttreatment in blood pressure or pulse rates. There was a trend toward decreased use of opioids in the intervention group. Comments by participants in the intervention group reflected the relaxing effects of HT treatment. The authors concluded Health Touch is an appropriate modality to decrease anxiety, may be appropriate for pain reduction, and may decrease the amount of opioid analgesics required postoperatively. The authors also concluded the findings support the use of HT as an effective complementary intervention for surgical outpatients.

Relevance to Nursing Practice

Nurses should collaborate with patients and their health care providers in integrating complementary health approaches as an additional intervention in pain management. Nurses should consider individual patient preferences when planning interventions for the management of pain. Integrated with nursing assessments, observations and traditional treatments for pain, HT provides an additional treatment modality as nurses strive to provide holistic care to their patients.

Refer to thePoint° for additional research on related nursing topics.

Skill 10-2 ▶ Giving a Back Massage

Massage has many benefits, including general relaxation and increased circulation. Massage can help alleviate pain (Westman & Blaisdell, 2016). A back massage can be incorporated into the patient's bath, as part of care before bedtime, or at any time to promote increased patient comfort. Some nurses do not always give back massages to patients because they do not think they have sufficient time. However, giving a back massage provides an opportunity for the nurse to observe the skin for signs of breakdown. It also improves circulation; decreases pain, symptom distress, and anxiety; improves sleep quality; and provides a means of communicating with the patient through the use of touch. A back massage also provides cutaneous stimulation as a method of pain relief.

Because some patients consider the back massage a luxury and may be reluctant to accept it, communicate its importance and value to the patient. An effective back massage should take 4 to 6 minutes to complete. A lotion is usually applied; warm it before applying to the back. Be aware of the patient's medical diagnosis when considering giving a back massage. A back massage is contraindicated, for example, when the patient has had back surgery or has fractured ribs. Position the patient on the abdomen or, if this is contraindicated, on the side for a back massage.

(*continued*)

Skill 10-2 ▶ Giving a Back Massage *(continued)*

DELEGATION CONSIDERATIONS	Providing a back massage may be delegated to nursing assistive personnel (NAP) or to unlicensed assistive personnel (UAP), as well as to licensed practical/vocational nurses (LPN/LVNs). The decision to delegate must be based on careful analysis of the patient's needs and circumstances, as well as the qualifications of the person to whom the task is being delegated. Refer to the Delegation Guidelines in Appendix A.

EQUIPMENT

- Pain assessment tool and pain scale
- Lotion or oil, to which the patient has no allergy or aversion (Westman & Blaisdell, 2016)
- Bath blanket
- Towel
- Nonsterile gloves, if indicated
- Additional PPE, as indicated

ASSESSMENT

Review the patient's health record and care plan for information about the patient's status and contraindications to back massage. Question the patient about any conditions that might require modifications or that might contraindicate a massage. Inquire about any allergies, such as to lotions or scents. Ask if the patient has any preferences for lotion or has his or her own lotion. Assess the patient's level of pain. Check the patient's medication administration record for the time an analgesic was last administered. If appropriate, administer an analgesic early enough so that it has time to take effect.

NURSING DIAGNOSIS

Determine the related factors for the nursing diagnoses based on the patient's current status. Appropriate nursing diagnoses may include:

- Acute pain
- Anxiety
- Disturbed sleep pattern

OUTCOME IDENTIFICATION AND PLANNING

The expected outcomes to achieve are that the patient reports increased comfort and/or decreased pain, and that the patient is relaxed. Other outcomes that may be appropriate include the patient displays decreased anxiety and improved relaxation; and patient verbalizes an understanding of the reasons for back massage.

IMPLEMENTATION

ACTION	**RATIONALE**
1. Perform hand hygiene and put on PPE, if indicated.	Hand hygiene and PPE prevent the spread of microorganisms. PPE is required based on transmission precautions.
2. Identify the patient.	Identifying the patient ensures the right patient receives the intervention and helps prevent errors.
3. Offer a back massage to the patient and explain the procedure.	Explanation encourages patient understanding and cooperation and reduces apprehension.
4. Put on gloves, if indicated.	Gloves are not usually necessary. Gloves prevent contact with blood and body fluid.
5. Close the room door and/or the curtain around the bed. Turn down the lights, if possible, and adjust the room temperature for patient comfort (Westman & Blaisdell, 2016).	Closing the door or curtain provides privacy, promotes relaxation, and reduces noise and stimuli that may aggravate pain and reduce comfort. Lowering the lights, reducing noise, and adjusting the temperature of the room create a calming environment (Westman & Blaisdell, 2016).

ACTION

6. Assess the patient's pain using an appropriate assessment tool and measurement scale (see Fundamentals Review 10-1 through 10-5). Ask the patient if he or she has any aversion to touch (Westman & Blaisdell, 2016).

7. Raise the bed to a comfortable working position, usually elbow height of the caregiver (VHA Center for Engineering & Occupational Safety and Health [CEOSH], 2016), and lower the side rail.

8. Assist the patient to a comfortable position, preferably the prone or side-lying position. Remove the covers and move the patient's gown just enough to expose the patient's back from the shoulders to sacral area. Drape the patient, as needed, with the bath blanket.

9. Warm the lubricant or lotion in the palm of your hand, or place the container in small basin of warm water. During massage, observe the patient's skin for reddened areas or injury. **Avoid areas of injury, such as wounds, burns, and pressure ulcers and areas with rashes, tubes, and IV lines** (Westman & Blaisdell, 2016) (see Chapter 8 for detailed information regarding skin assessment).

10. Using light, gliding strokes (*effleurage*), apply lotion to patient's shoulders, back, and sacral area (Figure 1).

11. Place your hands beside each other at the base of the patient's spine and stroke upward to the shoulders and back downward to the buttocks in slow, continuous strokes (Figure 2). Continue for several minutes.

12. Massage the patient's shoulders, entire back, areas over iliac crests, and sacrum with circular, stroking motions, keeping hands in contact with the patient's skin. Continue for several minutes, applying additional lotion, as necessary.

RATIONALE

Accurate assessment is necessary to guide treatment and pain relief interventions and to evaluate the effectiveness of pain control measures. Patients with posttraumatic stress disorder or previous negative experience with massage may not want to receive massage (Westman & Blaisdell, 2016).

Having the bed at the proper height prevents back and muscle strain.

This position exposes an adequate area for massage. Draping the patient provides privacy and warmth.

Cold lotion causes chilling and discomfort. Massage of these areas could result in further injury and is contraindicated (Westman & Blaisdell, 2016).

Effleurage relaxes the patient and lessens tension.

Continuous contact is soothing and stimulates circulation and muscle relaxation.

A firm stroke with continuous contact promotes relaxation.

FIGURE 1. Using light, gliding strokes to apply lotion.

FIGURE 2. Stroking upward to shoulders and back downward to the buttocks.

(continued)

Skill 10-2 ▶ Giving a Back Massage *(continued)*

ACTION	RATIONALE
13. Knead the patient's back by gently alternating grasping and compression motions (*pétrissage*) (Figure 3).	Kneading increases blood circulation.
14. Complete the massage with additional long, stroking movements that eventually become lighter in pressure (Figure 4).	Long, stroking motions are soothing and promote relaxation; continued stroking with gradual lightening of pressure helps extend the feeling of relaxation.

FIGURE 3. Kneading the patient's back.

FIGURE 4. Using long strokes with lessening pressure.

ACTION	RATIONALE
15. If excess lotion remains, use the towel to pat the patient dry.	Drying provides comfort and reduces the feeling of moisture on the back.
16. Remove gloves, if worn. Reposition patient's gown and covers. Raise side rail and lower bed. Assist patient to a position of comfort.	Repositioning bedclothes, linens, and the patient helps to promote patient comfort and safety.
17. Remove additional PPE, if used. Perform hand hygiene.	Proper removal of PPE reduces the risk for infection transmission and contamination of other items. Hand hygiene prevents transmission of microorganisms.
18. Evaluate the patient's response to this intervention. Reassess level of discomfort or pain using original assessment tools. Reassess and alter care plan, as appropriate.	Reassessment allows for individualization of the patient's care plan and promotes optimal patient comfort.

EVALUATION

The expected outcomes have been achieved when the patient reported increased comfort, decreased pain, and/or feelings of relaxation; the patient displayed decreased anxiety and improved relaxation; and patient verbalized an understanding of the reasons for back massage.

DOCUMENTATION

Guidelines

Document pain assessment and other significant assessments. Document massage use, length of time of massage, and patient response.

Sample Documentation

> 12/6/20 2330 Patient reports inability to sleep and increased pain at surgical site, rated 3/10. Medicated with acetaminophen 650 mg, as ordered. Back massage administered ×10 minutes. Skin intact without redness. Patient reports increased comfort and relaxation; "I feel like I could sleep now."
>
> —B. Black, RN
>
> 12/6/20 2400 Patient reports pain level 0/10.
>
> —B. Black, RN

UNEXPECTED SITUATIONS AND ASSOCIATED INTERVENTIONS	• *The patient cannot lie prone, so you are giving him a back massage while he is lying on his side. However, as you begin to massage the back, the patient cannot maintain the side-lying position:* If possible, have the patient hold on to the side rail on the side to which he is facing. If this is not possible or the patient cannot assist, use pillows and bath blankets to prevent the patient from rolling. If necessary, enlist the help of another person to maintain the patient's position. If possible, experiment with other positions based on the patient's condition and comfort, such as leaning forward against a pillow on the bedside table while sitting in a chair. • *While massaging the patient's back, you notice a 2-in reddened area on the patient's sacrum:* Note this observation in the patient's health record and report it to the health care provider. Do not massage the area. When the back massage is completed, position the patient off the sacral area, using pillows to maintain the patient's position, and institute a turning schedule.

SPECIAL CONSIDERATIONS

General Considerations

• Before giving a back massage, assess the patient's body structure and skin condition, and tailor the duration and intensity of the massage accordingly. If you are giving a back massage at bedtime, have the patient ready for bed beforehand so the massage can help him or her fall asleep.
• Massage only the hands, feet, or scalp of patients with sepsis; fever over 100°F, sickle cell or HIV crisis, thrombocytopenia or meningitis (Westman & Blaisdell, 2016).
• Check in frequently with the patient during the massage, asking how the massage feels and adjust the pressure and technique based on the patient's preferences (Westman & Blaisdell, 2016).

Infant and Child Considerations

• Hold infants and small children in a comfortable, well-supported position, such as against the chest or across the lap.

Older Adult Considerations

• Be gentle with massage. The skin on older adults is often fragile and dry.
• Reduce pressure, provide short massage sessions, and consider supine or seated positions for massage with older adults (American Massage Therapy Association, 2011).

EVIDENCE FOR PRACTICE ▶

MASSAGE AND FAMILY-CENTERED CARE

Patient- and family-centered care includes a focus on the patients' and families' needs related to and perspectives about what matters in the planning and delivery of health care. Hospitalization often results in emotional distress and stress for the patients' family members. Patients' families are often encouraged to participate in their loved one's care, but may feel anxious, depressed, and/or uncertain about how to help (Prichard & Newcomb, 2015).

Prichard, C., & Newcomb, P. (2015). Benefit to family members of delivering hand massage with essential oils to critically ill patients. *American Journal of Critical Care, 24*(5), 446–449.

This quasi-experimental pilot study evaluated the feasibility of teaching family members of patients in a trauma intensive care unit (ICU) to use hand massage with essential oils and the effect of the intervention on family members' feelings, specifically anxiety and depression. Fifteen adult family members of patients admitted to the trauma ICU were assigned to a control group and 15 were assigned to the treatment group. Each participant completed an anxiety and depression scale to obtain information describing participants' "current" feelings on the day of enrollment and again on the last study day, 4 days later. Participants were asked to visit their family member (patient) twice a day for 3 consecutive days. Nursing staff in the trauma ICU encouraged participants to provide usual family care, such as caressing and talking to the patient. The control group received no further instructions. Treatment group participants were screened for sensitivity to the essential oils and a patch test of the essential oil was performed on the patient and the participant. Each participant in the treatment group received written instructions for hand massage and a bottle of 5% bergamot oil mixed in almond oil. Participants were taught to administer hand massage in compliance with a method of simple

(continued)

Skill 10-2 ▶ Giving a Back Massage *(continued)*

structured touch, using repetitive stroking movements. Participants applied the intervention twice daily for 5 minutes per session for 3 consecutive days. The mean change in anxiety scores was significantly greater for the treatment group than for the control group in a positive direction. There was no significant difference in change in depression scores in the groups. Age was inversely related to the magnitude of change in anxiety scores; younger participants were more likely than older participants to experience relief from anxiety. The authors concluded that a brief, family-delivered touch/aroma intervention is feasible in an ICU and that gentle hand massage with essential oils may reduce the anxiety level of family members delivering the massage.

Relevance to Nursing

Nurses strive to provide holistic care for patients and families. Nurses must recognize and intervene to address the needs of patients and family members. Family-centered care and the use of complementary therapies delivered by family members can be used to help provide effective interventions to meet the emotional needs of family members and comfort patients.

EVIDENCE FOR PRACTICE ▶

MASSAGE PAIN RELIEF

Patient comfort is attained through management of many factors. Achieving pain relief and/or pain control is a large contributor to achieving patient comfort. Pharmacologic interventions alone may not address all of the factors involved in the pain experience. Do alternative approaches to managing pain that supplement medication administration help achieve effective pain management?

Related Research

Abbaspoor, Z., Akbari, M., & Najar, S. (2014). Effect of foot and hand massage in post-cesarean section pain control: A randomized control trial. *Pain Management Nursing, 15*(1), 132–136.

One of the problems for mothers in the post-cesarean section period is pain, which disturbs the early relationship between mothers and newborns. Timely pain management prevents the side effects of pain, facilitates the patient's recovery, reduces the costs of treatment by minimizing or eliminating the mother's distress, and increases mother–infant interactions. The aim of this study was to determine the effect of hand and foot massage on post-cesarean section pain. This study was carried out on 80 women who had an elective cesarean section. A visual analog scale was used to determine the pain intensity before, immediately, and 90 minutes after conducting 5 minutes of foot and hand massage. Vital signs were measured and recorded. Pain intensity was found to be significantly reduced after intervention, compared with the intensity before the intervention, in women who received the massage interventions when compared with women who did not receive massage interventions. There was also a significant difference between groups in terms of the pain intensity and requesting for analgesic. The authors concluded foot and hand massage can be considered as a complementary method to reduce the pain of cesarean section effectively and to decrease the amount of medications required, and their side effects.

Relevance to Nursing Practice

Massage is an economical intervention that is easily incorporated into nursing practice. As nursing activities and responsibilities have grown, however, the inclusion of patient massage has diminished in daily nursing care. Evidence indicates that massage can be an important part of decreasing pain and increasing comfort. Nurses should consider making time to incorporate this intervention into their practice.

Refer to thePoint® for additional research on related nursing topics.

Skill 10-3 ▶ Applying and Caring for a Patient Using a TENS Unit

Transcutaneous electrical nerve stimulation (TENS) is a noninvasive technique for providing pain relief that involves the use of low-voltage electrical stimulation of large-diameter fibers to inhibit the transmission of painful impulses carried over small-diameter fibers. The TENS unit consists of a battery-powered portable unit, lead wires, and cutaneous electrode pads that are applied to or around the painful area (Figure 1). TENS therapy is used to treat acute and chronic pain related to multiple health problems, including osteoporosis-related joint, bone or muscle problems, fibromyalgia-related problems, labor pain, cancer pain, and tendonitis (Cleveland Clinic, 2015).

TENS therapy requires an order/prescription from a health care provider. The TENS unit can be applied intermittently throughout the day or worn for extended periods.

FIGURE 1. TENS unit.

DELEGATION CONSIDERATIONS	The application of and care for a TENS unit is not delegated to nursing assistive personnel (NAP) or unlicensed assistive personnel (UAP). Depending on the state's nurse practice act and the organization's policies and procedures, the application of, and care for, a TENS unit may be delegated to licensed practical/vocational nurses (LPN/LVNs). The decision to delegate must be based on careful analysis of the patient's needs and circumstances, as well as the qualifications of the person to whom the task is being delegated. Refer to the Delegation Guidelines in Appendix A.

EQUIPMENT

- TENS unit
- Self-adhering electrodes
- Pain assessment tool and pain scale
- Disposable cleansing washcloths or skin cleanser, water, towel, and washcloth
- PPE, as indicated

ASSESSMENT

Review the patient's health record and care plan for specific instructions related to TENS therapy, including the order and conditions indicating the need for therapy. Review the patient's history for conditions that might contraindicate therapy, such as pacemaker insertion, cardiac monitoring, or electrocardiography. Determine the location of electrode placement in consultation with the ordering health care provider and based on the patient's report of pain. Assess the patient's understanding of TENS therapy and the rationale for its use.

Inspect the skin of the area designated for electrode placement for irritation, redness, or breakdown. Assess the patient's pain and level of discomfort using an appropriate assessment tool. Assess the characteristics of any pain. Assess for other symptoms that often occur with the pain, such as headache or restlessness. Ask the patient what interventions have and have not been successful in the past, to promote comfort and relieve pain. Assess the patient's vital signs. Check the patient's medication administration record for the time an analgesic was last administered. Assess the patient's response to a particular intervention to evaluate effectiveness and presence of any adverse effect.

Check the unit to ensure proper functioning and review the manufacturer's instructions for use.

(continued)

Skill 10-3 ▶ Applying and Caring for a Patient Using a TENS Unit   *(continued)*

NURSING DIAGNOSIS	Determine the related factors for the nursing diagnoses based on the patient's current status. Appropriate nursing diagnoses may include:

- Acute pain
- Chronic pain
- Deficient knowledge

OUTCOME IDENTIFICATION AND PLANNING	The expected outcome to achieve is that the patient verbalizes decreased discomfort and pain, without experiencing any injury or skin irritation or breakdown. Other appropriate outcomes may include patient verbalizing an understanding of the therapy, use of the device, and the reason for its use.

IMPLEMENTATION

ACTION	RATIONALE
1. Perform hand hygiene and put on PPE, if indicated.	Hand hygiene and PPE prevent the spread of microorganisms. PPE is required based on transmission precautions.
2. Identify the patient.	Identifying the patient ensures that the right patient receives the intervention and helps prevent errors.
3. Show the patient the TENS device, and explain its function and the reason for its use.	Explanation encourages patient understanding and cooperation and reduces apprehension.
4. Assess the patient's pain using an appropriate assessment tool and measurement scale (see Fundamentals Review 10-1 through 10-5).	Accurate assessment is necessary to guide treatment and relief interventions and evaluate the effectiveness of pain control measures.
5. Inspect the area where the electrodes are to be placed. Clean the patient's skin using the disposable cleansing wipe or skin cleanser and water. Dry the area thoroughly.	Inspection ensures that the electrodes will be applied to intact skin. Cleaning and drying help ensure that the electrodes will adhere.
6. Remove the adhesive backing from the self-adhering electrodes and apply them to the specified location (Figure 2).	Application to the proper location enhances the success of the therapy. Gel is necessary to promote conduction of the electrical current.

FIGURE 2. Applying TENS electrodes.

7. Check the placement of the electrodes; leave at least a 2-in (5-cm) space between them.	Proper spacing is necessary to reduce the risk of burns due to the proximity of the electrodes.

ACTION	RATIONALE
8. **Check the controls on the TENS unit to make sure that they are off.** Connect the wires to the electrodes (if not already attached) and plug them into the unit.	Having controls off prevents flow of electricity. This connection completes the electrical circuit necessary to stimulate the nerve fibers.
9. Turn on the unit and adjust the intensity setting to the lowest intensity and determine if the patient can feel a tingling, burning, or buzzing sensation (Figure 3). Then adjust the intensity to the prescribed amount or the setting most comfortable for the patient. Secure the unit to the patient.	Using the lowest setting at first introduces the patient to the sensations. Adjusting the intensity is necessary to provide the proper amount of stimulation.

FIGURE 3. Turning on TENS unit.

ACTION	RATIONALE
10. Set the pulse width (duration of the each pulsation) as indicated or recommended.	The pulse width determines the depth and width of the stimulation.
11. Assess the patient's pain level during therapy.	Pain assessment helps evaluate the effectiveness of therapy.
a. If intermittent use is ordered, turn the unit off after the specified duration of treatment and remove the electrodes. Clean the patient's skin at the electrode sites.	TENS therapy can be ordered for intermittent or continuous use. Skin care reduces the risk for irritation and breakdown.
b. If continuous therapy is ordered, periodically remove the electrodes from the skin (after turning off the unit) to inspect the area and clean the skin, according to facility policy. Reapply the electrodes and continue therapy. Change the electrodes according to manufacturer's directions.	Periodic removal of electrodes allows for skin assessment. Skin care reduces the risk for irritation and breakdown. Reapplication ensures continued therapy.
12. When therapy is discontinued, turn off the unit and remove the electrodes. Clean the patient's skin. Clean the unit and replace the batteries.	Turning off the unit and removing electrodes when therapy is discontinued reduces the risk of injury to the patient. Skin care reduces the risk for irritation and breakdown. Cleaning the unit and replacing the batteries ensures that the unit is ready for future use.
13. Remove PPE, if used. Perform hand hygiene.	Proper removal of PPE reduces the risk for infection transmission and contamination of other items. Hand hygiene prevents transmission of microorganisms.

EVALUATION
The expected outcomes have been achieved when the patient verbalizes decreased discomfort and pain, without injury or skin irritation or breakdown; and the patient verbalizes an understanding of the therapy, use of the device, and the reason for its use.

(*continued*)

Skill 10-3 ▶ Applying and Caring for a Patient Using a TENS Unit *(continued)*

DOCUMENTATION

Guidelines

Document the date and time of application; patient's initial pain assessment; skin assessment; electrode placement location; intensity and pulse width; duration of therapy; pain assessments during therapy and patient's response; and time of removal or discontinuation of therapy.

Sample Documentation

> 5/28/20 1105 Patient complaining of severe lower back pain, rating it as 9/10 on pain scale. Identified lower sacral area as site of pain. TENS therapy ordered for 30 to 45 minutes. Electrodes applied to right and left sides of sacral area. Intensity initially set at 80 pulses/sec with pulse width of 80 microseconds. Pain rating at 7/10 after 15 minutes of therapy. Intensity increased to 100 pulses/sec, with a pulse width increased to 100 microseconds. Pain rating at 5/10 after 15 minutes at increased settings. Therapy continued for an additional 15 minutes and discontinued. Patient rated pain at 3/10 at end of session. Skin on lower sacral area clean, dry, and intact without evidence of irritation or breakdown. Patient instructed to report increasing pain.
>
> —K. Lewin, RN

UNEXPECTED SITUATIONS AND ASSOCIATED INTERVENTIONS

- *While receiving TENS therapy, the patient reports pain and intolerable paresthesia:* Check the settings, connections, and placement of the electrodes. Adjust the settings and reposition the electrodes, as necessary.
- *During a TENS therapy session, the patient reports muscle twitching:* Assess the patient and check the intensity setting. Readjust the intensity to a lower setting, because the patient is most likely experiencing overstimulation.
- *While assessing the skin where the electrodes are placed for a patient receiving continuous TENS therapy, you notice some irritation and redness:* Clean and dry the area thoroughly. Reposition the electrodes in the same area, avoiding the irritated and reddened area.

SPECIAL CONSIDERATIONS

- Never place electrodes over the carotid sinus nerves, laryngeal or pharyngeal muscles (the front or sides of the neck); the eyes or temples; chest and upper back at the same time; irritated, infected, or broken skin; numb areas; or varicose veins (NHS Choices, 2015).
- Whenever electrodes are being repositioned or removed, first turn off the unit.

EVIDENCE FOR PRACTICE ▶

TENS AND POSTOPERATIVE PAIN

Patient comfort is attained through management of many factors. Achieving pain relief and/or pain control is a large contributor to achieving patient comfort. Pharmacologic interventions alone may not address all of the factors involved in the pain experience. Do alternative approaches to managing pain that supplement medication administration help achieve effective pain management?

Related Research

Erden, S., & Senol Celik, S. (2015). The effect of transcutaneous electrical nerve stimulation on post-thoracotomy pain. *Contemporary Nurse, 51*(2–3), 163–170.

This randomized controlled study examined the effect of TENS on postoperative pain and analgesic consumption in postoperative patients after posterolateral thoracotomy. Forty patients enrolled in the study, with 20 patients in the control group and 20 patients in the experimental group. Participants in the experimental group received TENS therapy. The participants in the control group received standard care without use of TENS therapy. Pain assessment and analgesic consumption were recorded for both groups. Reported pain levels and analgesic consumption of the participants in the experimental group were significantly lower than that of the control group ($p<0.05$). The researchers concluded the use of TENS reduced postoperative pain and analgesic consumption in patients who have undergone posterolateral thoracotomy. As a result, TENS can be recommended as a reliable analgesic method for postoperative patients after posterolateral thoracotomy.

Relevance to Nursing Practice
TENS has been shown to reduce pain and the use of analgesics and is an easily implemented analgesic (Erden & Senol Celik, 2015). Nurses have an important role in providing interventions to assist patients in controlling pain and educating patients about analgesic interventions. Nurses should consider the appropriateness of inclusion of nonpharmacologic interventions, such as TENS, in collaboration with health care providers and patients when planning care for patients experiencing or likely to experience pain. Nurses have a responsibility to be informed and knowledgeable regarding all methods of analgesia and work to provide a care plan that addresses individual patient needs.
Refer to thePoint° for additional research on related nursing topics.

Skill 10-4 ▶ Caring for a Patient Receiving Patient-Controlled Analgesia

Patient-controlled analgesia (PCA) allows patients to self-administer small doses of analgesic within a prescribed time interval, controlling the administration of their own medication within predetermined safety limits (Cooney et al., 2013). This approach can be used with oral analgesic agents as well as with infusions of opioid analgesic agents by intravenous, subcutaneous, sublingual, transdermal, **epidural**, and **perineural routes** (Golembiewski, Dasta, & Palmer, 2016; Hinkle & Cheever, 2018; Katz, Takyar, Palmer, & Liedgens, 2017; Shastay, 2017). PCA provides effective individualized analgesia and comfort. This drug delivery system can be used to manage acute and chronic pain in a health care facility or the home.

The PCA pump used to deliver an intravenous opioid analgesic permits the patient to self-administer medication (bolus doses) with episodes of increased pain or painful activities. A timing device electronically controls the PCA pump. The PCA system consists of a computerized, portable infusion pump containing a reservoir or chamber for a syringe or other reservoir that is prefilled with the prescribed medication, usually an opioid, or dilute anesthetic solution in the case of epidural administration (D'Arcy, 2013a; Hinkle & Cheever, 2018). When pain occurs, the patient pushes a button that activates the PCA device to deliver a small, preset bolus dose of the analgesic. A dose interval that is programmed into the PCA unit prevents reactivation of the pump and administration of another dose during that period of time (bolus; commonly 6 to 8 minutes). The pump mechanism can also be programmed to deliver only a specified amount of analgesic within a given time interval (basal rate; most commonly every hour or, occasionally, every 4 hours). These safeguards limit the risk for overmedication and allow the patient to evaluate the effect of the previous dose. PCA pumps also have a locked safety system that prohibits tampering with the device (Pasero & McCaffery, 2011).

The proper selection of patients for PCA is vital for a positive experience. Suitable candidates for this type of delivery system include people who are alert and capable of controlling the unit. The Joint Commission and Institute for Safe Medication Practices (ISMP) both identify people for whom this type of pain relief is not recommended. These include confused older adults, infants and very young children, cognitively impaired patients, patients with conditions for which oversedation poses a significant health risk (e.g., asthma and sleep apnea), and patients who are taking other medications that potentiate opioids (ISMP, 2016). PCA has proven safe for use in developmentally normal children as young as 4 to 6 years of age (DiGiusto et al., 2014; Pasero & McCaffery, 2011).

Nursing responsibilities for patients receiving medications via a PCA pump include collaboration with the health care provider to ensure appropriate patient selection criteria, patient/family teaching, initial device setup, monitoring the device to ensure proper functioning, and frequent assessment of the patient's response, including pain and discomfort control, respiratory status and sedation screening, and presence of adverse effects. Box 10-1 outlines guidelines for safe and effective use of PCA. Additional information related to epidural infusions is discussed in Skill 10-5.

(continued)

Skill 10-4 ▶ Caring for a Patient Receiving Patient-Controlled Analgesia *(continued)*

Box 10-1 Guidelines for Safe and Effective Use of Patient-Controlled Analgesia

Safe patient-controlled analgesia (PCA) use requires proper patient selection, education, assessment, and monitoring (ISMP, 2016). Use the following tips as guidelines to ensure optimal patient comfort and safety when caring for patients receiving PCA.

- Be aware of patient groups who generally are not good candidates for PCA, including infants and young children and patients with cognitive impairment.
- Caution is required when PCA is used in older adults; patients who are obese or have asthma, sleep apnea or other respiratory disease; patients taking other drugs that potentiate opioids, such as muscle relaxants, antiemetics, and sleeping medications; and patients who are morbidly obese.
- Use standard medical order sets and prefilled syringes with standard drug concentrations.
- Check PCA orders/prescriptions ensuring that they include the medication, the initial loading dose, demand (bolus) dose, lockout interval, and an hourly maximum administration rate. Some prescriptions include a continuous infusion rate.

- Be familiar with the particular PCA infusion device in use at a facility. Use smart infusion pump technology, when possible.
- Ensure that PCA pumps are programmed correctly. Check pump settings at least once every 4 hours. Two nurses should verify PCA programming when initiating infusion or making a change in infusion settings.
- Place warning signs on all PCA pumps that say "For patient use only."
- Assess pain level, alertness, sedation, pulse oximetry, capnography, and vital signs, including respiratory rate and quality, at least every 4 hours or more often as needed, such as during the first 24 hours of treatment and at night, when nocturnal hypoxia may develop.
- Teach patients and family members about the danger of PCA use by anyone other than the patient.

Source: Adapted from Casey, G. (2015). Capnography: Monitoring CO_2. *Nursing New Zealand (Wellington, N.Z.: 1995)*, *21*(9), 20–24; Cooney, M. F., Czarnecki, M., Dunwoody, C., et al. (2013). American Society for Pain Management nursing position statement with clinical practice guidelines: Authorized agent controlled analgesia. *Pain Management Nursing*, *14*(3), 176–181; D'Arcy, Y. (2013a). PCA by proxy: Taking the patient out of patient-controlled analgesia.This controversial practice can be done safely in carefully controlled circumstances. *Dimensions of Critical Care Nursing*, *32*(4), 200–203; Institute for Safe Medication Practices (ISMP). (2016). *Acute Care ISMP Medication Safety Alert!® Worth repeating… Recent PCA by proxy event suggests reassessment of practices that may have fallen by the wayside.* Retrieved https://www.ismp.org/Newsletters/acutecare/showarticle.aspx?id=1149; Institute for Safe Medication Practices (ISMP). (2003; updated 2017). *Acute Care ISMP Medication Safety Alert!® Part II: How to prevent errors. Safety issues with patient-controlled analgesia.* Retrieved http://www.ismp.org/newsletters/acutecare/articles/20030724.asp; Institute for Safe Medication Practices (ISMP). (2013). *Acute Care ISMP Medication Safety Alert!® Fatal PCA adverse events continue to happen…Better patient monitoring is essential to prevent harm.* Retrieved https://www.ismp.org/newsletters/acutecare/showarticle.aspx?id=50; and Lisi, D. M. (2013). Patient-controlled analgesia and the older patient. *US Pharmacist*, *38*(3), HS2–HS6. Retrieved https://www.uspharmacist.com/article/patient-controlled-analgesia-and-the-older-patient.

DELEGATION CONSIDERATIONS

The care related to PCA is not delegated to nursing assistive personnel (NAP) or to unlicensed assistive personnel (UAP). Depending on the state's nurse practice act and the organization's policies and procedures, specific aspects of the care related to PCA, such as monitoring the infusion and assessment of patient response, may be delegated to licensed practical/vocational nurses (LPN/LVNs). The decision to delegate must be based on careful analysis of the patient's needs and circumstances, as well as the qualifications of the person to whom the task is being delegated. Refer to the Delegation Guidelines in Appendix A.

EQUIPMENT

- PCA system, including infusion device
- Syringe (or appropriate reservoir for device) filled with medication
- PCA system tubing
- Antimicrobial swabs
- Appropriate label for syringe and tubing, based on facility policy and procedure
- Second nurse to verify medication and programmed pump information, if necessary, according to facility policy
- Pain assessment tool and pain scale
- Electronic medication administration record (eMAR) or medication administration record (MAR)
- Gloves
- Additional PPE, as indicated

ASSESSMENT

Review the patient's health record and care plan for specific instructions related to PCA therapy, including the health care provider's orders and conditions indicating the need for therapy. Check the health record for the prescribed drug, initial loading dose, dose for self-administration, and lockout interval. Check to ensure proper functioning of the unit. Assess the patient's level of consciousness and understanding of PCA therapy and the rationale for its use.

Review the patient's history for conditions that might contraindicate therapy, such as respiratory limitations, history of substance abuse, or psychiatric disorder. Review the patient's health record and assess for factors contributing to an increased risk for respiratory depression, such as the use of a basal infusion, the patient's age, obesity, upper abdominal or thoracic surgery, sleep apnea, history of smoking, concurrent CNS depressants, and impaired major organ functioning (Jarzyna et al., 2011; The Joint Commission, 2012). Determine the prescribed route for administration. Inspect the site to be used for the infusion for signs of infiltration or infection. If the route is via an IV infusion, ensure that the access is patent and the current solution is compatible with the drug ordered.

Assess the patient's level of consciousness and vital signs. Assess the patient's pain and level of discomfort using an appropriate assessment tool and pain scale (refer to Fundamentals Review 10-1 through 10-5). Assess the characteristics of any pain, and for other symptoms that often occur with the pain, such as headache or restlessness. Ask the patient what interventions have and have not been successful in the past to promote comfort and relieve pain. Assess the patient's vital signs. Assess the patient's respiratory status, including rate, depth, and rhythm; oxygen saturation level using pulse oximetry; and level of carbon dioxide concentration using capnography. Assess the patient's sedation score (Table 10-1). Determine the patient's response to the intervention to evaluate effectiveness and for the presence of adverse effects.

Table 10-1 — **Pasero Opioid-Induced Sedation Scale (POSS)**

PATIENT ASSESSMENT CHARACTERISTICS	SEDATION SCORE	ACTION
Sleeping, easy to arouse	S	
Awake and alert	1	No action needed
Slightly drowsy, easily aroused	2	No action needed
Frequently drowsy, arousable, drifts off during conversation	3	Requires action; decrease dose
Somnolent, minimal or no response to physical stimulation	4	Unacceptable, stop opioid, consider administering naloxone

Source: Used with permission. © 1994, Pasero C. Used with permission. As cited in Pasero C, McCaffery M. *Pain Assessment and Pharmacologic Management*, p. 510. St. Louis, Mosby/Elsevier, 2011.

NURSING DIAGNOSIS

Determine the related factors for the nursing diagnoses based on the patient's current status. Appropriate nursing diagnoses may include:

- Acute pain
- Ineffective breathing pattern
- Deficient knowledge

OUTCOME IDENTIFICATION AND PLANNING

The expected outcome to achieve is that the patient reports increased comfort and/or decreased pain, without adverse effects, oversedation, or respiratory depression. Other appropriate outcomes may include the patient verbalizes an understanding of the reason of use of the therapy; the patient verbalizes and demonstrates an understanding of the use of the therapy; and the patient's family verbalizes an understanding that the PCA is to be used only by the patient.

(continued)

Skill 10-4 ► Caring for a Patient Receiving Patient-Controlled Analgesia *(continued)*

IMPLEMENTATION

ACTION	RATIONALE
1. Gather equipment. Check the medication order against the original order in the health care record, according to facility policy. Clarify any inconsistencies. Check the patient's health record for allergies.	This comparison helps to identify errors that may have occurred when orders were transcribed. The health care provider's order/prescription is the legal record-of-medication order for each facility.
2. Know the actions, special nursing considerations, safe dose ranges, purpose of administration, and adverse effects of the medications to be administered. Consider the appropriateness of the medication for this patient.	This knowledge aids the nurse in evaluating the therapeutic effect of the medication in relation to the patient's disorder and can also be used to educate the patient about the medication.
3. Prepare the medication syringe or other reservoir for administration, based on facility policy (see Chapter 5 for additional information).	Proper preparation and administration procedures prevent errors.
4. Perform hand hygiene and put on PPE, if indicated.	Hand hygiene and PPE prevent the spread of microorganisms. PPE is required based on transmission precautions.
5. Identify the patient.	Identifying the patient ensures that the right patient receives the intervention and helps prevent errors.
6. Show the patient the device, and explain its function and the reason for use. Explain the purpose and action of the medication to the patient.	Explanation encourages patient understanding and cooperation and reduces apprehension.
7. Plug the PCA device into the electrical outlet, if necessary. Check status of battery power, if appropriate.	The PCA device requires a power source (electricity or battery) to run. Most units will alarm to acknowledge a low battery state.
8. Close the door to the room or pull the bedside curtain.	Closing the door or pulling the curtain provides for patient privacy.
9. Complete necessary assessments before administering medication. Check allergy bracelet or ask patient about allergies. Assess the patient's pain using an appropriate assessment tool and measurement scale (see Fundamentals Review 10-1 through 10-5).	Assessment is a prerequisite to medication administration. Accurate assessment is necessary to guide treatment and relief interventions and to evaluate the effectiveness of pain control measures.
10. Check the label on the prefilled drug syringe or reservoir with the medication record and patient identification (Figure 1). Obtain verification of information from a second nurse, according to facility policy.	This action verifies that the correct drug and dosage will be administered to the correct patient. Confirmation of information by a second nurse helps prevent errors.
11. Scan the patient's barcode on the identification band, if required.	This provides an additional check to ensure that the medication is given to the right patient.

FIGURE 1. Checking label on prefilled drug syringe with patient identification.

ACTION	RATIONALE
12. Connect tubing to prefilled syringe or other reservoir and place into the PCA device (Figure 2). **Prime the tubing.** Attach label to tubing, based on facility policy.	Doing so prepares the device to deliver the drug. Priming the tubing purges air from the tubing and reduces the risk for air embolism. Labeling tubing allows for identification of purpose of infusion, reducing confusion in the presence of multiple infusions.
13. Set the PCA device to administer the loading dose, if ordered, and then program the device based on the prescriber's order for medication dosage, dose interval, and lockout interval (Figure 3). Obtain verification of information from a second nurse, according to facility policy.	These actions ensure that the appropriate drug dosage will be administered. Confirmation of information by a second nurse helps prevent errors.

FIGURE 2. Placing syringe/reservoir into PCA device.

FIGURE 3. Programming PCA device.

ACTION	RATIONALE
14. Put on gloves. Depending on facility policy, remove the passive disinfection cap from the connection port on the IV infusion tubing or other access site, based on route of administration. Alternately, use an antimicrobial swab to clean the connection port. Connect the PCA tubing to the patient's IV infusion line or appropriate access site, based on the specific site used. Secure the site per facility policy and procedure. Remove gloves. Initiate the therapy by activating the appropriate button on the pump. Lock the PCA device, per facility policy.	Gloves prevent contact with blood and body fluids. Cleaning the connection port reduces the risk of infection. Connection and initiation are necessary to allow drug delivery to the patient. Locking the device prevents tampering with the settings.
15. Ensure the patient control (dosing button) is within the patient's reach. Attach the warning sign to the PCA control cord and/or PCA infusion device, per facility policy. Reinforce the steps for use with the patient and the need to press the button each time he or she needs relief from pain (Figure 4).	The patient control (dosing button) must be within reach to enable patient use. Warning sign/label provides warning/reinforcement for the patient, family members, and staff that the button is to be pressed only by the patient to reduce the risk for adverse effect (ISMP, 2016). Reinforcement of instructions promotes correct use of the device.

FIGURE 4. Reminding patient to press button to administer pain medication.

(continued)

Skill 10-4 ▶ Caring for a Patient Receiving Patient-Controlled Analgesia *(continued)*

ACTION	RATIONALE
16. Assess the patient's response to the medication: Assess the patient's pain at least every 4 hours or more often, as needed, based on patient's individual risk factors. Monitor vital signs, especially respiratory status, including respiratory rate, depth, and quality and oxygen saturation every 2 to 4 hours or more often, as needed, based on patient's individual risk factors and situation.	Continued assessment at frequent intervals helps evaluate the effectiveness of the drug and reduce the risk for complications (D'Arcy, 2013a; Jarzyna et al., 2011; Jungquist, Smith, Nicely, & Polomano, 2017; Jungquist, Vallerand, Sicoutris, Kwon, & Polomano, 2017).
17. Assess the patient's response to the medication: Assess the patient's sedation score (Table 10-1) and end-tidal carbon dioxide level (capnography) at least every 4 hours or more often, as needed, based on patient's individual risk factors.	Sedation occurs before clinically significant respiratory depression (D'Arcy, 2013b). Respiratory depression can occur with the use of opioid analgesics. Capnography is a more reliable indicator of respiratory depression (Casey, 2015; D'Arcy, 2013a; Jarzyna et al., 2011; Jungquist, Smith, et al., 2017; Jungquist, Vallerand, et al., 2017).
18. Assess the infusion site periodically, according to facility policy and nursing judgment. Assess the patient's use of the medication, noting number of attempts and number of doses delivered. Replace the drug syringe when it is empty.	Continued assessment of the infusion site is necessary for early detection of problems. Continued assessment of the patient's use of medication and effect is necessary to ensure adequate pain control without adverse effect. Replacing the syringe ensures continued drug delivery.
19. Make sure the patient control (dosing button) is within the patient's reach.	Easy access to the control is essential for the patients to use the device.
20. Remove gloves and additional PPE, if used. Perform hand hygiene.	Proper removal of PPE reduces the risk for infection transmission and contamination of other items. Hand hygiene prevents transmission of microorganisms.

EVALUATION

The expected outcomes have been achieved when the patient has reported increased comfort and/or decreased pain, without adverse effects, oversedation, and respiratory depression; the patient displayed an understanding of use of the therapy and the reason for its use; and the patient's family verbalized an understanding that the PCA is to be used only by the patient.

DOCUMENTATION

Guidelines

Document the date and time PCA therapy was initiated, initial assessments, drug and loading dose administered, if appropriate, and individual dosing and time interval. Document patient teaching and patient's response. Document continued pain, sedation level, vital signs and assessments, and patient's response to therapy.

Sample Documentation

> 6/1/20 0645 Patient returned from surgery with PCA therapy with morphine sulfate 1 mg/mL in place via IV infusion. Device programmed to deliver 0.1 mg at 10-minute lockout intervals. Patient complaining of moderate to severe abdominal pain, rating pain as 6 to 8/10 on a pain-rating scale. Patient instructed to press PCA button for pain relief. Vital signs within acceptable parameters. Respiratory rate 16 breaths/min, regular rhythm and depth. Oxygen saturation 96%; partial pressure end-tidal CO_2 ($PetCO_2$) 36%. IV of 1,000 mL D5LR infusing at 100 mL/min; IV site clean and dry without evidence of infiltration or infection.
>
> —P. Joyner, RN
>
> 6/1/20 0715 Patient rates pain at 4/10. Respirations 16 breaths/min, regular rhythm and depth. Encouraged patient to take deep breaths and cough. Lying on right side with the support of two pillows and head of bed elevated 30 degrees.
>
> —P. Joyner, RN

UNEXPECTED SITUATIONS AND ASSOCIATED INTERVENTIONS

- *While receiving PCA therapy, the patient's respiratory rate drops to 10 breaths/min, with a sedation score of 3 via sedation scale (Pasero Opioid-Induced Sedation Scale [POSS]):* Stop the PCA infusion if basal infusion is present. Notify the health care provider. Discontinue the basal infusion; if no basal infusion is being used, then reduce the medication dosage. Increase the frequency of sedation and respiratory rate monitoring to every 15 minutes. Arouse the patient every 15 minutes and encourage deep breathing (D'Arcy, 2008; Jarzyna et al., 2011; Jungquist, Smith, et al., 2017; Pasero & McCaffery, 2011).
- *While receiving PCA therapy, the patient is somnolent, with a sedation score of 4 via sedation scale (POSS):* Stop the medication infusion immediately. Stimulate the patient; raise the head of bed to seated position (if not contraindicated) and talk to patient (Jungquist, Smith, et al., 2017). Call the rapid response team (RRT) (Jungquist, Smith, et al., 2017). Notify the health care provider. Administer oxygen and an opioid antagonist, such as naloxone, based on facility policy (ISMP, 2017). Because naloxone reverses all analgesia, as well as the respiratory depression, patients will experience extremely severe pain once awake and alert (D'Arcy, 2008).
- *The patient's IV infusion line becomes infiltrated:* Stop the PCA infusion and IV infusion. Remove the IV catheter and restart the IV line in another site. Once the site is established, resume the IV and PCA infusion. Provide site care to the infiltration site based on facility policy.
- *The patient's subcutaneous infusion site becomes infiltrated:* Stop the PCA infusion. Remove the administration device. Obtain new administration equipment and restart the infusion at another site. Once the site is established, resume the PCA infusion. Provide site care to the infiltration site based on facility policy.

SPECIAL CONSIDERATIONS

General Considerations

- A wide variety of PCA devices are available on the market. Check the manufacturer's instructions before using the device.
- Adults and children who are cognitively and physically able to use the PCA equipment and are able to understand that pressing a button can result in pain relief are appropriate candidates for PCA therapy (DiGiusto et al., 2014; Pasero & McCaffery, 2011).
- Opioid analgesia via a continuous subcutaneous infusion (CSI) is a safe, effective alternative when IV access is not available and oral analgesia is no longer possible. Candidates for CSI are often patients requiring hospice and palliative care (Thomas & Barclay, 2015). Equipment consists of a small butterfly needle inserted subcutaneously and an infusion pump and administration set that is clearly labeled "Subcutaneous Infusion." This setup delivers the opioid in a small amount of fluid and can be programmed with a lockout feature and options for bolus dosing (Taylor et al., 2019).
- PCA by proxy refers to activation of the PCA dosing button by anyone other than the patient (Cooney et al., 2013; D'Arcy, 2013a). PCA by proxy is not recommended (ISMP, 2016; The Joint Commission, 2012; Wuhrman et al., 2007). PCA by proxy can cause serious analgesic overdoses resulting in oversedation, respiratory depression, and death (ISMP, 2016; The Joint Commission, 2012; Wuhrman et al., 2007).
- Some facilities have developed clinical practice guidelines for authorized agent-controlled analgesia (AACA). In these cases, one family member (**caregiver-controlled analgesia [CCA]**) or primary nurse (**nurse-controlled analgesia [NCA]**) is designated as the primary pain manager and *only* that person can press the PCA button for the patient. In the case of family members, the primary pain manager must be chosen carefully and taught to asses for pain and the adverse effect of the medication. Additionally, nursing staff must be vigilant in assessing the patient's need for and response to the medication, following the same assessment guidelines previously discussed. It is very important to follow facility guidelines to ensure safe administration (Cooney et al., 2013; D'Arcy, 2013a). Box 10-2 outlines guidelines for safe implementation of AACA.
- If using a device that provides continuous and bolus doses, the cumulative doses per hour should not exceed the total hourly dose ordered by the health care provider.
- Vital sign monitoring is crucial, especially when initiating therapy. Encourage the patient to practice coughing and deep breathing to promote ventilation and prevent pooling of secretions.

(continued)

Skill 10-4 ▶ Caring for a Patient Receiving Patient-Controlled Analgesia *(continued)*

Box 10-2 Guidelines for Safe Implementation of Authorized Agent-Controlled Analgesia

Authorized agent-controlled analgesia (AACA) can be implemented to provide prompt, safe, and effective pain relief for the patient who, because of cognitive or physical limitations, is unable to self-administer analgesics using an analgesic pump (Cooney et al., 2013). Use the following tips as guidelines to ensure optimal patient comfort and safety when caring for patients receiving AACA.

- Limit the number of authorized agents to one at a given time; alternative authorized agents may be designated to provide respite and/or coverage.
- Use standard AACA medical order sets.
- Provide patient and family education regarding the principles of AACA, requirements of an authorized agent, specific policies and procedures related to AACA, and the negative consequences of unauthorized activation of the analgesic infusion pump dosing button.

- Document the identity of the authorized agent(s) and caregiver-authorized agent, as well as education provided and feedback.
- Ensure that authorized agents only activate the dosing button if the patient is awake and/or the patient's words or behavior indicate that the patient is in pain or pain is anticipated. Authorized agents should verbalize an understanding of how to recognize pain, sedation, and respiratory depression.

Source: Adapted with permission from Cooney, M. F., Czarnecki, M., Dunwoody, C., et al. (2013). American Society for Pain Management nursing position statement with clinical practice guidelines: Authorized agent controlled analgesia. *Pain Management Nursing, 14*(3), 176–181.

- An opioid antagonist, such as naloxone, must be readily available in case the patient develops respiratory complications related to drug therapy.
- A fentanyl patient-controlled transdermal system (PCTS) is another patient-controlled delivery technique for pain medication and indicated for hospital treatment of acute postoperative pain (Polomano et al., 2017). The small device contains the medication in a reservoir in a patch that attaches to the patient's upper arm or chest with adhesive. When the patient pushes the button on the device, the medication is delivered by iontophoresis, an electrical current that introduces the medication into the tissues. The device is preprogrammed to deliver fixed doses of fentanyl and is restricted with a lockout interval between doses. The device will deliver the maximum number of doses or will operate for a specific period of time from the first dose, whichever occurs first (Lindley, Ding, Danesi, & Jones, 2017; Polomano et al.). The device then shuts off. If continued use is required, it is replaced with a new device, in another location, for up to three days (Polomano et al.).

Infant and Child Considerations

- PCA can be an effective method of pain control for a child. When determining the appropriateness of this therapy for a child, consider the child's chronologic age and developmental level, ability to understand (cognitive level), and motor skills (Pasero & McCaffery, 2011).
- Children who are cognitively and physically able to use the PCA equipment and are able to understand that pressing a button can result in pain relief are appropriate candidates for PCA therapy (DiGiusto et al., 2014; Pasero & McCaffery, 2011).

Home Care Considerations

- Be sure that the patient understands how to use the PCA device properly. Teach the patient how the device works, when to contact the health care provider, and signs and symptoms of adverse reactions and of drug tolerance.
- Advise the patient to change positions gradually to prevent orthostatic hypotension, which can result from use of an opioid analgesic.
- Ensure that a reliable adult is available who can provide backup assistance should the patient have difficulty.
- Collaborate to obtain a referral to a home health care provider to continue teaching and provide assessment of the therapy.

Skill 10-5 Caring for a Patient Receiving Epidural Analgesia

Epidural analgesia can be used to provide pain relief during the immediate postoperative period (particularly after thoracic, abdominal, orthopedic, and vascular surgery), procedural pain, trauma pain, and for chronic pain situations (Schrieber, 2015). Epidural pain management is also being used with infants and children (Kyle & Carman, 2017). The anesthesiologist or radiologist usually inserts the catheter in the mid-lumbar region into the epidural space that exists between the walls of the vertebral canal and the dura mater or outermost connective tissue membrane surrounding the spinal cord. For temporary therapy, the catheter exits directly over the spine, and the tubing is positioned over the patient's shoulder with the end of the catheter taped to the chest. For long-term therapy, the catheter may be tunneled subcutaneously and made to exit on the side of the body or on the abdomen (Figure 1).

The epidural analgesia can be administered using medications such as preservative-free fentanyl, hydromorphone, or morphine as a bolus dose (either one time or intermittently), via a continuous infusion pump, or by a patient-controlled epidural analgesia (PCEA) pump (Schrieber, 2015; Taylor et al., 2019). Epidural catheters used for the management of acute pain are typically removed within 36 to 72 hours after surgery, when oral medication can be substituted for pain relief (Schreiber). Additional information specific to PCA administration is discussed in Skill 10-4.

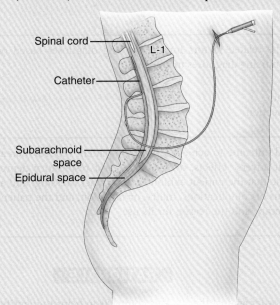

FIGURE 1. Placement of an epidural catheter for long-term use.

DELEGATION CONSIDERATIONS

The care related to epidural analgesia is not delegated to nursing assistive personnel (NAP) or to unlicensed assistive personnel (UAP). Depending on the state's nurse practice act and the organization's policies and procedures, specific aspects of the care related to epidural analgesia, such as monitoring the infusion and assessment of patient response, may be delegated to licensed practical/vocational nurses (LPN/LVNs). The decision to delegate must be based on careful analysis of the patient's needs and circumstances, as well as the qualifications of the person to whom the task is being delegated. Refer to the Delegation Guidelines in Appendix A.

EQUIPMENT

- Infusion device
- Epidural infusion tubing
- Prescribed epidural analgesic solutions
- Electronic medication administration record (eMAR) or medication administration record (MAR)
- Pain assessment tool and/or measurement scale
- Transparent dressing or gauze pads
- Labels for epidural infusion line
- Tape
- Emergency drugs and equipment, such as naloxone, oxygen, endotracheal intubation set, handheld resuscitation bag, per facility policy
- Gloves
- Additional PPE, as indicated

(continued)

Skill 10-5 ▶ Caring for a Patient Receiving Epidural Analgesia *(continued)*

ASSESSMENT

Review the patient's health record and care plan for specific instructions related to epidural analgesia therapy, including the health care provider's order for the drug and conditions indicating the need for therapy. Review the patient's history for conditions that might contraindicate therapy, such as local or systemic infections, increased intracranial pressure, coagulopathy, spinal instabilities/abnormalities or prior spinal surgery, hypovolemia, allergy to the prescribed medication, or thrombocytopenia (Schrieber, 2015). Check to ensure proper functioning of the infusion device. Assess the patient's level of consciousness and understanding of epidural analgesia therapy and the rationale for its use.

Assess the patient's level of consciousness and vital signs. Assess the patient's level of discomfort and pain using an appropriate assessment tool. Assess the characteristics of any pain. Assess for other symptoms that often occur with the pain, such as headache or restlessness. Ask the patient what interventions have and have not been successful in the past to promote comfort and relieve pain. Assess the patient's vital signs and respiratory status, including rate, depth, and rhythm, oxygen saturation level using pulse oximetry, and level of carbon dioxide concentration using capnography. Assess the patient's sedation score (see Table 10-1 in Skill 10-4). Assess the patient's response to the intervention to evaluate effectiveness and for the presence of adverse effects.

NURSING DIAGNOSIS

Determine the related factors for the nursing diagnoses based on the patient's current status. Appropriate nursing diagnoses may include:

- Acute pain
- Chronic pain
- Risk for infection

OUTCOME IDENTIFICATION AND PLANNING

The expected outcome to achieve is that the patient reports increased comfort and/or decreased pain, without adverse effects, oversedation, and respiratory depression. Other appropriate outcomes include that the patient exhibits a dry, intact dressing, and a catheter exit site free of signs and symptoms of complications, injury, or infection; and the patient displays an understanding of use of the therapy and the reason for its use.

IMPLEMENTATION

ACTION	**RATIONALE**
1. Gather equipment. Check the medication order against the original order in the health care record, according to facility policy. Clarify any inconsistencies. Check the patient's health record for allergies.	This comparison helps to identify errors that may have occurred when orders were transcribed. The health care provider's order/prescription is the legal record-of-medication order for each facility.
2. Know the actions, special nursing considerations, safe dose ranges, purpose of administration, and adverse effects of the medications to be administered. Consider the appropriateness of the medication for this patient.	This knowledge aids the nurse in evaluating the therapeutic effect of the medication in relation to the patient's disorder and can also be used to educate the patient about the medication.
3. Prepare the medication syringe or other reservoir for administration, based on facility policy (see Chapter 5 for additional information).	Proper preparation and administration prevents errors.
4. Perform hand hygiene and put on PPE, if indicated.	Hand hygiene and PPE prevent the spread of microorganisms. PPE is required based on transmission precautions.
5. Identify the patient.	Identifying the patient ensures that the right patient receives the intervention and helps prevent errors.

ACTION

6. Show the patient the device, and explain the function of the device and the reason for its use. Explain the purpose and action of the medication to the patient.

7. Close the door to the room or pull the bedside curtain.

8. Complete necessary assessments before administering the medication. Check allergy bracelet or ask the patient about allergies. Assess the patient's pain using an appropriate assessment tool and measurement scale (see Fundamentals Review 10-1 through 10-5). Put on gloves.

9. **Have an ampule of 0.4-mg naloxone and a syringe at the bedside, according to facility policy.**

10. After the catheter has been inserted and the infusion initiated by the anesthesiologist or radiologist, **identify the patient. Compare the label on the medication container and rate of infusion with the eMAR/MAR.** Obtain verification of information from a second nurse, according to facility policy. If using a barcode administration system, scan the barcode on the medication label, if required.

11. Tape all connection sites. **Label the bag, tubing, and pump apparatus "For Epidural Infusion Only." Do not administer any other opioid or adjuvant drugs without the approval of the clinician responsible for the epidural injection.**

12. Assess the catheter exit site and apply a transparent dressing over the catheter insertion site, if not already in place (Figure 2). Secure the catheter and tubing, based on facility policy. Remove gloves and additional PPE, if used. Perform hand hygiene.

13. Refer to Skill 10-4 for additional considerations if the epidural analgesia is being administered as PCA.

RATIONALE

Explanation encourages patient understanding and cooperation and reduces apprehension.

Closing the door or curtain provides for patient privacy.

Assessment is a prerequisite to administration of medications. Accurate assessment is necessary to guide treatment and relief interventions and to evaluate the effectiveness of pain control measures. Gloves are indicated for potential contact with blood or body fluids.

Naloxone reverses the respiratory depressant effect of opioids.

This action verifies that the correct drug and dosage will be administered to the correct patient. Confirmation of information by a second nurse helps prevent errors. Scanning the barcode provides an additional check to ensure that the medication is given to the right patient.

Taping prevents accidental dislodgement. Labeling prevents inadvertent administration of other IV medications through this setup. Additional medication may potentiate the action of the opioid, increasing the risk for respiratory depression.

The transparent dressing protects the site while still allowing assessment. Securing of catheter and tubing prevents accidental displacement and removal. Proper removal of PPE reduces the risk for infection transmission and contamination of other items. Hand hygiene reduces transmission of microorganisms.

Patient-controlled analgesia (PCA) requires additional patient education and nursing intervention to provide safe nursing care and promote optimal patient outcomes. Refer to Skill 10-4.

FIGURE 2. Assessing exit site.

(*continued*)

Skill 10-5 ▶ Caring for a Patient Receiving Epidural Analgesia *(continued)*

ACTION	RATIONALE
14. Monitor the infusion rate according to facility policy. Assess and record the patient's vital signs, sedation level (see Table 10-1 in Skill 10-4), and respiratory status, including the patient's oxygen saturation, continuously for the first 20 minutes after initiation, then at least every hour for the first 12 hours, every 2 hours up to 24 hours, then at 4-hour intervals (or according to facility policy) (Sawhney, 2012). **Notify the health care provider if the sedation rating is 3 or 4, the respiratory depth decreases, or the respiratory rate falls below 10 breaths/min.** Refer to Skill 10-4. Monitor end-tidal carbon dioxide level (capnography) for patients at high risk of respiratory depression (Schreiber, 2015).	Monitoring the infusion rate prevents incorrect administration of the medication. Opioids can depress the respiratory center in the medulla. A change in the level of consciousness is usually the first sign of altered respiratory function.
15. Keep the head of bed elevated 30 degrees unless contraindicated.	Elevation of the patient's head minimizes upward migration of the opioid in the spinal cord, thus decreasing the risk for respiratory depression.
16. Assess the patient's level of pain and the effectiveness of pain relief.	This information helps in determining the need for subsequent **breakthrough pain** medication.
17. Monitor the patient's blood pressure and pulse.	Hypotension can result from the use of epidural analgesia.
18. Monitor urinary output and assess for bladder distention.	Opioids can cause urinary retention.
19. Assess motor strength and sensation every 4 hours or as specified by facility policy.	The catheter may migrate into the intrathecal space and allow opioids to block the transmission of nerve impulses completely through the spinal cord to the brain.
20. Monitor for adverse effects (pruritus, nausea, decreased gastric motility, headache, and vomiting) (Schreiber, 2015).	Opioids may spread into the trigeminal nerve, causing itching, or resulting in nausea and vomiting owing to slowed gastrointestinal function or stimulation of a chemoreceptor trigger zone in the brain. Medications are available to treat these adverse effects.
21. Assess for signs of infection at the insertion site.	Inflammation or local infection can develop at the catheter insertion site.
22. Assess the catheter-site dressing for drainage, based on facility policy. Notify the anesthesia provider or pain management team immediately of any abnormalities. Change the dressing over the catheter exit site per facility policy using aseptic technique. Change the infusion tubing as specified by facility policy.	Catheter-site dressing should remain clean, dry, and intact. Abnormalities in the dressing may indicate leakage of cerebrospinal fluid or catheter dislodgement. Dressing and tubing changes using aseptic technique reduce the risk for infection.

EVALUATION

The expected outcomes have been achieved when the patient verbalizes pain relief and/or increased comfort; the patient exhibits a dry, intact dressing, and a catheter exit site free of signs and symptoms of complications, injury, or infection; and the patient verbalizes an understanding of use of the therapy and the reason for its use.

DOCUMENTATION

Guidelines

Document catheter patency; the condition of the insertion site and dressing; sedation score, oxygen saturation, vital signs, and other assessment information; the infusion rate and solution; any tubing change; any other analgesics administered; and the patient's response to the therapy.

Sample Documentation

> 6/3/20 0935 Continuous morphine infusion via epidural catheter in place; see medication administration record. Exit site clean and slightly moist. Transparent dressing in place. Patient rates pain 2/10. Temperature 98.2°F; pulse, 76 beats/min; respirations 16 breaths/min and effortless; blood pressure, 110/70 mm Hg. Pulse oximetry 96% on oxygen via nasal cannula at 2 L/min. Patient alert and quickly responds to verbal stimuli. Sedation score of 1. Bladder nonpalpable; urine output of 100 mL over the last 2 hours. Denies nausea, vomiting, or itching. Able to detect sensation of cold in lower extremities bilaterally. Able to wiggle toes and flex and dorsiflex feet bilaterally. Lower-extremity muscle strength equal and moderately strong bilaterally.
>
> *—T. James, RN*

UNEXPECTED SITUATIONS AND ASSOCIATED INTERVENTIONS

- *While receiving epidural analgesia, the patient's sedation score drops below 3 (Pasero Opioid-Induced Sedation Scale [POSS]) and/or has a respiratory rate of <10 breaths, or has shallow respirations:* Immediately notify the anesthesiologist. Stop the epidural infusion, if indicated, according to facility procedure. Encourage the patient to take deep, slow breaths, if possible. Prepare to administer oxygen and an opioid antagonist, such as naloxone, via a peripheral IV site.
- *The patient demonstrates weakness and loss of sensation in the lower extremities while receiving epidural analgesia:* Reassess the patient's lower extremities for motor and sensory function. If positive for sensorimotor loss, notify the health care provider and expect to decrease or stop the epidural infusion and possible removal of the catheter.
- *While receiving epidural analgesia, the patient suddenly develops a severe headache. Inspection of the catheter site reveals clear drainage on the dressing:* Stop the epidural infusion and notify the health care provider immediately. The catheter may have migrated and entered the dura.

SPECIAL CONSIDERATIONS

- Epidural infusion administration sets have no injection ports to prevent accidental infusion of other drugs via the infusion (Morton & Fontaine, 2018).
- Clearly label the medication infusion bag, tubing, and pump apparatus "For Epidural Infusion Only" to prevent accidental infusion of other drugs with preservatives that could cause neural damage, resulting in paralysis or death (Morton & Fontaine, 2018, p. 144).
- Notify the anesthesiologist or pain management team immediately if the patient exhibits any of the following: respiratory rate below 10 breaths/min, continued complaints of unmanaged pain, leakage at the insertion site, fever, inability to void, paresthesia, itching, or headache or any other questionable assessment findings (Schreiber, 2015).
- Do not administer other sedatives or analgesics, unless ordered by the anesthesiologist or pain management team, to avoid oversedation.
- Always ensure that the patient receiving epidural analgesia has a peripheral IV line in place, either as a continuous IV infusion or as an intermittent infusion device, to allow immediate administration of emergency drugs, if warranted.
- Keep in mind that drugs given via the epidural route diffuse slowly and can cause adverse reactions, including excessive sedation, for up to 12 hours after the infusion has been discontinued.
- PCEA catheter removal generally occurs within 3 days after insertion (Schreiber, 2015). Typically, an anesthesiologist orders analgesics and removes the catheter. However, facility policy may allow a specially trained nurse to remove the catheter.
- Be aware that no resistance should be felt during the removal of an epidural catheter. Assess the catheter to confirm the catheter tip is intact. Assess the exit site for bleeding and infection (Schreiber, 2015).
- Once the epidural catheter has been removed, alternative pain management measures must be readily available (Graber, 2015).

Infant and Child Considerations

- When epidural analgesia is administered, additional opioid analgesics are not administered in order to prevent complications such as respiratory depression, pruritus, nausea, vomiting, and urinary retention (Kyle & Carman, 2017, p. 432).

Skill 10-6 ▶ Caring for a Patient Receiving Continuous Wound Perfusion Pain Management

Continuous wound perfusion or infiltration management systems are one strategy often recommended as a component of multimodal analgesia (Polomano et al., 2017). **Continuous wound perfusion pain management systems** deliver a continuous infusion of local analgesia to intra-articular and wound sites (Polomano et al., 2017). These systems are used as an adjuvant in the management of postoperative pain in a wide range of surgical procedures, such as cardiothoracic and orthopedic procedures. The system consists of a balloon-type pump filled with local anesthetic and a catheter placed near an incision, in a nerve close to a surgical site, or in a wound bed (Figure 1). The catheter is placed during surgery and is not sutured into place; the site dressing holds it in place. The catheter delivers a consistent flow rate and uniform distribution to the surgical site. Continuous wound perfusion catheters decrease postoperative pain and opioid use and side effects, and have been associated with decreased postoperative nausea and vomiting, as well as increased and earlier patient mobility (D'Arcy, 2012; Reid et al., 2014).

FIGURE 1. Wound perfusion pain management system consists of a balloon (pump), filter, and catheter that deliver a specific amount of prescribed local anesthetic at the rate determined by the prescribing health care provider. (Redrawn from I-Flow Corporation, a Kimberly-Clark Health Care Company, with permission.)

DELEGATION CONSIDERATIONS	Care related to continuous wound perfusion pain management systems is not delegated to nursing assistive personnel (NAP) or to unlicensed assistive personnel (UAP). Depending on the state's nurse practice act and the organization's policies and procedures, specific aspects of the care related to continuous wound perfusion pain management systems, such as monitoring the infusion and assessment of patient response, may be delegated to licensed practical/vocational nurses (LPN/LVNs). The decision to delegate must be based on careful analysis of the patient's needs and circumstances, as well as the qualifications of the person to whom the task is being delegated. Refer to the Delegation Guidelines in Appendix A.

EQUIPMENT	• Electronic medication administration record (eMAR) or medication administration record (MAR) • Pain assessment tool and pain scale • Gauze and tape, or other dressing, based on facility policy • Gloves • Additional PPE, as indicated

ASSESSMENT	Review the patient's health record and care plan for specific instructions related to continuous perfusion analgesia therapy, including the health care provider's order for the drug and conditions indicating the need for therapy. Review the patient's history for allergy to the prescribed medication. Assess the patient's understanding of a continuous wound perfusion pain management system and the rationale for its use. Assess the patient's level of discomfort and pain using an appropriate assessment tool. Assess the characteristics of any pain. Assess for other symptoms that often occur with the pain, such as headache or restlessness. Assess the surgical site (see Chapter 8). Assess the catheter-insertion–site dressing. Assess the patient's vital signs and respiratory status, including rate, depth, and rhythm, and oxygen saturation level using pulse oximetry. Assess the patient's response to the intervention to evaluate its effectiveness and for the presence of adverse effects.
NURSING DIAGNOSIS	Determine the related factors for the nursing diagnoses based on the patient's current status. Appropriate nursing diagnoses may include: • Acute pain • Deficient knowledge • Risk for infection
OUTCOME IDENTIFICATION AND PLANNING	The expected outcome to achieve is that the patient reports increased comfort and/or decreased pain, without adverse effects. Other appropriate outcomes may include the patient exhibits a dry, intact dressing with continuous wound perfusion system catheter in place; patient remains free from infection; and patient demonstrates an understanding of the functioning of the wound perfusion system and the reason for its use.

IMPLEMENTATION

ACTION	RATIONALE
1. Check the medication order against the original health care provider's order, according to facility policy. Clarify any inconsistencies. Check the patient's health record for allergies.	This comparison helps to identify errors that may have occurred when orders were transcribed. The health care provider's order/prescription is the legal record-of-medication order for each facility.
2. Know the actions, special nursing considerations, safe dose ranges, purpose of administration, and adverse effects of the medications to be administered. Consider the appropriateness of the medication for this patient.	This knowledge aids the nurse in evaluating the therapeutic effect of the medication in relation to the patient's disorder and can also be used to educate the patient about the medication.
3. Perform hand hygiene and put on PPE, if indicated.	Hand hygiene and PPE prevent the spread of microorganisms. PPE is required based on transmission precautions.
4. Identify the patient.	Identifying the patient ensures that the right patient receives the intervention and helps prevent errors.
5. Close the door to the room or pull the bedside curtain.	Closing the door or curtain provides for patient privacy.
6. Assess the patient's pain. Administer postoperative analgesic, as ordered.	Continuous wound perfusion pain management is an adjuvant therapy; patients may require postoperative pain medication, with reduced frequency.
7. Check the medication label attached to the pain management system balloon. Compare it with the health care provider's order and eMAR or MAR, per facility policy. Assess the patient for perioral numbness or tingling, numbness or tingling of fingers or toes, blurred vision, ringing in the ears, metallic taste in the mouth, confusion, seizures, drowsiness, nausea and/or vomiting. Assess the patient's vital signs.	Checking the medication label with the order and MAR ensures correct therapy for the patient. These symptoms may indicate local anesthetic toxicity (I-Flow Corporation, 2015). Changes in vital signs may indicate adverse effect.

(continued)

Skill 10-6 ▶ Caring for a Patient Receiving Continuous Wound Perfusion Pain Management *(continued)*

8. Put on gloves. Assess the wound perfusion system. Inspect tubing for kinks; check that the white tubing clamps are open. If tubing appears crimped, massage area on tubing to facilitate flow. Check filter in tubing, which should be unrestricted and free from tape.

Gloves prevent contact with blood and body fluids. Tubing must be unclamped and free of kinks and/or crimping to maintain consistent flow of analgesic. Tape over filter interferes with properly functioning system.

9. Check the flow restrictor to ensure it is in contact with the patient's skin. Tape in place, as necessary (see Figure 1).

Checking the flow restrictor for adequate contact ensures accurate flow rate.

10. Check the insertion-site dressing. Ensure that it is intact. Assess for leakage and dislodgement. Assess for redness, warmth, swelling, pain at site, and drainage.

Transparent dressing holds the catheter in place. Dressing must stay in place to prevent accidental dislodgement or removal. These symptoms may indicate infection.

11. Review the device with the patient. Review the function of the device and reason for its use. Reinforce the purpose and action of the medication to the patient.

Explanation encourages patient understanding and cooperation and reduces apprehension.

To Remove the Catheter

12. Check to ensure that infusion is complete. Infusion is complete when the delivery time has passed and the balloon is no longer inflated.

Depending on the size and volume of the balloon, the infusion typically lasts 2 to 5 days. Infusion time should be recorded in the operative note or postoperative instructions. The balloon will no longer appear full, the outside bag will be flat, and a hard tube can be felt in the middle of the balloon (I-Flow Corporation, 2011a).

 13. Perform hand hygiene. Identify the patient. Put on gloves. Remove the catheter-site dressing. Loosen adhesive skin closure strips at the catheter site.

Hand hygiene and use of gloves reduce the risk of infection transmission. Identifying the patient ensures that the right patient receives the intervention and helps prevent errors. Loosening of materials allows the catheter to be free of constraints.

14. Grasp the catheter close to the patient's skin at the insertion site. Gently pull catheter to remove. Catheter should be easy to remove and not painful. Do not tug or quickly pull on the catheter during removal. Check the distal end of the catheter for the black marking.

Gentle removal prevents patient discomfort and accidental breakage of the catheter. Checking for the black mark at the distal end ensures the entire catheter was removed (I-Flow Corporation, 2011b).

15. Cover puncture site with a dry dressing, according to facility policy.

Covering the wound prevents contamination.

16. Dispose of the balloon, tubing, and catheter, according to facility policy.

Proper disposal reduces the risk for infection transmission and contamination of other items.

 17. Remove gloves and additional PPE, if used. Perform hand hygiene.

Proper removal of PPE reduces the risk for infection transmission and contamination of other items. Hand hygiene prevents transmission of microorganisms.

EVALUATION

The expected outcomes have been achieved when the patient reported increased comfort and/or decreased pain, without adverse effects; the patient exhibited a dry, intact dressing with continuous wound perfusion system catheter in place; patient remained free from infection; and patient demonstrated an understanding of the functioning of the wound perfusion system and the reason for its use.

DOCUMENTATION

Guidelines

Document system patency, the condition of the insertion site and dressing, vital signs and assessment information, analgesics administered, and the patient's response to the therapy.

Sample Documentation

> <u>6/3/20</u> 0935 Continuous wound perfusion pain management system in place. Exit site clean and dry. Transparent dressing in place. Temperature 98.7°F; pulse, 82 beats/min; respirations, 14 breaths/min and effortless; blood pressure, 112/74 mm Hg. Pulse oximetry 96% on room air. Patient alert and quickly responds to verbal stimuli. Denies nausea, vomiting, vision changes, paresthesias, dizziness, or ringing in ears. Patient rates pain in RLE 3/10. Ibuprofen 800 mg po given as ordered.
>
> *—T. James, RN*
>
> <u>6/3/20</u> 1035 Patient reports pain in RLE 1/10. OOB to ambulate length of hall with wife.
>
> *—T. James, RN*

UNEXPECTED SITUATIONS AND ASSOCIATED INTERVENTIONS

- *Patient reports and/or your assessment identifies the following symptoms: increase in pain; redness, swelling, pain, and/or discharge at the catheter site; dizziness, lightheadedness; blurred vision; ringing, buzzing in ears; metallic taste in mouth; numbness and/or tingling around the mouth, fingers, or toes; drowsiness; and/or confusion:* Close the clamp on the system tubing to stop the infusion. Report the symptoms to the patient's health care provider immediately. The presence of any of these symptoms may indicate local anesthetic toxicity (I-Flow Corporation, 2015).
- *The catheter and tubing are accidentally pulled out:* Check the distal end of the catheter for the black marking to ensure the entire catheter was removed. Assess the insertion site. Cover the site with a dry, sterile dressing. Notify the patient's health care provider. Assess the patient's level of pain and administer analgesic, as ordered.
- *Resistance is encountered and/or the catheter stretches during its removal:* Stop. Do not continue to try to remove the catheter. Wait 30 to 60 minutes and attempt to remove the catheter again. The patient's body movements may relieve constriction on the catheter to allow easier removal. If catheter is still difficult to remove, contact the patient's health care provider. Do not forcefully remove the catheter. Do not continue to apply tension if the catheter begins to stretch (I-Flow Corporation, 2011b).

SPECIAL CONSIDERATIONS

- During the infusion, the pump will gradually lose its shape and flatten. Be aware that a change in the appearance and size of the pump may not be evident for more than 24 hours after surgery, owing to the slow flow rate of the device (I-Flow Corporation, n.d.a.).
- Do not expect to observe a fluid level line in the balloon and fluid moving through the system tubing.
- Over time, expect to see the outside bag on the balloon becoming looser, with creases beginning to form in the bag.
- Know that as the medication is delivered, the pump will gradually become smaller.
- Do not tape or cover the filter (I-Flow Corporation, n.d.a.).
- Ensure the tubing clamp remains open and avoid kinks in the pump tubing (I-Flow Corporation, n.d.a.).
- Do not forcefully remove the catheter.
- Do not reuse or refill balloon. System is intended for one-time use.
- Protect the balloon and catheter site from water.
- Clip the balloon to the patient's clothing to prevent the application of tension on the system and site.
- Avoid placing cold therapy in the area of the flow restrictor. Contact with cold therapy will decrease flow rate.

Home Care Considerations

- Instruct patients to immediately close the clamp on the pump tubing and call their health care provider or 911 if they experience any of the following symptoms to prevent injury (I-Flow Corporation, 2015): increased pain; fever, chills, sweats; bowel or bladder changes; difficulty breathing; redness, warmth, discharge or excessive bleeding from the catheter site; pain, swelling or large bruise around the catheter site; dizziness, lightheadedness, blurred vision, ringing in the ears; numbness and/or tingling around the mouth; drowsiness or confusion.
- Patients may experience numbness at and around the surgical site and should take care to avoid injury at the site (I-Flow Corporation, 2015).

Enhance Your Understanding

Focusing on Patient Care: Developing Clinical Reasoning

Consider the case scenarios at the beginning of the chapter as you answer the following questions to enhance your understanding and apply what you have learned.

QUESTIONS

1. Since her surgery, Mildred Simpson has been spending most of her time in bed. A special pillow is placed between her legs to keep her hips in abduction. The nurse offers to give Mrs. Simpson a back massage. What areas would be **most** important for the nurse to address when performing this skill?

2. The health care provider decides to admit Joseph Watkins to the hospital for evaluation of his back pain. Intermittent TENS therapy is ordered and is to be started in the emergency department. How would the nurse initiate this therapy?

3. Jerome Batiste and his wife are concerned about using the PCA device at home. What information would the nurse provide to help alleviate their concerns?

You can find suggested answers after the Bibliography at the end of this chapter.

Integrated Case Study Connection

The case studies in the back of the book focus on integrating concepts. Refer to the following case studies to enhance your understanding of the concepts and skills in this chapter.

- Basic Case Studies: Claudia Tran, page 1106; Kate Townsend, 1109.
- Advanced Case Studies: Cole McKean, page 1128; Robert Espinoza, 1132.

Taylor Suite Resources

Explore these additional resources to enhance learning for this chapter:

- NCLEX-Style Questions and other resources on thePoint*, http://thePoint.lww.com/Lynn5e
- *Skill Checklists for Taylor's Clinical Nursing Skills*, 5e
- *Fundamentals of Nursing*: Chapter 35, Comfort and Pain Management

Bibliography

Abbaspoor, Z., Akbari, M., & Najar, S. (2014). Effect of foot and hand massage in post-cesarean section pain control: A randomized control trial. *Pain Management Nursing, 15*(1), 132–136.

American Holistic Nurses Association. (2016). Holistic stress management. *Guided imagery.* Retrieved http://www.ahna.org/Home/Resources/Stress-Management

American Massage Therapy Association. (2011). *Massage and the aging body.* Retrieved https://www.amtamassage.org/articles/3/MTJ/detail/2315

Booker, S. Q., & Haedtke, C. (2016). Assessing pain in verbal older adults. *Nursing, 46*(2), 65–68.

Casey, G. (2015). Capnography: Monitoring CO_2. *Nursing New Zealand (Wellington, N.Z.: 1995), 21*(9), 20–24.

Chou, R., Gordon, D. B., de Leon-Casasola, O. A., et al. (2016). Management of postoperative pain: A clinical practice guideline from the American Pain Society, the American Society of Regional Anesthesia and Pain Medicine, and the American Society of Anesthesiologists' Committee on Regional Anesthesia, Executive Committee, and Administrative Council. *The Journal of Pain, 17*(2), 131–157.

Chung, D., Lee, Y. J., Jo, M. H., et al. (2013). The ON-Q* pain management system in elective gynecology oncologic surgery: Management of postoperative surgical site pain compared to intravenous patient-controlled analgesia. *Obstetrics & Gynecology Science, 56*(2), 93–101.

Cleveland Clinic. (2015). *Transcutaneous electrical nerve stimulation (TENS).* Retrieved https://my.clevelandclinic.org/health/articles/tens

Cooney, M. F., Czarnecki, M., Dunwoody, C., et al. (2013). American Society for Pain Management nursing position statement with clinical practice guidelines: Authorized agent controlled analgesia. *Pain Management Nursing, 14*(3), 176–181.

D'Arcy, Y. (2008). Keep your patient safe during PCA. *Nursing, 38*(1), 50–55.

D'Arcy, Y. (2012). Treating acute pain in the hospitalized patient. *The Nurse Practitioner, 37*(8), 22–30.

D'Arcy, Y. (2013a). PCA by proxy: Taking the patient out of patient-controlled analgesia: This controversial practice can be done safely in carefully controlled circumstances. *Dimensions of Critical Care Nursing, 32*(4), 200–203.

D'Arcy, Y. (2013b). Turning the tide on respiratory depression. *Nursing, 43*(9), 38–45.

DiGiusto, M., Bhalla, T., Martin, D., Foerschler, D., Jones, M. J., & Tobias, J. (2014). Patient-controlled analgesia in the pediatric population: Morphine versus hydromorphone. *Journal of Pain Research, 7*, 471–475.

Dobbins, E. H. (2015). Sidestep the perils of PCA in post-op patients. *Nursing, 45*(4), 64–69.

Doenges, M. E., Moorhouse, M. F., & Murr, A. C. (Eds.). (2016). *Nursing diagnoses manual. Planning, individualizing, and documenting client care* (5th ed.). Philadelphia, PA: F.A. Davis Company.

Dossey, B. M., & Keegan, L. (2016). *Holistic nursing. A handbook for practice* (7th ed.). Burlington, MA: Jones & Bartlett Learning.

Eliopoulos, C. (2018). *Gerontological nursing* (9th ed.). Philadelphia, PA: Wolters Kluwer Health.

Epstein, H. M. (2017). Postoperative patient-controlled analgesia in the pediatric cardiac intensive care unit. *Critical Care Nurse, 37*(1), 55–61.

Erden, S., & Senol Celik, S. (2015). The effect of transcutaneous electrical nerve stimulation on post-thoracotomy pain. *Contemporary Nurse, 51*(2–3), 163–170.

Falzone, E., Hoffmann, C., & Keita, H. (2013). Postoperative analgesia in elderly patients. *Drugs & Aging, 30*(2), 81–90.

Golembiewski, J., Dasta, J., & Palmer, P. P. (2016). Evolution of patient-controlled analgesia: From intravenous to sublingual treatment. *Hospital Pharmacy, 51*(3), 214–229.

Graber, R. (2015). Regional anesthesia for postoperative pin control. *Medscape.* Retrieved http://emedicine.medscape.com/article/1268467-overview#showall

Grossman, S., & Porth, C. M. (2014). *Porth's pathophysiology: Concepts of altered health states* (9th ed.). Philadelphia, PA: Wolters Kluwer.

Hausladen Foley, M. K., Anderson, J., Mallea, L., Morrison, K., & Downey, M. (2016). Effects of Healing Touch on postsurgical adult outpatients. *Journal of Holistic Nursing, 34*(3), 271–279.

Herr, K., Coyne, P. J., McCaffery, M., Manworren, R., & Merkel, S; American Society for Pain Management Nursing. (2011). . Pain assessment in the patient unable to self-report: Position statement with clinical practice recommendations. *Pain Management Nursing, 12*(4), 230–250. Retrieved http://www.aspmn.org/Documents/PainAssessmentinthePatientUnabletoSelfReport.pdf#search = pain%20assessment%20in%20patients%20unable%20to%20self%20report

Hinkle, J. L., & Cheever, K. H. (2018). *Brunner & Suddarth's textbook of medical-surgical nursing* (14th ed.). Philadelphia, PA: Wolters Kluwer.

Hogan-Quigley, B., Palm, M. L., & Bickley, L. (2016). *Bates' nursing guide to physical examination and history taking* (2nd ed.). Philadelphia, PA: Wolters Kluwer.

Horgas, A. L. (2012). *Try this: Best practices in nursing care to older adults with dementia. Assessing pain in older adults with dementia.* Retrieved https://consultgeri.org/try-this/dementia/issue-d2.pdf

Horgas, A. L., Yoon, S. L., & Grall, M. (2012). *Pain. Nursing standard of practice protocol: Pain management in older adults.* Retrieved https://consultgeri.org/geriatric-topics/pain

I-Flow Corporation. (n.d.a.). *ON-Q* pain relief system. How it works. [Video].* Retrieved http://www.myon-q.com

I-Flow Corporation. (n.d.b.). *ON-Q* pain relief system. Why ON-Q* for post-op pain relief?* Retrieved http://www.myon-q.com/why-on-q.aspx

I-Flow Corporation. (2011a). *ON-Q* pain relief system. Patient guidelines.* Retrieved http://www.myon-q.com/media/60662/14-65-027-0-00_flap.pdf

I-Flow Corporation. (2011b). *ON-Q* catheter. Patient guideline insert.* Retrieved http://www.myon-q.com/media/56272/14-60-621-0-03.pdf

I-Flow Corporation. (2015). *ON-Q* pain relief system*. Retrieved http://www.myon-q.com/media/56275/patient-brochure-general-information.pdf

Institute for Safe Medication Practices (ISMP). (2013). *Acute Care ISMP Medication Safety Alert!* Fatal PCA adverse events continue to happen…Better patient monitoring is essential to prevent harm.* Retrieved https://www.ismp.org/newsletters/acutecare/showarticle.aspx?id=50

Institute for Safe Medication Practices (ISMP). (2016). *Acute Care ISMP Medication Safety Alert!* Worth repeating… Recent PCA by proxy event suggests reassessment of practices that may have fallen by the wayside.* Retrieved https://www.ismp.org/Newsletters/acutecare/showarticle.aspx?id=1149

Institute for Safe Medication Practices (ISMP). (2003; updated 2017). *Acute Care ISMP Medication Safety Alert!* Part II: How to prevent errors. Safety issues with patient-controlled analgesia.* Retrieved http://www.ismp.org/newsletters/acutecare/articles/20030724.asp

Institute for Safe Medication Practices (ISMP). (2017). *Targeted medication safety best practices for hospitals.* Retrieved https://www.ismp.org/tools/bestpractices

Institute of Medicine (IOM). (2011). *Relieving pain in America: A blueprint for transforming prevention, care, education, and research.* Washington, DC: The National Academies Press.

International Association for the Study of Pain (IASP). (2014). *Classification of chronic pain* (2nd ed.). Part III: Pain terms. Retrieved from http://www.iasp-pain.org/files/Content/ContentFolders/Publications2/ClassificationofChronicPain/Part_III-PainTerms.pdf

Jarvis, C. (2016). *Physical examination & health assessment* (7th ed.). St. Louis, MO: Elsevier.

Jarzyna, D., Jungquist, C. R., Pasero, C., et al. (2011). American Society for Pain Management nursing guidelines on monitoring for opioid-induced sedation and respiratory depression. *Pain Management Nursing, 12*(3), 118–145.

Jensen, S. (2015). *Nursing health assessment: A best practice approach* (2nd ed.). Philadelphia, PA: Wolters Kluwer.

The Joint Commission. (2012). *Sentinel Event Alert Issue 49: Safe use of opioids in hospitals.* Retrieved http://www.jointcommission.org/sea_issue_49

The Joint Commission. (2013a). *Pain management.* Retrieved https://www.jointcommission.org/topics/pain_management.aspx

The Joint Commission. (2013b). *Speak up: About your pain. [Online video].* Retrieved https://www.jointcommission.org/topics/speak_up_pain.aspx

Jungquist, C. R., Smith, K., Nicely, K. L., & Polomano, R. C. (2017). Monitoring hospitalized adult patients for opioid-induced sedation and respiratory depression. *The American Journal of Nursing, 117*(3 Suppl 1), S27–S35.

Jungquist, C. R., Vallerand, A. H., Sicoutris, C., Kwon, K. N., & Polomano, R. C. (2017). Assessing and managing acute pain: A call to action. *The American Journal of Nursing, 117*(3 Suppl 1), S4–S11.

Katz, P., Takyar, S., Palmer, P., & Liedgens, H. (2017). Sublingual, transdermal and intravenous patient-controlled analgesia for acute post-operative pain: Systematic literature review and mixed treatment comparison. *Current Medical Research and Opinion, 33*(5), 899–910.

Kyle, T., & Carman, S. (2017). *Essentials of pediatric nursing* (3rd ed.). Philadelphia, PA: Wolters Kluwer Health.

LeMone, P., Burke, K. M., Bauldoff, G., & Gubrud, P. (2015). *Medical-surgical nursing. Clinical reasoning in patient care* (6th ed.). New York: Pearson.

Lindley, P., Ding, L., Danesi, H., & Jones, J. B. (2017). Meta-analysis of the ease of care from a patient's perspective comparing fentanyl iontophoretic transdermal system versus morphine intravenous patient-controlled analgesia in postoperative pain management. *Journal of PeriAnesthesia Nursing 32*(4), 320–328.

Lisi, D. M. (2013). Patient-controlled analgesia and the older patient. *US Pharmacist, 38*(3), HS2–HS6. Retrieved https://www.uspharmacist.com/article/patient-controlled-analgesia-and-the-older-patient

Makris, U. E., Abrams, R. C., Gurland, B., Reid, M. C. (2014). Management of persistent pain in the older patient: A clinical review. *Journal of the American Medical Association, 312*(8), 825–836.

McCaffery, M. (1968). *Nursing practice theories related to cognition, bodily pain, and man-environment interactions.* Los Angeles, CA: UCLA Students' Store.

Merkel, S., Voepel-Lewis, T., & Malviya, S. (2002). Pain assessment in infants and young children: The FLACC Scale: A behavioral tool to measure pain in young children. *The American Journal of Nursing, 102*(10), 55–58.

Morton, P. G., & Fontaine, D. K. (2018). *Critical care nursing. A holistic approach* (11th ed.). Philadelphia, PA: Wolters Kluwer.

NANDA International, Inc. (2017). *Nursing diagnoses: Definitions & classification 2018–2020* © 2017 NANDA International, ISBN 978-1-62623-929-6. Used by arrangement with the Thieme Group, Stuttgart/New York.

National Health Service (NHS) (UK). NHS Choices. (2015). *TENS (transcutaneous electrical nerve stimulation).* Retrieved from http://www.nhs.uk/conditions/tens/Pages/Introduction.aspx

Pasero, C., & McCaffery, M. (2011). *Pain assessment and pharmacologic management.* St. Louis, MO: Elsevier.

Perry, S. E., Hockenberry, M. J., Lowdermilk, D. L., & Wilson, D. (2014). *Maternal child nursing care* (5th ed.). St. Louis, MO: Elsevier Mosby.

Polomano, R. C., Fillman, M., Giordano, N. A., Vallerand, A. H., Nicely, K. L., & Jungquist, C. R. (2017). Multimodal analgesia for acute postoperative and trauma-related pain. *The American Journal of Nursing, 117*(3 Suppl 1), S12–S26.

Prichard, C., & Newcomb, P. (2015). Benefit to family members of delivering hand massage with essential oils to critically ill patients. *American Journal of Critical Care, 24*(5), 446–449.

Ried, M., Schilling, C., Potzger, T., et al. (2014). Prospective, comparative study of the On-Q* PainBuster* postoperative pain relief system and thoracic epidural analgesia after thoracic surgery. *Journal of Cardiothoracic and Vascular Anesthesia, 28*(4), 973–978.

Sawhney, M. (2012). Epidural analgesia: What nurses need to know. *Nursing, 42*(8), 36–42.

Schreiber, M. L. (2015). Nursing care considerations: The epidural catheter. *MEDSURG Nursing, 24*(4), 273–276.

Shastay, A. (2017). Transdermal iontophoretic fentaNYL PCA. *Home Healthcare Now, 35*(3), 174–175.

Taylor, C., Lynn, P., & Bartlett, J. (2019). *Fundamentals of nursing: The art and science of person-centered care* (9th ed.). Philadelphia, PA: Wolters Kluwer.

Thomas, T., & Barclay, S. (2015). Continuous subcutaneous infusion in palliative care: A review of current practice. *International Journal of Palliative Nursing, 21*(2), 60, 62–64.

VHA Center for Engineering & Occupational Safety and Health (CEOSH). (2016). *Safe patient handling and mobility guidebook.* St. Louis, MO: Author. Retrieved http://www.tampavaref.org/safe-patient-handling.htm

Ward, C. W. (2015). A decision tree model for postoperative pain management. *MEDSURG Nursing, 24*(2), 77–88.

Ward, C. W. (2016). Non-pharmacologic methods of postoperative pain management. *MEDSURG Nursing, 25*(1), 9–10.

Weaver, M. (2017). Healing Touch: Positively sharing energy in a pediatric hospital. *Journal of Pain and Symptom Management, 54*(2), 259–261.

Westman, K. F., & Blaisdell, C. (2016). Many benefits, little risk: The use of massage in nursing practice. *The American Journal of Nursing, 116*(1), 34–39.

Wuhrman, E., Cooney, M. F., Dunwoody, C. J., Eksterowicz, N., Merkel, S., & Oakes, L. L.; American Society for Pain Management Nursing. (2007). Authorized and unauthorized ("PCA by proxy") dosing of analgesic infusion pumps: Position statement with clinical practice recommendations. *Pain Management Nursing, 8*(1), 4–11.

Xin, Y., Hong, Y., & Yong, L. Z. (2014). Efficacy of postoperative continuous wound infiltration with local anesthesia after open hepatectomy. *The Clinical Journal of Pain, 30*(7), 571–576.

SUGGESTED ANSWERS FOR FOCUSING ON PATIENT CARE: DEVELOPING CLINICAL REASONING

1. Review the patient's health record and care plan for information about the patient's status and contraindications to back massage, and review the health care provider's orders for the patient's activity level. Because of her surgery, it will probably be difficult for Mrs. Simpson to lie in a prone position; assess her ability to turn to her side for the massage. It will be necessary to maintain the position of the abductor pillow, to prevent adduction of her hip. Assess the patient's level of pain. Check the patient's medication administration record for the time an analgesic was last administered. If appropriate, administer an analgesic sufficiently early so it has time to take effect before beginning the massage. Assess for the need to obtain assistance of another caregiver to assist the patient to her side and maintain that position for the massage. Include an assessment of the patient's skin integrity, because of the increased risk for impaired skin integrity.

2. Review the patient's health record and care plan for specific instructions related to TENS therapy, including the order and conditions indicating the need for therapy, and prescribed settings. Review the patient's history for conditions that might contraindicate therapy, such as pacemaker insertion, cardiac monitoring, or electrocardiography. Determine the location of electrode placement in consultation with the ordering health care provider and based on the patient's report of pain. Assess the patient's understanding of TENS therapy and the rationale for its use. Explain the rationale for the use of TENS therapy and patient instructions.

   Before initiating therapy, inspect the skin of the area designated for electrode placement for irritation, redness, or breakdown. Assess the patient's pain and level of discomfort using an appropriate assessment tool. Check the unit to ensure proper functioning and review the manufacturer's instructions for use.

3. Provide teaching for Mr. Batiste and his wife concerning the rationale for the use of a PCA and how a PCA works. Show the patient and his wife the equipment as part of the explanation and provide a written copy of the information. Include information regarding safety mechanisms built into the device, as well as guidelines for adverse effects. Instruct the patient and his wife regarding symptoms that should be reported to the health care provider. They should be aware that a home care nurse will be consulted to continue support at home. The patient and/or his wife should be able to verbalize an understanding of information.

Nutrition

Focusing on Patient Care

This chapter will help you develop some of the skills related to nutrition needed to care for the following patients:

Paula Williams, age 78, who is recovering from a cerebrovascular accident (CVA), or stroke. The nurse needs to help her with breakfast.

Jack Mason, a 62-year-old man, has severe dysphagia related to progressive muscle weakness. He is NPO and receiving enteral nutrition through a nasogastric tube. He and his wife are considering the placement of a gastrostomy tube for long-term nutrition.

Cole Brenau, age 12, has cystic fibrosis and needs to increase his caloric intake through gastrostomy tube feedings at nighttime.

Refer to Focusing on Patient Care: Developing Clinical Reasoning at the end of the chapter to apply what you learn.

Learning Objectives

After completing the chapter, you will be able to accomplish the following:

1. Assist a patient with eating.
2. Confirm placement of a nasogastric feeding tube.
3. Administer a tube feeding.
4. Care for a gastrostomy tube.

Key Terms

aspiration: the misdirection of oropharyngeal secretions or gastric contents into the larynx and lower respiratory tract

calorie: measure of heat or energy; kilocalorie, commonly referred to as a calorie, is defined as the amount of heat required to raise 1 kg of water by 1°C

carbohydrate: organic compounds (commonly known as sugars and starches) that are composed of carbon, hydrogen, and oxygen; the most abundant and least expensive source of calories in the diet worldwide

dysphagia: difficulty swallowing or the inability to swallow

enteral nutrition: alternate form of feeding that involves passing a tube into the gastrointestinal (GI) tract to allow instillation of the appropriate formula

gastrostomy tube: a tube placed surgically (open or laparoscopically) into the stomach

jejunostomy tube: a tube placed surgically (open or laparoscopically) into the stomach

nasogastric (NG) tube: a tube inserted through the nose and into the stomach

nasointestinal (NI) tube: a tube inserted through the nose and into the upper portion of the small intestine

NPO (nothing by mouth): nothing can be consumed by mouth, including medications, unless ordered otherwise

nutrient: specific biochemical substance used by the body for growth, development, activity, reproduction, lactation, health maintenance, and recovery from illness or injury

nutrition: study of the nutrients and how they are handled by the body, as well as the impact of human behavior and environment on the process of nourishment

percutaneous endoscopic gastrostomy (PEG) tube: a gastrostomy tube placed percutaneously via endoscopy

percutaneous endoscopic jejunostomy (PEJ) tube: a jejunostomy tube placed percutaneously via endoscopy

residual: as applied to tube feeding, the amount of gastric contents in the stomach after the administration of a tube feeding

Good nutrition is vital for life and health. Important **nutrients**, found in food, are needed for the body to function. A varied diet is necessary to provide all of the essential nutrients that a person needs. Poor nutrition can seriously decrease a person's level of wellness. An adequate diet provides a balanced intake of all essential nutrients in appropriate amounts. Details related to appropriate dietary intake can be found in the *Dietary Guidelines for Americans 2015–2016* at http://health.gov/dietaryguidelines/2015/guidelines. Refer to information on thePoint, a fundamentals of nursing text, or a nutrition text for details related to sources, functions, and significance of carbohydrates, protein, and fat. Nurses incorporate nutrition into all aspects of person-centered nursing care and are involved in all aspects of nutritional care.

Because of the significant influence that adequate nutrition plays in restoring and maintaining health and disease prevention, the nurse integrates nutritional assessment into the care of the patient (Fundamentals Review 11-1). Ongoing data collection through various methods, such as history taking, the physical examination, and laboratory data analysis (Fundamentals Review 11-2), can provide pertinent information for directing the nursing care plan. Factors that may affect nutritional status are discussed in Fundamentals Review 11-3.

This chapter addresses skills necessary to care for patients with nutritional needs, including assisting a patient with eating, confirming the placement of a feeding tube, administering a tube feeding, and caring for a gastrostomy feeding tube.

Nasogastric tubes are also used to decompress or to drain unwanted fluid and air from the stomach, monitor bleeding in the GI tract, to remove undesirable substances (lavage), or to help treat an intestinal obstruction. Insertion and removal of nasogastric tubes for feeding and any of these other purposes is accomplished using essentially the same procedure and is discussed in Chapter 13.

Fundamentals Review 11-1

CLINICAL OBSERVATIONS FOR NUTRITIONAL ASSESSMENT

Body Area	Signs of Good Nutritional Status	Signs of Poor Nutritional Status
General appearance	Alert, responsive	Listless, apathetic, and cachexic
General vitality	Endurance, energetic, sleeps well, vigorous	Easily fatigued, no energy, falls asleep easily, looks tired, apathetic
Weight	Normal for height, age, body build	Overweight or underweight
Hair	Shiny, lustrous, firm, not easily plucked, healthy scalp	Dull and dry, brittle, loss of color, easily plucked, thin and sparse

(continued)

Fundamentals Review 11-1 continued

CLINICAL OBSERVATIONS FOR NUTRITIONAL ASSESSMENT

Body Area	Signs of Good Nutritional Status	Signs of Poor Nutritional Status
Face	Uniform skin color; healthy appearance, not swollen	Dark skin over cheeks and under eyes, flaky skin, facial edema (moon face), pale skin color
Eyes	Bright, clear, moist; no sores at corners of eyelids; membranes moist and healthy pink color; no prominent blood vessels	Pale eye membranes, dry eyes (xerophthalmia), increased vascularity, dull or scarred cornea
Lips	Good pink color, smooth, moist, not chapped or swollen	Swollen and puffy (cheilosis); angular lesion at corners of mouth or fissures or scars (stomatitis)
Tongue	Deep red, surface papillae present	Smooth appearance, beefy red or magenta colored, swollen, hypertrophy or atrophy
Teeth	Straight, no crowding, no cavities, no pain, bright, no discoloration, well-shaped jaw	Cavities, mottled appearance, malpositioned, missing teeth
Gums	Firm, good pink color, no swelling or bleeding	Spongy, bleed easily, marginal redness, recessed, swollen, and inflamed
Glands	No enlargement of the thyroid, face not swollen	Enlargement of the thyroid (goiter), enlargement of the parotid (swollen cheeks)
Skin	Smooth, good color, slightly moist; no signs of rashes, swelling, or color irregularities	Rough, dry, flaky, swollen, pale, pigmented, lack of fat under the skin, fat deposits around the joints, bruises, petechiae
Nails	Firm, pink	Spoon shaped (koilonychia), brittle, pale, ridged
Skeleton	Good posture, no malformations	Poor posture, beading of the ribs, bowed legs or knock-knees, prominent scapulas, chest deformity at diaphragm
Muscles	Well developed, firm, good tone, some fat under the skin	Flaccid, poor tone, wasted, underdeveloped, difficulty walking
Extremities	No tenderness	Weak and tender, presence of edema
Abdomen	Flat	Swollen
Nervous system	Normal reflexes, psychological stability	Decrease in or loss of ankle and knee reflexes, psychomotor changes, mental confusion, depression, sensory loss, motor weakness, loss of sense of position, loss of vibration, burning and tingling of the hands and feet (paresthesia)
Cardiovascular system	Normal heart rate and rhythm, no murmurs, normal blood pressure for age	Cardiac enlargement, tachycardia, elevated blood pressure
GI system	No palpable organs or masses (liver edge may be palpable in children)	Hepatosplenomegaly, enlarged liver or spleen

Source: Adapted from Dudek, S. G. (2018). *Nutrition essentials for nursing practice* (8th ed.). Philadelphia, PA: Wolters Kluwer; Jarvis, C. (2016). *Physical examination & health assessment* (7th ed.). St. Louis, MO: Elsevier.

Fundamentals Review 11-2

BIOCHEMICAL DATA WITH NUTRITIONAL IMPLICATIONS

- Hemoglobin (normal = 12 to 18 g/dL) decreased → anemia
- Hematocrit (normal = 40% to 50%) decreased → anemia increased → dehydration
- Serum albumin (normal = 3.3 to 5 g/dL) decreased → high risk for morbidity, mortality, and malnutrition (prolonged protein depletion), malabsorption
- Transferrin (normal = 240 to 480 mg/dL) decreased → anemia, protein deficiency

- Total lymphocyte count (normal = greater than 1,800) decreased → impaired nutritional intake, severe debilitating disease
- Blood urea nitrogen (normal = 17 to 18 mg/dL) increased → starvation, high protein intake, severe dehydration decreased → malnutrition, overhydration
- Creatinine (normal = 0.4 to 1.5 mg/dL) increased → dehydration decreased → reduction in total muscle mass, severe malnutrition

Source: From Dudek, S. (2018). *Nutrition essentials for nursing practice* (8th ed.). Philadelphia, PA: Wolters Kluwer; Fischbach, F., & Dunning, M. B. (2015). *A manual of laboratory and diagnostic tests* (9th ed.). Philadelphia, PA: Wolters Kluwer Health.

Fundamentals Review 11-3

FACTORS THAT MAY AFFECT NUTRITIONAL STATUS

- Socioeconomic status
- Psychosocial factors (meaning of food)
- Medical conditions that involve malabsorption, such as Crohn's disease or cystic fibrosis
- Age
- Medical conditions that may affect desire to eat, such as chemotherapy treatment or pregnancy accompanied by morning sickness
- Conditions that involve physical limitations, weakness, and/or fatigue
- Dysphagia

- Culture
- Medications
- Alcohol abuse
- Religion
- Megadoses of nutrient substances
- Alterations in mental status
- Illiteracy
- Language barriers
- Lack of caregiver or social support
- Knowledge of nutrition

Skill 11-1 ▶ Assisting a Patient With Eating

A variety of oral diets are available in health care settings and may be prescribed for use at home. A diet is prescribed based on the individual person's condition. Table 11-1 outlines several commonly prescribed modified consistency diets and therapeutic diets. Many patients can independently meet their nutritional needs by feeding themselves. Other patients, especially the very young and some older adult patients, such as people with arthritis of the hands, may have difficulty opening juice containers, for example. Patients with paralysis of the upper extremities or advanced dementia may be unable to feed themselves. The nurse should assist these patients, as needed.

The skill of assisting a patient with eating is frequently delegated to nursing assistants. However, the nurse is responsible for the initial and ongoing assessment of the patient for potential complications related to feeding. Before this skill can be delegated, it is paramount for the nurse to make sure that the nursing assistant has been educated to observe for any swallowing difficulties and has

(*continued*)

Skill 11-1 ▷ Assisting a Patient With Eating *(continued)*

Table 11-1 Modified Consistency and Selected Therapeutic Diets

DIET AND DESCRIPTION	INDICATIONS
Modified Consistency Diets	
Clear Liquid Diet: Composed only of clear fluids or foods that become fluid at body temperature. Requires minimal digestion and leaves minimal residue. Includes clear broth, coffee, tea, clear fruit juices (apple, cranberry, grape), gelatin, popsicles, commercially prepared clear liquid supplements.	Preparation for bowel surgery and lower endoscopy; acute gastrointestinal disorders; initial postoperative diet
Pureed Diet: Also known as a blenderized liquid diet because the diet is made up of liquids and foods blenderized to liquid form. All foods are allowed.	After oral or facial surgery; chewing and swallowing difficulties
Mechanically Altered Diet: Regular diet with modifications for texture. Excludes most raw fruits and vegetables and foods with seeds, nuts, and dried fruits. Foods are chopped, ground, mashed or soft.	Chewing and swallowing difficulties; after surgery to the head, neck, or mouth
Selected Therapeutic Diets	
Consistent-Carbohydrate **Diet:** Total daily carbohydrate content is consistent; emphasizes general nutritional balance. **Calories** based on attaining and maintaining healthy weight. High-fiber and heart-healthy fats encouraged; sodium and saturated fats are limited.	Type I and type 2 diabetes, gestational diabetes, impaired glucose tolerance
Fat-Restricted Diet: Low-fat diets are intended to lower the patient's total intake of fat.	Chronic cholecystitis (inflammation of the gallbladder) to decrease gallbladder stimulation; cardiovascular disease, to help prevent atherosclerosis
High fiber: Emphasis on increased intake of foods high in fiber.	Prevent or treat constipation; irritable bowel syndrome; diverticulosis
Low fiber: Fiber limited to <10 g/day.	Before surgery; ulcerative colitis; diverticulitis; Crohn's disease
Sodium restricted: Sodium limit may be set at 500–3,000 mg/day.	Hypertension; heart failure; acute and chronic renal disease, liver disease
Renal diet: Reduce workload on kidneys to delay or prevent further damage; control accumulation of uremic toxins. Protein restriction 0.6–1 g/kg/day; sodium restriction 1,000–3,000 mg/day; potassium and fluid restrictions dependent on patient situation	Nephrotic syndrome; chronic kidney disease; diabetic kidney disease

knowledge of **aspiration** precautions. Box 11-1 outlines special considerations and interventions for feeding patients with dementia or other alterations in cognition. Box 11-2 discusses special considerations and interventions for feeding patients with **dysphagia.**

DELEGATION CONSIDERATIONS	Assisting patients to eat may be delegated to nursing assistive personnel (NAP) or to unlicensed assistive personnel (UAP), as well as to licensed practical/vocational nurses (LPN/LVNs). See previous discussion. The decision to delegate must be based on careful analysis of the patient's needs and circumstances, as well as the qualifications of the person to whom the task is being delegated. Refer to the Delegation Guidelines in Appendix A.
EQUIPMENT	• Prepared food, based on prescribed diet • Wet wipes for hand hygiene, or access to hand gel/skin cleanser and water • Mouth care materials • Patient's dentures, eyeglasses, hearing aid, if needed • Special adaptive utensils, as needed • Napkins, protective covering, or towel • PPE, as indicated

Box 11-1 Special Considerations and Interventions for Feeding Patients With Dementia or Other Alterations in Cognition

- Change the environment in which meals occur.
- Assess the area where meals are served. Create a home-like environment by preparing food close to the place where it will be served to stimulate senses.
- Observe as many former rituals as possible, such as handwashing and saying a blessing.
- Avoid clutter and distractions.
- Maintain a pleasant, well-lighted room. Play calming music.
- Keep food as close to its original form as possible.
- Serve meals in the same place at the same time.
- Closely supervise mealtime.
- Check food temperatures to prevent accidental mouth burns.
- Assist as needed. Be alert for cues from the patient. Turning away may signal that the patient has had enough to eat or that the patient needs to slow down. Leaning forward with an open mouth usually means the patient is ready for more food.
- Stroking the underside of the chin may help promote swallowing.
- Provide one food item at a time. Offer small, frequent eating opportunities. A whole tray of food may be overwhelming.
- Ensure that the patient's glasses and hearing aid are working properly.
- Demonstrate what you want the patient to do. State the goal clearly, and then mimic the action with exaggerated motions.
- Provide foods and between-meal snacks that are easy to consume using the hands.
- Use adaptive feeding equipment, as needed, such as weighted utensils, large-handled cups, and larger or smaller silverware than standard.
- Promote family involvement to encourage eating.

Source: Adapted from Alzheimer's Association. Alzheimer's and Dementia Caregiver Center. (n.d.). *Food, eating and Alzheimer's.* Retrieved https://www.alz.org/care/alzheimers-food-eating.asp; Amella, E. J., & Batchelor-Aselage, M. B. (2014). Facilitating ADLs by caregivers of persons with dementia: The C3P model. *Occupational Therapy in Health Care, 28*(1), 51–61; Dudek, S. (2018). *Nutrition essentials for nursing practice* (8th ed.). Philadelphia, PA: Wolters Kluwer; and McGinley, E. (2015). Practical nutritional measures in patients with dementia. *Journal of Community Nursing, 29*(6), 36–40.

Box 11-2 Special Considerations and Interventions for Feeding Patients With Dysphagia

- Provide at least a 30-minute rest period prior to mealtime. A rested person will likely have less difficulty swallowing.
- Sit the patient upright, preferably in a chair. If bed rest is mandatory, elevate the head of the bed to a 90-degree angle.
- Provide mouth care immediately before meals to enhance the sense of taste.
- Avoid rushed or forced feeding. Adjust the rate of feeding and size of bites to the patient's tolerance. Allow patient to control the eating process if possible.
- Collaborate to obtain a speech therapy consult for swallowing evaluation.
- Initiate a nutrition consult for appropriate diet modification such as chopping, mincing, or pureeing of foods and liquid consistency (thin, nectar-thick, honey-like, spoon-thick).
- Keep in mind that some patients may find thickened liquids unpalatable and thus drink insufficient fluids.
- Reduce or eliminate distractions at mealtime so that the patient can focus attention on swallowing.
- Alternate solids and liquids.
- Assess for signs of aspiration during eating: sudden appearance of severe coughing; choking; cyanosis; voice change, hoarseness, and/or gurgling after swallowing; frequent throat clearing after meals; or regurgitation through the nose or mouth.
- Inspect oral cavity for retained food.
- Avoid or minimize the use of sedatives and hypnotics since these agents may impair the cough reflex and swallowing.

Source: Adapted from Dark, J., & Sander, R. (2014). Dysphagia: Helping vulnerable people to eat and drink. *Nursing & Residential Care, 16*(8), 438–441; Dudek, S. (2018). *Nutrition essentials for nursing practice* (8th ed.). Philadelphia, PA: Wolters Kluwer; and Metheny, N. (n.d.). *Preventing aspiration in older adults with dysphagia.* Retrieved https://consultgeri.org/try-this/general-assessment/issue-20

ASSESSMENT

Before assisting the patient, confirm the type of diet that has been ordered for the patient. Also, it is important to assess for any food allergies and religious or cultural preferences. Check to make sure the patient does not have any scheduled laboratory or diagnostic studies that may impact whether he or she is able to eat a meal. Before beginning the feeding, assess for any barriers to eating, such as swallowing difficulties or weakness and/or fatigue. Assess the patient's abdomen. Inspect the abdomen for distention and firmness; auscultate for bowel sounds or peristalsis and palpate the abdomen for distention and tenderness. If the abdomen is distended, consider measuring the abdominal girth at the umbilicus to establish a baseline.

(continued)

Skill 11-1 ► Assisting a Patient With Eating (continued)

NURSING DIAGNOSIS	Determine the related factors for the nursing diagnoses based on the patient's current status. Appropriate nursing diagnoses may include:

- Feeding self-care deficit
- Risk for aspiration
- Impaired swallowing

OUTCOME IDENTIFICATION AND PLANNING	The expected outcome to achieve when assisting a patient with feeding is that the patient consumes a variety of food consistent with the prescribed diet and individual circumstances to attain and maintain ideal body weight. Other outcomes include that the patient does not aspirate during or after the meal, and the patient expresses contentment related to eating, as appropriate.

IMPLEMENTATION

ACTION	RATIONALE
1. Check the medical order for the type of diet prescribed for the patient.	Ensures the correct diet for the patient.
2. Perform hand hygiene and put on PPE, if indicated.	Hand hygiene and PPE prevent the spread of microorganisms. PPE is required based on transmission precautions.
3. Identify the patient.	Identifying the patient ensures the right patient receives the intervention and helps prevent errors.
4. Explain the procedure to the patient.	Explanations provide reassurance and facilitate cooperation of the patient.
5. Assess level of consciousness, for any physical limitations, decreased hearing or visual acuity. If patient uses a hearing aid or wears glasses or dentures, provide, as needed. Ask if the patient has any cultural or religious preferences and food likes and dislikes, if possible.	Alertness is necessary for the patient to swallow and consume food. Using a hearing aid, glasses, and dentures for chewing facilitates the intake of food. Patient preferences should be considered in food selection as much as possible to increase the intake of food and maximize the benefit of the meal.
6. Pull the patient's bedside curtain. Assess the abdomen. Ask the patient if he or she has any nausea. Ask the patient if he or she has any difficulty swallowing. Assess the patient for nausea or pain and administer an antiemetic or analgesic, as needed.	Provides for privacy. A functioning GI tract is essential for digestion. The presence of pain or nausea will diminish appetite. If the patient is medicated, wait for the appropriate time for absorption of the medication before beginning the feeding.
7. Offer to assist the patient with any elimination needs.	Promotes comfort and may avoid interruptions for toileting during meals.
8. Provide hand hygiene and mouth care, as needed.	May improve appetite and promote comfort.
9. Remove any bedpans or undesirable equipment and odors, if possible, from the vicinity where the meal will be eaten. Perform hand hygiene.	Unpleasant odors and equipment may decrease the patient's appetite. Hand hygiene prevents the spread of microorganisms.
10. Open the patient's bedside curtain. Assist to, or position the patient in, a high-Fowler's or sitting position in the bed or chair. Position the bed in the low position if the patient remains in bed.	Proper positioning improves swallowing ability and reduces the risk of aspiration.
11. Place protective covering or towel over the patient if desired and as necessary.	Prevents soiling of the patient's gown.

ACTION

12. Check food tray to make sure that it is the correct tray before serving. Place tray on the overbed table so the patient can see the food, if able. Ensure that hot foods are hot and cold foods are cold. Use caution with hot beverages, allowing sufficient time for cooling, if needed. Ask the patient for his/her preference related to what foods are desired first. Cut food into small pieces, as needed. Observe swallowing ability throughout the meal.

13. If possible, sit facing the patient at the patient's eye level while eating is taking place (Figure 1). If the patient is able, encourage him or her to hold finger foods and feed self as much as possible. Converse with patient during the meal and make eye contact, as appropriate. If, however, the patient has **dysphagia**, limit questioning or conversation that would require patient response during eating. Play relaxation music if patient desires.

RATIONALE

Ensures that the correct tray is given to the patient. Encouraging the patient choice promotes patient dignity and respect. Close observation is necessary to assess for signs of aspiration or difficulty with meal.

Sitting at the patient's eye level and making eye contact create a more relaxed, person-centered atmosphere. In general, optimal mealtime involves social interaction and conversation. Talking during eating is contraindicated for patients with dysphagia because of increased risk for aspiration.

FIGURE 1. Sitting facing the patient at the patient's eye level and encouraging patient to feed herself.

14. Allow enough time for the patient to chew and swallow the food adequately. The patient may need to rest for short periods during eating.

15. When the meal is completed or the patient is unable to eat any more, remove the tray from the room. **Note the amount and types of food consumed. Note the volume of liquid consumed.**

16. Reposition the overbed table, remove the protective covering, offer hand hygiene, as needed, and offer the bedpan. Assist the patient to a position of comfort and relaxation.

 17. Remove PPE, if used. Perform hand hygiene.

Eating requires energy and many medical conditions can weaken patients. Rest can restore energy for eating.

Nutrition plays an important role in healing and overall health. If the patient is not eating enough to meet nutritional requirements, alternative methods need to be considered. Noting the amount and type of food and volume of liquids consumed allows for accurate documentation of intake.

Promotes the comfort of the patient, meets possible elimination needs, and facilitates digestion.

Proper removal of PPE reduces the risk for infection transmission and contamination of other items. Hand hygiene prevents the spread of microorganisms.

EVALUATION   The expected outcomes have been met when the patient consumes an adequate amount of nutrients consistent with the prescribed diet and individual circumstances to attain and maintain ideal body weight. In addition, the patient does not aspirate during or after the meal, and the patient expresses contentment related to eating.

(continued)

Skill 11-1 ▶ Assisting a Patient With Eating *(continued)*

DOCUMENTATION

Guidelines

Document the condition of the abdomen. Note that the head of bed (HOB) was elevated to at least 30 to 45 degrees. Note any swallowing difficulties and the patient's response to the meal. Document the percentage of the intake from the meal. If the patient had a poor intake, document the need for further consultation with the primary care provider and dietitian, as needed. Record any pertinent teaching that was conducted. Record liquids consumed on intake and output record, as appropriate.

Sample Documentation

> <u>12/23/20</u> 0730 Patient's abdomen soft, nondistended, positive bowel sounds. HOB elevated to 45 degrees. Gag reflex intact. Awake. Fed full liquid tray; consumed about 50%; ate most of the oatmeal, 120 mL of cranberry juice. Some conversation during the meal. Patient remains with HOB elevated, watching TV. Call bell in reach.
>
> —S. Essner, RN

UNEXPECTED SITUATIONS AND ASSOCIATED INTERVENTIONS

- *The patient states that he does not want to eat anything on the tray:* Explore with the patient the reason why he does not want to eat anything on the tray. Assess for psychological factors that impact nutrition. Malnutrition is sometimes found with depression in the older adult population. Mutually develop a plan to address the lack of nutritional intake and consult the dietitian, as needed.
- *The patient states that she feels nauseated and cannot eat:* Remove the tray from the patient's room. Explore with the patient the desirability of eating small amounts of foods or liquids, such as crackers or ginger ale, if the patient's diet permits. Administer antiemetic as prescribed, and encourage patient to retry small amounts of food after medication has had time to take effect.

SPECIAL CONSIDERATIONS

- Patients with arthritis of the hands may benefit from use of special utensils with modified handles that facilitate an easier grip. Contact an occupational therapist for guidance on adaptive equipment.
- A visually impaired patient may benefit from use of special plate guards, utensils, double handles, and compartmentalized plates. These patients may be guided to feed him- or herself through use of a "clock" pattern. For example, the chicken is placed at 6 o'clock; the vegetables at 3 o'clock.
- Refer to Box 11-1 for interventions and considerations related to assisting patients with alterations in cognition.
- For the patient with dysphagia, suggest small bites of food such as puddings, ground meat, or cooked vegetables. Advise the patient not to talk while swallowing and to swallow twice after each bite. Refer to Box 11-2 for additional considerations for this patient population.

EVIDENCE FOR PRACTICE ▶

NUTRITION SUPPORT STRATEGIES AND DEMENTIA

People living with dementia often lose some or all of the ability to feed themselves, which often is a source of significant challenges for caregivers. What are effective nutrition support strategies that have potential to be of assistance to these caregivers?

Related Research

Ball, L., Jansen, S., Desbrow, B., Morgan, K., Moyle, W., & Hughes, R. (2015). Experiences and nutrition support strategies in dementia care: Lessons from family carers. *Nutrition & Dietetics, 72*(1), 22–29.

This descriptive exploratory qualitative study examined the perceptions of caregivers of people with dementia living in the community. Interviews with 14 family caregivers were used to explore caregivers' perceptions of feeding and nutrition support, burdens related to care, and strategies used to address nutrition-related challenges. Caregivers described multiple physiologic, cognitive, emotional, functional and/or behavioral challenges, as well as multiple strategies used by the caregivers to address feeding challenges. Additional themes that emerged included feelings of being uninformed and unsupported in nutrition-related care by health care professionals and significant stress related to decreased food intake, weight loss, and wasting on the part of the person with dementia. The authors reported that most family caregivers experienced difficulty with nutrition care, and that this was a significant component of overall burden of care. Strategies used successfully by the participant caregivers included supervising meal-times, avoiding disagreements over food, and provision of regular snacks and finger foods. The authors concluded that caregivers of people with dementia feel unsupported and uninformed with respect to nutrition-related care.

Relevance for Nursing Practice

People with dementia are at risk for reduced nutritional intake with the potential for weight loss and malnutrition. This study suggests that health care professionals may not be providing sufficient education and support to people providing care for individuals with dementia. Nurses are involved in all aspects of nutritional care and have a responsibility to assist patients and their care givers in attaining and maintaining adequate nutritional intake. Nurses must utilize appropriate interventions to provide appropriate education and support to achieve this outcome.

Refer to thePoint° for additional research on related nursing topics.

Skill 11-2 ▶ Confirming Placement of a Nasogastric Tube

Verify correct placement of the nasogastric tube after the initial insertion, before beginning a feeding or instilling medications or liquids, and at 4-hour intervals during continuous feedings (Metheny, 2016b). This ensures that the tip of the tube is situated in the stomach or intestine, preventing inadvertent administration of substances into the wrong place. A misplaced feeding tube in the lungs or pulmonary tissue places the patient at risk for aspiration. Radiographic examination, measurement of tube length and measurement of tube marking, measurement of aspirate pH, visual assessment of aspirate, and monitoring of carbon dioxide have been suggested to confirm feeding tube placement. With the exception of radiographic examination, the use of two or more of these techniques in conjunction with each other increases the likelihood of correct tube placement (Bankhead et al., 2009; Metheny, 2016b; Rahimi, Farhadi, Ashtarian, & Changaei, 2015). An old technique of auscultation of air injected into a feeding tube has proved unreliable and may result in tragic consequences if used as an indicator of tube placement (Bankhead et al., 2009; Boeykens, Steeman, & Duysburgh, 2014; Metheny, 2016b). Therefore, do not use it to confirm feeding tube placement.

Allow 1-hour interval after patient has received medication or completed an intermittent feeding before testing pH of gastric fluid. If feeding is continuous, plan pH testing at a time when feeding can be withheld (Bankhead et al., 2009; Metheny, 2016b).

DELEGATION CONSIDERATIONS	The confirmation of placement of a nasogastric tube is not delegated to nursing assistive personnel (NAP) or to unlicensed assistive personnel (UAP). Depending on the state's nurse practice act and the organization's policies and procedures, confirmation of placement of a nasogastric tube may be delegated to licensed practical/vocational nurses (LPN/LVNs). The decision to delegate must be based on careful analysis of the patient's needs and circumstances, as well as the qualifications of the person to whom the task is being delegated. Refer to the Delegation Guidelines in Appendix A.
EQUIPMENT	• Nasogastric tube of appropriate size (8 to 18 Fr) • Normal saline solution or sterile water, for irrigation, depending on facility policy • Tongue blade • Irrigation set, including a Toomey (20 to 50 mL) • Bath towel or disposable pad • Nonsterile, disposable gloves • Additional PPE, as indicated • Tape measure, or other measuring device • pH paper or meter • Stethoscope

(continued)

Skill 11-2 ▶ Confirming Placement of a Nasogastric Tube *(continued)*

ASSESSMENT

Inspect the abdomen for distention and firmness; auscultate for bowel sounds or peristalsis and palpate the abdomen for distention and tenderness. If the abdomen is distended, consider measuring the abdominal girth at the umbilicus to establish a baseline. Assess the time when the patient last received medication or tube feeding.

NURSING DIAGNOSIS

Determine the related factors for the nursing diagnoses based on the patient's current status. Nursing diagnoses may vary depending on the reason for the NG tube insertion. Appropriate nursing diagnoses may include:

- Imbalanced nutrition, less than body requirements
- Risk for trauma
- Risk for aspiration

OUTCOME IDENTIFICATION AND PLANNING

The expected outcomes to achieve when confirming placement of an NG tube is that the tube is located in the patient's stomach without any complications and the patient does not exhibit signs and symptoms of aspiration.

IMPLEMENTATION

ACTION	RATIONALE
1. Gather equipment.	Assembling equipment provides for an organized approach to the task.
2. Perform hand hygiene and put on PPE, if indicated.	Hand hygiene and PPE prevent the spread of microorganisms. PPE is required based on transmission precautions.
3. Identify the patient.	Identifying the patient ensures the right patient receives the intervention and helps prevent errors.
4. Explain the procedure to the patient, including the rationale for confirming tube placement. Answer any questions as needed.	Explanation facilitates patient cooperation.
5. Assemble equipment on overbed table or other surface within reach.	Arranging items nearby is convenient, saves time, and avoids unnecessary stretching and twisting of muscles on the part of the nurse.
6. Close the patient's bedside curtain or door. Raise the bed to a comfortable working position, usually elbow height of the caregiver (VHA Center for Engineering & Occupational Safety and Health [CEOSH], 2016). Perform abdominal assessments as described above. Drape chest with bath towel or disposable pad.	Closing curtains or door provides for patient privacy. Having the bed at the proper height prevents back and muscle strain. Assessment is vital to detect changes in the patient's condition before initiating the intervention. Protective drape prevents accidental soiling of bed linens and patient clothing with stomach contents.
7. Confirm placement of the nasogastric tube in the patient's stomach using at least two methods. The first method utilized should be measurement of the exposed length of tube.	With the exception of radiographic examination, which is usually done immediately after insertion to verify initial tube placement, the use of two or more of these techniques in conjunction with each other increases the likelihood of correct tube placement (Bankhead et al., 2009; Metheny, 2016b; Rahimi et al., 2015). Any change in the length of the exposed tube may indicate dislodgement (Bankhead et al., 2009; Metheny, 2016b). If a significant change in the external length is observed, use other bedside tests to help determine if the tube has become dislocated (Bankhead et al., 2009; Best, 2013).

ACTION	RATIONALE
8. Put on gloves. Unsecure the tube from the patient's gown. Verify the position of the marking on the tube at the nostril. Measure length of exposed tube and compare with the documented length (Figure 1). Resecure the tube to the patient's gown.	Gloves prevent contact with blood and body fluids and transfer of microorganisms. The tube should be marked with an indelible marker at the nostril at the time it was placed. This marking should be assessed each time the tube is used to ensure the tube has not become displaced. Tube length should be checked and compared with this initial measurement, in conjunction with pH measurement and visual assessment of aspirate. An increase in the length of the exposed tube may indicate dislodgement (Bankhead et al., 2009; Metheny, 2016b).
9. Check to ensure a 1-hour interval has elapsed since the patient has received medication or completed an intermittent feeding before testing pH of gastric fluid. Attach syringe to end of tube and aspirate a small amount of stomach contents (Figure 2). If unable to obtain a specimen, reposition the patient and flush the tube with 30 mL of air in a large syringe. Slowly apply negative pressure to withdraw fluid.	The presence of medication or nutritional formula may affect the pH of gastrointestinal secretions and contribute to inaccurate readings (Bankhead et al., 2009; Metheny, 2016b). The tube is in the stomach if its contents can be aspirated: pH of aspirate can then be tested to determine gastric placement. Difficulty in aspiration may be due to a blocked tube, or the tip of the tube not being positioned in fluid. Injecting an air bolus will help remove the blockage, and repositioning the patient will help place the tip of the tube in fluid (Metheny, 2016b). This action may be necessary several times in order to obtain aspirate.

FIGURE 1. Measuring the length of the exposed nasogastric tube.

FIGURE 2. Aspirating gastric contents.

10. Measure the pH of aspirated fluid using pH paper or a meter. Place a drop of gastric secretions onto pH paper or place small amount in a plastic cup and dip the pH paper into it. Within 30 seconds, compare the color on the paper with the chart supplied by the manufacturer (Figure 3).	Testing of the pH and appearance of the aspirate may be helpful in determining tube location if feedings have been off for at least one hour (Bankhead et al., 2009; Metheny, 2016b). The pH of gastric contents is acidic (less than 5.5). If the patient is taking an acid-inhibiting agent, the range may be 4.0 to 6.0. The pH of intestinal fluid is 7.0 or higher. The pH of respiratory fluid is 6.0 or higher. This method will not effectively differentiate between intestinal fluid and pleural fluid.

FIGURE 3. Checking pH of gastric fluid.

(continued)

Skill 11-2 ▶ Confirming Placement of a Nasogastric Tube (continued)

ACTION	RATIONALE
11. Examine aspirated contents, checking for color and consistency.	Gastric fluid can be green with particles, off-white, or brown if old blood is present. Intestinal aspirate tends to look clear or straw-colored to a deep golden yellow color. Also, intestinal aspirate may be greenish brown if stained with bile. Respiratory or tracheobronchial fluid is usually off-white to tan and may be tinged with mucus. A small amount of blood-tinged fluid may be seen immediately after NG insertion.
12. If it is not possible to aspirate contents; assessments to check placement are inconclusive; the exposed tube length has changed; or there are any other indications that the tube is not in place, check placement by radiograph (x-ray) of placement of tube based on facility policy (and ordered by the primary health care provider).	The x-ray is considered the most reliable method for identifying the position of the NG tube.
13. Flush tube with 30 to 50 mL of water for irrigation. Disconnect syringe from tubing and cap end of tubing	Flushing tube prevents occlusion (Bankhead et al., 2009; Blumenstein, Shastri, & Stein, 2014; Bourgault, Ipe, Weaver, Swartz, & O'Dea, 2007; Metheny, 2008). Capping the tube deters the entry of microorganisms and prevents leakage onto the bed linens.
14. Clamp tube and remove the syringe. Cap the tube, reattach to the feeding delivery set, or attach tube to suction, based on the circumstances.	Capping or reattachment to feeding delivery set or reattachment to suction allows for appropriate treatment for individual patient.
15. Remove equipment and return patient to a position of comfort. Remove gloves. Raise side rail and lower bed.	Promotes patient comfort and safety. Removing gloves properly reduces the risk for infection transmission and contamination of other items.
16. Remove additional PPE, if used. Perform hand hygiene.	Proper removal of PPE reduces the risk for infection transmission and contamination of other items. Hand hygiene prevents transmission of microorganisms.

EVALUATION

The expected outcomes have been met when the tube is deemed to be located in the patient's stomach without complications, and the patient does not exhibit signs and symptoms of aspiration.

DOCUMENTATION

Guidelines

Document the type of nasogastric tube or gastrostomy/jejunostomy tube that is present. Record the criteria that were used to confirm proper placement, including the tube length in inches or centimeters compared to the length on initial insertion. Document the aspiration of gastric contents and pH of the gastric contents when intermittent feeding is used. Note the components of the abdominal assessment, such as observation of the abdomen, presence of distention or firmness, and presence of bowel sounds. Include subjective data, such as any reports from the patient of abdominal pain or nausea or any other patient response.

Sample Documentation

10/29/20 1015 Position of NG tube was compared with and matched initial measurement on insertion. Abdomen nondistended and soft; patient denies pain or nausea. Scant residual aspirated; yellow with dark flecks, pH 3.9. Tube flushed with 60-mL water with ease. Patient instructed to call for nurse for pain or nausea or other concerns related to feeding.

—S. Essner, RN

UNEXPECTED SITUATIONS AND ASSOCIATED INTERVENTIONS

- *No gastric contents can be aspirated*: If the patient is comatose, check oral cavity. If the tube is in a gastric area, small air boluses may need to be given until gastric contents can be aspirated. Refer to Step 9 above.

SPECIAL CONSIDERATIONS

General Considerations

- Check tube placement before administering any fluids, medications, or feedings. Use multiple techniques: x-ray, external length marking/measurement, pH testing, and aspirate characteristics.
- Sterile water should be used for tube flushes in immunocompromised or critically ill patients (Allen, 2015; Bankhead et al., 2009).
- Monitoring for carbon dioxide to determine NG tube position and/or dislodgement has been investigated (Gilbert & Burns, 2012; Irving, Lyman, Northington, Bartlett, & Kemper, 2014). This involves the use of a capnograph or a colorimetric end-tidal CO_2 detector to detect the presence of carbon dioxide, which would indicate tube positioning in the patient's airway instead of the stomach. Carbon dioxide detectors can be helpful in detecting when a feeding tube is in the tracheobronchial tree, but may not be sufficiently sensitive to detect misplacement (Metheny, 2016b).

EVIDENCE FOR PRACTICE ▶

VERIFICATION OF FEEDING TUBE PLACEMENT

Metheny, N. (2016a). AACN Practice Alert. Prevention of aspiration in adults. *Critical Care Nurse*, 36(1), e20–e24.

Metheny, N. (2016b). AACN Practice Alert. Initial and ongoing verification of feeding tube placement in adults (applies to blind insertions and placements with an electromagnetic device). *Critical Care Nurse*, 36(2), e8–e13.

Practice alerts are directives from AACN that are supported by authoritative evidence to ensure excellence in practice and a safe and humane work environment. These directives provide guidance and standardize practice, as well as identify/inform about new advances and trends. The AACN has provided directives addressing best practice for verification of feeding tube placement. Expected practice includes radiographic confirmation of correct tube placement on all critically ill patients who are to receive feedings or medications via blindly inserted gastric or small bowel tubes prior to initial use. The tube's exit site from the nose or mouth should be marked and length documented immediately after radiographic confirmation of correct tube placement. The mark should be observed routinely and the external tube measured to assess for a change in length of the external portion of the tube. Bedside techniques to assess tube location should be used at regular intervals to determine if the tube has remained in its intended position. These bedside techniques include measuring the pH and observing the appearance of fluid withdrawn from the tube.

Refer to thePoint° for additional research on related nursing topics.

  Skill 11-3 ▶ **Administering a Tube Feeding**

Depending on the patient's physical and psychosocial condition and nutritional requirements, a feeding through the NG tube or other GI tube might be ordered. The steps for administering feedings are similar regardless of the tube used. Feeding can be provided on an intermittent or continuous basis. Intermittent feedings are delivered at regular intervals, using gravity for instillation or a feeding pump to administer the formula over a set period of time. Intermittent feedings might also be given as a bolus, using a syringe to instill the formula quickly in one large amount. Intermittent feedings introducing the formula over a set period of time via gravity or pump, are the preferred method. If the order calls for continuous feeding, an external feeding pump is needed to regulate

(continued)

Skill 11-3 ▸ Administering a Tube Feeding *(continued)*

the flow of formula. Continuous feedings permit gradual introduction of the formula into the GI tract, promoting maximal absorption. However, there is a risk of both reflux and aspiration with this method. Feeding intolerance is less likely to occur with smaller volumes. Hanging smaller amounts of feeding also reduces the risk for bacteria growth and contamination of feeding at room temperature (when using open systems).

The procedure below describes using open systems and a feeding pump; the skill variation at the end of the skill describes using a closed system.

DELEGATION CONSIDERATIONS	The administration of a tube feeding is not usually delegated to nursing assistive personnel (NAP) or to unlicensed assistive personnel (UAP) in the acute care setting. The administration of a tube feeding in some settings may be delegated to NAP or UAP who have received appropriate training, after assessment of tube placement and patency by the registered nurse. Depending on the state's nurse practice act and the organization's policies and procedures, the administration of a tube feeding may be delegated to licensed practical/vocational nurses (LPN/LVNs). The decision to delegate must be based on careful analysis of the patient's needs and circumstances, as well as the qualifications of the person to whom the task is being delegated. Refer to the Delegation Guidelines in Appendix A.
EQUIPMENT	• Prescribed tube-feeding formula at room temperature • Feeding bag or prefilled tube-feeding set • Stethoscope • Nonsterile gloves • Additional PPE, as indicated • Alcohol preps • Disposable pad or towel • Large (Asepto or Toomey) syringe • Enteral feeding pump (if ordered) • Rubber band • Clamp (Hoffman or butterfly) • IV pole • Water for irrigation and hydration, as needed • pH paper • Tape measure, or other measuring device
ASSESSMENT	Assess the abdomen by inspecting for presence of distention, auscultate for bowel sounds, and palpate the abdomen for firmness or tenderness. If the abdomen is distended, consider measuring the abdominal girth at the umbilicus. If the patient reports any tenderness or nausea, exhibits any rigidity or firmness of the abdomen, and if bowel sounds are absent, confer with health care provider before administering the tube feeding. Assess for patient and/or family understanding, if appropriate, for the rationale for the tube feeding and address any questions or concerns expressed by the patient and family members.
NURSING DIAGNOSIS	Determine the related factors for the nursing diagnoses based on the patient's current status. Appropriate nursing diagnoses may include: • Risk for aspiration • Deficient knowledge • Imbalanced nutrition, less than body requirements
OUTCOME IDENTIFICATION AND PLANNING	The expected outcome to achieve when administering a tube feeding is that the patient will receive the tube feeding without complaints of nausea, episodes of vomiting, gastric distention, or diarrhea. Additional expected outcomes may include the following: the patient does not exhibit signs and symptoms of aspiration; the patient demonstrates an increase in weight; and the patient verbalizes knowledge related to tube feeding.

IMPLEMENTATION

ACTION	RATIONALE
1. Gather equipment. Check amount, concentration, type, and frequency of tube feeding in the patient's medical record. Check formula expiration date.	This provides for an organized approach to the task. Checking ensures that correct feeding will be administered. Outdated formula may be contaminated.

ACTION	**RATIONALE**
2. Perform hand hygiene and put on PPE, if indicated.	Hand hygiene and PPE prevent the spread of microorganisms. PPE is required based on transmission precautions.
3. Identify the patient.	Identifying the patient ensures the right patient receives the intervention and helps prevent errors.
4. Explain the procedure to the patient. Answer any questions, as needed.	Explanation facilitates patient cooperation.
5. Assemble equipment on overbed table or other surface within reach.	Organization facilitates performance of the task.
6. Close the patient's bedside curtain or door. Raise the bed to a comfortable working position, usually elbow height of the caregiver (VHACEOSH, 2016). Perform abdominal assessments as described above.	Closing curtains or door provides for patient privacy. Having the bed at the proper height prevents back and muscle strain. Assessment is vital to detect changes in the patient's condition before initiating the intervention.
7. **Position the patient with HOB elevated at least 30 to 45 degrees or as near normal position for eating as possible.**	This position minimizes possibility of reflux and aspiration into the trachea (Bankhead et al., 2009). Patients who are considered at high risk for aspiration should be assisted to at least a 45-degree position.
8. Confirm placement of the nasogastric tube in the patient's stomach using at least two methods (refer to Skill 11-2). The first method utilized should be measurement of the exposed length of tube.	With the exception of radiographic examination, which is usually done immediately after insertion to verify initial tube placement, the use of two or more of these techniques in conjunction with each other increases the likelihood of correct tube placement (Bankhead et al., 2009; Metheny, 2016b; Rahimi et al., 2015). Any change in the length of the exposed tube may indicate dislodgement (Bankhead et al., 2009; Metheny, 2016b). If a significant change in the external length is observed, use other bedside tests to help determine if the tube has become dislocated (Bankhead et al., 2009; Best, 2013).
9. Put on gloves. Unsecure the tube from the patient's gown. Verify the position of the marking on the tube at the nostril. Measure length of exposed tube and compare with the documented length.	Gloves prevent contact with blood and body fluids and transfer of microorganisms. The tube should be marked with an indelible marker at the nostril at the time it was placed. This marking should be assessed each time the tube is used to ensure the tube has not become displaced. Tube length should be checked and compared with the initial measurement, in conjunction with pH measurement and visual assessment of aspirate. An increase in the length of the exposed tube may indicate dislodgement (Bankhead et al., 2009; Metheny, 2016b).
10. Check the pH of and visualize aspirated contents, checking for color and consistency as described in Skill 11-2, Steps 9–12.	With the exception of radiographic examination, which is usually done immediately after insertion to verify initial tube placement, the use of two or more of these techniques in conjunction with each other increases the likelihood of correct tube placement (Bankhead et al., 2009; Metheny, 2016b; Rahimi et al., 2015).
11. If it is not possible to aspirate contents; assessments to check placement are inconclusive; the exposed tube length has changed; or there are any other indications that the tube is not in place, check placement by radiograph (x-ray) of placement of tube, based on facility policy (and ordered by the primary health care provider).	The x-ray is considered the most reliable method for identifying the position of the NG tube.

(continued)

Skill 11-3 ▶ Administering a Tube Feeding *(continued)*

ACTION	RATIONALE
12. After multiple steps have been taken to ensure that the feeding tube is located in the stomach or small intestine, **aspirate all gastric contents with the syringe and measure to check for gastric residual—the amount of feeding remaining in the stomach.** Return the residual based on facility policy. Proceed with feeding if amount of residual does not exceed facility policy or the limit indicated in the medical record.	Checking for **residual** before each feeding or every 4 to 6 hours during a continuous feeding according to institutional policy is implemented to identify delayed gastric emptying. High gastric residual volumes (200 to 250 mL or greater) can be associated with high risk for aspiration and aspiration-related pneumonia (Bourgault et al., 2007; Metheny, 2016a; Metheny, 2008). Some experts now recommend that the patient's pattern of residual is more important than the amount (Bankhead et al., 2009; Bourgault et al., 2007; Metheny, 2008). Research findings are inconclusive on the benefit of returning gastric volumes to the stomach or intestine to avoid fluid or electrolyte imbalance, which has been accepted practice. Consult facility policy concerning this practice. Some literature suggests repeated gastric residual aspiration should be minimized (Blumenstein et al., 2014).
13. Flush tube with 30 to 50 mL of water for irrigation. Disconnect syringe from tubing and cap end of tubing while preparing the formula feeding equipment. Remove gloves.	Flushing tube prevents occlusion (Bankhead et al., 2009; Blumenstein et al., 2014; Bourgault et al., 2007; Metheny, 2008). Capping the tube deters the entry of microorganisms and prevents leakage onto the bed linens.
14. Put on gloves before preparing, assembling, and handling any part of the feeding system.	Gloves prevent contact with blood and body fluids and deter transmission of contaminants to feeding equipment and/or formula.
15. Administer feeding.	
When Using a Feeding Bag Administration System (Open System)	
a. Label bag and/or tubing with date and time. Hang bag on IV pole and adjust to about 12 in above the stomach. Clamp tubing.	Labeling date and time of first use allows for disposal within 24 hours, to deter growth of microorganisms. Proper feeding bag height reduces risk of formula being introduced too quickly.
b. Check the expiration date of the formula. Cleanse top of feeding container with a disinfectant before opening it (Figure 1). Pour formula into feeding bag and allow solution to run through tubing. Close clamp.	Cleansing container top with alcohol minimizes risk for contaminants entering feeding bag. Formula displaces air in tubing.
c. Attach feeding administration set to feeding tube (Figure 2), open clamp, and regulate drip according to the medical order, or allow feeding to run in over 30 minutes.	Introducing formula at a slow, regular rate allows the stomach to accommodate to the feeding and decreases GI distress.

FIGURE 1. Cleaning top of feeding container with alcohol before opening it.

FIGURE 2. Attaching feeding administration set to NG tube.

ACTION

d. Add 30 to 60 mL (1 to 2 oz) of water for irrigation to feeding bag when feeding is almost completed (Figure 3) and allow it to run through the tube.

e. Clamp tubing immediately after water has been instilled. Disconnect feeding administration set from feeding tube. Clamp tube and cover end with cap (Figure 4).

RATIONALE

Water rinses the feeding from the tube and helps to keep it patent.

Clamping the tube prevents air from entering the stomach. Capping the tube deters entry of microorganisms and covering end of tube protects patient and linens from fluid leakage from tube.

FIGURE 3. Pouring water into feeding bag.

FIGURE 4. Capping NG tube after it is clamped.

When Using a Large Syringe (Open System)

a. Remove plunger from 30- or 60-mL syringe (Figure 5).

b. Attach syringe to feeding tube and pour premeasured amount of tube-feeding formula into syringe (Figure 6). Open the clamp on the feeding tube and allow formula to enter tube. Regulate rate, fast or slow, by height of the syringe. **Do not push formula with syringe plunger.**

Introducing the formula at a slow, regular rate allows the stomach to accommodate to the feeding and decreases GI distress. The higher the syringe is held, the faster the formula flows.

FIGURE 5. Removing plunger from a 60-mL syringe.

FIGURE 6. Pouring formula into syringe.

(*continued*)

Skill 11-3 ▶ Administering a Tube Feeding *(continued)*

ACTION	RATIONALE
c. When feeding is almost completed, **add 30 to 60 mL (1 to 2 oz) of water for irrigation to syringe (Figure 7)** and allow it to run through the tube.	Water rinses the feeding from the tube and helps to keep it patent.

FIGURE 7. Pouring water into almost-empty syringe.

ACTION	RATIONALE
d. When syringe has emptied, hold syringe high, clamp the tube, and disconnect from tube. Cover end with cap.	By holding syringe high, the formula will not backflow out of tube and onto patient. Clamping the tube prevents air from entering the stomach. Capping end of tube deters entry of microorganisms and prevents fluid leakage from tube.

When Using an Enteral Feeding Pump

ACTION	RATIONALE
a. Close flow-regulator clamp on tubing and fill feeding bag with prescribed formula, as described in Steps 15a and 15b. Amount used depends on facility policy. Place label on container with patient's name, date, and time the feeding was hung.	Closing clamp prevents formula from moving through tubing until nurse is ready. Labeling date and time of first use allows for disposal within 24 hours, to deter growth of microorganisms.
b. Hang feeding container on IV pole. Allow solution to flow through tubing.	This prevents air from being forced into the stomach or intestines.
c. Connect to feeding pump, following manufacturer's directions. Set rate (Figure 8). Maintain the patient in the upright position throughout the feeding. If the patient needs to lie flat temporarily, pause the feeding. Resume the feeding after the patient's position has been changed back to at least 30 to 45 degrees (Bankhead et al., 2009).	Feeding pumps vary. Some of the newer pumps have built-in safeguards that protect the patient from complications. Safety features include cassettes that prevent free flow of formula, automatic tube flush, safety tips that prevent accidental attachment to an IV setup, and various audible and visible alarms. Feedings are started at full strength rather than diluted. A smaller volume, 10 to 40 mL, of feeding infused per hour and gradually increased has been shown to be more easily tolerated by patients.

FIGURE 8. Setting infusion rate on pump.

ACTION

d. **Check placement of tube and gastric residual every 4 to 6 hours (Bankhead et al., 2009). Flush tube with 30 to 50 mL of water at least every 4 hours during continuous feeding.**

16. Observe the patient's response during and after tube feeding and assess the abdomen at least once a shift.

17. **Have patient remain in upright position for at least 1 hour after feeding.**

18. Remove equipment and return patient to a position of comfort. Remove gloves. Raise side rail and lower bed.

19. Put on gloves. Wash and clean equipment or replace according to facility policy. Remove gloves.

 20. Remove additional PPE, if used. Perform hand hygiene.

RATIONALE

Checking placement (Skill 11-2) verifies that the tube has not moved out of the stomach. Checking gastric residual (Step 12) monitors absorption of the feeding and prevents distention, which could lead to aspiration. Flushing at recommended intervals helps prevent clogging and obstruction of the feeding tube (Bankhead et al., 2009; Dudek, 2018).

Pain or nausea may indicate stomach distention, which may lead to vomiting. Physical signs, such as abdominal distention and firmness or regurgitation of tube feeding, may indicate intolerance.

This position minimizes risk for backflow and discourages aspiration, if any reflux or vomiting should occur.

Promotes patient comfort and safety. Removing gloves properly reduces the risk for infection transmission and contamination of other items.

This prevents contamination and deters spread of microorganisms. Reusable systems are cleansed with soap and water with each use and replaced every 24 hours. Refer to facility policy and manufacturer's guidelines for specifics on equipment care.

Proper removal of PPE reduces the risk for infection transmission and contamination of other items. Hand hygiene prevents transmission of microorganisms.

EVALUATION

The expected outcomes have been met when the patient receives the prescribed tube feeding without complaints of nausea, episodes of vomiting, gastric distention, or diarrhea; the patient does not exhibit signs and symptoms of aspiration; the patient demonstrates an increase in weight; and the patient voices knowledge related to tube feeding.

DOCUMENTATION

Guidelines

Document the type of NG tube or gastrostomy/jejunostomy tube that is present. Record the criteria that were used to confirm proper placement before feeding was initiated and during administration, as indicated, such as the tube length in inches or centimeters compared to the length on initial insertion. Document the aspiration of gastric contents and pH of the gastric contents when intermittent feeding is used. Note the components of the abdominal assessment, such as observation of the abdomen, presence of distention or firmness, and presence of bowel sounds. Include subjective data, such as any reports from the patient of abdominal pain or nausea or any other patient response. Record the amount of gastric residual volume that was obtained. Document the position of the patient, the type of feeding, and the method and the amount of feeding. Include any relevant patient teaching.

Sample Documentation

<u>10/29/20</u> 1815 Position of NG tube was compared with initial measurement on insertion; no change in measurement. Abdomen nondistended and soft; patient denies pain or nausea. HOB raised to 45 degrees. Thirty milliliters residual aspirated prior to feeding; pH 3.9. Aspirate returned to stomach; aspirate yellow with dark flecks. 150 mL of Jevity 1.2 Cal administered via bolus feeding. Tube flushed with 60-mL water with ease. Patient instructed to call for nurse for pain or nausea or other concerns related to feeding.

—S. Essner, RN

(continued)

Skill 11-3 ▶ Administering a Tube Feeding *(continued)*

UNEXPECTED SITUATIONS AND ASSOCIATED INTERVENTIONS	• *Nasogastric tube is found not to be in stomach or intestine:* Tube must be in the stomach before feeding. If the tube is in misplaced, the patient is at increased risk for aspiration. Refer to Skill 13-8 for steps to replace tube.

• *When checking for residual, the nurse aspirates a large amount:* Before discarding or replacing residual, check with the primary care provider and facility policy. Replacing a large amount may increase the patient's risk for vomiting and aspiration, whereas discarding a large amount may increase the patient's risk for metabolic alkalosis. At times, the primary care provider may instruct the nurse to replace half of the residual and recheck in a set amount of time.

• *Patient complains of nausea after tube feeding:* Ensure that the HOB remains elevated and that suction equipment is at the bedside. Check medication record to see if any antiemetics have been ordered for the patient. Consider notifying the primary care provider for an order of an antiemetic.

• *When attempting to aspirate contents, the nurse notes that tube is clogged:* Most obstructions are caused by coagulation of formula. Try using warm water or air and gentle pressure to remove the clog. Carbonated sodas, such as colas, and meat tenderizers have not been shown effective in removing clogs in feeding tubes. Never use a stylet to unclog tubes. Tube may have to be replaced. To prevent clogs, ensure that adequate flushing is completed after each feeding.

SPECIAL CONSIDERATIONS

• Sterile water should be used for tube flushes in immunocompromised or critically ill patients (Allen, 2015; Bankhead et al., 2009).

• Make sure the patient is as upright as possible during feeding. Keep the head of the bed elevated at 30 to 45 degrees at all times during administration of enteral feedings and for 1 hour afterward to prevent reflux and aspiration, unless contraindicated (Bankhead et al., 2009).

• Checking for the residual amount of feeding in the stomach is explained in Step 12. High gastric residual volumes (200 to 250 mL or greater) can be associated with high risk for aspiration and aspiration-related pneumonia (Bourgault et al., 2007; Metheny, 2008). Evaluate the significance of a single high gastric residual volume in relation to other indicators of GI intolerance, including abdominal distention, abdominal discomfort, nausea, and vomiting (Metheny, 2016a).

• Guidelines for holding feedings in relation to gastric residual volume vary (Bankhead et al., 2009; Mueller, Compher, & Ellen, 2011). Trends of increasing gastric residual volumes should be identified as a potential sign of GI intolerance and indicate the need for reassessment of the patient, reassessment of patient tolerance, and the potential need for promotility agents (Bankhead et al., 2009; Metheny, 2016a).

• If the gastric residual volume is 250 mL or greater for two consecutive residual checks, a promotility agent should be considered in adult patients (Bankhead et al., 2009).

• A gastric residual volume of greater than 500 mL in an adult patient should result in holding the **enteral nutrition** and reassessing patient tolerance (Bankhead et al., 2009).

• When the patient with dementia and/or family is deciding on whether to agree to tube-feeding nutrition, inform them that research is recommending that tube feedings need not be used for this population of patients because they do not increase survival or prevent malnutrition or aspiration. It is suggested to use such methods as increasing feeding assistance, removing dietary restrictions, and respecting patient preferences as a guide to type and amount of food provided (O'Sullivan Maillet et al., 2013).

• Some feeding equipment allows for the addition of water for flushes to a second feeding container, which enters the system through a second set of tubing. The feeding pump will automatically administer the preset volume of flush at the preset frequency.

Skill Variation ▶ Using a Prefilled Tube-Feeding Set (Closed System)

Prefilled tube-feeding sets, which are considered closed systems, are frequently used to provide patient nourishment (Figure A). Closed systems contain sterile feeding solutions in ready-to-hang containers. This method reduces the opportunity for bacterial contamination of the feeding formula. In general, these prefilled feedings are administered via an enteral pump.

1. Check amount, concentration, type, and frequency of tube feeding in the patient's medical record.
2. Gather all equipment, checking the feeding solution and container for correct solution and expiration date. Label with patient's name, type of solution, and prescribed rate.

Skill Variation ▶ Using a Prefilled Tube-Feeding Set (Closed System) *(continued)*

FIGURE A. Prefilled tube feedings in plastic containers and ready-to-use feeding in a can. (Reprinted with permission from Abbott Nutrition, a division of Abbott Laboratories.)

3. Perform hand hygiene. Put on PPE, as indicated.

4. Identify the patient and explain the procedure.

5. Put on gloves.

6. Ensure the correct placement of the feeding tube by checking marking on tube at nose (if NG tube), length of exposed tube, aspiration of stomach contents, and gastric or intestinal pH.
7. Check for residual amount of feeding in the stomach and return residual, as ordered.
8. Flush tube with 30 mL of water.
9. Put on nonsterile gloves; remove screw on cap and attach administration setup with drip chamber and tubing.
10. Hang feeding container on IV pole and connect to feeding pump, allowing solution to flow through tubing, following manufacturer's directions.
11. Attach the feeding setup to the patient's feeding tube.
12. Open the clamp of the patient's feeding tube.
13. Turn on the pump.
14. Set the pump at the prescribed rate of flow and remove the nonsterile gloves.
15. Observe the patient's response during the tube feeding.
16. Continue to assess the patient for signs and symptoms of GI distress, such as nausea, abdominal distention, or absence of bowel sounds.
17. Have the patient remain in the upright position throughout the feeding and for at least 1 hour after feeding. If patient's position needs to be changed to a supine position or turned in bed, pause the feeding pump during this time.
18. After the prescribed amount of feeding has been administrated (or according to facility policy), turn off the pump, put on nonsterile gloves, clamp the feeding tube, and disconnect it from the feeding set tube, capping the end of the feeding set.
19. Draw up 30 to 60 mL of water using a syringe.
20. Attach the syringe to the feeding tube; unclamp the feeding tube and instill the 30 to 60 mL of water into it.
21. Clamp the feeding tube.
22. Remove equipment according to facility policy.
23. Provide for any patient needs.

24. Remove gloves and additional PPE, if used. Perform hand hygiene.

EVIDENCE FOR PRACTICE ▶

VERIFICATION OF FEEDING TUBE PLACEMENT

Metheny, N. (2016a). AACN Practice Alert. Prevention of aspiration in adults. *Critical Care Nurse, 36*(1), e20–e24.

Metheny, N. (2016b). AACN Practice Alert. Initial and ongoing verification of feeding tube placement in adults. *Critical Care Nurse, 36*(2), e8–e13.

Refer to details in Skill 11-2, Evidence for Practice, and refer to thePoint* for additional research on related nursing topics.

Skill 11-4 ▶ Caring for a Gastrostomy Tube

When long-term enteral feeding is required, an enterostomal tube may be placed through an opening created into the stomach (**gastrostomy tube**) or into the jejunum (**jejunostomy tube**). Placement of a tube into the stomach or small intestine can be accomplished by a surgeon or gastroenterologist via endoscopy (**percutaneous endoscopic gastrostomy [PEG] tube** and **percutaneous endoscopic jejunostomy [PEJ] tube**) or via surgery (open or laparoscopically). PEG tube insertion is often used because, unlike a traditional, surgically placed gastrostomy tube, it usually does not require general anesthesia. Use of a PEG tube or other type of enterostomal tube requires an intact, functional GI tract. Providing care at the insertion site is a nursing responsibility and is important in the prevention of complications (Friginal-Ruiz & Lucendo, 2015). Site care is the same for a gastrostomy and a jejunostomy.

DELEGATION CONSIDERATIONS	The care of a gastrostomy tube, in the postoperative period, is not delegated to nursing assistive personnel (NAP) or to unlicensed assistive personnel (UAP) in the acute care setting. The care of a healed gastrostomy tube site in some settings may be delegated to NAP or UAP who have received appropriate training, after assessment of the tube by the registered nurse. Depending on the state's nurse practice act and the organization's policies and procedures, the care of a gastrostomy tube may be delegated to licensed practical/vocational nurses (LPN/LVNs). The decision to delegate must be based on careful analysis of the patient's needs and circumstances, as well as the qualifications of the person to whom the task is being delegated. Refer to the Delegation Guidelines in Appendix A.
EQUIPMENT	• Nonsterile gloves • Additional PPE, as indicated • Washcloth, towel, and skin cleanser or cotton-tipped applicators and sterile saline solution (depending on patient circumstances) • Gauze (if needed)
ASSESSMENT	Assess gastrostomy or jejunostomy tube site, noting any drainage, skin breakdown, or erythema. Measure the length of exposed tube, comparing it with the initial measurement after insertion. Alternately, mark the tube at the skin with indelible marker; mark should be at skin level at the insertion site. Check to ensure that the tube is securely stabilized and has not become dislodged. Also, assess the tension of the tube. If there is not enough tension, the tube may leak gastric or intestinal drainage around exit site. If the tension is too great, the internal anchoring device may erode into the gastric wall (Friginal-Ruiz & Lucendo, 2015).
NURSING DIAGNOSIS	Determine the related factors for the nursing diagnoses based on the patient's current status. Possible nursing diagnoses may include: • Imbalanced nutrition, less than body requirements • Impaired skin integrity • Risk for infection
OUTCOME IDENTIFICATION AND PLANNING	The expected outcome to achieve when caring for a gastrostomy tube is that the patient does not exhibit signs and symptoms of irritation, excoriation, or infection at the tube insertion site. In addition, the patient verbalizes little discomfort related to tube placement and verbalizes an understanding of the care needed for the gastrostomy tube, as appropriate.

IMPLEMENTATION

ACTION	**RATIONALE**
1. Gather equipment. Verify the medical order or facility policy and procedure regarding site care.	Assembling equipment provides for an organized approach to the task. Verification ensures the patient receives the correct intervention.
2. Perform hand hygiene and put on PPE, if indicated.	Hand hygiene and PPE prevent the spread of microorganisms. PPE is required based on transmission precautions.

ACTION	**RATIONALE**

3. Identify the patient.

Identifying the patient ensures the right patient receives the intervention and helps prevent errors.

4. Explain the procedure to the patient. Answer any questions, as needed.

Explanation facilitates patient cooperation.

5. Assess for presence of pain at the tube-insertion site. If pain is present, offer the patient analgesic medication per the medical order and wait for medication absorption before beginning insertion site care.

Feeding tubes can be uncomfortable, especially in the first few days after insertion. Analgesic medication may permit the patient to tolerate the insertion site care more easily. After the first few days, it has been reported that the need for pain medication decreases.

6. Pull the patient's bedside curtain. Assemble equipment on the bedside table, within reach. Raise bed to a comfortable working position, usually elbow height of the caregiver (VHACEOSH, 2016).

Provide for privacy. Assembling equipment provides for organized approach to the task. Appropriate working height facilitates comfort and proper body mechanics for the nurse.

7. Put on gloves. Assess the gastrostomy site, as described above.

Gloves prevent contact with blood and body fluids. Assessment is vital to detect changes in the patient's condition before initiating the intervention.

8. Measure the length of exposed tube, comparing it with the initial measurement after insertion. Alternately, examine the mark on the tube at the skin; mark should be at skin level at the insertion site.

Tube length should be checked and compared with the initial measurement or marking. Change in the length of the exposed tube may indicate displacement.

9. For the first 10 days when the gastrostomy tube is new and still has sutures holding it in place, dip a cotton-tipped applicator into sterile saline solution and gently clean around the insertion site, removing any crust or drainage (Figure 1). **Avoid adjusting or lifting the external disk for the first few days after placement, except to clean the area.** After the first 10 days, or when the gastric tube insertion site has healed and the sutures are removed, wet a washcloth and apply a small amount of skin cleanser onto washcloth. Gently cleanse around the insertion, removing any crust or drainage (Figure 2). Rinse site, removing all soap.

Cleaning new site with sterile saline solution prevents the introduction of microorganisms into the wound (O'Rear & Prahlow, 2015). Crust and drainage can harbor bacteria and lead to skin breakdown. Removing cleanser helps to prevent skin irritation. If able, the patient may shower and cleanse the site with soap and water.

FIGURE 1. Wiping gastric tube site with cotton-tipped applicator and sterile saline.

FIGURE 2. Cleaning site with skin cleanser, water, and washcloth.

10. Pat skin around insertion site dry.

Drying the skin thoroughly prevents skin breakdown.

(continued)

Skill 11-4 ▶ Caring for a Gastrostomy Tube *(continued)*

ACTION	**RATIONALE**
11. If the sutures have been removed, gently push the tube forward toward the abdomen and rotate the tube. Gently rotate the guard or external bumper 90 degrees at least once a day (Figure 3). Assess that the guard or external bumper is not digging into the surrounding skin. Avoid placing any tension on the tube.	Rotation of the tube prevents adherence to the tract (Friginal-Ruiz & Lucendo, 2015; O'Rear & Prahlow, 2015). Rotation of the guard or external bumper prevents skin breakdown and pressure injuries.
	The risk of dislodgement is decreased when the tube has an external anchoring or bumper device.

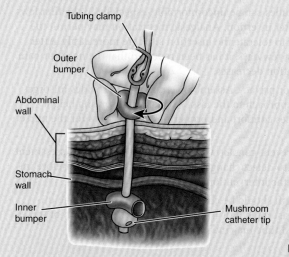

Tubing clamp
Outer bumper
Abdominal wall
Stomach wall
Inner bumper
Mushroom catheter tip

FIGURE 3. Gently turning or rotating guard or bumper 90 degrees.

12. Leave the site open to air unless there is drainage. If drainage is present, place one thickness of a precut gauze pad or drain sponge under the external bumper and change, as needed, to keep the area dry. Use a skin protectant or barrier cream to prevent skin breakdown.	The digestive enzymes from the gastric secretions may cause skin breakdown. Under normal conditions, expect only a minimal amount of drainage on a feeding tube dressing. Increased amounts of drainage should be explored for causes such as a possible gastric fluid leak.
13. If the tube is not in use, check that the cap is securely in place.	The cap should remain closed when the tube is not in use to deter entry of microorganisms and prevent leakage from the tube (Friginal-Ruiz & Lucendo, 2015).
14. Assess the integrity of the tape or device used to secure the tube to the stomach.	Securing tube prevents undue traction and pressure on the stoma site (Rollins, Nathwani, & Morrison, 2013).
15. Remove gloves. Lower the bed and assist the patient to a position of comfort, as needed.	Removing gloves reduces the risk for infection transmission and contamination of other items. Lowering bed and assisting patient ensure patient safety and comfort.
16. Remove additional PPE, if used. Perform hand hygiene.	Proper removal of PPE reduces the risk for infection transmission and contamination of other items. Hand hygiene prevents transmission of microorganisms.

EVALUATION   The expected outcomes have been met when the patient does not exhibit signs and symptoms of irritation, excoriation, or infection at the tube-insertion site; verbalizes little discomfort related to tube placement; and verbalizes an understanding of the care needed for the gastrostomy tube, as appropriate.

DOCUMENTATION

Guidelines   Document the care that was given, including the substance used to cleanse the tube site. Record the assessment of the site, including the surrounding skin and measurement of length of external tube and comparison to length on insertion. Note the presence of any drainage, recording the amount and color. Note the rotation of the tube and guard. Comment on the patient's response to the care, if the patient experienced any pain, and if an analgesic was administered. Record any patient instruction that was provided.

Sample Documentation

> <u>10/10/20</u> 1145 Gastrostomy tube site cleansed with skin cleanser and water. No change in measurement of tube length from initial measurement. Tube and guard rotated without difficulty. Site is of consistent tone with surrounding skin, without any signs of skin breakdown. Small amount of clear crust noted on tube. Patient tolerated without incident. Wife at bedside, actively participating in tube care.
>
> —S. Essner, RN

UNEXPECTED SITUATIONS AND ASSOCIATED INTERVENTIONS

- *Gastrostomy tube is leaking large amount of drainage:* Check tension of tube. If there is a large amount of slack between the internal guard and the external bumper, drainage can leak out of site. Apply gentle pressure to tube while pressing the external bumper closer to the skin. If the tube has an internal balloon holding it in place (similar to a urinary catheter balloon), check to make sure that the balloon is inflated properly.
- *Skin irritation is noted around insertion site:* If the skin is erythematous and appears to be broken down, gastric fluids may be leaking from the site. Gastric fluids have a low pH and are very acidic. Stop the leakage, as described above, and apply a skin barrier. If the skin has a patchy, red rash, the cause could be candidiasis (yeast). Notify the primary care provider for an order to apply an antifungal powder. Ensure that the site is kept dry.
- *Site appears erythematous and patient complains of pain at site:* Notify health care provider; patient could be developing cellulitis at the site.

SPECIAL CONSIDERATIONS

General Considerations

- Do not place a dressing between the skin and external fixation device unless drainage is present. Change the dressing immediately when soiled, to prevent skin complications.
- If length of exposed tube has changed or marking on tube is not visible, do not use the tube. Notify the patient's primary care provider of the finding.

Home Care Considerations

- Instruct patients on appropriate actions if the tube comes out. In the event the gastrostomy tube is pulled out, teach the patient to clean the area with water, cover the opening with a clean dressing, tape in place, and call the primary care provider immediately (Tracey & Patterson, 2006).
- Encourage patients to wear loose clothing to avoid applying pressure to the stoma (Friginal-Ruiz & Lucendo, 2015).

Enhance Your Understanding

Focusing on Patient Care: Developing Clinical Reasoning

Consider the case scenarios at the beginning of the chapter as you answer the following questions to enhance your understanding and apply what you have learned.

QUESTIONS

1. Ms. Williams tells the nurse that she hates hospital food and is too tired to eat. How can the nurse help Ms. Williams maintain her nutritional intake while recovering from her stroke?

2. Mr. Mason confides he is having "a lot of pain" in his throat and his nose feels "really sore." What assessments and nursing interventions should be a part of Mr. Mason's nursing care while he has the nasogastric tube?

3. The nurse is responsible for providing information to Cole and his family regarding home management of his gastrostomy tube and tube feedings. What information will the nurse include in the patient teaching?

You can find suggested answers after the Bibliography at the end of this chapter.

Enhance Your Understanding (Continued)

Integrated Case Study Connection

The case studies in the back of the book focus on integrating concepts. Refer to the following case studies to enhance your understanding of the concepts and skills in this chapter.

- Basic Case Studies: Claudia Tran, page 1106; Kate Townsend, page 1109.
- Advanced Case Studies: Cole McKean, page 1128; Robert Espinoza, page 1132.

Taylor Suite Resources

Explore these additional resources to enhance learning for this chapter:

- NCLEX-Style Questions and other resources on thePoint*, http://thePoint.lww.com/Lynn5e
- *Skill Checklists for Taylor's Clinical Nursing Skills,* 5e
- *Taylor's Video Guide to Clinical Nursing Skills:* Nutrition
- *Fundamentals of Nursing:* Chapter 36, Nutrition
- *Lippincott DocuCare* Fundamentals cases

Bibliography

Academy of Nutrition and Dietetics. (2013). Position paper. Position of the Academy of Nutrition and Dietetics: Ethical and legal issues in feeding and hydration. *Journal of the Academy of Nutrition and Dietetics, 113*(6), 828–833.

Allen, S. M. (2015). As a flushing agent for enteral nutrition, does sterile water compared to tap water affect the associated risk of infection in critically ill patients? *The Alabama Nurse, 42*(1), 5–6.

Alzheimer's Association. Alzheimer's and Dementia Caregiver Center. (n.d.). *Food, eating and Alzheimer's.* Retrieved https://www.alz.org/care/alzheimers-food-eating.asp

Amella, E. J., & Lawrence, J. F. (n.d.). *Eating and feeding issues in older adults with dementia. Part II: Interventions.* Retrieved https://consultgeri.org/try-this/dementia/issue-d11.2

Ball, L., Jansen, S., Desbrow, B., Morgan, K., Moyle, W., & Hughes, R. (2015). Experiences and nutrition support strategies in dementia care: Lessons from family carers. *Nutrition & Dietetics, 72*(1), 22–29.

Bankhead, R., Boullata, J., Brantley, S., et al; American Society for Parenteral and Enteral Nutrition (A.S.P.E.N.) Board of Directors. (2009). Enteral nutrition practice recommendations. *Journal of Parenteral and Enteral Nutrition, 33*(2), 122–167.

Best, C. (2013). Nasogastric feeding in the community: Safe and effective practice. *British Journal of Community Nursing, Nutrition Supplement,* S8–S12.

Blumenstein, I., Shastri, Y. M., & Stein, J. (2014). Gastroenteric tube feeding: Techniques, problems and solutions. *World Journal of Gastroenterology, 20*(26), 8505–8524.

Boeykens, K., Steeman, E., & Dyusburgh, I. (2014). Reliability of pH measurement and the auscultatory method to confirm the position of a nasogastric tube. *International Journal of Nursing Studies, 51*(11), 1427–1433.

Bourgault, A., Ipe, L., Weaver, J., Swartz, S., & O'Dea, P. J. (2007). Development of evidence-based guidelines and critical care nurses' knowledge of enteral feeding. *Critical Care Nurse, 27*(4), 17–29.

Brugnolli, A., Ambrosi, E., Canzan, F., & Saiani, L.; Naso-gastric Tube Group. (2014). Securing of nasogastric tubes in adult patients: A review. *International Journal of Nursing Studies, 51*(6), 943–950.

Catangui, E., Mejia, C., & Amorim, A. (2013). Development and implementation of a percutaneous endoscopic gastrostomy (PEG) nursing care plan. *British Journal of Neuroscience Nursing, 9*(6), 286–290.

Chapman, C., Barker, M., & Lawrence, W. (2015). Improving nutritional care: Innovation and good practice. *Journal of Advanced Nursing, 71*(4), 881–894.

Chau, J. P., Lo, S. H., Thompson, D. R., Fernandez, R., & Griffiths, R. (2011). Use of end-tidal carbon dioxide detection to determine correct placement of

nasogastric tube: A meta-analysis. *International Journal of Nursing Studies, 48*(4), 513–521.

Cheney, D. M., Siddiqui, T., Litts, J. K., Kuhn, M. A., & Belafsky, P. C. (2015). The ability of the 10-item Eating Assessment Tool (EAT-10) to predict aspiration risk in persons with dysphagia. *Annals of Otology, Rhinology, and Laryngology, 124*(5), 351–354.

Curtis, K. (2013). Caring for adult patients who require nasogastric feeding tubes. *Nursing Standard, 27*(38), 47–56.

Dark, J., & Sander, R. (2014). Dysphagia: Helping vulnerable people to eat and drink. *Nursing & Residential Care, 16*(8), 438–441.

Doenges, M. E., Moorhouse, M. F., & Murr, A. C. (2016). *Nursing diagnoses manual. Planning, individualizing, and documenting client care* (5th ed.). Philadelphia, PA: F.A. Davis Company.

Dudek, S. (2018). *Nutrition essentials for nursing practice* (8th ed.). Philadelphia, PA: Wolters Kluwer.

Edwards-Jones, V., & Leahy-Gilmartin, A. (2013). Care and maintenance of gastrostomy site infections. *Nursing & Residential Care, 15*(7), 470–475.

Eliopoulos, C. (2018). *Gerontological nursing* (9th ed.). Philadelphia, PA: Wolters Kluwer.

Fischbach, F., & Dunning, M. B. (2015). *A manual of laboratory and diagnostic tests* (9th ed.). Philadelphia, PA: Wolters Kluwer Health.

Fluids & electrolytes made incredibly easy (2015) (6th ed.). Philadelphia, PA: Wolters Kluwer Health.

Friginal-Ruiz, A. B., & Lucendo, A. J. (2015). Percutaneous endoscopic gastrostomy. A practical overview on its indications, placement conditions, management, and nursing care. *Gastroenterology Nursing, 38*(5), 354–366.

Gilbert, R. T., & Burns, S. M. (2012). Increasing the safety of blind gastric tube placement in pediatric patients: The design and testing of a procedure using a carbon dioxide detection device. *Journal of Pediatric Nursing, 27*(5), 528–532.

Grossman, S., & Porth, C. M. (2014). *Porth's pathophysiology: Concepts of altered health states* (9th ed.). Philadelphia, PA: Wolters Kluwer Health.

Hinkle, J. L., & Cheever, K. H. (2018). *Brunner & Suddarth's textbook of medical-surgical nursing* (14th ed.). Philadelphia, PA: Wolters Kluwer.

Irving, S. Y., Lyman, B., Northington, L., Bartlett, J. A., & Kemper, C.; Novel Project Work Group. (2014). Nasogastric tube placement and verification in children: Review of the current literature. *Critical Care Nurse, 34*(3), 67–78.

Jarvis, C. (2016). *Physical examination & health assessment* (7th ed.). St. Louis, MO: Elsevier.

Jensen, S. (2015). *Nursing Health Assessment: A best practice approach* (2nd ed.). Philadelphia, PA: Wolters Kluwer Health.

Kirk, L., Shelley, A., Battles, M., & Latty, C. (2014). Educating parents on gastrostomy devices: Necessary

components to achieve success. *Journal of Pediatric Nursing, 29*(5), 457–465.

Kyle, T., & Carman, S. (2017). *Essentials of pediatric nursing* (3rd ed.). Philadelphia, PA: Wolters Kluwer.

Liu, W., Galik, E., Bolz, M., Nahm, E. S., & Resnick, B. (2015). Optimizing eating performance of older adults with dementia living in long-term care: A systematic review. *Worldviews on Evidence-Based Nursing, 12*(4), 228–235.

McGinley, E. (2015). Practical nutritional measures in patients with dementia. *Journal of Community Nursing, 29*(6), 36–40.

Metheny, N. (n.d.). *Preventing aspiration in older adults with dysphagia.* Retrieved https://consultgeri.org/try-this/general-assessment/issue-20

Metheny, N. (2008). Residual volume measurement should be retained in enteral feeding protocols. *American Journal of Critical Care, 17*(1), 62–64.

Metheny, N. (2016a). AACN Practice Alert. Prevention of aspiration in adults. *Critical Care Nurse, 36*(1), e20–e24.

Metheny, N. (2016b). AACN Practice Alert. Initial and ongoing verification of feeding tube placement in adults (applies to blind insertions and placements with an electromagnetic device). *Critical Care Nurse, 36*(2), e8–e13.

Metheny, N. A., Mills, A. C., & Stewart, B. J. (2012). Monitoring for intolerance to gastric tube feedings: A national survey. *American Journal of Critical Care, 21*(2), e33–e40.

Morton, P. G., & Fontaine, D. K. (2018). *Critical care nursing. A holistic approach* (11th ed.). Philadelphia, PA: Wolters Kluwer.

Mueller, C., Compher, C., & Ellen, D. M.; American Society for Parenteral and Enteral Nutrition (A.S.P.E.N.) Board of Directors. (2011). A.S.P.E.N. clinical guidelines: Nutrition screening, assessment, and intervention in adults. *Journal of Parenteral and Enteral Nutrition, 35*(1), 16–24.

NANDA International, Inc.: Nursing Diagnoses - Definitions and Classification 2018–2020 © 2017 NANDA International, ISBN 978-1-62623-929-6. Used by arrangement with the Thieme Group, Stuttgart/New York.

O'Rear, J. M., & Prahlow, J. A. (2015). Early percutaneous endoscopic gastrostomy tube dislodgment. *American Journal of Nursing, 115*(6), 26–31.

Palmer, J., & Metheny, N. (2008). Preventing aspiration during nasogastric, nasointestinal, or gastrostomy tube feedings. *American Journal of Nursing, 108*(2), 40–48; quiz 49.

Perry, S. E., Hockenberry, M. J., Lowdermilk, D. L., & Wilson, D. (2014). *Maternal child nursing care* (5th ed.). St. Louis, MO: Elsevier Mosby.

Purnell, L. D. (2013). *Transcultural health care. A culturally competent approach* (4th ed.). Philadelphia, PA: F.A. Davis Company.

Rahimi, M., Farhadi, K., Ashtarian, H., & Changaei, F. (2015). Confirming nasogastric tube position: Methods and restrictions. A narrative review. *Journal of Nursing and Midwifery Sciences, 2*(1), 55–62.

Relph, W. L. (2015). Addressing the nutritional needs of older patients. *Nursing Older People, 28*(3), 16–19.

Riesenberg, L. A., Berg, K., Berg, D., et al. (2013). The development of a validated checklist for nasogastric tube insertion: Preliminary results. *American Journal of Medical Quality, 28*(5), 429–433.

Rollins, H., Nathwani, N., & Morrison, D. (2013). Optimising wound care in a child with an infected gastrostomy exit site. *British Journal of Nursing, 22*(22), 1275–1279.

Stepter, C. R. (2012). Maintaining placement of temporary enteral feeding tubes in adults: A critical appraisal of the evidence. *Medsurg Nursing, 21*(2), 61–68.

Taylor, C., Lynn, P., & Bartlett, J. (2019). *Fundamentals of nursing: The art and science of person-centered care* (9th ed.). Philadelphia, PA: Wolters Kluwer.

Taylor, S. J., Allan, K., McWilliam, H., & Toher, D. (2014). Nasogastric tube depth: The 'NEX' guideline is incorrect. *British Journal of Nursing, 23*(12), 641–644.

Tracey, D., & Patterson, G. (2006). Care of the gastrostomy tube in the home. *Home Healthcare Nurse, 24*(6), 381–386.

Turgay, A. S., & Khorshid, L. (2010). Effectiveness of the auscultatory and pH methods in predicting feeding tube placement. *Journal of Clinical Nursing, 19*(11–12), 1553–1559.

VHA Center for Engineering & Occupational Safety and Health (CEOSH). (2016). *Safe patient handling and mobility guidebook.* St. Louis, MO: Author. Retrieved http://www.tampavaref.org/safe-patient-handling.htm

SUGGESTED ANSWERS FOR FOCUSING ON PATIENT CARE: DEVELOPING CLINICAL REASONING

1. Explore the patient's usual food preferences and habits. Choose foods that the patient prefers from facility menus. In addition, encourage Ms. Williams' family to bring favorite foods from home. Food choices should focus on foods that are easy to eat and nutrient dense. Provide rest periods before mealtimes, so she is not overly tired. Assist the patient to a comfortable position for meals, help her with hand hygiene, and ensure she has clean dentures in place, and her glasses, as appropriate. Encourage her family to visit during mealtimes, to provide as normal a social environment as possible. Cut food and open packages as necessary, to limit the amount of exertion by the patient. Suggest she eat small portions, keeping some food items to snack on as the day progresses. Frequent small servings are not as tiring. Allow enough time for the patient to chew and swallow the food adequately. The patient may need to rest for short periods during eating. If Ms. Williams is agreeable, feed her a portion of the meal, to avoid overtiring.

2. Assess the patient's level of comfort every 4 hours and PRN. Offer analgesic as prescribed. Offer oral hygiene at least every 4 hours or more often. Discuss the potential for topical analgesic, such as analgesic throat spray, with the patient's health care provider. Reassess pain after interventions. Assess the patient's oral and nasal mucous membranes, as well as nasal skin, at least every shift. Ensure the tape anchoring the tube is not pulled taut, creating pressure on the nose. Retape/secure the NG tube with new commercially prepared device or tape every 24 hours; clean skin thoroughly and apply skin barrier. Retape in a slightly different position to prevent excessive pressure in one area of nostril.

3. Patients who are caring for a gastrostomy tube at home should understand the care of the tube, tube site, nutritional feeding routine, and potential adverse effects, with the accompanying actions. Provide Cole and his family with the date his tube was placed, the procedure used to place the tube, the tube size, how the tube is anchored, and the calibration measurement at skin level or the length of the external tube. Discuss, provide written information, and obtain a return demonstration for the care of the tube and tube site, as well as the feeding procedure. Teaching should include the formula type, frequency, rate of infusion, checking tube placement, and checking gastric residual, based on prescribed therapeutic regimen. Review infection control measures, such as handwashing before starting, refrigerating formula between use, disposing of unused formula after 24 hours, and measuring out only 4 hours of formula at a time. The length of the tube or calibration mark at the skin should be checked prior to each feeding or use of the tube. Cole should be in a sitting position for the feeding and for 1 hour afterward. Skin care for tube site includes washing the area with the cleansing agent identified by the health care provider or facility policy, rinsing, and patting dry. Cole should assess the site daily for swelling, redness, or yellow/green drainage. Cole and his family should verbalize an understanding of these instructions, as well as a knowledge of signs and symptoms that should be reported to their health care provider. These include the presence of nausea or vomiting, pain, fever, and residual in excess of identified limits. Cole and his family should also understand proper procedure if the gastrostomy tube should come out or become dislodged.

Urinary Elimination

Focusing on Patient Care

This chapter will help you develop some of the skills related to urinary elimination that may be necessary to care for the following patients:

Ralph Bellows, age 73, has been admitted with a stroke. Due to incontinence and skin breakdown, Ralph's nurse has decided to include the application of an external urinary sheath (condom catheter) in his plan of care.

Grace Halligan, age 24, is pregnant and has been placed on bed rest. She needs to void, but cannot get out of bed.

Mike Wimmer, age 36, receives peritoneal dialysis. Mike has noticed that the insertion site around his catheter is becoming tender and reddened.

Refer to Focusing on Patient Care: Developing Clinical Reasoning at the end of the chapter to apply what you learn.

Learning Objectives

After completing the chapter, you will be able to accomplish the following:

1. Assist with the use of a bedpan.
2. Assist with use of a urinal.
3. Assist with use of a bedside commode.
4. Assess bladder volume using an ultrasound bladder scanner.
5. Apply an external urinary sheath (condom catheter).
6. Catheterize a female patient's urinary bladder.
7. Catheterize a male patient's urinary bladder.
8. Remove an indwelling urinary catheter.
9. Administer intermittent closed catheter irrigation.
10. Administer continuous closed bladder irrigation.
11. Empty and change a stoma appliance on a urinary diversion.
12. Care for a suprapubic urinary catheter.
13. Care for a peritoneal dialysis catheter.
14. Care for hemodialysis access.

Key Terms

arteriovenous fistula: a surgically created passage connecting an artery and a vein; used in hemodialysis

arteriovenous graft: a surgically created connection between an artery and vein using synthetic material; used in hemodialysis

bruit: a sound caused by turbulent blood flow

external urinary sheath (condom catheter): soft, pliable sheath made of silicone material, applied externally to the penis, connected to drainage tubing and a collection bag

fenestrated: having a window-like opening

hemodialysis: removal from the body, by means of blood filtration, of toxins and fluid that are normally removed by the kidneys

ileal conduit: a surgical diversion formed by bringing the ureters to the ileum; urine is excreted through a stoma

indwelling urethral catheter (retention or Foley catheter): a catheter (tube) through the urethra into the bladder for the purpose of continuous drainage of urine; a balloon is inflated to ensure that the catheter remains in the bladder once it is inserted

intermittent urethral catheter (straight catheter): a catheter through the urethra into the bladder to drain urine for a short period of time (5 to 10 minutes)

peritoneal dialysis: removal of toxins and fluid from the body by the principles of diffusion and osmosis; accomplished by introducing a solution (dialysate) into the peritoneal cavity

peritonitis: inflammation of the peritoneal membrane

sediment: precipitate found at the bottom of a container of urine

stoma: artificial opening on the body surface

suprapubic urinary catheter: a urinary catheter surgically inserted through a small incision above the pubic area into the bladder

symphysis pubis: the anterior midline junction of the pubic bones; the bony projection under the pubic hair

thrill: palpable feeling caused by turbulent blood flow

U rine is excreted from the kidneys via the ureters to the bladder, where it is stored and eliminated via the urethra. Elimination from the urinary tract helps to rid the body of waste products and materials that exceed bodily needs. Numerous factors affect the amount and quality of urine produced by the body and the manner in which it is excreted. Some patients experience urinary elimination problems affecting fluid and electrolyte balance, hydration, skin integrity, comfort, and self-concept. Many health problems, medications, and health care interventions can affect urinary elimination. Nurses play an important role in preventing and managing urinary elimination problems.

This chapter covers skills that the nurse may use to promote urinary elimination. An assessment of the urinary system is required as part of providing interventions outlined in many of these skills. Refer to Fundamentals Review 12-1 for a review of the male and female genitourinary tract. Fundamentals Review 12-2 summarizes factors that may affect urinary elimination.

Fundamentals Review 12-1

ANATOMY OF THE GENITOURINARY TRACT

- The main components of the urinary tract are the kidneys, ureters, bladder, and urethra.
- The average female urethra is 1.5 to 2.5 in (3.7 to 6.2 cm) long; the average male urethra is 7 to 8 in (18 to 20 cm) long.

- The average age at which men begin to have prostatic enlargement is 50.

Female urinary tract

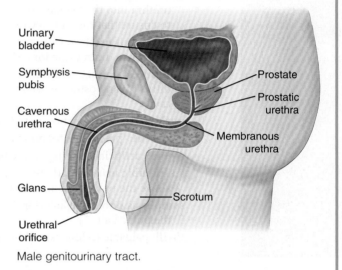

Male genitourinary tract.

Fundamentals Review 12-2

FACTORS AFFECTING URINARY ELIMINATION

Numerous factors affect the amount and quality of urine produced by the body and the manner in which it is excreted.

EFFECTS OF AGING

- Diminished ability of kidneys to concentrate urine may result in nocturia.
- Decreased bladder muscle tone may reduce the capacity of the bladder to hold urine, resulting in increased frequency of urination.
- Decreased bladder contractility leading to urine retention and stasis with an increased risk of urinary tract infection (UTI).
- Neuromuscular problems, degenerative joint problems, alterations in thought processes, and weakness may interfere with voluntary control of urination and the ability to reach a toilet in time.

FOOD AND FLUID INTAKE

- Dehydration leads to increased fluid reabsorption by the kidneys, leading to decreased and concentrated urine production.

- Fluid overload leads to excretion of a large quantity of dilute urine.
- Consumption of alcoholic beverages leads to increased urine production due to their inhibition of antidiuretic hormone release.
- Ingestion of foods high in water content may increase urine production.
- Ingestion of foods and beverages high in sodium content leads to decreased urine formation due to sodium and water reabsorption and retention.
- Ingestion of certain foods (e.g., asparagus, onions, beets) may lead to alterations in the odor or color of urine.

PSYCHOLOGICAL VARIABLES

- Individual, family, and sociocultural variables may influence voiding habits.
- Patients may view voiding as a personal and private act. The need to ask for assistance may lead to embarrassment and/or anxiety.
- Stress may lead to voiding of smaller amounts of urine at more frequent intervals.

Fundamentals Review 12-2 continued

FACTORS AFFECTING URINARY ELIMINATION

- Stress may lead to difficulty emptying the bladder due to its effects on relaxation of perineal muscles and the external urethral sphincter.

ACTIVITY AND MUSCLE TONE

- Regular exercise increases metabolism and optimal urine production and elimination.
- Prolonged periods of immobility may lead to poor urinary control and urinary stasis due to decreased bladder and sphincter tone.
- Use of indwelling urinary catheters leads to loss of bladder tone because the bladder muscle is not being stretched by filling with urine.
- Childbearing, muscle atrophy related to menopausal hormonal changes, and trauma-related muscle damage lead to decreased muscle tone.

PATHOLOGIC CONDITIONS

- Congenital urinary tract abnormalities, polycystic kidney disease, urinary tract infection, urinary calculi (kidney stones), hypertension, diabetes mellitus, gout, and certain connective tissue disorders lead to altered quantity and quality of urine.
- Diseases that reduce physical activity or lead to generalized weakness (e.g., arthritis, Parkinson's disease, degenerative joint disease) interfere with toileting.
- Cognitive deficits and psychiatric conditions may interfere with ability or desire to control urination voluntarily.
- Fever and diaphoresis (profuse perspiration) lead to conservation of body fluids.

- Other pathologic conditions, such as congestive heart failure, may lead to fluid retention and decreased urine output.
- High blood–glucose levels, such as with diabetes mellitus, may lead to increased urine output due to osmotic diuresis.

MEDICATIONS

- Abuse of analgesics, such as aspirin or ibuprofen, can cause kidney damage (nephrotoxic).
- Use of some antibiotics, such as gentamicin, can cause kidney damage.
- Use of diuretics can lead to moderate to severe increases in production and excretion of dilute urine, related to their prevention of water and certain electrolyte reabsorption in the renal tubules.
- Use of cholinergic medications may lead to increased urination due to stimulation of detrusor muscle contraction.
- Use of some analgesics, sedatives, and tranquilizers interferes with urination due to the diminished effectiveness of the neural reflex for voiding because of suppression of the central nervous system.
- Use of certain drugs causes changes to the color of urine. Anticoagulants may cause hematuria (blood in the urine) or a pink or red color. Diuretics can lighten the color of urine to pale yellow. Phenazopyridine can cause orange or orange-red urine. Amitriptyline and B-complex vitamins can cause green or blue-green urine. Levodopa (L-dopa) and injectable iron compounds can cause brown or black urine.

Skill 12-1 ▶ Assisting With the Use of a Bedpan

Patients who cannot get out of bed because of physical limitations or medical orders need to use a bedpan or urinal for voiding. Male patients confined to bed usually prefer to use the urinal for voiding (see Skill 12-2) and the bedpan for defecation; female patients usually prefer to use the bedpan for both. Many patients find it difficult and embarrassing to use the bedpan. When a patient uses a bedpan, promote comfort and normalcy and respect the patient's privacy as much as possible. Be sure to maintain a professional manner. In addition, provide skin care, perineal hygiene, and hand hygiene after bedpan use.

Regular bedpans have a rounded, smooth upper end and a tapered, open lower end. The upper end fits under the patient's buttocks toward the sacrum, with the open end toward the foot of the bed (Figure 1A). A special bedpan called a *fracture bedpan* is frequently used for patients with fractures of the femur or lower spine. Smaller and flatter than the ordinary bedpan, this type of bedpan

(continued)

Skill 12-1 ▶ Assisting With the Use of a Bedpan *(continued)*

is helpful for patients who cannot easily raise themselves onto the regular bedpan (see Figure 1B). The fracture pan has a shallow, narrow upper end with a flat wide rim, and a deeper, open lower end. The upper end fits under the patient's buttocks toward the sacrum, with the deeper, open lower end toward the foot of the bed.

A. Regular bedpan

B. Fracture pan

FIGURE 1. A. Standard bedpan. Position a standard bedpan like a regular toilet seat—the buttocks are placed on the wide, rounded shelf, with the open end pointed toward the foot of the bed. **B.** Fracture pan. Position a fracture pan with the thin edge toward the head of the bed.

DELEGATION CONSIDERATIONS	Assisting a patient with the use of a bedpan may be delegated to nursing assistive personnel (NAP) or to unlicensed assistive personnel (UAP), as well as to licensed practical/vocational nurses (LPN/LVNs). The decision to delegate must be based on careful analysis of the patient's needs and circumstances, as well as the qualifications of the person to whom the task is being delegated. Refer to the Delegation Guidelines in Appendix A.
EQUIPMENT	• Bedpan (regular or fracture) • Toilet tissue • Disposable clean gloves • Additional PPE, as indicated • Cover for bedpan or urinal (disposable waterproof pad or cover) • Disposable washcloths and skin cleanser • Moist towelettes, skin cleanser and water, or hand sanitizer
ASSESSMENT	Assess the patient's usual elimination habits. Determine why the patient needs to use a bedpan (e.g., a medical order for strict bed rest or immobilization). Also assess the patient's degree of limitation and ability to help with activity. Assess for health problems, such as hip surgery or spinal injury, which would contraindicate certain actions by the patient. Check for the presence of drains, dressings, intravenous fluid infusion sites/equipment, traction, or any other devices that could interfere with the patient's ability to help with the procedure or that could become dislodged. Assess the characteristics of the urine and the patient's skin.
NURSING DIAGNOSIS	Determine the related factors for the nursing diagnoses based on the patient's current status. Appropriate nursing diagnoses may include: • Risk for urge urinary incontinence • Toileting self-care deficit • Impaired urinary elimination

OUTCOME IDENTIFICATION AND PLANNING

The expected outcome to achieve when offering a bedpan is that the patient is able to void with assistance. Other appropriate outcomes may include the following: the patient maintains continence; the patient demonstrates how to use the bedpan with assistance; and the patient maintains skin integrity.

IMPLEMENTATION

ACTION	RATIONALE
1. Review the patient's medical record for any limitations in physical activity (see Skill Variation: Assisting With Use of a Bedpan When the Patient Has Limited Movement). Gather equipment.	Activity limitations may contraindicate certain actions by the patient. Assembling equipment provides for an organized approach to the task.
2. Perform hand hygiene and put on PPE, if indicated.	Hand hygiene and PPE prevent the spread of microorganisms. PPE is required based on transmission precautions.
3. Identify the patient.	Identifying the patient ensures the right patient receives the intervention and helps prevent errors.
4. Assemble equipment on a chair next to the bed within reach.	Arranging items nearby is convenient, saves time, and avoids unnecessary stretching and twisting of muscles on the part of the nurse.
5. Close curtains around the bed and close the door to the room, if possible. Discuss the procedure with the patient and assess the patient's ability to assist with the procedure, as well as personal hygiene preferences.	This ensures the patient's privacy. Discussion promotes reassurance and provides knowledge about the procedure. Dialogue encourages patient participation and allows for individualized nursing care.
6. Unless contraindicated, apply powder to the rim of the bedpan. Place bedpan and cover on a chair next to the bed. Put on gloves.	Powder helps keep the bedpan from sticking to the patient's skin and makes it easier to remove. Powder is not applied if the patient has respiratory problems, is allergic to powder, or if a urine specimen is needed (could contaminate the specimen). The bedpan on the chair allows for easy access. Gloves prevent contact with blood and body fluids.
7. Adjust the bed to a comfortable working height, usually elbow height of the caregiver (VHACEOSH, 2016). Place the patient in a supine position, with the head of the bed elevated about 30 degrees, unless contraindicated.	Having the bed at the proper height prevents back and muscle strain. Supine position is necessary for correct placement of the patient on the bedpan.
8. Fold top linen back just enough to allow placement of bedpan. If there is no waterproof pad on the bed and time allows, consider placing a waterproof pad under the patient's buttocks before placing the bedpan (Figure 2).	Folding back the linen in this manner minimizes unnecessary exposure while still allowing the nurse to place the bedpan. The waterproof pad will protect the bed should there be a spill.

FIGURE 2. Placing waterproof pad under patient's buttocks. (*Note: Covers should be folded back just enough to work, not expose patient unnecessarily. Covers in this series of photos have been pulled back to show action.*)

(*continued*)

Skill 12-1 ▶ Assisting With the Use of a Bedpan *(continued)*

ACTION	RATIONALE
9. Ask the patient to bend the knees. Have the patient lift his/her hips upward. Assist the patient, if necessary, by placing your hand that is closest to the patient palm up, under the lower back, and assist with lifting. Slip the bedpan into place with the other hand (Figure 3).	The nurse uses less energy when the patient can assist by placing some of his/her weight on the heels.
10. **Ensure that the bedpan is in proper position and the patient's buttocks are resting on the rounded shelf of the regular bedpan or the shallow rim of the fracture bedpan.**	Having the bedpan in the proper position prevents spills onto the bed, ensures patient comfort, and prevents injury to the skin from a misplaced bedpan.
11. Raise the head of the bed as near to sitting position as tolerated, unless contraindicated. Cover the patient with bed linens.	This position makes it easier for the patient to void or defecate, avoids strain on the patient's back, and allows gravity to aid in elimination. Covering promotes warmth and privacy.
12. **Place the call bell and toilet tissue within easy reach. Place the bed in the lowest position.** Leave the patient if it is safe to do so. Use side rails appropriately (Figure 4).	Falls can be prevented if the patient does not have to reach for items he or she needs. Placing the bed in the lowest position promotes patient safety. Leaving the patient alone, if possible, promotes self-esteem and shows respect for privacy. Side rails assist the patient in repositioning.

FIGURE 3. Assisting patient to raise hips upward and positioning the bedpan. (*Note: Covers should be folded back just enough to work, not expose patient unnecessarily. Covers in this series of photos have been pulled back to show action.*)

FIGURE 4. Placing call bell within patient's reach and handing patient toilet tissue.

13. Remove gloves and additional PPE, if used. Perform hand hygiene.

Proper removal of PPE prevents transmission of microorganisms. Hand hygiene deters the spread of microorganisms.

Removing the Bedpan

14. Perform hand hygiene and put on gloves and additional PPE, as indicated. Adjust the bed to a comfortable working height, usually elbow height of the caregiver (VHACEOSH, 2016). Have a receptacle, such as plastic trash bag, handy for discarding tissue.

Hand hygiene deters the spread of microorganisms. Gloves prevent exposure to blood and body fluids. Having the bed at the proper height prevents back and muscle strain. Proper disposal of soiled tissue prevents transmission of microorganisms.

15. Lower the head of the bed, if necessary, to about 30 degrees. Remove bedpan in the same manner in which it was offered, being careful to hold it steady. Ask the patient to bend the knees and lift the buttocks up from the bedpan. Assist the patient, if necessary, by placing your hand that is closest to the patient palm up, under the lower back, and assist with lifting. Place the bedpan on the bedside chair and cover it.

Holding the bedpan steady prevents spills. The nurse uses less energy when the patient can assist by placing some of his/her weight on the heels. Covering the bedpan helps to prevent the spread of microorganisms.

ACTION	**RATIONALE**
16. If the patient needs assistance with hygiene, wrap tissue around the hand several times, and wipe the patient clean, using one stroke from the pubic area toward the anal area. Discard tissue. Use warm, moist disposable washcloth and skin cleanser to clean the perineal area. Place the patient on his or her side and spread buttocks to clean the anal area.	Cleaning area from the front to back minimizes fecal contamination of the vagina and urinary meatus. Cleaning the patient after he or she has used the bedpan prevents offensive odors and skin irritation.
17. Do not place toilet tissue in the bedpan if a specimen is required or if output is being recorded. Place toilet tissue in an appropriate receptacle.	Mixing toilet tissue with a specimen makes laboratory examination more difficult and interferes with accurate output measurement.
18. Return the patient to a comfortable position. Make sure the linens under the patient are dry. Replace or remove the pad under the patient, as necessary. Remove your gloves and ensure that the patient is covered.	Positioning helps to promote patient comfort. Removing contaminated gloves prevents the spread of microorganisms.
19. Raise side rail. Lower bed height and adjust the head of the bed to a comfortable position. Reattach call bell.	These actions promote patient safety.
20. Offer patient supplies to wash and dry his/her hands, assisting as necessary.	Washing hands after using the urinal helps prevent the spread of microorganisms.
21. Put on clean gloves. Empty and clean the bedpan, measuring urine in graduated container, as necessary. Discard the trash receptacle with used toilet paper per facility policy.	Gloves prevent exposure to blood and body fluids. Cleaning reusable equipment helps prevent the spread of microorganisms.
22. Remove additional PPE, if used. Perform hand hygiene.	Proper removal of PPE reduces the risk for infection transmission and contamination of other items. Hand hygiene prevents the spread of microorganisms.

EVALUATION

The expected outcome has been met when the patient voids using the bedpan. Other outcomes have been met when the patient remains dry; the patient does not experience episodes of incontinence; the patient demonstrates measures to assist with using the bedpan; and the patient does not experience impaired skin integrity.

DOCUMENTATION

Guidelines

Document the patient's tolerance of the activity. Record the amount of urine voided on the intake and output record, if appropriate. Document any other assessments, such as unusual urine characteristics or alterations in the patient's skin.

Sample Documentation

12/06/20 0730 Patient placed on fracture bedpan with a two-person assist. Voided 400-mL dark yellow urine; strong odor noted. Perineal skin intact, without redness or irritation. Specimen sent for urinalysis as ordered.

—S. Barnes, RN

SPECIAL CONSIDERATIONS

- A fracture bedpan is usually more comfortable for the patient, but it does not hold as large a volume as the regular bedpan (see Figure 1).
- Very thin or older adult patients often find it easier and more comfortable to use the fracture bedpan.
- Bedpan should not be left in place for extended periods because this can result in excessive pressure and irritation to the patient's skin.

(continued)

Skill 12-1 ▶ Assisting With the Use of a Bedpan *(continued)*

Skill Variation ▶ Assisting With Use of a Bedpan When the Patient Has Limited Movement

Patients who are unable to lift themselves onto the bedpan or who have activity limitations that prohibit the required actions can be assisted onto the bedpan in an alternate manner using these actions:

1. Review patient's chart for any limitations in physical activity. Gather equipment.

2. Put on PPE, as indicated, and perform hand hygiene. Check the patient's identification band.

FIGURE A. Rolling patient on side to place bedpan. (*Note: Covers should be folded back just enough to work, not expose patient unnecessarily. Covers in photo pulled back to show action for photo.*)

3. Place bedpan and cover on chair next to bed. Close curtains around the bed and close the door to the room, if possible.
4. Discuss procedure with the patient and assess the patient's ability to assist with the procedure, as well as personal hygiene preferences.
5. Unless contraindicated, apply powder to the rim of the bedpan.
6. Adjust the bed to a comfortable working height, usually elbow height of the caregiver (VHACEOSH, 2016). Place the patient in a supine position, with the head of the bed elevated about 30 degrees, unless contraindicated. Put on disposable gloves.
7. Fold top linen just enough to turn the patient, while minimizing exposure. If no waterproof pad is on the bed and time allows, consider placing a waterproof pad under patient's buttocks before placing bedpan.
8. Assist the patient to roll to the opposite side or turn the patient into a side-lying position.
9. Hold the bedpan firmly against the patient's buttocks, with the upper end of the bedpan under the patient's buttocks toward the sacrum, and down into the mattress (Figure A).
10. Keep one hand against the bedpan. Apply gentle pressure to ensure the bedpan remains in place as you assist the patient to roll back onto the bedpan.
11. Ensure that the bedpan is in the proper position and the patient's buttocks are resting on rounded shelf of the regular bedpan or the shallow rim of the fracture bedpan.
12. Raise the head of bed as near to sitting position as tolerated, unless contraindicated. Cover the patient with bed linens.
13. Place call bell and toilet tissue within easy reach. Place the bed in the lowest position. Leave the patient if it is safe to do so. Use side rails appropriately.

14. Remove gloves, and PPE, if used. Perform hand hygiene.
15. To remove the bedpan, perform hand hygiene and put on disposable gloves, and additional PPE, as indicated. Raise the bed to a comfortable working height. Have a receptacle handy for discarding tissue.
16. Lower the head of the bed. Grasp the closest side of the bedpan. Apply gentle pressure to hold the bedpan flat and steady. Assist the patient to roll to the opposite side or turn the patient into a side-lying position with the assistance of a second caregiver. Remove the bedpan and set on chair. Cover the bedpan.
17. If patient needs assistance with hygiene, wrap tissue around the hand several times, and wipe patient clean, using one stroke from the pubic area toward the anal area. Discard tissue. Use warm, moist disposable washcloth and skin cleanser to clean perineal area. Place patient on his/her side and spread buttocks to clean anal area.
18. Return the patient to a comfortable position. Make sure the linens under the patient are dry and that the patient is covered.
19. Remove your gloves. Offer the patient supplies to wash and dry his/her hands, assisting as necessary.
20. Raise side rail. Lower bed height and adjust head of bed to a comfortable position. Reattach call bell.
21. Put on clean gloves. Empty and clean the bedpan, measuring urine in graduated container, as necessary. Remove gloves and additional PPE, if used. Perform hand hygiene.

EVIDENCE
FOR PRACTICE ▶

PATIENT EXPERIENCES WITH BEDPANS

Urinary and bowel elimination are intimate acts. The use of a bedpan to meet elimination needs impacts the privacy, dignity, and respect of patients. The use of bedpans in acute care and community settings remains common. What are the experiences of patients making use of bedpans?

Related Research

Gattinger, H., Werner, B., & Saxer, S. (2013). Patient experience with bedpans in acute care: A cross-sectional study. *Journal of Clinical Nursing, 22*(15–16), 2216–2224.

This descriptive quantitative study examined the individual experiences of patients using the bedpan in an acute care setting. A convenience sample of 78 patients completed a standardized questionnaire, collecting data related to frequency of bedpan use and the extent of inconvenient experiences related to bedpan use. The authors reported that most participants related feeling dependent on other people and no autonomous movement was possible while using the bedpan. Inconvenient experiences reported by participants included pain, unpleasant characteristics of the bedpan, including coldness and hardness, uncomfortable positions, lack of privacy, and hygiene inconveniences, such as wet skin and fears that urine would miss the bedpan. The authors concluded that nurses can address negative experiences associated with bedpan use by considering multiple courses of action when caring for patients who are dependent on use of a bedpan.

Relevance for Nursing Practice

Nurses and nursing staff are the primary providers of interventions related to meeting elimination needs in many health care settings. Nurses should consider the implementation of appropriate interventions to enhance patient experiences related to meeting urinary and bowel elimination and personal hygiene.

Refer to thePoint° for additional research on related nursing topics.

Skill 12-2 ▶ Assisting With the Use of a Urinal

Male patients confined to bed usually prefer to use the urinal (Figure 1) for voiding as a matter of convenience. Alternately, use of a urinal in the standing position facilitates emptying of the bladder. Patients who are unable to stand alone may benefit from assistance when voiding into a urinal. If the patient is unable to stand, the urinal may be used in bed. Patients may also use a urinal in the bathroom to facilitate measurement of urinary output. Many patients find it embarrassing to use the

FIGURE 1. Urinal.

(continued)

Skill 12-2 ▶ Assisting With the Use of a Urinal *(continued)*

urinal. Promote comfort and normalcy as much as possible, while respecting the patient's privacy. Provide skin care, perineal hygiene, and hand hygiene after urinal use and maintain a professional manner.

DELEGATION CONSIDERATIONS	Assisting a patient with the use of a urinal may be delegated to nursing assistive personnel (NAP) or to unlicensed assistive personnel (UAP), as well as to licensed practical/vocational nurses (LPN/LVNs). The decision to delegate must be based on careful analysis of the patient's needs and circumstances, as well as the qualifications of the person to whom the task is being delegated. Refer to the Delegation Guidelines in Appendix A.
EQUIPMENT	• Urinal with end cover (usually attached) • Toilet tissue • Clean gloves • Additional PPE, as indicated • Disposable washcloths and skin cleanser • Moist towelettes, skin cleanser and water, or hand sanitizer
ASSESSMENT	Assess the patient's usual elimination habits. Determine why the patient needs to use a urinal (e.g., a medical order for strict bed rest or immobilization). Also assess the patient's degree of limitation and ability to help with activity. Assess for health problems, such as hip surgery or spinal injury, which would contraindicate certain actions by the patient. Check for the presence of drains, dressings, intravenous fluid infusion sites/equipment, traction, or any other devices that could interfere with the patient's ability to help with the procedure or that could become dislodged. Assess the characteristics of the urine and the patient's skin.
NURSING DIAGNOSIS	Determine the related factors for the nursing diagnoses based on the patient's current status. Appropriate nursing diagnoses may include: • Urge urinary incontinence • Toileting self-care deficit • Impaired urinary elimination
OUTCOME IDENTIFICATION AND PLANNING	The expected outcome to achieve when offering a urinal is that the patient is able to void with assistance. Other appropriate outcomes may include the following: the patient maintains continence; the patient demonstrates how to use the urinal; and the patient maintains skin integrity.

IMPLEMENTATION

ACTION	RATIONALE
1. Review the patient's medical record for any limitations in physical activity. Gather equipment.	Activity limitations may contraindicate certain actions by the patient. Assembling equipment provides for an organized approach to the task.
2. Perform hand hygiene and put on PPE, if indicated.	Hand hygiene and PPE prevent the spread of microorganisms. PPE is required based on transmission precautions.
3. Identify the patient.	Identifying the patient ensures the right patient receives the intervention and helps prevent errors.
4. Assemble equipment on a chair next to the bed within reach.	Arranging items nearby is convenient, saves time, and avoids unnecessary stretching and twisting of muscles on the part of the nurse.

ACTION

5. Close the curtains around the bed and close the door to the room, if possible. Discuss the procedure with the patient and assess the patient's ability to assist with the procedure, as well as personal hygiene preferences.

6. Put on gloves.

7. Assist the patient to an appropriate position, as necessary: standing at the bedside, lying on one side or back, sitting in bed with the head elevated, or sitting on the side of the bed.

8. If the patient remains in the bed, fold the linens just enough to allow for proper placement of the urinal.

9. If the patient is not standing, have him spread his legs slightly. **Hold the urinal close to the penis and position the penis completely within the urinal (Figure 2). Keep the bottom of the urinal lower than the penis. If necessary, assist the patient to hold the urinal in place.**

RATIONALE

This ensures the patient's privacy. Discussion promotes reassurance and provides knowledge about the procedure. Dialogue encourages patient participation and allows for individualized nursing care.

Gloves prevent exposure to blood and body fluids.

These positions facilitate voiding and emptying of the bladder.

Folding back the linen in this manner minimizes unnecessary exposure while still allowing the nurse to place the urinal.

Slight spreading of the legs allows for proper positioning of the urinal. Placing the penis completely within the urinal and keeping the bottom lower than the penis avoids urine spills.

FIGURE 2. Positioning urinal in place for a male patient. (*Note: Covers should be folded back just enough to work, not expose patient unnecessarily. Covers have been pulled back to show action.*)

10. Cover the patient with the bed linens.

11. Place the call bell and toilet tissue within easy reach. Have a receptacle, such as a plastic trash bag, handy for discarding tissue. Ensure the bed is in the lowest position. Leave patient if it is safe to do so. Use side rails appropriately.

 12. Remove gloves and additional PPE, if used. Perform hand hygiene.

Covering promotes warmth and privacy.

Falls can be prevented if the patient does not have to reach for items he needs. Placing the bed in the lowest position promotes patient safety. Leaving the patient alone, if possible, promotes self-esteem and shows respect for privacy. Side rails assist the patient in repositioning.

Proper removal of PPE reduces transmission of microorganisms. Hand hygiene deters the spread of microorganisms.

Removing the Urinal

 13. Perform hand hygiene. Put on gloves and additional PPE, as indicated.

Hand hygiene and PPE prevent the spread of microorganisms. Gloves prevent exposure to blood and body fluids. PPE is required based on transmission precautions.

(continued)

Skill 12-2 ▶ Assisting With the Use of a Urinal *(continued)*

ACTION	RATIONALE
14. Pull back the patient's bed linens just enough to remove the urinal. Remove the urinal. Cover the open end of the urinal. Place on the bedside chair. If the patient needs assistance with hygiene, wrap tissue around the hand several times, and wipe the patient dry. Place tissue in a receptacle. Use warm, moist disposable washcloth and skin cleanser to clean perineal area, as necessary, and as per patient request.	Covering the end of the urinal helps to prevent the spread of microorganisms. Cleaning the patient after he has used the urinal prevents offensive odors and skin irritation.
15. Return the patient to a comfortable position. Make sure the linens under the patient are dry. Remove your gloves and ensure that the patient is covered.	Proper positioning promotes patient comfort. Removing contaminated gloves prevents the spread of microorganisms.
16. Ensure the patient call bell is in reach.	Promotes patient safety.
17. Offer patient supplies to wash and dry his hands, assisting as necessary.	Washing hands after using the urinal helps prevent the spread of microorganisms.
18. Put on clean gloves. Empty and clean the urinal, measuring urine in a graduated container, as necessary. Discard the trash receptacle with used toilet paper per facility policy.	Measurement of urine volume is required for accurate intake and output records.
19. Remove gloves and additional PPE, if used, and perform hand hygiene.	Gloves prevent exposure to blood and body fluids. Proper removal of PPE reduces the risk for infection transmission and contamination of other items. Hand hygiene prevents the spread of microorganisms.

EVALUATION

The expected outcome has been met when the patient voids using the urinal. Other outcomes have been met when the patient remains dry; the patient does not experience episodes of incontinence; the patient demonstrates measures to assist with using the urinal; and the patient does not experience impaired skin integrity.

DOCUMENTATION

Guidelines

Document the patient's tolerance of the activity. Record the amount of urine voided on the intake and output record, if appropriate. Document any other assessments, such as unusual urine characteristics or alterations in the patient's skin.

Sample Documentation

12/06/20 0730 Patient using urinal at bedside to void. Voided 600-mL yellow urine. Perineal skin intact, without redness or irritation. Reinforced need for continued use of urinal for recording accurate output. Patient verbalized an understanding of instructions.

—S. Barnes, RN

SPECIAL CONSIDERATIONS

- Urinal should not be left in place for extended periods because pressure and irritation to the patient's skin can result. If the patient is unable to use alone or with assistance, consider other interventions, such as assisting the patient to use a bedside commode or applying an external urinary sheath (condom catheter) (see Skills 12-3 and 12-5).
- It may be necessary to assist patients who have difficulty holding the urinal in place, such as those with limited upper extremity movement or alteration in mentation, to prevent spillage of urine.
- The urinal may also be used standing or sitting at the bedside or in the patient's bathroom, if patient is able to do so.

Skill 12-3 Assisting With the Use of a Bedside Commode

Patients who experience difficulty getting to the bathroom may benefit from the use of a bedside commode. Bedside commodes are portable toilet substitutes that can be used for voiding and defecation (Figure 1). A bedside commode can be placed close to the bed for easy use. Many have armrests attached to the legs that may interfere with ease of transfer. The legs usually have some type of end cap on the bottom to reduce movement, but care must be taken to prevent the commode from moving during transfer, resulting in patient injury or falls.

FIGURE 1. Bedside commode.

DELEGATION CONSIDERATIONS

Assisting a patient with the use of a commode may be delegated to nursing assistive personnel (NAP) or to unlicensed assistive personnel (UAP), as well as to licensed practical/vocational nurses (LPN/LVNs). The decision to delegate must be based on careful analysis of the patient's needs and circumstances, as well as the qualifications of the person to whom the task is being delegated. Refer to the Delegation Guidelines in Appendix A.

EQUIPMENT

- Commode with cover (usually attached)
- Toilet tissue
- Nonsterile gloves
- Additional PPE, as indicated
- Disposable washcloths and skin cleanser
- Moist towelettes, skin cleanser and water, or hand sanitizer

ASSESSMENT

Assess the patient's usual elimination habits. Determine why the patient needs to use a commode, such as weakness or unsteady gait. Assess the patient's degree of limitation and ability to help with the activity. Check for the presence of drains, dressings, intravenous fluid infusion sites/equipment, or other devices that could interfere with the patient's ability to help with the procedure or that could become dislodged. Assess the characteristics of the urine and the patient's skin.

NURSING DIAGNOSIS

Determine the related factors for the nursing diagnosis based on the patient's current status. Appropriate nursing diagnoses may include:

- Risk for falls
- Impaired urinary elimination
- Toileting self-care deficit

OUTCOME IDENTIFICATION AND PLANNING

The expected outcome to achieve when assisting with the use of a commode is that the patient is able to void with assistance. Other appropriate outcomes may include the following: the patient maintains continence; the patient demonstrates how to use the commode; the patient maintains skin integrity; and the patient remains free from injury.

(continued)

Skill 12-3 ▶ Assisting With the Use of a Bedside Commode *(continued)*

IMPLEMENTATION

ACTION	RATIONALE
1. Review the patient's chart for any limitations in physical activity. Gather equipment.	Physical limitations may require adaptations in performing the skill. Assembling equipment provides for an organized approach to the task.
2. Obtain assistance for patient transfer from another staff member and/or appropriate transfer equipment, as indicated (refer to Chapter 9).	Assistance from another person or use of appropriate transfer equipment may be required to transfer the patient safely to the commode.
3. Perform hand hygiene and put on PPE, if indicated.	Hand hygiene and PPE prevent the spread of microorganisms. PPE is required based on transmission precautions.
4. Identify the patient.	Identifying the patient ensures the right patient receives the intervention and helps prevent errors.
5. Close the curtains around the bed and close the door to the room, if possible. Discuss the procedure with the patient and assess the patient's ability to assist with the procedure, as well as personal hygiene preferences.	This ensures the patient's privacy. Discussion promotes reassurance and provides knowledge about the procedure. Dialogue encourages patient participation and allows for individualized nursing care.
6. Place the commode close to, and parallel with, the bed. Raise or remove the seat cover (refer to Figure 1, above).	Allows for easy access.
7. Assist the patient to a standing position and then help the patient pivot to the commode. **While bracing one commode leg with your foot, ask the patient to place his/her hands one at a time on the armrests. Assist the patient to lower himself/herself slowly onto the commode seat.**	Standing and then pivoting ensures safe patient transfer. Bracing the commode leg with a foot prevents the commode from shifting while the patient is sitting down.
8. Cover the patient with a blanket. Place call bell and toilet tissue within easy reach. Leave patient if it is safe to do so. Remove PPE, if used, and perform hand hygiene.	Covering the patient promotes warmth. Falls can be prevented if the patient does not have to reach for items he or she needs. Leaving patient alone, if possible, promotes self-esteem and shows respect for privacy. Proper removal of PPE reduces the risk for infection transmission and contamination of other items. Hand hygiene prevents the spread of microorganisms.

Assisting Patient Off Commode

ACTION	RATIONALE
9. Perform hand hygiene. Put on gloves and additional PPE, as indicated.	Hand hygiene deters the spread of microorganisms. Gloves prevent exposure to blood and body fluids.
10. Assist the patient to a standing position. If the patient needs assistance with hygiene, wrap toilet tissue around your hand several times, and wipe the patient clean, using one stroke from the pubic area toward the anal area. Discard tissue in an appropriate receptacle, according to facility policy, and continue with additional tissue until patient is dry. Place tissue in receptacle. Use warm, moist disposable washcloth and skin cleanser to clean perineal area, as necessary, and as per patient request.	Cleaning area from front to back minimizes fecal contamination of the vagina and urinary meatus. Cleaning the patient after he or she has used the commode prevents offensive odors and irritation to the skin.
11. Do not place toilet tissue in the commode if a specimen is required or if output is being recorded. Replace or lower the seat cover.	Mixing toilet tissue with a specimen makes laboratory examination more difficult and interferes with accurate output measurement. Covering the commode helps to prevent the spread of microorganisms.

ACTION	RATIONALE

12. Remove your gloves. Return the patient to the bed or chair. If the patient returns to the bed, raise side rails, as appropriate. Ensure that the patient is covered and call bell is readily within reach.

Removing contaminated gloves prevents spread of microorganisms. Returning the patient to the bed or chair promotes patient comfort. Side rails assist with patient movement in the bed. Having the call bell readily available promotes patient safety.

13. Offer patient supplies to wash and dry his or her hands, assisting as necessary.

Washing hands after using the commode helps prevent the spread of microorganisms.

14. Put on clean gloves. Empty and clean the commode, measuring urine in graduated container, as necessary.

Gloves prevent exposure to blood and body fluids. Accurate measurement of urine is necessary for accurate intake and output records.

 15. Remove gloves and additional PPE, if used. Perform hand hygiene.

Proper removal of PPE reduces the risk for infection transmission and contamination of other items. Hand hygiene prevents the spread of microorganisms.

EVALUATION

The expected outcome has been met when the patient successfully uses the bedside commode. Other outcomes have been met when the patient remains dry, does not experience episodes of incontinence, demonstrates measures to assist with using the commode, and does not experience impaired skin integrity or falls.

DOCUMENTATION

Guidelines

Document the patient's tolerance of the activity, including his/her ability to use the commode. Record the amount of urine voided and/or stool passed on the intake and output record, if appropriate. Document any other assessments, such as unusual urine or stool characteristics or alterations in the patient's skin.

Sample Documentation

07/06/20 0730 Patient using commode at bedside to void with assistance of one for transfer. Voided 325-mL yellow urine. Perineal skin intact and slightly red. Perineal hygiene provided and skin protectant applied. Reinforced need for continued use of commode related to patient's unsteady gait. Patient verbalized an understanding of instructions and states she will call for assistance when getting up to use commode.

—S. Barnes, RN

SPECIAL CONSIDERATIONS

- Commode can be left within patient's reach, to be used without assistance, if appropriate and safe to do so, based on patient's activity limitations and mobility. Adjust room door or curtain to provide privacy for the patient in the event the commode is used.

Skill 12-4 ▶ Assessing Bladder Volume Using an Ultrasound Bladder Scanner

A portable bladder ultrasound scanner is an accurate, reliable, and noninvasive device used to assess bladder volume. Bladder scanners do not pose a risk for the development of a urinary tract infection, unlike intermittent catheterization, which is also used to determine bladder volume (Widdall, 2015). A bladder scanner may be used when there is urinary frequency, absent or decreased urine output, bladder distention, or inability to void, and when establishing intermittent catheterization schedules. Protocols can be established to guide the decision to catheterize a patient. Some scanners offer the ability to print the scan results for documentation purposes.

(continued)

Skill 12-4 Assessing Bladder Volume Using an Ultrasound Bladder Scanner *(continued)*

Results are most accurate when the patient is in the supine position during the scanning. Ensure the biological sex setting on the device is set correctly. If a female patient has had a hysterectomy, the male button is pushed (Altschuler & Diaz, 2006). A postvoid residual (PVR) volume less than 50 mL indicates adequate bladder emptying. A PVR of greater than 150 mL is often recommended as the guideline for catheterization; a PVR of 100 mL or more indicates the bladder is not emptying completely (Bardsley, 2015b; National Institute of Diabetes and Digestive and Kidney Diseases [NIDDK], 2014).

DELEGATION CONSIDERATIONS	The assessment of bladder volume using an ultrasound bladder scanner is not delegated to nursing assistive personnel (NAP) or to unlicensed assistive personnel (UAP). Depending on the state's nurse practice act and the organization's policies and procedures, this procedure may be delegated to licensed practical/vocational nurses (LPN/LVNs). The decision to delegate must be based on careful analysis of the patient's needs and circumstances, as well as the qualifications of the person to whom the task is being delegated. Refer to the Delegation Guidelines in Appendix A.
EQUIPMENT	• Bladder scanner • Ultrasound gel or bladder scan gel pad • Alcohol wipe or other sanitizer recommended by the scanner manufacturer and/or facility policy • Clean gloves • Additional PPE, as indicated • Paper towel or washcloth
ASSESSMENT	Assess the patient for the need to check bladder volume, including signs of urinary retention, measurement of PVR volume, verification that the bladder is empty, identification of obstruction in an indwelling catheter, and evaluation of bladder distension to determine if catheterization is necessary. Verify medical order, if required by facility. Many facilities allow the use of a bladder scanner as a nursing judgment.
NURSING DIAGNOSIS	Determine the related factors for the nursing diagnoses based on the patient's current status. Appropriate nursing diagnoses may include: • Impaired urinary elimination • Urinary retention
OUTCOME IDENTIFICATION AND PLANNING	The expected outcome to achieve when using a bladder scanner is that the volume of urine in the bladder will be accurately measured. Other appropriate outcomes may include the following: the patient's urinary elimination will be maintained, with a urine output of at least 30 mL/hr; and the patient's bladder will not be distended.

IMPLEMENTATION

ACTION	RATIONALE
1. Review the patient's medical record for any limitations in physical activity. Gather equipment.	Physical limitations may require adaptations in performing the skill. Assembling equipment provides for an organized approach to the task.
2. Perform hand hygiene and put on PPE, if indicated.	Hand hygiene and PPE prevent the spread of microorganisms. PPE is required based on transmission precautions.
3. Identify the patient.	Identifying the patient ensures the right patient receives the intervention and helps prevent errors.

ACTION

4. Close the curtains around the bed and close the door to the room, if possible. Discuss the procedure with the patient and assess the patient's ability to assist with the procedure, as well as personal hygiene preferences.

5. Adjust the bed to a comfortable working height, usually elbow height of the caregiver (VHACEOSH, 2016). Place the patient in a supine position. Drape the patient. Stand on the patient's right side if you are right-handed, patient's left side if you are left-handed.

6. Put on clean gloves.

7. Press the ON button. Wait until the device warms up. Press the SCAN button to turn on the scanning screen.

8. Press the appropriate biological sex button. The appropriate icon for male or female will appear on the screen (Figure 1).

9. Clean the scanner head with the appropriate cleaner (Figure 2).

RATIONALE

This ensures the patient's privacy. Discussion promotes reassurance and provides knowledge about the procedure. Dialogue encourages patient participation and allows for individualized nursing care.

Having the bed at the proper height prevents back and muscle strain. Proper positioning allows accurate assessment of bladder volume. Keeping the patient covered as much as possible promotes patient comfort and privacy. Positioning allows for ease of use of dominant hand for the procedure.

Gloves prevent contact with blood and body fluids.

Many devices require a few minutes to prepare the internal programs.

The device must be programmed for the biological sex of the patient by pushing the correct button on it. If a female patient has had a hysterectomy, the male button is pushed (Altschuler & Diaz, 2006).

Cleaning the scanner head deters transmission of microorganisms.

FIGURE 1. Identifying icon for patient's biological sex. (*Photo by B. Proud.*)

FIGURE 2. Cleaning scanner head. (*Photo by B. Proud.*)

10. Gently palpate the patient's **symphysis pubis** (anterior midline junction of pubic bones). Place a generous amount of ultrasound gel (Figure 3A) or gel pad (Figure 3B) midline on the patient's abdomen, about 1 to 1.5 in above the symphysis pubis.

Palpation identifies the proper location and allows for correct placement of the scanner head over the patient's bladder.

A

B

FIGURE 3. **A.** Placing ultrasound gel about 1 to 1.5 in above symphysis pubis. (*Photo by B. Proud.*) **B.** Gel pad.

(*continued*)

Skill 12-4 ▶ Assessing Bladder Volume Using an Ultrasound Bladder Scanner *(continued)*

ACTION	RATIONALE
11. Place the scanner head on the gel or gel pad, **with the directional icon on the scanner head toward the patient's head. Aim the scanner head toward the bladder (point the scanner head slightly downward toward the coccyx) (Figure 4A). Press and release the scan button** (Figure 4B).	Proper placement allows for accurate reading of urine in the bladder (Widdall, 2015).

FIGURE 4. A. Positioning scanner head with directional icon toward patient's head and aiming the scanner head toward the bladder. **B.** Scan button. (*Photos by B. Proud.*)

12. Observe the image on the scanner screen. **Adjust the scanner head to center the bladder image on the crossbars (Figure 5).**	This action allows for accurate reading of urine in the bladder.

FIGURE 5. Centering image on crossbars.

13. Press and hold the DONE button until it beeps. Read the volume measurement on the screen. Print the results, if required, by pressing PRINT.	This action provides for accurate documentation of reading.

ACTION	RATIONALE
14. Use a washcloth or paper towel to remove remaining gel from the patient's skin. Alternately, gently remove gel pad from patient's skin. Return the patient to a comfortable position. Remove your gloves and ensure that the patient is covered.	Removal of the gel promotes patient comfort. Removing contaminated gloves prevents spread of microorganisms.
15. Lower bed height and adjust the head of the bed to a comfortable position. Reattach call bell, if necessary.	These actions promote patient safety.
16. Put on gloves. Clean the scanner head according to the manufacturer's instructions and/or facility policy.	Cleaning equipment prevents transmission of microorganisms.
17. Remove gloves and any additional PPE, if used. Perform hand hygiene.	Proper removal of PPE reduces the risk for infection transmission and contamination of other items. Hand hygiene prevents the spread of microorganisms.

EVALUATION

The expected outcome has been met when the volume of urine in the bladder is accurately measured; the patient's urinary elimination is maintained with a urine output of at least 30 mL/hr; and the patient's bladder is not distended.

DOCUMENTATION

Guidelines

Document the assessment data that led to the use of the bladder scanner, relevant symptoms, the urine volume measured, and the patient's response.

Sample Documentation

> 7/06/20 1130 Patient has not voided 8 hours after catheter removal. Patient denies feelings of discomfort, pressure, and pain. Bladder not palpable. Bladder scanned for 120 mL of urine. Patient encouraged to increase oral fluid intake to eight 6-oz glasses today. Dr. Liu notified of assessment. Orders received to rescan in 4 hours if patient does not void.
>
> —B. Clapp, RN

UNEXPECTED SITUATIONS AND ASSOCIATED INTERVENTIONS

- *You press wrong icon for the patient's biological sex when initiating the scanner:* Turn scanner off and back on. Reenter information using correct biological sex button.
- *You have reason to believe the bladder is full, based on assessment data, but scanner reveals little to no urine in bladder:* Ensure proper positioning of scanner head. Place a generous amount of ultrasound gel or gel pad midline on the patient's abdomen, about 1 to 1.5 in above the symphysis pubis. Place the scanner head on the gel or gel pad, with the directional icon on the scanner head toward the patient's head. Aim the scanner head toward the bladder (point the scanner head slightly downward toward the coccyx). Ensure that the bladder image is centered on the crossbars.

SPECIAL CONSIDERATIONS

- Ensure use of adequate amount of ultrasound gel. Do not use lubricant (Widdall, 2015).
- Ask or assist patients who are overweight or have larger abdominal tissue to hold abdomen up and away from area to be scanned to reduce risk for interference resulting in inaccurate measurement (Widdall, 2015).
- The use of bladder scanning can be used to reduce catheterization rates and associated complications (Institute for Healthcare Improvement [IHI], 2011).
- Bladder scanning in combination with intermittent catheterization may be beneficial in the management of postoperative urinary retention to avoid placement of an indwelling catheter (IHI, 2011).

Skill 12-5 ▶ Applying an External Urinary Sheath (Condom Catheter)

When voluntary control of urination is difficult or not possible for male patients, an alternative to an indwelling catheter is the **external urinary sheath (condom catheter)**. This soft, pliable sheath made of silicone material is applied externally to the penis and directs urine away from the body. Most devices are self-adhesive. The urinary sheath is connected to drainage tubing and a collection bag. The collection bag may be a leg bag. The risk for UTI with a urinary sheath is lower than the risk associated with an indwelling urinary catheter. Nursing care of a patient with a urinary sheath includes vigilant skin care to prevent excoriation. This includes removing the urinary sheath daily, washing the penis with skin cleanser and water and drying carefully, and inspecting the skin for irritation. In hot, humid weather, more frequent changing may be required. Always follow the manufacturer's instructions for applying the external urinary sheath because there are several variations. In all cases, take care to fasten the urinary sheath securely enough to prevent leakage, yet not so tightly as to constrict the blood vessels in the area. In addition, the tip of the tubing should be kept 1 to 2 in (2.5 to 5 cm) beyond the tip of the penis to prevent irritation to the sensitive glans area.

Maintaining free urinary drainage is another nursing priority. Institute measures to prevent the tubing from becoming kinked and urine from backing up in the tubing. Urine can lead to excoriation of the glans, so position the tubing that collects the urine from the external urinary sheath so that it draws urine away from the penis.

Always use a measuring or sizing guide supplied by the manufacturer to ensure the correct size of sheath is applied. Apply skin barriers, such as Cavilon or Skin-Prep, to the penis to protect penile skin from irritation and changes in integrity.

DELEGATION CONSIDERATIONS

The application of an external urinary sheath may be delegated to nursing assistive personnel (NAP) or to unlicensed assistive personnel (UAP), as well as to licensed practical/vocational nurses (LPN/LVNs). The decision to delegate must be based on careful analysis of the patient's needs and circumstances, as well as the qualifications of the person to whom the task is being delegated. Refer to the Delegation Guidelines in Appendix A.

EQUIPMENT

- External urinary sheath (condom catheter) in appropriate size
- Skin protectant, such as Cavilon or Skin-Prep
- Velcro leg strap, catheter-securing device, or tape
- Bath blanket
- Reusable leg bag with tubing or urinary drainage setup
- Premoistened disposable washcloths or
  - Basin with warm water
  - Skin cleanser, towel, washcloth
- Disposable gloves
- Additional PPE, as indicated
- Washcloth and towel
- Scissors

ASSESSMENT

Assess the patient's knowledge of the need for use of the urinary sheath. Ask the patient about any allergies, especially to latex or tape. Assess the size of the patient's penis to ensure that the appropriate-sized external urinary sheath is used. Inspect the skin in the groin and scrotal area, noting any areas of redness, irritation, or breakdown.

NURSING DIAGNOSIS

Determine the related factors for the nursing diagnoses based on the patient's current status. Appropriate nursing diagnoses may include:

- Impaired urinary elimination
- Functional urinary incontinence
- Risk for impaired skin integrity

| OUTCOME IDENTIFICATION AND PLANNING | The expected outcome to achieve when applying an external urinary sheath is that the patient's urinary elimination will be maintained, with a urine output of at least 30 mL/hr, and the bladder is not distended. Other outcomes may include the following: the patient's skin remains clean, dry, and intact, without evidence of irritation or breakdown. |

IMPLEMENTATION

ACTION	RATIONALE
1. Gather equipment.	Assembling equipment provides for an organized approach to the task.
2. Perform hand hygiene and put on PPE, if indicated.	Hand hygiene and PPE prevent the spread of microorganisms. PPE is required based on transmission precautions.
3. Identify the patient.	Identifying the patient ensures the right patient receives the intervention and helps prevent errors.
4. Close the curtains around the bed and close the door to the room, if possible. Discuss the procedure with the patient. Ask the patient if he has any allergies, especially to latex.	This ensures the patient's privacy. Discussion promotes reassurance and provides knowledge about the procedure. Dialogue encourages patient participation and allows for individualized nursing care. Some external urinary sheaths are made of latex.
5. Assemble equipment on overbed table or other surface within reach.	Arranging items nearby is convenient, saves time, and avoids unnecessary stretching and twisting of muscles on the part of the nurse.
6. Adjust the bed to a comfortable working height, usually elbow height of the caregiver (VHACEOSH, 2016). Stand on the patient's right side if you are right-handed, or on patient's left side if you are left-handed.	Having the bed at the proper height prevents back and muscle strain. Positioning on one side allows for ease of use of dominant hand for catheter application.
7. Prepare urinary drainage setup or reusable leg bag for attachment to the external urinary sheath.	Provides for an organized approach to the task.
8. Position the patient on his back with thighs slightly apart. Drape the patient so that only the area around the penis is exposed. Slide waterproof pad under the patient.	Positioning allows access to the site. Draping prevents unnecessary exposure and promotes warmth. The waterproof pad will protect bed linens from moisture.
9. Put on disposable gloves. Trim any long pubic hair that is in contact with the penis.	Gloves prevent contact with blood and body fluids. Trimming pubic hair prevents pulling of hair by adhesive, without the risk of infection associated with shaving.
10. Clean the genital area with washcloth, skin cleanser, and warm water. If patient is uncircumcised, retract foreskin and clean glans of penis. Replace foreskin. Clean the tip of the penis first, moving the washcloth in a circular motion from the meatus outward. Wash the shaft of the penis using downward strokes toward the pubic area. Rinse and dry. Remove gloves. Perform hand hygiene.	Washing removes urine, secretions, and microorganisms. The penis must be clean and dry to minimize skin irritation. If the foreskin is left retracted, it may cause venous congestion in the glans of the penis, leading to edema.
11. Put on gloves. Apply skin protectant to the penis and allow to dry.	Gloves prevent contact with blood and body fluids. Skin protectant minimizes the risk of skin irritation from adhesive and moisture and increases the adhesive's ability to adhere to skin.

(continued)

Skill 12-5 ▶ Applying an External Urinary Sheath (Condom Catheter) *(continued)*

ACTION	RATIONALE
12. Roll the external urinary sheath outward onto itself. Grasp the penis firmly with the nondominant hand. **Apply the external urinary sheath by rolling it onto the penis with the dominant hand (Figure 1). Leave 1 to 2 in (2.5 to 5 cm) of space between the tip of the penis and the end of the external urinary sheath.**	Rolling the external urinary sheath outward allows for easier application. The space prevents irritation to the tip of the penis and allows free drainage of urine.
13. **Apply pressure to the sheath at the base of the penis for 10 to 15 seconds.**	Application of pressure ensures good adherence of adhesive with skin.
14. Connect the external urinary sheath to drainage setup (Figure 2). Avoid kinking or twisting drainage tubing.	The collection device keeps the patient dry. Kinked tubing encourages backflow of urine.

FIGURE 1. Unrolling sheath onto penis.

FIGURE 2. Connecting external urinary sheath to drainage setup.

ACTION	RATIONALE
15. Remove gloves. Secure drainage tubing to the patient's inner thigh with Velcro leg strap or tape. Leave some slack in tubing for leg movement.	Proper attachment prevents tension on the sheath and potential inadvertent removal.
16. Assist the patient to a comfortable position. Cover the patient with bed linens. Place the bed in the lowest position.	Positioning and covering provide warmth and promote comfort. Bed in the lowest position promotes patient safety.
17. Secure the drainage bag below the level of the bladder. Check that drainage tubing is not kinked and that movement of side rails does not interfere with the drainage bag.	Facilitates drainage of urine and prevents the backflow of urine.
18. Remove equipment. Remove gloves and additional PPE, if used. Perform hand hygiene.	Proper disposal of equipment prevents transmission of microorganisms. Proper removal of PPE reduces the risk for infection transmission and contamination of other items. Hand hygiene prevents the spread of microorganisms.

EVALUATION

The expected outcome has been met when the external urinary sheath is applied without adverse effect; the patient's urinary elimination has been maintained, with a urine output of at least 30 mL/hr; and the patient's skin remains clean, dry, and intact, without evidence of irritation or breakdown.

DOCUMENTATION

Guidelines

Document the assessment data supporting the decision to use an external urinary sheath, the application of the external urinary sheath, and the condition of the patient's skin. Record urine output on the intake and output record.

Sample Documentation

> 7/12/20 1910 Patient incontinent of urine; states: "It just comes too fast. I can't get to the bathroom in time." Perineal skin slightly reddened. Discussed rationale for use of external urinary sheath. Patient and wife agreeable to trying external urinary sheath. Medium-sized external urinary sheath applied; 200 mL of clear urine returned. Leg bag in place for daytime use. Patient verbalized understanding of need to call for assistance to empty drainage bag.
>
> —B. Clapp, RN

UNEXPECTED SITUATIONS AND ASSOCIATED INTERVENTIONS

- *External urinary sheath leaks with every voiding:* Check the size of the external urinary sheath. If it is too big or too small, it may leak. Check the space between the tip of the penis and the end of the external urinary sheath. If this space is too small, the urine has no place to go and will leak out.
- *External urinary sheath will not stay on patient:* Ensure that the external urinary sheath is correct size and that the penis is thoroughly dried before applying the external urinary sheath. Remind the patient that the external urinary sheath is in place, so that he does not tug at the tubing. If the patient has a retracted penis, an external urinary sheath may not be the best choice; there are pouches made for patients with a retracted penis.
- *When assessing the patient's penis, you find a break in skin integrity:* Do not reapply the external urinary sheath. Allow skin to be open to air as much as possible. If your facility has a wound, ostomy, and continence nurse, arrange for a consult.

EVIDENCE FOR PRACTICE ▶

PREVENTION OF CATHETER-ASSOCIATED INFECTIONS

Centers for Disease Control and Prevention (CDC). (2015). *Healthcare-associated infections (HAIs). Catheter-associated urinary tract infections (CAUTI).* Retrieved https://www.cdc.gov/HAI/ca_uti/uti.html.

This site provides resources for health care providers and patients, including the CDC guidelines for prevention of catheter-associated infections. These guidelines recommend considering the use of alternatives to indwelling urethral catheterization in selected patients, when appropriate, such as the use of external urinary sheaths in cooperative male patients without urinary retention or bladder outlet obstruction.

Refer to thePoint® for additional research on related nursing topics.

Skill 12-6 ▶ Catheterizing the Female Urinary Bladder

Urinary catheterization is the introduction of a catheter (tube) through the urethra into the bladder for the purpose of withdrawing urine. Catheter-associated UTIs are the most common hospital-acquired infection in the United States and is one reason catheterization should be avoided whenever possible. When it is deemed necessary, it should be performed using strict aseptic technique and left in place for the shortest length of time possible (American Nurses Association [ANA], 2014; Gould, Umscheid, Agarwal, Kuntz, & Pegues, 2009; Society of Urologic Nurses and Associates [SUNA], 2015b).

(continued)

Skill 12-6 ▶ Catheterizing the Female Urinary Bladder *(continued)*

If a catheter is to remain in place for continuous drainage, an **indwelling urethral catheter (retention or Foley catheter)** is used. Indwelling catheters are also called *retention* or *Foley catheters*. The indwelling urethral catheter is designed so that it does not slip out of the bladder. A balloon is inflated to ensure that the catheter remains in the bladder once it is inserted (Figure 1A).

FIGURE 1. **A.** Indwelling urethral catheter. **B.** Intermittent urethral catheter.

Intermittent urethral catheters (straight catheters) are used to drain the bladder for shorter periods (5 to 10 minutes) (Figure 1B). Intermittent catheterization should be considered as an alternative to short- or long-term indwelling urethral catheterization to reduce catheter-associated UTIs (Hooton et al., 2010). Intermittent catheterization is becoming the gold standard for the management of bladder-emptying dysfunctions and following surgical interventions. Certain advantages to intermittent catheterization, including the lower risks of catheter-associated UTI and complications, may make it a more desirable and safer option than indwelling catheterization (Herter & Kazer, 2010; Panchisin, 2016; Wilson, 2015).

The following procedure reviews insertion of an indwelling catheter. The procedure for an intermittent catheter follows as a Skill Variation. Guidelines for caring for a patient with an indwelling catheter are summarized in Box 12-1.

Box 12-1 ▎ Guidelines for Care of the Patient With an Indwelling Catheter

- Use an indwelling catheter only when necessary. In addition, consider evidence-based practice guidelines and facility policy to ensure the catheter is removed at the earliest time possible, to limit use to the shortest duration possible (ANA, 2014; Gould et al., 2009; Hooton et al., 2010; SUNA, 2015a).
- Use strict hand hygiene principles.
- Use the smallest appropriate-size catheter.
- Use sterile technique when inserting a catheter.
- Secure the catheter properly to the patient's thigh or abdomen after insertion.
- Keep the drainage bag below the level of the patient's bladder to maintain drainage of urine and prevent the backflow of urine into the patient's bladder.
- Keep the drainage bag and tubing off the ground.
- Maintain a closed system whenever possible.

- If necessary, obtain urine samples using aseptic technique via a closed system.
- Keep the catheter free from obstruction to maintain free flow to the urine.
- Avoid irrigation, unless needed, to relieve or prevent obstruction (Gould et al., 2009; Herter & Kazer, 2010; SUNA, 2015a).
- Ensure that the patient maintains adequate fluid intake.
- Empty the drainage bag when one half to two thirds full or every 3 to 6 hours. (When emptying the drainage bag, do not touch drainage bag spout to the collection device.)
- Provide daily routine personal hygiene as outlined in Chapter 7. Do not use powders and lotions after cleaning. Do not use antibiotic or other antimicrobial cleaners or betadine at the urethral meatus (Herter & Kazer, 2010; SUNA, 2010a).

DELEGATION CONSIDERATIONS

The catheterization of the female urinary bladder is not delegated to nursing assistive personnel (NAP) or to unlicensed assistive personnel (UAP). Depending on the state's nurse practice act and the organization's policies and procedures, catheterization of the female urinary bladder may be delegated to licensed practical/vocational nurses (LPN/LVNs). The decision to delegate must be based on careful analysis of the patient's needs and circumstances, as well as the qualifications of the person to whom the task is being delegated. Refer to the Delegation Guidelines in Appendix A.

EQUIPMENT	• Sterile catheter kit that contains:

• Sterile catheter kit that contains:
  • Sterile gloves
  • Sterile drapes (one of which is **fenestrated**)
  • Sterile catheter (Use the smallest appropriate-size catheter, usually a 14F to 16F catheter with a 5- to 10-mL balloon [ANA, 2014; SUNA 2015b])
  • Antiseptic cleansing solution and cotton balls or gauze squares; antiseptic swabs
  • Lubricant
  • Forceps
  • Prefilled syringe with sterile water (sufficient to inflate indwelling catheter balloon)
  • Sterile specimen container (if specimen is required)
• Flashlight or lamp
• Waterproof, disposable pad
• Sterile, disposable urine collection bag and drainage tubing (may be connected to catheter in catheter kit)
• Catheter-securing device
• Disposable gloves
• Additional PPE, as indicated
• Washcloth, skin cleanser, and warm water to perform perineal hygiene before and after catheterization

ASSESSMENT

Assess the patient's usual elimination habits. Assess the patient's degree of limitations and ability to help with activity. Assess for health problems, such as hip surgery or spinal injury, which would contraindicate certain actions by the patient. Assess for the presence of any other conditions that may interfere with passage of the catheter or contraindicate insertion of the catheter, such as urethral strictures or bladder cancer. Check for the presence of drains, dressings, intravenous fluid infusion sites/equipment, traction, or any other devices that could interfere with the patient's ability to help with the procedure or that could become dislodged. Assess bladder fullness before performing the procedure, either by palpation or with a handheld bladder ultrasound device. Question patient about any allergies, especially to latex or iodine. Ask the patient if she has ever been catheterized. If she had an indwelling catheter previously, ask why and for how long it was used. The patient may have urethral strictures, which may make catheter insertion more difficult. Assess the characteristics of the urine and the patient's skin.

NURSING DIAGNOSIS

Determine the related factors for the nursing diagnoses based on the patient's current status. Appropriate nursing diagnoses may include:

• Impaired urinary elimination
• Urinary retention
• Risk for infection

OUTCOME IDENTIFICATION AND PLANNING

The expected outcome to achieve when catheterizing the female urinary bladder is that the catheter is successfully inserted without adverse effect; the patient's urinary elimination is maintained; and the patient's bladder is not distended. Other appropriate outcomes may include the following: the patient's skin remains clean, dry, and intact, without evidence of irritation or breakdown; and the patient verbalizes an understanding of the purpose for and care of the catheter, as appropriate.

IMPLEMENTATION

ACTION	RATIONALE
1. Review the patient's chart for any limitations in physical activity. Confirm the medical order for indwelling catheter insertion.	Physical limitations may require adaptations in performing the skill. Verifying the medical order ensures that the correct intervention is administered to the right patient.

(continued)

Skill 12-6 ▶ Catheterizing the Female Urinary Bladder *(continued)*

ACTION	RATIONALE
2. Gather equipment. Obtain assistance from another staff member, if necessary.	Assembling equipment provides for an organized approach to the task. Assistance from another person may be required to perform the intervention safely.
3. Perform hand hygiene and put on PPE, if indicated.	Hand hygiene and PPE prevent the spread of microorganisms. PPE is required based on transmission precautions.
4. Identify the patient.	Identifying the patient ensures the right patient receives the intervention and helps prevent errors.
5. Close the curtains around the bed and close the door to the room, if possible. Discuss the procedure with the patient and assess the patient's ability to assist with the procedure. Ask the patient if she has any allergies, especially to latex or iodine.	This ensures the patient's privacy. Discussion promotes reassurance and provides knowledge about the procedure. Dialogue encourages patient participation and allows for individualized nursing care. Some catheters and gloves in kits are made of latex. Some antiseptic solutions contain iodine.
6. Provide good lighting. Artificial light is recommended (use of a flashlight requires an assistant to hold and position it). Place a trash receptacle within easy reach.	Good lighting is necessary to see the meatus clearly. A readily available trash receptacle allows for prompt disposal of used supplies and reduces the risk of contaminating the sterile field.
7. Assemble equipment on overbed table or other surface within reach.	Arranging items nearby is convenient, saves time, and avoids unnecessary stretching and twisting of muscles on the part of the nurse.
8. Adjust the bed to a comfortable working height, usually elbow height of the caregiver (VHACEOSH, 2016). Stand on the patient's right side if you are right-handed, patient's left side if you are left-handed.	Having the bed at the proper height prevents back and muscle strain. Positioning allows for ease of use of dominant hand for catheter insertion.
9. Assist the patient to a dorsal recumbent position with knees flexed, feet about 2 ft apart, with her legs abducted. Drape the patient (Figure 2). Alternately, the Sims', or lateral, position can be used. Place the patient's buttocks near the edge of the bed with her shoulders at the opposite edge and her knees drawn toward her chest (Figure 3). Allow the patient to lie on either side, depending on which position is easiest for the nurse and best for the patient's comfort. Slide waterproof pad under the patient.	Proper positioning allows adequate visualization of the urinary meatus. Embarrassment, chilliness, and tension can interfere with catheter insertion; draping the patient will promote comfort and relaxation. The Sims' position may allow better visualization and be more comfortable for the patient, especially if hip and knee movements are difficult. The smaller area of exposure is also less stressful for the patient. The waterproof pad will protect bed linens from moisture.

FIGURE 2. Patient in dorsal recumbent position and draped properly.

FIGURE 3. Demonstration of side-lying position.

ACTION

10. Put on clean gloves. Clean the perineal area with washcloth, skin cleanser, and warm water, using a different corner of the washcloth with each stroke. Wipe from above orifice downward toward sacrum (front to back). Rinse and dry. Remove gloves. Perform hand hygiene again.

11. Prepare urine drainage setup if a separate urine collection system is to be used. Secure to bed frame, according to the manufacturer's directions.

12. Open sterile catheterization tray on a clean overbed table using sterile technique.

13. Put on sterile gloves. Grasp upper corners of drape and unfold drape without touching nonsterile areas. Fold back a corner on each side to make a cuff over gloved hands. Ask the patient to lift her buttocks and slide sterile drape under her with gloves protected by cuff.

14. Based on facility policy, position the fenestrated sterile drape. Place a fenestrated sterile drape over the perineal area, exposing the labia (Figure 4). (*Note:* The fenestrated drape is not shown in the remaining illustrations in order to provide a clear view of the procedure.)

RATIONALE

Gloves reduce the risk of exposure to blood and body fluids. Cleaning reduces microorganisms near the urethral meatus and provides an opportunity to visualize the perineum and landmarks before the procedure. Hand hygiene reduces the spread of microorganisms.

This facilitates connection of the catheter to the drainage system and provides for easy access.

Placement of equipment near the worksite increases efficiency. Sterile technique protects the patient and prevents transmission of microorganisms.

The drape provides a sterile field close to the meatus. Covering the gloved hands will help keep the gloves sterile while placing the drape.

The drape expands the sterile field and protects against contamination. Use of a fenestrated drape may limit visualization and is considered optional by some health care providers and/or facility policies.

FIGURE 4. Patient with fenestrated drape in place over perineum.

15. Place sterile tray on drape between the patient's thighs.

16. Open all the supplies. Remove cap from the prefilled sterile saline syringe and attach to the balloon inflation port on the catheter. Open the package of antiseptic swabs. Alternately, fluff cotton balls in a tray before pouring antiseptic solution over them. Open specimen container if specimen is to be obtained.

17. Lubricate 1 to 2 in of catheter tip.

18. With thumb and one finger of nondominant hand, spread labia and identify meatus (Figure 5). **Be prepared to maintain separation of labia with one hand until catheter is inserted and urine is flowing well and continuously.** If the patient is in the side-lying position, lift the upper buttock and labia to expose the urinary meatus (Figure 6).

Provides easy access to supplies.

It is necessary to open all supplies and prepare for the procedure while both hands are sterile.

Lubrication facilitates catheter insertion and reduces tissue trauma.

Smoothing the area immediately surrounding the meatus helps to make it visible. Allowing the labia to drop back into position may contaminate the area around the meatus, as well as the catheter. The nondominant hand is now contaminated.

(*continued*)

Skill 12-6 ▶ Catheterizing the Female Urinary Bladder *(continued)*

ACTION

RATIONALE

FIGURE 5. Using dominant hand to separate and hold labia open.

FIGURE 6. Exposing urinary meatus with patient in side-lying position.

19. Use the dominant hand to pick up an antiseptic swab or use forceps to pick up a cotton ball. **Clean one labial fold, top to bottom (from above the meatus down toward the rectum), then discard the cotton ball (Figure 7). Using a new cotton ball/swab for each stroke, continue to clean the other labial fold, then directly over the meatus.**

Moving from an area where there is likely to be less contamination to an area where there is more contamination helps prevent the spread of microorganisms. Cleaning the meatus last helps reduce the possibility of introducing microorganisms into the bladder.

20. With your noncontaminated, dominant hand, place the drainage end of the catheter in a receptacle. If the catheter is preattached to sterile tubing and drainage container (closed drainage system), position the catheter and setup within easy reach on sterile field. Ensure that the clamp on the drainage bag is closed.

This facilitates drainage of urine and minimizes risk of contaminating sterile equipment.

21. **Using your dominant hand, hold the catheter 2 to 3 in from the tip and insert slowly into the urethra (Figure 8). Advance the catheter until there is a return of urine (approximately 2 to 3 in [4.8 to 7.2 cm]). Once urine drains, advance the catheter another 2 to 3 in (4.8 to 7.2 cm). Do not force the catheter through the urethra into the bladder.** Ask the patient to breathe deeply, and rotate catheter gently if slight resistance is met as the catheter reaches the external sphincter.

The female urethra is about 1.5 to 2.5 in (3.6 to 6.0 cm) long. Applying force on the catheter is likely to injure mucous membranes. The sphincter relaxes and the catheter can enter the bladder easily when the patient relaxes. Advancing an indwelling catheter an additional 2 to 3 in (4.8 to 7.2 cm) ensures placement in the bladder and facilitates inflation of the balloon without damaging the urethra.

FIGURE 7. Wiping perineum with cotton ball held by forceps. Wipe in one direction—from top to bottom.

FIGURE 8. Inserting catheter with dominant hand while nondominant hand holds labia apart.

ACTION	**RATIONALE**
22. Hold the catheter securely at the meatus with your non-dominant hand. Use your dominant hand to inflate the catheter balloon (Figure 9). Inject the entire volume of sterile water supplied in a prefilled syringe. Remove the syringe from the port.	Bladder or sphincter contraction could push the catheter out. The balloon anchors the catheter in place in the bladder. The manufacturer provides appropriate amount of sterile water for the size of the catheter in the kit; as a result, use the entire syringe provided in the kit. Removal of the syringe from the injection port prevents the sterile water from pushing back into the syringe and resulting balloon deflation.

FIGURE 9. Inflating balloon of indwelling catheter.

23. Pull gently on the catheter after the balloon is inflated to feel resistance.	Improper inflation can cause patient discomfort and malpositioning of the catheter.
24. Attach the catheter to the drainage system if not already preattached (Figure 10).	Closed drainage system minimizes the risk for microorganisms being introduced into the bladder.
25. Remove equipment and dispose of it according to facility policy. Discard syringe in sharps container. Wash and dry the perineal area, as needed.	Proper disposal prevents the spread of microorganisms. Placing syringe in sharps container prevents reuse. Cleaning promotes comfort and appropriate personal hygiene.
26. Remove gloves. **Secure catheter tubing to the patient's inner thigh with a catheter-securing device (Figure 11).** Leave some slack in catheter for leg movement.	Proper attachment prevents trauma to the urethra and meatus from tension on the tubing. Whether to secure the drainage tubing over or under the leg depends on gravity flow, patient's mobility, and patient's comfort.

FIGURE 10. Attaching catheter to drainage bag.

FIGURE 11. Catheter secured to leg.

27. Assist the patient to a comfortable position. Cover the patient with bed linens. Place the bed in the lowest position.	Positioning and covering provides warmth and promotes comfort.

(continued)

Skill 12-6 ▶ Catheterizing the Female Urinary Bladder *(continued)*

ACTION	RATIONALE
28. Secure the drainage bag below the level of the bladder. Check that drainage tubing is not kinked and that movement of side rails does not interfere with the catheter or drainage bag.	This facilitates drainage of urine and prevents the backflow of urine.
29. Put on clean gloves. Obtain urine specimen immediately, if needed, from the drainage bag. Label specimen. Send urine specimen to the laboratory promptly or refrigerate it.	Catheter system is sterile. Obtaining a specimen immediately allows access to the sterile system. Keeping the urine at room temperature may cause microorganisms, if present, to grow and distort laboratory findings.
30. Remove gloves and additional PPE, if used. Perform hand hygiene.	Proper removal of PPE reduces the risk for infection transmission and contamination of other items. Hand hygiene prevents the spread of microorganisms.

EVALUATION

The expected outcomes have been met when the catheter is successfully inserted without adverse effect; the patient's urinary elimination is maintained; and the patient's bladder is not distended. Other outcomes have been met when the patient's skin remains clean, dry, and intact, without evidence of irritation or breakdown; and the patient verbalizes an understanding of the purpose for and care of the catheter, as appropriate.

DOCUMENTATION

Guidelines

Document the type and size of catheter and balloon inserted, as well as the amount of fluid used to inflate the balloon. Document the patient's tolerance of the activity. Record the amount of urine obtained through the catheter and any specimen obtained. Document any other assessments, such as unusual urine characteristics or alterations in the patient's skin. Record urine amount on intake and output record, if appropriate.

Sample Documentation

DocuCare Practice documenting catheterization of the female urinary bladder in *Lippincott DocuCare.*

> 7/14/20 0915 The primary care provider notified of palpable bladder (3 cm below umbilicus) and the patient's inability to void; 750 mL of urine noted with bladder scan. A 16F Foley catheter inserted without difficulty; 10 mL of sterile water injected into balloon port; 700-mL clear yellow urine returned. Patient states, "Oh, I feel much better now." Bladder is no longer palpable. Patient tolerated procedure without adverse event.
>
> —B. Clapp, RN

UNEXPECTED SITUATIONS AND ASSOCIATED INTERVENTIONS

- *No urine flow is obtained, and you note that the catheter is in the vaginal orifice:* Leave the catheter in place as a marker. Obtain new sterile gloves and catheter kit. Start the procedure over and attempt to place the new catheter directly above the misplaced catheter. Once the new catheter is correctly in place, remove the catheter in the vaginal orifice. Because of the risk of cross-infection, never remove a catheter from the vagina and insert it into the urethra.
- *Patient moves legs during procedure:* If no supplies have been contaminated, ask patient to hold still and continue with the procedure. If supplies have been contaminated, stop the procedure and start over. If necessary, get an assistant to remind the patient to hold still.
- *Urine flow is initially well established and urine is clear, but after several hours flow dwindles:* Check the tubing for kinking. If patient has changed position, the tubing and drainage bag may need to be moved to facilitate drainage of urine.
- *Urine leaks out of meatus around the catheter:* Do not increase the size of the indwelling catheter. Make sure the smallest-sized catheter with a 10-mL balloon is used. Large catheters cause bladder and urethral irritation and trauma. Large balloon-fill volumes occupy more space inside the bladder and put added weight on the base of the bladder. Irritation of the bladder wall and detrusor muscle can cause leakage. If leakage persists, consider an evaluation for urinary tract infection. Ensure that the correct amount of solution was used to inflate the balloon. Underfilling the balloon can cause the catheter to dislodge into the urethra, causing urethral spasm, pain, and discomfort. If you suspect underfill, do not attempt to push the catheter farther into the bladder. Remove the catheter and replace. Assess the patient for constipation. Bowel full of stool can cause pressure on the catheter lumen and prevent the drainage of urine. Implement interventions to prevent/treat constipation.

SPECIAL CONSIDERATIONS

General Considerations

- Be familiar with facility policy and/or primary health care provider guidelines for the maximum amount of urine to remove from the bladder at the time of insertion.
- If the patient is unable to lift buttocks or maintain the required position for the procedure, the assistance of another staff member may be necessary to place the drape under the patient and to help the patient maintain the required position.
- Supplies can be opened and prepared on the overbed table, moving the tray onto the bed just before cleansing the patient.
- If there is not an immediate flow of urine after the catheter has been inserted, several measures may prove helpful:
  - Have the patient take a deep breath, which helps to relax the perineal and abdominal muscles.
  - Rotate the catheter slightly, because a drainage hole may be resting against the bladder wall.
  - Raise the head of the patient's bed to increase pressure in the bladder area.
  - Assess the patient's intake to ensure adequate fluid intake for urine production.
  - Assess the catheter and drainage tubing for kinks and occlusion.
- If the catheter cannot be advanced, have the patient take several deep breaths. Rotate the catheter half a turn and try to advance it. If you are still unable to advance, remove the catheter. Notify the primary care provider.
- Some catheter kits do not contain the catheter. This allows you to select a catheter and balloon size separately.
- Lubricant may occlude the catheter lumen. If urine flow does not occur within a minute of catheter insertion, irrigate the catheter to free the lumen of lubricant (SUNA, 2015c).

Infant and Child Considerations

- Size 5F to 8F is used for infants and young children. Size 8F to 14F catheters are commonly used for older children (Perry, Hockenberry, Lowdermilk, & Wilson, 2014).
- Distraction, such as blowing bubbles, deep breathing, or singing a song, can help the child relax.
- Consider use of lidocaine jelly to anesthetize and lubricate the area before insertion of the catheter, decreasing the child's discomfort and anxiety.

Home Care Considerations

- Intermittent catheterization, performed by the patient or a caregiver in the home, may be necessary for patients with spinal cord injuries or other neurologic conditions. Although the risk for UTI is always present, most research supports the use of clean, rather than sterile, technique in the home environment (Bardsley, 2015a; Wilson, 2015). The procedure for self-intermittent catheterization is essentially the same as that used by the nurse to catheterize a patient. Box 12-2 outlines important information related to patient intermittent self-catheterization (ISC).
- Single-use catheters, reusable catheters that are cleaned between use, and no-touch catheters are options for use for intermittent self-catheterization (ISC) in the home setting (Holland & Fish, 2012).

Box 12-2 | Patient Intermittent Self-Catheterization

- Explain the reason for self-catheterization and corresponding health issues related to the need for catheterization.
- Explain the consequences of not doing intermittent self-catheterization, such as upper urinary tract problems, urinary tract infections, and incontinence.
- Explain potential complications, such as bleeding and the risk of urinary tract infections, and what to do if they occur.
- Ensure privacy and dignity.
- Include discussion regarding the frequency of intermittent catheterization and how to incorporate it into the patient's usual daily routine.
- Explain the anatomy of the urinary tract, hygiene, and preparation of the catheter.
- Demonstrate how to open, hold, and use the catheter.
- Explain catheterization process; demonstrate process; observe return demonstration by patient.
- Explore process to obtain supplies, cleaning of reusable catheters, and storage.
- Provide information in an appropriate format (such as written materials or video, in appropriate language) to reinforce instruction.
- Allow the patient adequate time to ask questions.
- Provide information about how to recognize a urinary tract infection and other signs/symptoms to report to the primary health care provider.
- Explain that aids are available to help meet the challenges of intermittent self-catheterization for patients with poor eyesight, reduced mobility, and/or reduced manual dexterity.

Source: Adapted from Bardsley, A. (2015b). Assessing and teaching female intermittent self-catheterization. *British Journal of Community Nursing,* *20*(7), 344–346; Logan, K. (2012). An overview of male intermittent self-catheterisation. *British Journal of Nursing (Mark Allen Publishing), 21*(18), S18–S22; Mangnall, J. (2015). Managing and teaching intermittent catheterisation. *British Journal of Community Nursing, 20*(2), 82–88; Rantell, A. (2012). Intermittent self-catheterisation in women. *Nursing Standard, 26*(42), 61–68; and Wilson, M. (2015). Clean intermittent self-catheterisation: Working with patients. *British Journal of Nursing (Mark Allen Publishing), 24*(2), 76–85.

Skill 12-6 ▶ Catheterizing the Female Urinary Bladder *(continued)*

Skill Variation ▶ Intermittent Female Urethral Catheterization

1. Check the medical record for the order for intermittent urethral catheterization. Review the patient's chart for any limitations in physical activity. Gather equipment. Obtain assistance from another staff member, if necessary.

2. Perform hand hygiene. Put on PPE, as indicated, based on transmission precautions.

3. Identify the patient. Discuss the procedure with the patient and assess the patient's ability to assist with the procedure. Ask the patient if she has any allergies, especially to latex or iodine.

4. Close the curtains around the bed and close the door to the room, if possible.

5. Provide good lighting. Artificial light is recommended (use of a flashlight requires an assistant to hold and position it). Place a trash receptacle within easy reach.

6. Assemble equipment on overbed table or other surface within reach.

7. Raise the bed to a comfortable working height. Stand on the patient's right side if you are right-handed, patient's left side if you are left-handed.

8. Put on disposable gloves. Assist the patient to dorsal recumbent position with knees flexed, feet about 2 ft apart, with her legs abducted. Drape the patient. Alternately, use the Sims, or lateral, position. Place the patient's buttocks near the edge of the bed with her shoulders at the opposite edge and her knees drawn toward her chest. Slide waterproof drape under patient.

9. Put on clean gloves. Clean the perineal area with washcloth, skin cleanser, and warm water, using a different corner of the washcloth with each stroke. Wipe from above the orifice downward toward the sacrum (front to back). Rinse and dry. Remove gloves. Perform hand hygiene again.

10. Open sterile catheterization tray on a clean overbed table using sterile technique.

11. Put on sterile gloves. Grasp upper corners of drape and unfold drape without touching nonsterile areas. Fold back a corner on each side to make a cuff over gloved hands. Ask the patient to lift her buttocks and slide the sterile drape under her with gloves protected by cuff.

12. Place a fenestrated sterile drape over the perineal area, exposing the labia, if appropriate.

13. Place the sterile tray on the drape between the patient's thighs.

14. Open all the supplies. Open package of antiseptic swabs. Alternately, fluff cotton balls in a tray before pouring antiseptic solution over them. Open specimen container if specimen is to be obtained.

15. Lubricate 1 to 2 in of catheter tip.

16. With thumb and one finger of nondominant hand, spread the labia and identify the meatus. If the patient is in the side-lying position, lift the upper buttock and labia to expose the urinary meatus. **Be prepared to maintain separation of the labia with one hand until the catheter is inserted and urine is flowing well and continuously.**

17. Use the dominant hand to pick up a cotton ball. **Clean one labial fold, top to bottom (from above the meatus down toward the rectum), then discard the cotton ball. Using a new cotton ball for each stroke, continue to clean the other labial fold, then directly over the meatus.**

18. With the noncontaminated, dominant hand, place the drainage end of the catheter in a receptacle. If a specimen is required, place the end into the specimen container in the receptacle.

19. **Using the dominant hand, hold the catheter 2 to 3 in from the tip and insert slowly into the urethra. Advance the catheter until there is a return of urine (approximately 2 to 3 in [4.8 to 7.2 cm]). Do not force the catheter through the urethra into the bladder.**
Ask the patient to breathe deeply, and rotate the catheter gently if slight resistance is met as the catheter reaches the external sphincter.

20. Hold the catheter securely at the meatus with the nondominant hand while the bladder empties. If a specimen is being collected, remove the drainage end of the tubing from the specimen container after required amount is obtained and allow urine to flow into the receptacle. Set the specimen container aside and place the lid on container.

21. Allow the bladder to empty. Withdraw the catheter slowly and smoothly after urine has stopped flowing. Remove equipment and dispose of it according to facility policy. Discard syringe in sharps container to prevent reuse. Wash and dry the perineal area, as needed.

22. Remove gloves. Assist the patient to a comfortable position. Cover the patient with bed linens. Place the bed in the lowest position.

23. Put on clean gloves. Secure the container lid and label specimen. Send urine specimen to the laboratory promptly or refrigerate it.

24. Remove gloves and additional PPE, if used. Perform hand hygiene.

Note: Intermittent catheterization in the home is performed using clean technique. The bladder's natural resistance to the microorganisms normally found in the home makes sterile technique unnecessary. Single-use catheters, reusable catheters, and no-touch catheters are options for use for intermittent self-catheterization (ISC) in the home setting (Holland & Fish, 2012). Reusable catheters are washed, dried, and stored for repeated use.

Box 12-2 outlines information related to patient intermittent self-catheterization.

**EVIDENCE
FOR PRACTICE ▶**

PREVENTION OF CATHETER-ASSOCIATED INFECTIONS

Centers for Disease Control and Prevention (CDC). (2015). *Healthcare-associated infections (HAIs). Catheter-associated urinary tract infections (CAUTI).* Retrieved https://www.cdc.gov/HAI/ca_uti/uti.html.

Institute for Healthcare Improvement (IHI). (2011). *How-to guide: Prevent catheter-associated urinary tract infection.* Cambridge, MA: Author. Retrieved http://www.ihi.org/resources/Pages/Tools/HowtoGuidePreventCatheterAssociatedUrinaryTractInfection.aspx.

Society of Urologic Nurses and Associates (SUNA). (2010a). *Clinical practice guidelines. Prevention & control of catheter-associated urinary tract infection (CAUTI). [Brochure].* Pitman, NJ: Author.

These guidelines provide evidence-based recommendations to guide care for patients requiring catheterization of the urinary bladder to prevent CAUTI.

Refer to thePoint® for additional research on related nursing topics.

**EVIDENCE
FOR PRACTICE ▶**

INDWELLING URINARY CATHETER TUBING AND DEPENDENT LOOPS

Preventing CAUTI is a health care priority. It is important to maintain a constant downward flow of urine to aid in the free flow of urine from the bladder to reduce the risk of urinary tract infection. Kinks and dependent loops (low points) in the tubing interfere with the free flow of urine from the bladder and contribute to backflow of urine in the drainage tubing into the bladder, contributing to the development of a urinary tract infection.

Related Research

Wuthier, P., Sublett, K., & Riehl, L. (2016). Urinary catheter dependent loops as a potential contributing cause of bacteriuria: An observational study. *Urologic Nursing, 36*(1), 7–16.

The objective of this observational, cross-sectional study was to determine the prevalence and nature of indwelling catheter-dependent loops in an acute care setting. Indwelling catheter tubing arrangements were noted and measured for 55 patients over 2 days. Catheter tubing with a dependent loop was defined as a configuration of tubing where the drainage tubing dips below the entry point into the catheter bag. Tubing with a dependent loop was noted in 48 (87%) of the patients, creating significant pressure differentials within the catheter tubing, interfering with the free flow of urine from the bladder. The authors concluded that dependent loops are very common in the acute care setting, and in spite of frequent education, are difficult to avoid.

Relevance to Nursing Practice

As caregivers who spend the most time with patients, nurses have a responsibility to use interventions to reduce the risk for catheter-associated UTI in patients with indwelling urinary catheters. Nurses must remain vigilant in caring for patients with indwelling catheters to prevent and take action to address dependent loops in urinary catheter drainage tubing. Manipulation of catheter drainage tubing to allow urine to flow freely into the drainage bag is a necessity.

Refer to thePoint® for additional research on related nursing topics.

Skill 12-7 ▶ Catheterizing the Male Urinary Bladder

Urinary catheterization is the introduction of a catheter (tube) through the urethra into the bladder for the purpose of withdrawing urine. Catheter-associated urinary tract infections are the most common hospital-acquired infection in the United States and is one reason catheterization should be avoided whenever possible. When it is deemed necessary, it should be performed using strict aseptic technique and left in place for the shortest length of time possible (Hooton et al., 2010). The duration of catheterization is the most important risk factor for the development of a UTI (ANA, 2014; Gould et al., 2009; SUNA, 2015c).

If a catheter is to remain in place for continuous drainage, an indwelling urethral catheter is used. Indwelling catheters are also called *retention* or *Foley catheters*. The indwelling urethral catheter is designed so that it does not slip out of the bladder. A balloon is inflated to ensure that the catheter remains in the bladder once it is inserted (Figure 1A).

Intermittent urethral catheters, or straight catheters, are used to drain the bladder for shorter periods (5 to 10 minutes) (Figure 1B). Intermittent catheterization should be considered as an alternative to short- or long-term indwelling urethral catheterization to reduce catheter-associated UTIs (Hooton et al., 2010). Intermittent catheterization is becoming the gold standard for the management of bladder-emptying dysfunctions and following surgical interventions. Certain advantages to intermittent catheterization, including the lower risks of catheter-associated UTI and complications, may make it a more desirable and safer option than indwelling catheterization (Herter & Kazer, 2010; Panchisin, 2016; Wilson, 2015).

The following procedure reviews insertion of an indwelling catheter into the male urinary bladder. The procedure for an intermittent catheter of a male bladder follows as a Skill Variation. Guidelines for caring for a patient with an indwelling catheter are summarized in Box 12-1, located within Skill 12-6.

DELEGATION CONSIDERATIONS	The catheterization of the male urinary bladder is not delegated to nursing assistive personnel (NAP) or to unlicensed assistive personnel (UAP). Depending on the state's nurse practice act and the organization's policies and procedures, catheterization of the male urinary bladder may be delegated to licensed practical/vocational nurses (LPN/LVNs). The decision to delegate must be based on careful analysis of the patient's needs and circumstances, as well as the qualifications of the person to whom the task is being delegated. Refer to the Delegation Guidelines in Appendix A.

EQUIPMENT	• Sterile catheter kit that contains:
	  • Sterile gloves
	  • Sterile drapes (one of which is fenestrated)
	  • Sterile catheter (Use the smallest appropriate-size catheter, usually a 14F to 16F catheter with a 5- to 10-mL balloon [ANA, 2014; SUNA, 2015c])
	  • Antiseptic cleansing solution and cotton balls or gauze squares; antiseptic swabs
	  • Lubricant
	  • Forceps
	  • Prefilled syringe with sterile water (sufficient to inflate indwelling catheter balloon)
	  • Sterile basin (usually base of kit serves as this)
	  • Sterile specimen container (if specimen is required)
	• Flashlight or lamp
	• Waterproof, disposable pad
	• Sterile, disposable urine collection bag and drainage tubing (may be connected to catheter in catheter kit)
	• Velcro leg strap, catheter-securing device, or tape
	• Disposable gloves
	• Additional PPE, as indicated
	• Washcloth, skin cleanser, and warm water to perform perineal hygiene before and after catheterization

ASSESSMENT

Assess the patient's usual elimination habits. Assess the patient's degree of limitations and ability to help with activity. Assess for health problems, such as hip surgery or spinal injury, which would contraindicate certain actions by the patient. Assess for the presence of any other conditions that may interfere with passage of the catheter or contraindicate insertion of the catheter, such as urethral strictures or bladder cancer. Check for the presence of drains, dressings, intravenous fluid infusion sites/equipment, traction, or any other devices that could interfere with the patient's ability to help with the procedure or that could become dislodged. Assess bladder fullness before performing the procedure, either by palpation or with a handheld bladder ultrasound device, and question the patient about any allergies, especially to latex or iodine. Ask the patient if he has ever been catheterized. If he had an indwelling catheter previously, ask why and for how long it was used. The patient may have urethral strictures, which may make catheter insertion more difficult. If the patient is 50 years of age or older, ask if he has had any prostate problems. Prostate enlargement typically is noted around the age of 50 years. Assess the characteristics of the urine and the patient's skin.

NURSING DIAGNOSIS

Determine the related factors for the nursing diagnoses based on the patient's current status. Appropriate nursing diagnoses may include:
- Impaired urinary elimination
- Risk for infection
- Urinary retention

OUTCOME IDENTIFICATION AND PLANNING

The expected outcome to achieve when catheterizing the male urinary bladder is that the catheter is successfully inserted without adverse effect; the patient's urinary elimination is maintained; and the patient's bladder is not distended. Other appropriate outcomes may include the following: the patient's skin remains clean, dry, and intact, without evidence of irritation or breakdown; and the patient verbalizes an understanding of the purpose for and care of the catheter, as appropriate.

IMPLEMENTATION

ACTION	RATIONALE
1. Review chart for any limitations in physical activity. Confirm the medical order for indwelling catheter insertion.	Physical limitations may require adaptations in performing the skill. Verifying the medical order ensures that the correct intervention is administered to the right patient.
2. Gather equipment. Obtain assistance from another staff member, if necessary.	Assembling equipment provides for an organized approach to the task. Assistance from another person may be required to perform the intervention safely.
3. Perform hand hygiene and put on PPE, if indicated.	Hand hygiene and PPE prevent the spread of microorganisms. PPE is required based on transmission precautions.
4. Identify the patient.	Identifying the patient ensures the right patient receives the intervention and helps prevent errors.
5. Close the curtains around the bed and close the door to the room, if possible. Discuss the procedure with the patient and assess the patient's ability to assist with the procedure. Ask the patient if he has any allergies, especially to latex or iodine.	This ensures the patient's privacy. Discussion promotes reassurance and provides knowledge about the procedure. Dialogue encourages patient participation and allows for individualized nursing care. Some catheters and gloves in kits are made of latex. Some antiseptic solutions contain iodine.
6. Provide good lighting. Artificial light is recommended (use of a flashlight requires an assistant to hold and position it). Place a trash receptacle within easy reach.	Good lighting is necessary to see the meatus clearly. A readily available trash receptacle allows for prompt disposal of used supplies and reduces the risk of contaminating the sterile field.

(continued)

Skill 12-7 ▶ Catheterizing the Male Urinary Bladder *(continued)*

ACTION	RATIONALE
7. Assemble equipment on overbed table or other surface within reach.	Arranging items nearby is convenient, saves time, and avoids unnecessary stretching and twisting of muscles on the part of the nurse.
8. Adjust the bed to a comfortable working height, usually elbow height of the caregiver (VHACEOSH, 2016). Stand on the patient's right side if you are right-handed, patient's left side if you are left-handed.	Having the bed at the proper height prevents back and muscle strain. Positioning allows for ease of use of dominant hand for catheter insertion.
9. Position the patient on his back with thighs slightly apart. Drape the patient so that only the area around the penis is exposed. Slide waterproof pad under the patient.	This prevents unnecessary exposure and promotes warmth. The waterproof pad will protect bed linens from moisture.
10. Put on clean gloves. Clean the genital area with washcloth, skin cleanser, and warm water. Clean the tip of the penis first, moving the washcloth in a circular motion from the meatus outward. Wash the shaft of the penis using downward strokes toward the pubic area. Rinse and dry. Remove gloves. Perform hand hygiene again.	Gloves reduce the risk of exposure to blood and body fluids. Cleaning the penis reduces microorganisms near the urethral meatus. Hand hygiene reduces the spread of microorganisms.
11. Prepare urine drainage setup if a separate urine collection system is to be used. Secure to bed frame according to the manufacturer's directions.	This facilitates connection of the catheter to the drainage system and provides for easy access.
12. Open sterile catheterization tray on a clean overbed table or other flat surface, using sterile technique.	Placement of equipment near worksite increases efficiency. Sterile technique protects patient and prevents spread of microorganisms.
13. Put on sterile gloves. Open sterile drape and place on patient's thighs. Place fenestrated drape with opening over the penis (Figure 1).	This maintains a sterile working area.

FIGURE 1. Patient lying supine with fenestrated drape over penis.

ACTION	RATIONALE
14. Place the catheter setup on or next to the patient's legs on sterile drape.	Sterile setup should be arranged so that the nurse's back is not turned to it, nor should it be out of the nurse's range of vision.
15. Open all the supplies. Remove cap from the prefilled sterile saline syringe and attach to the balloon inflation port on the catheter. Open package of antiseptic swabs. Alternately, fluff cotton balls in a tray before pouring antiseptic solution over them. Open specimen container if specimen is to be obtained. Remove cap from syringe prefilled with lubricant.	It is necessary to open all supplies and prepare for the procedure while both hands are sterile.
16. Place the drainage end of the catheter in a receptacle. If the catheter is preattached to sterile tubing and drainage container (closed drainage system), position catheter and setup within easy reach on sterile field. Ensure that the clamp on drainage bag is closed. Lubricate 1 to 2 in of catheter tip.	Facilitates drainage of urine and minimizes risk of contaminating sterile equipment. Lubrication facilitates catheter insertion and reduces tissue trauma.

ACTION

17. Lift the penis with the nondominant hand. Retract the foreskin in an uncircumcised patient. Be prepared to keep this hand in this position until the catheter is inserted and urine is flowing well and continuously. Use the dominant hand to pick up an antiseptic swab or use forceps to pick up a cotton ball. Using a circular motion, clean the penis, moving from the meatus down the glans of the penis (Figure 2). Repeat this cleansing motion two more times, using a new cotton ball/swab each time. Discard each cotton ball/swab after one use.

FIGURE 2. Lifting penis with gloved nondominant hand and cleaning meatus with cotton ball held with forceps in gloved dominant hand.

18. Hold the penis with slight upward tension and perpendicular to the patient's body. Use the dominant hand to pick up the lubricant syringe. Gently insert the tip of the syringe with a lubricant into the urethra and instill the 10 mL of lubricant (Figure 3).

FIGURE 3. Inserting syringe into urethra and instilling lubricant.

RATIONALE

The hand touching the penis becomes contaminated. Cleansing the area around the meatus and under the foreskin in the uncircumcised patient helps prevent infection. Moving from the meatus toward the base of the penis prevents bringing microorganisms to the meatus.

Most of the lubricant applied externally on the catheter may remain at the meatus, essentially allowing an unlubricated catheter to cause trauma to the lining of the urethra. As a result, the recommended procedure for urinary catheterization in male patients includes retrograde injection of a water-soluble lubricant before inserting the catheter (SUNA, 2015c). The lubricant causes the urethra to distend slightly and facilitates passage of the catheter without traumatizing the lining of the urethra. If the prepackaged kit does not contain a syringe with the lubricant, the nurse may need assistance in filling a syringe while keeping the lubricant sterile. Some facilities use lidocaine jelly for lubrication before catheter insertion. The jelly comes prepackaged in a sterile syringe and serves a dual purpose of lubricating and numbing the urethra. A medical order is necessary for the use of lidocaine jelly.

(continued)

Skill 12-7 ▶ Catheterizing the Male Urinary Bladder *(continued)*

ACTION	RATIONALE
19. Use the dominant hand to pick up the catheter and hold it an inch or two from the tip. Ask the patient to bear down as if voiding. **Insert the catheter tip into the meatus (Figure 4). Ask the patient to take deep breaths. Advance the catheter to the bifurcation or "Y" level of the ports. Do not use force to introduce the catheter. If the catheter resists entry, ask the patient to breathe deeply and rotate the catheter slightly.**	Bearing down eases the passage of the catheter through the urethra. The male urethra is about 20 cm long. Having the patient take deep breaths or twisting the catheter slightly may ease the catheter past resistance at the sphincters. Insert indwelling catheters for male patients to the catheter bifurcation (the "Y" level created by the balloon filling and urinary drainage ports) to assure the balloon is within the bladder and to avoid inadvertent inflation of the balloon in the urethra (ANA, 2014; SUNA, 2015c).
20. Hold the catheter securely at the meatus with your non-dominant hand. Use your dominant hand to inflate the catheter balloon. **Inject the entire volume of sterile water supplied in a prefilled syringe. Once the balloon is inflated, the catheter may be gently pulled back into place. Replace foreskin, if present, over the catheter. Lower the penis.**	Bladder or sphincter contraction could push the catheter out. The balloon anchors the catheter in place in the bladder. The manufacturer provides appropriate amount of solution for the size of the catheter in the kit; as a result, use the entire syringe provided in the kit.
21. Pull gently on the catheter after the balloon is inflated to feel resistance.	Improper inflation can cause patient discomfort and malpositioning of catheter.
22. Attach the catheter to drainage system, if necessary.	Closed drainage system minimizes the risk for microorganisms being introduced into the bladder.
23. Remove equipment and dispose of it according to facility policy. Discard syringe in sharps container. Wash and dry the perineal area, as needed.	Proper disposal prevents the spread of microorganisms. Placing syringe in sharps container prevents reuse. Promotes comfort and appropriate personal hygiene.
24. Remove gloves. Secure catheter tubing to the patient's inner thigh or lower abdomen (with the penis directed toward the patient's chest) with a catheter-securing device or tape (Figure 5). Leave some slack in the catheter for leg movement.	Proper attachment prevents trauma to the urethra and meatus from tension on the tubing. Whether to take the drainage tubing over or under the leg depends on gravity flow, patient's mobility, and comfort of the patient.

FIGURE 4. Inserting catheter using dominant hand.

FIGURE 5. Securing tubing to patient's abdomen.

ACTION	**RATIONALE**

25. Assist the patient to a comfortable position. Cover the patient with bed linens. Place the bed in the lowest position.

Positioning and covering provides warmth and promotes comfort.

26. Secure drainage bag below the level of the bladder. Check that drainage tubing is not kinked and that movement of side rails does not interfere with the catheter or drainage bag.

This facilitates drainage of urine and prevents the backflow of urine.

27. Put on clean gloves. Obtain urine specimen immediately, if needed, from drainage bag. Label specimen. Send urine specimen to the laboratory promptly or refrigerate it.

Catheter system is sterile. Obtaining specimen immediately allows access to sterile system. Keeping urine at room temperature may cause microorganisms, if present, to grow and distort laboratory findings.

28. Remove gloves and additional PPE, if used. Perform hand hygiene.

Proper removal of PPE reduces the risk for infection transmission and contamination of other items. Hand hygiene prevents the spread of microorganisms.

EVALUATION

The expected outcomes have been met when the catheter is successfully inserted without adverse effect; the patient's urinary elimination is maintained; and the patient's bladder is not distended. Other outcomes have been met when the patient's skin remains clean, dry, and intact, without evidence of irritation or breakdown; and the patient verbalizes an understanding of the purpose for and care of the catheter, as appropriate.

DOCUMENTATION

Guidelines

Document the type and size of catheter and balloon inserted, as well as the amount of fluid used to inflate the balloon. Document the patient's tolerance of the activity. Record the amount of urine obtained through the catheter and any specimen obtained. Document any other assessments, such as unusual urine characteristics or alterations in the patient's skin. Record urine amount on intake and output record, if appropriate.

Sample Documentation

DocuCare Practice documenting catheterization of the male urinary bladder in *Lippincott DocuCare*.

7/14/20 1830 Patient unable to void for 8 hours and reports, "I feel like I have to go to the bathroom." Bladder scanned for 540-mL urine. Primary care provider notified; 10-mL 2% lidocaine jelly instilled before catheterization per order; 14F Foley catheter inserted without difficulty; 10 mL of sterile water injected into 5-mL balloon port; 525-mL clear yellow urine returned. Patient reports decreased bladder pressure. Patient tolerated procedure without adverse event.

—B. Clapp, RN

UNEXPECTED SITUATIONS AND ASSOCIATED INTERVENTIONS

- *You cannot insert the catheter past 3 to 4 in; rotating the catheter and having the patient breathe deeply are of no help:* If still unable to place the catheter, notify the primary care provider. Repeated catheter placement attempts can traumatize the urethra. The primary care provider may order and insert a coudé catheter.
- *Patient is obese or has retracted penis:* Have an assistant available to place fingers on either side of the pubic area and press backward to bring the penis out of the pubic cavity. Hold the patient's penis up and forward. The catheter still needs to be inserted to the bifurcation; the length of the urethra has not changed.
- *Urine leaks out of the meatus around the catheter:* Do not increase the size of the indwelling catheter. Make sure the smallest-sized catheter with a 10-mL balloon is used. Large catheters cause bladder and urethral irritation and trauma. Large, balloon-fill volumes occupy more space inside the bladder and put added weight on the base of the bladder. Irritation of the bladder wall and detrusor muscle can cause leakage. If leakage persists, consider an evaluation for urinary tract

(continued)

infection. Ensure that the correct amount of solution was used to inflate the balloon. Underfilling the balloon can cause the catheter to dislodge into the urethra, causing urethral spasm, pain, and discomfort. If underfill is suspected, do not attempt to push the catheter farther into the bladder. Remove the catheter and replace it. Assess the patient for constipation. Bowel full of stool can cause pressure on the catheter lumen and prevent the drainage of urine. Implement interventions to prevent/treat constipation.

- *Urine flow is initially well established and urine is clear, but after several hours urine flow dwindles:* Check tubing for kinking. If the patient has changed position, the tubing and drainage bag may need to be moved to facilitate drainage of urine.

SPECIAL CONSIDERATIONS

General Considerations

- Be familiar with facility policy and/or primary health care provider guidelines for the maximum amount of urine to remove from the bladder at the time of insertion.
- Supplies can be opened and prepared on the overbed table, moving the tray onto the bed just before cleansing the patient.
- If there is not an immediate flow of urine after the catheter has been inserted, several measures may prove helpful:
  - Have the patient take a deep breath, which helps to relax the perineal and abdominal muscles.
  - Rotate the catheter slightly, because a drainage hole may be resting against the bladder wall.
  - Raise the head of the patient's bed to increase pressure in the bladder area.
  - Assess the patient's intake to ensure adequate fluid intake for urine production.
  - Assess the catheter and drainage tubing for kinks and occlusion.
  - Urethral strictures, false passages, prostatic enlargement, and postsurgical bladder-neck contractures can make urethral catheterization difficult and may require the services of a urologist. If there is any question to the location of the catheter, do not inflate the balloon. Remove the catheter and notify the health care provider (SUNA, 2015c).
- If the catheter cannot be advanced, having the patient take several deep breaths may be helpful. Rotate the catheter half a turn, and try to advance it. If you are still unable to advance it, remove the catheter. Notify the primary care provider.
- Some catheter kits do not contain the catheter. This allows you to select a catheter and balloon size separately.
- Lubricant may occlude the catheter lumen. If urine flow does not occur within a minute of catheter inserting use a syringe and irrigate, freeing the lumen of the lubricant (SUNA, 2015c).

Infant and Child Considerations

- Size 5F to 8F is used for infants and young children. Size 8F to 14F catheters are commonly used for older children (Perry et al., 2014).
- Distraction, such as blowing bubbles, deep breathing, or singing a song, can help the child relax.
- Consider use of lidocaine jelly to anesthetize and lubricate the area before insertion of the catheter, decreasing the child's discomfort and anxiety.

Older Adult Considerations

- If resistance is met while inserting a catheter and rotating does not help, it is important to never force the catheter. The resistance may be caused by enlargement of the prostate gland, which is commonly seen in men over age 50 years. A special crook-tipped catheter called a coudé catheter, inserted by the health care provider or advanced practice nurse, may be required to maneuver past the prostate gland.

Home Care Considerations

- Intermittent catheterization, performed by the patient or a caregiver in the home, may be necessary for patients with spinal cord injuries or other neurologic conditions. Although the risk for UTI is always present, most research supports the use of clean, rather than sterile, technique in the home environment (Bardsley, 2015a; Wilson, 2015). The procedure for self-intermittent catheterization is essentially the same as that used by the nurse to catheterize a patient. Box 12-2 outlines important information related to patient intermittent self-catheterization.
- Single-use catheters, reusable catheters that are cleaned between use, and no-touch catheters are options for use for intermittent self-catheterization (ISC) in the home setting (Holland & Fish, 2012).

Skill Variation ▶ Intermittent Male Urethral Catheterization

1. Check the medical record for the order for intermittent urethral catheterization. Review the patient's chart for any limitations in physical activity. Gather supplies. Obtain assistance from another staff member, if necessary.

2. Perform hand hygiene. Put on PPE, as indicated, based on transmission precautions.

3. Identify the patient. Discuss the procedure with the patient and assess the patient's ability to assist with the procedure. Ask the patient if he has any allergies, especially to latex or iodine.

4. Close the curtains around the bed and close the door to the room, if possible.

5. Provide good lighting. Artificial light is recommended (use of a flashlight requires an assistant to hold and position it). Place a trash receptacle within easy reach.

6. Assemble equipment on overbed table or other surface within reach.

7. Raise the bed to a comfortable working height. Stand on the patient's right side if you are right-handed, patient's left side if you are left-handed.

8. Position the patient on his back with thighs slightly apart. Drape the patient so that only the area around the penis is exposed. Slide waterproof pad under the patient.

9. Put on clean gloves. Clean the genital area with washcloth, skin cleanser, and warm water. Clean the tip of the penis first, moving the washcloth in a circular motion from the meatus outward. Wash the shaft of the penis using downward strokes toward the pubic area. Rinse and dry. Remove gloves. Perform hand hygiene again.

10. Open sterile catheterization tray on a clean overbed table using sterile technique.

11. Put on sterile gloves. Open sterile drape and place on the patient's thighs. Place fenestrated drape with opening over the penis.

12. Place catheter setup on or next to the patient's legs on sterile drape.

13. Open all the supplies. Open package of antiseptic swabs. Alternately, fluff cotton balls in a tray before pouring antiseptic solution over them. Open specimen container if specimen is to be obtained. Lubricate 1 to 2 in of the catheter tip.

14. Remove cap from syringe prefilled with lubricant.

15. Lift the penis with the nondominant hand. Retract foreskin in uncircumcised patient. **Be prepared to keep this hand in this position until catheter is inserted and urine is flowing well and continuously.**

16. Use the dominant hand to pick up an antiseptic swab or use forceps to pick up a cotton ball. Using a circular motion, clean the penis, moving from the meatus down the glans of the penis. Repeat this cleansing motion two more times, using a new cotton ball/swab each time. Discard each cotton ball/swab after one use.

17. Hold the penis with slight upward tension and perpendicular to the patient's body. Use the dominant hand to pick up the lubricant syringe. **Gently insert tip of syringe with lubricant into urethra and instill the 10 mL of lubricant.**

18. With the noncontaminated, dominant hand, place the drainage end of the catheter in a receptacle. If a specimen is required, place the end into the specimen container in the receptacle.

19. Use the dominant hand to pick up the catheter and hold it an inch or two from the tip. Ask the patient to bear down as if voiding. Insert the catheter tip into the meatus. Ask the patient to take deep breaths as you advance the catheter 6 to 8 in (14.4 to 19.2 cm) or until urine flows.

20. Hold the catheter securely at the meatus with the nondominant hand while the bladder empties. If a specimen is being collected, remove the drainage end of the tubing from the specimen container after the required amount is obtained and allow urine to flow into the receptacle. Set specimen container aside.

21. Allow the bladder to empty. Withdraw the catheter slowly and smoothly after urine has stopped flowing. Remove equipment and dispose of it according to facility policy. Discard syringe in sharps container to prevent reuse. Wash and dry the genital area, as needed. Replace foreskin in forward position, if necessary.

22. Remove gloves. Assist the patient to a comfortable position. Cover the patient with bed linens. Place the bed in the lowest position.

23. Put on clean gloves. Cover and label the specimen. Send the urine specimen to the laboratory promptly or refrigerate it.

24. Remove gloves and additional PPE, if used. Perform hand hygiene.

Note: Intermittent catheterization in the home is performed using clean technique. The bladder's natural resistance to the microorganisms normally found in the home makes sterile technique unnecessary. Single-use catheters, reusable catheters, and no-touch catheters are options for use for intermittent self-catheterization (ISC) in the home setting (Holland & Fish, 2012). Reusable catheters are washed, dried, and stored for repeated use.

Box 12-2 outlines important information related to patient intermittent self-catheterization.

(*continued*)

Skill 12-7 ▶ Catheterizing the Male Urinary Bladder *(continued)*

EVIDENCE FOR PRACTICE ▶ **PREVENTION OF CATHETER-ASSOCIATED INFECTIONS**

Centers for Disease Control and Prevention (CDC). (2015). *Healthcare-associated infections (HAIs). Catheter-associated urinary tract infections (CAUTI).* Retrieved https://www.cdc.gov/HAI/ca_uti/uti.html.

Institute for Healthcare Improvement (IHI). (2011). *How-to guide: Prevent catheter-associated urinary tract infection.* Cambridge, MA: Author. Retrieved http://www.ihi.org/resources/Pages/Tools/HowtoGuidePreventCatheterAssociatedUrinaryTractInfection.aspx.

Society of Urologic Nurses and Associates (SUNA). (2010a). *Clinical practice guidelines. Prevention & control of catheter-associated urinary tract infection (CAUTI).* [Brochure]. Pitman, NJ: Author.

These guidelines provide evidence-based recommendations to guide care for patients requiring catheterization of the urinary bladder to prevent CAUTI.

Refer to thePoint® for additional research on related nursing topics.

EVIDENCE FOR PRACTICE ▶ **INDWELLING URINARY CATHETER TUBING AND DEPENDENT LOOPS**

Preventing CAUTI is a health care priority. It is important to maintain a constant downward flow of urine to aid in the free flow of urine from the bladder to reduce the risk of urinary tract infection. Kinks and dependent loops (low points) in the tubing interfere with the free flow of urine from the bladder and contribute to backflow of urine in the drainage tubing into the bladder, contributing to the development of a urinary tract infection.

Related Research

Wuthier, P., Sublett, K., & Riehl, L. (2016). Urinary catheter dependent loops as a potential contributing cause of bacteriuria: An observational study. *Urologic Nursing, 36*(1), 7–16.

Refer to details in Skill 12-6, Evidence for Practice, and to thePoint® for additional research on related nursing topics.

Skill 12-8 ▶ Removing an Indwelling Urinary Catheter

Removal of an indwelling catheter is performed using clean technique. Take care to prevent trauma to the urethra during the procedure. Completely deflate the catheter balloon before catheter removal to avoid irritation and damage to the urethra and meatus. The patient may experience burning or irritation the first few times he or she voids after removal, due to urethral irritation. If the catheter was in place for more than a few days, decreased bladder muscle tone and swelling of the urethra may cause the patient to experience difficulty voiding or an inability to void. Monitor the patient for urinary retention. It is important to encourage adequate oral fluid intake to promote adequate urinary output. Check facility policy regarding the length of time the patient is allowed to accomplish successful voiding after catheter removal.

DELEGATION CONSIDERATIONS

Removal of an indwelling catheter is not delegated to nursing assistive personnel (NAP) or to unlicensed assistive personnel (UAP). Depending on the state's nurse practice act and the organization's policies and procedures, removal of an indwelling catheter may be delegated to licensed practical/vocational nurses (LPN/LVNs). The decision to delegate must be based on careful analysis of the patient's needs and circumstances, as well as the qualifications of the person to whom the task is being delegated. Refer to the Delegation Guidelines in Appendix A.

EQUIPMENT	• Syringe sufficiently large to accommodate the volume of solution used to inflate the balloon (balloon size/inflation volume is printed on the balloon inflation valve on the catheter at the bifurcation) • Waterproof, disposable pad	• Disposable gloves • Additional PPE, as indicated • Washcloth, skin cleanser, and warm water to perform perineal hygiene after catheter removal

ASSESSMENT	Check the medical record for an order to remove the catheter. Assess for discharge or encrustation around the urethral meatus. Assess urine output, including color and current amount in drainage bag.

NURSING DIAGNOSIS	Determine the related factors for the nursing diagnoses based on the patient's current status. Appropriate nursing diagnoses may include: • Impaired urinary elimination • Risk for injury • Urinary retention

OUTCOME IDENTIFICATION AND PLANNING	The expected outcome to achieve when removing an indwelling catheter is that the catheter will be removed without difficulty and with minimal patient discomfort. Other appropriate outcomes include the following: the patient voids without discomfort after catheter removal; the patient voids a minimum of 250 mL of urine within 6 to 8 hours of catheter removal; the patient's skin remains clean, dry, and intact, without evidence of irritation or breakdown; and the patient verbalizes an understanding of the need to maintain adequate fluid intake, as appropriate.

IMPLEMENTATION

ACTION	RATIONALE
1. Confirm the order for catheter removal in the medical record. Gather equipment.	Verifying the medical order ensures that the correct intervention is administered to the right patient. Assembling equipment provides for an organized approach to the task.
2. Perform hand hygiene and put on PPE, if indicated.	Hand hygiene and PPE prevent the spread of microorganisms. PPE is required based on transmission precautions.
3. Identify the patient.	Identifying the patient ensures the right patient receives the intervention and helps prevent errors.
4. Close the curtains around the bed and close the door to the room, if possible. Discuss the procedure with the patient and assess the patient's ability to assist with the procedure.	This ensures the patient's privacy. Discussion promotes reassurance and provides knowledge about the procedure. Dialogue encourages patient participation and allows for individualized nursing care.
5. Adjust the bed to a comfortable working height, usually elbow height of the caregiver (VHACEOSH, 2016). Stand on the patient's right side if you are right-handed, patient's left side if you are left-handed.	Having the bed at the proper height prevents back and muscle strain. Positioning allows for ease of use of dominant hand for catheter removal.
6. Position the patient as for catheter insertion. Drape the patient so that only the area around the catheter is exposed. Slide waterproof pad between the female patient's legs or over the male patient's thighs.	Positioning allows access to site. Draping prevents unnecessary exposure and promotes warmth. The waterproof pad will protect bed linens from moisture and serve as a receptacle for the used catheter after removal.

(continued)

Skill 12-8 ▶ Removing an Indwelling Urinary Catheter (continued)

ACTION	RATIONALE
7. Remove the device used to secure the catheter to the patient's thigh or abdomen.	This action permits removal of catheter.
8. Insert the syringe into the balloon inflation port. Allow the pressure within the balloon to force the syringe plunger back and fill the syringe with water. (Figure 1). Refer to manufacturer's instructions for deflation. **Do not cut the inflation port.**	Removal of sterile water deflates the balloon to allow for catheter removal. All of the sterile water must be removed to prevent injury to the patient. Aspiration by pulling on the syringe plunger may result in collapse of the inflation lumen; contribute to the formation of creases, ridges, or cuffing at the balloon area; and increase the catheter balloon diameter size on deflation, resulting in difficult removal and urethral trauma.

FIGURE 1. Removing fluid from balloon. (From Craven, RF. [2008]. Fundamentals of Nursing: Human Health and Function, 6th edition. P 1114; Wolters Kluwer Health | Lippincott Williams & Wilkins; Philadelphia, PA.)

ACTION	RATIONALE
9. Ask the patient to take several slow deep breaths. **Slowly and gently remove the catheter.** Place it on the waterproof pad and wrap it in the pad.	Slow deep breathing helps to relax the sphincter muscles. Slow gentle removal prevents trauma to the urethra. Using a waterproof pad prevents contact with the catheter.
10. Wash and dry the perineal area, as needed.	Cleaning promotes comfort and appropriate personal hygiene.
11. Remove gloves. Assist the patient to a comfortable position. Cover the patient with bed linens. Place the bed in the lowest position.	These actions provide warmth and promote comfort and safety.
12. Put on clean gloves. Remove equipment and dispose of it according to facility policy. Note characteristics and amount of urine in drainage bag.	Proper disposal prevents the spread of microorganisms. Observing the characteristics ensures accurate documentation.
13. Remove gloves and additional PPE, if used. Perform hand hygiene.	Proper removal of PPE reduces the risk for infection transmission and contamination of other items. Hand hygiene prevents the spread of microorganisms.

EVALUATION

The expected outcomes have been met when the catheter has been removed without difficulty and with minimal patient discomfort; the patient has voided without discomfort after catheter removal and a minimum of 250 mL of urine within 6 to 8 hours of catheter removal; the patient's skin remains clean, dry, and intact, without evidence of irritation or breakdown; and the patient verbalizes an understanding of the need to maintain adequate fluid intake, as appropriate.

DOCUMENTATION

Guidelines

Document the type and size of catheter removed and the amount of fluid removed from the balloon. Also document the patient's tolerance of the procedure. Record the amount of urine in the drainage bag. Note the time the patient is due to void. Document any other assessments, such as unusual urine characteristics or alterations in the patient's skin. Also record urine amount on intake and output record, if appropriate.

Sample Documentation

> 7/14/20 0800 Removed 15-mL fluid from catheter balloon; 14F Foley removed without difficulty; 500 mL of clear yellow urine noted in drainage bag at time of removal. Patient due to void by 1600. Patient instructed to drink six to eight 6-oz glasses of fluid in the course of the day, and that it may take some time for the passage of urine on his own; patient verbalized understanding of instructions. Urinal placed at bedside, with patient demonstrating appropriate use.
>
> —B. Clapp, RN

UNEXPECTED SITUATIONS AND ASSOCIATED INTERVENTIONS

- *Resistance is felt while attempting to pull out catheter:* Stop pulling the catheter. Reattach syringe to balloon inflation port and aspirate to make sure all the sterile water has been removed. Reattempt catheter removal. If resistance is still present, stop removal and notify the primary care provider.

SPECIAL CONSIDERATIONS

- Have alternate toileting measures available, as necessary, based on patient assessment. A bedside commode, urinal, or bedpan may be necessary if the patient is unable to get to the bathroom.
- Refer to facility policy and manufacturer's recommendation regarding balloon deflation. Aspiration by pulling on the syringe plunger may result in collapse of the inflation lumen; contribute to the formation of creases, ridges, or cuffing at the balloon area; and increase the catheter balloon diameter size on deflation, resulting in difficult removal and urethral trauma.

Skill 12-9 ▶ Performing Intermittent Closed Catheter Irrigation

Routine intermittent irrigation of long-term catheters is not recommended (Gould et al., 2009; SUNA, 2010a). Catheter irrigation should be avoided unless necessary to relieve or prevent obstruction (Gould et al., 2009; SUNA, 2015a). If obstruction is anticipated, continuous irrigation is suggested to prevent obstruction (SUNA, 2010a) (see Skill 12-10). However, intermittent irrigation is sometimes prescribed to restore or maintain the patency of the drainage system. **Sediment** or debris, as well as blood clots, might block the catheter, preventing the flow of urine out of the catheter. Irrigations might also be used to instill medications that will act directly on the bladder wall. Irrigating a catheter through a closed system is preferred to opening the catheter, because opening the catheter could lead to contamination and infection.

DELEGATION CONSIDERATIONS

Intermittent closed catheter irrigation is not delegated to nursing assistive personnel (NAP) or to unlicensed assistive personnel (UAP). Depending on the state's nurse practice act and the organization's policies and procedures, intermittent closed catheter irrigation may be delegated to licensed practical/vocational nurses (LPN/LVNs). The decision to delegate must be based on careful analysis of the patient's needs and circumstances, as well as the qualifications of the person to whom the task is being delegated. Refer to the Delegation Guidelines in Appendix A.

EQUIPMENT

- Sterile basin or container
- Sterile irrigating solution (at room temperature or warmed to body temperature)
- 30- to 60-mL syringe (with 18- or 19-gauge blunt-end needle, if catheter access port is not a needleless system)
- Clamp for drainage tubing
- Bath blanket
- Disposable gloves
- Additional PPE, as indicated
- Waterproof pad
- Alcohol or other disinfectant swab

(continued)

Skill 12-9 ► Performing Intermittent Closed Catheter Irrigation *(continued)*

ASSESSMENT	Check the medical record for an order to irrigate the catheter, including the type and amount of solution to use for the irrigation. Before performing the procedure, assess catheter drainage and amount of urine in drainage bag. Also assess for bladder fullness, either by palpation or with a handheld bladder ultrasound device. Assess for signs of adverse effects, which may include pain, bladder spasm, bladder distension/fullness, or lack of drainage from the catheter.
NURSING DIAGNOSIS	Determine related factors for the nursing diagnoses based on the patient's current status. Appropriate nursing diagnoses may include: • Impaired urinary elimination • Risk for infection
OUTCOME IDENTIFICATION AND PLANNING	The expected outcome to achieve when performing closed catheter irrigation is that the catheter is irrigated without adverse effect and the patient exhibits the free flow of urine through the catheter. Other outcomes may include the following: the patient's bladder is not distended; the patient remains free from pain; and the patient remains free of any signs and symptoms of infection.

IMPLEMENTATION

ACTION	**RATIONALE**
1. Confirm the order for catheter irrigation and prescribed solution in the medical record.	Verifying the medical order ensures that the correct intervention is administered to the right patient.
2. Gather equipment.	Assembling equipment provides for an organized approach to the task.
3. Perform hand hygiene and put on PPE, if indicated.	Hand hygiene and PPE prevent the spread of microorganisms. PPE is required based on transmission precautions.
4. Identify the patient.	Identifying the patient ensures the right patient receives the intervention and helps prevent errors.
5. Close the curtains around the bed and close the door to the room, if possible. Discuss the procedure with the patient.	This ensures the patient's privacy. Discussion promotes reassurance and provides knowledge about the procedure. Dialogue encourages patient participation and allows for individualized nursing care.
6. Assemble equipment on overbed table or other surface within reach.	Arranging items nearby is convenient, saves time, and avoids unnecessary stretching and twisting of muscles on the part of the nurse.
7. Adjust the bed to a comfortable working height, usually elbow height of the caregiver (VHACEOSH, 2016).	Having the bed at the proper height prevents back and muscle strain.
8. Put on gloves. Empty the catheter drainage bag and measure the amount of urine, noting the amount and characteristics of the urine. Remove gloves. Perform hand hygiene.	Gloves prevent contact with blood and body fluids. Emptying the drainage bag allows for accurate assessment of drainage after the irrigation solution is instilled. Assessment of urine provides a baseline for future comparison. Proper removal of PPE prevents transmission of microorganisms. Hand hygiene prevents the spread of microorganisms.

ACTION	RATIONALE
9. Assist the patient to a comfortable position and expose access port on catheter setup. Place waterproof pad under catheter and aspiration port. Remove catheter from device or tape anchoring catheter to the patient.	This provides adequate visualization. Waterproof pad protects patient and bed from leakage. Removing the catheter from the anchoring device or tape allows for manipulation of the catheter.
10. Open supplies, using aseptic technique. Pour sterile solution into sterile basin. Aspirate the prescribed amount of irrigant (usually 30 to 60 mL) into sterile syringe. Put on gloves.	Use of aseptic technique ensures sterility of irrigating fluid and prevents spread of microorganisms. Gloves prevent contact with blood and body fluids.
11. **Cleanse the access port on the catheter with antimicrobial swab (Figure 1).**	Cleaning the port reduces the risk of introducing organisms into the closed urinary system.
12. Clamp or fold catheter tubing below the access port (Figure 2).	This directs the irrigating solution into the bladder, preventing flow into the drainage bag.

FIGURE 1. Cleansing access port on catheter.

FIGURE 2. Clamping catheter below access port.

13. Attach the syringe to the access port on the catheter using a twisting motion (Figure 3). **Gently instill solution into catheter (Figure 4).**	Gentle irrigation prevents damage to bladder lining. Instillation of fluid dislodges material blocking the catheter.

FIGURE 3. Attaching syringe to access port with twisting motion.

FIGURE 4. Gently instilling irrigation solution.

(continued)

Skill 12-9 ▶ Performing Intermittent Closed Catheter Irrigation *(continued)*

ACTION	RATIONALE
14. Remove syringe from access port (Figure 5). **Unclamp or unfold tubing and allow irrigant and urine to flow into the drainage bag. Repeat procedure, as necessary.**	Gravity aids drainage of urine and irrigant from the bladder.

FIGURE 5. Removing syringe from access port.

ACTION	RATIONALE
15. Remove gloves. Secure catheter tubing to the patient's inner thigh or lower abdomen (if a male patient) with anchoring device or tape. Leave some slack in the catheter for leg movement.	Proper attachment prevents trauma to the urethra and meatus from tension on the tubing. Whether to take the drainage tubing over or under the leg depends on gravity flow and patient's mobility and comfort.
16. Assist the patient to a comfortable position. Cover the patient with bed linens. Place the bed in the lowest position.	Positioning and covering provide warmth and promote comfort. Lowering bed contributes to patient safety.
17. Secure drainage bag below the level of the bladder. Check that drainage tubing is not kinked and that movement of side rails does not interfere with catheter or drainage bag.	This facilitates drainage of urine and prevents the backflow of urine.
18. Remove equipment and discard syringe in appropriate receptacle. Remove gloves and additional PPE, if used. Perform hand hygiene.	Proper disposal of equipment prevents transmission of microorganisms. Proper removal of PPE reduces the risk for infection transmission and contamination of other items. Hand hygiene prevents the spread of microorganisms.
19. Assess the patient's response to the procedure and the quality and amount of drainage after the irrigation.	This provides accurate assessment of the patient's response to the procedure.

EVALUATION

The expected outcome has been met when the catheter is irrigated without adverse effect and the patient exhibits the free flow of urine through the catheter; the patient's bladder is not distended; the patient remains free from pain; and the patient remains free of any signs and symptoms of infection.

DOCUMENTATION

Guidelines

Document baseline assessment of the patient. Document the amount and type of irrigation solution used and the amount and characteristics of drainage returned after the procedure. Document the ease of irrigation and the patient's tolerance of the procedure. Record urine amount emptied from the drainage bag before the procedure and the amount of irrigant used on intake and output record. Subtract irrigant amount from the urine output when totaling output to provide accurate recording of urine output.

Sample Documentation

> 7/22/20 1630 Urinary catheter irrigated with 60 mL of normal saline without difficulty. All of irrigation returned plus 200 mL of cloudy yellow urine. Patient tolerated procedure without adverse effect. Order received to notify health care provider if urine output is less than 30 mL/hr.
>
> —B. Clapp, RN

UNEXPECTED SITUATIONS AND ASSOCIATED INTERVENTIONS

- *Irrigation solution will not enter the catheter:* Do not force the solution into the catheter. Notify primary care provider. Prepare to change catheter.
- *Tubing was not clamped before introducing irrigation solution:* Repeat irrigation, making sure to clamp the tube before introducing irrigation solution. If the tubing is not clamped, the irrigation solution will drain into the urinary drainage bag and not enter the catheter.

SPECIAL CONSIDERATIONS

- If irrigant is a medication intended for action in the bladder, be aware of specific dwell time included in the order or determined by the action of the medication. Allow the appropriate amount of time to lapse before unclamping the drainage tubing after instillation of the irrigant.

EVIDENCE FOR PRACTICE ▶

PREVENTION AND CONTROL OF CATHETER-ASSOCIATED URINARY TRACT INFECTIONS

Prevention of Catheter-Associated Infections

Centers for Disease Control and Prevention (CDC). (2015). *Healthcare-associated infections (HAIs). Catheter-associated urinary tract infections (CAUTI).* Retrieved https://www.cdc.gov/HAI/ca_uti/uti.html.

Institute for Healthcare Improvement (IHI). (2011). *How-to guide: Prevent catheter-associated urinary tract infection.* Cambridge, MA: Author. Retrieved http://www.ihi.org/resources/Pages/Tools/HowtoGuidePreventCatheterAssociatedUrinaryTractInfection.aspx.

Society of Urologic Nurses and Associates (SUNA). (2010a). *Clinical practice guidelines. Prevention & control of catheter-associated urinary tract infection (CAUTI). [Brochure].* Pitman, NJ: Author.

These guidelines provide evidence-based recommendations to guide care for patients requiring catheterization of the urinary bladder to prevent CAUTI.

Refer to thePoint® for additional research on related nursing topics.

Skill 12-10 ▶ Administering a Continuous Closed Bladder or Catheter Irrigation

Bladder irrigation is not recommended unless obstruction is anticipated, as might occur with bleeding after prostate or bladder surgery (SUNA, 2010a). Sediment or debris, as well as blood clots, might block the catheter, preventing the flow of urine out of the catheter. Indwelling catheters sometimes require continuous irrigation, or flushing, with solution to restore or maintain the patency of the drainage system. Catheter irrigation should be avoided, unless necessary, to relieve or prevent obstruction (Gould et al., 2009; SUNA, 2015a). If obstruction is anticipated, continuous irrigation is suggested to prevent obstruction (SUNA, 2010a). Irrigations might also be used to

(*continued*)

Skill 12-10

Administering a Continuous Closed Bladder or Catheter Irrigation *(continued)*

instill medications that will act directly on the bladder wall. Irrigating a catheter through a closed system is preferred to opening the catheter because opening the catheter could lead to contamination and infection. A triple-lumen or three-way catheter (Figure 1) is used for a continuous irrigation in order to maintain a closed system (Figure 2) to avoid contamination and resulting infection (SUNA, 2010a).

FIGURE 1. A triple-lumen catheter.

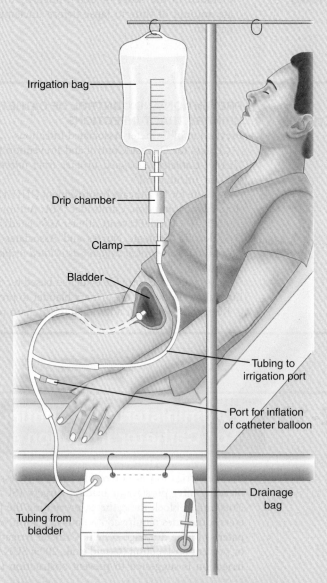

FIGURE 2. A continuous bladder irrigation (CBI) setup.

DELEGATION CONSIDERATIONS	The administration of continuous closed bladder irrigation is not delegated to nursing assistive personnel (NAP) or to unlicensed assistive personnel (UAP). Depending on the state's nurse practice act and the organization's policies and procedures, administration of continuous closed bladder irrigation may be delegated to licensed practical/vocational nurses (LPN/LVNs). The decision to delegate must be based on careful analysis of the patient's needs and circumstances, as well as the qualifications of the person to whom the task is being delegated. Refer to the Delegation Guidelines in Appendix A.
EQUIPMENT	• Sterile irrigating solution (at room temperature or warmed to body temperature) • Sterile tubing with drip chamber and clamp for connection to irrigating solution • IV pole • IV pump (if bladder is being irrigated with a solution containing medication) • Three-way indwelling catheter in place in patient's bladder • Indwelling catheter drainage setup (tubing and collection bag) • Alcohol or other disinfectant swab • Bath blanket • Disposable gloves • Additional PPE, as indicated
ASSESSMENT	Verify the order in the medical record for continuous bladder irrigation, including type and amount of irrigant or irrigation parameters. Assess the catheter to ensure that it has an irrigation port (if the patient has an indwelling catheter already in place). Assess the characteristics of urine present in tubing and drainage bag. Review the patient's medical record for, and ask the patient about, any allergies to medications. Before performing the procedure, assess the bladder for fullness either by palpation or with a handheld bladder ultrasound device. Assess for signs of adverse effects, which may include pain, bladder spasm, bladder distension/fullness, or lack of drainage from the catheter.
NURSING DIAGNOSIS	Determine related factors for the nursing diagnoses based on the patient's current status. Appropriate nursing diagnoses may include: • Impaired urinary elimination • Risk for infection
OUTCOME IDENTIFICATION AND PLANNING	The expected outcome to achieve is that the irrigation is administered without adverse effect and the patient exhibits free-flowing urine through the catheter. Initially, clots or debris may be noted. These should decrease over time, with the patient ultimately exhibiting urine that is free of clots or debris. Other outcomes may include the following: the continuous bladder irrigation continues without adverse effect; drainage is greater than the hourly amount of irrigation solution being placed in the bladder; and the patient exhibits no signs and symptoms of infection.

IMPLEMENTATION

ACTION	RATIONALE
1. Confirm the order for catheter irrigation in the medical record, including infusion parameters. If irrigation is to be implemented via gravity infusion, calculate the drip rate. Often, orders are to infuse to keep the urine clear of blood or clots.	Verifying the medical order ensures that the correct intervention is administered to the right patient. Solution must be administered via gravity at the appropriate rate as prescribed.
2. Gather equipment.	Assembling equipment provides for an organized approach to the task.

(continued)

Skill 12-10 ▶ Administering a Continuous Closed Bladder or Catheter Irrigation *(continued)*

ACTION	RATIONALE
3. Perform hand hygiene and put on PPE, if indicated.	Hand hygiene and PPE prevent the spread of microorganisms. PPE is required based on transmission precautions.
4. Identify the patient.	Identifying the patient ensures the right patient receives the intervention and helps prevent errors.
5. Close the curtains around the bed and close the door to the room, if possible. Discuss the procedure with the patient.	This ensures the patient's privacy. Discussion promotes reassurance and provides knowledge about the procedure. Dialogue encourages patient participation and allows for individualized nursing care.
6. Assemble equipment on overbed table or other surface within reach.	Arranging items nearby is convenient, saves time, and avoids unnecessary stretching and twisting of muscles on the part of the nurse.
7. Adjust the bed to a comfortable working height, usually elbow height of the caregiver (VHACEOSH, 2016).	Having the bed at the proper height prevents back and muscle strain.
8. Empty the catheter drainage bag and measure the amount of urine, noting the amount and characteristics of the urine.	Emptying the drainage bag allows for accurate assessment of drainage after the irrigation solution is instilled. Assessment of urine provides baseline for future comparison.
9. Assist the patient to a comfortable position and expose the irrigation port on the catheter setup. Place waterproof pad under the catheter and irrigation port.	This provides adequate visualization. Waterproof pad protects the patient and bed from leakage.
10. Prepare sterile irrigation bag for use as directed by manufacturer. Clearly label the solution as "Bladder Irrigant." Include the date and time on the label. Hang bag on IV pole 2.5 to 3 ft above the level of the patient's bladder. Close tubing clamp and insert sterile tubing with drip chamber to container using aseptic technique (Figure 3). Release clamp and remove protective cover on end of tubing without contaminating it. Allow solution to flush tubing and remove air (Figure 4). Clamp tubing and replace end cover.	Proper labeling provides accurate information for caregivers. Sterile solution not used within 24 hours of opening should be discarded. Aseptic technique prevents contamination of solution irrigation system. Priming the tubing before attaching irrigation clears air from the tubing that might cause bladder distention.

FIGURE 3. Inserting tubing into solution bag.

FIGURE 4. Removing air from irrigation tubing.

ACTION

RATIONALE

11. Put on gloves. **Cleanse the irrigation port on the catheter with an alcohol swab. Using aseptic technique, attach irrigation tubing to irrigation port of three-way indwelling catheter (Figure 5).**

Aseptic technique prevents the spread of microorganisms into the bladder.

12. Check the drainage tubing to make sure clamp, if present, is open.

An open clamp prevents accumulation of solution in the bladder.

13. **Release clamp on irrigation tubing and regulate flow at determined drip rate, according to the ordered rate (Figure 6). If the bladder irrigation is to be done with a medicated solution, use an electronic infusion device to regulate the flow.**

This allows for continual gentle irrigation without causing discomfort to the patient. An electronic infusion device regulates the flow of the medication.

FIGURE 5. Attaching irrigation tubing to irrigation port on catheter.

FIGURE 6. Regulating irrigation flow rate using flow clamp.

14. Remove gloves. Assist the patient to a comfortable position. Cover the patient with bed linens. Place the bed in the lowest position.

Positioning and covering provide warmth and promote comfort and safety.

15. Assess the patient's response to the procedure, and the quality and amount of drainage.

Assessment is necessary to determine the effectiveness of the intervention and to detect adverse effects.

 16. Remove equipment. Remove additional PPE, if used. Perform hand hygiene.

Proper disposal of equipment prevents transmission of microorganisms. Proper removal of PPE reduces the risk for infection transmission and contamination of other items. Hand hygiene prevents the spread of microorganisms.

17. As irrigation fluid container nears empty, clamp the administration tubing. Do not allow drip chamber to empty. Disconnect empty bag and attach a new full irrigation solution bag.

This eliminates the need to separate tubing from the catheter and clear air from the tubing. Opening the drainage system provides access for microorganisms.

18. Put on gloves and empty drainage collection bag as each new container is hung. Record initiation of new container and volume of drainage.

Gloves protect against exposure to blood, body fluids, and microorganisms. Accurate recording of volume of irrigation solution infused and catheter drainage allows for accurate calculation of urinary output.

EVALUATION

The expected outcome has been met when the irrigation has been administered without adverse effect and the patient exhibits free-flowing urine through the catheter; the continuous bladder irrigation continues without adverse effect; drainage from the catheter is greater than the hourly amount of irrigation solution being placed in the bladder; and the patient exhibits no signs and symptoms of infection.

(continued)

Skill 12-10 ▶ Administering a Continuous Closed Bladder or Catheter Irrigation *(continued)*

DOCUMENTATION

Guidelines

Document baseline assessment of the patient. Document the amount and type of irrigation solution used and the patient's tolerance of the procedure. Record urine amount emptied from the drainage bag before the procedure and the amount of irrigant used on intake and output record. Record the amount of urine and irrigant emptied from the drainage bag. **Subtract the amount of irrigant instilled from the total volume of drainage to obtain the volume of urine output.**

Sample Documentation

> 12/14/20 1330 Foley catheter replaced with 3-way Foley catheter. Bladder nonpalpable. Continuous bladder irrigation with normal saline initiated at 100 mL/hr. Patient tolerated procedure without adverse effect. Drainage from bladder slightly cloudy, light cherry colored. No evidence of clots.
>
> —B. Clapp, RN

UNEXPECTED SITUATIONS AND ASSOCIATED INTERVENTIONS

- *Continuous bladder irrigation begins and hourly drainage is less than amount of irrigation being given:* Palpate for bladder distention. If the patient is lying supine, rolling the patient onto his/her side may help increase the amount of drainage. Check to make sure that the tubing is not kinked. If return flow remains decreased, notify primary care provider.
- *Bladder irrigation is not flowing at ordered rate, even with clamp wide open:* Check the tubing for kinks or pressure points. Raise the bag 3 to 6 in and then check flow of irrigation solution. Frequently check flow rate of irrigation solution.

EVIDENCE FOR PRACTICE ▶

PREVENTION AND CONTROL OF CATHETER-ASSOCIATED URINARY TRACT INFECTIONS

Centers for Disease Control and Prevention (CDC). (2015). *Healthcare-associated infections (HAIs). Catheter-associated urinary tract infections (CAUTI).* Retrieved https://www.cdc.gov/HAI/ca_uti/uti.html.

Institute for Healthcare Improvement (IHI). (2011). *How-to guide: Prevent catheter-associated urinary tract infection.* Cambridge, MA: Author. Retrieved http://www.ihi.org/resources/Pages/Tools/HowtoGuidePreventCatheterAssociatedUrinaryTractInfection.aspx.

Society of Urologic Nurses and Associates (SUNA). (2010a). *Clinical practice guidelines. Prevention & control of catheter-associated urinary tract infection (CAUTI). [Brochure].* Pitman, NJ: Author.

These guidelines provide evidence-based recommendations to guide care for patients requiring catheterization of the urinary bladder to prevent CAUTI.

Refer to thePoint® for additional research on related nursing topics.

Skill 12-11 ▶ Emptying and Changing a Stoma Appliance on a Urinary Diversion

Urinary diversions may be used as part of the treatment for patients with obstructions or tumors in the urinary tract, a neurogenic bladder, radiation cystitis, or congenital anomalies of the lower urinary tract. An **ileal conduit** is a type of incontinent cutaneous urinary diversion. An ileal conduit involves a surgical resection of the small intestine, with transplantation of the ureters to the isolated segment of small bowel. This separated section of the small intestine is then brought to the abdominal wall, where urine is excreted through a **stoma**, a surgically created opening on the body surface. Such diversions are usually permanent, and the patient wears an external appliance to collect the urine because urine elimination from the stoma cannot be controlled voluntarily. Appliances are available in a one-piece (barrier backing already attached to the pouch) or two-piece (separate pouch that fastens to the barrier backing) system; they are usually changed every 3 to 7 days, although they could be changed more often. Proper application minimizes the risk for skin breakdown around the stoma. This skill addresses changing a one-piece appliance. A one-piece appliance consists of a pouch with an integral adhesive section that adheres to the patient's skin. The adhesive flange is generally made from hydrocolloid. The accompanying Skill Variation addresses changing a two-piece appliance.

The appliance usually is changed after a time of low fluid intake, such as in the early morning. Urine production is less at this time, making changing the appliance easier. Proper application minimizes the risk for skin breakdown around the stoma. Box 12-3 summarizes guidelines for care of the patient with a urinary diversion.

Box 12-3 Guidelines for Care of the Patient With a Urinary Diversion

- Keep the patient as free of odors as possible. If the patient has an external appliance, empty the appliance frequently.
- Inspect the patient's stoma regularly. It should be dark pink to red and moist. A pale stoma may indicate anemia, and a dark or purple-blue stoma may reflect compromised circulation or ischemia. Bleeding around the stoma and its stem should be minimal. Notify the primary care provider promptly if bleeding persists, is excessive, or if color changes occur in the stoma.
- Note the size of the stoma, which usually stabilizes within 6 to 8 weeks. Most stomas protrude 0.5 to 1 in from the abdominal surface and may initially appear swollen and edematous. After 6 weeks, the edema usually subsides. If an abdominal dressing is in place at the incision site after surgery, check it frequently for drainage and bleeding.
- Keep the skin around the stoma site (peristomal area) clean and dry. If care is not taken to protect the skin around the stoma, irritation or infection may occur. A leaking appliance frequently causes skin erosion. Candida or yeast infections can also occur around the stoma if the area is not kept dry.
- Measure the patient's fluid intake and output. Careful monitoring of the patient's urinary output is necessary to monitor fluid balance.

- Monitor the return of intestinal function and peristalsis. Initially after surgery, peristalsis is inhibited. Remember, the patient had a bowel resection as part of the urinary diversion procedure.
- Watch for mucus in the urine from an ileal conduit, which is a normal finding. The isolated segment of small intestine continues to produce mucus as part of its normal functioning.
- Explain each aspect of care to the patient and explain what his/her role will be when he or she begins self-care. Patient teaching is one of the most important aspects of ostomy care and should include family members, when appropriate. Teaching can begin before surgery so that the patient has adequate time to absorb the information.
- Encourage the patient to participate in care and to look at the stoma. Patients normally experience emotional depression during the early postoperative period. Help the patient to cope by listening, explaining, and being available and supportive. A visit from a representative of the local ostomy support group may be helpful. Patients usually begin to accept their altered body image when they are willing to look at the stoma, make neutral or positive statements concerning the ostomy, and express interest in learning self-care.

DELEGATION CONSIDERATIONS

The emptying of a stoma appliance on a urinary diversion may be delegated to nursing assistive personnel (NAP) or to unlicensed assistive personnel (UAP), as well as to licensed practical/vocational nurses (LPN/LVNs). The changing of a stoma appliance on a urinary diversion may be delegated to LPN/LVNs. The decision to delegate must be based on careful analysis of the patient's needs and circumstances, as well as the qualifications of the person to whom the task is being delegated. Refer to the Delegation Guidelines in Appendix A.

EQUIPMENT

- Premoistened disposable washcloths or
  - Basin with warm water
  - Skin cleanser, towel, washcloth
- Silicone-based adhesive remover
- Gauze squares
- Skin protectant, such as Skin-Prep
- Ostomy appliance

- Stoma-measuring guide
- Graduated container
- Ostomy belt (optional)
- Disposable gloves
- Additional PPE, as indicated
- Waterproof, disposable pad
- Small plastic trash bag

(*continued*)

Skill 12-11 ▷ Emptying and Changing a Stoma Appliance on a Urinary Diversion *(continued)*

ASSESSMENT	Assess current urinary diversion appliance, observing product style, condition of appliance, and stoma (if bag is clear). Note length of time the appliance has been in place. Determine the patient's knowledge of urinary diversion care, including level of self-care and ability to manipulate the equipment. After the appliance is removed, assess the skin surrounding the urinary diversion. Assess the condition of any abdominal scars or incisional areas, if surgery to create the urinary diversion was recent.
NURSING DIAGNOSIS	Determine the related factors for the nursing diagnoses based on the patient's current status. Appropriate nursing diagnoses may include: • Disturbed body image • Deficient knowledge • Risk for impaired skin integrity
OUTCOME IDENTIFICATION AND PLANNING	The expected outcome to achieve when changing a patient's urinary stoma appliance is that the stoma appliance is applied correctly to the skin to allow urine to drain freely. Other outcomes may include the following: the patient exhibits a moist red stoma with intact skin surrounding the stoma; the patient demonstrates knowledge of how to apply the appliance; and the patient verbalizes positive self-image.

IMPLEMENTATION

ACTION	RATIONALE
1. Gather equipment.	Assembling equipment provides for an organized approach to the task.
2. Perform hand hygiene and put on PPE, if indicated.	Hand hygiene and PPE prevent the spread of microorganisms. PPE is required based on transmission precautions.
3. Identify the patient.	Identifying the patient ensures the right patient receives the intervention and helps prevent errors.
4. Close the curtains around the bed and close the door to the room, if possible. Explain what you are going to do and why you are going to do it to the patient. Encourage the patient to observe or participate, if possible.	This ensures the patient's privacy. Explanation relieves anxiety and facilitates cooperation. Discussion promotes cooperation and helps to minimize anxiety. Having the patient observe or assist encourages self-acceptance.
5. Assemble equipment on overbed table or other surface within reach.	Arranging items nearby is convenient, saves time, and avoids unnecessary stretching and twisting of muscles on the part of the nurse.
6. Assist the patient to a comfortable sitting or lying position in bed or a standing or sitting position in the bathroom. If the patient is in bed, adjust the bed to a comfortable working height, usually elbow height of the caregiver (VHACEOSH, 2016). Place waterproof pad under the patient at the stoma site.	Either position should allow the patient to view the procedure in preparation for learning to perform it independently. Lying flat or sitting upright facilitates smooth application of the appliance. Having the bed at the proper height prevents back and muscle strain. A waterproof pad protects linens and the patient from moisture.

Emptying the Appliance

7. Put on gloves. Hold end of appliance over a bedpan, toilet, or measuring device. Remove the end cap from the spout. Open the spout and empty the contents into the bedpan, toilet, or measuring device (Figure 1).	Gloves protect the nurse from exposure to blood and body fluids. Emptying the pouch before handling it reduces the likelihood of spilling the excretions.

ACTION

RATIONALE

FIGURE 1. Emptying urine into graduated container.

8. Close the spout. Wipe the spout with toilet tissue. Replace the cap.

Drying the spout removes any urine.

9. Remove equipment. Remove gloves. Assist the patient to a comfortable position.

Proper removal of PPE prevents the transmission of microorganisms. Ensures patient comfort.

10. If appliance is not to be changed, place bed in lowest position. Remove additional PPE, if used. Perform hand hygiene.

Lowering the bed promotes patient safety. Proper removal of PPE reduces the risk for infection transmission and contamination of other items. Hand hygiene prevents the spread of microorganisms.

Changing the Appliance

11. Place a disposable waterproof pad on the overbed table or other work area. Open the premoistened disposable washcloths or set up the washbasin with warm water and the rest of the supplies. Place a trash bag within reach.

The pad protects the surface. Organization facilitates performance of the procedure.

12. Put on clean gloves. Place waterproof pad under the patient at the stoma site. Empty the appliance, if necessary, as described in Steps 6 to 8.

Waterproof pad protects linens and patient from moisture. Emptying the contents before removal prevents accidental spillage of fecal material.

13. Put on gloves. Gently remove the appliance faceplate, starting at the top and keeping the abdominal skin taut (Figure 2). Remove appliance faceplate from skin by pushing skin from appliance rather than pulling appliance from skin (Figure 3). Apply a silicone-based adhesive remover by spraying or wiping with the remover wipe, as needed.

Gloves prevent contact with blood and body fluids. The seal between the surface of the faceplate and the skin must be broken before the faceplate can be removed. Harsh handling of the appliance can damage the skin and impair the development of a secure seal in the future. Silicone-based adhesive remover allows for the rapid and painless removal of adhesives and prevents skin stripping (Rudoni, 2008; Stephen-Haynes, 2008).

FIGURE 2. Gently removing appliance faceplate from skin.

FIGURE 3. Pushing skin from appliance rather than pulling appliance from skin.

(continued)

Skill 12-11 ▶ Emptying and Changing a Stoma Appliance on a Urinary Diversion *(continued)*

ACTION	RATIONALE
14. Place the appliance in the trash bag, if disposable. If reusable, set aside to wash in lukewarm soap and water and allow to air dry after the new appliance is in place.	Thorough cleaning and airing of the appliance reduce odor and deterioration of appliance. For aesthetic and infection control purposes, used appliances should be discarded appropriately.
15. Clean skin around stoma with mild skin cleanser and water or a cleansing agent and a washcloth (Figure 4). Remove all old adhesive from the skin; additional adhesive remover may be used. Do not apply lotion to the peristomal area.	Cleaning the skin removes excretions and old adhesive and skin protectant. Excretions or a buildup of other substances can irritate and damage the skin. Lotion will prevent a tight adhesive seal.
16. Gently pat area dry. **Make sure skin around stoma is thoroughly dry.** Assess stoma and condition of surrounding skin.	Careful drying prevents trauma to skin and stoma. An intact, properly applied urinary collection device protects skin integrity. Any change in color and size of the stoma may indicate circulatory problems.
17. Place one or two gauze squares over the stoma opening (Figure 5).	Continuous drainage must be absorbed to keep skin dry during appliance change.

FIGURE 4. Cleaning stoma with cleansing agent and washcloth.

FIGURE 5. Placing one or two gauze squares over stoma opening.

18. Apply skin protectant to a 2-in (5-cm) radius around the stoma, and allow it to dry completely, which takes about 30 seconds.	The skin needs protection from the potentially excoriating effect of the appliance adhesive. The skin must be perfectly dry before the appliance is placed to get good adherence and to prevent leaks.
19. Lift the gauze squares for a moment and measure the stoma opening, using the measurement guide. Replace the gauze. Trace the same-size opening on the back center of the appliance. Cut the opening 1/8 in larger than the stoma size (Figure 6). Use a finger to gently smooth the wafer edges after cutting. Check that the spout is closed and the end cap is in place.	The appliance should fit snugly around the stoma, with only 1/8 in of skin visible around the opening. A faceplate opening that is too small can cause trauma to the stoma. If the opening is too large, exposed skin will be irritated by urine. Wafer edges may be uneven after cutting and could cause irritation to and/or pressure on the stoma. A closed spout and secured end cap prevent urine from leaking from the appliance.

FIGURE 6. Cutting the faceplate opening 1/8 in larger than stoma size.

ACTION

20. Remove the paper backing from the appliance faceplate. Quickly remove the gauze squares and discard appropriately; ease the appliance over the stoma. Gently press onto the skin while smoothing over the surface (Figure 7). Apply gentle, even pressure to the appliance for approximately 30 seconds.

RATIONALE

The appliance is effective only if it is properly positioned and adhered securely. Pressure on faceplate allows the faceplate to mold to the patient's skin and improves the seal.

FIGURE 7. Applying faceplate over stoma.

21. Secure optional belt to appliance and around the patient.

22. Remove gloves. Assist the patient to a comfortable position. Cover the patient with bed linens. Place the bed in the lowest position.

23. Put on clean gloves. Remove or discard any remaining equipment and assess the patient's response to the procedure.

24. Remove gloves and additional PPE, if used. Perform hand hygiene.

An elasticized belt helps support the appliance for some people.

Removing gloves reduces risk of transmission of microorganisms. Positioning and covering provide warmth and promote comfort. Bed in lowest position promotes patient safety.

The patient's response may indicate acceptance of the ostomy as well as the need for health teaching.

Proper removal of PPE reduces the risk for infection transmission and contamination of other items. Hand hygiene prevents the spread of microorganisms.

EVALUATION

The expected outcome has been met when the ileal conduit appliance is changed without trauma to the stoma or peristomal skin, or leaking; urine is draining freely into the appliance; the skin surrounding the stoma is clean, dry, and intact; and the patient shows an interest in learning to perform the pouch change and verbalizes positive self-image.

DOCUMENTATION

Guidelines

Document the procedure, including the appearance of the stoma, condition of the peristomal skin, characteristics of the urine, the patient's response to the procedure, and pertinent patient teaching.

Sample Documentation

> 7/23/20 1245 Ileal conduit appliance changed. Mr. Jones present. Mrs. Jones asking questions about care for ileal conduit, states, "I don't know if I'll ever be able to care for this thing at home." Tearful at times. Patient encouraged to express feelings. Patient agreed to talk with wound, ostomy, and continence nurse about concerns. Mr. Jones very supportive, also asking appropriate questions. Patient states she would like to watch change one more time before she attempts to do it. Stoma is moist and red, peristomal skin intact, draining yellow urine with small amount of mucus.
> —B. Clapp, RN

(continued)

Skill 12-11 ▶ Emptying and Changing a Stoma Appliance on a Urinary Diversion *(continued)*

UNEXPECTED SITUATIONS AND ASSOCIATED INTERVENTIONS

- *You remove appliance and find an area of skin excoriated:* Make sure that the appliance is not cut too large. Skin that is exposed inside of the ostomy appliance will become excoriated. Assess for the presence of a fungal skin infection. If present, consult with primary care provider to obtain appropriate treatment. Cleanse the skin thoroughly and pat dry. Apply products made for excoriated skin before placing appliance over stoma. Frequently check faceplate to ensure that a seal has formed and that there is no leakage. Confer with primary care provider for a wound, ostomy, and continence nurse consult to manage these issues. Document the excoriation in the patient's chart.
- *Faceplate is leaking after applying a new appliance:* Remove appliance, clean the skin, and start over.
- *You are ready to place the faceplate and notice that the opening is cut too large:* Discard appliance and begin over. A faceplate that is cut too big may lead to excoriation of the skin.
- *Stoma is dark brown or black:* Stoma should appear pink to red, shiny, and moist. Alterations indicate compromised circulation. If the stoma is dark brown or black, suspect ischemia and necrosis. Notify the primary care provider immediately.

SPECIAL CONSIDERATIONS

- Patients with urinary diversions created using a portion of the gastrointestinal tract will experience the presence of mucous in the urine (Schreiber, 2016). The segment of the gastrointestinal tract continues to produce mucous, as part of its normal functioning. This mucous production does not decrease over time, but is usually not a problem for patients with an ileal conduit (Stott & Fairbrother, 2015).

Skill Variation ▶ Applying a Two-Piece Appliance

A two-piece colostomy appliance is composed of a pouch and a separate adhesive faceplate that "click" together (Figure A). The faceplate is left in place for a period of time, usually 3 to 7 days. During this period, when the appliance requires changing, only the bag needs to be replaced.

FIGURE A. Two-piece appliances.

1. Gather necessary equipment.
2. Perform hand hygiene and put on PPE, if indicated.

3. Identify the patient.

4. Close the curtains around the bed and close the door to room, if possible. Explain what you are going to do and why you are going to do it to the patient. Encourage the patient to observe or participate, if possible.
5. Assemble equipment on overbed table or other surface within reach.
6. Assist the patient to a comfortable sitting or lying position in bed or a standing or sitting position in the bathroom.
7. Place a disposable pad on the work surface. Open the premoistened disposable washcloths or set up the washbasin with warm water and the rest of the supplies. Place a trash bag within reach.
8. Put on gloves. Place waterproof pad under the patient at the stoma site. Empty the appliance as described previously in Skill 12-11.
9. Gently remove pouch faceplate from skin by pushing skin from appliance rather than pulling appliance from skin. Start at the top of the appliance, while keeping the abdominal skin taut. Apply a silicone-based adhesive remover by spraying or wiping with the remover wipe.
10. Place the appliance in the trash bag, if disposable. If reusable, set aside to wash in lukewarm soap and water and allow to air dry after the new appliance is in place.
11. Clean skin around the stoma with a mild skin cleanser and water or a cleansing agent and a washcloth. Remove all old adhesive from skin; additional adhesive remover may be used. Do not apply lotion to peristomal area.

Skill Variation ▶ Applying a Two-Piece Appliance   *(continued)*

12. Gently pat area dry. Make sure skin around the stoma is thoroughly dry. Assess stoma and condition of surrounding skin. Place one or two gauze squares over stoma opening.
13. Apply skin protectant to a 2-in (5-cm) radius around the stoma, and allow it to dry completely, which takes about 30 seconds
14. Lift the gauze squares for a moment and measure the stoma opening, using the measurement guide. Replace the gauze. Trace the same-size opening on the back center of the appliance faceplate. Cut the opening 1/8 in larger than the stoma size. Use a finger to gently smooth the wafer edges after cutting.
15. Remove the backing from the faceplate. Quickly remove the gauze squares and ease the faceplate over the stoma. Gently press onto the skin while smoothing over the surface (Figure B). Apply gentle pressure to the faceplate for approximately 30 seconds.
16. Apply the appliance pouch to the faceplate following manufacturer's directions. Check that the spout is closed and the end cap is in place. If using a "click" system, lay the ring on the pouch over the ring on the faceplate. Ask the patient to tighten stomach muscles, if possible. Beginning at one edge of the ring, push the pouch ring onto the faceplate ring. A "click" should be heard when the pouch is secured onto the faceplate.

FIGURE B. Gently pressing faceplate to skin.

17. Remove gloves. Assist the patient to a comfortable position. Cover the patient with bed linens. Place the bed in the lowest position.
18. Put on clean gloves. Remove or discard equipment and assess the patient's response to the procedure.
19. Remove gloves and additional PPE, if used. Perform hand hygiene.

EVIDENCE FOR PRACTICE ▶

LIVING WITH A UROSTOMY

Urinary diversions may become part of the treatment for many health issues, with the aim to maintain or improve health-related quality of life. What is the impact of this treatment on patients' lives?

Related Research

Pazar, B., Yava, A., & Başal, Ş. (2015). Health-related quality of life in persons living with a urostomy. *Journal of Wound, Ostomy and Continence Nursing, 42*(3), 264–270.

The purpose of this prospective, descriptive study was to determine the life experiences and health-related quality of life of patients living with a urinary diversion (urostomy). The 24 participants had undergone a urostomy operation at least 4 months before participating in the study. Participants completed demographic and clinical information, as well as a widely used quality-of-life questionnaire. Most respondents stated that their urostomy affected their dressing habits (83%), sleep patterns (92%), family life (92%), participation in social activities (92%), and occupation (75%). All participants discussed problems with psychological health and sexual activity following the surgery as well. Analysis of scores on the quality-of-life questionnaire demonstrated that general wellness, functional condition, and symptomatic condition mean scores were lower than population-based norms associated with the instrument. The authors concluded creation of a urostomy negatively affected patients' lifestyle and health-related quality of life.

(continued)

Skill 12-11 ▶ Emptying and Changing a Stoma Appliance on a Urinary Diversion *(continued)*

Relevance to Nursing Practice

The creation of a urinary diversion can negatively affect every aspect of a person's life, including overall quality of life, sexual function, relationships with others, and body image. Determination and evaluation of patient experiences after the creation of a urinary diversion may assist nurses to provide appropriate support and intervention. Nurses need to consider the effect of this treatment on patients' lifestyles and health-related quality of life in order to provide person-centered nursing care.

Refer to thePoint® for additional research on related nursing topics.

Skill 12-12 ▶ Caring for a Suprapubic Urinary Catheter

A **suprapubic urinary catheter** may be used for long-term continuous urinary drainage. This type of catheter is surgically inserted through a small incision above the pubic area (Figure 1). Suprapubic bladder drainage diverts urine from the urethra when injury, stricture, prostatic obstruction, or gynecologic or abdominal surgery has compromised the flow of urine through the urethra. A suprapubic catheter is often preferred over indwelling urethral catheters for long-term urinary drainage. Suprapubic catheters are associated with decreased risk of contamination with organisms from fecal material, elimination of damage to the urethra; does not interfere with sexual activity; increased comfort for patients with limited mobility; and lower risk of catheter-associated UTIs on a short-term basis (Hooton et al., 2010; Rew & Smith, 2011; SUNA, 2010a). The drainage tube is secured with sutures or tape. Care of the patient with a suprapubic catheter includes skin care around the insertion site; care of the drainage tubing and drainage bag is the same as for an indwelling catheter (refer to Box 12-1 in Skill 12-6).

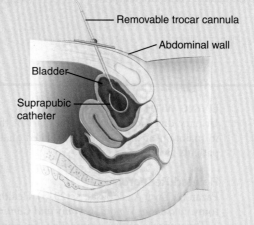

FIGURE 1. A suprapubic catheter positioned in bladder.

DELEGATION CONSIDERATIONS

The care of a suprapubic urinary catheter, in the postoperative period, is not delegated to nursing assistive personnel (NAP) or to unlicensed assistive personnel (UAP) in the acute care setting. The care of a healed suprapubic catheter site in some settings may be delegated to NAP or UAP who have received appropriate training, after assessment of the catheter by the registered nurse. Depending on the state's nurse practice act and the organization's policies and procedures, the care of a suprapubic urinary catheter may be delegated to licensed practical/vocational nurses (LPN/LVNs). The decision to delegate must be based on careful analysis of the patient's needs and circumstances, as well as the qualifications of the person to whom the task is being delegated. Refer to the Delegation Guidelines in Appendix A.

EQUIPMENT	• Premoistened disposable washcloths or
	  • Basin with warm water
	  • Skin cleanser, towel, washcloth
	• Disposable gloves
	• Additional PPE, as indicated
	• Velcro tube holder or tape to secure tube
	• Drainage sponge (if necessary)
	• Plastic trash bag
	• Sterile cotton-tipped applicators and sterile saline solution (if the patient has a new suprapubic catheter)

ASSESSMENT	Assess the suprapubic catheter and bag, observing the condition of the catheter and the drainage bag connected to the catheter, and the product style. If a dressing is in place at the insertion site, assess the dressing for drainage. Inspect the site around the suprapubic catheter, looking for drainage, erythema, or excoriation. Assess the method used to secure the catheter in place. If sutures are present, assess for intactness. Also, assess the characteristics of the urine in the drainage bag. Assess the patient's knowledge of caring for a suprapubic catheter.
NURSING DIAGNOSIS	Determine the related factors for the nursing diagnoses based on the patient's current status. Appropriate nursing diagnoses may include: • Impaired urinary elimination • Deficient knowledge • Risk for infection
OUTCOME IDENTIFICATION AND PLANNING	The expected outcomes to be achieved when caring for a suprapubic catheter are that the patient's skin remains clean, dry, and intact, without evidence of irritation or breakdown; and the patient verbalizes an understanding of the purpose for, and care of, the catheter, as appropriate. Other appropriate outcomes include the following: the patient's urinary elimination is maintained and the patient's bladder is not distended.

IMPLEMENTATION

ACTION	**RATIONALE**
1. Gather equipment.	Assembling equipment provides for an organized approach to task.
2. Perform hand hygiene and put on PPE, if indicated.	Hand hygiene and PPE prevent the spread of microorganisms. PPE is required based on transmission precautions.
3. Identify the patient.	Identifying the patient ensures the right patient receives the intervention and helps prevent errors.
4. Close the curtains around the bed and close the door to the room, if possible. Explain what you are going to do, and why you are going to do it, to the patient. Encourage the patient to observe or participate, if possible.	This ensures the patient's privacy. Explanation relieves anxiety and facilitates cooperation. Discussion promotes cooperation and helps to minimize anxiety. Having the patient observe or assist encourages self-acceptance.
5. Assemble equipment on overbed table or other surface within reach.	Arranging items nearby is convenient, saves time, and avoids unnecessary stretching and twisting of muscles on the part of the nurse.
6. Adjust the bed to a comfortable working height, usually elbow height of the caregiver (VHACEOSH, 2016). Assist the patient to a supine position. Place waterproof pad under the patient at the stoma site.	Having the bed at the proper height prevents back and muscle strain. The supine position is usually the best way to gain access to the suprapubic urinary catheter. A waterproof pad protects linens and patient from moisture.

(continued)

Skill 12-12 ▶ Caring for a Suprapubic Urinary Catheter *(continued)*

ACTION	RATIONALE

7. Put on clean gloves. Gently remove old dressing, if one is in place. Place dressing in trash bag. Remove gloves. Perform hand hygiene.

Gloves protect the nurse from blood, body fluids, and microorganisms. Proper disposal of contaminated dressing and hand hygiene deter the spread of microorganisms.

8. Assess the insertion site and surrounding skin.

Any changes in assessment could indicate potential infection.

9. Remove one disposable washcloth from package or wet washcloth with warm water and apply skin cleanser. **Gently cleanse around suprapubic exit site (Figure 2).** Remove any encrustations. Alternately, if this is a new suprapubic catheter, use sterile cotton-tipped applicators and sterile saline to clean the site until the incision has healed. Moisten the applicators with the saline. **Clean in circular motion from the insertion site outward (Figure 3).**

Using a gentle skin cleanser helps to protect the skin. The exit site is the most common area of skin irritation with a suprapubic catheter. If encrustations are left on the skin, they provide a medium for bacteria and an area of skin irritation.

FIGURE 2. Cleaning area around catheter site with skin cleanser and water.

FIGURE 3. Using sterile cotton-tipped applicators for cleaning.

10. Rinse area of all cleanser. Pat dry.

The skin needs to be kept dry to prevent any irritation.

11. If the exit site has been draining, place a small drain sponge around the catheter to absorb any drainage (Figure 4). Be prepared to change this sponge throughout the day, depending on the amount of drainage. Do not cut a 4 × 4 gauze to make a drain sponge.

A small amount of drainage from the exit site is normal. The sponge needs to be changed when it becomes soiled to prevent skin irritation and breakdown. The fibers from a cut 4 × 4 gauze may enter the exit site and cause irritation or infection.

12. Remove gloves. Form a loop in the tubing and anchor it on the patient's abdomen (Figure 5).

Anchoring the catheter and tubing absorbs any tugging, preventing tension on, and irritation to, the skin or bladder.

FIGURE 4. Applying small drain sponge around catheter.

FIGURE 5. Forming a loop in tubing and taping to abdomen.

ACTION	**RATIONALE**
13. Assist the patient to a comfortable position. Cover the patient with bed linens. Place the bed in the lowest position.	Positioning and covering provide warmth and promote comfort. Bed in lowest position promotes patient safety.
14. Put on clean gloves. Remove or discard equipment and assess the patient's response to the procedure.	Gloves prevent contact with blood and body fluids. The patient's response may indicate acceptance of the catheter or the need for health teaching.
15. Remove gloves and additional PPE, if used. Perform hand hygiene.	Proper removal of PPE reduces the risk for infection transmission and contamination of other items. Hand hygiene prevents the spread of microorganisms.

EVALUATION

The expected outcomes have been met when the patient's skin remains clean, dry, and intact, without evidence of irritation or breakdown; the patient verbalizes an understanding of the purpose for, and care of, the catheter, as appropriate; the patient's urinary elimination is maintained, with a urine output of at least 30 mL/hr; and the patient's bladder is not distended.

DOCUMENTATION

Guidelines

Document the appearance of catheter exit site and surrounding skin, urine amount and characteristics, as well as patient's reaction to the procedure.

Sample Documentation

> <u>7/12/20</u> 1845 Suprapubic catheter care performed. Patient assisted in care. Skin is slightly erythematous on R side where catheter was taped. Catheter taped to L side. Small amount of yellow, clear drainage noted on drain sponge. Patient would like to try to go without drain sponge at this time. Instructions given to call nurse if amount of drainage increases. Moderate amount of clear yellow urine continues to drain from catheter into collection bag.
>
> —B. Clapp, RN

UNEXPECTED SITUATIONS AND ASSOCIATED INTERVENTIONS

- *When cleaning the site, the catheter becomes dislodged and pulls out:* Notify primary care provider. It takes approximately 4 weeks for the suprapubic tract to become established, the time at which it can be safely changed (SUNA, 2016). The site of insertion can close fairly quickly prior to the establishment of the tract, so prompt attention is needed (Bullman, 2011). If this is a well-healed site, the health care provider or advanced practice nurse can replace a new catheter easily. If this is a new suprapubic tube, the primary care provider may want to assess for any trauma to the bladder wall.
- *Exit site is extremely excoriated:* Consult wound, ostomy, and incontinence nurse for evaluation. A skin protectant or barrier may need to be applied, as well as more frequent cleansing of the area and changing of the drain sponge (if applied).

SPECIAL CONSIDERATIONS

- Depending on the patient's situation, he or she may have both a suprapubic and indwelling urethral catheter. Urine will drain from both catheters; usually, drainage from the suprapubic catheter is the larger volume.
- If the suprapubic catheter is not draining into the bag but, instead, has a valve at the end of the catheter, open the valve at least every 6 hours (or more frequently depending on the order in the medical record or institutional policy) to drain the urine from the bladder.
- Remove dressings at the exit site when any oozing from the wound has diminished. Prolonged dressings around the site may harbor bacteria, increasing the risk of site infection, and contribute to overgranulation at the site (Rew & Smith, 2011).
- The use of antiseptics and petroleum-based ointments at the insertion site is not recommended (Bullman, 2011; Rew & Smith, 2011).
- Encourage patients to drink adequate fluids to keep the urine clear and free flowing; residual urine can lead to stone formation and infection (Bullman, 2011).

Skill 12-13 ▶ Caring for a Peritoneal Dialysis Catheter

Peritoneal dialysis is a method of removing fluid and wastes from the body of a patient with kidney failure. A catheter (a thin, soft silicone rubber tube) inserted through the abdominal wall into the peritoneal cavity allows a special fluid (dialysate) to be infused and then drained from the body, removing waste products and excess fluid (Figure 1). The exit site should be protected and kept clean and dry to allow for healing, which will take approximately 2 to 3 weeks (Lee & Park, 2012). Exit-site dressings are initially changed weekly, until the site is healed. Frequent dressing changes in the immediate postoperative period are not necessary unless there is excessive oozing, bleeding, or signs of infection, to decrease the risk of contamination and unnecessary movement of the catheter (Lee & Park, 2012). Once the exit site has healed, exit-site care is an important part of patient care. The catheter insertion site is a site for potential infection, possibly leading to catheter tunnel infection and **peritonitis**, therefore, meticulous care is needed. The incidence of exit-site infections can be reduced through a cleansing regimen by the patient or caregiver. Chronic exit-site care is performed daily or every other day (Hain & Chan, 2013). In the postoperative period, catheter care is performed using aseptic technique, to reduce the risk for a health care–acquired infection. At home, clean technique can be used by the patient and caregivers.

FIGURE 1. Position of catheter in peritoneal space. Patient is set up for peritoneal dialysis.

DELEGATION CONSIDERATIONS	The care of a peritoneal dialysis catheter is not delegated to nursing assistive personnel (NAP) or to unlicensed assistive personnel (UAP). Depending on the state's nurse practice act and the organization's policies and procedures, care of a peritoneal dialysis catheter may be delegated to licensed practical/vocational nurses (LPN/LVNs). The decision to delegate must be based on careful analysis of the patient's needs and circumstances, as well as the qualifications of the person to whom the task is being delegated. Refer to the Delegation Guidelines in Appendix A.

EQUIPMENT

- Face masks (2)
- Sterile gloves
- Nonsterile gloves
- Additional PPE, as indicated
- Antimicrobial cleansing agent, per facility policy
- Sterile gauze squares (4)
- Sterile basin
- Sterile drain sponge
- Transparent, occlusive site dressing
- Topical antibiotic, such as mupirocin or gentamicin, depending on order and policy
- Sterile applicator
- Plastic trash bag
- Bath blanket

ASSESSMENT	Inspect the peritoneal dialysis catheter exit site for any erythema, drainage, bleeding, tenderness, swelling, skin irritation or breakdown, or leakage. These signs could indicate exit-site or tunnel infection. Assess abdomen for tenderness, pain, and guarding. Assess the patient for nausea, vomiting, and fever, which could indicate peritonitis. Assess the patient's knowledge about measures used to care for the exit site.
NURSING DIAGNOSIS	Determine the related factors for the nursing diagnoses based on the patient's current status. Appropriate nursing diagnoses may include: • Risk for impaired skin integrity • Risk for infection • Deficient knowledge
OUTCOME IDENTIFICATION AND PLANNING	The expected outcomes to achieve when performing care for a peritoneal dialysis catheter are that the peritoneal dialysis catheter dressing change is completed using aseptic technique without trauma to the site or patient; the site is clean, dry, and intact, without evidence of inflammation or infection; and the patient participates in self-care, as appropriate.

IMPLEMENTATION

ACTION	RATIONALE
1. Review the patient's medical record for orders related to catheter site care. Gather equipment.	Ensures appropriate interventions for the patient. Assembling equipment provides for an organized approach to the task.
2. Perform hand hygiene and put on PPE, if indicated.	Hand hygiene and PPE prevent the spread of microorganisms. PPE is required based on transmission precautions.
3. Identify the patient.	Identifying the patient ensures the right patient receives the intervention and helps prevent errors.
4. Close the curtains around the bed and close the door to the room, if possible. Explain what you are going to do and why you are going to do it to the patient. Encourage the patient to observe or participate, if possible.	This ensures the patient's privacy. Explanation relieves anxiety and facilitates cooperation. Discussion promotes cooperation and helps to minimize anxiety. Having the patient observe or assist encourages self-acceptance.
5. Assemble equipment on overbed table or other surface within reach.	Arranging items nearby is convenient, saves time, and avoids unnecessary stretching and twisting of muscles on the part of the nurse.
6. Adjust the bed to a comfortable working height, usually elbow height of the caregiver (VHACEOSH, 2016). Assist the patient to a supine position. Expose the abdomen, draping the patient's chest with the bath blanket, exposing only the catheter site.	Having the bed at the proper height prevents back and muscle strain. The supine position is usually the best way to gain access to the peritoneal dialysis catheter. Use of bath blanket provides patient warmth and avoids unnecessary exposure.
7. Put on nonsterile gloves. Put on one of the facemasks; have patient put on the other mask.	Gloves protect the nurse from contact with blood and bodily fluids. Use of facemasks deters the spread of microorganisms.
8. Gently remove old dressing, noting odor, amount, and color of drainage; leakage and condition of skin around the catheter. Discard dressing in appropriate container.	Drainage, leakage, and skin condition can indicate problems with the catheter, such as infection.
9. Remove gloves and discard. Set up sterile field. Open packages. Using aseptic technique, place two sterile gauze squares in basin with antimicrobial agent. Leave two sterile gauze squares opened on sterile field. Alternately (based on facility's policy), place sterile antimicrobial swabs on the sterile field. Place sterile applicator on field. Squeeze a small amount of the topical antibiotic on one of the gauze squares on the sterile field.	Until catheter site has healed, aseptic technique is necessary for site care to prevent infection.

(continued)

Skill 12-13 ▶ Caring for a Peritoneal Dialysis Catheter *(continued)*

ACTION	RATIONALE
10. Put on sterile gloves. Pick up dialysis catheter with the nondominant hand. With the antimicrobial-soaked gauze/swab, cleanse the skin around the exit site using a circular motion, starting at the exit site and then slowly going outward 3 to 4 in. Gently remove crusted scabs, if necessary.	Aseptic technique is necessary to prevent infection. The antimicrobial agent cleanses the skin and removes any drainage or crust from the wound, reducing the risk for infection.
11. Continue to hold the catheter with your nondominant hand. After skin has dried, clean the catheter with an antimicrobial-soaked gauze, beginning at the exit site, going around catheter, and then moving up to end of the catheter. Gently remove crusted secretions on the tube, if necessary.	Antimicrobial agents cleanse the catheter and remove any drainage or crust from the tube, reducing the risk for infection.
12. Using the sterile applicator, apply the topical antibiotic to the catheter exit site, if prescribed.	Application of mupirocin or gentamicin at the catheter exit site prevents exit-site infection and peritonitis (Hain & Chan, 2013).
13. Place sterile drain sponge around the exit site. Then place a 4 × 4 gauze over the exit site. Cover with transparent, occlusive dressing. Remove gloves and then masks.	The drain sponge and 4 × 4 gauze are used to absorb any drainage from the exit site. Occlusion of the site with a dressing deters site contamination. Once the site is covered, masks and gloves are no longer necessary.
14. Label dressing with date, time of change, and initials.	Other personnel working with the catheter will know information related to site care.
15. Coil the exposed length of tubing and secure to the dressing or the patient's abdomen with tape.	Anchoring the catheter absorbs any tugging, preventing tension on, and irritation to, the skin or abdomen.
16. Assist the patient to a comfortable position. Cover the patient with bed linens. Place the bed in the lowest position.	Positioning and covering provide warmth and promote comfort. A bed in the low position promotes patient safety.
17. Put on clean gloves. Remove or discard equipment and assess the patient's response to the procedure.	These actions deter the spread of microorganisms. The patient's response may indicate acceptance of the catheter or the need for health teaching.
18. Remove gloves and additional PPE, if used. Perform hand hygiene.	Proper removal of PPE reduces the risk for infection transmission and contamination of other items. Hand hygiene prevents the spread of microorganisms.

EVALUATION

The expected outcomes have been met when the peritoneal dialysis catheter dressing change is completed using aseptic technique without trauma to the site or to the patient; the site is clean, dry, and intact, without evidence of redness, irritation, or excoriation; the patient's fluid balance is maintained; and the patient verbalizes appropriate measures to care for the site.

DOCUMENTATION

Guidelines

Document the dressing change, including condition of skin surrounding the exit site, drainage, or odor, as well as the patient's reaction to the procedure, and any patient teaching provided.

Sample Documentation

> 8/22/20 1530 Peritoneal dialysis catheter dressing changed; skin surrounding catheter slightly erythematous, but remains intact. Small amount of clear drainage, approximately the size of a dime without odor, noted on drain sponge. Patient asking appropriate questions regarding dressing change. Verbalized an understanding of explanations.
>
> —B. Clapp, RN

UNEXPECTED SITUATIONS AND ASSOCIATED INTERVENTIONS

- *Patient complains of pain when you palpate the abdomen; purulent or cloudy drainage is present, or foul odor is noted when old dressing is removed:* Notify primary care provider immediately. Any of these signs could indicate a site infection or peritonitis.
- *You note that the old dressing is saturated with clear fluid:* Replace dressing to prevent skin breakdown. Notify primary care provider. A frequent complication is leakage from the exit site. Frequently check dressing, especially after the patient has had solution placed in the abdominal cavity.

SPECIAL CONSIDERATIONS

General Considerations

- Instruct patients to avoid showering for 2 to 3 weeks, until the site has healed (Lee & Park, 2012).
- Instruct patients with a peritoneal dialysis catheter to avoid tub baths and public pools.
- Remind patients performing own site care of the importance of good handwashing before self-care. The use of alcohol-based hand gels or washing with antimicrobial soap is recommended (Hain & Chan, 2013).
- Discourage patients from wearing tight clothes and belts around the exit site.

Home Care Considerations

- Often, clean technique, instead of sterile technique, is used by the patient and caregivers in the home.
- Teach patients the signs of exit-site infection and encourage them to contact their primary care provider for prompt intervention.

Skill 12-14 ▶ Caring for a Hemodialysis Access (Arteriovenous Fistula or Graft)

Hemodialysis, a method of removing fluid and wastes from the body, requires access to the patient's vascular system. This is done via the insertion of a catheter into a large vein, typically a central venous catheter inserted into the chest (short- or long-term access) or the creation of a fistula or graft (long-term access). If a catheter is used (Figure 1), the site is cared for in the same manner as a central venous access device (see Skill 15-7). An **arteriovenous fistula** is a surgically created passage that connects an artery and vein (Figure 2). An **arteriovenous graft** is a surgically created connection between an artery and vein using a synthetic material (Figure 3). Accessing a hemodialysis arteriovenous graft or fistula should be done only by specially trained health care team members.

FIGURE 1. Central catheter for hemodialysis.

(continued)

Skill 12-14 ▶ Caring for a Hemodialysis Access (Arteriovenous Fistula or Graft) *(continued)*

FIGURE 2. Arteriovenous fistula for hemodialysis.

FIGURE 3. Arteriovenous graft for hemodialysis.

DELEGATION CONSIDERATIONS	The assessment of, and care for, a hemodialysis access is not delegated to nursing assistive personnel (NAP) or to unlicensed assistive personnel (UAP). Depending on the state's nurse practice act and the organization's policies and procedures, these procedures may be delegated to licensed practical/vocational nurses (LPN/LVNs). The decision to delegate must be based on careful analysis of the patient's needs and circumstances, as well as the qualifications of the person to whom the task is being delegated. Refer to the Delegation Guidelines in Appendix A.
EQUIPMENT	• Stethoscope • PPE, as indicated
ASSESSMENT	Ask the patient how much he or she knows about caring for the site. Ask the patient to describe important observations to be made. Note the location of the access site. Assess the site for signs of infection, including inflammation, edema, and drainage; and for healing of the incision. Assess for patency by assessing for presence of bruit and thrill (refer to explanation in Step 4, below).
NURSING DIAGNOSIS	Determine the related factors for the nursing diagnoses based on the patient's current status. Appropriate nursing diagnoses may include: • Deficient knowledge • Risk for injury
OUTCOME IDENTIFICATION AND PLANNING	The expected outcomes to achieve when caring for a hemodialysis catheter are that the graft or fistula remains patent, the patient verbalizes appropriate care measures and observations to be made, and the patient demonstrates appropriate care measures.

IMPLEMENTATION

ACTION

 1. Perform hand hygiene and put on PPE, if indicated.

 2. Identify the patient.

3. Close the curtains around the bed and close the door to the room, if possible. Explain what you are going to do, and why you are going to do it, to the patient.

4. Question the patient about the presence of muscle weakness and cramping; changes in temperature; sensations, such as numbness, tingling, pain, burning, itchiness; and pain.

5. Inspect the area over the access site for continuity of skin color. Inspect for any redness, warmth, tenderness, edema, rash, blemishes, bleeding, tremors, and twitches. Inspect the muscle strength, and the patient's ability to perform range of motion in the extremity/body part with the hemodialysis access.

6. Palpate over the access site, feeling for a **thrill** or vibration (Figure 4). Palpate pulses above and below the site. Palpate the continuity of the skin temperature along and around the extremity. Check capillary refill in fingers or toes of extremity with the fistula or graft.

FIGURE 4. Palpating access site for thrill.

7. Auscultate over the access site with bell of stethoscope, listening for a **bruit** or vibration.

8. Ensure that a sign is placed over the head of the bed informing the health care team which arm is affected. **Do not measure blood pressure, perform a venipuncture, or start an IV on the access arm.**

9. Instruct the patient not to sleep with the arm with the access site under the head or body.

10. Instruct the patient not to lift heavy objects with, or put pressure on, the arm with the access site. Advise the patient not to carry heavy bags (including purses) on the shoulder of that arm.

RATIONALE

Hand hygiene and PPE prevent the spread of microorganisms. PPE is required based on transmission precautions.

Identifying the patient ensures the right patient receives the intervention and helps prevent errors.

This ensures the patient's privacy. Explanation relieves anxiety and facilitates cooperation. Discussion promotes cooperation and helps to minimize anxiety.

Aids in determining the patency of the hemodialysis access, as well as the presence of complications.

Inspection aids in determining the patency of the hemodialysis access, as well as the status of the patient's circulatory, neurologic, and muscular function; and presence of infection. Compare with the opposite body area/part.

Palpation aids in determining the patency of the hemodialysis access, as well as the status of the patient's circulatory, neurologic, and muscular function; and presence of infection. Compare with the opposite body area/part.

Palpation aids in determining the patency of the hemodialysis access.

The affected arm should not be used for any other procedures, such as obtaining blood pressure, which could lead to clotting of the graft or fistula. Venipuncture or IV access could lead to an infection of the affected arm and could cause the loss of the graft or fistula.

This could lead to clotting of the fistula or graft.

This could lead to clotting of the fistula or graft.

(continued)

Skill 12-14 ▶ Caring for a Hemodialysis Access (Arteriovenous Fistula or Graft) *(continued)*

ACTION	RATIONALE

 11. Remove PPE, if used. Perform hand hygiene.

Proper removal of PPE reduces the risk for infection transmission and contamination of other items. Hand hygiene prevents the spread of microorganisms.

EVALUATION

The expected outcomes have been met when the access site has an audible bruit and a palpable thrill; the site is intact without signs of adverse complications, or pain; and the patient verbalizes appropriate information about caring for the access site and observations to report.

DOCUMENTATION

Guidelines

Document assessment findings, including the presence or absence of a bruit and thrill. Document any patient education and patient response.

Sample Documentation

> 5/10/20 0830 Arteriovenous fistula patent in left upper arm. Area without redness, pain, or edema; skin at site similar to surrounding skin tone. Patient denies pain and tenderness. Positive bruit and thrill noted. Patient verbalized understanding the importance of avoiding venipuncture in left arm.
>
> —B. Clapp, RN

Unexpected Situations and Associated Interventions

- *Thrill is diminished or not palpable and/or bruit is diminished or not audible:* Notify the primary care provider immediately. The thrill and bruit are caused by arterial blood flowing into the vein. If these signs are not present, the access may be clotting off.
- *Site is warm to touch, erythematous, or painful or has a skin blemish:* Notify the primary care provider. These signs can indicate a site infection.

EVIDENCE FOR PRACTICE ▶

HEMODIALYSIS AND PATIENT FATIGUE

Patients receiving chronic hemodialysis experience troubling symptoms that cause distress and adversely affect their quality of life. Fatigue is common and can be debilitating. What is the experience of patients receiving hemodialysis and how can nurses assist them in dealing with this issue?

Related Research

Horigan, A. E., & Barroso, J. V. (2016). A comparison of temporal patterns of fatigue in patients on hemodialysis. *Nephrology Nursing Journal, 43*(2), 129–138.

The aim of this qualitative descriptive study was to describe the experience and self-management of fatigue in patients on hemodialysis. One group of participants described postdialysis fatigue, an acute fatigue that occurred after hemodialysis session and required several hours of sleep or rest to recover. After resting, patients were able to ease back into and participate in activities of daily living. Another group of participants experienced continuous fatigue, a fatigue that was always present and became considerably worse after a hemodialysis session. After resting or sleeping for several hours after dialysis, some of this group of participants returned to their baseline level of fatigue; others had a prolonged recovery that lasted into the next day. Some participants identified functional limitations and decreased socialization on dialysis days, and the need to plan and organize activities for nonhemodialysis days. Participants in the continuous fatigue group experienced the need to limit activities in general.

Relevance to Nursing Practice

This information can be valuable to nurses caring for these patients and may be useful in planning appropriate nursing interventions, and in tailoring interventions to support patients with fatigue. The information can also be used to plan and implement appropriate patient education related to the fatigue associated with hemodialysis; devising ways to manage symptoms is important to improve quality of life.

Refer to thePoint® for additional research on related nursing topics.

Enhance Your Understanding

Focusing on Patient Care: Developing Clinical Reasoning

Consider the case scenarios at the beginning of the chapter as you answer the following questions to enhance your understanding and apply what you have learned.

QUESTIONS

1. When checking Ralph Bellow's external urinary sheath, you notice that, although the sheath is still in place, Mr. Bellow's bed is soaked with urine and there is very little urine in the catheter tubing. What should you do?

2. Grace Halligan is asking to go to the bathroom; she says, "I don't think I can go on a bedpan." You recheck the health care provider's orders and notice that Ms. Halligan is on strict bed rest. How can you help alleviate her concerns about using a bedpan?

3. Mike Wimmer notices that his peritoneal dialysis catheter insertion site is reddened and tender. He phones to ask what should be done. What should you tell Mike?

You can find suggested answers after the Bibliography at the end of this chapter.

Integrated Case Study Connection

The case studies in the back of the book focus on integrating concepts. Refer to the following case studies to enhance your understanding of the concepts and skills in this chapter.

- Basic Case Studies: Tiffany Jones, page 1100.
- Intermediate Case Studies: Lucille Howard, page 1123.
- Advanced Case Studies: Robert Espinoza, page 1132.

Taylor Suite Resources

Explore these additional resources to enhance learning for this chapter:

- NCLEX-Style Questions and other resources on thePoint*, http://thePoint.lww.com/Lynn5e
- *Skill Checklists for Taylor's Clinical Nursing Skills,* 5e
- *Taylor's Video Guide to Clinical Nursing Skills:* Urinary Elimination and Indwelling and Intermittent Catheters
- *Fundamentals of Nursing:* Chapter 37, Urinary Elimination
- *Lippincott DocuCare* Fundamentals cases

Bibliography

Altschuler, V., & Diaz, L. (2006). Bladder ultrasound. *Medsurg Nursing, 15*(5), 317–318.

American Association of Critical-Care Nurses (AACN). (2016). *Prevention of CAUTI in adults.* Retrieved https://www.aacn.org/clinical-resources/practice-alerts/prevention-of-cauti-in-adults

American Cancer Society. (2011). *Urostomy guide.* Retrieved http://www.cancer.org/treatment/treatmentsandsideeffects/physicalsideeffects/ostomies/urostomyguide/index

American Nephrology Nurses' Association. (2013). *Peritoneal dialysis fact sheet.* Pitman, NJ: Author. Retrieved https://www.annanurse.org/download/reference/practice/pdFactSheet.pdf

American Nurses Association (ANA). (2014). *Streamlined evidence-based RN tool: Catheter associated urinary tract infection (CAUTI) prevention.* Retrieved http://nursingworld.org/ANA-CAUTI-Prevention-Tool

Avent, Y. (2012). Understanding urinary diversions. *Nursing Made Incredibly Easy!, 10*(4), 47–52.

Bardsley, A. (2015a). Safe and effective catheterization for patients in the community. *British Journal of Community Nursing, 20*(4), 166–172.

Bardsley, A. (2015b). Assessing and teaching female intermittent self-catheterization. *British Journal of Community Nursing, 20*(7), 344–346.

Belizario, S. M. (2015). Preventing urinary tract infections with a two-person catheter insertion procedure. *Nursing, 45*(3), 67–69.

Bentley, A. (2012). Stoma care: Older adults. *PACEsetterS, 9*(1), 23–25.

Bernardini, J., Bender, F., Florio, T., et al. (2005). Randomized, double-blind trial of antibiotic exit site cream for prevention of exit site infection in peritoneal dialysis patients. *Journal of the American Society of Nephrology, 16*(2), 539–545.

Booth, F. (2014). Principles underlying urinary catheterization in the community. *Journal of Community Nursing, 28*(5), 72–77.

Bullman, S. (2011). Ins and outs of suprapubic catheters—a clinician's experience. *Urologic Nursing, 31*(5), 259–264.

Burch, J. (2011). Peristomal skin care and the use of accessories to promote skin health. *British Journal of Nursing (Mark Allen Publishing), 20*(7), S4–S10.

Burch, J. (2015). Troubleshooting stomas in the community setting. *Journal of Community Nursing, 29*(5), 93–96.

Carter, N. M., & Goodloe, L. R. (2014). An evidence-based approach to the prevention of catheter-associated urinary tract infections. *Urologic Nursing, 34*(5), 238–245.

Centers for Disease Control and Prevention (CDC). (2015). *Healthcare-associated infections (HAIs). Catheter-associated urinary tract infections (CAUTI).* Retrieved https://www.cdc.gov/HAI/ca_uti/uti.html

Chandler, P. (2015). Preventing and treating peristomal skin conditions in stoma patients. *British Journal of Community Nursing, 20*(8), 386–388.

Cohen, B. J., & Hull, K. L. (2015). *Memmler's structure and function of the human body* (11th ed.). Philadelphia: Wolters Kluwer.

Darbyshire, D., Rowbotham, D., Grayson, S., Taylor, J., & Shackley, D. (2016). Surveying patients about their experience with a urinary catheter. *International Journal of Urological Nursing, 10*(1), 14–20.

Davey, G. (2015). Troubleshooting indwelling catheter problems in the community. *Journal of Community Nursing, 29*(4), 67–74.

Doenges, M. E., Moorhouse, M. F., & Murr, A. C. (2016). *Nursing diagnoses manual. Planning, individualizing, and documenting client care* (5th ed.). Philadelphia, PA: F.A. Davis.

Eliopoulos, C. (2014). *Gerontological nursing* (8th ed.). Philadelphia, PA: Wolters Kluwer Health.

Evans, E. C., Hain, D., Kear, T. M., Dork, L. A., & Schrauf, C. (2014). Hemodialysis catheter outcomes pilot study: No dressing coverage with prescribed showering. *Nephrology Nursing Journal, 41*(1), 53–72.

Fischbach, F., & Dunning III, M. B. (2015). *A manual of laboratory and diagnostic tests* (9th ed.). Philadelphia, PA: Wolters Kluwer Health.

Gattinger, H., Werner, B., & Saxer, S. (2013). Patient experience with bedpans in acute care: A cross-sectional study. *Journal of Clinical Nursing, 22*(15–16), 2216–2224.

Goessaert, A. S., Antoons, S., Van Den Driessche, M., Tourchi, A., Pieters, R., & Everaert, K. (2013). No-touch intermittent catheterization: Caregiver point of view on sterility errors, duration, comfort and costs. *Journal of Advanced Nursing, 69*(9), 2000–2007.

Gould, C.V., Umscheid, C. A., Agarwal, R. K., Kuntz, G., & Pegues, D. A; Healthcare Infection Control Practices Advisory Committee (HICPAC). (2009). *Guideline for prevention of catheter-associated urinary tract infections 2009.* Retrieved https://www.cdc.gov/hicpac/pdf/CAUTI/CAUTIguideline2009final.pdf

Grossman, S., & Porth, C. M. (2014). *Porth's pathophysiology: Concepts of altered health states* (9th ed.). Philadelphia, PA: Wolters Kluwer Health/Lippincott Williams & Wilkins.

Hain, D. J., & Chan, J. (2013). Best available evidence for peritoneal dialysis catheter exit-site care. *Nephrology Nursing Journal, 40*(1), 63–69.

Herter, R., & Kazer, M. W. (2010). Best practices in urinary catheter care. *Home Healthcare Nurse, 28*(6), 342–349.

Hinkle, J. L., & Cheever, K. H. (2018). *Brunner & Suddarth's textbook of medical-surgical nursing* (14th ed.). Philadelphia, PA: Wolters Kluwer.

Holland, A. M., & Fish, D. (2012). *Benefits of the insertion tip and closed-system sleeve for intermittent catheterization.* Covington, GA: Bard Medical. Retrieved from http://www.bardmedical.com/media/135500/touchless_whitepaper.pdf

Holroyd, S. (2016). Innovation in catheter securement devices: Minimising risk of infection, trauma and pain. *British Journal of Community Nursing, 21*(5), 256–260.

Hooton, T. M., Bradley, S. F., Cardenas, D. D., et al. (2010). Diagnosis, prevention, and treatment of catheter-associated urinary tract infection in adults: 2009 international clinical practice guidelines from the Infectious Diseases Society of America. *Clinical Infectious Diseases, 50*(5), 625–663. Retrieved http://www.idsociety.org/uploadedFiles/IDSA/Guidelines-Patient_Care/PDF_Library/Comp%20UTI.pdf

Horigan, A. E., & Barroso, J. V. (2016). A comparison of temporal patterns of fatigue in patients on hemodialysis. *Nephrology Nursing Journal, 43*(2), 129–138.

Infusion Nurses Society (INS). (2016). Infusion therapy standards of practice. *Journal of Infusion Nursing, 39*(1S).

Institute for Healthcare Improvement (IHI). (2011). *How-to guide: Prevent catheter-associated urinary tract infection.* Cambridge, MA: Author. Retrieved http://www.ihi.org/resources/Pages/Tools/HowtoGuidePreventCatheterAssociatedUrinaryTractInfection.aspx

Jarvis, C. (2016). *Physical examination & health assessment* (7th ed.). St. Louis, MO: Elsevier.

Jensen, S. (2014). *Nursing health assessment: A best practice approach* (2nd ed.). Philadelphia, PA: Wolters Kluwer Health.

Kyle, T., & Carman, S. (2017). *Essentials of pediatric nursing* (3rd ed.). Philadelphia, PA: Wolters Kluwer.

Lawrence, J. A., Seiler, S., Wilson, B., & Harwood, L. (2014). Shower and no-dressing technique for tunneled central venous hemodialysis catheters: A quality improvement initiative. *Nephrology Nursing Journal, 41*(1), 67–72.

Lee, A., & Park, Y. (2012). Reducing peritoneal dialysis catheter exit site infections by implementing a standardized postoperative dressing protocol. *Renal Society of Australasia Journal, 8*(1), 18–22.

Lo, E., Nicolle, L. E., Coffin, S. E., et al. (2014). Strategies to prevent catheter-associated urinary tract infections in acute care hospitals: 2014 update. *Infection Control and Hospital Epidemiology, 35*(Suppl 2), S32–S47.

Logan, K. (2012). An overview of male intermittent self-catheterisation. *British Journal of Nursing (Mark Allen Publishing), 21*(18), S18–S22.

Mangnall, J. (2014). Urinary catheterization: Reducing the risk of infection. *Nursing & Residential Care, 16*(6), 310–318.

Mangnall, J. (2015). Managing and teaching intermittent catheterisation. *British Journal of Community Nursing, 20*(2), 82–88.

Mayo Clinic. (2013). *Tests and procedures. Hemodialysis.* Retrieved http://www.mayoclinic.org/tests-procedures/hemodialysis/basics/definition/prc-20015015

Mayo Clinic. (2016). *Tests and procedures. Peritoneal dialysis.* Retrieved http://www.mayoclinic.org/tests-procedures/peritoneal-dialysis/home/ovc-20202856

NANDA International, Inc. (2017). *Nursing diagnoses - Definitions and classification 2018–2020* © 2017 NANDA International, ISBN 978-1-62623-929-6. Used by arrangement with the Thieme Group, Stuttgart/New York.

National Institute of Diabetes and Digestive and Kidney Diseases (NIDDK). (2014). *Urodynamic testing.* Retrieved http://www.niddk.nih.gov/health-information/health-topics/diagnostic-tests/urodynamic-testing/Pages/Urodynamic%20Testing.aspx

National Kidney Foundation (NKF). (2013). *Peritoneal dialysis. What you need to know.* Retrieved https://www.kidney.org/sites/default/files/11-50-0215_peritonealdialysis.pdf

Nazarko, L. (2014). Urostomy management in the community. *British Journal of Community Nursing, 19*(9), 448–452.

Panchisin, T. L. (2016). Improving outcomes with the ANA CAUTI Prevention Tool. *Nursing, 46*(3), 55–59.

Pazar, B., Yava, A., & Başal, Ş. (2015). Health-related quality of life in persons living with a urostomy. *Journal of Wound, Ostomy and Continence Nursing, 42*(3), 264–270.

Perry, S. E., Hockenberry, M. J., Lowdermilk, D. L., & Wilson, D. (2014). *Maternal child nursing care* (5th ed.). St. Louis, MO: Elsevier.

Purnell, L. D. (2013). *Transcultural health care. A culturally competent approach* (4th ed.). Philadelphia, PA: F.A. Davis Company.

Rantell, A. (2012). Intermittent self-catheterisation in women. *Nursing Standard, 26*(42), 61–68.

Rew, M., & Smith, R. (2011). Reducing infection through the use of suprapubic catheters. *British Journal of Neuroscience Nursing, 7*(5), S13–S16.

Rudoni, C. (2008). A service evaluation of the use of silicone-based adhesive remover. *British Journal of Nursing (Mark Allen Publishing), 17*(2), S4, S6, S8–S9.

Schaepe, C., & Bergjan, M. (2015). Educational interventions in peritoneal dialysis: A narrative review of the literature. *International Journal of Nursing Studies, 52*(4), 882–898.

Schreiber, M. L. (2016). Ostomies: Nursing care and management. *Medsurg Nursing, 25*(2), 127–130.

Sheldon, P. (2013). Successful intermittent self-catheterisation teaching: One nurse's strategy of how and what to teach. *Urologic Nursing, 33*(3), 113–117.

Smart, C. (2014). Male urinary incontinence and the urinary sheath. *British Journal of Nursing (Mark Allen Publishing), 23*(9), S20–S25.

Society of Urologic Nurses and Associates (SUNA). (2010a). *Clinical practice guidelines. Prevention & control of catheter-associated urinary tract infection (CAUTI). [Brochure].* Pitman, NJ: Author.

Society of Urologic Nurses and Associates (SUNA). (2010b). *Adult intermittent self-catheterization. Patient fact sheet.* Pitman, NJ: Author.

Society of Urologic Nurses and Associates (SUNA). (2015a). *Clinical practice guidelines. Care of the patient with an indwelling catheter. [Brochure].* Pitman, NJ: Author.

Society of Urologic Nurses and Associates (SUNA). (2015b). *Clinical practice guidelines. Adult female urethral catheterization. [Brochure].* Pitman, NJ: Author.

Society of Urologic Nurses and Associates (SUNA). (2015c). *Clinical practice guidelines. Adult male urethral catheterization. [Brochure].* Pitman, NJ: Author.

Society of Urologic Nurses and Associates (SUNA). (2016). *Clinical practice guidelines. Suprapubic catheter replacement. [Brochure].* Pitman, NJ: Author.

Stelton, S., Zulkowski, K., & Ayello, E. A. (2015). Practice implications for peristomal skin assessment and care from the 2014 World Council of Enterostomal Therapists International Ostomy Guideline. *Advances in Skin and Wound Care, 28*(6), 275–284.

Stephen-Haynes, J. (2008). Skin integrity and silicone: Appeel 'no-sting' medical adhesive remover. *British Journal of Nursing (Mark Allen Publishing), 17*(12), 792–795.

Stott, C., & Fairbrother, G. (2015). Mucus and urinary diversions. *World Council of Enterostomal Therapists Journal, 35*(4), 36–41.

Strouse, A. C. (2015). Appraising the literature on bathing practices and catheter-associated urinary tract infection prevention. *Urologic Nursing, 35*(1), 11–17.

Stupak, D. M., Trubilla, J. A., & Groller, S. R. (2016). Hemodialysis catheter care: Identifying best cleansing agents. *Nephrology Nursing Journal, 43*(2), 153–155.

Taylor, C., Lynn, P., & Bartlett, J. (2019). *Fundamentals of nursing: The art and science of person-centered care* (9th ed.). Philadelphia, PA: Wolters Kluwer.

United Ostomy Associations of America, Inc. (2011). *Urostomy guide.* Retrieved http://www.ostomy.org/uploaded/files/ostomy_info/UrostomyGuide.pdf?direct =1

VHA Center for Engineering & Occupational Safety and Health (CEOSH). (2016). *Safe patient handling and mobility guidebook.* St. Louis, MO: Author. Retrieved http://www.tampavaref.org/safe-patient-handling.htm

Voegeli, D. (2010). Care or harm: Exploring essential components in skin care regimens. *British Journal of Nursing (Mark Allen Publishing), 19*(13), 812–819.

Voegeli, D. (2013). Moisture-associated skin damage: An overview for community nurses. *British Journal of Community Nursing, 18*(1), 6–12.

Whittle, A., & Black, K. (2014). Improving outcomes in peritoneal dialysis exit site care. *Renal Society of Australasia Journal, 10*(3), 126–132.

Widdall, D. A. (2015). Considerations for determining a bladder scan protocol. *Journal of the Australasian Rehabilitation Nurses' Association, 18*(3), 22–27.

Wilson, M. (2015). Clean intermittent self-catheterisation: Working with patients. *British Journal of Nursing (Mark Allen Publishing), 24*(2), 76–85.

Wuthier, P., Sublett, K., & Riehl, L. (2016). Urinary catheter dependent loops as a potential contributing cause of bacteriuria: An observational study. *Urologic Nursing 36*(1), 7–16.

Yates, A. (2016). Indwelling urinary catheterisation: What is best practice? *British Journal of Nursing (Mark Allen Publishing), 25*(9), S4–S13.

SUGGESTED ANSWERS FOR FOCUSING ON PATIENT CARE: DEVELOPING CLINICAL REASONING

1. Assess the patency of the external urinary sheath. Lack of adhesion of the sheath on the penis or resistance to gravity flow of urine would allow urine to leak around the sheath. You should assess for the presence of these conditions, as well as the condition of the patient's skin. Take care to fasten the external urinary sheath securely enough to prevent leakage, yet not so tightly as to constrict the blood vessels in the area. In addition, the tip of the tubing should be kept 1 to 2 in (2.5 to 5 cm) beyond the tip of the penis to prevent irritation to the sensitive glans area. Maintaining free urinary drainage is another nursing priority. Institute measures to prevent the tubing from becoming kinked and urine from backing up in the tubing. Urine can lead to excoriation of the glans, as well as separation of the sheath from the skin, so position the tubing that collects the urine from the external urinary sheath so that it draws urine away from the penis.

Always use a measuring or sizing guide supplied by the manufacturer to ensure the correct size of sheath is applied. Skin barriers, such as 3M or Skin-Prep, can be applied to the penis to protect penile skin from irritation and changes in integrity. In addition, nursing care of a patient with an external urinary sheath includes vigilant skin care to prevent excoriation. This includes removing the external urinary sheath daily, washing the penis with skin cleanser and water and drying carefully, and inspecting the skin for irritation. In hot and humid weather, more frequent changing may be required. Always follow the manufacturer's instructions for applying the external urinary sheath because there are several variations.

2. Begin by assessing what the patient understands about the reason she is required to use the bedpan for elimination. Based on this information, reinforce the rationale for the use of the bedpan. Promote comfort and normalcy as much as possible, while respecting the patient's privacy. Determine if a regular bedpan or a fracture pan would be most appropriate for Ms. Halligan. Also be sure to provide skin care and perineal hygiene after bedpan use and maintain a professional manner.

3. Obtain additional assessment data regarding the catheter site. Assessment data should include the presence of erythema, drainage, bleeding, tenderness, swelling, skin irritation or breakdown, or leakage. These signs could indicate exit-site or tunnel infection. In addition, inquire about any tenderness, pain, and guarding of the abdomen, as well as nausea, vomiting, and fever, which could indicate peritonitis. Assess the patient's knowledge about measures to care for the exit site. Remind Mr. Wimmer that exit-site and catheter care includes avoiding baths and public pools; the importance of good handwashing before self-care; and that he should be maintaining an occlusive dressing over the site.

Because he is experiencing site redness and tenderness, which could indicate an infection, instruct Mr. Wimmer to contact his primary care provider for an appointment to have his catheter and exit site evaluated.

Bowel Elimination

Focusing on Patient Care

This chapter will help you develop some of the skills related to bowel elimination necessary to care for the following patients:

Hugh Levens, a 64-year-old man, has been placed on a bowel program after a fall left him paralyzed from the waist down.

Isaac Greenberg, age 9, has been having blood in his stools. He is scheduled for a colonoscopy as an outpatient. He and his mother need teaching about the preparation for the procedure, which includes a small-volume cleansing enema.

Maria Blakely, age 26, has recently received an ileostomy. She is having problems with her appliance and is concerned about excoriation.

Refer to Focusing on Patient Care: Developing Clinical Reasoning at the end of the chapter to apply what you learn.

Learning Objectives

After completing the chapter, you will be able to accomplish the following:

1. Administer a large-volume cleansing enema.
2. Administer a small-volume cleansing enema.
3. Administer a retention enema.
4. Remove stool digitally.
5. Apply a fecal incontinence collection device.
6. Empty and change an ostomy appliance.
7. Irrigate a colostomy.
8. Insert a nasogastric tube.
9. Irrigate a nasogastric tube connected to suction.
10. Remove a nasogastric tube.

Key Terms

colostomy: artificial opening that permits feces from the colon to be eliminated through the stoma

constipation: dry, hard stool; persistently difficult passage of stool; and/or the incomplete passage of stool

defecation: emptying of the large intestine; also called a bowel movement

diarrhea: passage of more than three loose stools a day

enema: introduction of a solution into the large intestine

fecal impaction: prolonged retention or an accumulation of fecal material that forms a hardened mass in the rectum

fissure: linear break on the margin of the anus

flatus: intestinal gas; intestinal gas exiting anus

hemorrhoids: abnormally distended veins in the anal area

ileostomy: artificial opening created to allow liquid fecal content from the ileum to be eliminated through a stoma

ostomy: a surgically formed opening from the inside of an organ to the outside

stoma: the part of the ostomy that is attached to the skin; formed by suturing the mucosa to the skin

vagal response or stimulus: stimulation of the vagus nerve that causes an increase in parasympathetic stimulation, triggering a decrease in heart rate

Elimination of the waste products of digestion is a natural process critical for human functioning. Patients differ widely in their expectations about bowel elimination, their usual pattern of **defecation**, and the ease with which they speak about bowel elimination or bowel problems. Although most people have experienced minor acute bouts of **diarrhea** or **constipation**, some patients experience severe or chronic bowel elimination problems affecting their fluid and electrolyte balance, hydration, nutritional status, skin integrity, comfort, and self-concept. Moreover, many illnesses, diagnostic tests, medications, and surgical treatments can affect bowel elimination. Nurses play an integral role in preventing and managing bowel elimination problems.

This chapter covers skills the nurse may use to promote bowel elimination. Understanding the anatomy of the gastrointestinal (GI) system is integral to performing the skills in this chapter (Fundamentals Review 13-1). An abdominal assessment is required as part of providing the interventions outlined in many of these skills. Refer to Skill 3-7 in Chapter 3. Fundamentals Review 13-2 summarizes factors that may affect bowel elimination. Fundamentals Review 18-2 in Chapter 18 reviews the characteristics of stool.

Fundamentals Review 13-1

ANATOMY OF THE GASTROINTESTINAL TRACT

- The GI tract begins with the mouth and continues to the esophagus, the stomach, the small intestine, and the large intestine. It ends at the anus.
- From the mouth to the anus, the GI tract is approximately 9 m (30 ft) long.
- The small intestine consists of the duodenum, jejunum, and ileum.

- The large intestine consists of the cecum, colon (ascending, transverse, descending, and sigmoid), and rectum.
- Accessory organs of the GI tract include the teeth, salivary glands, gallbladder, liver, and pancreas.

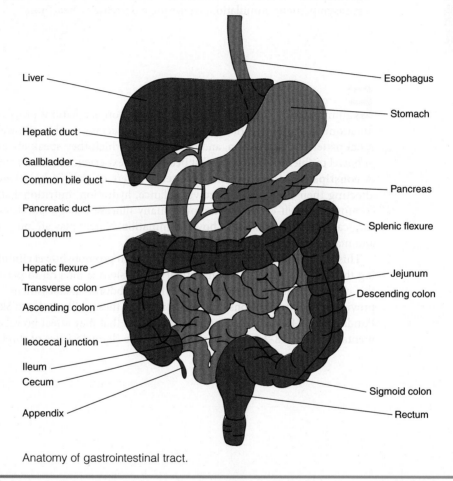

Liver

Hepatic duct

Gallbladder

Common bile duct

Pancreatic duct

Duodenum

Hepatic flexure

Transverse colon

Ascending colon

Ileocecal junction

Ileum

Cecum

Appendix

Esophagus

Stomach

Pancreas

Splenic flexure

Jejunum

Descending colon

Sigmoid colon

Rectum

Anatomy of gastrointestinal tract.

Fundamentals Review 13-2

FACTORS THAT AFFECT BOWEL ELIMINATION

- Mobility: Regular exercise improves GI motility and muscle tone, whereas inactivity decreases both. Adequate tone in the abdominal muscles, the diaphragm, and the perineal muscles is essential for ease of defecation.
- Diet: Foods high in fiber help keep stool moving through the intestines. High fluid intake keeps stools from becoming dry and hard. Adequate fluid also helps fiber to keep stool soft and bulky and prevents

dehydration from being a contributing factor to constipation.
- Medications: Antibiotics and laxatives may cause stool to become loose and more frequent. Diuretics may lead to dry, hard, and less frequent stools. Opioids decrease GI motility, leading to constipation.
- Intestinal diversions: Ileostomies normally have liquid, foul-smelling stool. Sigmoid colostomies normally have pasty, formed stool.

Skill 13-1 ▶ Administering a Large-Volume Cleansing Enema

Cleansing **enemas** are given to remove feces from the colon. Some of the reasons for administering a cleansing enema include relieving constipation or **fecal impaction**, preventing involuntary escape of fecal material during surgical procedures, promoting visualization of the intestinal tract by radiographic or instrument examination, and helping to establish regular bowel function during a bowel-training program. Cleansing enemas are classified as either large or small volume. This skill addresses administering a large-volume enema. (Small-volume enemas are addressed in Skill 13-2.)

Large-volume enemas are known as hypotonic or isotonic, depending on the solution used. Hypotonic (tap water) and isotonic (normal saline solution) enemas are large-volume enemas that result in rapid colonic emptying. However, using large volumes of solution (adults: 500 to 1,000 mL; infants: 150 to 250 mL) may be dangerous for patients with weakened intestinal walls, such as those with bowel inflammation or bowel infection. Large-volume enema solutions often require special preparation and equipment. See Table 13-1 for a list of commonly used enema solutions.

Table 13-1 Commonly Used Enema Solutions

SOLUTION	AMOUNT	ACTION	TIME TO TAKE EFFECT	ADVERSE EFFECTS
Tap water (hypotonic)	500–1,000 mL	Distends intestine, increases peristalsis, softens stool	15 minutes	Can lead to fluid and electrolyte imbalance, water intoxication. Should not be used in children
Normal saline (isotonic)	500–1,000 mL	Distends intestine, increases peristalsis, softens stool	15 minutes	
Soap	500–1,000 mL (concentrate at 3–5 mL/1,000 mL)	Distends intestine, irritates intestinal mucosa, which stimulates peristalsis, softens stool	10–15 minutes	Must only use Castile soap; other soaps will cause significant rectal mucosa irritation or damage
Hypertonic	70–130 mL	Draws fluids out of the interstitial space into the colon, leading to distention which stimulates peristalsis. Commonly used, commercially prepared (Fleet Enema)	5–10 minutes	Avoid in patients who are dehydrated or where sodium retention could be a concern. Can be irritating to rectum
Oil (mineral, olive, or cottonseed oil)	150–200 mL	Lubricates stool and intestinal mucosa. Often used as a retention enema. If able, patient may need to hold solution for 30–60 minutes	30 minutes	

DELEGATION CONSIDERATIONS

The administration of some types of enemas may be delegated to nursing assistive personnel (NAP) or to unlicensed assistive personnel (UAP) who have received appropriate training. The administration of a large-volume cleansing enema may be delegated to licensed practical/vocational nurses (LPN/LVNs). The decision to delegate must be based on careful analysis of the patient's needs and circumstances, as well as the qualifications of the person to whom the task is being delegated. Refer to the Delegation Guidelines in Appendix A.

(continued)

Skill 13-1 ▶ Administering a Large-Volume Cleansing Enema (continued)

EQUIPMENT	• Enema solution as ordered at a temperature of 105° to 110°F (40° to 43°C) for adults in the prescribed amount (amount will vary depending on the type of solution, patient's age, and patient's ability to retain the solution; average cleansing enema for an adult may range from 750 to 1,000 mL) • Disposable enema set, which includes a solution container and tubing • Water-soluble lubricant • IV pole • Necessary additives, as ordered • Waterproof pad • Bath thermometer (if available) • Bath blanket • Bedpan and toilet tissue • Disposable gloves • Additional PPE, as indicated • Paper towel • Washcloth, skin cleanser, and towel

ASSESSMENT

Ask the patient when he or she had the last bowel movement. Assess the patient's abdomen, including auscultating for bowel sounds, and palpating for tenderness and/or firmness. Because the goal of a cleansing enema is to increase peristalsis, which should increase bowel sounds, assess the abdomen before and after the enema. Assess the rectal area for any **fissures, hemorrhoids**, sores, or rectal tears. If any of these are present, take added care while inserting the tube. Assess the results of the patient's laboratory work, specifically the platelet count and white blood cell (WBC) count. An enema is contraindicated for patients with a low platelet count or low WBC count. An enema may irritate or traumatize the GI mucosa, causing bleeding, bowel perforation, or infection in these patients. Any unnecessary procedures that would place the patient with a low platelet count or low WBC count at risk for bleeding or infection should not be performed. Assess for dizziness, lightheadedness, diaphoresis, and clammy skin. The enema may stimulate a **vagal response or stimulus**, which increases parasympathetic stimulation, causing a decrease in heart rate. Do not administer enemas to patients who have severe abdominal pain, bowel obstruction, bowel inflammation or bowel infection, or after rectal, prostate, or colon surgery.

NURSING DIAGNOSIS

Determine the related factors for the nursing diagnoses based on the patient's current status. Appropriate nursing diagnoses may include:

• Acute pain
• Constipation
• Risk for constipation

OUTCOME IDENTIFICATION AND PLANNING

The expected outcome to achieve when administering a cleansing enema is that the patient expels feces. Other appropriate outcomes may include the following: the patient verbalizes decreased discomfort; abdominal distention is absent; and the patient remains free of any evidence of trauma to the rectal mucosa or other adverse effects.

IMPLEMENTATION

ACTION	RATIONALE
1. Verify the order for the enema. Gather equipment.	Verifying the medical order is crucial to ensuring that the proper enema is administered to the right patient. Assembling equipment provides for an organized approach to the task.
2. Perform hand hygiene and put on PPE, if indicated.	Hand hygiene and PPE prevent the spread of microorganisms. PPE is required based on transmission precautions.
3. Identify the patient.	Identifying the patient ensures the right patient receives the intervention and helps prevent errors.

ACTION	RATIONALE
4. Explain the procedure to the patient and provide the rationale as to why the enema is needed. Discuss the associated discomforts that may be experienced and possible interventions that may allay this discomfort. Answer any questions, as needed.	Explanation facilitates patient cooperation and reduces anxiety.
5. Assemble equipment on overbed table or other surface within reach.	Arranging items nearby is convenient, saves time, and avoids unnecessary stretching and twisting of muscles on the part of the nurse.
6. Close the curtains around the bed and close the door to the room, if possible. Discuss where the patient will defecate. Have a bedpan, commode, or nearby bathroom ready for use.	This ensures the patient's privacy. Explanation relieves anxiety and facilitates cooperation. The patient is better able to relax and cooperate if he or she is familiar with the procedure and knows everything is in readiness when the urge to defecate is felt. Defecation usually occurs within 5 to 15 minutes.
7. Warm the enema solution in the amount ordered, and check the temperature with a thermometer, if available. If a thermometer is not available, warm to room temperature or slightly higher, and test on inner wrist. If tap water is used, adjust the temperature as it flows from the faucet.	Warming the solution prevents chilling the patient, adding to the discomfort of the procedure. Cold solution could cause cramping; a too-warm solution could cause trauma to intestinal mucosa.
8. Add enema solution to a container. Release clamp and allow fluid to progress through the tube before reclamping.	This causes any air to be expelled from the tubing. Although allowing air to enter the intestine is not harmful, it may further distend the intestine.
9. Adjust the bed to a comfortable working height, usually elbow height of the caregiver (VHACEOSH, 2016). Position the patient on the left side (Sims position), with the upper thigh pulled toward the abdomen, if possible, or the knee–chest position, as dictated by patient comfort and condition. Fold top linen back just enough to allow access to the patient's rectal area. Drape the patient with the bath blanket, as necessary, to maintain privacy and warmth. Place a waterproof pad under the patient's hip.	Having the bed at the proper height prevents back and muscle strain. Sims position or knee–chest position facilitates flow of solution via gravity into the rectum and colon, optimizing solution retention. Folding back the linen in this manner minimizes unnecessary exposure and promotes the patient's comfort and warmth. The waterproof pad will protect the bed.
10. Put on gloves.	Gloves prevent contact with contaminants and body fluids.
11. Elevate solution so that it is no higher than 18 in (45 cm) above level of anus (Figure 1). Plan to give the solution slowly over a period of 5 to 10 minutes. Hang the container on an IV pole or hold it at the proper height.	Gravity forces the solution to enter the intestine. The amount of pressure determines the rate of flow and pressure exerted on the intestinal wall. Giving the solution too quickly causes rapid distention and pressure, poor defecation, or damage to the mucous membrane.

FIGURE 1. Adjusting height of solution container until it is no more than 18 in above patient.

(continued)

Skill 13-1 ▶ Administering a Large-Volume Cleansing Enema *(continued)*

ACTION	RATIONALE
12. Generously lubricate end of the rectal tube 2 to 3 in (5 to 7 cm). A disposable enema set may have a prelubricated rectal tube.	Lubrication facilitates passage of the rectal tube through the anal sphincter and prevents injury to the mucosa.
13. Lift buttock to expose anus. Ask patient to take several deep breaths. Slowly and gently insert the enema tube 3 to 4 in (7 to 10 cm) for an adult. Direct it at an angle pointing toward the umbilicus, not the bladder (Figure 2).	Good visualization of the anus helps prevent injury to tissues. Deep breathing helps relax the anal sphincters. The anal canal is about 1 to 2 in (2.5 to 5 cm) long. Insertion 3 to 4 in ensures the tube is inserted past the external and internal anal sphincters; further insertion may damage intestinal mucous membrane. The suggested angle follows the normal intestinal contour and thus will help to prevent perforation of the bowel. Slow insertion of the tube minimizes spasms of the intestinal wall and sphincters.
14. If resistance is met while inserting the tube, permit a small amount of solution to enter, withdraw the tube slightly, and then continue to insert it. **Do not force entry of the tube.** Ask the patient to take several deep breaths.	Resistance may be due to spasms of the intestine or failure of the internal sphincter to open. The solution may help to reduce spasms and relax the sphincter, thus making continued insertion of the tube safe. Forcing a tube may injure the intestinal mucosa wall. Taking deep breaths helps relax the anal sphincter.
15. Introduce solution slowly over a period of 5 to 10 minutes. Hold tubing all the time that solution is being instilled. Assess for dizziness, lightheadedness, nausea, diaphoresis, and clammy skin during administration. **If the patient experiences any of these symptoms, stop the procedure immediately, monitor the patient's heart rate and blood pressure, and notify the primary care provider.**	Introducing the solution slowly helps prevent rapid distention of the intestine and a desire to defecate. Assessment allows for detection of a vagal response. The enema may stimulate a vagal response, which increases parasympathetic stimulation, causing a decrease in heart rate.
16. Clamp tubing or lower container if the patient has the urge to defecate or cramping occurs (Figure 3). Instruct the patient to take small, fast breaths or to pant.	These techniques help relax muscles and prevent premature expulsion of the solution.

FIGURE 2. Inserting enema tip into anus, directing tip toward umbilicus.

FIGURE 3. Holding bag lower to slow flow of enema solution.

ACTION	**RATIONALE**
17. After the solution has been given, clamp tubing (Figure 4) and remove the tube. Have paper towel ready to receive the tube as it is withdrawn.	Wrapping the tube in a paper towel prevents dripping of solution.
18. Return the patient to a comfortable position. Encourage the patient to hold the solution until the urge to defecate is strong, usually in about 5 to 15 minutes. Make sure the linens under the patient are dry. Remove your gloves and ensure that the patient is covered.	This amount of time usually allows muscle contractions to become sufficient to produce good results. Promotes patient comfort. Removing contaminated gloves prevents spread of microorganisms.
19. Raise side rail. Lower bed height and adjust head of bed to a comfortable position.	Promotes patient safety.
20. Remove additional PPE, if used. Perform hand hygiene.	Proper removal of PPE reduces the risk for infection transmission and contamination of other items. Hand hygiene prevents the spread of microorganisms.
21. When patient has a strong urge to defecate, place him or her in a sitting position on a bedpan or assist to a commode or bathroom. Offer toilet tissues, if not in the patient's reach (Figure 5). Stay with the patient or have call bell readily accessible.	The sitting position is most natural and facilitates defecation. Fall prevention is a high priority due to the urgency of reaching the commode.

FIGURE 4. Clamping tubing before removing.

FIGURE 5. Offering toilet tissue to patient on bedside commode.

22. Remind the patient not to flush the commode before you inspect results of enema.	The results need to be observed and recorded. Additional enemas may be necessary if the health care provider has ordered enemas "until clear." Refer to "Special Considerations" below.
23. Put on gloves and assist patient, if necessary, with cleaning anal area. Offer washcloths, skin cleanser, and water for handwashing. Remove gloves.	Cleaning the anal area and proper hygiene deter the spread of microorganisms. Gloves prevent contact with contaminants and body fluids.
24. Leave the patient clean and comfortable. Care for equipment properly.	Bacteria that grow in the intestine can be spread to others if equipment is not properly cleaned.
25. Perform hand hygiene.	Hand hygiene deters the spread of microorganisms.

EVALUATION   The expected outcome has been met when the patient expels feces; the patient verbalizes decreased discomfort; abdominal distention is absent; and the patient remains free of any evidence of trauma to the rectal mucosa or other adverse effect.

(continued)

Skill 13-1 ▶ Administering a Large-Volume Cleansing Enema *(continued)*

DOCUMENTATION

Guidelines

Document the amount and type of enema solution used; amount, consistency, and color of stool; pain assessment rating; assessment of perineal area for any irritation, tears, or bleeding; and the patient's reaction to the procedure.

Sample Documentation

> <u>7/22/20</u> 1310 800-mL warm tap water enema given via rectum. Large amount of soft, brown stool returned. No irritation, tears, or bleeding noted in perineal area. Patient complained of "stomach cramping" relieved when enema was released. Rates pain as 0 after evacuation of enema.
>
> —K. Sanders, RN

UNEXPECTED SITUATIONS AND ASSOCIATED INTERVENTIONS

- *Solution does not flow into rectum:* Reposition rectal tube. If solution will still not flow, remove the tube and check for any fecal contents.
- *Patient cannot retain enema solution for adequate amount of time:* Patient may need to be placed on bedpan in the supine position while receiving the enema. The head of the bed may be elevated 30 degrees for the patient's comfort.
- *Patient cannot tolerate large amount of enema solution:* Amount and length of administration may have to be modified if patient begins to complain of pain.
- *Patient complains of severe cramping with introduction of enema solution:* Lower solution container and check the temperature and flow rate. If the solution is too cold or flow rate too fast, severe cramping may occur.

SPECIAL CONSIDERATIONS

General Considerations

- Do not use rectal agents and rectal manipulation, including enemas, with patients who are myelosuppressed and/or patients at risk for myelosuppression and mucositis. These interventions can lead to development of bleeding, anal fissures, or abscesses, which are portals for infection (National Cancer Institute [NCI], 2016).
- If the patient experiences fullness or pain or if fluid escapes around the tube, stop administration. Wait 30 seconds to a minute and then restart the flow at a slower rate. If symptoms persist, stop administration and contact the patient's primary health care provider.
- If the order states the enema is to be given "until clear," check with the primary care provider before administering more than three enemas. Severe fluid and electrolyte imbalances may occur if the patient receives more than three cleansing enemas. Results are considered clear whenever there are no more pieces of stool in enema return. The solution may be colored but still considered a clear return.

Infant and Child Considerations

- When administering an enema to a child, use isotonic solutions. Plain water is not used because it is hypotonic and can cause rapid fluid shift and fluid overload (Perry, Hockenberry, Lowdermilk, & Wilson, 2014).
- Appropriate fluid volume for an enema (Perry et al., 2014):
  - Infant: 120 to 240 mL
  - 2 to 4 years: 240 to 360 mL
  - 4 to 10 years: 360 to 480 mL
  - 11 years: 480 to 720 mL
- Position the infant or toddler on the abdomen with knees bent. Position the child or adolescent on the left side with the right leg flexed toward the chest (Kyle & Carman, 2017).
- Insert tubing into the rectum 2 to 3 in for children (2 to 10 years); 1 in for infants (Perry et al., 2014).

Older Adult Considerations

- If the older adult cannot retain the enema solution, administer the enema with the patient on the bedpan in the supine position. For comfort, elevate the head of the bed 30 degrees, if necessary, and use pillows appropriately.

Skill 13-2 ▶ Administering a Small-Volume Cleansing Enema

Cleansing enemas are given to remove feces from the colon. Some of the reasons for administering a cleansing enema include relieving constipation or fecal impaction, preventing involuntary escape of fecal material during surgical procedures, promoting visualization of the intestinal tract by radiographic or instrument examination, and helping to establish regular bowel function during a bowel-training program. Cleansing enemas are classified as either large or small volume. This skill addresses administering a small-volume enema. (Large-volume enemas are addressed in Skill 13-1.) Small-volume enemas (adult: 70 to 130 mL) are also known as hypertonic enemas. These hypertonic solutions work by drawing water into the colon, which stimulates the defecation reflex. They may be contraindicated in patients for whom sodium retention is a problem. They are also contraindicated for patients with renal impairment or reduced renal clearance, because these patients have compromised ability to excrete phosphate adequately, with resulting hyperphosphatemia (Jacobson, Peery, Thompson, Kanapka, & Caswell, 2010).

DELEGATION CONSIDERATIONS	The administration of some types of enemas may be delegated to nursing assistive personnel (NAP) or to unlicensed assistive personnel (UAP) who have received appropriate training. The administration of a small-volume cleansing enema may be delegated to licensed practical/vocational nurses (LPN/LVNs). The decision to delegate must be based on careful analysis of the patient's needs and circumstances, as well as the qualifications of the person to whom the task is being delegated. Refer to the Delegation Guidelines in Appendix A.
EQUIPMENT	• Commercially prepared enema with rectal tip • Water-soluble lubricant • Waterproof pad • Bath blanket • Bedpan and toilet tissue • Disposable gloves • Additional PPE, as indicated • Paper towel • Washcloth, skin cleanser, and towel
ASSESSMENT	Assess the patient's abdomen, including auscultating for bowel sounds, and palpating the abdomen. Because the goal of a cleansing enema is to increase peristalsis, which should increase bowel sounds, assess the abdomen before and after the enema. Inspect the rectal area for any fissures, hemorrhoids, sores, or rectal tears. If any of these are noted, take added care while administering the enema. Check the results of the patient's laboratory work, specifically the platelet count and white blood cell (WBC) count. A low platelet count may seriously compromise the patient's ability to clot blood. A low WBC count places the patient at risk for infection. Therefore, do not perform any unnecessary procedures that would place the patient at risk for bleeding or infection. Rectal agents and manipulation, including enemas, are discouraged for use with myelosuppressed patients and/or patients at risk for myelosuppression and mucositis, because they can lead to development of bleeding, anal fissures, or abscesses, which are portals for infection (NCI, 2016). Assess for dizziness, lightheadedness, diaphoresis, nausea, and clammy skin. The enema may stimulate a vagal response, which increases parasympathetic stimulation, causing a decrease in heart rate. Do not administer enemas to patients who have severe abdominal pain, bowel obstruction, bowel inflammation or bowel infection, or after rectal, prostate, and colon surgery.
NURSING DIAGNOSIS	Determine the related factors for the nursing diagnoses based on the patient's current status. Appropriate nursing diagnoses may include: • Acute pain • Constipation • Risk for constipation
OUTCOME IDENTIFICATION AND PLANNING	The expected outcome to achieve when administering a cleansing enema is that the patient expels feces and reports a decrease in pain and discomfort. In addition, the patient remains free of any evidence of trauma to the rectal mucosa.

(continued)

Skill 13-2 ▶ Administering a Small-Volume Cleansing Enema *(continued)*

IMPLEMENTATION

ACTION	RATIONALE
1. Verify the order for the enema. Gather equipment.	Verifying the medical order is crucial to ensuring that the proper enema is administered to the right patient. Assembling equipment provides for an organized approach to the task.
2. Perform hand hygiene and put on PPE, if indicated.	Hand hygiene and PPE prevent the spread of microorganisms. PPE is required based on transmission precautions.
3. Identify the patient.	Identifying the patient ensures the right patient receives the intervention and helps prevent errors.
4. Explain the procedure to the patient and provide the rationale why the tube is needed. Discuss the associated discomforts that may be experienced and possible interventions that may allay this discomfort. Answer any questions, as needed.	Explanation facilitates patient cooperation and reduces anxiety.
5. Assemble equipment on overbed table or other surface within reach.	Arranging items nearby is convenient, saves time, and avoids unnecessary stretching and twisting of muscles on the part of the nurse.
6. Close the curtains around the bed and close the door to the room, if possible. Discuss where the patient will defecate. Have a bedpan, commode, or nearby bathroom ready for use.	This ensures the patient's privacy. Explanation relieves anxiety and facilitates cooperation. The patient is better able to relax and cooperate if he or she is familiar with the procedure and knows everything is in readiness when the urge to defecate is felt. Defecation usually occurs within 5 to 15 minutes.
7. Adjust the bed to a comfortable working height, usually elbow height of the caregiver (VHACEOSH, 2016). Position the patient on the left side (Sims position), with the upper thigh pulled toward the abdomen, if possible, or the knee–chest position, as dictated by patient comfort and condition. Fold top linen back just enough to allow access to the patient's rectal area. Drape the patient with the bath blanket, as necessary, to maintain privacy and provide warmth. Place a waterproof pad under the patient's hip.	Having the bed at the proper height prevents back and muscle strain. Sims or knee–chest position facilitates flow of solution via gravity into the rectum and colon, optimizing retention of solution. Folding back the linen in this manner minimizes unnecessary exposure and promotes the patient's comfort and warmth. The waterproof pad will protect the bed.
8. Put on gloves.	Gloves prevent contact with contaminants and body fluids.
9. Remove the cap (Figure 1) and generously lubricate end of rectal tube 2 to 3 in (5 to 7 cm).	Lubrication facilitates passage of the rectal tube through the anal sphincter and prevents injury to the mucosa.

FIGURE 1. Removing cap from prepackaged enema solution container.

ACTION

10. Lift buttock to expose anus. Ask the patient to take several deep breaths. Slowly and gently insert the rectal tube 3 to 4 in (7 to 10 cm) for an adult. Direct it at an angle pointing toward the umbilicus, not bladder (Figure 2). **Do not force entry of the tube.**

11. Compress the container with your hands (Figure 3). Roll the end up on itself, toward the rectal tip. Administer all the solution in the container. Assess for dizziness, lightheadedness, nausea, diaphoresis, and clammy skin during administration. **If the patient experiences any of these symptoms, stop the procedure immediately, monitor the patient's heart rate and blood pressure, and notify the primary care provider.**

FIGURE 2. Inserting tube into rectum, directing toward umbilicus.

12. After the solution has been given, remove the tube, **keeping the container compressed.** Have paper towel ready to receive tube as it is withdrawn. Encourage the patient to hold the solution until the urge to defecate is strong, usually in about 5 to 15 minutes.

13. Remove gloves. Return the patient to a comfortable position. Make sure the linens under the patient are dry. Ensure that the patient is covered.

14. Raise side rail. Lower bed height and adjust head of bed to a comfortable position.

 15. Remove additional PPE, if used. Perform hand hygiene.

16. When the patient has a strong urge to defecate, place him or her in a sitting position on a bedpan or assist to commode or bathroom. Stay with patient or have call bell readily accessible.

17. Remind the patient not to flush the toilet or empty the commode before you inspect the results of the enema.

RATIONALE

Good visualization of the anus helps prevent injury to tissues. Deep breathing helps relax the anal sphincters. The anal canal is about 1 to 2 in (2.5 to 5 cm) long. Insertion 3 to 4 in ensures the tube is inserted past the external and internal anal sphincters; further insertion may damage intestinal mucous membrane. The suggested angle follows the normal intestinal contour, helping prevent perforation of the bowel. Forcing a tube may injure the intestinal mucosa wall.

Rolling the container aids administration of all its contents. Assessment allows for detection of a vagal response. The enema may stimulate a vagal response, which increases parasympathetic stimulation, causing a decrease in heart rate.

FIGURE 3. Compressing container.

If the container is released, a vacuum will form, allowing some of the enema solution to reenter the container. This amount of time usually allows muscle contractions to become sufficient to produce good results.

Promotes patient comfort. Removing contaminated gloves prevents spread of microorganisms.

Promotes patient safety.

Proper removal of PPE reduces the risk for infection transmission and contamination of other items. Hand hygiene prevents the spread of microorganisms.

The sitting position is most natural and facilitates defecation. Fall prevention is a high priority due to the urgency of reaching the commode.

The results need to be observed and recorded. Additional enemas may be necessary if the health care provider has ordered enemas "until clear." Refer to "Special Considerations" on the following page.

(continued)

Skill 13-2 ▶ Administering a Small-Volume Cleansing Enema *(continued)*

ACTION	RATIONALE
18. Put on gloves and assist patient, if necessary, with cleaning of anal area. Offer washcloths, skin cleanser, and water for handwashing. Remove gloves.	Cleaning the anal area and proper hygiene deter the spread of microorganisms.
19. Leave the patient clean and comfortable. Care for equipment properly.	Bacteria that grow in the intestine can be spread to others if equipment is not properly cleaned.
20. Perform hand hygiene.	Hand hygiene deters the spread of microorganisms.

EVALUATION

The expected outcome has been met when the patient expels feces; the patient verbalizes decreased discomfort; abdominal distention is absent; and the patient remains free of any evidence of trauma to the rectal mucosa or other adverse effect.

DOCUMENTATION

Guidelines

Document the amount and type of enema solution used; amount, consistency, and color of stool; pain assessment rating; assessment of perineal area for any irritation, tears, or bleeding; and patient's reaction to the procedure.

Sample Documentation

> <u>7/22/20</u> 1310 210-mL Fleet enema given via rectum. Large amount of soft, brown stool returned. No irritation, tears, or bleeding noted in perineal area. Patient stated "stomach fullness" relieved when enema was released. Rates pain as 0 after evacuation of enema.
> —*K. Sanders, RN*

UNEXPECTED SITUATIONS AND ASSOCIATED INTERVENTIONS

- *Patient cannot retain enema solution for adequate amount of time:* Patient may need to be placed on bedpan in the supine position while receiving the enema. The head of the bed may be elevated 30 degrees for the patient's comfort.

SPECIAL CONSIDERATIONS

General Considerations

- In patients who are myelosuppressed and/or patients at risk for myelosuppression and mucositis, rectal agents and manipulation, including enemas, are discouraged because they can lead to development of bleeding, anal fissures, or abscesses, which are portals for infection (NCI, 2016).
- If the enema has been ordered to be given "until clear," check with the primary care provider before administering more than three enemas. Severe fluid and electrolyte imbalances may occur if the patient receives more than three cleansing enemas. Results are considered clear whenever there are no more pieces of stool in enema return. The solution may be colored but still considered a clear return.

Infant and Child Considerations

- Position the infant or toddler on the abdomen with knees bent. Position the child or adolescent on the left side with the right leg flexed toward chest (Kyle & Carman, 2017).
- Insert tubing into the rectum 1 to 1.5 in (2.5 to 4 cm) for infants and 2 to 3 in (5 to 7.5 cm) for children (Kyle & Carman, 2017).
- Hold the child's buttocks together for 5 to 10 minutes, if needed, to encourage retention of the enema (Kyle & Carman, 2017).

Older Adult Considerations

- Use caution when giving enemas containing phosphates to frail older adults due to the potential for dehydration, electrolyte imbalances, and sodium phosphate toxicity (Niv, Grinberg, Dickman, Wasserberg, & Niv, 2013).

Skill 13-3 ▶ Administering a Retention Enema

Retention enemas are ordered for various reasons. *Oil-retention* enemas help to lubricate the stool and intestinal mucosa, making defecation easier. *Carminative* enemas help to expel **flatus** from the rectum and relieve distention secondary to flatus. *Medicated* enemas are used to administer a medication rectally. *Anthelmintic* enemas are administered to destroy intestinal parasites.

DELEGATION CONSIDERATIONS

The administration of some types of enemas may be delegated to nursing assistive personnel (NAP) or to unlicensed assistive personnel (UAP) who have received appropriate training. The administration of a retention enema may be delegated to licensed practical/vocational nurses (LPN/LVNs). The decision to delegate must be based on careful analysis of the patient's needs and circumstances, as well as the qualifications of the person to whom the task is being delegated. Refer to the Delegation Guidelines in Appendix A.

EQUIPMENT

- Enema solution (varies depending on reason for enema), often prepackaged, commercially prepared solutions
- Nonsterile gloves
- Additional PPE, as indicated
- Waterproof pad
- Bath blanket
- Washcloth, skin cleanser, and towel
- Bedpan or commode
- Toilet tissue
- Water-soluble lubricant

ASSESSMENT

Ask the patient when he or she had the last bowel movement. Assess the patient's abdomen, including auscultating for bowel sounds, and palpating. Because the goal of a cleansing enema is to increase peristalsis, which should increase bowel sounds, assess the abdomen before and after the enema. Assess the rectal area for any fissures, hemorrhoids, sores, or rectal tears. If present, added care should be taken while inserting the tube. Check the results of the patient's laboratory work, specifically the platelet count and white blood cell (WBC) count. A low platelet count may seriously compromise the patient's ability to clot blood. A low WBC count places the patient at risk for infection. Therefore, do not perform any unnecessary procedures that would place the patient at risk for bleeding or infection. Rectal agents and manipulation, including enemas, are discouraged for use with myelosuppressed patients and/or patients at risk for myelosuppression and mucositis, because they can lead to development of bleeding, anal fissures, or abscesses, which are portals for infection (NCI, 2016). Assess for dizziness, lightheadedness, diaphoresis, nausea, and clammy skin. The enema may stimulate a vagal response, which increases parasympathetic stimulation, causing a decrease in heart rate. Do not administer enemas to patients who have severe abdominal pain, bowel obstruction, bowel inflammation or bowel infection, or after rectal, prostate, and colon surgery.

NURSING DIAGNOSIS

Determine the related factors for the nursing diagnoses based on the patient's current status. Appropriate nursing diagnoses may include:

- Constipation
- Acute pain
- Risk for injury

OUTCOME IDENTIFICATION AND PLANNING

The expected outcome to achieve when administering a retention enema is that the patient retains the solution for the prescribed, appropriate length of time and experiences the expected therapeutic effect of the solution. Other appropriate outcomes may include the following: the patient verbalizes decreased discomfort; abdominal distention is absent; the patient demonstrates signs and symptoms indicative of a resolving infection; and the patient remains free of any evidence of trauma to the rectal mucosa or other adverse effect.

IMPLEMENTATION

ACTION	RATIONALE
1. Verify the order for the enema. Gather equipment.	Verifying the medical order is crucial to ensuring that the proper enema is administered to the right patient. Assembling equipment provides for an organized approach to the task.

(continued)

Skill 13-3 ▶ Administering a Retention Enema *(continued)*

ACTION	RATIONALE
2. Perform hand hygiene and put on PPE, if indicated.	Hand hygiene and PPE prevent the spread of microorganisms. PPE is required based on transmission precautions.
3. Identify the patient.	Identifying the patient ensures the right patient receives the intervention and helps prevent errors.
4. Explain the procedure to the patient and provide the rationale as to why the tube is needed. Discuss the associated discomforts that may be experienced and possible interventions that may allay this discomfort. Answer any questions, as needed.	Explanation facilitates patient cooperation and reduces anxiety.
5. Assemble equipment on overbed table or other surface within reach.	Arranging items nearby is convenient, saves time, and avoids unnecessary stretching and twisting of muscles on the part of the nurse.
6. Close the curtains around the bed and close the door to the room, if possible. Discuss where the patient will defecate. Have a bedpan, commode, or nearby bathroom ready for use.	This ensures the patient's privacy. Explanation relieves anxiety and facilitates cooperation. The patient is better able to relax and cooperate if he or she is familiar with the procedure and knows everything is in readiness if the urge to dispel the enema is felt.
7. Adjust the bed to a comfortable working height, usually elbow height of the caregiver (VHACEOSH, 2016). Position the patient on the left side (Sims position), with the upper thigh pulled toward the abdomen, if possible, or the knee–chest position, as dictated by patient comfort and condition. Fold top linen back just enough to allow access to the patient's rectal area. Drape the patient with the bath blanket, as necessary, to maintain privacy and provide warmth. Place a waterproof pad under the patient's hip.	Having the bed at the proper height prevents back and muscle strain. Sims or knee–chest position facilitates flow of solution via gravity into the rectum and colon, optimizing retention of the solution. Folding back the linen in this manner minimizes unnecessary exposure and promotes the patient's comfort and warmth. The waterproof pad will protect the bed.
8. Put on gloves.	Gloves prevent contact with blood and body fluids.
9. Remove cap of prepackaged enema solution. Apply a generous amount of lubricant to the tube.	Lubrication is necessary to minimize trauma on insertion.
10. Lift buttock to expose anus. Ask the patient to take several deep breaths. Slowly and gently insert the rectal tube 3 to 4 in (7 to 10 cm) for an adult. Direct it at an angle pointing toward the umbilicus (Figure 1).	Good visualization of the anus helps prevent injury to tissues. Deep breathing helps relax the anal sphincters. The anal canal is about 1 to 2 in (2.5 to 5 cm) long. Inserting 3 to 4 in ensures the tube is inserted past the external and internal anal sphincters; further insertion may damage intestinal mucous membrane. The suggested angle follows the normal intestinal contour and thus will help to prevent perforation of the bowel. Slow insertion of the tube minimizes spasms of the intestinal wall and sphincters. Deep breathing helps relax the anal sphincters.

FIGURE 1. Inserting tube into rectum, directing toward umbilicus.

ACTION

11. Compress the container with your hands (Figure 2). Roll the end up on itself, toward the rectal tip. Administer all the solution in the container. Assess for dizziness, light-headedness, nausea, diaphoresis, and clammy skin during administration. **If the patient experiences any of these symptoms, stop the procedure immediately, monitor the patient's heart rate and blood pressure, and notify the primary care provider.**

FIGURE 2. Compressing container.

12. **Remove the container while keeping it compressed. Have paper towel ready to receive tube as it is withdrawn.**

13. **Instruct the patient to retain the enema solution for at least 30 minutes or as indicated, per manufacturer's direction.**

14. Remove gloves. Return the patient to a comfortable position. Make sure the linens under the patient are dry and ensure that the patient is covered.

15. Raise side rail. Lower bed height and adjust head of bed to a comfortable position.

16. Remove additional PPE, if used. Perform hand hygiene.

17. When the patient has a strong urge to dispel the solution, place him or her in a sitting position on bedpan or assist to commode or bathroom. Stay with the patient or have call bell readily accessible.

18. Remind the patient not to flush the commode before you inspect the results of the enema, if used for bowel evacuation. Record character of stool, as appropriate, and patient's reaction to the enema.

19. Put on gloves and assist patient, if necessary, with cleaning of anal area. Offer washcloths, skin cleanser, and water for handwashing. Remove gloves.

20. Leave patient clean and comfortable. Care for equipment properly.

21. Perform hand hygiene.

RATIONALE

Rolling the container aids administration of all of the contents of the container. Assessment allows for detection of a vagal response. The enema may stimulate a vagal response, which increases parasympathetic stimulation, causing a decrease in heart rate.

If container is released, a vacuum will form, allowing some of the enema solution to reenter the container.

Solution needs to dwell for at least 30 minutes, or per manufacturer's direction, to allow for its optimal action.

Removing contaminated gloves prevents spread of microorganisms. Promotes patient comfort.

Promotes patient safety.

Proper removal of PPE reduces the risk for infection transmission and contamination of other items. Hand hygiene prevents the spread of microorganisms.

The sitting position is most natural and facilitates defecation. Fall prevention is a high priority due to the urgency of reaching the commode.

The results need to be observed and recorded.

Cleaning the anal area and proper hygiene deter the spread of microorganisms. Proper removal of PPE reduces the risk for infection transmission and contamination of other items.

Bacteria that grow in the intestine can be spread to others if equipment is not properly cleaned.

Hand hygiene deters the spread of microorganisms.

(continued)

Skill 13-3 ▶ Administering a Retention Enema *(continued)*

EVALUATION

The expected outcome has been met when the patient expels feces without evidence of trauma to the rectal mucosa. Depending on the reason for the retention enema, other outcomes met may include the patient verbalizing a decrease in pain after the enema; and the patient demonstrating signs and symptoms indicative of a resolving infection.

DOCUMENTATION

Guidelines

Document the amount and type of enema solution used; length of time retained by the patient; amount, consistency, and color of stool, as appropriate; pain assessment rating; assessment of perineal area for any irritation, tears, or bleeding; and the patient's reaction to the procedure.

Sample Documentation

> 6/26/20 2030 100 mL of mineral oil administered as enema via rectum. Small amount of firm, black stool returned. Small (approx. 1 cm) tear noted at 2 o'clock position on anus. No erythema or bleeding noted. Physician notified of tear and stool color. Reports pain as 2 on a 0-to-10 rating scale after enema evacuated.
>
> —K. Sanders, RN

UNEXPECTED SITUATIONS AND ASSOCIATED INTERVENTIONS

- *Solution does not flow into rectum:* Reposition rectal tube; if solution still will not flow, remove and check for any fecal contents.
- *Patient cannot retain enema solution for adequate amount of time:* Place patient on bedpan in supine position while receiving enema. Elevate the head of the bed 30 degrees for the patient's comfort. If still unable to retain, notify primary care provider.

SPECIAL CONSIDERATIONS

General Considerations

- In patients who are myelosuppressed and/or patients at risk for myelosuppression and mucositis, rectal agents and manipulation, including enemas, are discouraged because they can lead to development of bleeding, anal fissures, or abscesses, which are portals for infection (NCI, 2016).

Infant and Child Considerations

- Position the infant or toddler on the abdomen with knees bent. Position the child or adolescent on the left side with the right leg flexed toward chest (Kyle & Carman, 2017).
- Insert tubing into the rectum 1 to 1.5 in (2.5 to 4 cm) for infants and 2 to 3 in (5 to 7.5 cm) for children (Kyle & Carman, 2017).
- Hold the child's buttocks together for 5 to 10 minutes, if needed, to encourage retention of the enema (Kyle & Carman, 2017).

Skill 13-4 ▶ Digital Removal of Stool

Fecal impaction (prolonged retention or an accumulation of fecal material that forms a hardened mass in the rectum), most often caused by constipation, prevents the passage of normal stools. If a patient with a fecal impaction cannot expel the fecal mass voluntarily and oil and cleansing enemas fail to break up the mass, the impaction may need to be removed manually. However, before digital removal of feces is considered, dietary interventions, adequate fluids, and medication adjustment should be included in the patient's care plan (Rey, Barcelo, Jiménez-Cebrián, Alvarez-Sanchez, Diaz-Rubio, & Rocha, 2014). Digital removal of stool is very uncomfortable and may cause great discomfort to the patient as well as irritation of the rectal mucosa and bleeding. An order from the primary health care provider is required. The primary care provider may order an oil-retention enema to be given before the procedure to soften stool (refer to Skill 13-3). In addition, many patients find that a sitz bath or tub bath after this procedure soothes the irritated perineal area.

DELEGATION CONSIDERATIONS	Digital removal of stool is not delegated to nursing assistive personnel (NAP) or to unlicensed assistive personnel (UAP). Depending on the state's nurse practice act and the organization's policies and procedures, the digital removal of stool may be delegated to licensed practical/vocational nurses (LPN/LVNs). The decision to delegate must be based on careful analysis of the patient's needs and circumstances, as well as the qualifications of the person to whom the task is being delegated. Refer to the Delegation Guidelines in Appendix A.

EQUIPMENT

- Disposable gloves
- Additional PPE, as indicated
- Water-soluble lubricant
- Waterproof pad
- Bath blanket
- Bedpan
- Toilet paper, washcloth, skin cleanser, and towel
- Sitz bath (optional)

ASSESSMENT

Verify the time of the patient's last bowel movement by asking the patient and checking the patient's medical record. Assess the abdomen, including auscultating for bowel sounds, and palpating for tenderness and/or firmness. Inspect the rectal area for any fissures, hemorrhoids, sores, or rectal tears. If any of these are noted, consult the prescriber for the appropriateness of the intervention. Check the results of the patient's laboratory work, specifically the platelet count and white blood cell (WBC) count. A low platelet count may seriously compromise the patient's ability to clot blood. A low WBC count places the patient at risk for infection. Therefore, do not perform any unnecessary procedures that would place the patient at risk for bleeding or infection. Rectal agents and manipulation, such as digital removal of stool, are discouraged for use with myelosuppressed patients and/or patients at risk for myelosuppression and mucositis, because they can lead to development of bleeding, anal fissures, or abscesses, which are portals for infection (NCI, 2016). Digital removal of stool may irritate or traumatize the GI mucosa, causing bleeding, bowel perforation, or infection. Assess for dizziness, lightheadedness, diaphoresis, and clammy skin. Assess pulse rate and blood pressure before and after the procedure. The procedure may stimulate a vagal response, which increases parasympathetic stimulation, causing a decrease in heart rate and blood pressure. Do not perform digital removal of stool on patients who have bowel inflammation or bowel infection, or after rectal, prostate, and colon surgery.

NURSING DIAGNOSIS

Determine the related factors for the nursing diagnoses based on the patient's current status. Appropriate nursing diagnoses may include:

- Constipation
- Acute pain
- Risk for injury

OUTCOME IDENTIFICATION AND PLANNING

The expected outcome to achieve when digitally removing stool is that the patient will expel feces with assistance. Other appropriate outcomes may include: the patient verbalizes decreased discomfort; abdominal distention is absent; and the patient remains free of any evidence of trauma to the rectal mucosa or other adverse effect.

IMPLEMENTATION

ACTION	**RATIONALE**
1. Verify the order for digital removal of stool. Gather equipment.	Digital removal of stool is considered an invasive procedure and requires a medical order. Verifying the medical order is crucial to ensuring that the proper procedure is administered to the right patient. Assembling equipment provides for an organized approach to the task.
2. Perform hand hygiene and put on PPE, if indicated.	Hand hygiene and PPE prevent the spread of microorganisms. PPE is required based on transmission precautions.

(continued)

Skill 13-4 ▶ Digital Removal of Stool *(continued)*

ACTION	RATIONALE
3. Identify the patient.	Identifying the patient ensures the right patient receives the intervention and helps prevent errors.
4. Explain the procedure to the patient and provide the rationale why the procedure is needed. Discuss the associated discomforts that may be experienced. Discuss signs and symptoms of a slow heart rate. Instruct the patient to alert you if any of these symptoms are felt during the procedure. Have a bedpan ready for use.	Explanation relieves anxiety and facilitates cooperation. The patient is better able to relax and cooperate if he or she is familiar with the procedure.
5. Assemble equipment on overbed table or other surface within reach.	Arranging items nearby is convenient, saves time, and avoids unnecessary stretching and twisting of muscles on the part of the nurse.
6. Close the curtains around the bed and close the door to the room, if possible. Discuss where the patient will defecate, if necessary. Have a bedpan, commode, or nearby bathroom ready for use.	This ensures the patient's privacy. Explanation relieves anxiety and facilitates cooperation. The patient is better able to relax and cooperate if he or she is familiar with the procedure and knows everything is in readiness if the urge to defecate is felt.
7. Adjust the bed to a comfortable working height, usually elbow height of the caregiver (VHACEOSH, 2016). Position the patient on the left side (Sims position), with the upper thigh pulled toward the abdomen, if possible, or the knee–chest position, as dictated by patient comfort and condition. Fold top linen back just enough to allow access to the patient's rectal area. Drape the patient with the bath blanket, as necessary, to maintain privacy and provide warmth. Place a waterproof pad under the patient's hip.	Having the bed at the proper height prevents back and muscle strain. Sims or knee–chest position facilitates access into the rectum and colon. Folding back the linen in this manner minimizes unnecessary exposure and promotes the patient's comfort and warmth. The waterproof pad will protect the bed.
8. Put on nonsterile gloves.	Gloves prevent contact with blood and body fluids, as well as feces.
9. Generously lubricate index finger of dominant hand with water-soluble lubricant and insert finger gently into anal canal, pointing toward the umbilicus (Figure 1).	Lubrication reduces irritation of the rectum. The presence of the finger added to the mass tends to cause discomfort for the patient if the work is not done slowly and gently.
10. Gently work the finger around and into the hardened mass to break it up (Figure 2) and then remove pieces of it. Instruct patient to bear down, if possible, while extracting feces to ease in removal. Place extracted stool in bedpan.	Fecal mass may be large and may need to be removed in smaller pieces.

FIGURE 1. Inserting lubricated forefinger of dominant hand into anal canal, pointing toward umbilicus.

FIGURE 2. Gently working finger around to break up stool mass.

ACTION	RATIONALE
11. Remove impaction at intervals if it is severe. **Instruct the patient to alert you if he or she begins to feel lightheaded or nauseated. If patient reports either symptom, stop removal and assess the patient.**	Removal of stool in intervals helps to prevent discomfort and irritation, and vagal nerve stimulation. Assessment allows for detection of a vagal response. The enema may stimulate a vagal response, which increases parasympathetic stimulation, causing a decrease in heart rate.
12. When the procedure is completed, put on clean gloves. Assist the patient, if necessary, with cleaning of anal area (Figure 3). Offer washcloth, skin cleanser, and water for handwashing. If the patient is able, offer sitz bath.	Cleaning deters the transmission of microorganisms and promotes hygiene. Sitz bath may relieve the irritated perianal area.

FIGURE 3. Cleaning anal area with washcloth and skin cleanser.

ACTION	RATIONALE
13. Remove gloves. Return the patient to a comfortable position. Make sure the linens under the patient are dry. Ensure that the patient is covered.	Removing contaminated gloves prevents spread of microorganisms. The other actions promote patient comfort.
14. Raise side rail. Lower bed height and adjust head of bed to a comfortable position.	These promote patient safety.
15. Remove additional PPE, if used. Perform hand hygiene.	Proper removal of PPE reduces the risk for infection transmission and contamination of other items. Hand hygiene prevents the spread of microorganisms.

EVALUATION

The expected outcome has been met when the fecal impaction is removed and the patient expels feces with assistance; the patient verbalizes decreased discomfort; abdominal distention is absent; and the patient remains free of any evidence of trauma to the rectal mucosa or other adverse effect.

DOCUMENTATION

Guidelines

Document the following: abdominal assessment; color, consistency, and amount of stool removed; condition of perianal area after the procedure; pain assessment rating; and the patient's reaction to the procedure.

Sample Documentation

> <u>6/29/20</u> 1030 Digital removal of large amount of hard, brown stool. Abdomen soft, nondistended. Perineal area remains free from tears, erythema, or bleeding. Patient denied any lightheadedness or nausea during procedure. Rates pain as 1 on a 0-to-10 scale.
>
> —*K. Sanders, RN*

(continued)

Skill 13-4 ▶ Digital Removal of Stool *(continued)*

UNEXPECTED SITUATIONS AND ASSOCIATED INTERVENTIONS	• *Patient complains of being dizzy, lightheaded, or nauseated or begins to vomit:* Stop digital stimulation immediately. Vagal nerve might have been stimulated. Assess heart rate and blood pressure. Notify primary care provider. • *Patient experiences a large amount of pain during procedure:* Stop procedure and notify primary care provider.
SPECIAL CONSIDERATIONS	• In patients who are myelosuppressed and/or patients at risk for myelosuppression and mucositis, rectal agents and manipulation, such as digital removal of stool, are discouraged because they can lead to development of bleeding, anal fissures, or abscesses, which are portals for infection (NCI, 2016). • Recurrence of fecal impaction is common. It is important to help prevent and manage this condition by increasing dietary fiber content to 30 g/day, increasing water intake, and discontinuation of medications that can contribute to colonic hypomotility (Obokhare, 2012).

Skill 13-5 ▶ Applying a Fecal Incontinence Collection Device

A fecal incontinence device is an external collection system used to protect the perianal and perineal skin from excoriation due to repeated exposure to liquid stool. This device reduces skin damage by diverting liquid stool into a collection bag (Powers & Zimmaro Bliss, 2012). A skin barrier may be applied before the device to protect the patient's skin and improve adhesion. If excoriation is already present, the skin barrier should be applied before applying a device.

DELEGATION CONSIDERATIONS	Application of a fecal incontinence collection device may be delegated to nursing assistive personnel (NAP) or to unlicensed assistive personnel (UAP) who have received appropriate training. Application of a fecal incontinence collection device may be delegated to licensed practical/vocational nurses (LPN/LVNs). The decision to delegate must be based on careful analysis of the patient's needs and circumstances, as well as the qualifications of the person to whom the task is being delegated. Refer to the Delegation Guidelines in Appendix A.
EQUIPMENT	• Fecal incontinence device • Disposable gloves • Additional PPE, as indicated • Washcloth, skin cleanser, and towel • Drainage (Foley) bag • Scissors (optional) • Skin protectant or barrier • Bath blanket
ASSESSMENT	Assess the amount and consistency of stool being passed. Also assess the frequency of bowel movements. Inspect the perianal area for any excoriation, wounds, or hemorrhoids.
NURSING DIAGNOSIS	Determine the related factors for the nursing diagnoses based on the patient's current status. Appropriate nursing diagnoses may include: • Bowel incontinence • Risk for impaired skin integrity • Impaired skin integrity
OUTCOME IDENTIFICATION AND PLANNING	The expected outcome to achieve when applying a fecal incontinence device is that the patient expels feces into the device and maintains intact perianal skin. Other outcomes may include the following: the patient demonstrates a decrease in the amount and severity of excoriation; and the patient verbalizes decreased discomfort.

IMPLEMENTATION

ACTION	RATIONALE

1. Gather equipment.

Assembling equipment provides for an organized approach to the task.

2. Perform hand hygiene and put on PPE, if indicated.

Hand hygiene and PPE prevent the spread of microorganisms. PPE is required based on transmission precautions.

3. Identify the patient.

Identifying the patient ensures the right patient receives the intervention and helps prevent errors.

4. Close the curtains around the bed and close the door to the room, if possible. Explain what you are going to do and why you are going to do it to the patient.

This ensures the patient's privacy. Explanation relieves anxiety and facilitates cooperation. Discussion promotes cooperation and helps to minimize anxiety.

5. Assemble equipment on overbed table or other surface within reach.

Arranging items nearby is convenient, saves time, and avoids unnecessary stretching and twisting of muscles on the part of the nurse.

6. Adjust the bed to a comfortable working height, usually elbow height of the caregiver (VHACEOSH, 2016). Position the patient on the left side (Sims position), as dictated by patient comfort and condition. Fold top linen back just enough to allow access to the patient's rectal area. Drape the patient with the bath blanket, as necessary, to maintain privacy and provide warmth. Place a waterproof pad under the patient's hip.

Having the bed at the proper height prevents back and muscle strain. Sims position facilitates access into the rectum. Folding back the linen in this manner minimizes unnecessary exposure and promotes the patient's comfort and warmth. The waterproof pad will protect the bed.

7. Put on gloves. Cleanse perianal area. Pat dry thoroughly.

Gloves protect the nurse from microorganisms in feces. Skin must be dry for device to adhere securely.

8. Trim perianal hair with scissors, if needed.

It may be uncomfortable if the perianal hair is pulled by adhesive from the fecal device. Trimming with scissors minimizes the risk for infection compared with shaving.

9. Apply the skin protectant or barrier and allow it to dry. Skin protectant may be contraindicated for use with some devices. Check manufacturer's recommendations before use.

Skin protectant aids in device adhesion and protects skin from irritation and injury from the adhesive. Skin must be dry for device to adhere securely.

10. If necessary, enlarge the opening in the adhesive skin barrier to fit the patient's anatomy. Do not cut beyond the printed line on the barrier. Remove paper backing from adhesive of device (Figure 1).

Cutting away too much of the adhesive backing will result in poor adhesion to the patient's skin. Removing the paper backing is necessary so that the device can adhere to the skin.

FIGURE 1. Removing paper backing from adhesive of rectal device.

(continued)

Skill 13-5 ▶ Applying a Fecal Incontinence Collection Device *(continued)*

ACTION	RATIONALE

11. With nondominant hand, separate buttocks. Apply fecal device to anal area with dominant hand, ensuring that the bag opening is over anus (Figure 2). Hold the device in place for 30 seconds to achieve good adhesion.

Opening should be over anus so that stool empties into bag and does not stay on patient's skin, which could lead to skin breakdown. The device is effective only if it is properly positioned and adhered securely.

FIGURE 2. Applying device over anal opening.

12. Release buttocks. Attach connector of fecal incontinence device to drainage bag (Figure 3). Hang drainage bag below level of the patient (Figure 4).

Bag must be dependent for stool to drain into bag.

FIGURE 3. Attaching connector of fecal device to tubing of drainage bag.

FIGURE 4. Checking that drainage bag is below level of patient.

13. Remove gloves. Return the patient to a comfortable position. Make sure the linens under the patient are dry. Ensure that the patient is covered.

Removing contaminated gloves prevents spread of microorganisms. Promotes patient comfort.

14. Raise side rail. Lower bed height and adjust head of bed to a comfortable position.

Promotes patient safety.

15. Remove additional PPE, if used. Perform hand hygiene.

Proper removal of PPE reduces the risk for infection transmission and contamination of other items. Hand hygiene prevents the spread of microorganisms.

EVALUATION	The expected outcome has been met when the patient expels feces into the device and maintains intact perianal skin; the patient demonstrates a decrease in the amount and severity of excoriation; and the patient verbalizes decreased discomfort.
DOCUMENTATION	
Guidelines	Document the date and time the fecal device was applied; appearance of perianal area; color of stool; intake and output (amount of stool out); and the patient's reaction to the procedure.
Sample Documentation	

> 8/13/20 1210 Perianal area slightly erythematous. Fecal incontinence bag applied due to incontinence of large amounts of liquid stool and potential skin breakdown. Approximately 90 mL of liquid brown stool noted in drainage bag.
>
> —*K. Sanders, RN*

UNEXPECTED SITUATIONS AND ASSOCIATED INTERVENTIONS	• *Perianal area becomes excoriated:* Remove device. Thoroughly cleanse skin and apply skin barrier. Allow to dry completely. Reapply device. Monitor device adhesion and change device as soon as there is a break in adhesion. Confer with primary care provider for a wound, ostomy, and continence nurse consult to manage these issues. • *Stool is leaking from around sides of fecal device:* Remove device. Thoroughly cleanse skin and apply skin barrier. Allow to dry completely. Reapply device. Monitor device adhesion and change device as soon as there is a break in adhesion.
SPECIAL CONSIDERATIONS	• Fecal collector may be left in place for up to 7 days as long as skin barrier is intact and adherent (Hollister, 2005). Remove fecal device based on manufacturer's recommendations.

 Skill 13-6 | **Emptying and Changing an Ostomy Appliance**

Patients sometimes undergo a bowel diversion (surgical procedure) to create an opening into the abdominal wall for fecal elimination. The word **ostomy** is a term for a surgically formed opening from the inside of an organ to the outside. The intestinal mucosa is brought out to the abdominal wall, and a **stoma**, the part of the ostomy that is attached to the skin, is formed by suturing the mucosa to the skin. An **ileostomy** allows liquid fecal content from the ileum of the small intestine to be eliminated through the stoma. A **colostomy** permits formed feces in the colon to exit through the stoma. Colostomies are further classified by the part of the colon from which they originate.

Ostomy appliances or pouches are applied to the opening to collect stool. Nurses should empty an ostomy appliance that can be drained when it is approximately one third full; remove and change nondrainable pouches when they are half full. These actions reduce the risk of leakage and potential odor (Schreiber, 2016). Ostomy appliances are available in a one-piece (barrier backing already attached to the pouch) or two-piece (separate pouch that fastens to the barrier backing) system. Appliances are usually changed every 3 to 7 days, although they could be changed more often. Proper application minimizes the risk for skin breakdown around the stoma. The skill outlined below addresses changing a one-piece appliance. A one-piece appliance consists of a pouch with an integral adhesive section that adheres to the patient's skin. The adhesive flange is generally made from hydrocolloid. The accompanying Skill Variation addresses changing a two-piece appliance. Box 13-1 summarizes guidelines for care of the patient with a bowel diversion.

(continued)

Skill 13-6 ▶ Emptying and Changing an Ostomy Appliance *(continued)*

Box 13-1 Guidelines for Ostomy Care

The patient with an ostomy needs physical and psychological support both preoperatively and postoperatively. Support can come from the patient's significant others, members of the health care team, and people who have had similar experiences. Patients who receive consultation preoperatively and care postoperatively from an enterostomal therapy nurse or a wound ostomy continence nurse (WOCN) experience better long-term outcomes (Schreiber, 2016). Even when a WOCN is involved in the patient's care, the ostomy requires specific physical care for which the nurse is responsible initially. Use the following guidelines to help promote the physical and psychological comfort of the patient with an ostomy:

- Keep the patient as free of odors as possible. Empty an ostomy appliance that can be drained when it is approximately one third full, reducing the risk of leakage and potential odor (Landmann, 2015). Remove and change nondrainable pouches when they are half full.
- Inspect the patient's stoma regularly. It should be dark pink to red in color and moist. A pale stoma may indicate anemia, and a dark or purple-blue stoma may reflect compromised circulation or ischemia. Bleeding around the stoma and its stem should be minimal. Notify the primary care provider promptly if bleeding persists or is excessive, or if color changes occur in the stoma.
- Note the size of the stoma, which usually stabilizes within 6 to 8 weeks. Most stomas protrude 0.5 to 1 in from the abdominal surface and may initially appear swollen and edematous. After 6 weeks, the edema has usually subsided. Depending on the surgical technique, the final stoma may be flush with the skin. Erosion of skin around the stoma area can also lead to a flush stoma. If an abdominal dressing is in place at the surgical incision, check it frequently for drainage and bleeding. The dressing is usually removed after 24 hours.

- Keep the skin around the stoma site (peristomal area) clean and dry. If care is not taken to protect the skin around the stoma, irritation or infection may occur. A leaking appliance frequently causes skin erosion. Candida or yeast infections can also occur around the stoma if the area is not kept dry.
- Measure the patient's fluid intake and output. Check the ostomy appliance for the quality and quantity of discharge. Initially after surgery, peristalsis may be inhibited. As peristalsis returns, stool will be eliminated from the stoma. Record intake and output every 4 hours for the first 3 days after surgery. If the patient's output decreases while intake remains stable, report the condition promptly.
- Explain each aspect of care to the patient and explain what his or her role will be when beginning self-care. Patient teaching is one of the most important aspects of colostomy care and should include family members and/or people identified by the patient to include in care, when appropriate. Teaching can begin before surgery, if possible, so that the patient has adequate time to absorb the information.
- Appliances can be either drainable or closed. A pouch that can be drained is emptied when it is one third full and replaced every 3 to 7 days, or whenever the seal comes away from the skin. Nondrainable pouches require removal and changing when they are half full.
- Encourage the patient to participate in care and to look at the ostomy. Patients normally experience emotional depression during the early postoperative period. Help the patient cope by listening, explaining, and being available and supportive. A visit from a representative of the local ostomy support group may be helpful. Patients usually begin to accept their altered body image when they are willing to look at the stoma, make neutral or positive statements concerning the ostomy, and express interest in learning self-care.

DELEGATION CONSIDERATIONS	Emptying a stoma appliance on an ostomy may be delegated to nursing assistive personnel (NAP) or to unlicensed assistive personnel (UAP), as well as to licensed practical/vocational nurses (LPN/LVNs). Changing a stoma appliance on an ostomy may be delegated to an LPN/LVN. The decision to delegate must be based on careful analysis of the patient's needs and circumstances, as well as the qualifications of the person to whom the task is being delegated. Refer to the Delegation Guidelines in Appendix A.

EQUIPMENT	• Basin with warm water

- Basin with warm water
- Skin cleanser, towel, washcloth
- Toilet tissue or paper towel
- Silicone-based adhesive remover
- Gauze squares
- Washcloth
- Skin protectant, such as Skin-Prep
- One-piece ostomy appliance
- Closure clamp, if required, for appliance
- Stoma measuring guide
- Graduated container, toilet or bedpan
- Ostomy belt (optional)
- Disposable gloves
- Additional PPE, as indicated
- Small plastic trash bag
- Waterproof disposable pad

ASSESSMENT

Assess current appliance, looking at product style, condition of appliance, and stoma (if bag is clear). Note length of time the appliance has been in place. Determine the patient's knowledge of ostomy care. After removing the appliance, assess the stoma and the skin surrounding the stoma. The stoma should be dark pink to red in color and moist. A pale stoma may indicate anemia, and a dark or purple-blue stoma may reflect compromised circulation or ischemia. Bleeding around the stoma and its stem should be minimal. Promptly notify the primary care provider if bleeding persists, is excessive, or if color changes occur in the stoma. Note the size of the stoma, which usually stabilizes within 6 to 8 weeks. Most stomas protrude ½ to 1 in from the abdominal surface and may initially appear swollen and edematous. After 6 weeks, the edema has usually subsided. Depending on the surgical technique, the final stoma may be flush with the skin. Erosion of skin around the stoma area can also lead to a flush stoma. If an abdominal dressing is in place at the surgical incision, check it frequently for drainage and bleeding. The dressing is usually removed after 24 hours. Assess any abdominal scars, if surgery was recent. Assess the amount, color, consistency, and odor of stool from the ostomy.

NURSING DIAGNOSIS

Determine the related factors for the nursing diagnoses based on the patient's current status. Appropriate nursing diagnoses may include:

- Risk for impaired skin integrity
- Deficient knowledge
- Disturbed body image

OUTCOME IDENTIFICATION AND PLANNING

The expected outcome to be met when changing and emptying a bowel diversion appliance is that the stoma appliance is applied correctly to the skin to allow stool to drain freely. Other outcomes may include the following: the patient exhibits a moist red stoma with intact skin surrounding the stoma; the patient demonstrates knowledge of how to apply the appliance; the patient demonstrates positive coping skills; the patient expels stool that is appropriate in consistency and amount for the ostomy location; and the patient verbalizes positive self-image.

IMPLEMENTATION

ACTION	RATIONALE
1. Gather equipment.	Assembling equipment provides for an organized approach to the task.
2. Perform hand hygiene and put on PPE, if indicated.	Hand hygiene and PPE prevent the spread of microorganisms. PPE is required based on transmission precautions.
3. Identify the patient.	Identifying the patient ensures the right patient receives the intervention and helps prevent errors.
4. Close the curtains around the bed and close the door to the room, if possible. Explain what you are going to do and why you are going to do it to the patient. Encourage the patient to observe or participate, if possible.	This ensures the patient's privacy. Explanation relieves anxiety and facilitates cooperation. Discussion promotes cooperation and helps to minimize anxiety. Having the patient observe or assist encourages self-acceptance.
5. Assemble equipment on overbed table or other surface within reach.	Arranging items nearby is convenient, saves time, and avoids unnecessary stretching and twisting of muscles on the part of the nurse.
6. Assist the patient to a comfortable sitting or lying position in bed or a standing or sitting position in the bathroom. If the patient is in bed, adjust the bed to a comfortable working height, usually elbow height of the caregiver (VHACEOSH, 2016). Place waterproof pad under the patient at the stoma site.	Either position should allow the patient to view the procedure in preparation to learn to perform it independently. Lying flat or sitting upright facilitates smooth application of the appliance. Having the bed at the proper height prevents back and muscle strain. A waterproof pad protects linens and patient from moisture.

(continued)

Skill 13-6 ▶ Emptying and Changing an Ostomy Appliance *(continued)*

ACTION	RATIONALE

Emptying an Appliance

7. Put on gloves. Remove clamp and fold end of appliance or pouch upward like a cuff (Figure 1).

Gloves prevent contact with blood, body fluids, and microorganisms. Creating a cuff before emptying prevents additional soiling and odor.

8. Empty contents into bedpan, toilet, or measuring device (Figure 2).

Appliances do not need rinsing because rinsing may reduce appliance's odor barrier.

FIGURE 1. Removing clamp, getting ready to empty pouch.

FIGURE 2. Emptying contents of appliance into a measuring device.

9. Wipe the lower 2 in of the appliance or pouch with toilet tissue or paper towel (Figure 3).

Drying the lower section removes any additional fecal material, thus decreasing odor problems.

FIGURE 3. Wiping lower 2 in of pouch with paper towel.

10. Uncuff edge of appliance or pouch and apply clip or clamp, or secure Velcro closure. Ensure the curve of the clamp follows the curve of the patient's body. Remove gloves. Assist the patient to a comfortable position.

The edge of the appliance or pouch should remain clean. The clamp secures closure. Hand hygiene deters spread of microorganisms. Ensures patient comfort.

11. If appliance is not to be changed, place bed in lowest position. Remove additional PPE, if used. Perform hand hygiene.

Proper removal of PPE reduces the risk for infection transmission and contamination of other items. Hand hygiene prevents the spread of microorganisms.

Changing an Appliance

12. Place a disposable pad on the work surface. Open the premoistened disposable washcloths or set up the washbasin with warm water and the rest of the supplies. Place a trash bag within reach.

Protects surface. Organization facilitates performance of the procedure.

ACTION	RATIONALE
13. Put on clean gloves. Place waterproof pad under the patient at the stoma site. Empty the appliance as described in Steps 7–10.	Protect linens and patient from moisture. Emptying the contents before removal prevents accidental spillage of fecal material.
14. Put on gloves. Start at the top of the appliance and keep the abdominal skin taut. Gently remove pouch faceplate from skin by pushing skin from the appliance rather than pulling the appliance from skin (Figure 4). Apply a silicone-based adhesive remover by spraying or wiping with the remover wipe.	Gloves prevent contact with blood and body fluids. The seal between the surface of the faceplate and the skin must be broken before the faceplate can be removed. Harsh handling of the appliance can damage the skin and impair the development of a secure seal in the future. Silicone-based adhesive remover allows for the rapid and painless removal of adhesives and prevents skin stripping (Chandler, 2015; Rudoni, 2011; Stephen-Haynes, 2008).

FIGURE 4. Gently removing appliance.

15. Place the appliance in the trash bag, if disposable. If reusable, set aside to wash in lukewarm soap and water and allow to air dry after the new appliance is in place.	Thorough cleaning and airing of the appliance reduce odor and deterioration of the appliance. For aesthetic and infection control purposes, discard used appliances appropriately.
16. Use toilet tissue to remove any excess stool from the stoma (Figure 5). Cover the stoma with gauze pad. Clean the skin around the stoma with skin cleanser and water or a cleansing agent and a washcloth. Remove all old adhesive from the skin; use an adhesive remover, as necessary. Do not apply lotion to the peristomal area.	Toilet tissue, used gently, will not damage the stoma. The gauze absorbs any drainage from the stoma while the skin is being prepared. Cleaning the skin removes excretions and old adhesive and skin protectant. Excretions or a buildup of other substances can irritate and damage the skin. Lotion will prevent a tight adhesive seal.
17. Gently pat area dry. **Make sure the skin around the stoma is thoroughly dry.** Assess the stoma and the condition of the surrounding skin (Figure 6).	Careful drying prevents trauma to the skin and stoma. An intact, properly applied fecal collection device protects skin integrity. Any change in color and size of the stoma may indicate circulatory problems. Refer to Box 13-1.

FIGURE 5. Using toilet tissue to wipe around stoma.

FIGURE 6. Assessing stoma and peristomal skin.

(*continued*)

Skill 13-6 ▶ Emptying and Changing an Ostomy Appliance (continued)

ACTION	RATIONALE
18. Apply skin protectant to a 2-in (5 cm) radius around the stoma, and allow it to dry completely, which takes about 30 seconds.	The skin needs protection from the excoriating effect of the excretion and appliance adhesive. The skin must be perfectly dry before the appliance is placed, to get good adherence and to prevent leaks.
19. Lift the gauze squares for a moment and measure the stoma opening, using the measurement guide (Figure 7). Replace the gauze. Trace the same-size opening on the back center of the appliance (Figure 8). Cut the opening 1/8 in larger than the stoma size (Figure 9). Using a finger, gently smooth the wafer edges after cutting.	The appliance should fit snugly around the stoma, with only 1/8 in of skin visible around the opening. A faceplate opening that is too small can cause trauma to the stoma. If the opening is too large, exposed skin will be irritated by stool. Wafer edges may be uneven after cutting and could cause irritation to, and/or pressure on, the stoma.

FIGURE 7. Using measurement guide to measure size of stoma.

FIGURE 8. Tracing the same-sized circle on back and center of skin barrier.

FIGURE 9. Cutting the opening 1/8 in larger than stoma size.

20. Remove the paper backing from the appliance faceplate (Figure 10). Quickly remove the gauze squares and ease the appliance over the stoma (Figure 11). Gently press onto the skin while smoothing over the surface. Apply gentle, even pressure to the appliance for approximately 30 seconds.	The appliance is effective only if it is properly positioned and adhered securely. Pressure on the appliance faceplate allows it to mold to the patient's skin and improve seal (Jones, Springfield, Brudwich, & Ladd, 2011).

ACTION

RATIONALE

FIGURE 10. Removing paper backing on faceplate.

FIGURE 11. Easing appliance over stoma.

21. Close the bottom of the appliance or pouch by folding the end upward and using the clamp or clip that comes with the product (Figure 12), or secure the Velcro closure. Ensure the curve of the clamp follows the curve of the patient's body.

A tightly sealed appliance will not leak and cause embarrassment and discomfort for the patient.

FIGURE 12. Using clip to close bottom of appliance.

22. Remove gloves. Assist the patient to a comfortable position. Cover the patient with bed linens. Place the bed in the lowest position.

Provides warmth and promotes comfort and safety.

23. Put on clean gloves. Remove or discard equipment and assess the patient's response to the procedure.

Gloves prevent contact with blood, body fluids, and microorganisms that contaminate the used equipment. The patient's response may indicate acceptance of the ostomy as well as the need for health teaching.

 24. Remove gloves and additional PPE, if used. Perform hand hygiene.

Proper removal of PPE reduces the risk for infection transmission and contamination of other items. Hand hygiene prevents the spread of microorganisms.

EVALUATION

The expected outcomes have been met when the patient tolerates the procedure without pain and the peristomal skin remains intact without excoriation; odor is contained within the closed system; and the patient participates in ostomy appliance care, demonstrates positive coping skills, and expels stool that is appropriate in consistency and amount for the location of the ostomy.

(*continued*)

Skill 13-6 ▶ Emptying and Changing an Ostomy Appliance *(continued)*

DOCUMENTATION

Guidelines

Document appearance of stoma, condition of peristomal skin, characteristics of drainage (amount, color, consistency, unusual odor), the patient's reaction to procedure, and pertinent patient teaching.

Sample Documentation

DocuCare Practice documenting changing and emptying an ostomy appliance in *Lippincott DocuCare*.

> 7/22/20 1630 Colostomy appliance changed due to leakage. Stoma is pink, moist, and flat against abdomen. No erythema or excoriation of surrounding skin. Moderate amount of pasty, brown stool noted in bag. Patient asking appropriate questions during appliance application; states, "I'm ready to try changing the next one."
>
> —B. Clapp, RN

UNEXPECTED SITUATIONS AND ASSOCIATED INTERVENTIONS

- *Peristomal skin is excoriated or irritated:* Make sure that the appliance is not cut too large. Skin that is exposed inside of the ostomy appliance will become excoriated. Assess for the presence of a fungal skin infection. If present, consult with the primary care provider to obtain appropriate treatment. Thoroughly cleanse skin and apply skin barrier. Allow to dry completely. Reapply pouch. Monitor pouch adhesion and change pouch as soon as there is a break in adhesion. Confer with primary care provider for a wound, ostomy, and continence nurse consult to manage these issues. Document the excoriation in the patient's chart.
- *Patient continues to notice odor:* Check system for any leaks or poor adhesion. Clean outside of bag thoroughly when emptying.
- *Bag continues to come loose or fall off:* Thoroughly cleanse skin and apply skin barrier. Allow to dry completely. Reapply pouch. Monitor pouch adhesion and change pouch as soon as there is a break in adhesion.
- *Stoma is protruding into bag:* This is called a prolapse. Have the patient rest for 30 minutes. If the stoma is not back to normal size within that time, notify primary care provider. If stoma stays prolapsed, it may twist, resulting in impaired circulation to the stoma.
- *Stoma is dark brown or black:* Stoma should appear pink to red, shiny and moist. Alterations indicate compromised circulation. If the stoma is dark brown or black, suspect ischemia and necrosis. Notify the primary care provider immediately.

Skill Variation ▶ Applying a Two-Piece Appliance

A two-piece colostomy appliance is composed of a pouch and a separate adhesive faceplate (Figure A). The faceplate is left in place for a period of time, usually 3 to 7 days. During this period, when the colostomy appliance requires changing, only the bag needs to be replaced. The two main types of two-piece appliances are (1) those that "click" together, and (2) those that "adhere" together. The clicking Tupperware-type joining action provides extra security because there is a sensation when the appliance is secured, which the patient can feel. One problem with this type of system is that those with reduced manual dexterity may find it difficult to secure. Another disadvantage is that it is less discreet because the parts of the appliance that click together are more bulky than the one-piece system. Two-piece appliances with an adhesive system have the advantage that they are more discreet than conventional two-piece systems. They may also be simpler to use for those with poor manual dexterity. A potential disadvantage is that if the adhesive is not joined correctly and forms a crease, then feces or flatus may leak out, causing odor and embarrassment. Regardless of the type of two-piece appliance in use, the procedure to change is basically the same.

FIGURE A. Two-piece appliances. (Courtesy of Hollister, Incorporated, Libertyville, Illinois.)

Skill Variation ▶ Applying a Two-Piece Appliance *(continued)*

1. Gather necessary equipment.
2. Perform hand hygiene and put on PPE, if indicated.

3. Identify the patient.

4. Close the curtains around the bed and close the door to the room, if possible. Explain what you are going to do and why you are going to do it to the patient. Encourage the patient to observe or participate, if possible.
5. Assemble equipment on overbed table or other surface within reach.
6. Assist the patient to a comfortable sitting or lying position in bed or a standing or sitting position in the bathroom.
7. Place a disposable pad on the work surface. Set up the washbasin with warm water and the rest of the supplies. Place a trash bag within reach.
8. Put on gloves. Place waterproof pad under the patient at the stoma site. Empty the appliance as described previously in Skill 13-6.
9. Starting at the top of the appliance, gently remove the pouch faceplate while keeping the abdominal skin taut. Apply a silicone-based adhesive remover by spraying or wiping with the remover wipe. Push the skin from the appliance rather than pulling the appliance from the skin.
10. Place the appliance in the trash bag, if disposable. If reusable, set aside to wash in lukewarm soap and water and allow to air dry after the new appliance is in place.
11. Use toilet tissue to remove any excess stool from the stoma. Cover the stoma with gauze pad. Clean skin around the stoma with skin cleanser and water or a cleansing agent and a washcloth. Remove all old adhesive from skin; use an adhesive remover as necessary. Do not apply lotion to peristomal area.
12. Gently pat area dry. Make sure skin around the stoma is thoroughly dry. Assess the stoma and condition of surrounding skin.
13. Apply skin protectant to a 2-in (5 cm) radius around the stoma, and allow it to dry completely, which takes about 30 seconds.
14. Lift the gauze squares for a moment and measure the stoma opening, using the measurement guide. Replace the gauze. Trace the same-size opening on the back center of the appliance faceplate. Cut the opening 1/8 in larger than the stoma size. Use a finger to gently smooth the wafer edges after cutting.
15. Remove the backing from the faceplate. Quickly remove the gauze squares and ease the faceplate over the stoma. Gently press onto the skin while smoothing over the

surface. Apply gentle pressure to the faceplate for approximately 30 seconds (Figure B).

FIGURE B. Gently press faceplate to skin.

16. Apply the appliance pouch to the faceplate following manufacturer's directions. If using a "click" system, lay the ring on the pouch over the ring on the faceplate. Ask the patient to tighten stomach muscles, if possible. Beginning at one edge of the ring, push the pouch ring onto the faceplate ring (Figure C). A "click" should be heard when the pouch is secured onto the faceplate.

FIGURE C. Applying appliance pouch to faceplate.

17. If using an "adhere" system, remove the paper backing from the faceplate and pouch. Starting at one edge, carefully match the pouch adhesive with the faceplate adhesive. Press firmly and smooth the pouch onto the faceplate, taking care to avoid creases.
18. Close bottom of pouch by folding the end upward and using the clamp or clip that comes with the product, or secure Velcro closure. Ensure the curve of the clamp follows the curve of the patient's body.
19. Remove gloves. Assist the patient to a comfortable position. Cover the patient with bed linens. Place the bed in the lowest position.
20. Put on clean gloves. Remove or discard equipment and assess the patient's response to the procedure.
21. Remove gloves and additional PPE, if used. Perform hand hygiene.

Skill 13-6 ▶ Emptying and Changing an Ostomy Appliance *(continued)*

EVIDENCE FOR PRACTICE ▶

LIVING WITH A COLOSTOMY

A stoma operation causes major changes in a patient's life because of the resulting physical damage, disfigurement, loss of bodily function, and change in personal hygiene. Such changes are a cause of major concern for patients and raise important issues for the provision of quality care.

Related Research

Claessens, I., Probert, R., Tielemans, C., et al. (2015). The Ostomy Life Study: The everyday challenges faced by people living with a stoma in a snapshot. *Gastrointestinal Nursing, 13*(5), 18–25.

This survey explored users' experiences and worries, and related impact on daily living in relation to ostomy leakage, ballooning, discretion and appearance of the stoma bag, as well as challenges related to coupling and two-piece appliances. The survey was developed by 193 stoma care nurses from 10 countries. The online survey included responses from more than 4,138 participants from 11 countries, spanning all age groups, stoma types, stoma products, and a variety of cultures. The results showed that the majority of ostomates have issues related to leakage and ballooning. Seventy-six percent of participants experienced leakage during the previous 6 months and 91% of participants worried about leakage. Ninety-one percent of respondents experienced ballooning during the past 6 months and 94% worried about it. For approximately 40% of the respondents, problems with leakage and ballooning had a negative effect on sleep or led to unplanned appliance changes. Data revealed factors contributing to an ostomate's sense of feeling different, including the appearance of the stoma appliance. Only 25% of respondents did not worry about the appearance of the stoma appliance. Data revealed a significant correlation ($p < 0.001$) between age and concern about appearance, with a higher percentage of people below 70 years of age worrying about appearance than people over the age of 70. Similarly, people who had their stoma for more than 12 years worried significantly less about its appearance compared with those who had their stoma for a shorter time. The authors concluded concerns relating to the use of a stoma appliance, such as leakage, ballooning, and appearance may limit social and physical activities and have a negative impact on sleep for those living with an ostomy.

Relevance for Nursing Practice

Patients experiencing life-altering surgeries, such as colostomies and ileostomies, require much information and support to adapt and achieve an adequate standard of living. Nurses are the members of the health care team who typically spend the most time in direct contact with these patients. Nurses have a unique opportunity to provide the education and support these patients need, and improve the care provided to these patients. In addition to assisting patients to learn the physical care needs related to a stoma, nurses must address the psychosocial concerns of patients with ostomies as part of their nursing interventions. Nurses should use this information to gain a better understanding of the challenges that patients living with a stoma face on a daily basis and to guide the provision of appropriate nursing care to best support these patients.

Refer to thePoint® for additional research on related nursing topics.

Skill 13-7 ▶ Irrigating a Colostomy

Colostomy irrigation is a way of achieving fecal continence and control (Kent, Arnold Long, & Bauer, 2015). Irrigations are used to promote regular evacuation of some colostomies. Colostomy irrigation may be indicated in patients who have a left-sided end colostomy in the descending or sigmoid colon, are mentally alert, have adequate vision, and have adequate manual dexterity needed to perform the procedure. Contraindications to colostomy irrigation include irritable bowel syndrome, peristomal hernia, postradiation damage to the bowel, diverticulitis, and Crohn's disease (Kent et al., 2015). Ileostomies are not irrigated because the fecal content of the ileum is liquid and cannot be controlled.

Once the patient has established a routine and bowel continence has been established, a small appliance can be worn over the stoma. These "stoma caps" are small-capacity appliances with a pad to soak up discharge and a flatus filter (Kent et al., 2015). If a colostomy irrigation is to be implemented, the nurse should consult facility policy regarding the accepted procedure and, ideally, consult with a wound, ostomy, and continence nurse for patient education and support.

DELEGATION CONSIDERATIONS	Colostomy irrigation is not delegated to nursing assistive personnel (NAP) or to unlicensed assistive personnel (UAP). Depending on the state's nurse practice act and the organization's policies and procedures, the administration of a small-volume cleansing enema may be delegated to licensed practical/vocational nurses (LPN/LVNs). The decision to delegate must be based on careful analysis of the patient's needs and circumstances, as well as the qualifications of the person to whom the task is being delegated. Refer to the Delegation Guidelines in Appendix A.

EQUIPMENT

- Disposable irrigation system and irrigation sleeve
- Waterproof pad
- Bedpan or toilet
- Water-soluble lubricant
- IV pole
- Disposable gloves

- Additional PPE, as indicated
- Solution at a temperature of 98.6°F (37°C) (normally tap water)
- Washcloth, skin cleanser, and towels
- Paper towel
- New ostomy appliance, if needed, or stoma cover

ASSESSMENT

Ask patient if he or she has been experiencing any abdominal discomfort. Ask the patient about the date of the last irrigation and whether there have been any changes in stool pattern or consistency. If the patient irrigates his or her colostomy at home, ask if he or she has any special routines during irrigation, such as reading the newspaper or listening to music. Also determine how much solution the patient typically uses for irrigation. The normal amount of irrigation fluid varies, but is usually around 500 to 1,000 mL for an adult. If this is a first irrigation, the normal irrigation volume is around 500 mL. Assess the ostomy, ensuring that the diversion is a colostomy. Note placement of colostomy on abdomen, color and size of ostomy, color and condition of stoma, and amount and consistency of stool.

NURSING DIAGNOSIS

Determine the related factors for the nursing diagnoses based on the patient's current status. Possible nursing diagnoses may include:

- Deficient knowledge
- Anxiety

- Disturbed body image

OUTCOME IDENTIFICATION AND PLANNING

The expected outcome to be met when irrigating a colostomy is that the patient expels soft, formed stool. Other appropriate outcomes include the patient remains free of any evidence of trauma to the stoma and intestinal mucosa; the patient demonstrates the ability to participate in care; and the patient voices increased confidence with ostomy care.

IMPLEMENTATION

ACTION	**RATIONALE**
1. Verify the order for the irrigation. Gather equipment (Figure 1).	Verifying the medical order is crucial to ensuring that the proper treatment is administered to the right patient. Assembling equipment provides for an organized approach to the task.

Irrigation bag

Irrigation sleeve

Stoma cone

FIGURE 1. Irrigation sleeve and bag.

(continued)

Skill 13-7 ▶ Irrigating a Colostomy *(continued)*

ACTION	RATIONALE
2. Perform hand hygiene and put on PPE, if indicated.	Hand hygiene and PPE prevent the spread of microorganisms. PPE is required based on transmission precautions.
3. Identify the patient.	Identifying the patient ensures the right patient receives the intervention and helps prevent errors.
4. Close the curtains around the bed and close the door to the room, if possible. Explain what you are going to do and why you are going to do it to the patient. Plan where the patient will receive irrigation. Assist the patient onto bedside commode or into nearby bathroom.	Closing the curtains and door ensures the patient's privacy. Explanation relieves anxiety and facilitates cooperation. Discussion promotes cooperation and helps to minimize anxiety. The patient cannot hold the irrigation solution. A large immediate return of irrigation solution and stool usually occurs.
5. Assemble equipment on overbed table or other surface within reach.	Arranging items nearby is convenient, saves time, and avoids unnecessary stretching and twisting of muscles on the part of the nurse.
6. Warm solution in amount ordered and check temperature with a bath thermometer, if available. If bath thermometer is not available, warm to room temperature or slightly higher, and test on inner wrist. Water should feel lukewarm (Clow, Disley, Greening, & Harker, 2015). If tap water is used, adjust temperature as it flows from faucet.	If the solution is too cool, the patient may experience cramps or nausea. Solution that is too warm or too hot can cause irritation and trauma to intestinal mucosa.
7. Add irrigation solution to container. Release clamp and allow fluid to progress through tube before reclamping.	This process causes any air to be expelled from the tubing. Although allowing air to enter the intestine is not harmful, it may further distend the intestine.
8. Hang container on IV pole so that bottom of bag will be at the patient's shoulder level when seated.	Gravity forces the solution to enter the intestine. The amount of pressure determines the rate of flow and pressure exerted on the intestinal wall.
9. Put on gloves.	Gloves prevent contact with blood, body fluids, and microorganisms.
10. Remove ostomy appliance and attach irrigation sleeve (Figure 2). Place drainage end into toilet bowl or commode.	The irrigation sleeve directs all irrigation fluid and stool into the toilet or bedpan for easy disposal.
11. Lubricate end of cone with water-soluble lubricant.	The lubricant facilitates passage of the cone into the stoma opening.

FIGURE 2. Positioning of irrigation sleeve on abdomen.

ACTION	**RATIONALE**

12. Insert the cone through the top of the irrigation sleeve and into the stoma (Figure 3A). Introduce solution slowly over a period of 5 to 10 minutes. Hold cone and tubing (or if patient is able, allow patient to hold) all the time that solution is being instilled (Figure 3B). Control rate of flow by closing or opening the clamp.

If the irrigation solution is administered too quickly, the patient may experience nausea and cramps due to rapid distention and increased pressure in the intestine.

FIGURE 3. Colostomy irrigation. **A.** Inserting irrigation cone. **B.** Instilling irrigating fluid with sleeve in place.

13. Hold cone in place for an additional 10 seconds after the fluid is infused.

The additional time allows a small amount of dwell time for the irrigation solution.

14. Remove cone. Patient should remain seated on toilet or bedside commode.

An immediate return of solution and stool will usually occur, followed by a return in spurts for up to 45 more minutes.

15. After majority of solution has returned, allow the patient to clip (close) the bottom of irrigating sleeve and continue with daily activities.

Leaving the sleeve in place allows the patient to continue with daily activities until return of solution is complete. Solution may return in spurts for up to 45 minutes.

16. After solution has stopped flowing from stoma, put on clean gloves. Remove irrigating sleeve and cleanse skin around stoma opening with skin cleanser and water. Gently pat peristomal skin dry.

Gloves prevent contact with blood and body fluids. Peristomal skin must be clean and free of any liquid or stool before application of a new appliance.

17. Attach new appliance to stoma or stoma cover (see Skill 13-6), as needed.

Some patients will not require an appliance, but may use a stoma cover. Protects stoma.

18. Remove gloves. Return the patient to a comfortable position. Make sure the linens under the patient are dry, if appropriate. Ensure that the patient is covered.

Removing contaminated gloves prevents spread of microorganisms. Promotes patient comfort.

19. Raise side rail. Lower bed height and adjust head of bed to a comfortable position, as necessary.

Promotes patient safety.

20. Remove additional PPE, if used. Perform hand hygiene.

Proper removal of PPE reduces the risk for infection transmission and contamination of other items. Hand hygiene prevents the spread of microorganisms.

EVALUATION

The expected outcome has been achieved when the irrigation solution flows easily into the stoma opening and the patient expels soft, formed stool; the patient remains free of any evidence of trauma to the stoma and intestinal mucosa; the patient demonstrates the ability to participate in care; and the patient voices increased confidence with ostomy care.

(continued)

Skill 13-7 ▶ Irrigating a Colostomy *(continued)*

DOCUMENTATION

Guidelines

Document the procedure, including the amount of irrigating solution used; color, amount, and consistency of stool returned; condition of stoma; degree of patient participation; and patient's reaction to irrigation.

Sample Documentation

> 8/1/20 0945 1,000 mL of warmed tap water used to irrigate colostomy. Large amount of soft, dark brown stool returned. Patient performed procedure with small amount of assistance from nurse. Stoma is pink and moist with no signs of bleeding. Patient tolerated procedure without incident. New ostomy appliance applied.
>
> —B. Clapp, RN

UNEXPECTED SITUATIONS AND ASSOCIATED INTERVENTIONS

- *Irrigation solution is not flowing or is flowing at a slow rate:* Check clamp on tubing to make sure that the tubing is open. Gently manipulate cone in stoma to alter the direction of the cone; if stool or tissue is blocking cone opening, this may block flow of fluid. Remove cone from stoma, clean the area, and gently reinsert. Alternately, assist the patient to a side-lying or sitting position in bed. Place a waterproof pad under the irrigation sleeve. Place the drainage end of the sleeve in a bedpan.
- *Patient experiences abdominal cramping:* Check the temperature of the irrigation fluid; decrease rate of irrigation fluid.
- *Patient experiences breakthrough evacuation of stool:* This is not uncommon in the beginning. The bowel needs to get used to the procedure over a period of 2 or 3 weeks (Clow et al., 2015). Once irrigation is established, irrigate at approximately the same time on each occasion and do not hurry the procedure (Clow et al.).

SPECIAL CONSIDERATIONS

- Irrigation is contraindicated for patients who are myelosuppressed and/or patients at risk for myelosuppression and mucositis. The stoma of a patient who is neutropenic should not be manipulated (NCI, 2016).

EVIDENCE FOR PRACTICE ▶

COLOSTOMY IRRIGATION AND QUALITY OF LIFE

Colostomy irrigation stimulates emptying of the colon at regularly scheduled times and offers the patient some control over bowel function. Colostomy irrigation is not always easy or successful (Clow et al., 2015). Is this an intervention that should be considered an important part of patient care?

Related Research

Kent, D. J., Arnold Long, M., Bauer, C. (2015). Does colostomy irrigation affect functional outcomes and quality of life in persons with a colostomy? *Journal of Wound, Ostomy and Continence Nursing, 42*(2), 155–161.

This systematic review of the literature examined studies that evaluated health-related quality of life in people aged 18 years or older with colostomies of the sigmoid or descending left colon and who perform colostomy irrigations. The resulting research revealed four studies that met the inclusion criteria. Findings indicated colostomy irrigation reduces the frequency of bowel evacuations when compared to spontaneous evacuation and containment using a pouching system. Regular irrigation is associated with reductions in pouch usage. Colostomy irrigation frequently resulted in absence of bowel evacuations for 24 hours or longer, with some subjects discontinuing ongoing use of a pouching system. Participants reported reductions in flatus and odors associated with the presence of a colostomy. One study in the review reported higher health-related quality of life for participants using colostomy irrigation, measured using the Digestive Disease Quality of Life-15; however, no differences were found when health-related quality of life was measured using a more generic instrument. Based on the review of the related literature, the authors concluded that instruction on principles and techniques of colostomy irrigation should be considered when managing patients with a permanent, left-sided colostomy.

Relevance to Nursing Practice
Nurses have a responsibility to update and maintain relevant knowledge and skills to maintain competence in providing care options to patients. The creation of a bowel diversion can negatively affect every aspect of a person's life, including overall quality of life. Nurses need to consider the effect of this treatment on patients' lifestyles and health-related quality of life in order to provide person-centered nursing care. Colostomy irrigation is not always easy, straightforward, or successful, but it provides a management option that has the potential to contribute to patient-focused and person-centered care.

Refer to thePoint®for additional research on related nursing topics.

 Skill 13-8 ▶ **Inserting a Nasogastric Tube**

A nasogastric (NG) tube is a pliable single- or double-lumen (inner open space) tube that is hollow, allowing for the removal of gastric secretions and instillation of solutions such as medications or feedings into the stomach. The NG tube is passed through the nose and into the stomach. NG tubes are used to decompress or to drain unwanted fluid and air from the stomach, monitor bleeding in the gastrointestinal (GI) tract, to remove undesirable substances (lavage), or to help treat an intestinal obstruction. Tubes for decompression typically are attached to suction. Suction can be applied intermittently or continuously. When the underlying condition has been resolved and/or the NG tube is no longer indicated, the tube is removed (Refer to Skill 13-10).

NG tubes are also used to provide short-term nutrition, using the stomach as a natural reservoir for food. The use of NG tubes for nutritional purposes is discussed in Chapter 11.

Radiographic examination, measurement of tube length and measurement of tube marking, measurement of aspirate pH, visual assessment of aspirate, and monitoring of carbon dioxide have been suggested to confirm tube placement in the stomach. With the exception of radiographic examination, the use of two or more of these techniques in conjunction with each other increases the likelihood of correct tube placement (Bankhead et al., 2009; Metheny, 2016b; Rahimi, Farhadi, Ashtarian, & Changaei, 2015). An old technique of auscultation of air injected into a tube has proved unreliable and may result in tragic consequences if used as an indicator of tube placement (Bankhead et al., 2009; Boeykens, Steeman, & Duysburgh, 2014; Metheny, 2016b). Therefore, do not use it to confirm tube placement.

DELEGATION CONSIDERATIONS	The insertion of an NG tube is not delegated to nursing assistive personnel (NAP) or to unlicensed assistive personnel (UAP). Depending on the state's nurse practice act and the organization's policies and procedures, insertion of an NG tube may be delegated to licensed practical/vocational nurses (LPN/LVNs). The decision to delegate must be based on careful analysis of the patient's needs and circumstances, as well as the qualifications of the person to whom the task is being delegated. Refer to the Delegation Guidelines in Appendix A.

EQUIPMENT

- NG tube of appropriate size (8 to 18 Fr)
- Stethoscope
- Water-soluble lubricant
- Normal saline solution or sterile water, for irrigation, depending on facility policy
- Tongue blade
- Irrigations set, including a Toomey (20 to 50 mL)
- Flashlight
- Nonallergenic tape (1 in wide)
- Tissues
- Glass of water with straw

- Topical anesthetic—lidocaine spray or gel (optional)
- Clamp
- Suction apparatus (if ordered)
- Bath towel or disposable pad
- Emesis basin
- Safety pin and rubber band
- Nonsterile, disposable gloves
- Additional PPE, as indicated
- Tape measure, or other measuring device
- Skin barrier
- pH paper

(continued)

Skill 13-8 ▶ Inserting a Nasogastric Tube *(continued)*

ASSESSMENT

Assess the patency of the patient's nares by asking the patient to occlude one nostril and breathe normally through the other. Select the nostril through which air passes more easily. Also, assess the patient's history for any recent facial trauma, polyps, blockages, or surgeries. Patients with facial fractures or facial surgeries present a higher risk for misplacement of the tube into the brain. Many facilities require a health care provider to place NG tubes in these patients. Inspect the abdomen for distention and firmness; auscultate for bowel sounds or peristalsis and palpate the abdomen for distention and tenderness. If the abdomen is distended, consider measuring the abdominal girth at the umbilicus to establish a baseline.

NURSING DIAGNOSIS

Determine the related factors for the nursing diagnoses based on the patient's current status. Nursing diagnoses may vary depending on the reason for the NG tube insertion. Appropriate nursing diagnoses may include:

- Imbalanced nutrition: Less than body requirements
- Impaired swallowing
- Risk for aspiration

OUTCOME IDENTIFICATION AND PLANNING

The expected outcome to achieve when inserting an NG tube is that the tube is passed into the patient's stomach without any complications. Other outcomes may include the following: the patient exhibits no signs and symptoms of aspiration; the patient rates pain as decreased from prior to insertion; the patient demonstrates weight gain, indicating improved nutrition; and the patient verbalizes an understanding of the reason for NG tube insertion.

IMPLEMENTATION

ACTION	RATIONALE
1. Verify the medical order for insertion of an NG tube. Gather equipment, including selection of the appropriate NG tube.	Ensures the patient receives the correct treatment. Assembling equipment provides for an organized approach to the task. NG tubes should be radiopaque, contain clearly visible markings for measurement, and may have multiple ports for aspiration.
2. Perform hand hygiene and put on PPE, if indicated.	Hand hygiene and PPE prevent the spread of microorganisms. PPE is required based on transmission precautions.
3. Identify the patient.	Identifying the patient ensures the right patient receives the intervention and helps prevent errors.
4. Explain the procedure to the patient, including the rationale for why the tube is needed. Discuss the associated discomforts that may be experienced and possible interventions that may allay this discomfort. Answer any questions, as needed.	Explanation facilitates patient cooperation. Some patient surveys report that of all routine procedures, the insertion of an NG tube is considered the most painful. Lidocaine gel or sprays are possible options to decrease discomfort during NG tube insertion.
5. Assemble equipment on overbed table or other surface within reach.	Arranging items nearby is convenient, saves time, and avoids unnecessary stretching and twisting of muscles on the part of the nurse.
6. Close the patient's bedside curtain or door. Raise the bed to a comfortable working position, usually elbow height of the caregiver (VHACEOSH, 2016). Assist the patient to high-Fowler's position or elevate the head of the bed 45 degrees if the patient is unable to maintain an upright position. Drape chest with a bath towel or disposable pad. Have emesis basin and tissues within reach.	Closing curtains or door provides for patient privacy. Having the bed at the proper height prevents back and muscle strain. Upright position is more natural for swallowing and protects against bronchial intubation aspiration, if the patient should vomit. Passage of the tube may stimulate gagging and tearing of eyes.

ACTION	RATIONALE

7. **Measure the distance to insert the tube by placing the tube tip at the patient's nostril and extending it to the tip of the earlobe (Figure 1) and then to tip of the xiphoid process (Figure 2). Add any extra length based on facility policy. Mark the tube with an indelible marker.**

Measurement ensures that the tube will be long enough to enter the patient's stomach (Curtis, 2013). Some research suggests the need for additional tube length to safely reach the gastric body with recommendations to add 10 cm to the measurement of distance (Riesenberg et al., 2013).

FIGURE 1. Measuring NG tube from nostril to tip of earlobe.

FIGURE 2. Measuring NG tube from tip of earlobe to xiphoid process.

8. Put on gloves. Lubricate the tip of the tube (at least 2 to 4 in) with water-soluble lubricant. Apply topical anesthetic to the nostril and oropharynx, as appropriate.

Lubrication reduces friction and facilitates passage of the tube into the stomach. Water-soluble lubricant will not cause pneumonia if the tube accidentally enters the lungs. Topical anesthetics act as local anesthetics, reducing discomfort. Consult the health care provider for an order for a topical anesthetic, such as lidocaine gel or spray, if needed.

9. After selecting the appropriate nostril, ask the patient to flex the head slightly back against the pillow. Gently insert the tube into the nostril while directing the tube upward and backward along the floor of the nose (Figure 3). The patient may gag when the tube reaches the pharynx. Provide tissues for tearing or watering of eyes. Offer comfort and reassurance to the patient.

Following the normal contour of the nasal passage while inserting the tube reduces irritation and the likelihood of mucosal injury. The tube stimulates the gag reflex readily. Tears are a natural response as the tube passes into the nasopharynx. Many patients report that gagging and throat discomfort can be more painful than the tube passing through the nostrils.

FIGURE 3. Beginning insertion with patient positioned with head slightly flexed back.

(*continued*)

Skill 13-8 ▶ Inserting a Nasogastric Tube *(continued)*

ACTION	RATIONALE
10. When pharynx is reached, instruct the patient to touch chin to chest. Encourage the patient to sip water through a straw or swallow (Figure 4). Advance the tube in downward and backward direction when patient swallows. Stop when the patient breathes. **If gagging and coughing persist, stop advancing the tube and check placement of the tube with a tongue blade and flashlight. If the tube is curled, straighten the tube and attempt to advance again. Keep advancing the tube until pen marking is reached. Do not use force.** Rotate the tube if it meets resistance.	Bringing the head forward helps close the trachea and open the esophagus. Swallowing helps advance the tube, causes the epiglottis to cover the opening of the trachea, and helps to eliminate gagging and coughing. Excessive coughing and gagging may occur if the tube has curled in the back of throat. Forcing the tube may injure mucous membranes.

FIGURE 4. Advancing tube after patient drops chin to chest and while swallowing.

ACTION	RATIONALE
11. **Discontinue the procedure and remove the tube if there are signs of distress, such as gasping, coughing, cyanosis, and inability to speak or hum.**	The tube is in the airway if the patient shows signs of distress and cannot speak or hum. If after three attempts, NG insertion is unsuccessful, another nurse may try or the patient should be referred to another health care professional.
12. Secure the tube loosely to the nose or cheek until it is determined that the tube is in the patient's stomach. Confirm placement of the NG tube in the patient's stomach using at least two methods, based on the type of tube in place.	Tube placement must be verified before administration of any fluids or medications. This ensures that the tip of the tube is situated in the stomach or intestine, preventing inadvertent administration of substances into the wrong place. A misplaced feeding tube in the lungs or pulmonary tissue places the patient at risk for aspiration. With the exception of radiographic examination, which is usually done immediately after insertion to verify initial tube placement, the use of two or more of these techniques in conjunction with each other increases the likelihood of correct tube placement (Bankhead et al., 2009; Metheny, 2016b; Rahimi et al., 2015). Aspiration of gastric contents may not be possible with some small-bore feeding tubes.
a. Obtain radiograph (x-ray) of placement of the tube, based on facility policy and as ordered by the primary care provider.	The x-ray is considered the most reliable method for identifying the position of the NG tube.

ACTION

b. Put on gloves. Attach the syringe to end of the tube and aspirate a small amount of stomach contents. If unable to obtain a specimen, reposition the patient and flush the tube with 30 mL of air in a large syringe. Slowly apply negative pressure to withdraw fluid.

c. Measure the pH of aspirated fluid using pH paper or a meter. Place a drop of gastric secretions onto pH paper or place small amount in a plastic cup and dip the pH paper into it. Within 30 seconds, compare the color on the paper with the chart supplied by the manufacturer.

d. Visualize aspirated contents, checking for color and consistency.

e. Measure the length of the exposed tube at the nostril. Mark the tube with an indelible marker.

13. After confirmation of the tube placement, secure the tube. Apply skin barrier to the tip and end of the nose and allow to dry. Remove gloves and secure the tube with a commercially prepared device (follow manufacturer's directions) or tape to the patient's nose. To secure with tape:

a. Cut a 4-in piece of tape and split bottom 2 in (Figure 5) or use packaged nose tape for NG tubes.

RATIONALE

Gloves prevent contact with blood and body fluids and transfer of microorganisms. The tube is in the stomach if its contents can be aspirated: pH of aspirate can then be tested to determine gastric placement. Difficulty in aspiration may be due to a blocked tube or the tip of the tube may not be positioned in fluid. Injecting an air bolus will help remove the blockage and repositioning the patient will help place the tip of the tube in fluid (Metheny, 2016b). This action may be necessary several times in order to obtain aspirate.

Current research demonstrates that the use of pH is predictive of correct placement. The pH of gastric contents is acidic (less than 5.5). If the patient is taking an acid-inhibiting agent, the range may be 4.0 to 6.0. The pH of intestinal fluid is 7.0 or higher. The pH of respiratory fluid is 6.0 or higher. This method will not effectively differentiate between intestinal fluid and pleural fluid.

Gastric fluid can be green with particles, off-white, or brown if old blood is present. Intestinal aspirate tends to look clear or straw-colored to a deep golden-yellow color. Also, intestinal aspirate may be greenish-brown if stained with bile. Respiratory or tracheobronchial fluid is usually off-white to tan and may be tinged with mucus. A small amount of blood-tinged fluid may be seen immediately after NG insertion.

The tube should be marked with an indelible marker at the nostril at the time it was placed. This marking should be assessed each time the tube is used to ensure the tube has not become displaced. Tube length should be checked and compared with this initial measurement, in conjunction with pH measurement and visual assessment of aspirate, at regular intervals. An increase in the length of the exposed tube may indicate dislodgement (Bankhead et al., 2009; Hinkle & Cheever, 2018; Metheny, 2016b).

Securing the tube prevents migration of the tube inward and outward. Skin barrier improves adhesion and protects skin. Constant pressure of the tube against the skin and mucous membranes may cause tissue injury.

FIGURE 5. Making a 2-in cut into a 4-in strip of tape.

(*continued*)

Skill 13-8 ▶ Inserting a Nasogastric Tube *(continued)*

ACTION	RATIONALE

b. Place unsplit end over the bridge of the patient's nose (Figure 6).

c. Wrap split ends under and around the NG tube (Figure 7). **Be careful not to pull the tube too tightly against the nose.**

FIGURE 6. Applying tape to patient's nose.

FIGURE 7. Wrapping split ends around NG tube.

14. Put on gloves. Clamp the tube and remove the syringe. Cap or attach the tube to suction (Figure 8) according to the medical orders. Remove gloves.

Gloves prevent contact with blood and body fluids and transfer of microorganisms. Suction provides for decompression of stomach and drainage of gastric contents.

15. Measure the length of the exposed tube. Reinforce marking on the tube at the nostril with indelible ink. Ask the patient to turn his/her head to the side opposite the nostril in which the tube is inserted. Secure the tube to the patient's gown by using rubber band or tape and safety pin. For additional support, tape the tube onto the patient's cheek using a piece of tape. **If a double-lumen tube (e.g., Salem sump) is used, secure the vent above stomach level.** Attach the vent at shoulder level (Figure 9).

The tube should be marked with an indelible marker at the nostril. This marking should be assessed each time the tube is used to ensure the tube has not become displaced. Tube length should be checked and compared with this initial measurement, in conjunction with pH measurement and visual assessment of aspirate, at regular intervals. An increase in the length of the exposed tube may indicate dislodgement (Bankhead et al., 2009; Hinkle & Cheever, 2018; Metheny, 2016b). Securing prevents tension and tugging on the tube. Turning the head ensures adequate slack in the tubing to prevent tension when the patient turns the head. Securing the double-lumen tube above stomach level prevents seepage of gastric contents and keeps the lumen clear for venting air.

FIGURE 8. NG tube attached to wall suction.

FIGURE 9. Patient with Salem sump tube (NG) secured. Note blue vent at patient's shoulder.

ACTION	**RATIONALE**
16. Put on gloves. Assist with or provide oral hygiene at 2- to 4-hour intervals. Lubricate the lips generously and clean nares and lubricate, as needed. Offer analgesic throat lozenges or anesthetic spray for throat irritation, if needed.	Gloves prevent contact with blood and body fluids and transfer of microorganisms. Oral hygiene keeps mouth clean and moist, promotes comfort, and reduces thirst.
17. Remove equipment and return patient to a position of comfort. Remove gloves. Raise side rail and lower bed.	Promotes patient comfort and safety. Removing gloves properly reduces the risk for infection transmission and contamination of other items.
18. Remove additional PPE, if used. Perform hand hygiene.	Proper removal of PPE reduces the risk for infection transmission and contamination of other items. Hand hygiene prevents transmission of microorganisms.

EVALUATION

The expected outcome has been met when patient exhibits an NG tube placed into the stomach without any complications. In addition, other outcomes are met when patient demonstrates weight gain, indicating improved nutrition; the patient remains free of any signs and symptoms of aspiration; the patient rates pain as decreased from prior to insertion; and the patient verbalizes an understanding of the reason for NG tube insertion.

DOCUMENTATION

Guidelines

Document the size and type of the NG tube that was inserted and the measurement from the tip of the nose to the end of the exposed tube. Also, document the results of the x-ray that was taken to confirm the tube position, if applicable. Record a description of the gastric contents, including the pH of the contents. Document the naris where the tube is placed and the patient's response to the procedure. Include assessment data related to the abdomen. Record the patient teaching that was discussed.

Sample Documentation

DocuCare Practice documenting NG tube insertion in *Lippincott DocuCare.*

> 10/4/20 0945 Abdomen slightly distended and taut; hypoactive bowel sounds. Patient reports transient nausea. 14-Fr Levin tube inserted via R naris, 20 cm of tube from naris to end of tube; gastric contents aspirated, pH 4, contents light green; patient tolerated without incident.
>
> —S. Essner, RN

UNEXPECTED SITUATIONS AND ASSOCIATED INTERVENTIONS

- *As a tube is passing through the pharynx, the patient begins to retch and gag:* This is common during placement of an NG tube. Ask the patient if he or she wants the nurse to stop the procedure, which will allow the patient to gain composure from the gagging episode. Continue to advance the tube when the patient relates that he or she is ready. Have the emesis basin nearby in case the patient begins to vomit.
- *The nurse is unable to pass the tube after trying a second time down the one nostril:* If the patient's condition permits, inspect the other nostril and attempt to pass the NG tube down this nostril. If unable to pass down this nostril, consult another health professional.
- *As the tube is passing through the pharynx, the patient begins to cough and shows signs of respiratory distress:* **Stop advancing the tube.** The tube is most likely entering the trachea. Pull the tube back into the nasal area. Support the patient as he or she regains normal breathing ability and composure. If the patient feels that he or she can tolerate another attempt, ask the patient to keep chin on chest and swallow as the tube is advanced to help prevent the tube from entering the trachea. Begin to advance the tube, watching for any signs of respiratory distress.
- *No gastric contents can be aspirated:* Reposition the patient and flush the tube with 30 mL of air in a large syringe. Slowly apply negative pressure to withdraw fluid.

(continued)

Skill 13-8 ▶ Inserting a Nasogastric Tube *(continued)*

SPECIAL CONSIDERATIONS

General Considerations

To promote patient safety when administering a tube feeding, be sure to do the following:

- Check tube placement before administering any fluids, medications, or feedings. Use multiple techniques: x-ray, external length marking/measurement, pH testing, and aspirate characteristics.
- Sterile water should be used for tube flushes in immunocompromised or critically ill patients (Allen, 2015; Bankhead et al., 2009).
- Some patients require a nasointestinal tube. To insert a nasointestinal tube:
  - Measure the tube from the tip of the nose to the earlobe and from the earlobe to the xiphoid process. Add 8 to 10 in for intestinal placement. Mark tubing at the desired point.
  - Place the patient on his/her right side. The nasointestinal tube is usually placed in the stomach and allowed to advance through peristalsis through the pyloric sphincter (may take up to 24 hours).
  - Administer medications to enhance GI motility, such as metoclopramide, if ordered.
  - Test the pH of aspirate when the tube has advanced to the marked point to confirm placement in the intestine. Confirm position by radiograph. Secure with tape once placement is confirmed.
  - Monitoring for carbon dioxide to determine NG tube position and/or dislodgement has been investigated (Gilbert & Burns, 2012; Irving, Lyman, Northington, Bartlett, & Kemper, 2014; Mordiffi, Goh, Phua, & Chan, 2016; Rahimi et al., 2015). This involves the use of a capnograph or a colorimetric end-tidal CO_2 detector to detect the presence of carbon dioxide, which would indicate tube positioning in the patient's airway instead of the stomach.

Infant and Child Considerations

- Infants are obligate nose breathers; insertion of the tube via the mouth may be appropriate (orogastric tube) (Perry et al., 2014).
- Age-specific equations are available to predict insertion distance and are the best method to determine insertion distance based on age and height for infants and children, 8 years, 4 months of age, or younger (Perry et al., 2014). Other methods to determine insertion distance include the nose or mouth to ear–mid-xiphoid–umbilicus span. The accuracy of these methods has been challenged and further investigation is needed (Freeman, Saxton, & Holberton, 2012; Irving et al., 2014).

Skill 13-9 ▶ Irrigating a Nasogastric Tube Connected to Suction

Nasogastric (NG) tubes are used to decompress or to drain unwanted fluid and air from the stomach, monitor bleeding in the gastrointestinal (GI) tract, remove undesirable substances (lavage), or to help treat an intestinal obstruction. Tubes for decompression typically are attached to suction or the tube may be clamped. Suction can be applied intermittently or continuously. When the underlying condition has been resolved and/or the NG tube is no longer indicated, the tube is removed (Refer to Skill 13-10). The tube must be kept free from obstruction or clogging and is usually irrigated every 4 to 8 hours.

To promote patient safety when instilling solutions into an NG tube, tube placement must be verified before administration of any fluids or medications. This ensures that the tip of the tube is situated in the stomach or intestine, preventing inadvertent administration of substances into the wrong place. A misplaced feeding tube in the lungs or pulmonary tissue places the patient at risk for aspiration. Radiographic examination, measurement of tube length and measurement of tube marking, measurement of aspirate pH, visual assessment of aspirate, and monitoring of carbon dioxide have been suggested to confirm feeding tube placement. With the exception of radiographic examination, the use of two or more of these techniques in conjunction with each other increases the likelihood of correct tube placement (Bankhead et al., 2009; Metheny, 2016b; Rahimi et al., 2015). An old technique of auscultation of air injected into a feeding tube has proved unreliable and may result in tragic consequences if used as an indicator of tube placement (Bankhead et al., 2009; Boeykens et al., 2014; Metheny, 2016b). Therefore, do not use to confirm feeding tube placement (Hodin & Bordeianou, 2015).

DELEGATION CONSIDERATIONS	The irrigation of an NG tube is not delegated to nursing assistive personnel (NAP) or to unlicensed assistive personnel (UAP). Depending on the state's nurse practice act and the organization's policies and procedures, irrigation of an NG tube may be delegated to licensed practical/vocational nurses (LPN/LVNs). The decision to delegate must be based on careful analysis of the patient's needs and circumstances, as well as the qualifications of the person to whom the task is being delegated. Refer to the Delegation Guidelines in Appendix A.

EQUIPMENT

- NG tube connected to continuous or intermittent suction
- Water, sterile water, or normal saline solution for irrigation (based on facility policy)
- Nonsterile gloves
- Additional PPE, as indicated
- Irrigation set (or a 60-mL catheter-tip syringe and cup for irrigating solution)
- Clamp
- Disposable waterproof pad or bath towel
- Emesis basin
- Tape measure, or other measuring device
- pH paper and measurement scale

ASSESSMENT	Assess abdomen by inspecting for presence of distention, auscultating for bowel sounds, and palpating the abdomen for firmness or tenderness. If the abdomen is distended, consider measuring the abdominal girth at the umbilicus. If the patient reports any tenderness or nausea, or exhibits any rigidity or firmness of the abdomen, confer with the primary care provider. If the NG tube is attached to suction, assess suction to ensure that it is running at the prescribed pressure. Also, inspect drainage from NG tube, including color, consistency, and amount.

NURSING DIAGNOSIS	Determine the related factors for the nursing diagnoses based on the patient's current status. Nursing diagnoses may vary depending on the reason for the NG tube insertion. Appropriate nursing diagnoses may include:

- Imbalanced nutrition: Less than body requirements
- Risk for injury
- Risk for deficient fluid volume

OUTCOME IDENTIFICATION AND PLANNING	The expected outcome to achieve when irrigating a patient's NG tube is that the tube will maintain patency with irrigation. In addition, the patient will not experience any trauma or injury.

IMPLEMENTATION

ACTION	**RATIONALE**
1. Gather equipment. Verify the medical order or facility policy and procedure regarding frequency of irrigation, solution type, and amount of irrigant. Check expiration dates on irrigating solution and irrigation set.	Assembling equipment provides for an organized approach to the task. Verification ensures the patient receives the correct intervention. Facility policy dictates safe interval for reuse of equipment.
2. Perform hand hygiene and put on PPE, if indicated.	Hand hygiene and PPE prevent the spread of microorganisms. PPE is required based on transmission precautions.
3. Identify the patient.	Identifying the patient ensures the right patient receives the intervention and helps prevent errors.
4. Explain the procedure to the patient and why this intervention is needed. Answer any questions, as needed. Perform key abdominal assessments as described above.	Explanation facilitates patient cooperation. Due to potential changes in a patient's condition, assessment is vital before initiating intervention.

(continued)

Skill 13-9 ▸ Irrigating a Nasogastric Tube Connected to Sudlion *(continued)*

ACTION	RATIONALE
5. Assemble equipment on overbed table or other surface within reach.	Organization facilitates performance of the task.
6. Pull the patient's bedside curtain. Raise bed to a comfortable working position, usually elbow height of the caregiver (VHACEOSH, 2016). Assist the patient to 30- to 45-degree position, unless this is contraindicated. Pour the irrigating solution into container.	Provides for privacy. Appropriate working height facilitates comfort and proper body mechanics for the nurse. This position minimizes risk for aspiration. Preparing the irrigation provides for an organized approach to the task.
7. Put on gloves. Place waterproof pad on the patient's chest, under connection of the NG tube and suction tubing. **Check placement of the NG tube.** (Refer to Skill 13-8.)	Gloves prevent contact with body fluids. Waterproof pad protects patient's clothing and bed linens from accidental leakage of gastric fluid. Checking placement before the instillation of fluid is necessary to prevent accidental instillation into the respiratory tract if the tube has become dislodged.
8. Draw up 30 mL of irrigation solution (or amount indicated in the order or policy) into the syringe (Figure 1).	This delivers measured amount of irrigant through the tube. Saline solution (isotonic) may be used to compensate for electrolytes lost through NG drainage.

FIGURE 1. Preparing syringe with 30 mL of irrigation solution.

9. Clamp the NG tube near connection site. Disconnect the tube from the suction apparatus (Figure 2) and lay on a disposable pad or towel, or hold both tubes upright in nondominant hand (Figure 3).	Clamping prevents leakage of gastric fluid.

FIGURE 2. Clamping nasogastric tube while disconnecting.

FIGURE 3. Holding both tubes upright to prevent leakage of gastric fluid.

ACTION	RATIONALE
10. Place tip of the syringe in the tube. **If Salem sump or double-lumen tube is used, make sure that the syringe tip is placed in the drainage port and not in blue air vent.** Hold the syringe upright and gently insert the irrigant (Figure 4) (or allow solution to flow in by gravity if facility policy or medical order indicates). **Do not force solution into the tube.**	Gentle insertion of saline solution (or gravity insertion) is less traumatic to gastric mucosa. The blue air vent acts to decrease pressure built up in the stomach when the Salem sump is attached to suction. It is not to be used for irrigation.

FIGURE 4. Gently instilling irrigation.

ACTION	RATIONALE
11. **If unable to irrigate the tube, reposition patient and attempt irrigation again. Inject 10 to 20 mL of air and aspirate again. If repeated attempts to irrigate the tube fail, consult with primary care provider or follow facility policy.**	Tube may be positioned against gastric mucosa, making it difficult to irrigate. Injection of air may reposition end of the tube.
12. After irrigant has been instilled, hold the end of the NG tube over irrigation tray or emesis basin. Observe for return flow of NG drainage into an available container. Alternately, you may reconnect the NG tube to suction and observe the return drainage as it drains into the suction container.	Return flow may be collected in an irrigating tray or other available container and measured. This amount will need to be subtracted from the irrigant to record the true NG drainage. A second method involves subtracting the total irrigant from the shift from the total NG drainage emptied over the entire shift, to find the true NG drainage. Check facility policy for guidelines. Observation determines tube patency and correct operation of suction apparatus.
13. If not already done, reconnect drainage port to suction, if ordered.	Allows for continued removal of gastric contents, as ordered.
14. Inject air into blue air vent after irrigation is complete. Position the blue air vent above the patient's stomach.	Following irrigation, the blue air vent is injected with air to keep it clear. Positioning the blue air vent above the stomach prevents the stomach contents from leaking from the NG tube.
15. Remove gloves. Lower the bed and raise side rails, as necessary. Assist the patient to a position of comfort. Perform hand hygiene.	Lowering bed and assisting the patient to a comfortable position promote safety and comfort.
16. Put on gloves. Measure returned solution, if collected outside of suction apparatus. Rinse equipment if it will be reused. Label with the date, patient's name, room number, and purpose (for NG tube/irrigation).	Gloves prevent contact with blood and body fluids. Irrigant placed in the tube is considered intake; solution returned is recorded as output. Record on the intake and output record. Rinsing promotes cleanliness, infection control, and prepares equipment for next irrigation.
17. Remove gloves and additional PPE, if used. Perform hand hygiene.	Proper removal of PPE reduces the risk for infection transmission and contamination of other items. Hand hygiene prevents transmission of microorganisms.

EVALUATION   The expected outcome has been met when the patient demonstrates a patent and functioning NG tube. In addition, the patient reports no distress with the irrigation. The patient remains free of any signs and symptoms of injury or trauma.

(continued)

Skill 13-9 ▶ Irrigating a Nasogastric Tube Connected to Suction *(continued)*

DOCUMENTATION

Guidelines

Document assessment of the patient's abdomen. Record if the patient's NG tube is clamped or connected to suction, including the type of suction. Document the color and consistency of the NG drainage. Record the solution type and amount used to irrigate the NG tube, as well as ease of irrigation or any difficulty related to the procedure. Record the amount of returned irrigant, if collected outside of the suction apparatus. Alternately, record irrigant amount so it can be subtracted from total NG drainage amount at the end of the shift. Record the patient's response to the procedure and any pertinent teaching points that were reviewed, such as instructions for the patient to contact the nurse for any feelings of nausea, bloating, or abdominal pain.

Sample Documentation

> <u>10/15/20</u> 1100 Abdomen slightly distended but soft; absent bowel sounds, denies nausea. NG tube placement confirmed; gastric contents clear with brown flecks, pH 4; exposed NG tube 20 cm, consistent with documented length. NG tube irrigated with 30 mL of normal saline. NG tube reconnected to low intermittent suction. Clear drainage with brown flecks noted from tube. Patient tolerated irrigation without incident.
>
> —S. Essner, RN

UNEXPECTED SITUATIONS AND ASSOCIATED INTERVENTIONS

- *Flush solution is meeting a lot of force when plunger is pushed:* Inject 20 to 30 mL of free air through the NG tube into the stomach in an attempt to reposition the tube and enable flushing of the tube.
- *The tube is connected to suction as ordered, but nothing is draining from the tube:* First, check the suction canister to ensure that the suction is working appropriately. Disconnect the NG tube from suction and place your gloved thumb over the end of the suction tubing. If there is suction present, the problem lies in the tube itself. Next, attempt to flush the tube to ensure its patency.
- *After flushing the tube, the tube is not reconnected to suction as ordered:* Reconnect the tube to suction as soon as error is noticed. Assess the abdomen for distention and ask the patient if he or she is experiencing any nausea or any abdominal discomfort. Complete any paperwork per institutional policy, such as a variance report.

SPECIAL CONSIDERATIONS

- A one-way, anti-reflux valve may be used in the airflow lumen to prevent reflux of gastric contents through the airflow lumen (Figure 5). When pressure from gastric contents enters the airflow tubing, the valve closes to prevent secretions from exiting the tube. This valve is removed before flushing the lumen with air, and then replaced.
- Monitoring for carbon dioxide to determine the NG tube position and/or dislodgement has been investigated (Gilbert & Burns, 2012; Irving et al., 2014; Mordiffi et al., 2016; Rahimi et al., 2015). This involves the use of a capnograph or a colorimetric end-tidal CO_2 detector to detect the presence of carbon dioxide, which would indicate tube positioning in the patient's airway instead of the stomach.

FIGURE 5. One-way antireflux valve for Salem sump tube.

Skill 13-10 ▶ Removing a Nasogastric Tube

When the nasogastric (NG) tube is no longer necessary for treatment, the primary care provider will order the tube to be removed. The NG tube is removed as carefully as it was inserted, to provide as much comfort as possible for the patient and to prevent complications. When the tube is removed, the patient must hold his/her breath to prevent aspiration of any secretions or fluid left in the tube as it is removed.

DELEGATION CONSIDERATIONS	The removal of an NG tube is not delegated to nursing assistive personnel (NAP) or to unlicensed assistive personnel (UAP). Depending on the state's nurse practice act and the organization's policies and procedures, removal of an NG tube may be delegated to licensed practical/vocational nurses (LPN/LVNs). The decision to delegate must be based on careful analysis of the patient's needs and circumstances, as well as the qualifications of the person to whom the task is being delegated. Refer to the Delegation Guidelines in Appendix A.
EQUIPMENT	• Tissues • 50-mL syringe • Nonsterile gloves • Additional PPE, as indicated • Stethoscope • Disposable plastic bag • Bath towel or disposable pad • Normal saline solution for irrigation (optional) • Emesis basin
ASSESSMENT	Perform an abdominal assessment by inspecting for presence of distention, auscultating for bowel sounds, and palpating the abdomen for firmness or tenderness. If the abdomen is distended, consider measuring the abdominal girth at the umbilicus. If the patient reports any tenderness or nausea, exhibits any rigidity or firmness with distention, and if bowel sounds are absent, confer with the health care provider before discontinuing the NG tube. Assess any output from the NG tube, noting amount, color, and consistency.
NURSING DIAGNOSIS	Determine the related factors for the nursing diagnoses based on the patient's current status. Appropriate nursing diagnoses may include: • Readiness for enhanced nutrition • Risk for aspiration
OUTCOME IDENTIFICATION AND PLANNING	The expected outcome to achieve when removing an NG tube is that the tube is removed with minimal discomfort to the patient; the patient does not aspirate; and the patient maintains an adequate nutritional intake. In addition, the abdomen remains free from distention and tenderness.

IMPLEMENTATION

ACTION	RATIONALE
1. Check medical record for the order for removal of the NG tube.	This ensures correct implementation of primary care provider's order.
2. Perform hand hygiene and put on PPE, if indicated.	Hand hygiene and PPE prevent the spread of microorganisms. PPE is required based on transmission precautions.
3. Identify the patient.	Identifying the patient ensures the right patient receives the intervention and helps prevent errors.
4. Explain the procedure to the patient and why this intervention is warranted. Describe that it will entail a quick few moments of discomfort. Perform key abdominal assessments as described above.	Patient cooperation is facilitated when explanations are provided. Due to changes in a patient's condition, assessment is vital before initiating intervention.

(continued)

Skill 13-10 ▶ Removing a Nasogastric Tube *(continued)*

ACTION	RATIONALE
5. Pull the patient's bedside curtain. Raise the bed to a comfortable working position; usually elbow height of the caregiver (VHACEOSH, 2016). Assist the patient to a 30- to 45-degree position. Place a towel or disposable pad across the patient's chest (Figure 1). Give tissues and emesis basin to the patient.	Provides for privacy. Appropriate working height facilitates comfort and proper body mechanics for the nurse. Towel or pad protects the patient from contact with gastric secretions. Emesis basin is helpful if the patient vomits or gags. Tissues are necessary if the patient wants to blow his/her nose when the tube is removed.
6. Put on gloves. Discontinue suction and separate the tube from suction. Detach the tube from the patient's gown and carefully remove adhesive tape from the patient's nose.	Gloves prevent contact with blood and body fluids. Disconnecting the tube from suction and the patient allows for its unrestricted removal.
7. Check placement (as outlined in Skill 13-8) and flush with 10 mL of water or normal saline solution (optional) or clear with 30 to 50 mL of air (Figure 2).	Air or saline solution clears the tube of secretions, feeding, or debris.

FIGURE 1. Placing towel or disposable pad across patient's chest.

FIGURE 2. Flushing NG tube with 10-mL water.

8. Clamp the tube with fingers by doubling the tube on itself (Figure 3). Instruct the patient to take a deep breath and hold it. Quickly and carefully remove the tube while the patient holds breath. Coil the tube in the disposable pad as you remove it from the patient.	Clamping prevents drainage of gastric contents into the pharynx and esophagus. The patient holds breath to prevent accidental aspiration of gastric secretions in the tube. Careful removal minimizes trauma and discomfort for the patient. Containing the tube in a towel while removing it prevents leakage onto the patient.

FIGURE 3. Doubling tube on itself.

9. Dispose of the tube per facility policy. Remove gloves. Perform hand hygiene.	This prevents contamination with microorganisms.

ACTION	**RATIONALE**
10. Offer mouth care to the patient and facial tissue to blow nose. Lower the bed and assist the patient to a position of comfort, as needed.	These interventions promote patient comfort.
11. Remove equipment and raise side rail and lower bed.	Promotes patient comfort and safety.
12. Put on gloves and measure the amount of NG drainage in the collection device. Record the measurement on the output flow record, subtracting irrigant fluids if necessary (Figure 4). Add solidifying agent to NG drainage and dispose of drainage according to facility policy.	Irrigation fluids are considered intake. To obtain the true NG drainage, irrigant fluid amounts are subtracted from the total NG drainage. NG drainage is recorded as part of the output of fluids from the patient. Solidifying agents added to liquid NG drainage facilitate safe biohazard disposal.

FIGURE 4. Measuring the amount of nasogastric drainage in collection device.

| 13. Remove additional PPE, if used. Perform hand hygiene. | Proper removal of PPE reduces the risk for infection transmission and contamination of other items. Hand hygiene prevents transmission of microorganisms. |

EVALUATION

The expected outcome has been met when the patient experiences minimal discomfort and pain on NG tube removal and does not aspirate. In addition, the patient's abdomen remains free from distention and tenderness, and the patient verbalizes measures to maintain an adequate nutritional intake.

DOCUMENTATION

Guidelines

Document assessment of the abdomen. If an abdominal girth reading was obtained, record this measurement. Document the removal of the NG tube from the naris where it had been placed. Note if there is any irritation to the skin of the naris. Record the amount of NG drainage in the suction container on the patient's intake-and-output record as well as the color of the drainage. Record any pertinent teaching, such as instruction to the patient to notify the nurse if he or she experiences any nausea, abdominal pain, or bloating.

Sample Documentation

> 10/29/20 1320 NG tube removed from L naris without incident. 600 mL of dark brown liquid emptied from NG tube. Patient's abdomen is 66 cm; abdomen is soft, nontender with hypoactive bowel sounds in all four quadrants.
>
> —S. Essner, RN

UNEXPECTED SITUATIONS AND ASSOCIATED INTERVENTIONS

- *Within 2 hours after NG tube removal, the patient's abdomen is showing signs of distention:* Notify primary care provider. Anticipate order to reinsert the NG tube.
- *Epistaxis occurs with removal of the NG tube:* Occlude both nares until bleeding has subsided. Ensure that patient is in upright position. Document epistaxis in patient's medical record.

Enhance Your Understanding

Focusing on Patient Care: Developing Clinical Reasoning

Consider the case scenarios at the beginning of the chapter as you answer the following questions to enhance your understanding and apply what you have learned.

QUESTIONS

1. While you are digitally removing feces from Hugh Levens, he suddenly complains of feeling lightheaded. You note that he is now diaphoretic. What should you do?

2. Isaac Greenberg is afraid that the enema is going to hurt. His mother worries about being able to prepare properly for his colonoscopy. What information should you include when teaching the steps to administer a small-volume enema? What interventions should you include to promote Isaac's comfort and safety?

3. Maria Blakely has noted that an area of peristomal skin is becoming erythematous and excoriated. She asks you whether she should cut her ostomy bag bigger so that the adhesive does not irritate this skin. How should you reply?

You can find suggested answers after the Bibliography at the end of this chapter.

Integrated Case Study Connection

The case studies in the back of the book focus on integrating concepts. Refer to the following case studies to enhance your understanding of the concepts and skills in this chapter.

- Intermediate Case Studies: Victoria Holly, page 1115.

Taylor Suite Resources

Explore these additional resources to enhance learning for this chapter:

- NCLEX-Style Questions and other resources on thePoint®, http://thePoint.lww.com/Lynn5e
- *Skill Checklists for Taylor's Clinical Nursing Skills,* 5e
- *Taylor's Video Guide to Clinical Nursing Skills:* Bowel Elimination
- *Fundamentals of Nursing:* Chapter 38, Bowel Elimination
- *Lippincott DocuCare* Fundamentals cases

Bibliography

Allen, S. M. (2015). As a flushing agent for enteral nutrition, does sterile water compared to tap water affect the associated risk of infection in critically ill patients? *The Alabama Nurse, 42*(1), 5–6.

A-Rahim, Y. I., & Falchuk, M. (2018). UpToDate. *Bowel preparation before colonoscopy in adults.* Wolters Kluwer. Retrieved https://www.uptodate.com/contents/bowel-preparation-before-colonoscopy-in-adults

Avent, Y. (2012). Understanding fecal diversions. *Nursing Made Incredibly Easy!, 10*(5), 11–16.

Bankhead, R., Boullata, J., Brantley, S., et al.; The American Society for Parenteral and Enteral Nutrition (A.S.P.E.N.) Board of Directors. (2009). Enteral nutrition practice recommendations. *Journal of Parenteral and Enteral Nutrition, 33*(2), 122–167.

Bardsley, A. (2015). Approaches to managing chronic constipation in older people within the community setting. *British Journal of Community Nursing, 20*(9), 444–450.

Bauer, C. (2016). Colostomy irrigation to maintain continence: An old method revived. *Nursing, 46*(8), 59–62.

Beeckman, S., Campbell, J., Campbell, K., et al. (2015). *Proceedings from the Global IAD Expert Panel. Incontinence-associated dermatitis: Moving prevention forward. Wounds International.* Retrieved http://www.woundsinternational.com/media/other-resources/_/1154/files/iad_web.pdf

Boeykens, K., Steeman, E., & Dyusburgh, I. (2014). Reliability of pH measurement and the auscultatory method to confirm the position of a nasogastric tube. *International Journal of Nursing Studies, 51*(11), 1427–1433.

Borowitz, S. (2016). *Pediatric constipation. Medscape.* Retrieved http://emedicine.medscape.com/article/928185-overview#a5

Brugnolli, A., Ambrosi, E., Canzan, F., Saiani, L.; Naso-gastric Tube Group. (2014). Securing of naso-gastric tubes in adult patients: A review. *International Journal of Nursing Studies, 51*(6), 943–950.

Burch, J. (2014). Care of patients with peristomal skin complications. *Nursing Standard, 28*(37), 51–57.

Chandler, P. (2015). Preventing and treating peristomal skin conditions in stoma patients. *British Journal of Community Nursing, 20*(8), 386–388.

Chau, J. P., Lo, S. H., Thompson, D. R., Fernandez, R., & Griffiths, R. (2011). Use of end-tidal carbon dioxide detection to determine correct placement of nasogastric tube: A meta-analysis. *International Journal of Nursing Studies, 48*(4), 513–521.

Claessens, I., Probert, R., Tielemans, C., et al. (2015). The Ostomy Life Study: The everyday challenges faced by people living with a stoma in a snapshot. *Gastrointestinal Nursing, 13*(5), 18–25.

Clow, T., Disley, H., Greening, L., & Harker, G. (2015). Professional guidance for teaching colostomy irrigation. *World Council of Enterostomal Therapists Journal, 35*(2), 15–19.

Cobb, M. D., Grant, M., Tallman, N. J., et al. (2015). Colostomy irrigation. Current knowledge and practice of WOC nurses. *Journal of Wound, Ostomy and Continence Nursing, 42*(1), 65–70.

Cohen, B. J., & Hull, K. L. (2015). *Memmler's structure and function of the human body* (11th ed.). Philadelphia, PA: Wolters Kluwer.

Cronin, E. (2016). Silicone-based stoma accessories in clinical practice. *British Journal of Nursing (Mark Allen Publishing), 25*(5), S28–S34.

Curtis, K. (2013). Caring for adult patients who require nasogastric feeding tubes. *Nursing Standard, 27*(38), 47–56.

Doenges, M. E., Moorhouse, M. F., & Murr, A. C. (2016). *Nursing diagnoses manual. Planning, individualizing, and documenting client care* (5th ed.). Philadelphia, PA: F.A. Davis Company.

Dudek, S. (2017). *Nutrition essentials for nursing practice* (8th ed.). Philadelphia, PA: Wolters Kluwer.

Eliopoulos, C. (2018). *Gerontological nursing* (9th ed.). Philadelphia, PA: Wolters Kluwer.

Freeman, D., Saxton, V., & Holberton, J. (2012). Estimation of gastric tube insertion length in newborns. *Advances in Neonatal Care, 12*(3), 179–182.

Gilbert, R. T., & Burns, S. M. (2012). Increasing the safety of blind gastric tube placement in pediatric patients: The design and testing of a procedure using a carbon dioxide detection device. *Journal of Pediatric Nursing, 27*(5), 528–532.

Gray, M., Colwell, J. C., Doughty, D., et al. (2013). Peristomal moisture-associated skin damage in adults with fecal ostomies. *Journal of Wound, Ostomy and Continence Nursing, 40*(4), 389–399.

Grossman, S., & Porth, C. M. (2014). *Porth's pathophysiology: Concepts of altered health states* (9th ed.). Philadelphia, PA: Wolters Kluwer Health.

Gump, K., & Schmelzer, M. (2016). Gaining control over fecal incontinence. *MEDSURG Nursing, 25*(2), 97–102.

Hester, S. (Ed.). (2015). PL Detail-Document #310604, Treatment of constipation in adults. *Pharmacist's Letter, 22*(6), 1–4. Retrieved http://pharmacistsletter.therapeuticresearch.com/pl/ArticleDD.aspx?nidchk=1&cs=&s=PL&pt=2&fpt=31&dd=290410&pb=PL&cat=3980&segment=5478

Hinkle, J. L., & Cheever, K. H. (2018). *Brunner & Suddarth's textbook of medical-surgical nursing* (14th ed.). Philadelphia, PA: Wolters Kluwer.

Hodin, R. A., & Bordeianou, L. (2015). *Nasogastric and nasoenteric tubes*. UpToDate Wolters Kluwer. Retrieved http://www.uptodate.com/contents/nasogastric-and-nasoenteric-tubes?source = search_result&search = salem+sump&selectedTitle = 1~1

Hoffmire Heideman, B. (2015). Helping patients overcome ostomy challenges. *Wound Care Advisor, 4*(5), 12–16.

Holland, A., Smith, F., Penny, K. (2013). Carbon dioxide detection for testing nasogastric tube placement in adults (Protocol). *Cochrane Database of Systematic Reviews,* 10. Art. No.: CD010773. doi: 10.1002/14651858.CD010773.

Hollister. (n.d.). *Fecal collector.* Retrieved http://www.hollister.com/en/products/critical-care-products/bowel-care/fecal-collectors/fecal-collector

Hollister. (2005). *Drainable fecal incontinence collector. Protocol.* Libertyville, IL: Author. Retrieved http://www.hollister.com/~/media/files/pdfs%E2%80%93for%E2%80%93download/critical%E2%80%93care/fecal_collector_care_tips_1907278-405.pdf

Holroyd, S. (2015). How can community nurses manage chronic constipation? *Journal of Community Nursing, 29*(5), 74–82.

Irving, S. Y., Lyman, B., Northington, L., Bartlett, J. A., & Kemper, C. (2014). Nasogastric tube placement and verification in children: Review of the current literature. *Critical Care Nurse, 34*(3), 67–78.

Jacobson, R. M., Peery, J., Thompson, W. O., Kanapka, J. A., & Caswell, M. (2010). Serum electrolyte shifts following administration of sodium phosphates enema. *Gastroenterology Nursing, 33*(3), 191–201.

Jarvis, C. (2016). *Physical examination and health assessment* (7th ed.). St. Louis, MO: Elsevier.

Jensen, S. (2015). *Nursing health assessment: A best practice approach* (2nd ed.). Philadelphia, PA: Wolters Kluwer Health.

Jones, T., Springfield, T., Brudwich, M., & Ladd, A. (2011). Fecal ostomies. Practical management for the home health clinician. *Home Healthcare Nurse, 29*(5), 306–317.

Karch, A. M. (2017). *Focus on nursing pharmacology* (7th ed.). Philadelphia, PA: Wolters Kluwer.

Kent, D. J., Arnold Long, M ., Bauer, C. (2015). Does colostomy irrigation affect functional outcomes and quality of life in persons with a colostomy? *Journal of Wound, Ostomy and Continence Nursing, 42*(2), 155–161.

Kyle, T., & Carman, S. (2017). *Essentials of pediatric nursing* (3rd ed.). Philadelphia, PA: Wolters Kluwer.

Lafon, C., & Lawson, L. (2012). Postoperative ileus in GI surgical patients: Pathogenesis and interventions. *Gastrointestinal Nursing, 10*(2), 45–49.

Landmann, R. G. (2015). UpToDate. *Routine care of patients with an ileostomy or colostomy and management of ostomy complications.* Wolters Kluwer. Retrieved http://www.uptodate.com/contents/routine-care-of-patients-with-an-ileostomy-or-colostomy-and-management-of-ostomy-complications?source=search_result&search=colostomy+care&selectedTitle=1~150

Massey, R. L. (2012). Return of bowel sounds indicating an end of postoperative ileus: Is it time to cease this long-standing nursing tradition? *MEDSURG Nursing, 21*(3), 146–150.

Mayo Foundation for Medical Education and Research (MFMER). (2013a). *Constipation. Symptoms.* Retrieved http://www.mayoclinic.org/diseases-conditions/constipation/basics/symptoms/con-20032773

Mayo Foundation for Medical Education and Research (MFMER). (2013b). *Constipation. Treatment.* Retrieved http://www.mayoclinic.org/diseases-conditions/constipation/basics/treatment/con-20032773

Metheny, N. (2016a). AACN Practice Alert. Prevention of aspiration in adults. *Critical Care Nurse, 36*(1), e20–e24.

Metheny, N. (2016b). AACN Practice Alert. Initial and ongoing verification of feeding tube placement in adults. *Critical Care Nurse, 36*(2), e8–e13.

Mordiffi, S. Z., Goh, M. L., Phua, J., & Chan, Y. H. (2016). Confirming nasogastric tube placement: Is the colorimeter as sensitive and specific as x-ray? A diagnostic accuracy study. *International Journal of Nursing Studies, 61,* 248–257.

NANDA International, Inc. (2014). *Nursing diagnoses: Definitions & classification 2018–2020* © 2017 NANDA International, ISBN 978-1-62623-929-6. Used by arrangement with the Thieme Group, Stuttgart/New York.

National Cancer Institute (NCI). (2016). *Gastrointestinal complications (PDQ®)—health professional version. Constipation: Contraindications.* Retrieved http://www.cancer.gov/about-cancer/treatment/side-effects/constipation/gi-complications-hp-pdq#link/_332_toc

National Institute of Diabetes and Digestive and Kidney Diseases (NIDDK). (2014). *Ostomy surgery of the bowel.* Retrieved https://www.niddk.nih.gov/health-information/health-topics/digestive-diseases/ostomy-surgery-bowel/Pages/ez.aspx

Ness, W., Hibberts, F., & Miles, S. (2012). *Management of lower bowel dysfunction, including DRE and DRF. RCN guidance for nurses.* London, UK: Royal College of Nursing.

Niv, G., Grinberg, T., Dickman, R., Wasserberg, N., & Niv, Y. (2013). Perforation and mortality after cleansing enema for acute constipation are not rare but preventable. *International Journal of General Medicine, 26*(6), 323–328.

Obokhare, I. (2012). Fecal impaction: A cause for concern? *Clinics in Colon and Rectal Surgery, 25*(1), 53–57.

Peart, J., & Richardson, A. (2015). Developing a critical care bowel management assessment tool to manage faecal incontinence. *Nursing in Critical Care, 20*(1), 34–40.

Peate, I. (2014). How to administer an enema. *Nursing Standard, 30*(14), 30–33.

Perry, S. E., Hockenberry, M. J., Lowdermilk, D. L., & Wilson, D. (2014). *Maternal child nursing care* (5th ed.). St. Louis, MO: Elsevier.

Powers, J., & Zimmaro Bliss, D. (2012). Product options for faecal incontinence management in acute care. *World Council of Enterostomal Therapists Journal, 32*(1), 20–23.

Rahimi, M., Farhadi, K., Ashtarian, H., & Changaei, F. (2015). Confirming nasogastric tube position: Methods and restrictions. A narrative review. *Journal of Nursing and Midwifery Sciences, 2*(1), 55–62.

Readding, L. (2016). Practical guidance for nurses caring for stoma patients with long-term conditions. *British Journal of Community Nursing, 21*(2), 90–92, 94, 96–98.

Rey, E., Barcelo, M., Jiménez-Cebrián, M. J., Alvarez-Sanchez, A., Diaz-Rubio, M., & Rocha, A. L. (2014). A nation-wide study of prevalence and risk factors for fecal impaction in nursing homes. *PLoS One, 9*(8), e105281.

Riesenberg, L. A., Berg, K., Berg, D., et al. (2013). The development of a validated checklist for nasogastric tube insertion: Preliminary results. *American Journal of Medical Quality, 28*(5), 429–433.

Rudoni, C. (2011). Peristomal skin irritation and the use of a silicone-based barrier film. *British Journal of Nursing (Mark Allen Publishing), 20*(16), S12–S18.

Schreiber, M. L. (2016). Ostomies: Nursing care and management. *MEDSURG Nursing, 25*(2), 127–130.

Simons, S. R., & Abdallah, L. M. (2012). Bedside assessment of enteral tube placement: Aligning practice with evidence. *American Journal of Nursing, 112*(2), 40–46.

Solomons, J., & Woodward, S. (2013). Digital removal of faeces in the bowel management of patients with spinal cord injury: A review. *British Journal of Neuroscience Nursing, 9*(5), 216–222.

Southgate, G., & Bradbury, S. (2016). Management of incontinence-associated dermatitis with a skin barrier protectant. *British Journal of Nursing (Mark Allen Publishing), 25*(9), S20–S29.

Stephen-Haynes, J. (2008). Skin integrity and silicone: Appeel 'no-sting' medical adhesive remover. *British Journal of Nursing (Mark Allen Publishing), 17*(12), 792–795.

Taylor, C., Lynn, P., & Bartlett, J. (2019). *Fundamentals of nursing: The art and science of person-centered care* (9th ed.). Philadelphia, PA: Wolters Kluwer.

U.S. National Library of Medicine, National Institutes of Health. (2014). Bowel retraining. *MedlinePlus.* Retrieved https://medlineplus.gov/ency/article/003971.htm

Van Leeuwen, A. M., & Bladh, M. L. (2015). *Davis's comprehensive handbook of laboratory & diagnostic tests with nursing implications* (5th ed.). Philadelphia, PA: F.A. Davis Company.

VHA Center for Engineering & Occupational Safety and Health (CEOSH). (2016). *Safe patient handling and mobility guidebook.* St. Louis, MO: Author. Retrieved http://www.tampavaref.org/safe-patient-handling.htm

Voegeli, D. (2016). Incontinence-associated dermatitis: New insights into an old problem. *British Journal of Nursing (Mark Allen Publishing), 25*(5), 256, 258, 260–262.

Watson, A. J., Nicol, L., Donaldson, S., Fraser, C., & Silversides, A. (2013). Complications of stomas: Their aetiology and management. *British Journal of Community Nursing, 18*(3), 111–116.

White, M. (2014). Using silicone technology to maintain healthy skin in stoma care. *British Journal of Nursing (Mark Allen Publishing), 23*(22), 16–21.

Whiteley, I., & Sinclair, G. (2014). Faecal management systems for disabling incontinence or wounds. *British Journal of Nursing (Mark Allen Publishing), 23*(16), 881–885.

SUGGESTED ANSWERS FOR FOCUSING ON PATIENT CARE: DEVELOPING CLINICAL REASONING

1. This procedure is very uncomfortable and may cause great discomfort to the patient as well as irritation of the rectal mucosa and bleeding. Digital removal of a fecal mass can stimulate the vagus nerve, resulting in a slowed heart rate, as well as nausea, diaphoresis, lightheadedness, and/or dizziness. If the patient experiences any of these symptoms, stop the procedure immediately; monitor the patient's heart rate, blood pressure, and symptoms. Maintain the patient in a supine position, provide reassurance, and notify the primary care provider.

2. Hypertonic solution preparations are available commercially and are administered in smaller volumes (adult, 70 to 130 mL). These solutions draw water into the colon, which stimulates the defecation reflex. This enema is packaged in a flexible bottle containing hypertonic solution with an attached prelubricated firm tip about 2 to 3 in (5 to 7.5 cm) long, and is easy to use. Explain the purpose and what they can expect. Use developmentally appropriate terms for a 9 year old. Isaac and his mother should plan to administer the enema in or near the bathroom, so Isaac is not worried about being incontinent or getting to the toilet in time. Reinforce that the procedure will not hurt. Isaac will feel some pressure from the tube in his rectum, and in his belly. Explain that a child or adolescent should be positioned on the left side

with the right leg flexed toward chest (Kyle & Carman, 2017). Explain to Isaac's mother that she should generously lubricate the end of the rectal tube 2 to 3 in before administering. She should direct it at an angle pointing toward the umbilicus, not the bladder. She should ask Isaac to take several deep breaths when inserting it to help relax the anal sphincter. She should encourage Isaac to hold the solution until the urge to defecate is strong. Finally, the mother should hold the child's buttocks together, if needed, to encourage retention of the enema.

3. Explain that she should cut the opening only 1/8 in larger than the stoma size. Creating a larger opening will expose the already irritated peristomal skin to further irritation from stool. Advise Maria to contact her ostomy nurse specialist or her physician to rule out a superimposed fungal infection, which would require treatment with an antifungal medication. Reinforce basic teaching with Maria. Ensure she understands the routine care of her ostomy. Explain that she should empty the ostomy appliance frequently. This prevents excess pressure on the adhesive that could pull the adhesive plate off her skin and allow fecal material to come in contact with peristomal skin. Instruct Maria to keep the skin around the stoma site (peristomal area) clean and dry. If care is not taken to protect the skin around the stoma, irritation or infection may occur. A leaking appliance frequently causes skin erosion. Candida or yeast infections can also occur around the stoma if the area is not kept dry. If an appliance is leaking from underneath the skin barrier, ring, or wafer, the bag will have to be removed, the skin cleaned, and a new bag applied. The act of removing an appliance from the skin can result in skin stripping, removal of the outer, loosely bound, epidermal cell layers. This can be uncomfortable for the patient or, at worst, very painful. The cumulative effects of skin stripping over time can result in peristomal skin breakdown. The use of a silicone-based adhesive remover allows for the easy, rapid, and painless removal of a stoma pouch without the associated problems of skin stripping (Chandler, 2015; Rudoni, 2011; Stephen-Haynes, 2008). Instruct Maria to use adhesive remover when removing her appliance, to prevent further skin damage. Explain that she should thoroughly cleanse the peristomal skin with a gentle cleanser, and then thoroughly dry it. The use of a skin barrier is important, as well as ensuring good adhesion when the appliance is replaced.

Oxygenation

Focusing on Patient Care

This chapter will help you develop some of the skills related to oxygenation necessary to care for the following patients:

Scott Mingus, age 35, who has a chest drain after thoracic surgery.

Saranam Srivastava, age 58, with a history of smoking, who is scheduled for a bowel resection and needs preoperative teaching regarding an incentive spirometer.

Paula Cunningham, age 72, who is intubated and requires suctioning through her endotracheal tube.

Refer to Focusing on Patient Care: Developing Clinical Reasoning at the end of the chapter to apply what you learn.

Learning Objectives

After completing the chapter, you will be able to accomplish the following:

1. Use a pulse oximeter.
2. Teach a patient to use an incentive spirometer.
3. Administer oxygen by nasal cannula.
4. Administer oxygen by mask.
5. Use an oxygen hood.
6. Suction the oropharynx and nasopharynx.
7. Insert an oropharyngeal airway.
8. Insert a nasopharyngeal airway.
9. Suction an endotracheal tube using an open system.
10. Suction an endotracheal tube using a closed system.
11. Secure an endotracheal tube.
12. Suction a tracheostomy.
13. Provide care of a tracheostomy tube.
14. Provide care of a chest drainage system.
15. Assist with chest tube removal.
16. Use a manual resuscitation bag and mask to deliver oxygen.

Key Terms

alveoli: small air sacs at the end of the terminal bronchioles that are the site of gas exchange

atelectasis: incomplete expansion or collapse of a part of the lungs

cardiopulmonary system: the respiratory and cardiovascular systems

cilia: microscopic, hair-like projections that propel mucus toward the upper airway so it can be expectorated

dyspnea: difficult or labored breathing

endotracheal tube: polyvinylchloride airway that is inserted through the nose or mouth into the trachea, using a laryngoscope

expiration: act of breathing out

extubation: removal of a tube (in this case, an endotracheal tube)

hemothorax: blood in the pleural space, potentially disrupting the negative pressure in the pleural space

hyperventilation: condition in which more than the normal amount of air is entering and leaving the lungs as a result of an increase in rate or depth of respiration or both

hypoventilation: decreased rate or depth of air movement into the lungs

hypoxia: inadequate amount of oxygen available to the cells

inspiration: act of breathing in

nasal cannula: disposable plastic device with two protruding prongs for insertion into the nostrils; used to administer oxygen

nasopharyngeal airway: a curved, soft rubber or plastic tube inserted into the back of the pharynx through the nose

oropharyngeal airway: a semicircular tube of plastic or rubber inserted into the back of the pharynx through the mouth

pneumothorax: air in the pleural space

pulse oximetry: noninvasive technique that measures the oxygen saturation (SpO_2) of arterial blood

respiration: gas exchange between the atmospheric air in the alveoli and the blood in the capillaries

spirometer: instrument used to measure lung capacity and volume; one type is used to encourage deep breathing (incentive spirometry)

subcutaneous emphysema: small pockets of air trapped in the subcutaneous tissue; usually found around chest tube insertion sites

tachypnea: rapid breathing

tracheostomy tube: curved tube inserted into an artificial opening made into the trachea (tracheostomy); comes in varied angles and multiple sizes

ventilation (breathing): the movement of air into and out of the lungs

Life depends on a constant supply of oxygen. This demand for oxygen is met by the function of the respiratory and cardiovascular systems, together known as the **cardiopulmonary system**. Gas exchange, the intake of oxygen and the release of carbon dioxide, is made possible by the respiratory system (Fig. 14-1). The cardiovascular system (Fig. 14-2) delivers oxygen to the cells. Oxygenation of body tissues depends on essentially three factors:

- Integrity of the airway system to transport air to and from the lungs
- A properly functioning alveolar system in the lungs to oxygenate venous blood and to remove carbon dioxide from the blood
- A properly functioning cardiovascular system and blood supply to carry nutrients and wastes to and from body cells.

The air passages must remain patent (open) for oxygen to enter the system. Any condition that interferes with normal functioning must be minimized or eliminated to prevent pulmonary distress, which could lead to death. This chapter covers the skills necessary for the nurse to promote oxygenation. While performing skills related to oxygenation, keep in mind factors that affect cardiopulmonary function, leading to impaired oxygenation, and how these factors might affect a particular patient (Fundamentals Review 14-1).

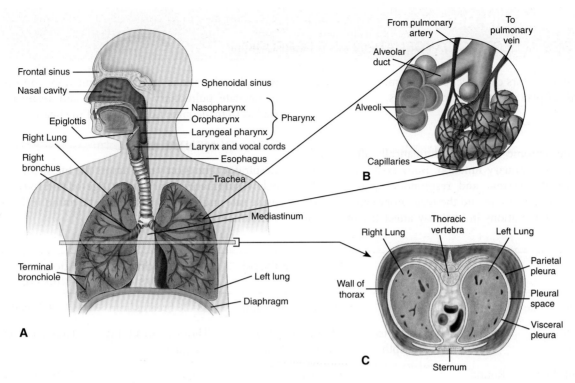

FIGURE 14-1. Organs of respiratory tract. **A.** Overview. **B.** Alveoli (air sacs) of lungs and blood capillaries. **C.** Transverse section through lungs.

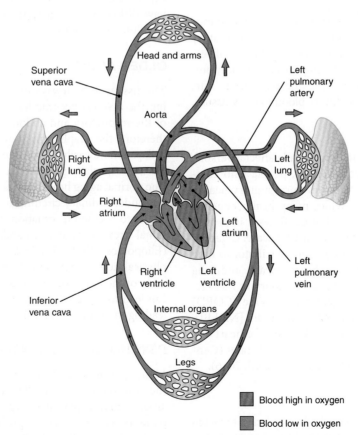

FIGURE 14-2. The right side of the heart pumps deoxygenated blood to the lungs, where oxygen is picked up and carbon dioxide released. The left side of the heart pumps oxygenated blood out to all other parts of the body. (Reprinted with permission from Taylor, J. J., & Cohen, B. J. [2013]. *Memmler's structure and function of the human body* [10th ed.]. Philadelphia, PA: Wolters Kluwer Health/Lippincott Williams & Wilkins.)

Fundamentals Review 14-1

FACTORS AFFECTING OXYGENATION AND PERFUSION

A variety of factors can affect cardiopulmonary functioning. This display reviews common factors.

LEVEL OF HEALTH

Acute and chronic illness can dramatically affect a person's cardiopulmonary function. Body systems (e.g., the cardiovascular system and respiratory system or the musculoskeletal system and the respiratory system) work together, so alterations in one may affect the other. For example, alterations in muscle function contribute to inadequate pulmonary **ventilation** and **respiration**, as well as to inadequate functioning of the heart.

DEVELOPMENTAL LEVEL

Respiratory function varies across the life span. The table below summarizes variations. Age-related variations in pulse rate and blood pressure can be found in Chapter 2, Fundamentals Review 2-1.

	Infant (Birth–1 year)	Early Childhood (1–5 years)	Late Childhood (6–12 years)	Adolescent and Adult (18+ years)
Respiratory rate	20–40 breaths/min	20–32 breaths/min	18–26 breaths/min	12–20 breaths/min
Respiratory pattern	Abdominal breathing, irregular in rate and depth	Abdominal breathing, irregular	Thoracic breathing, regular	Thoracic, regular
Shape of thorax	Round	Elliptical	Elliptical	Elliptical or barrel-shaped

MEDICATIONS

Many medications affect the function of the cardiopulmonary system. Many medications depress the respiratory system. The nurse should monitor rate and depth of respirations in patients who are taking certain medications, such as opioids. Other medications decrease heart rate, with the potential to alter the flow of blood to body tissues.

LIFESTYLE

Activity levels and habits can dramatically affect a person's cardiopulmonary status. For example, people who exercise can better respond to stressors to respiratory health. Regular physical activity provides many health benefits, including increased heart and lung fitness, improved muscle fitness, and reduced risk of heart disease. Cigarette smoking (active or passive) is a major contributor to lung disease and respiratory distress, heart disease, and lung cancer. Cigarette smoking is the most important risk factor for chronic obstructive pulmonary disease (COPD) (National Heart, Lung, and Blood Institute [NHLBI], 2013). Smoking is one of the key risk factors for heart disease, the leading cause of death in the United States (Centers for Disease Control and Prevention [CDC], 2016).

ENVIRONMENT

Research indicates that there is a high correlation between air pollution and occupational exposure to certain chemicals and lung disease. Additionally, people who have experienced an alteration in respiratory functioning often have difficulty continuing to perform self-care activities in a polluted environment.

OLDER ADULTS

The tissues and airways of the respiratory tract (including the **alveoli**) become less elastic with age. The power of the respiratory and abdominal muscles is reduced, and therefore the diaphragm moves less efficiently. Airways collapse more easily. These alterations increase the risk for disease, especially pneumonia and other chest infections. The normal aging heart can maintain adequate cardiac output under ordinary circumstances, but may have a limited ability to respond to situations that cause physical or emotional stress, when the demands on the heart are increased (Eliopoulos, 2014; Hinkle & Cheever, 2018). Decreased physical activity, physical deconditioning, decreased elasticity of the blood vessels, and stiffening of the heart valves can lead to a decrease in the overall function of the heart, leading to decreased oxygenation of body tissues.

PSYCHOLOGICAL HEALTH

Many psychological factors can have an impact on the respiratory system. People responding to stress or anxiety may experience **hyperventilation**. In addition, patients with respiratory problems often develop some anxiety as a result of the **hypoxia** caused by the respiratory problem.

Skill 14-1 ▶ Using a Pulse Oximeter

Pulse oximetry is a noninvasive technique that measures the arterial oxyhemoglobin saturation (SpO_2) of arterial blood. The reported result is a ratio, expressed as a percentage, between the actual oxygen content of the hemoglobin and the potential maximum oxygen-carrying capacity of the hemoglobin (Van Leeuwen & Bladh, 2015). A sensor, or probe, uses a beam of red and infrared light that travels through tissue and blood vessels. One part of the sensor emits the light and another part receives the light. The oximeter then calculates the amount of light that has been absorbed by arterial blood. Oxygen saturation is determined by the amount of each light absorbed; nonoxygenated hemoglobin absorbs more red light and oxygenated hemoglobin absorbs more infrared light.

Sensors are available for use on a finger, a toe, a foot (infants), an earlobe, forehead, and the bridge of the nose. It is important to use the appropriate sensor for the intended site; use of a sensor on a site other than what it is intended can result in inaccurate or unreliable readings (Johnson, Anderson, & Hill, 2012). Circulation to the sensor site must be adequate to ensure accurate readings. Pulse oximeters also display a measured pulse rate.

It is important to know the patient's hemoglobin level before evaluating oxygen saturation because the test measures only the percentage of oxygen carried by the available hemoglobin. Thus, even a patient with a low hemoglobin level could appear to have a normal SpO_2 because most of that hemoglobin is saturated. However, the patient may not have enough oxygen to meet body needs. Also, take into consideration the presence of pre-existing health conditions, such as COPD. Parameters for acceptable oxygen saturation readings may be different for these patients. For patients with chronic lung disease, a level of 88% to 92% may be considered within normal limits (Mitchell, 2015). Be aware of any medical orders regarding acceptable ranges and/or check with the patient's primary care provider. A range of 95% to 100% is considered normal SpO_2. Values ≤90% are abnormal, indicating that oxygenation to the tissues is inadequate. It is important to investigate these low values for potential hypoxia or technical error.

Pulse oximetry is useful for monitoring patients receiving oxygen therapy, titrating oxygen therapy, monitoring those at risk for hypoxia, monitoring those at risk of hypoventilation (opioids use, neurologic compromise), and postoperative patients. Pulse oximeter measurements are less accurate at SpO_2 less than 80%, but the clinical importance of this is questionable (Hess, MacIntyre, Galvin, & Mishoe, 2016, p. 24). Pulse oximetry does not replace arterial blood gas analysis. Desaturation (decreased level of SpO_2) indicates gas exchange abnormalities. Oxygen desaturation is considered a late sign of respiratory compromise in patients with reduced rate and depth of breathing (Johnson, Schweitzer, & Ahrens, 2011).

DELEGATION CONSIDERATIONS	The measurement of oxygen saturation using a pulse oximeter may be delegated to nursing assistive personnel (NAP) or to unlicensed assistive personnel (UAP), as well as to licensed practical/vocational nurses (LPN/LVNs). The decision to delegate must be based on careful analysis of the patient's needs and circumstances, as well as the qualifications of the person to whom the task is being delegated. Refer to the Delegation Guidelines in Appendix A.
EQUIPMENT	• Pulse oximeter with an appropriate sensor or probe • Alcohol wipe(s) or disposable cleansing cloth • Nail polish remover (if necessary) • PPE, as indicated
ASSESSMENT	Assess for the presence of health problems that may impact oxygenation. Assess the patient's respiratory rate and depth and mental status. Significant changes from baseline may indicate an alteration in oxygenation. Assess the patient's skin temperature and color, including the color of the nail beds. Temperature is a good indicator of blood flow. Warm skin indicates adequate circulation. In a well-oxygenated patient, the skin and nail beds are usually pink. Skin that is bluish or dusky indicates hypoxia (inadequate amount of oxygen available to the cells). Also check capillary refill; prolonged capillary refill indicates a reduction in blood flow. Assess the quality of the pulse proximal to the sensor application site. Assess for edema of the sensor site. Avoid placing a sensor on edematous tissue; the presence of edema can interfere with readings. Auscultate the lungs (see Skill 3-5). Note the amount of oxygen and delivery method if the patient is receiving supplemental oxygen.

(continued)

Skill 14-1 ▶ Using a Pulse Oximeter *(continued)*

NURSING DIAGNOSIS	Determine the related factors for the nursing diagnoses based on the patient's current status. Appropriate nursing diagnoses may include:

- Impaired gas exchange
- Ineffective airway clearance
- Activity intolerance

OUTCOME IDENTIFICATION AND PLANNING	The expected outcome to achieve when measuring oxygen saturation with a pulse oximeter is that the patient will exhibit oxygen saturation within a range of 95% to 100%, or within acceptable parameters for the person, and the heart rate displayed on the oximeter will correlate with the pulse measurement.

IMPLEMENTATION

ACTION	RATIONALE
1. Review health record for any health problems that would affect the patient's oxygenation status. Gather equipment.	Identifying influencing factors aids in interpretation of results. Assembling equipment provides for an organized approach to the task.
2. Perform hand hygiene and put on PPE, if indicated.	Hand hygiene and PPE prevent the spread of microorganisms. PPE is required based on transmission precautions.
3. Identify the patient.	Identifying the patient ensures the right patient receives the intervention and helps prevent errors.
4. Assemble equipment to the bedside stand or overbed table or other surface within reach.	Bringing everything to the bedside conserves time and energy. Arranging items nearby is convenient, saves time, and avoids unnecessary stretching and twisting of muscles on the part of the nurse.
5. Close the curtains around the bed and close the door to the room, if possible. Explain what you are going to do and why you are going to do it to the patient.	This ensures the patient's privacy. Explanation relieves anxiety and facilitates cooperation.
6. Select an appropriate site for application of the sensor.	Inadequate circulation can interfere with the oxygen saturation (SpO_2) reading.
a. Use the patient's index, middle, or ring finger (Figure 1).	Fingers are easily accessible.

FIGURE 1. Selecting an appropriate finger.

ACTION

b. Check the proximal pulse (Figure 2) and capillary refill (Figure 3) closest to the site.

c. If circulation to the site is inadequate, consider using the earlobe, forehead, or bridge of the nose. Use the appropriate oximetry sensor for the chosen site.

d. Use a toe only if lower extremity circulation is not compromised.

FIGURE 2. Assessing pulse.

7. Select proper equipment:

a. If one finger is too large for the probe, use a smaller finger.

b. Use probes appropriate for the patient's age and size. Use a pediatric probe for a small adult, if necessary.

c. Check if the patient is allergic to adhesive. A nonadhesive finger clip or reflectance sensor is available.

8. Prepare the monitoring site. Cleanse the selected area with the alcohol wipe or disposable cleansing cloth, as necessary (Figure 4). Allow the area to dry. If necessary, remove the nail polish and artificial nails after checking pulse oximeter's manufacturer's instructions.

RATIONALE

Brisk capillary refill and a strong pulse indicate adequate circulation to the site.

These alternate sites are highly vascular alternatives. Correct use of appropriate equipment is vital for accurate results. The appropriate ear oximetry sensor should be used to obtain measurements from a patient's ear. The use of a finger sensor should be limited to use on the finger (Johnson et al., 2012).

Peripheral vascular disease is common in lower extremities.

FIGURE 3. Assessing capillary refill.

Inaccurate readings can result if the probe or sensor is not attached correctly.

Probes come in adult, pediatric, and infant sizes.

A reaction may occur if the patient is allergic to an adhesive substance.

Skin oils, dirt, or grime on the site can interfere with the passage of light waves. Research is conflicting regarding the effect of dark color nail polish and artificial nails. It is prudent to remove the nail polish (World Health Organization [WHO], 2011; Yönt, Korhan, & Dizer, 2014). Refer to facility policy and pulse oximeter's manufacturer's instructions regarding nail polish and artificial nails for additional information.

FIGURE 4. Cleaning area.

(continued)

Skill 14-1 ▶ Using a Pulse Oximeter *(continued)*

ACTION	**RATIONALE**
9. Attach the probe securely to the skin (Figure 5). **Make sure that the light-emitting sensor and the light-receiving sensor are aligned opposite each other (not necessary to check if placed on the forehead or bridge of the nose).**	Secure attachment and proper alignment promote satisfactory operation of the equipment and an accurate recording of the SpO_2.
10. Connect the sensor probe to the pulse oximeter (Figure 6), turn the oximeter on, and check operation of the equipment (audible beep, fluctuation of the bar of light or waveform on the face of the oximeter).	Audible beep represents the arterial pulse, and fluctuating waveform or light bar indicates the strength of the pulse. A weak signal will produce an inaccurate recording of the SpO_2. Tone of the beep reflects SpO_2 reading. If SpO_2 drops, the tone becomes lower in pitch.

FIGURE 5. Attaching probe to patient's finger.

FIGURE 6. Connecting sensor probe to unit.

11. Set alarms on the pulse oximeter. Check the manufacturer's alarm limits for high and low pulse rate settings (Figure 7).	Alarm provides additional safeguard and signals when high or low limits have been surpassed.

FIGURE 7. Checking alarms.

12. Check oxygen saturation at regular intervals, as ordered by the primary care provider, nursing assessment, and signaled by alarms. Monitor the hemoglobin level.	Monitoring SpO_2 provides ongoing assessment of the patient's condition. A low hemoglobin level may be satisfactorily saturated yet inadequate to meet a patient's oxygen needs.
13. Remove the sensor on a regular basis and check for skin irritation or signs of pressure (every 2 hours for spring-tension sensor or every 4 hours for adhesive finger or toe sensor).	Prolonged pressure may lead to tissue necrosis. Adhesive sensor may cause skin irritation.

ACTION	**RATIONALE**

 14. Clean nondisposable sensors according to the manufacturer's directions. Remove PPE, if used. Perform hand hygiene.

Cleaning equipment between each patient use reduces the spread of microorganisms. Proper removal of PPE reduces the risk for infection transmission and contamination of other items. Hand hygiene prevents the spread of microorganisms.

EVALUATION

The expected outcome has been met when the patient exhibits an oxygen saturation within a range of 95% to 100%, or within acceptable parameters for the person, and the heart rate displayed on the oximeter correlates with the pulse measurement.

DOCUMENTATION

Guidelines

Documentation should include the type of sensor and location used; assessment of the proximal pulse and capillary refill; pulse oximeter reading; the amount of oxygen and delivery method if the patient is receiving supplemental oxygen; lung assessment, if relevant; and any other relevant interventions required as a result of the reading.

Sample Documentation

> 9/03/20 Pulse oximeter placed on patient's index finger on right hand. Radial pulse present with brisk capillary refill. Pulse oximeter reading 98% on oxygen at 2 L/min via nasal cannula. Heart rate measured by oximeter correlates with the radial pulse measurement.
> —C. Bausler, RN

UNEXPECTED SITUATIONS AND ASSOCIATED INTERVENTIONS

- *Absent or weak signal:* Check vital signs and patient condition. If satisfactory, check connections and circulation to site. Hypotension makes an accurate recording difficult. Equipment such as a restraint or blood pressure cuff may compromise circulation to site and cause venous blood to pulsate, giving an inaccurate reading. If extremity is cold, cover with a warm blanket and/or use another site.
- *Potentially inaccurate reading:* Check prescribed medications and history of circulatory disorders. Try the device on a healthy person to see if the problem is equipment related or patient related. Drugs that cause vasoconstriction interfere with accurate recording of oxygen saturation.
- *A bright light (sunlight or fluorescent light) is suspected of causing equipment malfunction:* Turn off light or cover the probe with a dry washcloth. Bright light can interfere with operation of light sensors and cause an unreliable report.

SPECIAL CONSIDERATIONS

General Considerations

- Review facility procedures for obtaining pulse oximetry readings if the patient's fingers are not suitable. Correct use of appropriate equipment is vital for accurate results. The appropriate ear oximetry sensor should be used to obtain measurements from a patient's ear. A finger sensor should be limited to use on the finger. The oximetry measurement obtained during clinical assessment should include a record of the type of sensor used.
- Accuracy of readings can be influenced by conditions that decrease arterial blood flow, such as peripheral edema, hypotension, and peripheral vascular disease.
- Pulse oximetry may be less reliable in patients with chronic bronchitis and emphysema (Amalakanti & Pentakota, 2016).
- Inexpensive, portable pulse oximeters may be less reliable and should be used with caution in acutely ill patients (Jones et al., 2015).
- Correlate the pulse reading on the pulse oximeter with the patient's heart rate. Variation between pulse and heart rate may indicate that not all pulsations are being detected and another sensor site may be required.
- Excessive motion of the sensor probe site, such as with extremity tremors or shivering, can also interfere with obtaining an accurate reading.
- Bradycardia and irregular cardiac rhythms may also cause inaccurate readings.
- In patients with low cardiac output, the forehead sensor may be better than the digit sensor for pulse oximetry.

(continued)

Skill 14-1 ▶ Using a Pulse Oximeter *(continued)*

Infant and Child Considerations

- For infants, the oximeter probe may be placed on the toe or foot (Figure 8).

FIGURE 8. Oximetry probe on infant's toe.

Older Adult Considerations

- Careful attention to the patient's skin integrity and condition is necessary to prevent injury. Pressure or tension from the probe, as well as any adhesive used, can damage older, dry, thin skin.

Home Care Considerations

- Portable units are available for use in the home or in an outpatient setting.

EVIDENCE FOR PRACTICE ▶

PULSE OXIMETRY

Monitoring oxygen saturation by using pulse oximetry is a common method for assessing respiratory status in various clinical and home care situations. It is imperative that the nurse has adequate knowledge to use the equipment appropriately, correctly interpret the resulting data, and take appropriate action based on the information.

Related Research

Seeley, M. C., McKenna, L., & Hood, K. (2015). Graduate nurses' knowledge of the functions and limitations of pulse oximetry. *Journal of Clinical Nursing, 24*(23–24), 3538–3549.

   In this study, graduate nurses entering professional practice and novice nurses completing their first year of professional practice were surveyed to assess knowledge of pulse oximetry. The survey instrument was designed to assess pulse oximetry knowledge, including factors that affect pulse oximetry application and interpretation, as well as the participants' ability to translate knowledge and apply to common clinical scenarios. The results identified a satisfactory level of knowledge pertaining to practical factors affecting the function and limiting the clinical application of pulse oximetry. However, the results also identified significant deficits relating to the theoretical factors that affect pulse oximetry application and interpretation. These deficits have the potential to contribute to patient mismanagement. The researchers suggested nurse educators should examine curriculum content related to the appropriate use of pulse oximetry in prelicensure programs and make changes to strengthen this content to improve understanding.

Relevance for Nursing Practice

Inappropriate use and interpretation of pulse oximetry increase the risk of mismanagement and potentially undetected alterations in the respiratory status of patients. Nurse educators should work to ensure adequate inclusion of related content in nursing education curriculum as well as orientation curriculum for new graduate nurses. Nurses themselves have a responsibility to take action to ensure adequate levels of knowledge to support best practices in professional practice, participating in continuing education to support up-to-date practice knowledge.

   Refer to thePoint® for additional research on related nursing topics.

Skill 14-2 ▶ Teaching a Patient to Use an Incentive Spirometer

Incentive spirometry provides visual reinforcement for deep breathing by the patient. It assists the patient to breathe slowly and deeply, and to sustain maximal **inspiration**, while providing immediate positive reinforcement. Incentive spirometry encourages the patient to maximize lung inflation and prevent or reduce **atelectasis**. Optimal gas exchange is supported and secretions can be cleared and expectorated.

DELEGATION CONSIDERATIONS	Patient teaching related to the use of an incentive **spirometer** is not delegated to nursing assistive personnel (NAP), to unlicensed assistive personnel (UAP), or to licensed practical/vocational nurses (LPN/LVNs). Depending on the state's nurse practice act and the organization's policies and procedures, the LPN/LVN may reinforce and encourage the use of the incentive spirometer by the patient. The decision to delegate must be based on careful analysis of the patient's needs and circumstances, as well as the qualifications of the person to whom the task is being delegated. Refer to the Delegation Guidelines in Appendix A.

EQUIPMENT
- Incentive spirometer
- Stethoscope
- Folded blanket or pillow for splinting of chest or abdominal incision, if appropriate
- PPE, as indicated

ASSESSMENT

Assess the patient for pain and administer pain medication, as prescribed, if deep breathing may cause pain. Presence of pain may interfere with learning and performing required activities. Assess lung sounds before and after use to establish a baseline and to determine the effectiveness of incentive spirometry. Incentive spirometry encourages patients to take deep breaths, and lung sounds may be diminished before using the incentive spirometer. Assess vital signs and oxygen saturation to provide baseline data to evaluate patient response. Oxygen saturation may increase due to reinflation of alveoli.

NURSING DIAGNOSIS

Determine the related factors for the nursing diagnoses based on the patient's current status. Appropriate nursing diagnoses may include:

- Impaired gas exchange
- Acute pain
- Deficient knowledge

OUTCOME IDENTIFICATION AND PLANNING

The expected outcome to achieve when teaching a patient to use an incentive spirometer is that the patient accurately demonstrates the procedure for using the spirometer. Other outcomes that may be appropriate include the following: the patient demonstrates increased oxygen saturation level; the patient reports adequate control of pain during use; and the patient demonstrates increased lung expansion with clear breath sounds.

IMPLEMENTATION

ACTION	RATIONALE
1. Review the patient's health record for any health problems that would affect the patient's oxygenation status. Gather equipment.	Identifying influencing factors aids in interpretation of results. Assembling equipment provides for an organized approach to the task.
2. Perform hand hygiene and put on PPE, if indicated.	Hand hygiene and PPE prevent the spread of microorganisms. PPE is required based on transmission precautions.
3. Identify the patient.	Identifying the patient ensures the right patient receives the intervention and helps prevent errors.

(*continued*)

Skill 14-2 ▶ Teaching a Patient to Use an Incentive Spirometer *(continued)*

ACTION	RATIONALE
4. Assemble equipment on the overbed table or other surface within reach.	Bringing everything to the bedside conserves time and energy. Arranging items nearby is convenient, saves time, and avoids unnecessary stretching and twisting of muscles on the part of the nurse.
5. Close the curtains around the bed and close the door to the room, if possible. Explain what you are going to do and why you are going to do it to the patient. Using the chart provided with the device by the manufacturer, note the patient's inspiration target, based on the patient's height and age.	This ensures the patient's privacy. Explanation relieves anxiety and facilitates cooperation. Target for inspiration is based on the patient's height and age and provides an individualized target for each patient.
6. Assist the patient to an upright or semi-Fowler's position, if possible. Remove dentures if they fit poorly. Assess the patient's level of pain. Administer pain medication, as prescribed, if needed. Wait the appropriate amount of time for the medication to take effect. **If the patient has recently undergone abdominal or chest surgery, place a pillow or folded blanket over a chest or abdominal incision for splinting.**	Upright position facilitates lung expansion. Dentures may inhibit the patient from taking deep breaths if the patient is concerned that dentures may fall out. Pain may decrease the patient's ability to take deep breaths. Deep breaths may cause the patient to cough. Splinting the incision supports the area and helps reduce pain from the incision (refer to Chapter 6, Skill 6-1).
7. Demonstrate how to steady the device with one hand and hold the mouthpiece with the other hand (Figure 1). If the patient cannot use hands, assist the patient with the incentive spirometer.	This allows the patient to remain upright, visualize the volume of each breath, and stabilize the device.

FIGURE 1. Patient using incentive spirometer.

8. Instruct the patient to exhale normally and then place lips securely around the mouthpiece.	Patient should fully empty lungs so that maximum volume may be inhaled. A tight seal allows for maximum use of the device.
9. **Instruct the patient to inhale slowly and as deeply as possible through the mouthpiece without using nose (if desired, a nose clip may be used).** Note the movement of the inhalation indicator on the spirometer.	Inhaling through the nose would provide an inaccurate measurement of inhalation volume. The inhalation indicator on the spirometer moves during inhalation, to gauge lung expansion.
10. When the patient cannot inhale anymore, **the patient should hold his or her breath and count to three.** Check position of gauge to determine progress and level attained. If patient begins to cough, splint an abdominal or chest incision.	Holding breath for 3 seconds helps the alveoli to reexpand. Volume on incentive spirometry should increase with practice.

ACTION

RATIONALE

11. Instruct the patient to remove lips from mouthpiece and exhale normally. **If patient becomes lightheaded during the process, tell him or her to stop and take a few normal breaths before resuming incentive spirometry.**

Deep breaths may change the CO_2 level, leading to lightheadedness.

12. Encourage the patient to perform incentive spirometry 5 to 10 times every 1 to 2 hours, if possible.

This helps to reinflate the alveoli and prevent atelectasis due to **hypoventilation.**

13. Clean the mouthpiece with water and shake to dry. Remove PPE, if used. Perform hand hygiene.

Cleaning equipment deters the spread of microorganisms and contaminants. Proper removal of PPE reduces the risk for infection transmission and contamination of other items. Hand hygiene prevents the spread of microorganisms.

EVALUATION

The expected outcome has been met when the patient demonstrates the steps for use of the incentive spirometer correctly and exhibits lung sounds that are clear and equal in all lobes; the patient demonstrates an increase in oxygen saturation levels, and verbalizes adequate pain control and the importance of, and need for, incentive spirometry.

DOCUMENTATION

Guidelines

Document that the incentive spirometer was used by the patient, the number of repetitions, and the average volume reached. Document patient teaching and patient response, if appropriate. If the patient coughs, document whether the cough is productive or nonproductive. If productive cough is present, include the characteristics of the sputum, including consistency, amount, and color.

Sample Documentation

> 9/8/20 Incentive spirometry performed × 10, volume 1,500 mL obtained. Patient with nonproductive cough during incentive spirometry.
>
> —C. Bausler, RN

UNEXPECTED SITUATIONS AND ASSOCIATED INTERVENTIONS

- *Volume inhaled is decreasing*: Assess the patient's pain and anxiety level. Patient may have pain and not be inhaling fully, or patient may have experienced pain previously during incentive spirometry and have an increased anxiety level. If ordered, medicate patient when pain is present. Discuss fears with patient and encourage him or her to inhale fully or to increase the volume by 100 each time incentive spirometry is performed.
- *Patient attempts to blow into incentive spirometer*: Compare the incentive spirometer to a straw. Remind patient to exhale before beginning each time.

SPECIAL CONSIDERATIONS

General Considerations

- Incentive spirometers are not recommended for routine prophylactic use in postoperative adult and pediatric patients (Strickland et al., 2013).

Older Adult Considerations

- Older adults have decreased muscle function and fatigue more easily. Encourage rest periods between repetitions.

Skill 14-3 ▶ Administering Oxygen by Nasal Cannula

A variety of devices are available for delivering oxygen to the patient. Each has a specific function and oxygen concentration. Device selection is based on the patient's condition and oxygen needs. A **nasal cannula**, also called nasal prongs, is the most commonly used oxygen delivery device. Oxygen may be administered using nasal cannula by a low- or high-flow system. High-flow systems aerosolize oxygen and warmed normal saline, providing the ability for higher flow rates, which results in higher oxygen concentrations (LeMone, Burke, Bauldoff, & Gubrud, 2015; Nishimura, 2016).

The cannula is a disposable plastic device with two protruding prongs for insertion into the nostrils. The cannula connects to an oxygen source with a flow meter and, as appropriate, a humidifier. Table 14-1 compares various oxygen delivery systems.

Table 14-1   Oxygen Delivery Systems

METHOD	AMOUNT DELIVERED FiO$_2$ (FRACTION OF INSPIRED OXYGEN)	PRIORITY NURSING INTERVENTIONS
Nasal cannula	*Low flow* 1–2 L/min = 24–28% 3–5 L/min = 32–40% 6 L/min = 44%	Check frequently that both prongs are in the patient's nares. For patients with chronic lung disease, limit rate to the minimum needed to raise arterial oxygen saturation to maintain a level of 88–92% (Mitchell, 2015).
Nasal cannula	*High flow* Maximum flow 60 L/min 10 L/min = 65% 15 L/min = 90%	Closely monitor the patient's respiratory status for changes indicating impending respiratory failure. Pharyngeal pressure is affected by mouth opening or closing, delivered flow, and size of nasal prongs (Nishimura, 2016). High-flow nasal cannula oxygen delivery is often better tolerated by children than other noninvasive delivery methods (Mayfield, Jauncey-Cooke, Hough, Schibler, Gibbons, & Bogossian, 2014).
Simple mask	*Low flow* 5–8 L/min = 40–60% (5 L/min is minimum setting)	Monitor patient frequently to check mask placement. Support patient if claustrophobia is a concern. Secure health care provider's order to replace mask with nasal cannula during mealtime.
Partial rebreather mask	*Low flow* 8–11 L/min = 50–75%	Set flow rate so that mask remains two thirds full during inspiration. Keep reservoir bag free of twists or kinks.
Nonrebreather mask	*Low flow* 10–15 L/min = 80–95%	Maintain flow rate so reservoir bag collapses only slightly during inspiration. Check that valves and rubber flaps are functioning properly (open during **expiration** and closed during inhalation). Monitor Sao$_2$ with pulse oximeter.
Venturi mask	*High flow* 4–10 L/min = 24–40%	Requires careful monitoring to verify FiO$_2$ at flow rate ordered. Check that air intake valves are not blocked.

Source: Reprinted with permission from Hinkle, J. L., & Cheever, K. H. (2018). *Brunner & Suddarth's textbook of medical-surgical nursing* (14th ed.). Philadelphia, PA: Wolters Kluwer and additional information adapted from Mayfield, S., Jauncey-Cooke, J., Hough, J. L., Schibler, A., Gibbons, K., & Bogossian, F. (2014). High-glow nasal cannula therapy for respiratory support in children. *Cochrane Database of Systematic Reviews*, 3. Art. No.: CD009850. doi: 10.1002/14651858.CD009850.pub2; Nishimura, M. (2016). High-flow nasal cannula oxygen therapy in adults: Physiological benefits, indication, clinical benefits, and adverse effects. *Respiratory Care*, 61(4), 529–541.

DELEGATION CONSIDERATIONS

The administration of oxygen by nasal cannula is not delegated to nursing assistive personnel (NAP) or to unlicensed assistive personnel (UAP). Reapplication of the nasal cannula during nursing care activities, such as during bathing, may be performed by NAP or UAP. Depending on the state's nurse practice act and the organization's policies and procedures, administration of oxygen by nasal cannula may be delegated to licensed practical/vocational nurses (LPN/LVNs). The decision to delegate must be based on careful analysis of the patient's needs and circumstances, as well as the qualifications of the person to whom the task is being delegated. Refer to the Delegation Guidelines in Appendix A.

EQUIPMENT	
	• Flow meter connected to oxygen supply • Humidifier with sterile, distilled water (optional for low-flow system) • Nasal cannula and tubing • Gauze to pad tubing over ears (optional) • PPE, as indicated
ASSESSMENT	Assess the patient's oxygen saturation level before starting oxygen therapy to provide a baseline for evaluating the effectiveness of oxygen therapy. Assess the patient's respiratory status, including respiratory rate, rhythm, effort, and lung sounds. Note any signs of respiratory distress, such as **tachypnea**, nasal flaring, use of accessory muscles, or **dyspnea**.
NURSING DIAGNOSIS	Determine the related factors for the nursing diagnoses based on the patient's current status. Appropriate nursing diagnoses may include: • Impaired gas exchange • Ineffective breathing pattern • Risk for activity intolerance
OUTCOME IDENTIFICATION AND PLANNING	The expected outcome to achieve when administering oxygen by nasal cannula is that the patient will exhibit an oxygen saturation level within acceptable parameters. Other outcomes that may be appropriate include the following: the patient will not experience dyspnea; and the patient will demonstrate effortless respirations within an acceptable and appropriate range, without evidence of nasal flaring or use of accessory muscles.

IMPLEMENTATION

ACTION	RATIONALE
1. Review the medical order to verify the use of the nasal cannula, flow rate, and administration parameters. Gather equipment.	Reviewing orders ensures the patient receives prescribed amount of oxygen. Assembling equipment provides for an organized approach to the task.
2. Perform hand hygiene and put on PPE, if indicated.	Hand hygiene and PPE prevent the spread of microorganisms. PPE is required based on transmission precautions.
3. Identify the patient.	Identifying the patient ensures the right patient receives the intervention and helps prevent errors.
4. Assemble equipment on the overbed table or other surface within reach.	Bringing everything to the bedside conserves time and energy. Arranging items nearby is convenient, saves time, and avoids unnecessary stretching and twisting of muscles on the part of the nurse.
5. Close the curtains around the bed and close the door to the room, if possible.	This ensures the patient's privacy.
6. Explain what you are going to do and the reason for doing it to the patient. Review safety precautions necessary when oxygen is in use.	Explanation relieves anxiety and facilitates cooperation. Oxygen supports combustion; a small spark could cause a fire.

(*continued*)

Skill 14-3 ▶ Administering Oxygen by Nasal Cannula *(continued)*

ACTION	RATIONALE
7. Connect the nasal cannula to the oxygen source, with humidification, if appropriate (Figure 1). Adjust the flow rate as ordered (Figure 2). Check that oxygen is flowing out of prongs.	Oxygen forced through a water reservoir is humidified before it is delivered to the patient, thus preventing dehydration of the mucous membranes. Low-flow oxygen does not require humidification.

FIGURE 1. Connecting cannula to oxygen source.

FIGURE 2. Adjusting flow rate.

8. Place prongs in the patient's nostrils (Figure 3). Place tubing over and behind each ear with adjuster comfortably under chin. Alternatively, the tubing may be placed around the patient's head, with the adjuster at the back or base of the head. Place gauze pads at ear beneath the tubing or commercially available ear pads, as necessary (Figure 4).	Correct placement of the prongs and fastener facilitates oxygen administration and patient comfort. Pads reduce irritation and pressure and protect the skin.

FIGURE 3. Applying cannula to nares.

FIGURE 4. Placing gauze pad at ears.

9. Adjust the fit of the cannula, as necessary (Figure 5). Tubing should be snug but not tight against the skin.	Proper adjustment maintains the prongs in the patient's nose. Excessive pressure from tubing could cause irritation and pressure to the skin.
10. **Encourage patients to breathe through the nose, with the mouth closed.**	Nose breathing provides for optimal delivery of oxygen to the patient. The percentage of oxygen delivered can be reduced in patients who breathe through the mouth.
11. Reassess the patient's respiratory status, including the respiratory rate, effort, and lung sounds. Note any signs of respiratory distress, such as tachypnea, nasal flaring, use of accessory muscles, or dyspnea.	Assesses the effectiveness of oxygen therapy.

ACTION	**RATIONALE**

 12. Remove PPE, if used. Perform hand hygiene.

Proper removal of PPE reduces the risk for infection transmission and contamination of other items. Hand hygiene prevents the spread of microorganisms.

13. Put on clean gloves. Remove and clean the cannula and assess nares at least every 8 hours, or according to facility recommendations (Figure 6). Check nares for evidence of irritation or bleeding.

The continued presence of the cannula causes irritation and dryness of the mucous membranes.

FIGURE 5. Adjusting cannula, if needed.

FIGURE 6. Cleaning cannula, when indicated.

EVALUATION

The expected outcome has been met when the patient demonstrates an oxygen saturation level within acceptable parameters; the patient remains free of dyspnea; and demonstrates effortless respirations within an acceptable and appropriate range, without evidence of nasal flaring or use of accessory muscles.

DOCUMENTATION

Guidelines

Document your assessment before and after intervention. Document the amount of oxygen applied, and the patient's respiratory rate, oxygen saturation, and lung sounds.

Sample Documentation

DocuCare Practice documenting the administration of oxygen by nasal cannula in *Lippincott DocuCare.*

9/17/20 1300 Oxygen via nasal cannula applied at 2 L/min. Humidification in place. Pulse oximeter before placing oxygen 92%; after oxygen at 2 L/min 98%. Respirations even and unlabored. Chest rises symmetrically. No nasal flaring or retractions noted. Lung sounds clear and equal in all lobes.

—C. Bausler, RN

UNEXPECTED SITUATIONS AND ASSOCIATED INTERVENTIONS

- *Patient was fine on oxygen delivered by nasal cannula but now states she is short of breath, and the pulse oximeter reading is less than 93%:* Check to see that the oxygen tubing is still connected to the flow meter and the flow meter is still on the previous setting. Someone may have stepped on the tubing, pulling it from the flow meter, or the oxygen may have accidentally been turned off. Assess lung sounds to note any changes. Report changes and assessment findings to primary care provider.
- *Areas over ear or back of head are reddened:* Ensure that areas are adequately padded and that tubing is not pulled too tight. If available, a skin care team may be able to offer some suggestions.

(continued)

Skill 14-3 ▶ Administering Oxygen by Nasal Cannula *(continued)*

SPECIAL CONSIDERATIONS

Home Care Considerations

- Oxygen administration may need to be continued in the home setting. Portable oxygen concentrators are used frequently in home situations. Instruct caregivers about safety precautions with oxygen use and make sure they understand the rationale for the specific liter flow of oxygen.
- Oxygen supports combustion. To prevent fires and injuries, take the following precautions:
  - Do not smoke in a home where oxygen is in use. Place "No Smoking" signs in conspicuous places in the patient's home. Instruct the patient and family about the hazard of smoking when oxygen is in use.
  - Keep oils, grease, alcohol, and other liquids that can burn away from oxygen.
  - Keep oxygen at least 6 ft away from any source of fire, such as a stove, fireplace, or candle (MedlinePlus, 2016).
  - Keep oxygen 6 ft away from toys with electric motors, electric baseboard or space heaters, hairdryers, electric razors, and electric toothbrushes (MedlinePlus, 2016).
  - Do not use electrical equipment near oxygen administration set (e.g., space heaters, blow dryers).
  - Use caution with gas or electric appliances.
  - Ground oxygen concentrators.
  - Secure the oxygen tank in a holder and away from direct sunlight or heat.
  - Allow adequate airflow around the oxygen concentrator (avoid placing flush against the wall).
  - Notify the local fire department of the use of oxygen in the home.

EVIDENCE FOR PRACTICE ▶

OXYGEN THERAPY AND TUBING LENGTH

Although patients using long-term oxygen therapy are provided portable oxygen reservoirs for short-term use, stationary oxygen delivery systems provide oxygen to the patient for the majority of each day. Shorter lengths of tubing are sometimes suggested as necessary to maintain adequate flow, but often result in limitations of patient mobility. Does the length of the oxygen delivery tubing affect the flow of oxygen delivered to the patient?

Related Research

Aguiar, C., Davidson, J., Carvalho, A. K., et al. (2015). Tubing length for long-term oxygen therapy. *Respiratory Care, 60*(2), 179–182.

This study evaluated whether 98.42 ft (30 m) oxygen tubing affects oxygen flow and FiO_2 delivery from one stationary oxygen cylinder and two oxygen concentrators. The three oxygen delivery systems were randomly chosen. Oxygen delivery at 1, 3, and 5 L/min and FiO_2 were measured five times at each flow at the proximal and distal outlets of the tubing. The difference between flows and at each of the locations was analyzed. Flows were similar for 1 and 3 L/min; distal flow was higher than proximal flow at 5 L/min, but was not statistically significant. FiO_2 was lower at distal than proximal outlet tubing at flows 1, 3, and 5 L/min, but the mean difference between measurements was less than 1%. The authors concluded there was no important change in flow and tubing length of up to 98.42 ft (30 m) may be used by patients for oxygen delivery in the home with flows up to 5 L/min.

Relevance for Nursing Practice

Nurses need to make use of evidence-based knowledge to provide appropriate care and assist patients to maintain a desired quality of life. Use of a length of tubing to provide prescribed oxygen therapy and to allow sufficient freedom of movement will enable patients to maintain desired mobility and contribute to an improved quality of life.

Refer to thePoint® for additional research on related nursing topics.

Skill 14-4 ▶ Administering Oxygen by Mask

When a patient requires a higher concentration of oxygen than a nasal cannula can deliver (6 L or 44% oxygen concentration), or is unable or unwilling to maintain a nasal cannula, an oxygen mask may be used (see Table 14-1 in Skill 14-3 for a comparison of different types of oxygen delivery systems). Fit the mask carefully to the patient's face to avoid oxygen leakage. The mask should be comfortably snug, but not tight against the face. Disposable and reusable face masks are available. The most commonly used types of masks are the simple face mask, the partial rebreather mask, the nonrebreather mask, and the Venturi mask. Figure 1 illustrates different types of oxygen masks.

FIGURE 1. Types of oxygen masks. **A.** Venturi mask. **B.** Nonrebreather mask. **C.** Partial rebreather mask. **D.** Simple face mask. **E.** High-flow oxygen face mask and bottle.

(*continued*)

Skill 14-4 ▶ Administering Oxygen by Mask *(continued)*

DELEGATION CONSIDERATIONS

The administration of oxygen by a mask is not delegated to nursing assistive personnel (NAP) or to unlicensed assistive personnel (UAP). Reapplication of the mask during nursing care activities, such as during bathing, may be performed by NAP or UAP. Depending on the state's nurse practice act and the organization's policies and procedures, administration of oxygen by a mask may be delegated to licensed practical/vocational nurses (LPN/LVNs). The decision to delegate must be based on careful analysis of the patient's needs and circumstances, as well as the qualifications of the person to whom the task is being delegated. Refer to the Delegation Guidelines in Appendix A.

EQUIPMENT

- Flow meter connected to oxygen supply
- Humidifier with sterile distilled water, if necessary, for the type of mask prescribed
- Face mask, specified by medical order
- Gauze to pad elastic band (optional)
- PPE, as indicated

ASSESSMENT

Assess the patient's oxygen saturation level before starting oxygen therapy to provide a baseline for determining the effectiveness of therapy. Assess the patient's respiratory status, including respiratory rate, rhythm, effort, and lung sounds. Note any signs of respiratory distress, such as tachypnea, nasal flaring, use of accessory muscles, or dyspnea.

NURSING DIAGNOSIS

Determine the related factors for the nursing diagnoses based on the patient's current status. Appropriate nursing diagnoses may include:

- Impaired gas exchange
- Ineffective breathing pattern
- Activity intolerance

OUTCOME IDENTIFICATION AND PLANNING

The expected outcome to achieve when administering oxygen by mask is that the patient will exhibit an oxygen saturation level within acceptable parameters. Other outcomes that may be appropriate include the following: the patient will not experience dyspnea; and the patient will demonstrate effortless respirations within an acceptable and appropriate range, without evidence of nasal flaring or use of accessory muscles.

IMPLEMENTATION

ACTION	RATIONALE
1. Review the medical order to verify the use of the particular mask, flow rate/concentration, and administration parameters. Gather equipment.	Reviewing orders ensures the patient receives prescribed amount of oxygen. Assembling equipment provides for an organized approach to the task.
2. Perform hand hygiene and put on PPE, if indicated.	Hand hygiene and PPE prevent the spread of microorganisms. PPE is required based on transmission precautions.
3. Identify the patient.	Identifying the patient ensures the right patient receives the intervention and helps prevent errors.
4. Assemble equipment on the overbed table or other surface within reach.	Bringing everything to the bedside conserves time and energy. Arranging items nearby is convenient, saves time, and avoids unnecessary stretching and twisting of muscles on the part of the nurse.
5. Close the curtains around the bed and close the door to the room, if possible.	This ensures the patient's privacy.
6. Explain what you are going to do and the reason for doing it to the patient. Review safety precautions necessary when oxygen is in use.	Explanation relieves anxiety and facilitates cooperation. Oxygen supports combustion; a small spark could cause a fire.

ACTION

7. Attach the face mask to the oxygen source (with humidification, if appropriate, for the specific mask) (Figure 2). Start the flow of oxygen at the specified rate. For a mask with a reservoir, be sure to allow oxygen to fill the bag (Figure 3) before proceeding to the next step.

RATIONALE

Oxygen forced through a water reservoir is humidified before it is delivered to the patient, thus preventing dehydration of the mucous membranes. A reservoir bag must be inflated with oxygen because the bag is the oxygen supply source for the patient.

FIGURE 2. Connecting face mask to oxygen source.

FIGURE 3. Allowing oxygen to fill bag.

8. Position face mask over the patient's nose and mouth (Figure 4). **Adjust the elastic strap so that the mask fits snugly but comfortably on the face (Figure 5).** Adjust to the prescribed flow rate (Figure 6).

A loose or poorly fitting mask will result in oxygen loss and decreased therapeutic value. Masks may cause a feeling of suffocation, and the patient needs frequent attention and reassurance.

FIGURE 4. Applying face mask over nose and mouth.

FIGURE 5. Adjusting elastic straps.

(continued)

Skill 14-4 ▶ Administering Oxygen by Mask *(continued)*

| ACTION | RATIONALE |

FIGURE 6. Adjusting flow rate.

9. If the patient reports irritation or you note redness, use gauze pads under the elastic strap at pressure points to reduce irritation to ears and scalp.

Pads reduce irritation and pressure and protect the skin.

10. Reassess the patient's respiratory status, including respiratory rate, effort, and lung sounds. Note any signs of respiratory distress, such as tachypnea, nasal flaring, use of accessory muscles, or dyspnea.

This helps assess the effectiveness of oxygen therapy.

11. Remove PPE, if used. Perform hand hygiene.

Proper removal of PPE reduces the risk for infection transmission and contamination of other items. Hand hygiene prevents the spread of microorganisms.

12. **Remove the mask and dry the skin every 2 to 3 hours if the oxygen is running continuously. Do not use powder around the mask.**

The tight-fitting mask and moisture from condensation can irritate the skin on the face. There is a danger of inhaling powder if it is placed on the mask.

EVALUATION

The expected outcome has been met when the patient demonstrates an oxygen saturation level within acceptable parameters; the patient remains free of dyspnea; and demonstrates effortless respirations within an acceptable and appropriate range, without evidence of nasal flaring or use of accessory muscles.

DOCUMENTATION

Guidelines

Document type of mask used, amount of oxygen used, oxygen saturation level, lung sounds, and rate/pattern of respirations. Document your assessment before and after intervention.

Sample Documentation

DocuCare Practice documenting the administration of oxygen by mask in *Lippincott DocuCare*.

9/22/20 Patient reports feeling short of breath. Skin pale, respirations 30 breaths/min and labored. Lung sounds decreased throughout. Oxygen saturation via pulse oximeter 88%. Findings reported to Dr. Lu. Oxygen via nonrebreather face mask applied at 12 L/min as ordered. Patient's skin is pink after O₂ applied. Oxygen saturation increased to 98%. Respirations even and unlabored. Chest rises symmetrically. Respiratory rate 18 breaths/min. Lungs remain with decreased breath sounds throughout. Patient denies dyspnea.

—C. Bausler, RN

UNEXPECTED SITUATIONS AND ASSOCIATED INTERVENTIONS

- *Patient was previously fine but is now short of breath, and the pulse oximeter reading is less than 93%:* Check to see that the oxygen tubing is still connected to the flow meter and the flow meter is still on the previous setting. Someone may have stepped on the tubing, pulling it from the flow meter, or the oxygen may have accidentally been turned off. Assess lung sounds for any changes. Report changes and assessment findings to primary care provider. .
- *Areas over ear or back of head are reddened:* Ensure that areas are adequately padded and that tubing is not pulled too tight. If available, a skin care team may be able to offer some suggestions.

SPECIAL CONSIDERATIONS

General Considerations

- Different types of face masks are available for use (refer to Table 14-1 in Skill 14-3 for more information).
- It is important to ensure the mask fits snugly around the patient's face. If it is loose, it will not effectively deliver the right amount of oxygen.
- The mask may be removed for the patient to eat, drink, and take medications. If appropriate, obtain an order for oxygen via nasal cannula for use during mealtimes and limit the amount of times the mask is removed to maintain adequate oxygenation.

Skill Variation ▶ Using an Oxygen Hood

Oxygen hoods are generally used to deliver oxygen to infants. They can supply an oxygen concentration up to 80% to 90% (Kyle & Carman, 2017). The oxygen hood, a clear plastic cover, is placed over the infant's head and neck; it allows easy access to the chest and lower body. Continuous pulse oximetry allows for monitoring oxygenation and making adjustments according to the infant's condition (Perry, Hockenberry, Lowdermilk, & Wilson, 2014). The infant must be removed from the hood for feeding; obtain an order for oxygen delivery for use during feeding times. Assessment of an infant should include assessment of skin color. A pale or cyanotic patient may not be receiving sufficient oxygen. Assess the patient's respiratory status, including respiratory rate, rhythm, effort, and lung sounds. Assessment should also include assessing the patient for any signs of respiratory distress, such as nasal flaring, grunting, or retractions; oxygen-depleted patients often exhibit these signs. Additional equipment required includes the oxygen hood, oxygen analyzer, and a humidification device.

1. Perform hand hygiene and put on PPE, if indicated.

2. Identify the patient.

3. Assemble equipment to the bedside stand or overbed table.
4. Close the curtains around the bed and close the door to the room, if possible.
5. Explain what you are going to do and the reason for doing it to the patient and parents/guardians. Review safety precautions necessary when oxygen is in use.
6. Calibrate the oxygen analyzer according to manufacturer's directions.
7. Place hood on crib. Connect humidifier to oxygen source in the wall. Connect the oxygen tubing to the hood.

Adjust flow rate as ordered by health care provider. Check that oxygen is flowing into the hood.

8. Turn on analyzer. **Place oxygen analyzer probe in hood.**
9. Adjust oxygen flow, as necessary, based on sensor readings. Once oxygen levels reach the prescribed amount, place hood over patient's head (Figure A). The hood should not rub against the infant's neck, chin, or shoulder.

FIGURE A. Placing oxygen hood over infant's head.

10. **Do not block hole in top of hood, if present.**
11. Instruct family members not to raise edges of the hood.
12. Reassess the patient's respiratory status, including respiratory rate, effort, oxygen saturation, and lung sounds. Note any signs of respiratory distress, such as tachypnea, nasal flaring, grunting, retractions, or dyspnea.
13. Remove PPE, if used. Perform hand hygiene.
14. **Check bedding and patient's head frequently for moisture. Change linen and dry the patient's skin, as needed, to keep the patient dry.**
15. **Monitor the patient's body temperature at regular intervals.**

Skill 14-5 ▶ Suctioning the Oropharyngeal and Nasopharyngeal Airways

Suctioning of the pharynx is indicated to maintain a patent airway and to remove saliva, pulmonary secretions, blood, vomitus, or foreign material from the pharynx. Suctioning helps a patient who cannot successfully clear his or her airway by coughing. When performing suctioning, position yourself on the appropriate side of the patient. If you are right-handed, stand on the patient's right side; if left-handed, stand on the patient's left side. This allows for comfortable use of the dominant hand to manipulate the suction catheter. The following skill describes suctioning of the **oropharyngeal airway**. See the accompanying Skill Variation for a description of suctioning of the **nasopharyngeal airway**.

DELEGATION CONSIDERATIONS

Suctioning of the oropharyngeal airway may be delegated to nursing assistive personnel (NAP) or to unlicensed assistive personnel (UAP) who have received appropriate training. Depending on the state's nurse practice act and the organization's policies and procedures, the suctioning of the oropharyngeal and nasopharyngeal airways may be delegated to licensed practical/vocational nurses (LPN/LVNs). The decision to delegate must be based on careful analysis of the patient's needs and circumstances, as well as the qualifications of the person to whom the task is being delegated. Refer to the Delegation Guidelines in Appendix A.

EQUIPMENT

- Portable or wall suction unit with tubing
- A commercially prepared suction kit with an appropriate-size catheter or
  - Sterile suction catheter with Y-port in the appropriate size (Adult: 10 to 16 Fr)
  - Sterile disposable container
  - Sterile gloves
- Sterile water or saline
- Towel or waterproof pad
- Goggles and mask or face shield
- Disposable, clean gloves
- Water-soluble lubricant
- Additional PPE, as indicated

ASSESSMENT

Assess lung sounds. Patients who need to be suctioned may have crackles or gurgling present. Assess oxygen saturation level. Oxygen saturation usually decreases when a patient needs to be suctioned. Assess respiratory status, including respiratory rate, rhythm, and depth. Patients may become tachypneic when they need to be suctioned. Assess the patient for signs of respiratory distress, such as nasal flaring, retractions, or grunting. Assess effectiveness of coughing and expectoration. Suctioning of the airway may be necessary for patients with an ineffective cough who are unable to expectorate secretions. Assess for history of deviated septum, nasal polyps, nasal obstruction, nasal injury, epistaxis (nasal bleeding), or nasal swelling. Assess for pain. Assess the characteristics and amount of secretions while suctioning.

NURSING DIAGNOSIS

Determine the related factors for the nursing diagnoses based on the patient's current status. Appropriate nursing diagnoses may include:

- Ineffective airway clearance
- Ineffective breathing pattern
- Risk for aspiration

OUTCOME IDENTIFICATION AND PLANNING

The expected outcome to achieve when suctioning the patient's oropharyngeal airway is that the patient will exhibit improved breath sounds and a clear, patent airway. Other outcomes that may be appropriate include the following: the patient will exhibit an oxygen saturation level within acceptable parameters; the patient will demonstrate effortless respirations within an acceptable and appropriate range, without evidence of respiratory distress.

IMPLEMENTATION

ACTION	**RATIONALE**
1. Gather equipment.	Assembling equipment provides for an organized approach to the task.
2. Perform hand hygiene and put on PPE, if indicated.	Hand hygiene and PPE prevent the spread of microorganisms. PPE is required based on transmission precautions.
3. Identify the patient.	Identifying the patient ensures the right patient receives the intervention and helps prevent errors.
4. Assemble equipment on the overbed table or other surface within reach.	Bringing everything to the bedside conserves time and energy. Arranging items nearby is convenient, saves time, and avoids unnecessary stretching and twisting of muscles on the part of the nurse.
5. Close the curtains around the bed and close the door to the room, if possible.	This ensures the patient's privacy.
6. Determine the need for suctioning. Verify the suction order in the patient's medical record, if necessary. **Assess for pain or the potential to cause pain. Administer pain medication, as prescribed, before suctioning.**	To minimize trauma to airway mucosa, suctioning should be done only when secretions have accumulated or adventitious breath sounds are audible. Some facilities require an order for naso- and oropharyngeal suctioning. Suctioning stimulates coughing, which is painful for patients with surgical incisions and other conditions.
7. Explain what you are going to do and the reason for suctioning to the patient, even if the patient does not appear to be alert. Reassure the patient you will interrupt the procedure if he or she indicates respiratory difficulty.	Explanation alleviates fears. Even if the patient appears unconscious, explain what is happening. Any procedure that compromises respiration is frightening for the patient.
8. Adjust the bed to a comfortable working height, usually elbow height of the caregiver (VHACEOSH, 2016). Lower the side rail closest to you. **If conscious, place the patient in a semi-Fowler's position. If unconscious, place the patient in the lateral position, facing you.** Move the bedside table close to your work area and raise it to waist height.	Having the bed at the proper height prevents back and muscle strain. A sitting position helps the patient to cough and makes breathing easier. Gravity also facilitates catheter insertion. The lateral position prevents the airway from becoming obstructed and promotes drainage of secretions. The bedside table provides a work surface and helps maintain sterility of objects on the work surface.
9. Place towel or waterproof pad across the patient's chest.	This protects bed linens.
10. **Adjust suction to appropriate pressure (Figure 1).**	Higher pressures can cause excessive trauma, hypoxemia, and atelectasis.

FIGURE 1. Adjusting wall suction.

(*continued*)

Skill 14-5 ▸ Suctioning the Oropharyngeal and Nasopharyngeal Airways *(continued)*

ACTION	RATIONALE

- Using a wall unit for adults and adolescents: no more than 150 mm Hg; neonates: no more than 80 mm Hg; infants: no more than 100 mm Hg; children: no more than 125 mm Hg (Hess et al., 2016).

- For a portable unit for an adult: 10 to 15 cm Hg; neonates: 6 to 8 cm Hg; infants: 8 to 10 cm Hg; children: 8 to 10 cm Hg; adolescents: 8 to 15 cm Hg. **Put on a disposable, clean glove and occlude the end of the connecting tubing to check suction pressure.** Place the connecting tubing in a convenient location.

Higher pressures can cause excessive trauma, hypoxemia, and atelectasis.

11. Open sterile suction package using aseptic technique. The open wrapper or container becomes a sterile field to hold other supplies. Carefully remove the sterile container, touching only the outside surface. Set it up on the work surface and pour sterile saline into it.

Sterile normal saline or water is used to lubricate the outside of the catheter, minimizing irritation of mucosa during introduction. It is also used to clear the catheter between suction attempts.

12. Place a small amount of water-soluble lubricant on the sterile field, taking care to avoid touching the sterile field with the lubricant package.

Lubricant facilitates passage of the catheter and reduces trauma to mucous membranes.

13. Increase the patient's supplemental oxygen level or apply supplemental oxygen per facility policy or primary care provider order.

Suctioning removes air from the patient's airway and can cause hypoxemia. Hyperoxygenation can help prevent suction-induced hypoxemia.

14. Put on face shield or goggles and mask. Put on sterile gloves. **The dominant hand will manipulate the catheter and must remain sterile. The nondominant hand is considered clean rather than sterile and will control the suction valve (Y-port) on the catheter.** In the home setting and other community-based settings, maintenance of sterility is not necessary.

Gloves and other PPE protect the nurse from microorganisms. Handling the sterile catheter using a sterile glove helps prevent introducing organisms into the respiratory tract. In the home setting and other community-based settings, clean (instead of sterile) technique is used because the patient is not exposed to disease-causing organisms that may be found in health care settings, such as hospitals.

15. With the dominant gloved hand, pick up the sterile catheter. Pick up the connecting tubing with the nondominant hand and connect the tubing and suction catheter (Figure 2).

Sterility of the suction catheter is maintained.

16. Moisten the catheter by dipping it into the container of sterile saline (Figure 3). Occlude Y-tube to check suction.

Lubricating the inside of the catheter with saline helps move secretions in the catheter. Checking suction ensures equipment is working properly.

FIGURE 2. Connecting suction catheter to tubing.

FIGURE 3. Dipping catheter into sterile saline.

ACTION	**RATIONALE**

17. Encourage the patient to take several deep breaths.

Hyperventilation can help prevent suction-induced hypoxemia.

18. Apply lubricant to the first 2 to 3 in of the catheter, using the lubricant that was placed on the sterile field.

Lubricant facilitates passage of the catheter and reduces trauma to mucous membranes.

19. Remove the oxygen delivery device, if appropriate. Do not apply suction as the catheter is inserted. Hold the catheter between your thumb and forefinger.

Suctioning removes air from the patient's airway and can cause hypoxemia. Using suction while inserting the catheter can cause trauma to the mucosa and remove excessive oxygen from the respiratory tract.

20. Insert the catheter:

Correct distance for insertion ensures proper placement of the catheter. The general guideline for determining insertion distance for nasopharyngeal suctioning for an individual patient is to estimate the distance from the patient's earlobe to the nose.

    a. **For nasopharyngeal suctioning**, gently insert the catheter through the naris and along the floor of the nostril toward the trachea (Figure 4). Roll the catheter between your fingers to help advance it. Advance the catheter approximately 5 to 6 in to reach the pharynx.

    b. **For oropharyngeal suctioning**, insert catheter through the mouth, along the side of the mouth toward the trachea. Advance the catheter 3 to 4 in to reach the pharynx (for nasotracheal suctioning, see the accompanying Skill Variation).

21. **Apply suction by intermittently occluding the Y-port on the catheter with the thumb of your nondominant hand and gently rotating the catheter as it is being withdrawn (Figure 5). Do not suction for more than 10 to 15 seconds at a time.**

Turning the catheter as it is withdrawn minimizes trauma to the mucosa. Suctioning for longer than 10 to 15 seconds robs the respiratory tract of oxygen, which may result in hypoxemia. Suctioning too quickly may be ineffective at clearing all secretions.

FIGURE 4. Inserting catheter into naris.

FIGURE 5. Suctioning nasopharynx.

22. Replace the oxygen delivery device using your nondominant hand, if appropriate, and have the patient take several deep breaths.

Suctioning removes air from the patient's airway and can cause hypoxemia. Hyperventilation can help prevent suction-induced hypoxemia.

(continued)

Skill 14-5 ▶ Suctioning the Oropharyngeal and Nasopharyngeal Airways *(continued)*

ACTION	**RATIONALE**

23. Flush the catheter with saline (Figure 6). Assess the effectiveness of suctioning and repeat, as needed, and according to the patient's tolerance. Wrap the suction catheter around your dominant hand between attempts.

Flushing clears the catheter and lubricates it for next insertion. Reassessment determines the need for additional suctioning. Wrapping prevents inadvertent contamination of the catheter.

FIGURE 6. Rinsing catheter.

24. **Allow at least a 30-second to 1-minute interval if additional suctioning is needed. No more than three suction passes should be made per suctioning episode. Alternate the naris, unless contraindicated, if repeated suctioning is required. Do not force the catheter through the naris.** Encourage the patient to cough and deep breathe between suctioning. **Suction the oropharynx after suctioning the nasopharynx.**

The interval allows for reventilation and reoxygenation of airways. Excessive suction passes contribute to complications. Alternating the naris reduces trauma. Suctioning the oropharynx after the nasopharynx clears the mouth of secretions. More microorganisms are usually present in the mouth, so it is suctioned last to prevent transmission of contaminants.

25. When suctioning is completed, remove gloves from the dominant hand over the coiled catheter, pulling them off inside out. Remove the glove from the nondominant hand and dispose of gloves, catheter, and container with solution in the appropriate receptacle. Assist the patient to a comfortable position. Raise bed rail and place bed in the lowest position.

This technique reduces transmission of microorganisms. Proper positioning with raised side rails and proper bed height provide for patient comfort and safety.

26. Turn off suction. Remove supplemental oxygen placed for suctioning, if appropriate. Remove face shield or goggles and mask. Perform hand hygiene.

Proper removal of PPE and hand hygiene reduce the risk of transmission of microorganisms.

27. Perform oral hygiene after suctioning.

Respiratory secretions that are allowed to accumulate in the mouth are irritating to mucous membranes, pose a risk for aspiration, and are unpleasant for the patient. Oral hygiene care can limit the growth of pathogens in the oropharyngeal secretions, decreasing the incidence of aspiration pneumonia, community-acquired pneumonia, hospital-acquired nonventilator-associated pneumonia, and ventilator-associated pneumonia (American Association of Critical-Care Nurses [AACN], 2010; Coker, Ploeg, Kaasalainen, & Fisher, 2013; Hillier, Wilson, Chamberlain, & King, 2013; Quinn & Baker, 2015).

28. Reassess the patient's respiratory status, including respiratory rate, effort, oxygen saturation, and lung sounds.

This assesses effectiveness of suctioning and the presence of complications.

29. Remove additional PPE, if used. Perform hand hygiene.

Proper removal of PPE reduces the risk for infection transmission and contamination of other items. Hand hygiene prevents the spread of microorganisms.

EVALUATION

The expected outcome has been met when the patient demonstrates improved breath sounds and a clear, patent airway; exhibits an oxygen saturation level within acceptable parameters; and demonstrates effortless respirations within an acceptable and appropriate range, without evidence of respiratory distress.

DOCUMENTATION

Guidelines

Document the time of suctioning, assessments before and after intervention, reason for suctioning, route used, and the characteristics and amount of secretions.

Sample Documentation

> 9/17/20 1440 Patient with gurgling on inspiration and weak cough; unable to clear secretions. Lungs with rhonchi (sonorous wheezes) in upper airways. Nasopharyngeal suction completed with 12-Fr catheter. Large amount of thick, yellow secretions obtained. After suctioning, lung sounds clear in all lobes, respirations 18 breaths/min, no gurgling noted.
>
> —C. Bausler, RN

UNEXPECTED SITUATIONS AND ASSOCIATED INTERVENTIONS

- *The catheter or sterile glove touches an unsterile surface:* Stop the procedure. If the gloved hand is still sterile, call for assistance and have someone open another catheter or remove the gloves and restart the procedure.
- *Patient vomits during suctioning:* If the patient gags or becomes nauseated, remove the catheter; it has probably entered the esophagus inadvertently. If the patient needs to be suctioned again, change catheters, because it is probably contaminated. Turn the patient to the side and elevate the head of the bed to prevent aspiration.
- *Epistaxis (bleeding) is noted with continued suctioning:* Notify the primary care provider and anticipate the need for a nasal trumpet (see Skill Variation in Skill 14-6: Inserting a Nasopharyngeal Airway). The nasal trumpet will protect the nasal mucosa from further trauma related to suctioning.

SPECIAL CONSIDERATIONS

Infant and Child Considerations

- For infants, use a 5- to 6-Fr catheter.
- For children, use a 6- to 10-Fr catheter.

Skill Variation ▶ Nasotracheal Suctioning

Nasotracheal suctioning is indicated to maintain a patent airway and remove saliva, pulmonary secretions, blood, vomitus, or foreign material from the trachea. Tracheal suctioning can lead to hypoxemia, cardiac dysrhythmias, trauma, atelectasis, infection, bleeding, and pain. It is imperative to be diligent in maintaining aseptic technique and following facility guidelines and procedures to prevent potential hazards. In the home setting and other community-based settings, clean technique is used because the patient is not exposed to disease-causing organisms that may be found in health care settings, such as hospitals. When performing suctioning, position yourself on the appropriate side of the patient. If you are right-handed, stand on the patient's right side; if left-handed, stand on the patient's left side.

This allows for comfortable use of the dominant hand to manipulate the suction catheter. To perform nasotracheal suctioning:

1. Perform hand hygiene. Put on PPE, as indicated.

2. Identify the patient.

3. Assemble equipment to the bedside stand or overbed table or other surface within reach.

(continued)

Skill 14-5 Suctioning the Oropharyngeal and Nasopharyngeal Airways *(continued)*

Skill Variation Nasotracheal Suctioning *(continued)*

4. Close the curtains around the bed and close the door to the room, if possible.
5. Determine the need for suctioning. **Assess for pain or the potential to cause pain. Administer pain medication, as prescribed, before suctioning.**
6. Explain to the patient what you are going to do and the reason for doing it, even if the patient does not appear to be alert.
7. Adjust bed to a comfortable working position. Lower the side rail closest to you. **If the patient is conscious, place him or her in a semi-Fowler's position. If the patient is unconscious, place him or her in the lateral position, facing you.** Move the overbed table close to your work area and raise to waist height.
8. Place a towel or waterproof pad across the patient's chest.
9. **Turn suction to appropriate pressure. Put on a disposable, clean glove and occlude the end of the connecting tubing to check suction pressure.** Place the connecting tubing in a convenient location.
10. Open sterile suction package using aseptic technique. The open wrapper becomes a sterile field to hold other supplies. Carefully remove the sterile container, touching only the outside surface. Set it up on the work surface and pour sterile saline into it.
11. Place a small amount of water-soluble lubricant on the sterile field, taking care to avoid touching the sterile field with the lubricant package.
12. Increase the patient's supplemental oxygen level or apply supplemental oxygen per facility policy or medical order.
13. Put on face shield or goggles and mask. Put on sterile gloves. **The dominant hand will manipulate the catheter and must remain sterile.** The nondominant hand is considered clean rather than sterile and will control the suction valve.
14. With dominant gloved hand, pick up the sterile catheter. Pick up the connecting tubing with the nondominant hand and connect the tubing and suction catheter.
15. Moisten the catheter by dipping it into the container of sterile saline. Occlude the Y-tube to check suction.
16. Encourage the patient to take several deep breaths.
17. Apply lubricant to the first 2 to 3 in of the catheter, using the lubricant that was placed on the sterile field.
18. Remove the oxygen delivery device, if appropriate. Do not apply suction as the catheter is inserted. Hold the catheter in your thumb and forefinger. Gently insert the catheter through the naris and along the floor of the

nostril toward the trachea. Roll the catheter between your fingers to help advance it. Advance the catheter approximately 8 to 9 in to reach the trachea. Resistance should not be met. If resistance is met, the carina or tracheal mucosa has been hit. Withdraw the catheter at least 1-2 in before applying suction.
19. Apply suction by intermittently occluding the Y-port on the catheter with the thumb of your nondominant hand, and gently rotating the catheter as it is being withdrawn. **Do not suction for more than 10 to 15 seconds at a time.**
20. Replace the oxygen delivery device using your nondominant hand and have the patient take several deep breaths.
21. Flush the catheter with saline. Assess effectiveness of suctioning and repeat, as needed, and according to patient's tolerance. Wrap the suction catheter around your dominant hand between attempts.
22. **Allow at least a 30-second to 1-minute interval if additional suctioning is needed. No more than three suction passes should be made per suctioning episode.** Alternate the naris, unless contraindicated, if repeated suctioning is required. Do not force catheter through the naris. Encourage the patient to cough and deep breathe between suctioning. Suction the oropharynx after suctioning the trachea.
23. When suctioning is completed, remove glove from dominant hand over the coiled catheter, pulling it off inside out. Remove glove from nondominant hand and dispose of gloves, catheter, and container with solution in the appropriate receptacle. Remove face shield or goggles and mask. Perform hand hygiene.
24. Turn off suction. Remove supplemental oxygen placed for suctioning, if appropriate. Assist the patient to a comfortable position.
25. Offer oral hygiene after suctioning.
26. Reassess the patient's respiratory status, including respiratory rate, effort, oxygen saturation, and lung sounds.
27. Remove additional PPE, if used. Perform hand hygiene.
28. Document the time of suctioning, your assessments before and after intervention, the reason for suctioning, route used, and the characteristics and amount of secretions.

Skill 14-6 ▷ Inserting an Oropharyngeal Airway

An oropharyngeal airway is a semicircular tube of plastic inserted into the back of the pharynx through the mouth in a patient who is breathing spontaneously. The oropharyngeal airway can help protect the airway of an unconscious patient by preventing the tongue from falling back against the posterior pharynx and blocking it. Once the patient regains consciousness, the oropharyngeal airway is removed. Tape is not used to hold the airway in place because the patient should be able to expel the airway once he or she becomes alert. The nurse can insert this device at the bedside with little to no trauma to the unconscious patient. Oropharyngeal airways may also be used to aid in ventilation during a code situation and to facilitate suctioning an unconscious or semiconscious patient. Alternatively, airway support may be provided with a nasopharyngeal airway (Refer to the accompanying Skill Variation.)

DELEGATION CONSIDERATIONS

The insertion of an oropharyngeal airway is not delegated to nursing assistive personnel (NAP) or to unlicensed assistive personnel (UAP). Depending on the state's nurse practice act and the organization's policies and procedures, the insertion of an oropharyngeal airway may be delegated to licensed practical/vocational nurses (LPN/LVNs). The decision to delegate must be based on careful analysis of the patient's needs and circumstances, as well as the qualifications of the person to whom the task is being delegated. Refer to the Delegation Guidelines in Appendix A.

EQUIPMENT

- Oropharyngeal airway of appropriate size
- Disposable gloves
- Suction equipment
- Goggles and mask or face shield (optional)
- Flashlight (optional)
- Additional PPE, as indicated

ASSESSMENT

Assess patient's level of consciousness and ability to protect the airway. Assess amount and consistency of oral secretions. Auscultate lung sounds. If the tongue is occluding the airway, lung sounds may be diminished. Assess for loose teeth or recent oral surgery, which may contraindicate the use of an oropharyngeal airway.

NURSING DIAGNOSIS

Determine related factors for the nursing diagnoses based on the patient's current status. Appropriate nursing diagnoses may include:

- Risk for aspiration
- Ineffective airway clearance
- Risk for injury

OUTCOME IDENTIFICATION AND PLANNING

The expected outcome is that the patient will maintain a patent airway and exhibit oxygen saturation within acceptable parameters. Another outcome that may be appropriate is that the patient remains free from aspiration and injury.

IMPLEMENTATION

ACTION	RATIONALE
1. Gather equipment.	Assembling equipment provides for an organized approach to the task.
2. Perform hand hygiene and put on PPE, if indicated.	Hand hygiene and PPE prevent the spread of microorganisms. PPE is required based on transmission precautions.
3. Identify the patient.	Identifying the patient ensures the right patient receives the intervention and helps prevent errors.

Skill 14-6 ▶ Inserting an Oropharyngeal Airway *(continued)*

ACTION	**RATIONALE**
4. Assemble equipment on the overbed table or other surface within reach.	Arranging items nearby is convenient, saves time, and avoids unnecessary stretching and twisting of muscles on the part of the nurse.
5. Close the curtains around the bed and close the door to the room, if possible.	This ensures the patient's privacy.
6. Explain to the patient what you are going to do and the reason for doing it, even if the patient does not appear to be alert.	Explanation alleviates fears. Even if a patient appears unconscious, the nurse should explain what is happening.
7. Put on disposable gloves; put on goggles and mask or face shield, as indicated.	Gloves and other PPE prevent contact with contaminants and body fluids.
8. Measure the oropharyngeal airway for correct size (Figure 1). Measure the oropharyngeal airway by holding the airway on the side of the patient's face. The airway should reach from the opening of the mouth to the back angle of the jaw.	Correct size ensures correct insertion and fit, allowing for conformation of the airway to the curvature of the palate.
9. **Check mouth for any loose teeth, dentures, or other foreign material. Remove dentures or material, if present.**	Prevents aspiration or swallowing of objects. During insertion, the airway may push any foreign objects in the mouth to the back of the throat.
10. Position patient in semi-Fowler's position.	This position facilitates airway insertion and helps prevent the tongue from moving back against the posterior pharynx.
11. Suction the patient, if necessary.	This removes excess secretions and helps maintain a patent airway.
12. Open the patient's mouth by using your thumb and index finger to gently pry teeth apart. **Insert the airway with the curved tip pointing up toward the roof of the mouth (Figure 2).**	This is done to advance the tip of the airway past the tongue, toward the back of the throat.

FIGURE 1. Measuring for oropharyngeal airway.

FIGURE 2. Inserting airway.

13. Slide the airway across the tongue to the back of the mouth. Rotate the airway 180 degrees as it passes the uvula (Figure 3). The tip should point down and the curvature should follow the contour of the roof of the mouth. Use a flashlight to confirm the position of the airway with the curve fitting over the tongue.	This is done to shift the tongue anteriorly, thereby allowing the patient to breathe through and around the airway.
14. Ensure accurate placement and adequate ventilation by auscultating breath sounds (Figure 4).	If the airway is placed correctly, lung sounds should be audible and equal in all lobes.
15. Position the patient on his or her side when the airway is in place.	This position helps keep the tongue out of the posterior pharynx area and helps to prevent aspiration if the unconscious patient should vomit.

ACTION	**RATIONALE**

FIGURE 3. Rotating airway.

FIGURE 4. Auscultating breath sounds.

16. Remove gloves and additional PPE, if used. Perform hand hygiene.

Proper removal of PPE reduces the risk for infection transmission and contamination of other items. Hand hygiene prevents the spread of microorganisms.

17. Remove the airway for a brief period every 4 hours, or according to facility policy. Assess mouth; provide mouth care and clean the airway according to facility policy before reinserting it.

Tissue irritation and ulceration can result from prolonged use of an airway. Mouth care provides moisture to mucous membranes and helps maintain tissue integrity.

EVALUATION

The expected outcome has been met when the patient exhibits a patent airway with oxygen saturation within acceptable parameters, and remains free from injury and aspiration.

DOCUMENTATION

Guidelines

Document the placement of the airway, airway size, removal/cleaning, assessment before and after intervention, and oxygen saturation level.

Sample Documentation

> 9/22/20 1210 Patient noted to have gurgling with respirations, tongue back in posterior pharynx. Difficult to suction oropharynx. Size 4 oropharyngeal airway inserted. Patient placed on left side. Lung sounds clear and equal in all lobes. Pulse oximeter 98% on room air.
> —C. Bausler, RN

UNEXPECTED SITUATIONS AND ASSOCIATED INTERVENTIONS

- *The patient awakens:* Remove the oral airway once the patient is awake because it may be uncomfortable and cause vomiting. Conscious patients can usually protect their airway.
- *The tongue is sliding back into the posterior pharynx, causing respiratory difficulties:* Put on disposable gloves and remove the airway. Make sure the airway is the appropriate size for the patient.
- *Patient vomits as oropharyngeal airway is inserted:* Quickly position patient onto his or her side to prevent aspiration. Remove oral airway. Suction mouth, if needed.

SPECIAL CONSIDERATIONS

General Considerations

- Wearing gloves, remove the airway briefly every 4 hours to provide mouth care. Assess the mouth and tongue for tissue irritation, tooth damage, bleeding, and ulceration. Ensure that the lips and tongue are not between the teeth and the airway to prevent injury.
- When reinserting the oropharyngeal airway, attempt to insert it on the other side of the mouth. This helps to prevent irritation to the tongue and mouth.
- Suction secretions, as needed, by manipulating around and through the oropharyngeal airway.

(continued)

Skill 14-6 ▶ Inserting an Oropharyngeal Airway *(continued)*

Skill Variation ▶ Inserting a Nasopharyngeal Airway

Nasopharyngeal airways (nasal trumpets) are curved, uncuffed, soft plastic tubes inserted into the back of the pharynx through the nose in patients who are breathing spontaneously. The nasal trumpet provides a route from the nares to the pharynx to help maintain a patent airway. These airways may be indicated if the teeth are clenched, the tongue is enlarged, or the patient needs frequent nasopharyngeal suctioning. The appropriate-size range for a nasal trumpet for adolescents to adults is 24 to 36 Fr. Additional assessments include assessing for the presence of nasal conditions, such as a deviated septum or recent nasal or oral surgery, traumatic brain injury, central facial fractures, basilar skull or cribriform fractures, and increased risk for bleeding, such as anticoagulant therapy, which would contraindicate the use of a nasopharyngeal airway.

1. Perform hand hygiene and put on PPE, if indicated.

2. Identify the patient.

3. Assemble equipment on the overbed table or other surface within reach.
4. Close the curtains around the bed and close the door to the room, if possible.
5. Explain what you are going to do and the reason you are doing it to the patient, even if the patient does not appear to be alert.
6. Put on disposable gloves. If the patient is coughing or has copious secretions, also wear a mask and goggles.
7. Measure the nasopharyngeal airway for correct size (Figure A). Measure the nasopharyngeal airway length by holding the airway on the side of the patient's face. The airway should reach from the tip of the nose to the earlobe. The airway with the largest outer diameter that fits the patient's nostril should be used (Morton & Fontaine, 2018).

8. Adjust the bed to a comfortable working level, usually elbow height of the caregiver (VHACEOSH, 2016). Lower the side rail closest to you. **If the patient is awake and alert, position in semi-Fowler's position. If the patient is not conscious or alert, position in a side-lying position.**
9. Suction patient, if necessary.
10. Lubricate the nasopharyngeal airway generously with the water-soluble lubricant, covering the airway from the tip to the guard rim (Figure B).

FIGURE B. Lubricating nasopharyngeal airway.

11. **Gently insert the airway into the naris (Figure C), narrow end first, pointing it down, toward the back of the throat, until the rim is touching the naris (Figure D). If resistance is met, stop and try the other naris.**

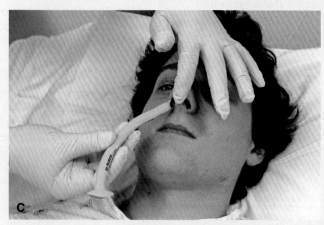

FIGURE C. Inserting nasopharyngeal airway.

FIGURE A. Measuring nasopharyngeal airway.

Skill Variation > Inserting a Nasopharyngeal Airway *(continued)*

FIGURE D. Nasopharyngeal airway inserted until the rim is touching the naris.

12. Check placement by closing the patient's mouth and placing your fingers in front of the tube opening to check for air movement. Assess the pharynx to visualize the tip of the airway behind the uvula. Assess the nose for blanching or skin stretching.

13. Remove gloves and raise the bed rail. Place bed in the lowest position. Remove additional PPE, if used. Perform hand hygiene.

14. Remove the airway, clean in warm soapy water, and place in other naris at least every 8 hours, or according to facility policy. If the patient coughs or gags on insertion, the nasal trumpet may be too long. Assess the pharynx. You should be able to visualize the tip of the airway behind the uvula.

Skill 14-7 > Suctioning an Endotracheal Tube: Open System

The purpose of suctioning is to maintain a patent airway and remove pulmonary secretions, blood, vomitus, or foreign material from the airway. When suctioning via an **endotracheal tube,** the goal is to remove secretions that are not accessible to **cilia** bypassed by the tube itself. Tracheal suctioning can lead to hypoxemia, cardiac dysrhythmias, trauma, atelectasis, infection, bleeding, and pain. Therefore, it is imperative to be diligent in maintaining aseptic technique and in following facility guidelines and procedures to prevent potential hazards. Tracheal suctioning should be performed only when clinically indicated and not routinely (American Association for Respiratory Care (AARC) Clinical Practice Guidelines, 2010; Morton & Fontaine, 2018; Sole, Bennet, & Ashworth, 2015).

Because suctioning removes secretions not accessible to bypassed cilia, the recommendation is to insert the catheter only as far as the end of the endotracheal tube. Catheter contact and suction can cause tracheal mucosal damage, loss of cilia, edema, and fibrosis, and increase the risk of infection and bleeding for the patient. Insertion of the suction catheter to a predetermined distance, no more than 1 cm past the length of the endotracheal tube (adults) and 0.5 cm (pediatric patients) (Boroughs & Dougherty, 2015), avoids contact with the trachea and carina, reducing the effects of tracheal mucosal damage (Boroughs & Dougherty, 2015; Hahn, 2010; Ireton, 2007; Pate & Zapata, 2002). Box 14-1 outlines several methods for determining appropriate suction catheter depth. The suction catheter should be small enough not to occlude the airway being suctioned but large enough to remove secretions; in adults, use a suction catheter that occludes less than 50% of the lumen of the tracheostomy or endotracheal tube and a catheter with a diameter one half the diameter of the tube in pediatric patients (AARC, 2010; Hockenberry & Wilson, 2015).

Tracheal suctioning is an uncomfortable procedure at minimum, and it can be a very painful and/or distressing experience. Therefore, anticipate assessing for the need for the administration of analgesic medication to a patient before suctioning (Arroyo-Novoa et al., 2008; Düzkaya & Kuğuoğlu, 2015). As mentioned previously, perform suctioning only when clinically necessary because of the many potential risks, including hypoxia, infection, tracheal tissue damage, dysrhythmias, and atelectasis.

Some consider open-system suctioning to be the most efficient way to suction the endotracheal tube, arguing that there are no limitations to the movement of the suction catheter while suctioning. However, the nurse may unknowingly contaminate an open system during the procedure. In addition, with the open system, the patient must be removed from the ventilator during suctioning. Closed-system suction, recommended for use with patients who are mechanically ventilated, may be used routinely or when a patient must be suctioned frequently and quickly due to an excess of secretions, depending on the policies of the facility (AARC, 2010; Morton and Fontaine, 2018). Refer to Skill 14-8.

(continued)

Skill 14-7 ▶ Suctioning an Endotracheal Tube: Open System (continued)

Box 14-1 Methods to Determine Suction Catheter Depth

Open Suction System

Method 1 (Endotracheal Tubes)

- Using a suction catheter with centimeter increments on it, insert the suction catheter into the endotracheal tube until the centimeter markings on both the endotracheal tube and catheter align.
- Insert the suction catheter no further than an additional 1 cm.

Method 2 (Endotracheal Tubes)

- Combine the length of the endotracheal tube and any adapter being used, and add an additional 1 cm.
- Document the determined length at the bedside or on the care plan, according to facility policy.

Method 3 (Endotracheal and Tracheostomy Tubes)

- Using a spare endotracheal or tracheostomy tube of the same size as being used for the patient, insert the suction catheter to the end of the tube.

- Note the length of catheter used to reach the end of the tube.
- Document the determined length at the bedside or on the care plan. Alternately, mark the distance on the suction catheter with permanent ink or tape and place the catheter at the bedside for reference. Refer to facility policy.

Closed Suction System (Endotracheal and Tracheostomy Tubes)

- Combine the length of the endotracheal or **tracheostomy tube** and any adapter being used, and add an additional 1 cm.
- Advance the catheter until the appropriate length can be seen through the catheter sheath or window.
- Document the depth of the catheter at the bedside or on the care plan.

Source: Adapted from Hahn, M. (2010). 10 considerations for endotracheal suctioning. *The Journal for Respiratory Care Practitioners, 23*(7), 32–33; Republished with permission of American Association of Critical Care Nurses from Pate, M., & Zapata, T. (2002). Ask the experts: How deeply should I go when I suction an endotracheal or tracheostomy tube? Critical Care Nurse, 22(2), 130–131, permission conveyed through Copyright Clearance Center, Inc.

DELEGATION CONSIDERATIONS	Suctioning an endotracheal tube is not delegated to nursing assistive personnel (NAP) or to unlicensed assistive personnel (UAP). Depending on the state's nurse practice act and the organization's policies and procedures, suctioning of an endotracheal tube in a stable situation, such as long-term care and other community-based care settings, may be delegated to licensed practical/vocational nurses (LPN/LVNs). The decision to delegate must be based on careful analysis of the patient's needs and circumstances, as well as the qualifications of the person to whom the task is being delegated. Refer to the Delegation Guidelines in Appendix A.
EQUIPMENT	• Portable or wall suction unit with tubing • A commercially prepared suction kit with an appropriate-size catheter (see General Considerations) or • Sterile suction catheter with Y-port in the appropriate size • Sterile, disposable container • Sterile gloves • Towel or waterproof pad • Goggles and mask or face shield • Additional PPE, as indicated • Disposable, clean gloves • Resuscitation bag connected to 100% oxygen • Assistant (optional)
ASSESSMENT	Assess for coarse crackles over the trachea, the most common indicator for endotracheal suctioning (Sole et al., 2015). Assess lung sounds. Wheezes, crackles, gurgling or diminished breath sounds may indicate the need for suctioning. Assess for the presence of visualized secretions in the artificial airway, audible secretions, and ineffective coughing (Morton & Fontaine, 2018; Sole et al.). Assess oxygen saturation level. Deterioration in oxygen desaturation may be an indication of the need for suctioning (AARC, 2010). Assess respiratory status, including respiratory rate and depth. Patients may become tachypneic when they need to be suctioned. Assess the patient for signs of respiratory distress, such as nasal flaring, retractions, or grunting. Additional indications for suctioning via an endotracheal tube include acute respiratory distress, and frequent or sustained coughing. Also assess for pain and the potential to cause pain during the intervention. Perform individualized pain management in response to the patient's needs (Arroyo-Novoa et al., 2008;

Dükaya & Kuğuoğlu, 2015). Administer pain medication, as prescribed, before suctioning. Assess appropriate suction catheter depth. Refer to Box 14-1. Assess the characteristics and amount of secretions while suctioning.

NURSING DIAGNOSIS	Determine the related factors for the nursing diagnoses based on the patient's current status. Appropriate nursing diagnoses may include: • Ineffective airway clearance • Risk for infection • Impaired gas exchange
OUTCOME IDENTIFICATION AND PLANNING	The expected outcome is that the patient will exhibit a clear, patent airway. Other outcomes that may be appropriate include the following: the patient will exhibit an oxygen saturation level within acceptable parameters; the patient will demonstrate a respiratory rate and depth within acceptable parameters; and the patient will remain free from any signs of respiratory distress.

IMPLEMENTATION

ACTION	RATIONALE
1. Gather equipment.	Assembling equipment provides for an organized approach to the task.
2. Perform hand hygiene and put on PPE, if indicated.	Hand hygiene and PPE prevent the spread of microorganisms. PPE is required based on transmission precautions.
3. Identify the patient.	Identifying the patient ensures the right patient receives the intervention and helps prevent errors.
4. Assemble equipment on the overbed table or other surface within reach.	Arranging items nearby is convenient, saves time, and avoids unnecessary stretching and twisting of muscles on the part of the nurse.
5. Close the curtains around the bed and close the door to the room, if possible.	This ensures the patient's privacy.
6. Determine the need for suctioning. Verify the suction order in the patient's medical record. **Assess for pain or the potential to cause pain. Administer pain medication, as prescribed, before suctioning.**	Tracheal suctioning should be performed only when clinically indicated and not routinely (AARC, 2010; Morton & Fontaine, 2018; Sole et al., 2015). Suctioning can cause moderate to severe pain for patients. Individualized pain management is imperative (Arroyo-Novoa et al., 2008; Düzkaya & Kuğuoğlu, 2015). Suctioning stimulates coughing, which is painful for patients with surgical incisions.
7. Explain what you are going to do and the reason for doing it to the patient, even if the patient does not appear to be alert. Reassure the patient you will interrupt the procedure if he or she indicates respiratory difficulty.	Explanation alleviates fears. Even if the patient appears unconscious, the nurse should explain what is happening. Any procedure that compromises respiration is frightening for the patient.
8. Adjust the bed to a comfortable working position, usually elbow height of the caregiver (VHACEOSH, 2016). Lower the side rail closest to you. **If conscious, place in a semi-Fowler's position. If unconscious, place the patient in the lateral position, facing you.** Move the overbed table close to your work area and raise it to waist height.	Having the bed at the proper height prevents back and muscle strain. A sitting position helps the patient to cough and makes breathing easier. Gravity also facilitates catheter insertion. The lateral position prevents the airway from becoming obstructed and promotes drainage of secretions. The overbed table provides a work surface and maintains sterility of objects on work surface.

(continued)

Skill 14-7 ▶ Suctioning an Endotracheal Tube: Open System *(continued)*

ACTION	RATIONALE
9. Place towel or waterproof pad across the patient's chest.	This protects bed linens and the patient.
10. **Adjust suction to appropriate pressure (Figure 1).**	Higher pressures can cause excessive trauma, hypoxemia, and atelectasis.

- Using a wall unit for adults and adolescents: no more than 150 mm Hg; neonates: no more than 80 mm Hg; infants: no more than 100 mm Hg; children: no more than 125 mm Hg (Hess et al., 2016).
- For a portable unit for an adult: 10 to 15 cm Hg; neonates: 6 to 8 cm Hg; infants: 8 to 10 cm Hg; children: 8 to 10 cm Hg; adolescents: 8 to 15 cm Hg.

FIGURE 1. Turning suction unit to appropriate pressure.

ACTION	RATIONALE
11. Put on a disposable, clean glove and occlude the end of the connecting tubing to check suction pressure. Place the connecting tubing in a convenient location. Place the resuscitation bag connected to oxygen within convenient reach, if using.	Glove prevents contact with blood and body fluids. Checking pressure ensures equipment is working properly. Allows for an organized approach to the procedure.
12. Open sterile suction package using aseptic technique. The open wrapper becomes a sterile field to hold other supplies. Carefully remove the sterile container, touching only the outside surface. Set it up on the work surface and pour sterile saline into it.	Sterile normal saline or water is used to lubricate the outside of the catheter, minimizing irritation of mucosa during introduction. It is also used to clear the catheter between suction attempts.
13. Put on face shield or goggles and mask. Put on sterile gloves. **The dominant hand will manipulate the catheter and must remain sterile. The nondominant hand is considered clean rather than sterile and will control the suction valve (Y-port) on the catheter.**	Handling the sterile catheter using a sterile glove helps prevent introducing organisms into the respiratory tract; the clean glove protects the nurse from microorganisms.
14. With dominant gloved hand, pick up sterile catheter. Pick up the connecting tubing with the nondominant hand and connect the tubing and suction catheter.	Sterility of the suction catheter is maintained.
15. Moisten the catheter by dipping it into the container of sterile saline, unless it is a silicone catheter. Occlude Y-tube to check suction.	Lubricating the inside of the catheter with saline helps move secretions in the catheter. Silicone catheters do not require lubrication. Checking suction ensures equipment is working properly.

ACTION

16. Using your nondominant hand, remove the ventilator tubing from the endotracheal tube and attach the manual resuscitation bag. Hyperventilate the patient using your nondominant hand and the manual resuscitation bag, delivering three to six breaths (Figure 2). Alternatively, use the sigh mechanism on a mechanical ventilator.

RATIONALE

Hyperventilation and hyperoxygenation aids in preventing hypoxemia during suctioning.

FIGURE 2. Removing ventilator tubing from endotracheal tube to hyperventilate the patient using a manual resuscitation bag.

17. Open the adapter on the mechanical ventilator tubing or remove the manual resuscitation bag with your nondominant hand.

This exposes the endotracheal tube without contaminating sterile gloved hand.

18. Using your dominant hand, gently and quickly insert the catheter into the endotracheal tube (Figure 3). **Advance the catheter to the predetermined length. Do not occlude Y-port when inserting the catheter.**

Catheter contact and suction cause tracheal mucosal damage, loss of cilia, edema, and fibrosis, and increase the risk of infection and bleeding for the patient. Insertion of the suction catheter to a predetermined distance, no more than 1 cm past the length of the endotracheal tube, avoids contact with the trachea and carina, reducing the effects of tracheal mucosal damage (Boroughs & Dougherty, 2015; Hahn, 2010; Ireton, 2007). If resistance is met, the carina or tracheal mucosa has been hit. Withdraw the catheter at least 0.5 in before applying suction. Occluding the Y-port (i.e., suctioning) when inserting the catheter increases the risk for trauma to the airway mucosa and increases the risk of hypoxemia.

FIGURE 3. Inserting suction catheter into endotracheal tube.

(continued)

Skill 14-7 ▶ Suctioning an Endotracheal Tube: Open System *(continued)*

ACTION	RATIONALE
19. Apply suction by intermittently occluding the Y-port on the catheter with the thumb of your nondominant hand, and gently rotate the catheter as it is being withdrawn (Figure 4). **Do not suction for more than 10 to 15 seconds at a time.**	Turning the catheter as it is withdrawn minimizes trauma to the mucosa. Suctioning for longer than 15 seconds robs the respiratory tract of oxygen, which may result in hypoxemia (AARC, 2010). Suctioning too quickly may be ineffective at clearing all secretions.

FIGURE 4. Withdrawing suction catheter and intermittently occluding Y-port with thumb to apply suction.

ACTION	RATIONALE
20. Hyperventilate the patient using your nondominant hand and a manual resuscitation bag and deliver three to six breaths. Replace the oxygen delivery device, if applicable, using your nondominant hand and have the patient take several deep breaths. If the patient is mechanically ventilated, close the adapter on the mechanical ventilator tubing or replace the ventilator tubing and use the sigh mechanism on a mechanical ventilator.	Suctioning removes air from the patient's airway and can cause hypoxemia. Hyperventilation and hyperoxygenation can help prevent suction-induced hypoxemia.
21. Flush catheter with saline. Assess the effectiveness of suctioning and repeat, as needed, and according to patient's tolerance. Wrap the suction catheter around your dominant hand between attempts.	Flushing clears the catheter and lubricates it for next insertion. Reassessment determines need for additional suctioning. Wrapping the catheter prevents inadvertent contamination of the catheter.
22. **Allow at least a 30-second to 1-minute interval if additional suctioning is needed. Do not make more than three suction passes per suctioning episode.** Suction the oropharynx after suctioning the trachea. Do not reinsert in the endotracheal tube after suctioning the mouth.	The interval allows for reventilation and reoxygenation of airways. Excessive suction passes contribute to complications. Suctioning the oropharynx clears the mouth of secretions. More microorganisms are usually present in the mouth, so it is suctioned last to prevent transmission of contaminants.
23. Perform oral hygiene after tracheal suctioning.	Respiratory secretions that are allowed to accumulate in the mouth are irritating to mucous membranes, pose a risk for aspiration, and are unpleasant for the patient. Oral hygiene care can limit the growth of pathogens in the oropharyngeal secretions, decreasing the incidence of aspiration pneumonia, community-acquired pneumonia, hospital-acquired nonventilator-associated pneumonia, and ventilator-associated pneumonia (AACN, 2010; Coker et al., 2013; Hillier et al., 2013; Quinn & Baker, 2015).
24. When suctioning is completed, remove gloves from dominant hand over the coiled catheter, pulling off inside out. Remove glove from nondominant hand and dispose of gloves, catheter, and container with solution in the appropriate receptacle. Assist patient to a comfortable position. Raise bed rail and place bed in the lowest position.	This technique of glove removal and disposal of equipment reduces transmission of microorganisms. Proper positioning with raised side rails and proper bed height provide for patient comfort and safety.
25. Turn off suction. Remove face shield or goggles and mask. Perform hand hygiene.	Removing face shield or goggles and mask properly reduces the risk for infection transmission and contamination of other items. Hand hygiene prevents transmission of microorganisms.

ACTION

26. Reassess the patient's respiratory status, including respiratory rate, effort, oxygen saturation, lung sounds, tracheal sounds, and presence/absence of secretions in artificial airway.

27. Remove additional PPE, if used. Perform hand hygiene.

RATIONALE

These assess effectiveness of suctioning and the presence of complications.

Proper removal of PPE reduces the risk for infection transmission and contamination of other items. Hand hygiene prevents the spread of microorganisms.

EVALUATION

The expected outcome has been met when performing endotracheal suctioning when the patient exhibits a clear, patent airway; an oxygen saturation level within acceptable parameters; a respiratory rate and depth within acceptable parameters; and the patient remains free from any signs of respiratory distress.

DOCUMENTATION

Guidelines

Document the time of suctioning, assessments before and after interventions, reason for suctioning, oxygen saturation levels, and the characteristics and amount of secretions.

Sample Documentation

> <u>9/1/20</u> 1850 Tan secretions noted in ET tube; coarse crackles noted to auscultation over trachea. Lung sounds coarse in lower lobes. Respirations 24 breaths/min, regular rhythm. Intercostal retractions noted. Endotracheal tube suctioning completed with 12-Fr catheter. Small amount of thin, tan secretions obtained. Specimen for culture collected and sent. After suctioning, no secretions noted in ET tube, auscultation over trachea clear, lung sounds clear, respirations 18 breaths/min, no intercostal retractions noted.
>
> —C. Bausler, RN

UNEXPECTED SITUATIONS AND ASSOCIATED INTERVENTIONS

- *Catheter or sterile glove is contaminated:* Reconnect patient to ventilator, if in use. Discard gloves and suction catheter. Gather supplies and begin procedure again.
- *When suctioning, your eye becomes contaminated with respiratory secretions:* After attending to the patient, perform hand hygiene and flush your eye with a large amount of sterile water. Contact employee health or house supervisor immediately for further treatment. Wear goggles or a face shield when suctioning to prevent exposure to body fluids.
- *Patient is extubated during suctioning:* Remain with patient. Call for help to notify the primary care provider. Assess patient's vital signs, ability to breathe without assistance, and oxygen saturation. Be ready to deliver assisted breaths with a bag-valve mask (see Skill 14-14) or administer oxygen. Anticipate the need for reintubation.
- *Oxygen saturation level decreases after suctioning:* Hyperoxygenate patient. Auscultate lung sounds. If lung sounds are absent over one lobe, alert staff to notify primary care provider. Remain with patient. Patient may have **pneumothorax** or malplaced endotracheal tube. Anticipate an order for a stat chest x-ray and possible chest tube placement or reintubation.
- *Patient develops signs of intolerance to suctioning; oxygen saturation level decreases and remains low after hyperoxygenation; patient becomes cyanotic or patient becomes bradycardic:* Stop suctioning. Auscultate lung sounds. Consider hyperventilating patient with manual resuscitation device. Remain with patient. Alert staff to notify primary care provider.

SPECIAL CONSIDERATIONS

General Considerations

Determine the size of catheter to use by the size of the endotracheal tube. The external diameter of the suction catheter should occlude less than 50% of the lumen of the tracheostomy or endotracheal

(continued)

Skill 14-7 ▶ Suctioning an Endotracheal Tube: Open System   *(continued)*

tube and 50% in pediatric patients (AARC, 2010; Hockenberry & Wilson, 2015). Larger catheters can contribute to trauma and hypoxemia.

- The practice of instillation of saline solution directly into the airway is not supported by evidence and is not recommended for inclusion as part of evidence-based practice and suctioning (AARC, 2010; Boroughs & Dougherty, 2015; Khimani, Ali, Ratani, & Awan, 2015; Leddy & Wilkinson, 2015; Owen et al., 2016).
- Make sure emergency equipment is easily accessible at the bedside. Keep a bag-valve mask, oxygen, and suction equipment at the bedside of a patient with an endotracheal tube at all times.

Infant and Child Considerations

- Insertion of the suction catheter to a predetermined distance, no more than 0.5 cm past the length of the endotracheal tube avoids contact with the trachea and carina, reducing the effects of tracheal mucosal damage (Boroughs & Dougherty, 2015).
- Maximal time for application of negative pressure (suction) for neonates, children, and adolescents should be less than 5 seconds (Boroughs & Dougherty, 2015).

EVIDENCE FOR PRACTICE ▶

ENDOTRACHEAL TUBES AND PATIENT COMMUNICATION

Placement of an endotracheal tube results in the inability to speak, which can be frightening and frustrating for the patient and may contribute to ineffective responses to patient concerns and needs.

Related Research

Guttormson, J. L., Bremer, K. L., & Jones, R. M. (2015). "Not being able to talk was horrid": A descriptive, correlational study of communication during mechanical ventilation. *Intensive and Critical Care Nursing, 31*(3), 179–186.

   The purpose of this descriptive analysis was to describe the patient experience of communication during mechanical ventilation. This study was a secondary analysis of data collected to study the relationship between sedation and the mechanically ventilated patients' recall of the intensive care unit (ICU). During initial data analysis for the primary study, communication emerged as an important component of the patients' ICU experience. Structured interviews were conducted with patients after extubation using the Intensive Care Experience Questionnaire, and included follow-up questions to patient comments and open-ended questions related to the ICU experience. Seven items from the questionnaire were used for this secondary analysis. Participants identified that the inability to communicate needs was associated with helplessness, and the perceived lack of information received was associated with not feeling in control and helplessness. Ineffective communication impacted negatively on satisfaction with care. Participants expressed frustration with failed communication and a lack of information received. Participants also verbalized a desire for a better system of communication during intubation and mechanical ventilation. The authors concluded that communication effectiveness impacts patients' sense of safety and well-being during intubation and mechanical ventilation.

Relevance for Nursing Practice

Effective communication is a cornerstone of professional nursing care. Communication strategies for patients who are unable to communicate verbally are a critical part of the provision of care. Good communication enables nurses to provide appropriate and person-centered nursing care. Nurses have a responsibility to develop and implement communication strategies to meet the needs of all patients in their care.

   Refer to thePoint® for additional research on related nursing topics.

EVIDENCE FOR PRACTICE ▶

ENDOTRACHEAL SUCTIONING

Sole, M. L., Bennet, M. B., & Ashworth, S. (2015). Clinical indicators for endotracheal suctioning in adult patients receiving mechanical ventilation. *American Journal of Critical Care, 24*(4), 318–324.

   Refer to details in Skill 14-8, Evidence for Practice, and refer to thePoint® for additional research on related nursing topics.

Skill 14-8 ▶ Suctioning an Endotracheal Tube: Closed System

The purpose of suctioning is to maintain a patent airway and remove pulmonary secretions, blood, vomitus, or foreign material from the airway. When suctioning via an endotracheal tube, the goal is to remove secretions that are not accessible to cilia bypassed by the tube itself. Tracheal suctioning can lead to hypoxemia, cardiac dysrhythmias, trauma, atelectasis, infection, bleeding, and pain. Therefore, it is imperative to be diligent in maintaining aseptic technique and in following facility guidelines and procedures to prevent potential hazards. Tracheal suctioning should be performed only when clinically indicated and not routinely (AARC, 2010; Morton & Fontaine, 2018; Sole et al., 2015).

Because suctioning removes secretions not accessible to bypassed cilia, the recommendation is to insert the catheter only as far as the end of the endotracheal tube. Catheter contact and suction can cause tracheal mucosal damage, loss of cilia, edema, and fibrosis, and increase the risk of infection and bleeding for the patient. Insertion of the suction catheter to a predetermined distance, no more than 1 cm past the length of the endotracheal tube (adults) and 0.5 cm (pediatric patients) (Boroughs & Dougherty, 2015), avoids contact with the trachea and carina, reducing the effects of tracheal mucosal damage (Boroughs & Dougherty, 2015; Hahn, 2010; Ireton, 2007). Box 14-1 in Skill 14-7 outlines several methods for determining appropriate suction catheter depth. The suction catheter should be small enough not to occlude the airway being suctioned but large enough to remove secretions; in adults, use a suction catheter that occludes less than 50% of the lumen of the tracheostomy or endotracheal tube and a catheter with a diameter one half the diameter of the tube in pediatric patients (AARC, 2010; Hockenberry & Wilson, 2015).

Tracheal suctioning is an uncomfortable procedure at minimum, and it can be a very painful and/or distressing experience. Therefore, anticipate assessing for the need for the administration of analgesic medication to a patient before suctioning (Arroyo-Novoa et al., 2008; Düzkaya & Kuğuoğlu, 2015). As mentioned previously, perform suctioning only when clinically necessary because of the many potential risks, including hypoxia, infection, tracheal tissue damage, dysrhythmias, and atelectasis.

Closed-system suction (Figure 1), recommended for use with patients who are mechanically ventilated, may be used routinely or when a patient must be suctioned frequently and quickly due to an excess of secretions, depending on the policies of the facility (AARC, 2010; Morton and Fontaine, 2018). One drawback of closed suctioning may be the hindrance of the sheath when rotating the suction catheter upon removal.

FIGURE 1. Closed suction device.

DELEGATION CONSIDERATIONS

Suctioning an endotracheal tube is not delegated to nursing assistive personnel (NAP) or to unlicensed assistive personnel (UAP). Depending on the state's nurse practice act and the organization's policies and procedures, suctioning of an endotracheal tube in a stable situation, such as long-term care and other community-based care settings, may be delegated to licensed practical/vocational nurses (LPN/LVNs). The decision to delegate must be based on careful analysis of the patient's needs and circumstances, as well as the qualifications of the person to whom the task is being delegated. Refer to the Delegation Guidelines in Appendix A.

(*continued*)

Skill 14-8 ▶ Suctioning an Endotracheal Tube: Closed System *(continued)*

EQUIPMENT
- Portable or wall suction unit with tubing
- Closed suction device of appropriate size for patient
- 3- or 5-mL normal saline solution in dosette or syringe
- Sterile gloves
- Additional PPE, as indicated

ASSESSMENT

Assess for coarse crackles over the trachea, the most common indicator for endotracheal suctioning (Sole et al., 2015). Assess lung sounds. Wheezes, crackles, gurgling or diminished breath sounds may indicate the need for suctioning. Assess for the presence of visualized secretions in the artificial airway, audible secretions, and ineffective coughing (Morton & Fontaine, 2018; Sole et al., 2015). Assess oxygen saturation level. Deterioration in oxygen desaturation may be an indication of the need for suctioning (AARC, 2010). Assess respiratory status, including respiratory rate and depth. Patients may become tachypneic when they need to be suctioned. Assess the patient for signs of respiratory distress, such as nasal flaring, retractions, or grunting. Additional indications for suctioning via an endotracheal tube include acute respiratory distress, and frequent or sustained coughing. Also assess for pain and the potential to cause pain during the intervention. Perform individualized pain management in response to the patient's needs (Arroyo-Novoa et al., 2008; Dükaya & Kuğuoğlu, 2015). Administer pain medication, as prescribed, before suctioning. Assess appropriate suction catheter depth. Refer to Box 14-1 in Skill 14-7. Assess the characteristics and amount of secretions while suctioning.

NURSING DIAGNOSIS

Determine the related factors for the nursing diagnoses based on the patient's current status. Appropriate nursing diagnoses may include:
- Ineffective airway clearance
- Risk for infection
- Impaired gas exchange

OUTCOME IDENTIFICATION AND PLANNING

The expected outcome is that the patient will exhibit a clear, patent airway. Other outcomes that may be appropriate include the following: the patient will exhibit an oxygen saturation level within acceptable parameters; the patient will demonstrate a respiratory rate and depth within acceptable parameters; and the patient will remain free from any signs of respiratory distress.

IMPLEMENTATION

ACTION	RATIONALE
1. Gather equipment.	Assembling equipment provides for an organized approach to the task.
2. Perform hand hygiene and put on PPE, if indicated.	Hand hygiene and PPE prevent the spread of microorganisms. PPE is required based on transmission precautions.
3. Identify the patient.	Identifying the patient ensures the right patient receives the intervention and helps prevent errors.
4. Assemble equipment on the overbed table or other surface within reach.	Arranging items nearby is convenient, saves time, and avoids unnecessary stretching and twisting of muscles on the part of the nurse.
5. Close the curtains around the bed and close the door to the room, if possible.	This ensures the patient's privacy.

ACTION	RATIONALE

6. Determine the need for suctioning. Verify the suction order in the patient's medical record. **Assess for pain or the potential to cause pain. Administer pain medication, as prescribed, before suctioning.**

Tracheal suctioning should be performed only when clinically indicated and not routinely (AARC, 2010; Morton & Fontaine, 2018; Sole et al., 2015). Suctioning can cause moderate to severe pain for patients. Individualized pain management is imperative (Arroyo-Novoa et al., 2008; Düzkaya & Kuğuoğlu, 2015). Suctioning stimulates coughing, which is painful for patients with surgical incisions.

7. Explain what you are going to do and the reason for doing it to the patient, even if the patient does not appear to be alert. Reassure the patient you will interrupt the procedure if he or she indicates respiratory difficulty.

Explanation alleviates fears. Even if the patient appears unconscious, the nurse should explain what is happening. Any procedure that compromises respiration is frightening for the patient.

8. Adjust the bed to a comfortable working position, usually elbow height of the caregiver (VHACEOSH, 2016). Lower the side rail closest to you. **If conscious, place the patient in a semi-Fowler's position. If unconscious, place the patient in the lateral position, facing you.** Move the overbed table close to your work area and raise to waist height.

Having the bed at the proper height prevents back and muscle strain. A sitting position helps the patient to cough and makes breathing easier. Gravity also facilitates catheter insertion. The lateral position prevents the airway from becoming obstructed and promotes drainage of secretions. The overbed table provides work surface and maintains sterility of objects on work surface.

9. **Adjust suction to appropriate pressure (Figure 2).**

Higher pressures can cause excessive trauma, hypoxemia, and atelectasis.

- Using a wall unit for adults and adolescents: no more than 150 mm Hg; neonates: no more than 80 mm Hg; infants: no more than 100 mm Hg; children: no more than 125 mm Hg (Hess et al., 2016).

- For a portable unit for an adult: 10 to 15 cm Hg; neonates: 6 to 8 cm Hg; infants: 8 to 10 cm Hg; children: 8 to 10 cm Hg; adolescents: 8 to 15 cm Hg.

FIGURE 2. Turning suction device to appropriate pressure.

10. Open the package of the closed suction device using aseptic technique. Make sure that the device remains sterile.

The device must remain sterile to prevent a nosocomial infection.

11. Put on sterile gloves.

Gloves deter the spread of microorganisms.

(continued)

Skill 14-8 ▶ Suctioning an Endotracheal Tube: Closed System *(continued)*

ACTION	**RATIONALE**
12. If a closed suctioning device is not in place, continue with Step 13. If this device is already in place, continue with Step 16.	
13. Using nondominant hand, disconnect ventilator from endotracheal tube. Place ventilator tubing in a convenient location so that the inside of the tubing remains sterile, or continue to hold the tubing in your nondominant hand.	This provides access to the endotracheal tube while keeping one hand sterile. The inside of the ventilator tubing should remain sterile to prevent a nosocomial infection.
14. **Using dominant hand and keeping device sterile, connect the closed suctioning device so that the suctioning catheter is in line with the endotracheal tube.**	Keeping the device sterile decreases the risk for a nosocomial infection.
15. **Keeping the inside of the ventilator tubing sterile, attach ventilator tubing to port perpendicular to the endotracheal tube.** Attach suction tubing to suction catheter.	The inside of the ventilator tubing must remain sterile to prevent a nosocomial infection. By connecting the ventilator tubing to the port, the patient does not need to be disconnected from the ventilator to be suctioned.
16. Pop top off sterile normal saline dosette. Open plug to port by suction catheter and insert saline dosette or syringe.	The saline will help to clean the catheter between suctioning.
17. Hyperventilate the patient by using the sigh button on the ventilator before suctioning. Turn safety cap on suction button of catheter so that button is depressed easily.	Hyperoxygenating and hyperventilating before suctioning helps to decrease the effects of oxygen removal during suctioning. The safety button keeps the patient from accidentally depressing the button and decreasing the oxygen saturation.
18. Grasp suction catheter through protective sheath, about 6 in (15 cm) from the endotracheal tube. Gently insert the catheter into the endotracheal tube (Figure 3). Release the catheter while holding on to the protective sheath. Move hand farther back on catheter. **Grasp catheter through sheath and repeat movement, advancing the catheter to the predetermined length. Do not occlude Y-port when inserting the catheter.**	The sheath keeps the suction catheter sterile. Catheter contact and suction cause tracheal mucosal damage, loss of cilia, edema, and fibrosis, and increase the risk of infection and bleeding for the patient. Insertion of the suction catheter to a predetermined distance, no more than 1 cm past the length of the endotracheal tube, avoids contact with the trachea and carina, reducing the effects of tracheal mucosal damage (Boroughs & Dougherty, 2015; Hahn, 2010; Ireton, 2007). If resistance is met, the carina or tracheal mucosa has been hit. Withdraw the catheter at least 0.5 in before applying suction. Suctioning when inserting the catheter increases the risk for trauma to airway mucosa and increases the risk of hypoxemia.
19. Apply intermittent suction by depressing the suction button with thumb of nondominant hand (Figure 4). Gently rotate the catheter with thumb and index finger of dominant hand as catheter is being withdrawn. **Do not suction for more than 10 to 15 seconds at a time.** Hyperoxygenate or hyperventilate with sigh button on ventilator, as ordered.	Turning the catheter while withdrawing it helps clean surfaces of the respiratory tract and prevents injury to tracheal mucosa. Suctioning for longer than 15 seconds robs the respiratory tract of oxygen, which may result in hypoxemia (AARC, 2010). Suctioning too quickly may be ineffective at clearing all secretions. Hyperoxygenation and hyperventilation reoxygenate the lungs.

FIGURE 3. Grasping the catheter through the protective sheath and inserting into endotracheal tube.

FIGURE 4. Depressing suction button.

ACTION	**RATIONALE**

20. Once the catheter is withdrawn back into the sheath (Figure 5), depress the suction button while gently squeezing the normal saline dosette until the catheter is clean. **Allow at least a 30-second to 1-minute interval if additional suctioning is needed. No more than three suction passes should be made per suctioning episode.**

Flushing cleans and clears the catheter and lubricates it for next insertion. Allowing time interval and replacing oxygen delivery setup help compensate for hypoxia induced by the suctioning. Excessive suction passes contribute to complications.

FIGURE 5. Removing suction catheter by pulling back into sheath.

21. When the procedure is completed, **ensure that the catheter is withdrawn into the sheath,** and turn the safety button. Remove normal saline dosette and apply cap to port.

By turning the safety button, the suction is blocked at the catheter so the suction cannot remove oxygen from the endotracheal tube.

22. Suction the oral cavity with a separate single-use, disposable catheter and perform oral hygiene. Remove gloves. Turn off suction.

Suctioning of the oral cavity removes secretions that may be stagnant in the mouth and pharynx, reducing the risk for infection. Respiratory secretions that are allowed to accumulate in the mouth are irritating to mucous membranes, pose a risk for aspiration, and are unpleasant for the patient. Oral hygiene care can limit the growth of pathogens in the oropharyngeal secretions, decreasing the incidence of aspiration pneumonia, community-acquired pneumonia, hospital-acquired nonventilator-associated pneumonia, and ventilator-associated pneumonia (AACN, 2010; Coker et al., 2013; Hillier et al., 2013; Quinn & Baker, 2015). Proper removal of PPE reduces the risk for infection transmission and contamination of other items.

23. Assist the patient to a comfortable position. Raise the bed rail and place the bed in the lowest position.

Ensures patient comfort. Proper positioning with raised side rails and proper bed height provide for patient comfort and safety.

24. Reassess the patient's respiratory status, including respiratory rate, effort, oxygen saturation, lung sounds, tracheal sounds, and presence/absence of secretions in artificial airway.

These assess effectiveness of suctioning and the presence of complications.

 25. Remove additional PPE, if used. Perform hand hygiene.

Proper removal of PPE reduces the risk for infection transmission and contamination of other items. Hand hygiene prevents the spread of microorganisms.

EVALUATION

The expected outcomes have been met when the patient exhibits a clear, patent airway; an oxygen saturation level within acceptable parameters; a respiratory rate and depth within acceptable parameters; and the patient remains free from any signs of respiratory distress.

(continued)

Skill 14-8 ▶ Suctioning an Endotracheal Tube: Closed System *(continued)*

DOCUMENTATION

Guidelines

Document the time of suctioning, your assessments before and after intervention, reason for suctioning, oxygen saturation levels, and the characteristics and amount of secretions.

Sample Documentation

9/1/20 1850 Tan secretions noted in ET tube; coarse crackles noted to auscultation over trachea. Lung sounds coarse in lower lobes. Respirations 24 breaths/min, regular rhythm. Intercostal retractions noted. Endotracheal tube suctioning completed with 12-Fr catheter. Small amount of thin, tan secretions obtained. Specimen for culture collected and sent. After suctioning, no secretions noted in ET tube, auscultation over trachea clear, lung sounds clear, respirations 18 breaths/min, no intercostal retractions noted.

—C. Bausler, RN

UNEXPECTED SITUATIONS AND ASSOCIATED INTERVENTIONS

- *Patient is extubated during suctioning:* Remain with patient. Call for help to notify the primary care provider. Assess patient's vital signs, ability to breathe without assistance, and oxygen saturation. Be ready to deliver assisted breaths with a bag-valve mask (see Skill 14-14) or administer oxygen. Anticipate the need for reintubation.
- *Oxygen saturation level decreases after suctioning:* Hyperoxygenate patient. Auscultate lung sounds. If lung sounds are absent over one lobe, alert staff to notify primary care provider. Remain with patient. Patient may have pneumothorax or malplaced endotracheal tube. Anticipate an order for a stat chest x-ray and possible chest tube placement or reintubation.
- *Patient develops signs of intolerance to suctioning; oxygen saturation level decreases and remains low after hyperoxygenation; patient becomes cyanotic or patient becomes bradycardic:* Stop suctioning. Auscultate lung sounds. Consider hyperventilating patient with manual resuscitation device. Remain with patient. Alert staff to notify primary care provider.

SPECIAL CONSIDERATIONS

General Considerations

- The practice of instillation of saline solution directly into the airway is not supported by evidence and is not recommended for inclusion as part of evidence-based practice and suctioning (AARC, 2010; Boroughs & Dougherty, 2015; Khimani et al., 2015; Leddy & Wilkinson, 2015; Owen et al., 2016).
- Determine the size of catheter to use by the size of the endotracheal tube. The external diameter of the suction catheter should occlude less than 50% of the lumen of the tracheostomy or endotracheal tube and 50% in pediatric patients (AARC, 2010; Hockenberry & Wilson, 2015). Larger catheters can contribute to trauma and hypoxemia.
- Make sure emergency equipment is easily accessible at the bedside. Keep bag-valve mask, oxygen, and suction equipment at the bedside of a patient with an endotracheal tube at all times.

Infant and Child Considerations

- Insertion of the suction catheter to a predetermined distance, no more than 0.5 cm past the length of the endotracheal tube avoids contact with the trachea and carina, reducing the effects of tracheal mucosal damage (Boroughs & Dougherty, 2015).
- Maximal time for application of negative pressure (suction) for neonates, children, and adolescents should be less than 5 seconds (Boroughs & Dougherty, 2015).

EVIDENCE FOR PRACTICE ▶

ENDOTRACHEAL SUCTIONING

Patients with endotracheal and tracheostomy tubes often require suctioning via the tube to remove secretions from the airway. Tracheal suctioning should be performed only when clinically indicated and not routinely (AARC, 2010; Morton & Fontaine, 2018). What are appropriate clinical indications?

Related Research

Sole, M. L., Bennet, M. B., & Ashworth, S. (2015). Clinical indicators for endotracheal suctioning in adult patients receiving mechanical ventilation. *American Journal of Critical Care, 24*(4), 318–324.

The purpose of this descriptive study was to determine clinical cues for endotracheal suctioning in patients who have endotracheal tubes and require mechanical ventilation. Participants included a convenience sample of 42 adult patients receiving mechanical ventilation in critical care units. Physiologic data were recorded immediately before and after baseline endotracheal suctioning. Baseline endotracheal suctioning using a closed-system device was completed. Participants were then assessed hourly for up to 4 hours for guideline-based cues for endotracheal suctioning. In addition, lung sounds were auscultated. Guideline-based cues were based on guidelines from the American Association for Respiratory Care. Tracheal auscultation was done above the sternum, and lung sounds were also auscultated. Participants received endotracheal suctioning when cues were detected or 4 hours after baseline suctioning. Secretions were collected, measured, and weighed. The mean time to endotracheal suctioning was 2 hours and a mean 4.4 mL of secretions was removed. The most frequent suctioning cues included crackles over the trachea (88%), sawtooth waveform on ventilator (33%) (indicating obstruction to flow in the airways), coughing (29%), and visible secretions (5%). Cues resolved and physiologic parameters improved after suctioning. Coarse lung sounds did not improve. The researchers concluded that the most common indicator for the need for endotracheal suctioning is the presence of coarse crackles over the trachea and suggested patients receiving mechanical ventilation should be routinely assessed for coarse crackles over the trachea as an indicator for the need for suctioning of the airway. It was also concluded that despite common practice, assessment of lung sounds to identify the need for suctioning is not supported.

Relevance for Nursing Practice
Tracheal suctioning should be performed only when clinically indicated and not routinely (AARC, 2010; Morton & Fontaine, 2018; Sole et al., 2015). Nurses have a responsibility to use appropriate assessment techniques to support clinical decision making and to implement evidence-based strategies to meet the needs of patients in their care.
Refer to thePoint® for additional research on related nursing topics.

EVIDENCE FOR PRACTICE ▶

ENDOTRACHEAL TUBES AND PATIENT COMMUNICATION
Guttormson, J. L., Bremer, K. L., & Jones, R. M. (2015). "Not being able to talk was horrid": A descriptive, correlational study of communication during mechanical ventilation. *Intensive and Critical Care Nursing, 31*(3), 179–186.
Refer to details in Skill 14-7, Evidence for Practice, and refer to thePoint® for additional research on related nursing topics.

Skill 14-9 ▶ Securing an Endotracheal Tube

Endotracheal tubes provide an airway for patients who cannot maintain a sufficient airway on their own. A tube is passed through the mouth or nose into the trachea. Patients who have an endotracheal tube have a high risk for skin breakdown related to the securing of the endotracheal tube, compounded by the risk of increased secretions. The endotracheal tube is often held in place with adhesive tape and should be retaped every 24 hours to prevent skin breakdown and to ensure that the tube is secured properly. Retaping an endotracheal tube requires two people. There are other ways of securing an endotracheal tube besides using tape. Figure 1 shows an example of a commercially available endotracheal tube holder. To secure with another device, follow the

(*continued*)

Skill 14-9 ▶ Securing an Endotracheal Tube *(continued)*

manufacturer's recommendations. The literature suggests noncommercial airway holders, such as adhesive tape, exert less force on a patient's face than commercial devices (Fisher, Chenelle, Marchese, Kratohvil, & Kacmarek, 2014; Shimizu, Mizutani, Yamahita, Hagiya, & Tanaka, 2011). Commercial holders may allow for a more rapid and secure movement of the airway from one side of the mouth to the other (Fisher et al., 2014). One example of a method of taping an endotracheal tube is provided below, but this skill might be performed differently in your facility. Always refer to specific facility policy.

FIGURE 1. Commercially available endotracheal tube holder.

DELEGATION CONSIDERATIONS	Securing an endotracheal tube is not delegated to nursing assistive personnel (NAP) or to unlicensed assistive personnel (UAP). Depending on the state's nurse practice act and the organization's policies and procedures, securing of an endotracheal tube in a stable situation, such as long-term care and other community-based care settings, may be delegated to licensed practical/vocational nurses (LPN/LVNs). The decision to delegate must be based on careful analysis of the patient's needs and circumstances, as well as the qualifications of the person to whom the task is being delegated. Refer to the Delegation Guidelines in Appendix A.

EQUIPMENT

- Assistant (nurse or respiratory therapist)
- Portable or wall suction unit with tubing
- Sterile suction catheter with Y-port
- 1-in tape (adhesive or waterproof tape)
- Disposable gloves
- Mask and goggles or face shield
- Additional PPE, as indicated
- Sterile suctioning kit
- Oral suction catheter
- Two 3-mL syringes or tongue blade

- Scissors
- Washcloth and cleaning agent
- Skin barrier (e.g., 3M or Skin-Prep)
- Adhesive remover swab
- Towel
- Razor (optional)
- Shaving cream (optional)
- Sterile saline or water
- Handheld pressure gauge

ASSESSMENT

Assess for the need for retaping, which may include loose or soiled tape, pressure on mucous membranes, or repositioning of tube. Assess endotracheal tube length. The tube has markings on the side to ensure it is not moved during the retaping. Note the centimeter (cm) marking at the patient's lip or naris. Assess lung sounds to obtain a baseline. Ensure that the lung sounds are still heard throughout the lobes. Assess oxygen saturation level. If the tube is dislodged, the oxygen saturation level may change. Assess the chest for symmetric rise and fall during respiration. If the tube is dislodged, the rise and fall of the chest will change. Assess the patient's need for pain medication or sedation. Assess pain. The patient should be calm, free of pain, and relaxed during the retaping so as not to move and cause an accidental **extubation**. Inspect the area on the posterior portion of the neck for any skin breakdown that may result from irritation or pressure from tape or endotracheal tube holder.

| NURSING DIAGNOSIS | Determine the related factors for the nursing diagnoses based on the patient's current status. Appropriate nursing diagnoses may include: |

- Risk for impaired skin integrity
- Impaired oral mucous membrane
- Risk for injury

| OUTCOME IDENTIFICATION AND PLANNING | The expected outcome to achieve is that the tube remains in place, and the patient maintains bilaterally equal and clear lung sounds. Other outcomes may include the following: the patient demonstrates understanding about the reason for the endotracheal tube; skin remains intact; oxygen saturation remains within acceptable parameters; chest rises symmetrically; the patient's airway remains clear; and cuff pressure does not exceed 24 to 30 cm H_2O (Chenelle, Oto, Dulemanji, Fisher, & Kacmarek, 2015; Grant, 2013). |

IMPLEMENTATION

ACTION	**RATIONALE**
1. Gather equipment.	Assembling equipment provides for an organized approach to the task.
2. Perform hand hygiene and put on PPE, if indicated.	Hand hygiene and PPE prevent the spread of microorganisms. PPE is required based on transmission precautions.
3. Identify the patient.	Identifying the patient ensures the right patient receives the intervention and helps prevent errors.
4. Assemble equipment on the overbed table or other surface within reach.	Arranging items nearby is convenient, saves time, and avoids unnecessary stretching and twisting of muscles on the part of the nurse.
5. Close the curtains around the bed and close the door to the room, if possible.	This ensures the patient's privacy.
6. Assess the need for endotracheal tube retaping. **Administer pain medication or sedation, as prescribed, before attempting to retape endotracheal tube.** Explain what you are going to do and the reason for doing it to the patient, even if the patient does not appear to be alert.	Retaping the endotracheal tube can stimulate coughing, which may be painful for patients, particularly those with surgical incisions. Explanation alleviates fears, facilitates cooperation, and provides reassurance for the patient. Any procedure that may compromise respiration is frightening for the patient. Even if the patient appears unconscious, the nurse should explain what is happening.
7. Obtain the assistance of a second person to hold the endotracheal tube in place while the old tape is removed and the new tape is placed.	This prevents accidental extubation.
8. Adjust the bed to a comfortable working position, usually elbow height of the caregiver (VHACEOSH, 2016). Lower the side rail closest to you. **If conscious, place the patient in a semi-Fowler's position. If unconscious, place the patient in the lateral position, facing you.** Move the overbed table close to your work area and raise to waist height. Place a trash receptacle within easy reach of the work area.	Having the bed at the proper height prevents back and muscle strain. A sitting position helps the patient to cough and makes breathing easier. Gravity also facilitates catheter insertion. The lateral position prevents the airway from becoming obstructed and promotes drainage of secretions. The overbed table provides work surface and maintains sterility of objects on the work surface. Placing the trash receptacle within reach allows for an organized approach to care.
9. Put on face shield or goggles and mask. Suction patient as described in Skill 14-7 or 14-8.	PPE prevents exposure to contaminants. Suctioning decreases the likelihood of the patient coughing during the retaping of the endotracheal tube. If the patient coughs, the tube may become dislodged.

(continued)

Skill 14-9 ▶ Securing an Endotracheal Tube *(continued)*

ACTION	RATIONALE
10. Measure a piece of tape for the length needed to reach around the patient's neck to the mouth plus 8 in. Cut tape. Lay it adhesive side up on the table.	Extra length is needed so that tape can be wrapped around the endotracheal tube.
11. Cut another piece of tape long enough to reach from one jaw around the back of the neck to the other jaw. Lay this piece on the center of the longer piece on the table, matching the tapes' adhesive sides together.	This prevents the tape from sticking to the patient's hair and the back of the neck.
12. Take one 3-mL syringe or tongue blade and wrap the sticky tape around the syringe until the nonsticky area is reached. Do this for the other side as well.	This helps the nurse or respiratory therapist to manage the tape without it sticking to the sheets or the patient's hair.
13. Take one of the 3-mL syringes or tongue blades and pass it under the patient's neck so that there is a 3-mL syringe on either side of the patient's head.	This makes the tape easy to access when retaping the tube.
14. Put on disposable gloves. Have the assistant put on gloves as well.	Gloves protect hands from exposure to contaminants.
15. Provide oral care, including suctioning the oral cavity.	This helps to decrease secretions in the oral cavity and pharynx region.
16. Take note of the "cm" position markings on the tube. Begin to unwrap old tape from around the endotracheal tube. After one side is unwrapped, have assistant hold the endotracheal tube as close to the lips or naris as possible to offer stabilization.	Assistant should hold the tube to prevent accidental extubation. Holding the tube as close to lips or naris as possible prevents accidental dislodgement of tube.
17. Carefully remove the remaining tape from the endotracheal tube (Figure 2). **After tape is removed, have assistant gently and slowly move endotracheal tube (if orally intubated) to the other side of the mouth (Figure 3). Assess mouth for any skin breakdown. Before applying new tape, make sure that markings on endotracheal tube are at same spot as when retaping began.**	The endotracheal tube may cause pressure injuries if left in the same place over time. By moving the tube, the risk for pressure injury is reduced.

FIGURE 2. Ensuring endotracheal tube is stabilized and removing old tape.

FIGURE 3. Moving endotracheal tube to other side of mouth.

18. Remove old tape from cheeks and side of face. Use adhesive remover to remove excess adhesive from tape (Figure 4). Clean the face and neck with washcloth and cleanser. If patient has facial hair, consider shaving cheeks. Pat cheeks dry with the towel.	To prevent skin breakdown, remove old adhesive. Shaving helps to decrease pain when tape is removed. Cheeks must be dry before new tape is applied to ensure that it sticks.

ACTION	RATIONALE

FIGURE 4. Cleaning cheeks at site of tape.

19. Apply the skin barrier to the patient's face (under nose, on cheeks, and lower lip) where the tape will sit. Unroll one side of the tape. Ensure that nonstick part of tape remains behind the patient's neck while pulling firmly on the tape. Place adhesive portion of tape snugly against the patient's cheek. Keep track of the pilot balloon from the endotracheal tube, to avoid taping it to the patient's face. Split the tape in half from the end to the corner of the mouth.

Skin barrier protects the skin from injury with subsequent tape removal and helps the tape adhere better to the skin. The tape should be snug to the side of the patient's face to prevent accidental extubation.

20. Place the top-half piece of tape under the patient's nose (Figure 5). Wrap the lower half around the tube in one direction, such as over and around the tube. Fold over tab on end of tape.

By placing one piece of tape on the lip and the other piece of tape on the tube, the tube remains secure. Tab makes tape removal easier.

21. Unwrap second side of tape. Split to corner of the mouth. Place the bottom-half piece of tape along the patient's lower lip. Wrap the top half around the tube in the opposite direction, such as below and around the tube. Fold over tab on end of tape. Apply pressure to the tape on the endotracheal tube to ensure the tape is secure (Figure 6). Remove gloves.

Alternating the placement of the top and bottom pieces of tape provides more anchorage for the tube. Wrapping the tape in an alternating manner ensures that the tape will not accidentally be unwound.

FIGURE 5. Placing the top-half of the tape under the patient's nose.

FIGURE 6. Applying pressure to the tape on the endotracheal tube to ensure the tape is secure.

22. Auscultate lung sounds. Assess for cyanosis, oxygen saturation, chest symmetry, and endotracheal tube stability. Again check to ensure that the tube is at the correct depth.

If the tube has been moved from original place, the lung sounds may change, as well as oxygen saturation and chest symmetry. The tube should be stable and should not move with each respiration cycle.

(*continued*)

Skill 14-9 ▶ Securing an Endotracheal Tube *(continued)*

ACTION	**RATIONALE**
23. If the endotracheal tube is cuffed, check pressure of the balloon by attaching a handheld pressure gauge to the pilot balloon of the endotracheal tube.	Maximal cuff pressures should not exceed 24 to 30 cm H_2O to prevent excessive pressure on tracheal mucosal wall and surrounding structures and resulting tracheal ischemia and necrosis (Chenelle et al., 2015; Grant, 2013).
24. Assist the patient to a comfortable position. Raise the bed rail and place the bed in the lowest position.	Ensures patient comfort. Proper positioning with raised side rails and proper bed height provide for patient comfort and safety.
25. Remove face shield or goggles and mask. Remove additional PPE, if used. Perform hand hygiene.	Proper removal of PPE reduces the risk for infection transmission and contamination of other items. Hand hygiene prevents the spread of microorganisms.

EVALUATION

The expected outcome has been met when the endotracheal tube tape is changed without dislodgement or a depth change of the tube; lung sounds remain equal; no pressure injury is noted; airway remains clear; oxygen saturation remains within acceptable parameters; the patient's chest rises symmetrically; and cuff pressure does not exceed 24 to 30 cm H_2O (Chenelle et al., 2015; Grant, 2013).

DOCUMENTATION

Guidelines

Document the procedure, including the depth of the endotracheal tube from teeth, lips, or naris; the amount, consistency, and color of secretions suctioned; presence of any skin or mucous membrane changes or pressure injury; and your before and after assessments, including lung sounds, oxygen saturation, cuff pressure, and chest symmetry.

Sample Documentation

> <u>9/27/20</u> 1305 Endotracheal tube tape changed; tube remains 12 cm at lips; suctioned for tenacious, yellow secretions, copious in amount; 2-cm pressure injury noted on left side of tongue. Tube moved to right side of mouth; lung sounds clear and equal after retaping; pulse oximeter remains 98% on 35% FiO_2, cuff pressure 22 cm H_2O; chest rises symmetrically.
>
> —C. Bausler, RN

UNEXPECTED SITUATIONS AND ASSOCIATED INTERVENTIONS

- *Patient is accidentally extubated during tape change:* Stay with patient. Instruct assistant to notify primary care provider. Assess patient's vital signs, ability to breathe without assistance, and oxygen saturation. Be ready to deliver assisted breaths with a bag-valve mask (Skill 14-14) or administer oxygen. Anticipate the need for reintubation.
- *Tube depth changes during retaping:* Tube depth should be maintained at the same level unless otherwise ordered by the primary care provider. Remove tape around tube, adjust tube to ordered depth, and reapply tape.
- *Air leak (air escaping around the balloon) is heard on inspiration cycle of ventilator:* Auscultate lung sounds and check depth of endotracheal tube to ensure that it has not dislodged. Obtain handheld pressure gauge and check pressure. Air may need to be added to the balloon to prevent air leak. If pressure is already 24 to 30 cm H_2O, you may need to contact the primary care provider before adding more air to balloon. Sometimes, a change in the patient's position will resolve air leaks.
- *Patient is biting on endotracheal tube:* Obtain a bite block. With the help of an assistant, place the bite block around the endotracheal tube or in patient's mouth. If ordered, consider sedating the patient.
- *Depth of endotracheal tube changes with respiratory cycle:* Remove old tape. Repeat taping of the endotracheal tube, ensuring that tape is snug against the patient's face.
- *Patient has trauma to face that prevents the use of tape when securing the endotracheal tube:* You may need to obtain a commercially prepared endotracheal tube holder. There are various types on the market; check with your facility for availability.
- *Lung sounds are greater on one side:* Check the depth of the endotracheal tube. If the tube has been advanced, the lung sounds will appear greater on the side on which the tube is further down.

Remove tape and move tube so that it is placed properly. If the depth has not changed, assess patient's oxygen saturation, and respiratory rate. Notify primary care provider. Anticipate the need for a chest x-ray.

- *Pressure injury is noted in the mouth or naris (if patient is intubated via naris):* If the ulcer is painful, you may obtain an order for a topical numbing medication, such as lidocaine viscous jelly. Apply topically with cotton-tipped applicator. Keep area clean by performing more frequent oral or nasal care. Ensure that ventilator or oxygen tubing is not pulling on the endotracheal tube, thus applying pressure on the patient's skin.
- *Pilot balloon is accidentally cut while caring for endotracheal tube:* Notify primary care provider. Obtain a 22-gauge IV catheter and thread it into the pilot balloon tubing, being careful not to puncture the tubing with the needle, below the cut. Remove the needle from the catheter and apply a stopcock or needleless Luer-Lok to the catheter. If air is needed to reinflate the balloon, a syringe can be attached to the stopcock or Luer-Lok so that air may be added. Anticipate the need for an endotracheal tube change.

SPECIAL CONSIDERATIONS

- Make sure emergency equipment is easily accessible at the bedside. Keep bag-valve mask, oxygen, an extra endotracheal tube of the same size, and suction equipment at the bedside of a patient with an endotracheal tube at all times.

EVIDENCE FOR PRACTICE ▶

SECURING ENDOTRACHEAL TUBES

Maintenance of the airway is imperative for patients who are intubated. Oral tracheal intubation is a commonly performed intervention for critically ill patients who need ventilatory support. Unplanned removal or displacement of the tube can be a life-threatening event. Various methods, including tape and commercially marketed devices, are available to prevent accidental removal or displacement.

Related Research

Fisher, D. F., Chenelle, C. T., Marchese, A. D., Kratohvil, J. P., & Kacmarek, R. M. (2014). Comparison of commercial and noncommercial endotracheal tube-securing devices. *Respiratory Care, 59*(9), 1315–1323.

This study examined 16 commercially available endotracheal tube holders and a noncommercial device (adhesive tape) in simulated clinical conditions. The security of the endotracheal tubes (16 of the 16) was tested by measuring distance displaced after tugging on the tube. The holders were also evaluated for speed of moving the endotracheal tube to the opposite side of the mouth (9 of the 16). The force applied by the holder to the patient's skin and face was calculated with a sensor located on a mannequin and measured when the head was rotated vertically or horizontally. A weight was attached to the endotracheal tube using nylon line and dropped to simulate a tug on the tube. Tube displacement distance as a result of the tug test was the same for both commercial and noncommercial devices. Seventeen extubations occurred during testing, all with the commercial devices. It took less time to move the endotracheal tube using the commercial devices compared with noncommercial devices. The commercially available holders exerted more pressure than noncommercial devices. The researchers suggested that noncommercial airway holders exert less force on a patient's face than commercial devices, and the type of securing method affects airway stability. Many commercial holders allow for rapid but secure movement of the artificial airway. The authors concluded that neither type of securement method is superior in all characteristics and situations.

Relevance for Nursing Practice

Nurses are in an important position to influence patient care practices. It is also important to provide cost-efficient and effective care, because this is becoming an increasingly important issue in health care. There may be no one ideal device or method for securing an endotracheal tube; nurses must be aware of the specifics for the available methods and facility policy to guide patient care decisions to provide individualized, patient-centered care.

Refer to thePoint® for additional research on related nursing topics.

Skill 14-10 ▶ Suctioning a Tracheostomy: Open System

The purpose of suctioning is to maintain a patent airway and remove pulmonary secretions, blood, vomitus, or foreign material from the airway. When suctioning via a tracheostomy tube, the goal is to remove secretions that are not accessible to cilia bypassed by the tube itself. Tracheal suctioning can lead to hypoxemia, cardiac dysrhythmias, trauma, atelectasis, infection, bleeding, and pain. Therefore, it is imperative to be diligent in maintaining aseptic technique and in following facility guidelines and procedures to prevent potential hazards. In the home setting and other community-based settings, clean technique is used, as the patient is not exposed to disease-causing organisms that may be found in health care settings, such as hospitals (Sterni et al., 2016). Tracheal suctioning should be performed only when clinically indicated and not routinely (AARC, 2010; Morton & Fontaine, 2018; Sole et al., 2015).

Because suctioning removes secretions not accessible to bypassed cilia, the recommendation is to insert the catheter only as far as the end of the endotracheal tube. Catheter contact and suction can cause tracheal mucosal damage, loss of cilia, edema, and fibrosis, and increase the risk of infection and bleeding for the patient. Insertion of the suction catheter to a predetermined distance, no more than 1 cm past the length of the tracheostomy tube (adults) and 0.5 cm (pediatric patients), avoids contact with the trachea and carina, reducing the effects of tracheal mucosal damage (Boroughs & Dougherty, 2015; Hahn, 2010; Ireton, 2007). Box 14-1 in Skill 14-7 discusses several methods for determining appropriate suction catheter depth. The suction catheter should be small enough not to occlude the airway being suctioned but large enough to remove secretions; in adults, use a suction catheter that occludes less than 50% of the lumen of the tracheostomy or endotracheal tube and 50% in pediatric patients (AARC, 2010; Hockenberry & Wilson, 2015).

Tracheal suctioning is an uncomfortable procedure at minimum, and it can be a very painful and/or distressing experience. Therefore, anticipate assessing for the need for the administration of analgesic medication to a patient before suctioning (Arroyo-Novoa et al., 2008; Düzkaya & Kuğuoğlu, 2015). As mentioned previously, perform suctioning only when clinically necessary because of the many potential risks, including hypoxia, infection, tracheal tissue damage, dysrhythmias, and atelectasis.

Note: In-line, closed suction systems are available to suction mechanically ventilated patients. The use of closed suction catheter systems may avoid some of the infection control issues and other complications associated with open suction techniques. The closed suctioning procedure is the same for patients with tracheostomy tubes and endotracheal tubes connected to mechanical ventilation. See Skill 14-8.

DELEGATION CONSIDERATIONS

Suctioning a tracheostomy is not delegated to nursing assistive personnel (NAP) or to unlicensed assistive personnel (UAP). Depending on the state's nurse practice act and the organization's policies and procedures, suctioning of a tracheostomy in a stable situation, such as long-term care and other community-based care settings, may be delegated to licensed practical/vocational nurses (LPN/LVNs). The decision to delegate must be based on careful analysis of the patient's needs and circumstances, as well as the qualifications of the person to whom the task is being delegated. Refer to the Delegation Guidelines in Appendix A.

EQUIPMENT

- Portable or wall suction unit with tubing
- A commercially prepared suction kit with an appropriate-size catheter (see General Considerations) or
- Sterile suction catheter with Y-port in the appropriate size
- Sterile, disposable container
- Sterile gloves
- Towel or waterproof pad
- Goggles and mask or face shield
- Additional PPE, as indicated
- Disposable, clean gloves
- Resuscitation bag connected to 100% oxygen

ASSESSMENT	Assess for coarse crackles over the trachea, the most common indicator for endotracheal suctioning (Sole et al., 2015). Assess lung sounds. Wheezes, crackles, gurgling or diminished breath sounds may indicate the need for suctioning. Assess for the presence of visualized secretions in the artificial airway, audible secretions, and ineffective coughing (Morton & Fontaine, 2018; Sole et al.). Assess oxygen saturation level. Deterioration in oxygen desaturation may be an indication of the need for suctioning (AARC, 2010). Assess respiratory status, including respiratory rate and depth. Patients may become tachypneic when they need to be suctioned. Assess the patient for signs of respiratory distress, such as nasal flaring, retractions, or grunting. Additional indications for suctioning via a tracheostomy tube include acute respiratory distress, and frequent or sustained coughing. Also assess for pain and the potential to cause pain during the intervention. Perform individualized pain management in response to the patient's needs (Arroyo-Novoa et al., 2008; Dükaya & Kuğuoğlu, 2015). Administer pain medication, as prescribed, before suctioning. Assess appropriate suction catheter depth. Refer to Box 14-1 in Skill 14-7. Assess the characteristics and amount of secretions while suctioning.
NURSING DIAGNOSIS	Determine the related factors for the nursing diagnoses based on the patient's current status. Appropriate nursing diagnoses may include: • Ineffective airway clearance • Impaired gas exchange • Risk for aspiration
OUTCOME IDENTIFICATION AND PLANNING	The expected outcome is that the patient will exhibit a clear, patent airway. Other outcomes that may be appropriate include the following: the patient will exhibit an oxygen saturation level within acceptable parameters; the patient will demonstrate a respiratory rate and depth within acceptable parameters; and the patient will remain free from any signs of respiratory distress.

IMPLEMENTATION

ACTION	**RATIONALE**
1. Gather equipment.	Assembling equipment provides for an organized approach to the task.
2. Perform hand hygiene and put on PPE, if indicated.	Hand hygiene and PPE prevent the spread of microorganisms. PPE is required based on transmission precautions.
3. Identify the patient.	Identifying the patient ensures the right patient receives the intervention and helps prevent errors.
4. Assemble equipment on the overbed table or other surface within reach.	Arranging items nearby is convenient, saves time, and avoids unnecessary stretching and twisting of muscles on the part of the nurse.
5. Close the curtains around the bed and close the door to the room, if possible.	This ensures the patient's privacy.
6. Determine the need for suctioning. Verify the suction order in the patient's medical record. **Assess for pain or the potential to cause pain. Administer pain medication, as prescribed, before suctioning.**	Tracheal suctioning should be performed only when clinically indicated and not routinely (AARC, 2010; Morton & Fontaine, 2018; Sole et al., 2015). Suctioning can cause moderate to severe pain for patients. Individualized pain management is imperative (Arroyo-Novoa et al., 2008; Düzkaya & Kuğuoğlu, 2015). Suctioning stimulates coughing, which is painful for patients with surgical incisions.

(continued)

Skill 14-10 ▶ Suctioning a Tracheostomy: Open System *(continued)*

ACTION	**RATIONALE**
7. Explain to the patient what you are going to do and the reason for doing it, even if the patient does not appear to be alert. Reassure the patient you will interrupt the procedure if he or she indicates respiratory difficulty.	Explanation alleviates fears. Even if the patient appears unconscious, the nurse should explain what is happening. Any procedure that compromises respiration is frightening for the patient.
8. Adjust the bed to a comfortable working position, usually elbow height of the caregiver (VHACEOSH, 2016). Lower the side rail closest to you. **If conscious, place the patient in a semi-Fowler's position (Figure 1). If unconscious, place the patient in the lateral position, facing you.**	Having the bed at the proper height prevents back and muscle strain. A sitting position helps the patient to cough and makes breathing easier. Gravity also facilitates catheter insertion. The lateral position prevents the airway from becoming obstructed and promotes drainage of secretions.
9. Place a towel or waterproof pad across the patient's chest.	This protects bed linens and the patient.
10. **Adjust suction to appropriate pressure (Figure 2).**	Higher pressures can cause excessive trauma, hypoxemia, and atelectasis.
• Using a wall unit for adults and adolescents: no more than 150 mm Hg; neonates: no more than 80 mm Hg; infants: no more than 100 mm Hg; children: no more than 125 mm Hg (Hess et al., 2016).	
• For a portable unit for an adult: 10 to 15 cm Hg; neonates: 6 to 8 cm Hg; infants: 8 to 10 cm Hg; children: 8 to 10 cm Hg; adolescents: 8 to 15 cm Hg. Put on a disposable, clean glove and occlude the end of the connecting tubing to check suction pressure. Place the connecting tubing in a convenient location. If using, place the resuscitation bag connected to oxygen within convenient reach.	Higher pressures can cause excessive trauma, hypoxemia, and atelectasis. Glove prevents contact with blood and body fluids. Checking pressure ensures equipment is working properly. Preparation allows for an organized approach to the procedure.

FIGURE 1. Patient in semi-Fowler's position.

FIGURE 2. Turning suction unit to appropriate pressure.

11. Open the sterile suction package using aseptic technique. The open wrapper or container becomes a sterile field to hold other supplies. Carefully remove the sterile container, touching only the outside surface. Set it up on the work surface and pour sterile saline into it.	Sterile normal saline or water is used to lubricate the outside of the catheter, minimizing irritation of mucosa during introduction. It is also used to clear the catheter between suction attempts.

ACTION	RATIONALE

12. Put on face shield or goggles and mask (Figure 3). Put on sterile gloves. **The dominant hand will manipulate the catheter and must remain sterile. The nondominant hand is considered clean rather than sterile and will control the suction valve (Y-port) on the catheter.**

Handling the sterile catheter using a sterile glove helps prevent introducing organisms into the respiratory tract; the clean glove protects the nurse from microorganisms.

13. With the dominant gloved hand, pick up the sterile catheter. Pick up the connecting tubing with the nondominant hand and connect the tubing and suction catheter (Figure 4).

Suction catheter sterility is maintained.

FIGURE 3. Putting on goggles and mask.

FIGURE 4. Connecting suction catheter to suction tubing.

14. Moisten the catheter by dipping it into the container of sterile saline, unless it is a silicone catheter (Figure 5). Occlude Y-tube to check suction (Figure 6).

Lubricating the inside of the catheter with saline helps move secretions in the catheter. Silicone catheters do not require lubrication. Checking ensures equipment is working properly.

FIGURE 5. Moistening catheter in saline solution.

FIGURE 6. Occluding Y-port to check for proper suction.

15. Using your nondominant hand and a manual resuscitation bag, hyperventilate the patient, delivering three to six breaths or use the sigh mechanism on a mechanical ventilator.

Hyperoxygenation and hyperventilation aid in preventing hypoxemia during suctioning.

16. Remove the manual resuscitation bag or open the adapter on the mechanical ventilator tubing with your nondominant hand.

This exposes the tracheostomy tube without contaminating sterile gloved hand.

(continued)

Skill 14-10 ▶ Suctioning a Tracheostomy: Open System *(continued)*

ACTION	RATIONALE
17. Using your dominant hand, gently and quickly insert the catheter into the trachea. **Advance the catheter to the predetermined length. Do not occlude the Y-port when inserting the catheter.**	Catheter contact and suction cause tracheal mucosal damage, loss of cilia, edema, and fibrosis, and increase the risk of infection and bleeding for the patient. Insertion of the suction catheter to a predetermined distance, no more than 1 cm past the length of the endotracheal tube, avoids contact with the trachea and carina, reducing the effects of tracheal mucosal damage (Boroughs & Dougherty, 2015; Hahn, 2010; Ireton, 2007). If resistance is met, the carina or tracheal mucosa has been hit. Withdraw the catheter at least 0.5 in before applying suction. Suctioning when inserting the catheter increases the risk for trauma to airway mucosa and increases the risk of hypoxemia.
18. Apply suction by intermittently occluding the Y-port on the catheter with the thumb of your nondominant hand, and gently rotate the catheter as it is being withdrawn (Figure 7). **Do not suction for more than 10 to 15 seconds at a time.**	Turning the catheter as it is withdrawn minimizes trauma to the mucosa. Suctioning for longer than 15 seconds robs the respiratory tract of oxygen, which may result in hypoxemia (AARC, 2010). Suctioning too quickly may be ineffective at clearing all secretions.

FIGURE 7. Intermittently occluding the Y-port on the catheter to apply suction while withdrawing catheter.

ACTION	RATIONALE
19. Hyperventilate the patient using your nondominant hand and a manual resuscitation bag, delivering three to six breaths. Replace the oxygen delivery device, if applicable, using your nondominant hand and have the patient take several deep breaths. If the patient is mechanically ventilated, close the adapter on the mechanical ventilator tubing and use the sigh mechanism on a mechanical ventilator.	Suctioning removes air from the patient's airway and can cause hypoxemia. Hyperventilation can help prevent suction-induced hypoxemia.
20. Flush the catheter with saline. Assess the effectiveness of suctioning and repeat, as needed, according to the patient's tolerance. Wrap the suction catheter around your dominant hand between attempts.	Flushing clears the catheter and lubricates it for next insertion. Reassessment determines the need for additional suctioning. Wrapping the catheter around the hand prevents inadvertent contamination of the catheter.
21. **Allow at least a 30-second to 1-minute interval if additional suctioning is needed. Do not make more than three suction passes per suctioning episode. Encourage the patient to cough and deep breathe between suctioning attempts.** Suction the oropharynx after suctioning the trachea. Do not reinsert in the tracheostomy after suctioning the mouth.	The interval allows for reventilation and reoxygenation of airways. Excessive suction passes contribute to complications. Clears the mouth of secretions. More microorganisms are usually present in the mouth, so it is suctioned last to prevent transmission of contaminants.

ACTION	**RATIONALE**

22. Perform oral hygiene after tracheal suctioning.

Respiratory secretions that are allowed to accumulate in the mouth are irritating to mucous membranes, pose a risk for aspiration, and are unpleasant for the patient. Oral hygiene care can limit the growth of pathogens in the oropharyngeal secretions, decreasing the incidence of aspiration pneumonia, community-acquired pneumonia, hospital-acquired nonventilator-associated pneumonia, and ventilator-associated pneumonia (AACN, 2010; Coker et al., 2013; Hillier et al., 2013; Quinn & Baker, 2015).

23. When suctioning is completed, coil the catheter in one hand. Remove the glove from the hand over the coiled catheter (catheter remains inside glove), pulling the glove off inside out (Figure 8). Remove the glove from the other hand, pulling inside out, and dispose of gloves, catheter, and container with solution in the appropriate receptacle. Assist the patient to a comfortable position. Raise the bed rail and place the bed in the lowest position.

This technique reduces transmission of microorganisms. Ensures patient comfort. Proper positioning with raised side rails and proper bed height provide for patient comfort and safety.

FIGURE 8. Removing gloves while keeping catheter inside.

 24. Turn off suction. Remove supplemental oxygen placed for suctioning, if appropriate. Remove face shield or goggles and mask. Perform hand hygiene.

Proper removal of PPE reduces the risk for infection transmission and contamination of other items. Hand hygiene prevents transmission of microorganisms.

25. Reassess the patient's respiratory status, including respiratory rate, effort, oxygen saturation, and lung sounds.

Assesses the effectiveness of suctioning and the presence of complications.

 26. Remove additional PPE, if used. Perform hand hygiene.

Proper removal of PPE reduces the risk for infection transmission and contamination of other items. Hand hygiene prevents the spread of microorganisms.

EVALUATION

The expected outcomes have been met when the patient exhibits a clear, patent airway; an oxygen saturation level within acceptable parameters; a respiratory rate and depth within acceptable parameters; and the patient remains free from any signs of respiratory distress.

DOCUMENTATION

Guidelines

Document the time of suctioning, your assessments before and after intervention, reason for suctioning, and the characteristics and amount of secretions.

(continued)

Skill 14-10 ▶ Suctioning a Tracheostomy: Open System *(continued)*

Sample Documentation

> <u>9/1/20</u> 1515 Yellow secretions noted in opening of tracheostomy tube; coarse crackles noted to auscultation over trachea. Lungs auscultated for wheezes in upper and lower lobes bilaterally. Respirations at 24 breaths/min. Weak, ineffective cough noted. Tracheal suction completed with 12-Fr catheter. Large amount of thick, yellow secretions obtained. Specimen for culture collected and sent, as ordered. After suctioning, no secretions noted in tracheostomy tube, auscultation over trachea clear, faint wheezing persists, oxygen saturation at 97%, respirations 18 breaths/min.
>
> —C. Bausler, RN

UNEXPECTED SITUATIONS AND ASSOCIATED INTERVENTIONS

- *Patient coughs hard enough to dislodge tracheostomy:* Keep a spare tracheostomy and obturator at the bedside. Insert obturator into tracheostomy tube and reinsert tracheostomy into stoma. Remove obturator. Secure ties and auscultate lung sounds. Palpate for any **subcutaneous emphysema.**
- *Tracheostomy becomes dislodged and is not easily replaced:* Notify the primary care provider immediately. This is an emergency situation. Cover the tracheostomy stoma. Assess the patient's respiratory status. Anticipate the possible need for maintaining ventilation using a manual resuscitation device and mask, and for possible oro- or nasotracheal intubation.
- *Lung sounds do not improve greatly and oxygen saturation remains low after three suctioning attempts:* Allow the patient time to recover from previous suctioning. If needed, hyperoxygenate again. Suction the patient again and assess whether the oxygen saturation increases, lung sounds improve, and secretion amount decreases.

SPECIAL CONSIDERATIONS

General Considerations

- Determine the size of the catheter to use by the size of the tracheostomy. The external diameter of the suction catheter should occlude less than 50% of the lumen of the tracheostomy or endotracheal tube and 50% in pediatric patients (AARC, 2010; Hockenberry & Wilson, 2015). Larger catheters can contribute to trauma and hypoxemia.
- The practice of instillation of saline solution directly into the airway is not supported by evidence and is not recommended for inclusion as part of evidence-based practice and suctioning (AARC, 2010; Boroughs & Dougherty, 2015; Khimani et al., 2015; Leddy & Wilkinson, 2015; Owen et al., 2016).
- Make sure emergency equipment is easily accessible at the bedside. Keep a bag-valve mask, oxygen, the obturator from the current tracheostomy, spare tracheostomy of the same size, spare tracheostomy one size smaller, and suction equipment at the bedside of a patient with a tracheostomy tube at all times.
- If the patient is currently using a tracheostomy without a cuff, keep a spare tracheostomy of the same size with a cuff at the bedside for emergency use.

Skill 14-11 ▶ Providing Care of a Tracheostomy Tube

The nurse is responsible for either replacing a disposable inner cannula or cleaning a nondisposable inner cannula. The inner cannula requires replacement or cleaning to prevent accumulation of secretions that can interfere with respiration and occlude the airway. Because soiled tracheostomy dressings place the patient at risk for the development of skin breakdown and infection, regularly change dressings and tracheostomy collar or ties. Use gauze dressings that are not filled with cotton to prevent aspiration of foreign bodies (e.g., lint or cotton fibers) into the trachea. Clean the skin around a tracheostomy to prevent buildup of dried secretions and skin breakdown. Exercise care when changing the tracheostomy collar or ties to prevent accidental decannulation or expulsion of the tube. Have an assistant hold the tube in place during the changing of a collar. When changing a tracheostomy tie, keep the soiled tie in place until a clean one is securely attached. Facility policy and patient condition determine specific procedures and schedules, but a newly inserted tracheostomy may require attention every 1 to 2 hours. Because the respiratory tract is sterile and the tracheostomy provides a direct opening, meticulous care is necessary when using aseptic technique. Once the tracheostomy site is healed, in the home setting and other community-based settings, clean technique is used, as the patient is not exposed to disease-causing organisms that may be found in health care settings, such as hospitals.

DELEGATION CONSIDERATIONS

Care of a tracheostomy tube is not delegated to nursing assistive personnel (NAP) or to unlicensed assistive personnel (UAP). Depending on the state's nurse practice act and the organization's policies and procedures, care of a tracheostomy tube in a stable situation, such as long-term care and other community-based care settings, may be delegated to licensed practical/vocational nurses (LPN/LVNs). The decision to delegate must be based on careful analysis of the patient's needs and circumstances, as well as the qualifications of the person to whom the task is being delegated. Refer to the Delegation Guidelines in Appendix A.

EQUIPMENT

- Disposable gloves
- Sterile gloves
- Goggles and mask or face shield
- Additional PPE, as indicated
- Sterile normal saline
- Sterile cup or basin
- Sterile cotton-tipped applicators
- Sterile gauze sponges

- Disposable inner tracheostomy cannula, appropriate size for the patient
- Sterile suction catheter and glove set
- Commercially prepared tracheostomy or drain dressing
- Commercially prepared tracheostomy holder
- Plastic disposal bag
- Additional nurse

ASSESSMENT

Assess for signs and symptoms of the need to perform tracheostomy care, which include soiled dressings and holder or ties, secretions in the tracheostomy tube, and diminished airflow through the tracheostomy, or in accordance with facility policy. Assess insertion site for any redness or purulent drainage; if present, these may signify an infection. Assess patient for pain. If the tracheostomy is new, pain medication may be needed before performing tracheostomy care. Assess lung sounds and oxygen saturation levels. Lung sounds should be equal in all lobes, with an oxygen saturation level within acceptable parameters. If tracheostomy is dislodged, lung sounds and oxygen saturation level will diminish. Inspect the area on the posterior portion of the neck for any skin breakdown that may result from irritation or pressure from tracheostomy holder or ties.

NURSING DIAGNOSIS

Determine the related factors for the nursing diagnoses based on the patient's current status. Appropriate nursing diagnoses may include:

- Impaired skin integrity
- Risk for infection

- Ineffective airway clearance

OUTCOME IDENTIFICATION AND PLANNING

The expected outcome to achieve when performing tracheostomy care is that the patient will exhibit a tracheostomy tube and site free from drainage, secretions, and skin irritation or breakdown and a patent airway. Other outcomes that may be appropriate include the following: oxygen saturation levels will be within acceptable parameters, and the patient will have no evidence of respiratory distress.

IMPLEMENTATION

ACTION	RATIONALE
1. Gather equipment.	Assembling equipment provides for an organized approach to the task.
2. Perform hand hygiene and put on PPE, if indicated.	Hand hygiene and PPE prevent the spread of microorganisms. PPE is required based on transmission precautions.

(continued)

Skill 14-11 ▶ Providing Care of a Tracheostomy Tube *(continued)*

ACTION	RATIONALE

3. Identify the patient.

Identifying the patient ensures the right patient receives the intervention and helps prevent errors.

4. Assemble equipment on the overbed table or other surface within reach.

Arranging items nearby is convenient, saves time, and avoids unnecessary stretching and twisting of muscles on the part of the nurse.

5. Close the curtains around the bed and close the door to the room, if possible.

This ensures the patient's privacy.

6. Determine the need for tracheostomy care. **Assess the patient's pain and administer pain medication, if indicated.**

If tracheostomy is new, pain medication may be needed before performing tracheostomy care.

7. Explain what you are going to do and the reason for doing it to the patient, even if the patient does not appear to be alert. Reassure the patient you will interrupt the procedure if he or she indicates respiratory difficulty.

Explanation alleviates fears. Even if the patient appears unconscious, the nurse should explain what is happening. Any procedure that compromises respiration is frightening for the patient.

8. Adjust the bed to a comfortable working position, usually elbow height of the caregiver (VHACEOSH, 2016). Lower the side rail closest to you. **If conscious, place the patient in a semi-Fowler's position. If unconscious, place the patient in the lateral position, facing you.** Move the overbed table close to your work area and raise it to waist height. Place a trash receptacle within easy reach of the work area.

Having the bed at the proper height prevents back and muscle strain. A sitting position helps the patient to cough and makes breathing easier. Gravity also facilitates catheter insertion. The lateral position prevents the airway from becoming obstructed and promotes drainage of secretions. The overbed table provides a work surface and maintains sterility of objects on the work surface. Trash receptacle within reach prevents reaching over the sterile field or turning back to the field to dispose of trash.

9. Put on face shield or goggles and mask. Suction tracheostomy, if necessary. If tracheostomy has just been suctioned, remove soiled site dressing and discard before removal of gloves used to perform suctioning.

PPE prevents contact with contaminants. Suctioning removes secretions to prevent occluding the outer cannula while the inner cannula is removed.

Cleaning the Tracheostomy: Disposable Inner Cannula

(See the accompanying Skill Variation for steps for cleaning a non-disposable inner cannula.)

10. Carefully open the package with the new disposable inner cannula, taking care not to contaminate the cannula or the inside of the package (Figure 1). Carefully open the package with the sterile cotton-tipped applicators, taking care not to contaminate them. Open the sterile cup or basin and fill 0.5 in deep with saline. Open the plastic disposable bag and place within reach on work surface.

Inner cannula must remain sterile. Saline and applicators will be used to clean the tracheostomy site. Plastic disposable bag will be used to discard removed inner cannula.

FIGURE 1. Carefully opening package with new disposable inner cannula. (*Photo by B. Proud.*)

ACTION	**RATIONALE**
11. Put on disposable gloves.	Gloves protect against exposure to blood and body fluids.
12. Remove the oxygen source if one is present. Stabilize the outer cannula and faceplate of the tracheostomy with your nondominant hand. Grasp the locking mechanism of the inner cannula with your dominant hand. Press the tabs and release the lock (Figure 2). Gently remove the inner cannula and place in disposal bag. If not already removed, remove site dressing and dispose of it in the trash.	Stabilizing the faceplate prevents trauma to, and pain from, the stoma. Releasing the lock permits removal of the inner cannula.
13. Working quickly, discard gloves and put on sterile gloves. Pick up the new inner cannula with your dominant hand; stabilize the faceplate with your nondominant hand and gently insert the new inner cannula into the outer cannula. Press the tabs to allow the lock to grab the outer cannula (Figure 3). Reapply oxygen source, if needed.	Sterile gloves are necessary to prevent contamination of the new inner cannula. Locking to outer cannula secures the inner cannula in place. Maintains oxygen supply to the patient.

FIGURE 2. Releasing lock on inner cannula.

FIGURE 3. Locking new inner cannula in place.

Applying Clean Dressing and Holder

(See accompanying Skill Variations for steps for an alternate site dressing if a commercially prepared sponge is not available and to secure a tracheostomy with tracheostomy ties/tape instead of a collar.)

14. Remove oxygen source, if necessary. Dip cotton-tipped applicator or gauze sponge in cup or basin with sterile saline and clean stoma under faceplate. Use each applicator or sponge only once, moving from stoma site outward (Figure 4).	Saline is nonirritating to tissue. Cleansing from stoma outward and using each applicator only once promotes aseptic technique.

FIGURE 4. Cleaning from stoma site, outward.

15. Pat skin gently with dry 4 × 4 gauze sponge.	Gauze removes excess moisture.

(*continued*)

Skill 14-11 ▶ Providing Care of a Tracheostomy Tube *(continued)*

ACTION	RATIONALE
16. Slide commercially prepared tracheostomy dressing or prefolded non–cotton-filled 4 × 4-in dressing under the faceplate.	Lint or fiber from a cut cotton-filled gauze pad can be aspirated into the trachea, causing respiratory distress, or can embed in the stoma and cause irritation or infection.
17. Change the tracheostomy holder:	
a. Obtain the assistance of a second person to hold the tracheostomy tube in place while the old collar is removed and the new collar is placed.	Holding the tracheostomy tube in place ensures that the tracheostomy will not inadvertently be expelled if the patient coughs or moves. Doing so provides attachment for one side of the faceplate.
b. Open the package for the new tracheostomy collar.	Allows access to the new collar.
c. Both nurses should put on clean gloves.	Gloves prevent contact with blood, body fluids, and contaminants.
d. One nurse holds the faceplate while the other pulls up the Velcro tabs. Gently remove the collar.	Holding the tracheostomy tube in place ensures that the tracheostomy will not inadvertently be expelled if the patient coughs or moves. Pulling up the Velcro tabs loosens the collar.
e. The first nurse continues to hold the tracheostomy faceplate.	Prevents accidental extubation.
f. The other nurse places the collar around the patient's neck and inserts first one tab, then the other, into the openings on the faceplate and secures the Velcro tabs on the tracheostomy holder (Figure 5).	Securing the Velcro tabs holds the tracheostomy in place and prevents accidental expulsion of the tracheostomy tube.
g. Check the fit of the tracheostomy collar. You should be able to fit one finger between the neck and the collar. Check to make sure that the patient can flex the neck comfortably. Reapply the oxygen source, if necessary (Figure 6).	Allowing one fingerbreadth under the collar permits neck flexion that is comfortable and ensures that the collar will not compromise circulation to the area. Maintains oxygen supply to the patient.

FIGURE 5. Securing tabs on tracheostomy holder.

FIGURE 6. Reapplying oxygen source.

18. Remove gloves. Remove face shield or goggles and mask. Assist the patient to a comfortable position. Raise the bed rail and place the bed in the lowest position.	Proper removal of PPE reduces the risk for infection transmission and contamination of other items. Ensures patient comfort. Proper positioning with raised side rails and proper bed height provide for patient comfort and safety.
19. Reassess the patient's respiratory status, including respiratory rate, effort, oxygen saturation, and lung sounds.	Assessments determine the effectiveness of interventions and for the presence of complications.
20. Remove additional PPE, if used. Perform hand hygiene.	Proper removal of PPE reduces the risk for infection transmission and contamination of other items. Hand hygiene prevents the spread of microorganisms.

EVALUATION

The expected outcome has been met when the patient exhibits a tracheostomy tube and site that are free from drainage, secretions, and skin irritation or breakdown; oxygen saturation level is within acceptable parameters; airway is patent; and the patient is without evidence of respiratory distress. In addition, the patient verbalizes that the site is free of pain and exhibits no evidence of skin breakdown on the posterior portion of the neck.

DOCUMENTATION

Guidelines

Document your assessments before and after interventions, including site assessment, presence of pain, lung sounds, and oxygen saturation levels. Document presence of skin breakdown that may result from irritation or pressure from the tracheostomy collar. Document care given.

Sample Documentation

> <u>9/26/20</u> 1300 Tracheostomy care completed; lung sounds clear in all lobes; respirations even/unlabored; site without erythema or edema; small amount of thick, yellow secretions noted at site, oxygen saturation 95% on O_2 35% via trach collar.
>
> —*C. Bausler, RN*

UNEXPECTED SITUATIONS AND ASSOCIATED INTERVENTIONS

- *Patient coughs hard enough to dislodge tracheostomy:* Keep a spare tracheostomy and obturator at bedside. Insert obturator into the new tracheostomy and insert tracheostomy into stoma. Remove obturator. Secure ties and auscultate lung sounds. Palpate for any subcutaneous emphysema.
- *Tracheostomy becomes dislodged and is not easily replaced:* Notify the primary care provider immediately. This is an emergency situation. Cover the tracheostomy stoma. Assess the patient's respiratory status. Anticipate the possible need for maintaining ventilation using a manual resuscitation device and mask, and for possible oro- or nasotracheal intubation.
- *On palpating around the insertion site, you note a moderate amount of subcutaneous emphysema in tissue:* Assess for dislodgement of the tracheostomy tube. If the tube has become displaced, a buildup of air in the subcutaneous portion of the skin is likely. Notify the primary care provider if the subcutaneous emphysema is a change in the status of the tracheostomy.

SPECIAL CONSIDERATIONS

General Considerations

- One nurse working alone should always place new tracheostomy ties before removing old ties to prevent accidental extubation of the tracheostomy. If it is necessary to remove old ties first, obtain the assistance of a second person to hold the tracheostomy tube in place while the old tie is removed and the new tie is replaced.
- Make sure emergency equipment is easily accessible at the bedside. Keep a bag-valve mask, oxygen, the obturator from the current tracheostomy, spare tracheostomy of the same size, spare tracheostomy one size smaller, and suction equipment at the bedside of a patient with a tracheostomy tube at all times.
- If the patient is currently using a tracheostomy without a cuff, keep a spare tracheostomy of the same size with a cuff at the bedside for emergency use.

Home Care Considerations

- Instruct the patient and home caregiver on how to perform tracheostomy care. Observe a return demonstration and provide feedback.
- Clean, rather than sterile, technique can be used in the home setting.
- Sterile saline can be made by mixing 1 teaspoon of table salt in 1 quart of water and boiling for 15 minutes. The solution is cooled and stored in a clean, dry container. Discard saline at the end of each day to prevent growth of bacteria.
- Instruct the patient who is performing self-care to use a mirror to view the steps in the procedure.

(*continued*)

Skill 14-11 ▶ Providing Care of a Tracheostomy Tube *(continued)*

Skill Variation ▶ Cleaning a Nondisposable Inner Cannula

Some tracheostomies use nondisposable inner cannulas, requiring the nurse to clean the inner cannula. Aseptic technique is maintained during the procedure. Clean, rather than sterile, technique can be used in the home setting. Additional equipment includes the following: sterile tracheostomy cleaning kit, if available, or three sterile basins; sterile brush/pipe cleaners; and sterile cleaning solutions (hydrogen peroxide and normal saline solution).

1. Perform hand hygiene and put on PPE, if indicated.

2. Identify the patient.

3. Assemble equipment to the bedside stand or overbed table or other surface within reach.
4. Close the curtains around the bed and close the door to the room, if possible.
5. Determine the need for tracheostomy care. **Assess the patient's pain and administer pain medication, if indicated.** Explain what you are going to do and the reason for doing it to the patient, even if the patient does not appear to be alert. Reassure the patient that you will interrupt the procedure if he or she indicates respiratory difficulty.
6. Adjust the bed to a comfortable working position, usually elbow height of the caregiver (VHACEOSH, 2016). Lower the side rail closest to you. **If conscious, place the patient in a semi-Fowler's position. If unconscious, place the patient in the lateral position, facing you.** Move the overbed table close to your work area and raise it to waist height. Place a trash receptacle within easy reach of the work area.
7. Put on face shield or goggles and mask. Suction tracheostomy, if necessary. If tracheostomy has just been suctioned, remove soiled site dressing and discard before removal of gloves used to perform suctioning.
8. Prepare supplies: Open the tracheostomy care kit and separate basins, touching only the edges. If kit is not available, open three sterile basins. Fill one basin 0.5 in deep with hydrogen peroxide or half hydrogen peroxide and half saline, based on facility policy. Fill other two basins 0.5 in with saline. Open sterile brush or pipe cleaners, cotton-tipped applicators, and gauze pads, if they are not already available in the cleaning kit.
9. Put on disposable gloves.
10. Remove the oxygen source if one is present. If not already removed, remove site dressing and dispose

of it in the trash can. Stabilize the outer cannula and faceplate of the tracheostomy with your nondominant hand. Rotate the inner cannula in a counterclockwise motion with your dominant hand to release the lock (Figure A).

FIGURE A. Rotating inner cannula while stabilizing outer cannula.

11. Continue to hold the faceplate. Gently remove the inner cannula (Figure B) and carefully drop it in the basin with the hydrogen peroxide. Replace the oxygen source over the outer cannula.

FIGURE B. Removing inner cannula for cleaning.

Skill Variation ▶ Cleaning a Nondisposable Inner Cannula *(continued)*

12. Discard gloves and put on sterile gloves. Remove the inner cannula from the soaking solution. Moisten the brush or pipe cleaner in saline and insert into tube, using a back-and-forth motion to clean (Figure C).

FIGURE C. Using brush to clean inner cannula.

13. Agitate the cannula in saline solution. Remove and tap against the inner surface of the basin. Place on sterile gauze pad. If secretions have accumulated in outer cannula during cleaning of inner cannula, suction outer cannula using sterile technique.

14. Stabilize the outer cannula and faceplate with nondominant hand. Replace inner cannula into outer cannula with dominant hand. Turn clockwise and check that the inner cannula is secure (Figure D). Reapply oxygen source, if needed.

FIGURE D. Replacing inner cannula.

15. Continue with site care as detailed above in Skill 14-11.

Skill Variation ▶ Using Alternate Site Dressing if Commercially Prepared Sponge is Not Available

If a commercially prepared site dressing or drain sponge is not available, do not cut a gauze sponge to use at the tracheostomy site. Cutting the gauze can cause loose fibers, which can become lodged in the stoma, causing irritation or infection. Loose fibers could also be inhaled into the trachea, causing respiratory distress.

1. Bring necessary equipment to the bedside stand or over-bed table.

2. Perform hand hygiene and put on PPE, if indicated.

3. Identify the patient.

4. Close the curtains around the bed and close the door to the room, if possible.

5. Determine the need for tracheostomy care. **Assess the patient's pain and administer pain medication, if indicated.**

6. Explain what you are going to do and the reason for doing it to the patient, even if the patient does not appear to be alert. Reassure the patient that you will interrupt the procedure if he or she indicates respiratory difficulty.

7. Adjust the bed to a comfortable working position, usually elbow height of the caregiver (VHACEOSH, 2016). Lower the side rail closest to you. **If conscious, place the patient in a semi-Fowler's position. If unconscious, place the patient in the lateral position, facing you.** Move the overbed table close to your work area and raise it to waist height. Place a trash receptacle within easy reach of the work area.

(continued)

Skill 14-11 ▶ Providing Care of a Tracheostomy Tube *(continued)*

Skill Variation ▶ Using Alternate Site Dressing if Commercially Prepared Sponge Is Not Available *(continued)*

8. Remove oxygen source. Dip cotton-tipped applicator or gauze sponge in second basin with sterile saline and clean stoma under faceplate. Use each applicator or sponge only once, moving from stoma site outward.
9. Pat skin gently with dry 4 × 4 gauze sponge.

10. Fold two gauze sponges on the diagonal, to form triangles. Slide one triangle under the faceplate on each side of the stoma, with the longest side of the triangle against the tracheostomy tube.

Skill Variation ▶ Securing a Tracheostomy With Ties/Tape

A tracheostomy may be secured in place using twill ties or tape. One nurse working alone should always place new tracheostomy ties in place before removing old ties to prevent accidental extubation of tracheostomy. If it is necessary to remove old ties first, obtain the assistance of a second person to hold the tracheostomy tube in place while the old tie is removed and the new tie is replaced.

1. Perform hand hygiene and put on PPE, if indicated.

2. Identify the patient.

3. Assemble equipment to the bedside stand or overbed table or other surface within reach.
4. Close the curtains around the bed and close the door to the room, if possible.
5. Determine the need for tracheostomy care. **Assess the patient's pain and administer pain medication, if indicated.** Explain what you are going to do and the reason for doing it to the patient, even if the patient does not appear to be alert. Reassure the patient that you will interrupt the procedure if he or she indicates respiratory difficulty.
6. Adjust the bed to a comfortable working position, usually elbow height of the caregiver (VHACEOSH, 2016). Lower the side rail closest to you. **If conscious, place the patient in a semi-Fowler's position. If unconscious, place the patient in the lateral position, facing you.** Move the overbed table close to your work area and raise to waist height. Place a trash receptacle within easy reach of the work area.
7. Put on clean gloves. If another nurse is assisting, both nurses should put on clean gloves.
8. Cut a piece of the tape twice the length of the neck circumference plus 4 in. Trim ends of tape on the diagonal.

9. Insert one end of the tape through the faceplate opening alongside the old tie. Pull through until both ends are even length (Figure E).

FIGURE E. Pulling tape through faceplate opening alongside old tie until ends are an even length

10. Slide both ends of the tape under the patient's neck and insert one end through the remaining opening on other side of the faceplate. Pull snugly and tie ends in double square knot to the side of the patient's neck. You should be able to fit one finger between the neck and the ties. Avoid tying knot at the back of patient's neck, as this can cause excess pressure and skin breakdown. In addition, the ties could be confused with the patient's gown and mistakenly untied. Check to make sure the patient can flex his or her neck comfortably.
11. Carefully cut and remove old ties. Reapply oxygen supply, if necessary.

Skill 14-12 ▶ Providing Care of a Chest Drainage System

A chest tube is indicated when negative pressure in the pleural space is disrupted, as from thoracic surgery or unanticipated trauma (Muzzy & Butler, 2015). Chest tubes may be inserted to drain fluid (pleural effusion), blood (**hemothorax**), or air (pneumothorax) from the pleural space. A chest tube is a firm plastic tube with drainage holes in the proximal end that is inserted in the pleural space. Once inserted, the tube is secured with a suture and tape, covered with an airtight dressing, and attached to a drainage system that may or may not be attached to suction. Other components of the system may include a closed water seal drainage system that prevents air from reentering the chest once it has escaped, and a suction control chamber that prevents excess suction pressure from being applied to the pleural cavity. The suction chamber may be a water-filled or a dry chamber. A water-filled suction chamber is regulated by the amount of water in the chamber, whereas dry suction is automatically regulated to changes in the patient's pleural pressure. There are also portable drainage systems that use gravity for drainage. Table 14-2 compares different types of chest drainage systems. The following procedure is based on the use of a traditional water seal, three-compartment chest drainage system. Figure 1 is an example of this system. The Skill Variation following the procedure describes a technique for caring for a chest drainage system using dry seal or suction.

Table 14-2 Comparison of Chest Drainage Systems

TYPE	DESCRIPTION	COMMENTS
Traditional water seal (also referred to as wet-suction) chamber	Has three chambers: a collection chamber, water seal chamber (middle chamber), and wet-suction control chamber. Generally used to provide 20 cm H_2O of suction (Kane et al., 2013).	• Requires that sterile fluid be instilled into water seal and suction chambers. • Has positive and negative pressure–release valves. • Intermittent bubbling indicates that system is functioning properly. • Additional suction can be added by connecting system to a suction source.
Dry-suction water seal (also referred to as dry suction)	Has three chambers: a collection chamber, water seal chamber (middle chamber), and dry-suction control chamber. Provides between 10 and 40 cm H_2O of suction (Kane et al., 2013).	• Requires that sterile fluid be instilled in water seal chamber at 2-cm level. • No need to fill suction chamber with fluid. • Suction pressure is set with a regulator. • Has positive and negative pressure–release valves. • Has an indicator to signify that the suction pressure is adequate. • Quieter than traditional water seal systems.
Dry-suction (also referred to as one-way valve system)	Has a one-way mechanical valve that allows air to leave the chest and prevents air from moving back into the chest	• No need to fill suction chamber with fluid; can be set up quickly in an emergency. • Works even if knocked over, making it ideal for patients who are ambulatory.

Source: Adapted from Hinkle, J. L., & Cheever, K. H. (2018). *Brunner & Suddarth's textbook of medical-surgical nursing* (14th ed.). Philadelphia, PA: Wolters Kluwer; Kane, C. J., York, N. L., & Minton, L. A. (2013). Chest tubes in the critically ill patient. *Dimensions of Critical Care Nursing, 32*(3), 111–117.

DELEGATION CONSIDERATIONS	Care of a chest tube is not delegated to nursing assistive personnel (NAP) or to unlicensed assistive personnel (UAP). Depending on the state's nurse practice act and the organization's policies and procedures, care of a chest tube may be delegated to licensed practical/vocational nurses (LPN/LVNs). The decision to delegate must be based on careful analysis of the patient's needs and circumstances, as well as the qualifications of the person to whom the task is being delegated. Refer to the Delegation Guidelines in Appendix A.

(continued)

Skill 14-12 ▸ Providing Care of a Chest Drainage System *(continued)*

FIGURE 1. Chest drainage system.

EQUIPMENT	• Bottle of sterile normal saline or water • Two pairs of padded or rubber-tipped Kelly clamps (if a clamp is not in place on the drainage system tubing) • Pair of clean scissors • Disposable gloves • Additional PPE, as indicated • Foam tape • Prescribed drainage system, if changing is required

EQUIPMENT
- Bottle of sterile normal saline or water
- Two pairs of padded or rubber-tipped Kelly clamps (if a clamp is not in place on the drainage system tubing)
- Pair of clean scissors
- Disposable gloves
- Additional PPE, as indicated
- Foam tape
- Prescribed drainage system, if changing is required

ASSESSMENT

Assess the patient's vital signs and mental status. Significant changes from baseline may indicate complications. Assess for restlessness and shortness of breath. Assess the patient's respiratory status, including oxygen saturation level. If the chest tube is not functioning appropriately, the patient may become tachypneic and hypoxic. Assess the patient's lung sounds. The lung sounds over the chest tube site may be diminished due to the presence of fluid, blood, or air. Also assess the patient for pain. Sudden pressure or increased pain indicates potential complications. In addition, many patients report pain at the chest tube insertion site and request medication for the pain. Assess the patient's knowledge of the chest tube to ensure that he or she understands the rationale for the chest tube.

NURSING DIAGNOSIS

Determine the related factors for the nursing diagnoses based on the patient's current status. Appropriate nursing diagnoses may include:

- Impaired gas exchange
- Deficient knowledge
- Acute pain

OUTCOME IDENTIFICATION AND PLANNING

The expected outcome to achieve is that the patient will not experience any complications related to the chest drainage system or respiratory distress. Other outcomes that may be appropriate include the following: the patient understands the need for the chest tube; the patient will have adequate pain control at the chest tube insertion site; lung sounds will be clear and equal bilaterally; and the patient will be able to increase activity tolerance gradually.

IMPLEMENTATION

ACTION	RATIONALE

1. Gather equipment.

Assembling equipment provides for an organized approach to the task.

2. Perform hand hygiene and put on PPE, if indicated.

Hand hygiene and PPE prevent the spread of microorganisms. PPE is required based on transmission precautions.

3. Identify the patient.

Identifying the patient ensures the right patient receives the intervention and helps prevent errors.

4. Assemble equipment on the overbed table or other surface within reach.

Arranging items nearby is convenient, saves time, and avoids unnecessary stretching and twisting of muscles on the part of the nurse.

5. Close the curtains around the bed and close the door to the room, if possible.

This ensures the patient's privacy.

6. Explain what you are going to do, and the reason for doing it, to the patient.

Explanation relieves anxiety and facilitates cooperation.

7. **Assess the patient's level of pain. Administer prescribed medication, as needed.**

Regular pain assessments are required to maintain adequate analgesic relief from the discomfort and pain caused by chest drains (Kane, York, & Minton, 2013; Muzzy & Butler, 2015).

8. Put on clean gloves.

Gloves prevent contact with contaminants and body fluids.

Assessing the Drainage System

9. Move the patient's gown to expose the chest tube insertion site. Keep the patient covered as much as possible, using a bath blanket to drape the patient, if necessary. Observe the dressing at the chest tube insertion site and confirm that it is dry, intact, and occlusive (Figure 2).

Keeping the patient as covered as possible maintains the patient's privacy and limits unnecessary exposure of the patient. If the dressing is not intact and occlusive, air can leak into the space, causing displacement of the lung tissue, and the site could be contaminated. Some patients experience significant drainage or bleeding at the insertion site. If this occurs, the dressing needs to be replaced to maintain occlusion of the site.

FIGURE 2. Assessing chest tube insertion site.

10. Check that all connections are securely taped. Gently palpate around the insertion site, feeling for crepitus, a result of air or gas collecting under the skin (subcutaneous emphysema). This may feel crunchy or spongy, or like "popping" under your fingers.

The body will absorb small amounts of subcutaneous emphysema after the chest tube is removed. If larger amounts or increasing amounts are present, it could indicate improper placement of the tube or an air leak and can cause discomfort to the patient.

(continued)

Skill 14-12 ▶ Providing Care of a Chest Drainage System *(continued)*

ACTION	**RATIONALE**
11. Check drainage tubing to ensure that there are no dependent loops or kinks. Position the drainage collection device below the tube insertion site.	Dependent loops or kinks in the tubing can prevent the tube from draining appropriately (Kane et al., 2013). The drainage collection device must be positioned below the tube insertion site so that drainage can move out of the tubing and into the collection device.
12. If the chest tube is ordered to be connected to suction, note the fluid level in the suction chamber and check it with the amount of ordered suction. Look for bubbling in the suction chamber. Temporarily disconnect the suction to check the level of water in the chamber. Add sterile water or saline, if necessary, to maintain correct amount of suction.	Some fluid is lost due to evaporation. If suction is set too low, the amount needs to be increased to ensure that enough negative pressure is placed in the pleural space to drain the pleural space sufficiently. If suction is set too high, the amount needs to be decreased to prevent any damage to the fragile lung tissue. Gentle bubbling in the suction chamber indicates that suction is being applied to assist drainage.
13. Observe the water seal chamber for fluctuations of the water level with the patient's inspiration and expiration (tidaling). If suction is used, temporarily disconnect the suction to observe for fluctuation. Assess for the presence of bubbling in the water seal chamber. Add water, if necessary, to maintain the level at the 2-cm mark, or the mark recommended by the manufacturer.	Fluctuation of the water level in the water seal chamber with inspiration and expiration is an expected and normal finding. Bubbles in the water seal chamber, after the initial insertion of the tube or when air is being removed, are a normal finding. Constant bubbles in the water seal chamber after initial insertion period indicate an air leak in the system. Leaks can occur within the drainage unit, or at the insertion site.
14. Assess the amount and type of fluid drainage. Measure drainage output at the end of each shift by marking the level on the container or placing a small piece of tape at the drainage level to indicate date and time (Figure 3). The amount should be a running total, because the drainage system is never emptied. If the drainage system fills, remove and replace it (see Guidelines below).	Measurement allows for accurate intake and output measurement and assessment of the effectiveness of therapy, and it contributes to the decision to remove the tube. The drainage system would lose its negative pressure if it were opened.

FIGURE 3. Drainage marked on device.

15. Remove gloves. Assist the patient to a comfortable position. Raise the bed rail and place the bed in the lowest position, as necessary.	Proper removal of PPE reduces the risk for infection transmission and contamination of other items. Placing the patient in a comfortable position ensures patient comfort. Proper positioning with raised side rails and proper bed height provide for patient comfort and safety.
16. Remove additional PPE, if used. Perform hand hygiene.	Proper removal of PPE reduces the risk for infection transmission and contamination of other items. Hand hygiene prevents the spread of microorganisms.

ACTION

Changing the Drainage System

17. Some drainage systems have a clamp on the drainage tubing. If present, there is no need to use other clamps. Otherwise, obtain two-padded Kelly clamps, a new drainage system, and a bottle of sterile water. Add water to the water seal chamber in the new system until it reaches the 2-cm mark or the mark recommended by the manufacturer. Follow manufacturer's directions to add water to the suction system, if suction is ordered.

18. Put on clean gloves and additional PPE, as indicated.

19. **Engage the clamp on the drainage tubing. Alternatively, apply Kelly clamps 1.5 to 2.5 in from insertion site and 1 in apart, going in opposite directions (Figure 4).**

RATIONALE

Gathering equipment provides for an organized approach. Appropriate level of water in the water seal chamber is necessary to prevent air from entering the chest. Appropriate level of water in the suction chamber provides the ordered suction.

Gloves prevent contact with contaminants and body fluids.

Clamps provide a more complete seal and prevent air from entering the pleural space through the chest tube.

FIGURE 4. Padded clamps on chest tube.

20. Remove the suction from the current drainage system by unrolling (Figure 5) or use scissors to carefully cut away (Figure 6) any foam tape on the connection of the chest tube and drainage system. Using a slight twisting motion, remove the drainage system. **Do not pull on the chest tube.**

Removing suction permits application of new system. In many facilities, bands or foam tape are placed where the chest tube meets the drainage system to ensure that the chest tube and the drainage system remain connected. Due to the negative pressure, a slight twisting motion may be needed to separate the tubes. The chest tube is sutured in place; do not tug on the chest tube and dislodge it.

FIGURE 5. Unrolling foam tape.

FIGURE 6. Carefully cutting foam tape.

(continued)

Skill 14-12 ▶ Providing Care of a Chest Drainage System *(continued)*

ACTION	RATIONALE
21. Keeping the end of the chest tube sterile, insert the end of the new drainage system into the chest tube (Figure 7). **Unclamp the tubing clamp or remove Kelly clamps.** Reconnect suction, if ordered. Apply foam tape to chest tube/drainage system connection site.	Chest tube is sterile. Tube must be reconnected to suction to form a negative pressure and allow for reexpansion of lung or drainage of fluid. Prolonged clamping can result in a pneumothorax. Bands or foam tape help prevent the separation of the chest tube from the drainage system.

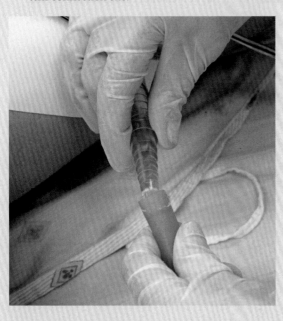

FIGURE 7. Inserting the end of the new drainage system into the chest tube.

22. Assess the patient and the drainage system as outlined (Steps 5 to 15).	Assess for changes related to the manipulation of the system and placement of a new drainage system.
23. Remove additional PPE, if used. Perform hand hygiene.	Proper removal of PPE reduces the risk for infection transmission and contamination of other items. Hand hygiene prevents the spread of microorganisms.

EVALUATION

The expected outcome has been met when the chest drainage system is patent and functioning. In addition, the patient remains free of signs and symptoms of respiratory distress and complications related to the chest drainage system; the patient verbalizes adequate pain relief, gradually increases activity tolerance, and demonstrates an understanding of the need for the chest tube.

DOCUMENTATION

Guidelines

Document the site of the chest tube, amount and type of drainage, amount of suction applied, and presence of any bubbling, tidaling, or subcutaneous emphysema noted. Document the type of dressing in place and the patient's pain level, as well as any measures performed to relieve the patient's pain. Document changing of drainage system, if completed.

Sample Documentation

> <u>9/10/20</u> 1805 Chest tube present in right lower portion of rib cage at the axillary line. Draining moderate amount of serosanguinous fluid. Suction at 20 cm H$_2$O noted; gentle bubbling noted in suction chamber. Tidaling present in water seal chamber, no air leak noted. Small amount of subcutaneous emphysema noted around insertion site, unchanged from previous assessment; patient denies any pain; occlusive dressing remains intact.
>
> —*C. Bausler, RN*

UNEXPECTED SITUATIONS AND ASSOCIATED INTERVENTIONS

- *The chest tube becomes separated from the drainage device:* Put on gloves. Open the normal saline solution or sterile water and submerge the chest tube into the bottle 1 to 2 in below the surface of the solution, taking care to avoid contaminating the chest tube. This creates a water seal until a new drainage unit can be attached. Assess the patient for any signs of respiratory distress. Notify the primary care provider. Do not leave the patient. Anticipate the need for a new drainage system and a chest x-ray.
- *The chest tube becomes dislodged:* Put on gloves. Immediately apply an occlusive dressing to the site. There is a controversy in the literature over whether the occlusive dressing should be a sterile Vaseline-impregnated gauze covered with an occlusive tape or a sterile 4 × 4 gauze folded and covered with an occlusive tape. (An example of an occlusive tape would be foam tape or the clear dressing used to cover IV insertion sites.) Assess the patient for any signs of respiratory distress. Notify the primary care provider. Anticipate the need for a chest x-ray. The primary care provider will determine whether the chest tube needs to be replaced.
- *While assessing the chest tube, you notice a lack of drainage when there had been drainage previously:* Check for kinked tubing or a clot in the tubing. Note the amount of suction on which the chest tube is set. **Do not** perform "milking" of the tubing (squeezing and releasing small segments of tubing between the fingers) and "stripping" of the tubing (squeezing the length of the tube without releasing it) (Makic, Rauen, Jones, & Fisk, 2015; Kane et al., 2013; Muzzy & Butler, 2015). Bruising and trauma of lung tissue can occur as a result, as well as dangerously increased negative pressure in the pleural space. If the suction is not set appropriately, adjust until the ordered amount is achieved. Keeping the tubing horizontal across the bed or chair before dropping vertically into the drain device, and avoiding dependent loops optimize drainage. Notify the primary care provider if the lack of drainage persists.
- *Drainage dramatically increases or becomes bright red:* Notify the primary care provider immediately. This can indicate fresh bleeding.
- *Chest tube drainage suddenly decreases and the water seal chamber is not tidaling:* Notify the primary care provider immediately. This could signal that the tube is blocked. Assess the patient's respiratory status.

SPECIAL CONSIDERATIONS

General Considerations

- Ensure that a bottle of sterile water or normal saline is at the bedside at all times. Never clamp chest tubes except to change the drainage system, or when there is a medical order, such as for a trial before chest tube removal. If the chest tube becomes accidentally disconnected from the drainage system, place the end of the chest tube into the sterile solution (see Unexpected Situations above). This prevents more air from entering the pleural space through the chest tube, but allows for any air that does enter the pleural space, through respirations, to escape once pressure builds up.
- Keep two rubber-tipped clamps and additional dressing material at the bedside for quick access, if needed.
- **Do not** perform "milking" of the tubing (squeezing and releasing small segments of tubing between the fingers) and "stripping" of the tubing (squeezing the length of the tube without releasing it) to promote drainage. This creates excessive negative pressure that can damage delicate lung tissue. Stripping and milking are not necessary to maintain chest tube patency and probably do more harm than good (Makic et al., 2015, p. 44).
- If the patient has a small pneumothorax with little or no drainage and suction is not used, the tube may be connected to a Heimlich valve. A Heimlich valve is a water seal chamber that allows air to exit from, but not enter, the chest tube. Check to assure that the valve is pointing in the correct direction. The blue end should be connected to the chest tube and the clear end is open as the vent. The arrow on the casing points away from the patient.
- Maintain the chest drainage system in an upright position and lower than the level of the tube insertion site. This is necessary for proper function of the system and to aid drainage.
- Encourage the use of an incentive spirometer, if ordered, and/or frequent deep breathing and coughing by the patient. This helps drain the lungs, promotes lung expansion, and prevents atelectasis.

Infant and Child Considerations

- Illness and hospitalization alone can be a source of overwhelming distress and anxiety for children and their families. The presence and discomfort related to equipment that prevents children from freely moving and invades their body may add to the situation. Provide age-appropriate activities and distraction to help decrease discomfort and promote the child's coping abilities (Crawford, 2011).

(continued)

Skill 14-12 ▶ Providing Care of a Chest Drainage System *(continued)*

Skill Variation ▶ Caring for a Chest Drainage System Using Dry Seal or Suction

1. Perform hand hygiene and put on PPE, if indicated.

2. Identify the patient.

3. Assemble equipment to the bedside stand or overbed table or other surface within reach.
4. Close the curtains around the bed and close the door to the room, if possible.
5. Explain what you are going to do and the reason for doing it to the patient.
6. **Assess the patient's level of pain. Administer prescribed medication, as needed.**
7. Put on clean gloves. Move the patient's gown to expose the chest tube insertion site. Keep the patient covered as much as possible, using a bath blanket to drape the patient, if necessary. Observe the dressing around the chest tube insertion site and ensure that it is dry, intact, and occlusive.
8. Check that all connections are taped securely. Gently palpate around the insertion site, feeling for subcutaneous emphysema, a collection of air or gas under the skin. This may feel crunchy or spongy, or like "popping" under your fingers.
9. Check drainage tubing to ensure that there are no dependent loops or kinks. The drainage collection device must be positioned below the tube insertion site.

10. If the chest tube is ordered to be to suctioned, assess the amount of suction set on the chest tube against the amount of suction ordered. Assess for the presence of the suction control indicator, which is a bellows or float device, when adjusting the regulator to the desired level of suction, if prescribed.
11. Assess for fluctuations in the diagnostic indicator with the patient's inspiration and expiration.
12. Check the air-leak indicator for leaks in dry systems with a one-way valve.
13. Assess the amount and type of fluid drainage. Measure drainage output at the end of each shift by marking the level on the container or placing a small piece of tape at the drainage level to indicate date and time. The amount should be a running total, because the drainage system is never emptied. If the drainage system fills, it is removed and replaced.
14. Some portable chest drainage systems require manual emptying of the collection chamber. Follow the manufacturer's recommendations for timing of emptying. Typically, the unit should not be allowed to fill completely because drainage could spill out. Wear gloves, clean the syringe port with an alcohol wipe, use a 60-mL Luer-Lok syringe, screw the syringe into the port, and aspirate to withdraw fluid. Repeat, as necessary, to empty the chamber. Dispose of the fluid according to facility policy.
15. Remove gloves and additional PPE, if used. Perform hand hygiene.

Skill 14-13 ▶ Assisting With Removal of a Chest Tube

Chest tubes are removed after the lung is reexpanded and drainage is minimal. An advanced practice professional usually performs chest tube removal. The practitioner will determine when the chest tube is ready for removal by evaluating the chest x-ray, assessing the patient, and the amount of drainage from the tube. Some facilities are developing programs to train, support, and ensure continued competency of nurses to remove chest tubes to improve control of the timing of the procedure and allow for appropriate preprocedural analgesia, reducing associated pain and anxiety (Hood, Henderson, & Pasero, 2014; Muzzy & Butler, 2015).

DELEGATION CONSIDERATIONS

Assisting with the removal of a chest tube is not delegated to nursing assistive personnel (NAP) or to unlicensed assistive personnel (UAP). Depending on the state's nurse practice act and the organization's policies and procedures, assisting with the removal of a chest tube may be delegated to licensed practical/vocational nurses (LPN/LVNs). The decision to delegate must be based on careful analysis of the patient's needs and circumstances, as well as the qualifications of the person to whom the task is being delegated. Refer to the Delegation Guidelines in Appendix A.

(continued)

EQUIPMENT	• Disposable gloves • Additional PPE, as indicated • Suture removal kit (tweezers and scissors)	• Sterile Vaseline-impregnated gauze and 4 × 4 gauze dressings or other occlusive dressings, based on facility policy • Occlusive tape, such as foam tape

ASSESSMENT

Assess the patient's respiratory status, including respiratory rate and oxygen saturation level. This provides a baseline for comparison after the tube is removed. If the patient begins to have respiratory distress, he or she will usually become tachypneic and hypoxic. Assess the patient's lung sounds. The lung sounds over the chest tube site may be diminished due to the tube. Assess the patient for pain. Many patients report pain at the chest tube insertion site and request medication for the pain. If the patient has not recently received pain medication, give it before the chest tube removal to decrease the pain felt with the procedure and ease anxiety (Ertuğ & Ülker, 2011; Hood et al., 2014; Kane et al., 2013; Muzzy & Butler, 2015).

NURSING DIAGNOSIS

Determine the related factors for the nursing diagnoses based on the patient's current status. Appropriate nursing diagnoses may include:

- Deficient knowledge
- Acute pain
- Risk for injury

OUTCOME IDENTIFICATION AND PLANNING

The expected outcomes to achieve when caring for a patient after removal of a chest tube is that the tube is removed without patient injury and the patient remains free from respiratory distress. Other outcomes that may be appropriate include the following: the insertion site will remain clean and dry without evidence of infection; the patient will experience adequate pain control during the chest tube removal; and lung sounds will be clear and equal bilaterally.

IMPLEMENTATION

ACTION	RATIONALE
1. Gather equipment.	Assembling equipment provides for an organized approach to the task.
2. Perform hand hygiene and put on PPE, if indicated.	Hand hygiene and PPE prevent the spread of microorganisms. PPE is required based on transmission precautions.
3. Identify the patient.	Identifying the patient ensures the right patient receives the intervention and helps prevent errors.
4. Assemble equipment on the overbed table or other surface within reach.	Arranging items nearby is convenient, saves time, and avoids unnecessary stretching and twisting of muscles on the part of the nurse.
5. Administer pain medication, as prescribed. **Premedicate patient before the chest tube removal, at a sufficient interval to allow for the medication to take effect, based on the medication prescribed.**	Most patients report discomfort during chest tube removal (Ertuğ & Ülker, 2011; Hood et al., 2014; Kane et al., 2013; Muzzy & Butler, 2015).
6. Close the curtains around the bed and close the door to the room, if possible.	This ensures the patient's privacy.
7. Explain what you are going to do and the reason for doing it to the patient. Explain any nonpharmacologic pain interventions the patient may use to decrease discomfort during tube removal.	Explanation relieves anxiety and facilitates cooperation. Nonpharmacologic pain management interventions, such as relaxation exercises and the application of cold, have been shown to help decrease pain during chest tube removal (Ertuğ & Ülker, 2011).

(continued)

Skill 14-13 ▶ Assisting With Removal of a Chest Tube (continued)

ACTION	RATIONALE
8. Explain that the patient will be required to take and hold a deep breath or exhale during chest tube removal. Instruct the patient to practice taking deep breaths and holding them. Alternately, the patient may be asked to take a deep breath and hum during removal of the tube (Muzzy & Butler, 2015).	The chest tube must be removed during breath holding or expiration to prevent air from reentering the pleural space (Hood et al., 2014; Kane et al., 2013; Muzzy & Butler, 2015).
9. Put on clean gloves.	Gloves prevent contact with contaminants and body fluids.
10. Provide reassurance to the patient while the practitioner removes the dressing and then the tube.	The removal of the dressing and the tube can increase the patient's anxiety level. Offering reassurance will help the patient feel more secure and help decrease anxiety.
11. **After the practitioner has removed the chest tube and secured the occlusive dressing, assess patient's lung sounds, vital signs, oxygen saturation, and pain level.**	In most facilities, advanced practice professionals remove chest tubes, but some facilities have developed programs to train and support nurses to remove chest tubes (Hood et al., 2014; Muzzy & Butler, 2015). Once the tube is removed, the patient's respiratory status will need to be assessed to ensure that no distress is present.
12. Anticipate an order for a chest x-ray.	A chest x-ray is performed to evaluate the status of the lungs after chest tube removal, to ensure that the lung is still fully inflated.
13. Dispose of equipment appropriately.	This reduces the risk for transmission of microorganisms and contamination of other items.
14. Remove gloves and additional PPE, if used. Perform hand hygiene.	Proper removal of PPE reduces the risk for infection transmission and contamination of other items. Hand hygiene prevents the spread of microorganisms.
15. Continue to monitor the patient's cardiopulmonary status and comfort level. Monitor the site and dressing.	Continued monitoring allows for assessment of possible respiratory distress if lung does not remain inflated. Checking dressing ensures the assessment of changes in patient condition and enables timely intervention to prevent complications.

EVALUATION

The expected outcomes have been met when the tube has been removed without patient injury and the patient remains free from respiratory distress; the insertion site remains clean and dry without evidence of infection; the patient verbalizes adequate pain control; and lung sounds are clear and equal bilaterally.

DOCUMENTATION

Guidelines

Document the patient's respiratory rate, oxygen saturation, lung sounds, total chest tube output, pain assessment, and status of the insertion site and dressing.

Sample Documentation

9/16/20 1950 Procedure explained to patient. Morphine sulfate 2 mg IV given, as ordered. Health care provider at bedside, and right mid-axillary lower lobe chest tube removed. Vaseline gauze and gauze dressings applied over insertion site covered by foam tape. Lung sounds clear, slightly diminished over right lower lobe. Respirations unlabored at 16 breaths/min, pulse 88, blood pressure 118/64. Oxygen saturation 97% on room air; 322 mL of serosanguinous drainage noted in drainage device. Patient denies pain or respiratory distress.

—C. Bausler, RN

UNEXPECTED SITUATIONS AND ASSOCIATED INTERVENTIONS	• *Patient experiences respiratory distress after chest tube removal:* Auscultate lung sounds. Diminished or absent lung sounds could be a sign that the lung has not fully reinflated or that the fluid has returned. Notify the primary care provider immediately. Anticipate an order for a chest x-ray and possible reinsertion of a chest tube. • *Chest tube dressing becomes loosened:* Change the chest tube dressing at least every 24 hours or per facility policy in order to assess the site for erythema and drainage. Replace the occlusive dressing using a sterile technique. The dressing should remain occlusive for at least 3 days.
SPECIAL CONSIDERATIONS *Infant and Child Considerations*	• It may be difficult to gain the cooperation of the child when performing the deep breathing during tube removal. Distraction may be helpful. Ask child to blow up a balloon or blow bubbles (Crawford, 2011).

Skill 14-14 ▶ Using a Manual Resuscitation Bag and Mask

If the patient is not breathing with an adequate rate and depth, or if the patient has lost the respiratory drive, a bag and mask may be used to deliver oxygen until the patient is resuscitated or can be intubated with an endotracheal tube. Bag and mask devices are frequently referred to as Ambu bags ("air mask bag unit") or BVM ("bag-valve-mask" device). The bags come in infant, pediatric, and adult sizes. The bag consists of an oxygen reservoir (commonly referred to as the tail), oxygen tubing, the bag itself, a one-way valve to prevent secretions from entering the bag, an exhalation port, an elbow so that the bag can lie across the patient's chest, and a mask.

DELEGATION CONSIDERATIONS	The use of a BVM may be delegated to nursing assistive personnel (NAP) or to unlicensed assistive personnel (UAP) in an emergency situation. The use of a BVM may be delegated to licensed practical/vocational nurses (LPN/LVNs). The decision to delegate must be based on careful analysis of the patient's needs and circumstances, as well as the qualifications of the person to whom the task is being delegated. Refer to the Delegation Guidelines in Appendix A.
EQUIPMENT	• Handheld resuscitation device with a mask • Face shield or goggles and mask • Oxygen source • Additional PPE, as indicated • Disposable gloves
ASSESSMENT	Assess the patient's respiratory effort and drive. If the patient is breathing less than 10 breaths/min, is breathing too shallowly, or is not breathing at all, assistance with a BVM may be needed. Assess the oxygen saturation level. Patients who have decreased respiratory effort and drive may also have a decreased oxygen saturation level. Assess heart rate and rhythm. Bradycardia may occur with a decreased oxygen saturation level, leading to a cardiac dysrhythmia. Many times, a BVM is used in a crisis situation. Manual ventilation is also used during airway suctioning.
NURSING DIAGNOSIS	Determine the related factors for the nursing diagnoses based on the patient's current status. Appropriate nursing diagnoses may include: • Ineffective breathing pattern • Impaired gas exchange
OUTCOME IDENTIFICATION AND PLANNING	The expected outcome is that the patient will exhibit signs and symptoms of adequate respirations and oxygenation. Other outcomes that may be appropriate include the following: the patient will receive adequate volume of respirations with the BVM; and the patient will maintain oxygen saturation within acceptable parameters.

(*continued*)

Skill 14-14 ▶ Using a Manual Resuscitation Bag and Mask *(continued)*

IMPLEMENTATION

ACTION	RATIONALE

 1. If not a crisis situation, perform hand hygiene.

Hand hygiene prevents the spread of microorganisms.

2. Put on PPE, as indicated.

PPE prevents the spread of microorganisms. PPE is required based on transmission precautions.

 3. If not a crisis situation, identify the patient.

Identifying the patient ensures the right patient receives the intervention and helps prevent errors.

4. Explain what you are going to do and the reason for doing it to the patient, even if the patient does not appear to be alert.

Explanation alleviates fears. Even if the patient appears unconscious, the nurse should explain what is happening.

5. Put on disposable gloves. Put on face shield or goggles and mask.

Using gloves deters the spread of microorganisms. PPE protects the nurse from pathogens.

6. **Ensure that the mask is connected to the bag device (Figure 1), the oxygen tubing is connected to the oxygen source (Figure 2), and the oxygen is turned on, at a flow rate of 10 to 15 L/min.** This may be done by visualizing or by listening to the open end of the reservoir or tail: if air is heard flowing, the oxygen tubing is attached and on.

Expected results might **not** be accomplished if the oxygen tubing is not attached and on.

FIGURE 1. Connecting mask to bag-valve device.

FIGURE 2. Connecting oxygen tubing on bag to oxygen source.

7. Initiate CPR, if indicated. Refer to Skill 16-1.

Start CPR in any situation in which either breathing alone or breathing and a heartbeat are absent. The brain is sensitive to hypoxia and will sustain irreversible damage after 4 to 6 minutes of no oxygen. The faster CPR is initiated, the greater the chance of survival.

8. If possible, get behind head of bed and remove headboard. **Slightly hyperextend the patient's neck (unless contraindicated). If unable to hyperextend, use jaw-thrust maneuver to open airway.**

Standing at head of bed makes positioning easier when obtaining seal of mask to face. Hyperextending the neck opens the airway.

ACTION

9. Place mask over the patient's face with opening over oral cavity. If mask is teardrop-shaped, the narrow portion should be placed over the bridge of the nose.

10. Use the thumb and index finger of one hand to make a "C" on the side of the mask, pressing the edges of the mask to the face to form a seal around the patient's face. Use the remaining three fingers on the same hand to lift the angles of the jaw to open the airway and press the mask to the face.

11. Using the remaining hand, squeeze the bag to give a breath over 1 second (Figure 3), watching the chest for symmetric rise.

12. Deliver the breaths with the patient's own inspiratory effort, if present. Avoid delivering breaths when the patient exhales. Deliver one breath every 5 to 6 seconds (about 10 to 12 breaths/min, adults) (American Heart Association [AHA], 2015a), if the patient's own respiratory drive is absent. Continue delivering breaths until the patient's drive returns or until the patient is intubated and attached to mechanical ventilation.

13. When use of the manual resuscitation bag and mask is no longer required, dispose of equipment appropriately.

 14. Remove face shield or goggles and mask. Remove gloves and additional PPE, if used. Perform hand hygiene.

RATIONALE

This helps ensure an adequate seal so that oxygen can be forced into the lungs.

This helps ensure that an adequate seal is formed so that oxygen can be forced into the lungs.

Volume of air needed is based on patient's size. Enough has been delivered if the chest is rising. If air is introduced rapidly, it may enter the stomach.

FIGURE 3. Creating a seal between mask and patient's face and squeezing the bag.

If a patient has spontaneous inspiratory effort, breaths delivered to the patient must be timed to coincide with the spontaneous breaths to avoid the discomfort of dyssynchronous breathing, anxiety, and resistance to ventilation (Morton & Fontaine, 2018).

Once patient's airway has been stabilized or patient is breathing on own, bag-mask delivery can be stopped.

Reduces the risk for transmission of microorganisms and contamination of other items.

Proper removal of PPE reduces the risk for infection transmission and contamination of other items. Hand hygiene prevents the spread of microorganisms.

EVALUATION

The expected outcomes have been met when the patient exhibits signs and symptoms of adequate respirations and oxygenation (absence of cyanosis); the patient receives adequate volume of respirations with the BVM; and the patient maintains oxygen saturation within acceptable parameters.

DOCUMENTATION

Guidelines

Document the incident, including the patient's respiratory effort before initiation of bag-mask breaths, lung sounds, oxygen saturation, chest symmetry, and resolution of incident (i.e., intubation or patient's respiratory drive returns).

(continued)

Skill 14-14 ▶ Using a Manual Resuscitation Bag and Mask *(continued)*

Sample Documentation

> 9/1/20 2015 Patient arrived to emergency department with respiratory rate of 4 breaths/min; respirations shallow; manual breaths delivered using adult bag with mask and 100% oxygen, oxygen saturation increased from 78% to 100% after eight breaths delivered; Dr. Alsup at bedside; patient sedated with 5 mg midazolam before intubation with 7.5-mm oral endotracheal tube, taped 10 cm at lips; lung sounds clear and equal in all lobes; see graphics for ventilator settings. Nasogastric tube placed via R naris to low intermittent suction, small amount of dark green drainage noted, chest x-ray obtained.
>
> —C. Bausler, RN

UNEXPECTED SITUATIONS AND ASSOCIATED INTERVENTIONS

- *Breaths become increasingly difficult to deliver due to resistance:* Obtain order for placement of naso- or orogastric tube to remove air from the stomach (many facilities have policies that allow placement of a gastric tube during resuscitation). If air is delivered too fast, it may be introduced into the stomach. When the stomach fills with air, it decreases the space available for the lungs to inflate.
- *Chest is not rising when breaths are delivered, and resistance is felt:* Reposition the head or perform the jaw-thrust maneuver. If the chest is not rising at all and resistance is being met, the tongue or another object may be obstructing the airway. If repositioning does not resolve the effort, consider performing the Heimlich maneuver.
- *Chest is rising asymmetrically:* Instruct assistant to listen to lung sounds bilaterally. Patient may need a chest tube placed due to pneumothorax. Anticipate the need for chest tube placement.
- *Oxygen saturation decreases from 100% to 80%:* Assess whether the chest is rising. If the chest is rising asymmetrically, the patient may have a pneumothorax. Anticipate the need for a chest tube. Check oxygen tubing. Someone may have stepped on the tubing, either kinking the tubing or pulling the tubing from the oxygen device.
- *A seal cannot be formed around the patient's face, and a large amount of air is escaping around mask:* Assess face and mask. Is the mask the correct size for the patient? If the mask size is correct, reposition fingers, or have a second person hold the mask while you compress the bag.

SPECIAL CONSIDERATIONS

- If a patient has spontaneous inspiratory effort, breaths delivered to the patient must be timed to coincide with the spontaneous breaths to avoid the discomfort of dyssynchronous breathing, anxiety, and resistance to ventilation (Morton & Fontaine, 2018).
- If three or more rescuers are present, two rescuers can provide more effective bag-mask ventilation than one rescuer (AHA, 2015b). One rescuer maintains a seal on the mask and an open airway with two hands using the technique described above, while the other squeezes the bag to deliver the ventilation and oxygenation.
- Have equipment to suction airway readily available when using a BVM. Air can be forced into the stomach during manual ventilation with a mask, causing abdominal distention. This distention can cause vomiting and possible aspiration. Be alert for vomiting; watch through the mask. If the patient starts to vomit, stop ventilating immediately, remove the mask, wipe and suction vomitus as needed, then resume ventilation.

Infant and Child Considerations

- Deliver the breaths with the patient's own inspiratory effort, if present. Deliver one breath every 3 to 5 seconds (about 12 to 20 breaths/min, adults) (AHA, 2015b), if the patient's own respiratory drive is absent.

EVIDENCE FOR PRACTICE ▶

CARDIOPULMONARY RESUSCITATION AND EMERGENCY CARDIAC CARE
The American Heart Association provides guidelines for cardiopulmonary resuscitation and emergency cardiac care and has incorporated these guidelines into the Basic Life Support and Advanced Life Support education for health care providers who respond to respiratory and cardiovascular emergencies.

American Heart Association (AHA). (2015b). *2015 American Heart Association Guidelines for CPR & Emergency Cardiovascular Care.* Retrieved https://eccguidelines.heart.org/index.php/circulation/cpr-ecc-guidelines-2

Refer to thePoint® for additional research on related nursing topics.

Enhance Your Understanding

Focusing on Patient Care: Developing Clinical Reasoning

Consider the case scenarios at the beginning of the chapter as you answer the following questions to enhance your understanding and apply what you have learned.

QUESTIONS

1. Scott Mingus has a chest drain in place after thoracic surgery. The chest tube has been draining 20 to 30 mL of serosanguinous fluid every hour. Suddenly, the chest tube output is 110 mL/hr and the drainage is bright red. What should the nurse do?

2. Saranam Srivastava has a history of smoking and is scheduled for abdominal surgery. She needs to learn how to use an incentive spirometer. What should the nurse include in patient education regarding the use of an incentive spirometer?

3. The nurse caring for Paula Cunningham determines that Ms. Cunningham needs to be suctioned via her endotracheal tube. What assessment findings might lead to this conclusion? How would the nurse determine if the suctioning of Ms. Cunningham's airway was effective?

You can find suggested answers after the Bibliography at the end of this chapter.

Integrated Case Study Connection

The case studies in the back of the book focus on integrating concepts. Refer to the following case studies to enhance your understanding of the concepts and skills in this chapter.

- Basic Case Studies: Kate Townsend, page 1109.
- Intermediate Case Studies: Olivia Greenbaum, page 1113; George Patel, page 1126.
- Advanced Case Studies: Cole McKean, page 1128; Damian Wallace, page 1130; George Patel, Gwen Galloway, Claudia Tran, and James White, page 1134.

Taylor Suite Resources

Explore these additional resources to enhance learning for this chapter:

- NCLEX-Style Questions and other resources on thePoint*, http://thePoint.lww.com/Lynn5e
- *Skill Checklists for Taylor's Clinical Nursing Skills,* 5e
- *Taylor's Video Guide to Clinical Nursing Skills:* Oxygenation and Tracheostomy Care
- *Fundamentals of Nursing:* Chapter 39, Oxygenation and Perfusion
- *Lippincott DocuCare* Fundamentals cases

Bibliography

Aguiar, C., Davidson, J., Carvalho, A. K., et al. (2015). Tubing length for long-term oxygen therapy. *Respiratory Care, 60*(2), 179–182.

Amalakanti, S., & Pentakota, M. R. (2016). Pulse oximetry overestimates oxygen saturation in COPD. *Respiratory Care, 61*(4), 423–427.

American Association for Respiratory Care (AARC) Clinical Practice Guidelines. (2010). Endotracheal suctioning of mechanically ventilated patients with artificial airways 2010. *Respiratory Care, 55*(6), 758–764.

American Association of Critical-Care Nurses (AACN). (2010). Practice Alert: Oral care in the critically ill. Retrieved http://www.aacn.org/wd/practice/content/oral-care-practice-alert.pcms?menu=practice

American Heart Association (AHA). (2015a). *Highlights of the 2015 American Heart Association Guidelines Update for CPR and ECC.* Dallas, TX: Author. Retrieved https://eccguidelines.heart.org/wp-content/uploads/2015/10/2015-AHA-Guidelines-Highlights-English.pdf

American Heart Association (AHA). (2015b). *2015 American Heart Association Guidelines for CPR & Emergency Cardiovascular Care.* Retrieved https://eccguidelines.heart.org/index.php/circulation/cpr-ecc-guidelines-2

American Heart Association (AHA). (2016). *Hands-only CPR.* Retrieved http://cpr.heart.org/AHAECC/CPRAndECC/Programs/HandsOnlyCPR/UCM_473196_Hands-Only-CPR.jsp

Arroyo-Novoa, C., Figueroa-Ramos, M., Puntillo, K., et al. (2008). Pain related to tracheal suctioning in awake acutely and critically ill adults: A descriptive study. *Intensive & Critical Care Nursing, 24*(1), 20–27.

Boroughs, D. S., & Dougherty, J. M. (2015). Pediatric tracheostomy care: What home care nurses need to know. *American Nurse Today, 10*(3), 8–10.

Buckley, T., Dudley, J., Eberhart, M., et al. (2007). AARC clinical practice guideline: Oxygen therapy in the home or alternate site health care facility—2007 revision & update. *Respiratory Care, 52*(1), 1063–1068.

Centers for Disease Control and Prevention (CDC). (2016). *Heart disease fact sheet.* Retrieved http://www.cdc.gov/dhdsp/data_statistics/fact_sheets/fs_heart_disease.htm

Chenelle, C. T., Oto, J., Dulemanji, D., Fisher, D. F., & Kacmarek, R. M. (2015). Evaluation of an automated endotracheal tube cuff controller during simulated mechanical ventilation. *Respiratory Care, 60*(2), 183–190.

Coker, E., Ploeg, J., Kaasalainen, S., & Fisher, A. (2013). A concept analysis of oral hygiene care in dependent older adults. *Journal of Advanced Nursing, 69*(10), 2360–2371.

Crawford, D. (2011). Care and nursing management of a child with a chest drain. *Nursing Children and Young People, 23*(10), 27–33.

Darr, A., Siddiq, S., Jolly, K., & Spinou, C. (2016). Neck stoma patients: Is vital information displayed at the bedside? *British Journal of Nursing, 25*(5), 242–247.

Dawson, D. (2014). Essential principles: Tracheostomy care in the adult patient. *British Association of Critical Care Nurses, 19*(2), 63–72.

Doenges, M. E., Moorhouse, M. F., & Murr, A. C. (2016). *Nursing diagnoses manual. Planning,*

individualizing, and documenting client care (5th ed.). Philadelphia, PA: F.A. Davis Company.

Düzkaya, D. S., & Kuğuoğlu, S. (2015). Assessment of pain during endotracheal suction in the pediatric intensive care unit. *Pain Management Nursing, 16*(1), 11–19.

Eliopoulos, C. (2014). *Gerontological nursing* (8th ed.). Philadelphia, PA: Wolters Kluwer Health.

Ertuğ, N., & Ülker, S. (2011). The effect of cold application on pain due to chest tube removal. *Journal of Clinical Nursing, 21*(5–6), 784–790.

Fisher, D. F., Chenelle, C. T., Marchese, A. D., Kratohvil, J. P., & Kacmarek, R. M. (2014). Comparison of commercial and noncommercial endotracheal tube-securing devices. *Respiratory Care, 59*(9), 1315–1323.

Grant, T. (2013). Do current methods for endotracheal tube cuff inflation create pressures above the recommended range? A review of the evidence. *Journal of Perioperative Practice, 23*(12), 292–295.

Grossman, S., & Porth, C. M. (2014). *Porth's pathophysiology: Concepts of altered health states* (9th ed.). Philadelphia, PA: Wolters Kluwer Health.

Guttormson, J. L., Bremer, K. L., & Jones, R. M. (2015). "Not being able to talk was horrid": A descriptive, correlational study of communication during mechanical ventilation. *Intensive and Critical Care Nursing, 31*(3), 179–186.

Hahn, M. (2010). 10 considerations for endotracheal suctioning. *The Journal for Respiratory Care Practitioners, 23*(7), 32–33.

Hess, D. R., MacIntyre, N. R., Galvin, W. F., & Mishoe, S. C. (2016). *Respiratory care. Principles and practice* (3rd ed.). Sudbury, MA: Jones & Bartlett Learning.

Higginson, R., Jones, B., & Davies, K. (2010). Airway management for nurses: Emergency assessment and care. *British Journal of Nursing, 19*(16), 1006–1014.

Higginson, R., & Parry, A. (2013). Emergency airway management: Common ventilation techniques. *British Journal of Nursing, 22*(7), 366–371.

Higginson, R., Parry, A. & Williams, M. (2016). Airway management in the hospital environment. *British Journal of Nursing, 25*(2), 94–100.

Hillier, B., Wilson, C., Chamberlain, D., & King, L. (2013). Preventing ventilator-associated pneumonia through oral care, product selection, and application method. *AACN Advanced Critical Care, 24*(1), 38–58.

Hinkle, J. L., & Cheever, K. H. (2018). *Brunner & Suddarth's textbook of medical-surgical nursing* (14th ed.). Philadelphia, PA: Wolters Kluwer.

Hockenberry, M. J., & Wilson, D. (2015). *Wong's nursing care of infants and children* (10th ed.). St. Louis, MO: Elsevier.

Hood, B. S., Henderson, W., & Pasero, C. (2014). Chest tube removal: An expanded role for the bedside nurse. *Journal of PeriAnesthesia Nursing, 29*(1), 53–59.

Ireton, J. (2007). Tracheostomy suction: A protocol for practice. *Paediatric Nursing, 19*(10), 14–18.

Jarvis, C. (2016). *Physical examination and health assessment* (7th ed.). St. Louis, MO: Elsevier.

Jensen, S. (2015). *Nursing health assessment: A best practice approach* (2nd ed.). Philadelphia, PA: Wolters Kluwer Health.

Johnson, C. L., Anderson, M. A., & Hill, P. D. (2012). Comparison of pulse oximetry measures in a healthy population. *Medsurg Nursing, 21*(2), 70–76.

Johnson, A., Schweitzer, D., & Ahrens, T. (2011). Time to throw away your stethoscope? Capnography: Evidence-based patient monitoring technology. *Journal of Radiological Nursing, 30*(1), 25–34.

Jones, M., Olorvida, E., Monger, K., et al. (2015). How well do inexpensive, portable pulse oximeter values agree with arterial oxygenation saturation in acutely ill patients? *Medsurg Nursing, 24*(6), 391–396.

Kane, C. J., York, N. L., & Minton, L. A. (2013). Chest tubes in the critically ill patient. *Dimensions of Critical Care Nursing, 32*(3), 111–117.

Karch, A. M. (2017). *Focus on nursing pharmacology* (7th ed.). Philadelphia, PA: Wolters Kluwer.

Khimani, R., Ali, F., Ratani, S., & Awan, S. (2015). Practices of tracheal suctioning technique among health care professionals: Literature review. *International Journal of Nursing Education, 7*(1), 179–183.

Kyle, T., & Carman, S. (2017). *Essentials of pediatric nursing* (3rd ed.). Philadelphia, PA: Wolters Kluwer Health.

Leddy, R., & Wilkinson, J. M. (2015). Endotracheal suctioning practices of nurses and respiratory therapists: How well do they align with clinical practice guidelines? *Canadian Journal of Respiratory Therapy, 51*(3), 60–64.

LeMone, P., Burke, K. M., Bauldoff, G., & Gubrud, P. (2015). *Medical-surgical nursing. Clinical reasoning in patient care* (6th ed.). New York: Pearson.

Levy, S. D., Alladina, J. W., Higgert, K. A., Harris, R. S., Bajwa, E. K., & Hess, D. R. (2016). High-flow oxygen therapy and other inhaled therapies in intensive care units. *Lancet, 387*(10030), 1867–1878.

Makic, M. B., Rauen, C., Jones, K., & Fisk, A. C. (2015). Continuing to challenge practice to be evidence based. *Critical Care Nurse, 35*(2), 39–50.

Mayfield, S., Jauncey-Cooke, J., Hough, J. L., Schibler, A., Gibbons, K., & Bogossian, F. (2014). High-glow nasal cannula therapy for respiratory support in children. *Cochrane Database of Systematic Reviews*, 3. Art. No.: CD009850. doi: 10.1002/14651858.CD009850. pub2.

McCoy, R. (2016). Home oxygen therapy: Delivery options and clinical issues. *RT: The Journal for Respiratory Care Practitioners, 29*(6), 18–20.

McDonald, C. F. (2014). Oxygen therapy for COPD. *Journal of Thoracic Disease, 6*(11), 1632–1639.

MedlinePlus. (2016). *Oxygen safety*. Retrieved https://medlineplus.gov/ency/patientinstructions/000049.htm

Mitchell, J. (2015). Pathophysiology of COPD: Part 2. *Practice Nursing, 26*(9), 444–449.

Morris, L. L., McIntosh, E., & Whitmer, A. (2014). The importance of tracheostomy progression in the intensive care unit. *Critical Care Nurse, 34*(1), 40–49.

Morris, L. L., Whitmer, A., & McIntosh, E. (2013). Tracheostomy care and complications in the intensive care unit. *Critical Care Nurse, 33*(5), 18–30.

Morton, P. G., & Fontaine, D. K. (2018). *Critical care nursing. A holistic approach* (11th ed.). Philadelphia, PA: Wolters Kluwer.

Murphie, P. (2015). Home oxygen therapy: An update for community nurses. *Journal of Community Nursing, 29*(4), 55–59.

Muzzy, A. C., & Butler, A. K. (2015). Managing chest tubes: Air leaks and unplanned tube removal. *American Nurse Today, 10*(5), 10–13.

NANDA International, Inc. *Nursing Diagnoses - Definitions and Classification 2018–2020* © 2017 NANDA International, ISBN 978-1-62623-929-6. Used by arrangement with the Thieme Group, Stuttgart/New York.

National Fire Protection Association (NFPA). (2013). *Public education: Medical oxygen*. Retrieved http://www.nfpa.org/public-education/by-topic/safety-in-the-home/medical-oxygen

National Heart, Lung, and Blood Institute (NHLBI). (2013). *COPD*. Retrieved http://www.nhlbi.nih.gov/health/health-topics/topics/copd/atrisk

Nishimura, M. (2016). High-flow nasal cannula oxygen therapy in adults: Physiological benefits, indication, clinical benefits, and adverse effects. *Respiratory Care, 61*(4), 529–541.

Owen, E. B., Woods, C. R., O'Flynn, J. A., Boone, M. C., Calhoun, A. W., & Montgomery V. L. (2016). A bedside decision tree for use of saline with endotracheal tube suctioning in children. *Critical Care Nurse, 36*(1), e1–e10.

Pate, M., & Zapata, T. (2002). Ask the experts: How deeply should I go when I suction an endotracheal or tracheostomy tube? *Critical Care Nurse, 22*(2), 130–131.

Perry, S. E., Hockenberry, M. J., Lowdermilk, D. L., & Wilson, D. (2014). *Maternal child nursing care* (5th ed.). St. Louis, MO: Elsevier.

Philip, K., Richardson, R., & Cohen, J. (2013). Staff perceptions of respiratory rate measurement in a general hospital. *British Journal of Nursing, 22*(10), 570–574.

Purnell, L. D. (2013). *Transcultural health care. A culturally competent approach* (4th ed.). Philadelphia, PA: F.A. Davis Company.

Quinn, B., & Baker, D. L. (2015). Comprehensive oral care helps prevent hospital-acquired nonventilator pneumonia. *American Nurse Today, 10*(3), 18–22.

Schreiber, M. L. (2015). Tracheostomy: Site care, suctioning, and readiness. *Medsurg Nursing, 24*(2), 121–124.

Schuman, A. J. (2014). Pulse oximetry. The fifth vital sign. *Contemporary Pediatrics, 31*(10), 44–46.

Seeley, M. C., McKenna, L., & Hood, K. (2015). Graduate nurses' knowledge of the functions and limitations of pulse oximetry. *Journal of Clinical Nursing, 24*(23–24), 3538–3549.

Shimizu, T., Mizutani, T., Yamahita, S., Hagiya, K., & Tanaka, M. (2011). Endotracheal tube extubation force: Adhesive tape versus endotracheal tube holder. *Respiratory Care, 56*(11), 1825–1829.

Sole, M. L., Bennet, M. B., & Ashworth, S. (2015). Clinical indicators for endotracheal suctioning in adult patients receiving mechanical ventilation. *American Journal of Critical Care, 24*(4), 318–324.

Sterni, L. M., Collaco, J. M., Baker, C. D., et al. (2016). An official American Thoracic Society Clinical Practice Guideline: Pediatric chronic home invasive ventilation. *American Journal of Respiratory and Critical Care Medicine, 193*(8), e16–e35.

Strickland, S. L., Rubin, B. K., Drescher, G. S., et al. (2013). AARC clinical practice guideline: Effectiveness of nonpharmacologic airway clearance therapies in hospitalized patients. *Respiratory Care, 58*(12), 2187–2193.

Taylor, C., Lynn, P., & Bartlett, J. (2019). *Fundamentals of nursing: The art and science of person-centered care* (9th ed.). Philadelphia, PA: Wolters Kluwer.

Taylor, J. J., & Cohen, B. J. [2013]. *Memmler's structure and function of the human body* [10th ed.]. Philadelphia, PA: Wolters Kluwer Health/Lippincott Williams & Wilkins.

VHA Center for Engineering & Occupational Safety and Health (CEOSH). (2016). *Safe patient handling and mobility guidebook*. St. Louis, MO: Author. Retrieved http://www.tampavaref.org/safe-patient-handling.htm

Van Leeuwen, A. M., & Bladh, M. L. (2015). *Davis's comprehensive handbook of laboratory & diagnostic tests with nursing implications* (5th ed.). Philadelphia, PA: F.A. Davis Company.

Vottier, G., Matrot, B., Jones, P., & Dauger, S. (2016). A cross-over study of continuous tracheal cuff pressure monitoring in critically-ill children. *Intensive Care Medicine, 42*(1), 132–133.

Ward, J. J. (2013). High-flow oxygen administration by nasal cannula for adult and perinatal patients. *Respiratory Care, 58*(1), 98–122.

Wiles, K. S. (2016). Oxygen therapy in the home. *AARC Times, 40*(5), 24–26.

World Health Organization (WHO). (2011). *Patient Safety. Using the pulse oximeter*. Retrieved http://www.who.int/patientsafety/safesurgery/pulse_oximetry/who_ps_pulse_oxymetry_tutorial2_advanced_en.pdf

Yönt, G. H., Korhan, E. A., & Dizer, B. (2014). The effect of nail polish on pulse oximetry readings. *Intensive and Critical Care Nursing, 30*(2), 111–115.

SUGGESTED ANSWERS FOR FOCUSING ON PATIENT CARE: DEVELOPING CLINICAL REASONING

1. Notify the primary care provider immediately. This can indicate fresh bleeding. Assess the patient's vital signs and level of consciousness. Significant changes from baseline may indicate complications. Assess the patient's respiratory status, including oxygen saturation level. The patient may become tachypneic and hypoxic. Assess the patient's lung sounds. The lung sounds over the chest tube site may be diminished due to the presence of increased blood. Also assess the patient for pain. Sudden pressure or increased pain indicates potential complications. Reassure the patient, as necessary, to decrease anxiety. Maintain the patient on bed rest and monitor closely. Anticipate the need for additional IV fluids or blood transfusions, as well as the potential for surgery to control the bleeding.

2. Assess the patient's level of knowledge regarding the use of an incentive spirometer. Assess the patient's level of pain. Administer pain medication, as prescribed, if needed. Wait the appropriate amount of time for the medication to take effect. Explain the rationale for use of an incentive spirometer and the goal of the activity. If the patient has recently undergone abdominal or chest surgery,

place a pillow or folded blanket over a chest or abdominal incision for splinting. Demonstrate how to steady the device with one hand and hold the mouthpiece with the other hand. If the patient cannot use hands, assist the patient with the incentive spirometer. Instruct the patient to exhale normally and then place lips securely around the mouthpiece. Instruct the patient to inhale slowly and as deeply as possible through the mouthpiece without using the nose (if desired, a nose clip may be used). When the patient cannot inhale anymore, the patient should hold her breath and count to three. Check the position of gauge to determine progress and level attained. If the patient begins to cough, splint an abdominal or chest incision. Instruct the patient to remove lips from mouthpiece and exhale normally. If the patient becomes lightheaded during the process, tell her to stop and take a few normal breaths before resuming incentive spirometry. Encourage the patient to perform incentive spirometry 5 to 10 times every 1 to 2 hours, if possible. Clean the mouthpiece with water and shake to dry. Patient should verbalize an understanding of the rationale, procedure, and cleaning of equipment and be able to give a return demonstration of the use of the incentive spirometer.

3. Assess lung sounds. Patients who need to be suctioned may have crackles or gurgling present. Assess oxygen saturation level. Oxygen saturation usually decreases when a patient needs to be suctioned. Assess respiratory status, including respiratory rate and depth. Patients may become tachypneic when they need to be suctioned. Assess patient for signs of respiratory distress, such as nasal flaring, retractions, or grunting. Additional indications for suctioning via an endotracheal tube include secretions in the tube, acute respiratory distress, and frequent or sustained coughing. Also assess for pain and the potential to cause pain during the intervention. Perform individualized pain management in response to the patient's needs (Arroyo-Novoa et al., 2008; Düzkaya & Kuğuoğlu, 2015). If the patient has had abdominal surgery or other procedures, administer pain medication before suctioning. Assess appropriate suction catheter depth (refer to Box 14-1 in Skill 14-7). Determine if suctioning the patient's airway was effective by reassessing the patient. The symptoms that indicated the need for airway suctioning should be absent or greatly diminished. The patient should not exhibit signs of respiratory distress, and should have an oxygen saturation level within normal limits.

Fluid, Electrolyte, and Acid–Base Balance

15

Focusing on Patient Care

This chapter will help you develop some of the skills related to fluid, electrolyte, acid–base balance necessary to care for the following patients:

Simon Lawrence, age 3 years, has been admitted to the pediatric floor with dehydration after vomiting for 2 days. He will be treated with intravenous fluids to assist in rehydration.

Melissa Cohen, age 32, was just involved in a motor vehicle crash. She has lost a large amount of blood and needs a blood transfusion.

Jack Tracy, age 67, is undergoing chemotherapy at the outpatient chemotherapy center. His recently implanted port will be deaccessed prior to leaving the center.

Refer to Focusing on Patient Care: Developing Clinical Reasoning at the end of the chapter to apply what you learn.

Learning Objectives

After completing the chapter, you will be able to accomplish the following:

1. Initiate a peripheral venous access IV infusion.
2. Change an IV solution container and administration set.
3. Monitor an IV site and infusion.
4. Change a peripheral venous access site dressing.
5. Cap for intermittent use and flush a peripheral venous access device.
6. Administer a blood transfusion.
7. Change the site dressing and flush a central venous access device.
8. Access an implanted port.
9. Deaccess an implanted port.
10. Remove a peripherally inserted central catheter (PICC).

Key Terms

autologous transfusion: a blood transfusion donated by the patient in anticipation that he or she may need the transfusion during a hospital stay

blood typing: determining a person's blood type (A, B, AB, or O)

central venous access device (CVAD): a venous access device in which the tip of the catheter terminates in the central venous circulation, usually in the superior vena cava just above the right atrium

crossmatching: determining the compatibility of two blood specimens

dehydration: the loss or deprivation of water from the body or tissues

edema: accumulation of fluid in body tissues

hypertonic: having a greater concentration of solutes than the solution with which it is being compared

hypervolemia (fluid volume excess): excess of isotonic fluid (water and sodium) in the extracellular space

hypotonic: having a lesser concentration than the solution with which it is being compared

hypovolemia (fluid volume deficit): deficiency of isotonic fluid (water and sodium) from the extracellular space

implanted port: a type of CVAD; subcutaneous injection port attached to a catheter; distal catheter tip dwells in the lower one third of the superior vena cava to the junction of the superior vena cava and the right atrium (Infusion Nurses Society [INS], 2016a), and the proximal end or port is usually implanted in a subcutaneous pocket of the upper chest wall. Implanted ports placed in the antecubital area of the arm are referred to as *peripheral access system ports.*

isotonic: having about the same solute concentration as the solution with which it is being compared

nontunneled percutaneous central venous catheter: a type of CVAD that has a short dwell time (3 to 10 days); may have double, triple, or quadruple lumens; are more than 8 cm, depending on patient size; introduced through the skin into the internal jugular, subclavian, or femoral veins and sutured into place; and are mainly used in critical care and emergency settings

peripheral venous access device: a short (less than 3 in) peripheral catheter placed in a peripheral vein for short-term therapy. This device is not appropriate for certain therapies, such as vesicant chemotherapy, drugs that are classified as irritants, or parenteral nutrition.

peripherally inserted central catheter (PICC): a type of CVAD, more than 20 cm, depending on patient size, that can be introduced into a peripheral vein (usually the basilic, brachial, or cephalic vein), and advanced so the distal tip dwells in the lower one third of the superior vena cava to the junction of the superior vena cava and the right atrium (INS, 2016a)

tunneled percutaneous central venous catheter: a type of CVAD; intended for long-term use; implanted into the internal or external jugular or subclavian vein; length of this catheter is more than 8 cm (approximately 90 cm on average), depending on patient size; tunneled in subcutaneous tissue under the skin (usually the midchest area) for 3 to 6 in to its exit site

T his chapter discusses the skills needed to care for patients with fluid, electrolyte, and acid–base balance needs. Body fluid makes up approximately 50% to 60% of body weight in a healthy person and the primary body fluid is water. The balance, or homeostasis, of fluid, electrolytes, and acid–base is interrelated and maintained through the functions of almost every organ of the body. In a healthy person, fluid intake and fluid losses are about equal. Fundamentals Review 15-1 lists the average adult daily fluid sources and losses. Abnormalities in fluid, electrolyte, and acid–base balance are also interrelated and may occur together.

The use of infused intravenous (IV) solutions may be prescribed as part of patient care related to fluid, electrolyte, and acid–base disturbances. The health care provider with prescriptive privileges is responsible for prescribing the kind and amount of solution to be used. The nurse is responsible for critically evaluating all patient orders prior to administration, as well as for initiating, monitoring, and discontinuing the therapy. Any concerns regarding the type or amount of therapy prescribed should be immediately and clearly communicated to the prescribing health care provider. The contents of selected IV solutions are listed, along with comments about their use, in Fundamentals Review 15-2. As with other therapeutic agents, the nurse must understand the rationale for the use of IV therapy for the individual patient, the type of solution being used, its desired effect, and potential adverse reactions and effects (Fundamentals Review 15-3).

Fundamentals Review 15-1

AVERAGE ADULT DAILY FLUID SOURCES AND LOSSES

Fluid Intake (mL)		Fluid Output (mL)	
Ingested water	1,300	Kidneys	1,500
Ingested food	1,000	Skin	600
Metabolic oxidation	300	Lungs	300
		Gastrointestinal	200
Total	2,600	*Total*	2,600

Fundamentals Review 15-2

SELECTED INTRAVENOUS SOLUTIONS

Solution	Comments
ISOTONIC	
0.9% NaCl (normal saline)	Not desirable as a routine maintenance solution because it provides only Na^+ and Cl^-, which are provided in excessive amounts.
	May be used to expand temporarily the extracellular compartment if circulatory insufficiency is a problem; also used to treat hypovolemia, metabolic alkalosis, hyponatremia, and hypochloremia.
	Used with administration of blood transfusions.
Lactated Ringer's solution	Contains multiple electrolytes in about the same concentrations as found in plasma (note that this solution is lacking in Mg^{2+} and PO_4^{3-}).
	Used in the treatment of hypovolemia, burns, and fluid lost from gastrointestinal sources.
	Useful in treating metabolic acidosis.
HYPOTONIC	
0.33% NaCl (¹⁄₃-strength normal saline)	Provides Na^+, Cl^-, and free water.
	Na^+ and Cl^- allow kidneys to select and retain needed amounts.
	Free water is desirable as aid to kidneys in elimination of solutes.
	Used in treating hypernatremia.
0.45% NaCl (½-strength normal saline)	A hypotonic solution that provides Na^+, Cl^-, and free water.
	Used as a basic fluid for maintenance needs.
	Often used to treat hypernatremia (because this solution contains a small amount of Na^+, it dilutes the plasma sodium while not allowing it to drop too rapidly).
HYPERTONIC	
5% dextrose in lactated Ringer's solution	Supplies fluid and calories to the body
	Replaces electrolytes; shifts fluid from the intracellular compartment into the intravascular space, expanding vascular volume
5% dextrose in 0.9% NaCl (normal saline)	Used to treat syndrome of inappropriate antidiuretic hormone (SIADH).
	Can temporarily be used to treat hypovolemia if plasma expander is not available.

Source: Adapted from Hale, A., & Hovey, M. J. (2014). *Fluid, electrolyte, and acid–base imbalances.* Philadelphia, PA: F.A. Davis Company; Hinkle, J. L., & Cheever, K. H. (2018). *Brunner & Suddarth's textbook of medical-surgical nursing* (14th ed.). Philadelphia, PA: Wolters Kluwer; and Willis L. M. (2015). *Fluids & electrolytes made incredibly easy!* (6th ed.). Philadelphia, PA: Wolters Kluwer.

Fundamentals Review 15-3

COMPLICATIONS ASSOCIATED WITH INTRAVENOUS INFUSIONS

Complication/Cause	Signs and Symptoms	Nursing Considerations
Infiltration: the escape of fluid into the subcutaneous tissue Dislodged needle Penetrated vessel wall	Swelling, pallor, coldness, or pain around the infusion site; significant decrease in the flow rate	Check infusion site every hour for signs/symptoms. Discontinue the infusion if symptoms occur. Restart the infusion at a different site. Use site-stabilization device.
Venous access device–related infection: Improper hand decontamination/hand hygiene Frequent disconnection of tubing, access ports, and/or access caps Poor insertion technique, multiple insertion attempts Multilumen catheters Long-term catheter insertion Frequent dressing changes Inadequate/improper decontamination of hub prior to use An IV solution that becomes contaminated when solutions are changed, a medication is added, or the solution is allowed to infuse for too long a period Inappropriate administration set changes	Erythema, edema, induration, drainage at the insertion site Fever, malaise, chills, other vital sign changes	Perform hand hygiene before and after palpating catheter insertion sites; before and after inserting, replacing, accessing, and dressing a venous access device. Assess catheter site routinely. Notify primary care provider immediately if any signs of infection. Use scrupulous aseptic technique when starting an infusion. Follow best-practice guidelines for site care, changing of administration tubing sets, connectors, caps, and other administration equipment. Follow facility protocol for culture of drainage. Consider use of 2% chlorhexidine wash for daily skin cleansing.
Phlebitis: an inflammation of a vein Mechanical trauma from needle or catheter Chemical trauma from solution	Local, acute tenderness; redness, warmth, and slight edema of the vein above the insertion site	Discontinue the infusion immediately. Apply warm compresses to the affected site. Avoid further use of the vein. Restart the infusion in another vein.
Thrombus: a blood clot Tissue trauma from needle or catheter	Symptoms similar to phlebitis IV fluid flow may cease if clot obstructs needle	Stop the infusion immediately. Apply warm compresses as ordered by the primary care provider. Restart the IV at another site. *Do not rub or massage the affected area.*
Speed shock: the body's reaction to a substance that is injected into the circulatory system too rapidly Too rapid a rate of fluid infusion into circulation	Pounding headache, fainting, rapid pulse rate, apprehension, chills, back pains, and dyspnea	Use the proper IV tubing. Carefully monitor the rate of fluid flow. Check the rate frequently for accuracy. A time tape is useful for this purpose.
Fluid overload: the condition caused when too large a volume of fluid infuses into the circulatory system Too large a volume of fluid infused into circulation	Engorged neck veins, increased blood pressure, and difficulty in breathing (dyspnea)	If symptoms develop, slow the rate of infusion. Notify the primary care provider immediately. Monitor vital signs. Carefully monitor the rate of fluid flow. Check the rate frequently for accuracy.
Air embolus: air in the circulatory system Break in the IV system above the heart level allowing air in the circulatory system as a bolus	Respiratory distress Increased heart rate Cyanosis Decreased blood pressure Change in level of consciousness	Pinch off catheter or secure system to prevent entry of air. Place patient on left side in Trendelenburg position. Call for immediate assistance. Monitor vital signs and pulse oximetry.

Skill 15-1 ▶ Initiating a Peripheral Venous Access IV Infusion

Administering and monitoring intravenous (IV) fluids is an essential part of routine patient care. The primary care provider often orders IV therapy to prevent or correct problems in fluid and electrolyte balance. For IV fluid and other therapies to be administered, an IV access must be established. The nurse initiating a peripheral venous access needs to assess for the safest, most appropriate location for each particular patient. Refer to the Assessment section of this skill. Figure 1 illustrates potential infusion sites for peripheral venous catheters. Consider the use of methods to reduce pain and discomfort of catheter insertion, such as local anesthetic agents and adjunctive therapies (cognitive, behavioral, and complementary therapies) (INS, 2016a).

Verify the amount and type of solution to be administered, as well as the prescribed infusion rate. Critically evaluating all patient orders prior to administration. Any concerns regarding the type or amount of therapy prescribed should be immediately and clearly communicated to the prescribing health care provider. Evaluate the patient's need for IV therapy, the type of solution being used, its desired effect, and potential adverse reactions and effects. Follow the facility's policies and guidelines to determine if the infusion should be administered by electronic infusion device or by gravity. Refer to Box 15-1 for guidelines to calculate the flow rate for gravity infusion.

FIGURE 1. Infusion sites. **A.** Ventral and dorsal aspects of lower arm and hand. **B.** Scalp.

Box 15-1   Regulating IV Flow Rate

Follow facility guidelines to determine if infusion should be administered by electronic infusion device or by gravity.

- Check medical order for IV solution.
- Check patency of IV access.

If the infusion is to be administered by gravity infusion:

- Verify drop factor (number of drops in 1 mL) of the equipment in use.
- Calculate the flow rate:

  EXAMPLE—Administer 1,000 mL D$_5$W over 10 hours (set delivers 60 gtt drops/1 mL).

  a. Standard formula

  $$\text{gtt (drops)/min} = \frac{\text{volume (mL)} \times \text{drop factor (gtt (drops)/mL)}}{\text{time (in minutes)}}$$

  $$\text{gtt (drops)/min} = \frac{1000 \text{ mL} \times 60}{600 \ (60 \text{ min} \times 10 \text{ h})}$$

  $$= \frac{60,000}{600}$$

  $$= 100 \text{ gtt (drops)/min}$$

b. Short formula using milliliters per hour

$$\text{gtt (drops)/min} = \frac{\text{milliliters per hour} \times \text{drop factor (gtt (drops)/mL)}}{\text{time (60 min)}}$$

Find milliliters per hour by dividing 1,000 mL by 10 hours:

$$\frac{1000}{10} = 100 \text{ mL/60}$$

$$\text{gtt (drops)/min} = \frac{100 \text{ mL} \times 60}{60 \text{ min}}$$

$$= \frac{6000}{60}$$

$$= 100 \text{ drops/min}$$

DELEGATION GUIDELINES

The initiation of a peripheral venous access IV infusion is not delegated to nursing assistive personnel (NAP) or to unlicensed assistive personnel (UAP). Depending on the state's nurse practice act and the organization's policies and procedures, initiation of a peripheral venous access IV infusion may be delegated to licensed practical/vocational nurses (LPN/LVNs). The decision to delegate must be based on careful analysis of the patient's needs and circumstances, as well as the qualifications of the person to whom the task is being delegated. Refer to the Delegation Guidelines in Appendix A.

EQUIPMENT

- IV solution, as prescribed
- Electronic MAR (eMAR) or medication administration record (MAR)
- Towel or disposable pad
- Nonallergenic tape
- IV administration set
- Label for infusion set (for next change date)
- Transparent site dressing
- Electronic infusion device (if appropriate)
- Tourniquet
- Time tape and/or label (for IV container)
- Cleansing swabs (>0.5% chlorhexidine preferred; tincture of iodine, an iodophor [povidone-iodine], or 70% alcohol may also be used) (INS, 2016b; Mimoz et al., 2015; O'Grady et al., 2011)
- IV securement/stabilization device, as appropriate
- Clean gloves
- Additional PPE, as indicated
- IV pole
- Local anesthetic (based on facility policy and/or if prescribed)
- IV catheter
- Short extension tubing, if not permanently attached to the IV catheter
- Needleless connector or end cap for extension tubing
- Alcohol or other disinfectant wipes
- Passive disinfection caps (based on facility policy)
- Skin protectant wipe (e.g., Skin-Prep)
- Single-use clippers or scissors for hair removal (as indicated)
- Prefilled 2-mL syringe with sterile normal saline for injection

(continued)

Skill 15-1 ▶ Initiating a Peripheral Venous Access IV Infusion *(continued)*

ASSESSMENT

Review the patient's record for baseline data, such as vital signs, intake and output balance, and pertinent laboratory values, such as serum electrolytes. Assess the appropriateness of the solution for the patient. Inspect the IV infusion solution for any particulates and check the IV label. Confirm it is the solution prescribed. Review assessment and laboratory data that may influence solution administration. The suitability of particular veins for peripheral IV infusions varies with individual circumstances. Determine site selection after considering the accessibility of a vein; the condition of a vein; and the type of fluid to be infused. Assess arms and hands for potential sites for initiating the IV. Keep in mind the following guidelines related to peripheral venous catheters and access sites:

- Determine the most desirable accessible vein. Use the venous site most likely to last the full length of the prescribed therapy, using the forearm to increase dwell time, promote self-care, and prevent accidental removal and occlusions (INS, 2016b). The dorsal and ventral surfaces of the upper extremities, including the metacarpal, cephalic, basilic, and median veins, are appropriate sites for infusion (INS, 2016b). Avoid the ventral surface of the wrist because of the potential risk for nerve damage (INS, 2016b). Figure 15-1.1A illustrates infusion sites on the arm and hand for adult patients.
- Generally, either arm may be used for IV therapy. Usually the nondominant arm is selected for patient comfort and to limit movement in the impacted extremity. For example, if the patient is right-handed, the IV is preferably placed on the left extremity to improve the patient's ability to complete activities of daily living. This is particularly important if the duration of infusion is expected to be prolonged.
- Determine accessibility based on the patient's condition. The use of an extremity for IV therapy may be contraindicated in some circumstances. For example, patients with a history of breast cancer with same-side surgical axillary lymph node removal; patients with burns, infections, or traumatic injury to the extremity; and patients with an upper extremity arteriovenous fistula or graft or other catheters for dialysis treatment will not be able to have an IV catheter placed on the impacted extremity.
- Do not use the antecubital veins if another vein is available. They are not a good choice for infusion because flexion of the patient's arm can displace the IV catheter over time. By avoiding the antecubital veins for peripheral venous catheters, a PICC line may be inserted at a later time, if needed.
- Do not use veins in the leg of an adult, unless other sites are inaccessible, because of the danger of stagnation of peripheral circulation and possible serious complications. The cannulation of the lower extremities is associated with risk of tissue damage, thrombophlebitis, and ulceration (INS, 2016b). Some facilities require a medical order to insert an IV catheter in an adult patient's lower extremity.

NURSING DIAGNOSIS

Determine the related factors for the nursing diagnoses based on the patient's current status. Appropriate nursing diagnoses may include:

- Deficient fluid volume
- Risk for shock
- Risk for imbalanced fluid volume

OUTCOME IDENTIFICATION AND PLANNING

The expected outcome to achieve when initiating a peripheral venous access IV infusion is that the access device is inserted using sterile technique on the first attempt. Also, the patient experiences minimal discomfort, and the IV solution infuses without difficulty.

IMPLEMENTATION

ACTION	RATIONALE
1. Verify the IV solution order on the eMAR/MAR with the medical order. Consider the appropriateness of the prescribed therapy in relation to the patient. Clarify any inconsistencies. Check the patient's chart for allergies. Check solution for color, leaking, and expiration date. Know techniques for IV insertion, precautions, and purpose of the IV solution administration, if ordered. Gather necessary supplies.	This ensures that the correct IV solution and rate of infusion, and/or medication will be administered. The nurse is responsible for critically evaluating all patient orders prior to administration. Any concerns regarding the type or amount of therapy prescribed should be immediately and clearly communicated to the prescribing health care provider. This knowledge and skill is essential for safe and accurate IV and medication administration. Preparation promotes efficient time management and an organized approach to the task.

ACTION	RATIONALE

2. Perform hand hygiene and put on PPE, if indicated.

Hand hygiene and PPE prevent the spread of microorganisms. PPE is required based on transmission precautions.

3. Identify the patient.

Identifying the patient ensures the right patient receives the intervention and helps prevent errors.

4. Assemble equipment to the bedside stand or overbed table or other surface within reach.

Bringing everything to the bedside conserves time and energy. Arranging items nearby is convenient, saves time, and avoids unnecessary stretching and twisting of muscles on the part of the nurse.

5. Close the curtains around the bed and close the door to the room, if possible. Explain what you are going to do and why you are going to do it to the patient. Ask the patient about allergies to medications, tape, or skin antiseptics, as appropriate. If considering using a local anesthetic, inquire about allergies for these substances as well.

This ensures the patient's privacy. Explanation relieves anxiety and facilitates cooperation. Possible allergies may exist related to medications, tape, or local anesthetic. Injectable anesthetic can result in allergic reactions and tissue damage.

6. If using a local anesthetic, explain the rationale and procedure to the patient. Apply the anesthetic to a few potential insertion sites. Allow sufficient time for the anesthetic to take effect.

Explanations provide reassurance and facilitate the patient's cooperation. Local anesthetic decreases the degree of pain felt at the insertion site. Some of the anesthetics take up to an hour to become effective.

Prepare the IV Solution and Administration Set

7. Compare the IV container label with the eMAR/MAR. Remove IV bag from outer wrapper, if indicated. Check expiration dates. Scan bar code on container, if necessary. Compare patient identification band with the eMAR/MAR. Alternately, label the solution container with the patient's name, solution type, additives, date, and time. Complete a time strip for the infusion and apply to IV container.

Checking the label with eMAR/MAR ensures the correct IV solution will be administered. Identifying the patient ensures the right patient receives the medications and helps prevent errors. Time strip allows for quick visual reference by the nurse to monitor infusion accuracy.

8. Maintain aseptic technique when opening sterile packages and IV solution. Remove administration set from the package (Figure 2). Apply label to the tubing reflecting the day/date for next set change, per facility guidelines.

Asepsis is essential for preventing the spread of microorganisms. Labeling the tubing ensures adherence to facility policy regarding administration set changes and reduces the risk of spread of microorganisms. Refer to Box 15-2 in Skill 15-2 for recommended administration set change guidelines.

Connector   Spike   Slide clamp

Drip chamber

Injection port

Roller clamp

FIGURE 2. Basic administration set for gravity infusion.

(*continued*)

Skill 15-1 ▶ Initiating a Peripheral Venous Access IV Infusion *(continued)*

ACTION	RATIONALE
9. Close the roller clamp or slide the clamp on the IV administration set (Figure 3). Invert the IV solution container and remove the cap on the entry site, taking care not to touch the exposed entry site. Remove the cap from the spike on the administration set. Using a twisting and pushing motion, insert the administration set spike into the entry site of the IV container (Figure 4). Alternately, follow the manufacturer's directions for insertion.	Clamping the IV tubing prevents air and fluid from entering the IV tubing at this time. Inverting the container allows easy access to the entry site. Touching the opened entry site on the IV container and/or the spike on the administration set results in contamination and the container/administration set would have to be discarded. Inserting the spike punctures the seal in the IV container and allows access to the contents.

FIGURE 3. Closing clamp on administration set.

FIGURE 4. Inserting administration set spike into entry site of IV fluid container.

10. Hang the IV container on the IV pole. Squeeze the drip chamber and fill at least halfway (Figure 5).	Suction causes fluid to move into the drip chamber. Fluid prevents air from moving down the tubing.

FIGURE 5. Squeezing drip chamber to fill at least halfway.

ACTION	RATIONALE

11. Open the IV tubing clamp, and allow fluid to move through the tubing. Follow the additional manufacturer's instructions for specific electronic infusion pump, as indicated. **Allow fluid to flow until all air bubbles have disappeared and the entire length of the tubing is primed (filled) with IV solution (Figure 6).** Close the clamp. Alternately, some brands of tubing may require removal of the cap at the end of the IV tubing to allow fluid to flow. Maintain its sterility. After fluid has filled the tubing, recap the end of the tubing.

This technique prepares for IV fluid administration and removes air from the tubing. If not removed from the tubing, large amounts of air can act as an embolus. Touching the open end of the tubing results in contamination and the administration set would have to be discarded.

12. If an electronic device is to be used, follow the manufacturer's instructions for inserting the tubing into the device (Figure 7).

This ensures proper use of equipment.

FIGURE 6. Priming administration set.

FIGURE 7. Inserting administration set into electronic infusion device.

Initiate Peripheral Venous Access

13. Place the patient in low-Fowler's position in bed. Place a protective towel or pad under the patient's arm.

The supine position permits either arm to be used and allows for good body alignment. The towel protects the underlying surface from blood contamination.

14. Provide emotional support, as needed.

The patient may experience anxiety because he/she may, in general, fear needlestick or IV infusion.

15. Open the short extension tubing package. Attach the needleless connector or end cap, if not in place. Clean the needleless connector or end cap with alcohol wipe. Insert a syringe with normal saline into the extension tubing. Fill the extension tubing with normal saline and place the extension tubing and syringe back on the package, within easy reach.

Priming the extension tubing removes air from the tubing and prevents administration of air when connected to venous access. Having the tubing within easy reach facilitates accomplishment of procedure.

16. Select and palpate for an appropriate vein. Refer to the guidelines in the previous Assessment section. If the intended insertion site is visibly soiled, clean the area with soap and water.

The use of an appropriate vein decreases discomfort for the patient and reduces the risk for damage to body tissues.

17. If the site is hairy and facility policy permits, clip a 2-in area around the intended entry site.

Hair can harbor microorganisms and inhibit adhesion of site dressing. Shaving causes microabrasions and increases risk for infection (INS, 2016b, p. S44).

18. Put on gloves.

Gloves prevent contact with blood and body fluids.

(continued)

Skill 15-1 ▶ Initiating a Peripheral Venous Access IV Infusion *(continued)*

ACTION	RATIONALE
19. Apply a tourniquet 3 to 4 in above the venipuncture site to obstruct venous blood flow and distend the vein (Figure 8). Direct the ends of the tourniquet away from the entry site. Make sure the radial pulse is still present.	Impeding venous blood flow causes the vein to distend while maintaining arterial circulation. Distended veins are easy to see, palpate, and enter. The end of the tourniquet could contaminate the area of injection if directed toward the entry site. Tourniquet may be applied too tightly, so assessment for radial pulse is important. Checking radial pulse ensures arterial supply is not compromised.

FIGURE 8. Applying tourniquet.

ACTION	RATIONALE
20. Instruct the patient to hold the arm lower than the heart.	Lowering the arm below the heart level helps distend the veins by filling them.
21. Ask the patient to open and close the fist. Observe and palpate for a suitable vein. Try the following techniques if a vein cannot be felt:	Contracting the muscles of the forearm forces blood into the veins, thereby distending them further.
a. Lightly stroke the vein downward.	Stroking the vein helps distend the vein by filling it with blood.
b. Remove tourniquet and place warm, dry compresses over intended vein for 10 to 15 minutes.	Warm compresses help dilate veins. The use of dry heat increases the likelihood of successful peripheral catheter insertion (INS, 2016b).
22. **Cleanse the site with >5% chlorhexidine, or according to facility policy. Press the applicator against the skin and apply chlorhexidine using a gentle back and forth motion. Do not wipe or blot. Allow to dry completely for at least 30 seconds (INS, 2016a).**	Cleansing is necessary because organisms on the skin can be introduced into the tissues or the bloodstream with the needle. Use of >0.5% chlorhexidine in alcohol solution is preferred for skin antisepsis. If there is a contraindication to alcoholic chlorhexidine solution, tincture of iodine, an iodophor (povidone-iodine), or 70% alcohol may also be used (INS, 2016b; Mimoz et al., 2015; O'Grady et al., 2011). Iodophor (povidone-iodine) must remain on the skin for 1½ to 2 minutes or longer to completely dry for adequate antisepsis (INS, 2016a).
23. Using the nondominant hand placed about 1 or 2 in below the entry site, hold the skin taut against the vein. Avoid touching the prepared site. Ask the patient to remain still while performing the venipuncture.	Pressure on the vein and surrounding tissues stabilizes the vein and helps prevent movement of the vein as the needle or catheter is being inserted. The planned IV insertion site is not palpated after skin cleansing unless sterile gloves are worn to prevent contamination (INS, 2016b). Patient movement may prevent proper technique for IV insertion.

ACTION	RATIONALE

24. Align the IV catheter on top of the vein; enter the skin gently, holding the catheter by the hub in your dominant hand, bevel side up, at a 10- to 15-degree angle (Figure 9). Insert the catheter from directly over the vein or from the side of the vein. While following the course of the vein, advance the needle or catheter into the vein. A sensation of "give" can be felt when the needle enters the vein.

This allows the needle or catheter to enter the vein with minimal trauma and deters passage of the needle through the vein.

25. Continue to hold the skin taut. When blood returns through the catheter and/or the flashback chamber of the catheter, use the push-off tab to separate the catheter from the needle stylet and advance the catheter into the vein until the hub is at the venipuncture site. The exact technique depends on the type of device used.

The tourniquet causes increased venous pressure, resulting in automatic backflow. Placing the access device well into the vein helps to prevent dislodgement.

26. Release the tourniquet. Activate the safety mechanism on the needle stylet. Compress the skin well above the catheter tip to stop the flow of blood. Quickly remove the protective cap from the extension tubing and attach it to the catheter hub and tighten the Luer lock. Stabilize the catheter or needle with your nondominant hand.

Bleeding is minimized and the patency of the vein is maintained if the connection is made smoothly between the catheter and extension tubing.

27. Continue to stabilize the catheter or needle and pull back on the syringe to assess for blood return, then, flush gently with the saline, observing the site for infiltration and leaking. Remove the syringe from the end cap.

Infiltration and/or leaking and the patient reports of pain and/or discomfort indicate that the insertion into the vein is not successful and should be discontinued. The syringe is no longer needed once flushing is complete.

28. Open the skin protectant wipe. Apply the skin protectant to the site, making sure to apply—at minimum—the area to be covered with the dressing. Place a sterile transparent dressing and/or catheter securing/stabilization device over the venipuncture site. Loop the tubing near the entry site, and anchor with tape (nonallergenic) close to the site.

Skin protectant aids in adhesion of the dressing and decreases the risk for skin trauma when the dressing is removed. Transparent dressing allows easy visualization and protects the site. Stabilization/securing devices preserve the integrity of the access device, minimize catheter movement at the hub, and prevent catheter dislodgement and loss of access (INS, 2016b). Some stabilization devices act as a site dressing also. The weight of the tubing is sufficient to pull it out of the vein if it is not well anchored. Nonallergenic tape is less likely to tear fragile skin.

29. Label the IV dressing with the date, time, site, and type and size of the catheter placed (Figure 10).

Other personnel working with the infusion will know the site, type of device being used, and when it was inserted.

FIGURE 9. Stretching skin taut and inserting needle.

FIGURE 10. Venous access site with labeled dressing.

(continued)

Skill 15-1 ▶ Initiating a Peripheral Venous Access IV Infusion *(continued)*

ACTION

30. Using an antimicrobial swab, vigorously scrub the needleless connector or end cap on the extension tubing and allow to dry. Remove the end cap from the administration set. Insert the end of the administration set into the needleless connector or end cap (Figure 11). Loop the administration set tubing near the entry site, and anchor with tape (nonallergenic) close to the site. Remove gloves.

RATIONALE

Venous access device administration set entry points, end caps, and needleless connectors must be vigorously scrubbed and disinfected prior to each access to reduce the risk for introduction of microorganisms and prevent venous access device–related infection (Frimpong, Caguioa, & Octavo, 2015; Harper, 2014; INS, 2016b; The Joint Commission, 2018; Loveday et al., 2014). Friction is needed to physically remove microorganisms from the top, sides, and threads of the needleless connector or end cap. Allow the antiseptic to dry completely (15 to 30 seconds) to ensure complete effectiveness (Harper). Inserting the administration set allows initiation of the fluid infusion. The weight of the tubing is sufficient to pull it out of the vein if it is not well anchored. Nonallergenic tape is less likely to tear fragile skin. Removing gloves properly reduces the risk for infection transmission and contamination of other items.

FIGURE 11. Inserting administration set into the end cap of venous access device.

31. Open the clamp on the administration set. Set the flow rate and begin the fluid infusion (Figure 12). Alternately, start the flow of solution by releasing the clamp on the tubing and counting the drops. Adjust until the correct drop rate is achieved. Assess the flow of the solution and function of the infusion device. Inspect the insertion site for signs of infiltration (Figure 13).

Verifying the rate and device settings ensures the patient receives the correct volume of solution. If the catheter slips out of the vein, the solution will accumulate (infiltrate) into the surrounding tissue.

FIGURE 12. Initiating IV fluid infusion.

FIGURE 13. Inspecting insertion site.

ACTION	**RATIONALE**
32. Apply an IV securement/stabilization device if not already in place as part of the dressing, as indicated, based on facility policy. Explain to the patient the purpose of the device and the importance of safeguarding the site when using the extremity.	These systems are recommended for use on all venous access sites, and particularly central venous access sites, to preserve the integrity of the access device, minimize catheter movement at the hub, and prevent catheter dislodgement and loss of access (INS, 2016b). Some devices act as a site dressing also and may already have been applied.
33. Apply a passive disinfection cap to each access site on the administration set. Using an antimicrobial swab, vigorously scrub each access site cap on the administration set tubing and allow to dry. Attach a passive disinfection cap to each site (Figure 14).	Passive disinfection caps contain an antiseptic-impregnated sponge that dispenses the antiseptic over the connector's top and threads, and protect the hub from contamination by touch or airborne sources (Stango, Runyan, Stern, Macri, & Vacca, 2014). Venous access device administration set entry points, end caps, and needleless connectors must be vigorously scrubbed and disinfected prior to each access to reduce the risk for introduction of microorganisms and prevent venous access device–related infection (Frimpong et al., 2015; Harper, 2014; INS, 2016b; The Joint Commission, 2018; Loveday et al., 2014). Friction is needed to physically remove microorganisms from the top, sides, and threads of the needleless connector or end cap. Allow the antiseptic to dry completely (15 to 30 seconds) to ensure complete effectiveness (Harper).

FIGURE 14. Attaching a passive disinfection cap to each access site.

34. Remove equipment and return the patient to a position of comfort. Lower the bed, if not in the lowest position.	Promotes patient comfort and safety.
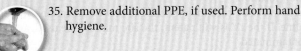 35. Remove additional PPE, if used. Perform hand hygiene.	Proper removal of PPE reduces the risk for infection transmission and contamination of other items. Hand hygiene prevents transmission of microorganisms.
36. Return to check the flow rate and observe the IV site for infiltration and/or other complications 30 minutes after starting infusion, and at least hourly thereafter. Ask the patient if he/she is experiencing any pain or discomfort related to the IV infusion.	Continued monitoring is important to maintain the correct flow rate. Early detection of problems ensures prompt intervention.

EVALUATION   The expected outcome has been met when the IV access is initiated on the first attempt; fluid flows easily into the vein without any sign of infiltration; and the patient verbalizes minimal discomfort related to insertion and demonstrates an understanding of the reasons for the IV.

(continued)

Skill 15-1

Initiating a Peripheral Venous Access IV Infusion   *(continued)*

DOCUMENTATION

Guidelines

Document the location where the IV access was placed, as well as the size of the IV catheter or needle, the type of IV solution, and the rate of the IV infusion, as well as the use of a securing or stabilization device. In addition, document the condition of the site. Record the patient's reaction to the procedure and pertinent patient teaching, such as alerting the nurse if the patient experiences any pain from the IV or notices any swelling at the site. Document the IV fluid solution on the intake and output record.

Sample Documentation

DocuCare Practice documenting peripheral venous access infusion in *Lippincott DocuCare.*

> 11/02/20 0830 20-gauge IV started in L hand via the dorsal metacarpal vein. Transparent dressing and peripheral stabilization device applied. Site without redness, drainage, or edema; patient denies discomfort. $D_5$1/2 NS with 20 mEq KCl begun at 110 mL/hr. Patient instructed to call with any pain, discomfort, or swelling and verbalizes an understanding of instructions.
>
> —*S. Barnes, RN*

UNEXPECTED SITUATIONS AND ASSOCIATED INTERVENTIONS

- *An artery is inadvertently accessed or the patient complains of paresthesias, numbness, or tingling upon insertion:* Immediately remove the catheter, apply pressure to the insertion site, and notify the primary care provider. Rapid attention may prevent permanent injury; nerves and arteries are often located in very close proximity to the venipuncture site (INS, 2016b, p. S44).
- *Fluid does not easily flow into the vein:* Reposition the extremity because certain positions that the patient may assume may prevent the IV from infusing properly. If the IV is a free-flowing IV, raise the height of the IV pole. This may promote an increase in IV flow. Attempt to flush the IV with 2 to 3 mL of saline in a syringe. Check the IV connector to ensure that the clamp is fully open. If fluid still does not flow easily, or if resistance is met while flushing, the IV may be against a valve and may need to be restarted in a different location.
- *Fluid does not flow easily into the vein and the skin around the insertion site is edematous and cool to the touch:* IV has infiltrated. Put on gloves and remove the catheter. Use a skin marker to outline the area with visible signs of infiltration to allow for assessment of changes. Secure gauze with tape over the insertion site without applying pressure. Assess the area distal to the venous access device for capillary refill, sensation, and motor function (INS, 2016a). Restart the IV in a new location. Estimate the volume of fluid that escaped into the tissue based on the rate of infusion and length of time since the last assessment. Notify the primary health care provider and use an appropriate method for clinical management of the infiltrate site, based on the infused solution and facility guidelines (INS, 2016b). Record site assessment and interventions, as well as the site for new venous access.
- *A small hematoma is forming at the site while you are inserting the catheter:* The vein is "blowing," which means a small hole has been made in the vein and blood is leaking out into the tissues. Remove and discard the catheter and choose an alternate insertion site.
- *Fluids are leaking around the insertion site:* Change the dressing on the IV. If the site continues to leak, remove IV and restart it in a new location.
- *IV infusion set becomes disconnected from IV:* Discard the IV tubing to prevent infection. Attempt to flush IV with 3 mL of normal saline. If the IV is still patent, the site may still be used, as long as the catheter hub has not been contaminated.
- *IV catheter is partially pulled out of insertion site (migrates externally):* Do not reinsert the catheter. Whether the IV is salvageable depends on how much of the catheter remains in the vein. Assess for proper placement in the vein before further use (INS, 2016b). If this catheter is not removed, monitor it closely for signs of infiltration and infection.

SPECIAL CONSIDERATIONS

General Considerations

- A 20- to 24-gauge catheter is recommended for most infusions in adult patients (INS, 2016b).
- An individual nurse should not make more than two attempts at vascular access placement when initiating venous access for a patient. If unsuccessful after two attempts, a colleague with advanced skills, such as a member of the nurse IV team, should attempt to initiate the venous

access, limiting total attempts to no more than four (INS, 2016b). Multiple unsuccessful attempts cause the patient pain and result in delayed treatment, limited future vascular access, increased costs, and increased risk for complications (INS, 2016b).

- Factors that may interfere with successful placement of a peripheral catheter include increased patient age, obesity, hypovolemia, injection drug use, the presence of multiple chronic diseases, and/or multiple hospitalizations requiring IV access (Dougherty, 2013; Dychter, Gold, Carson, & Haller, 2012; Fields, Piela, Au, & Ku, 2014; Partovi-Deilami, Nielsen, Møller, Nesheim, & Jørgensen, 2016). These patients lack easy access using the traditional techniques of direct visualization, anatomic landmarks, and palpation (Houston, 2013).
- Ultrasound-guided peripheral IV placement is a safe, efficient intervention for difficult-to-access patients (Houston, 2013; INS, 2016b). The Infusion Nurses Society recommends the use of ultrasound for placement of peripheral venous access devices in patients with difficult venous access and/or after failed venipuncture attempts (INS, 2016b).
- Closed IV catheter systems are available. These systems have the short extension tubing integrated into the catheter, eliminating the need to attach the extension tubing to the IV catheter before insertion, which reduces potential contamination.

Infant and Child Considerations

- Potential sites for pediatric patients include veins in the hand (should not be first choice), forearm, and upper arm below the axilla; avoid the antecubital area, which has a higher failure rate (INS, 2016b).
- Additional sites for infants and toddlers include veins of the scalp and, if not walking, the foot; avoid the use of the hand or fingers (INS, 2016b). Scalp arteries in infants are visible (see Fig. 40-17B). Carefully palpate the site before insertion. If the site is pulsating, do not use.
- Do not choose hand insertion sites as the first choice for children because their nerve endings are very close to the surface of the skin, and such an insertion is more painful. Once the child can walk, do not use the feet as insertion sites.
- A 22- to 24-gauge catheter is recommended for neonates and pediatric patients to minimize insertion-related trauma (INS, 2016b).
- Use chlorhexidine with caution in infants under 2 months of age and premature infants due to the risk of skin irritation and chemical burns (INS, 2016b).

Older Adult Considerations

- A 22- to 24-gauge catheter is recommended for older adults to minimize insertion-related trauma (INS, 2016b).
- To decrease the risk for trauma to the vessel, experienced nurses may omit use of a tourniquet if the patient has prominent but especially fragile veins.

EVIDENCE FOR PRACTICE ▶

INFUSION NURSING STANDARDS OF PRACTICE

Infusion Nurses Society (INS). (2016b). Infusion therapy. Standards of practice. *Journal of Infusion Nursing, 39*(Suppl 1), S1–S159.

The Infusion Nurses Society is recognized as the global authority in infusion therapy. The *Infusion Nursing Standards of Practice* is an evidence-based document, providing guidelines for nurses related to infusion therapy for use in all patient settings and addressing all patient populations.

Refer to thePoint° for additional research on related nursing topics.

EVIDENCE FOR PRACTICE ▶

INFUSION NURSING POLICIES AND PROCEDURES FOR INFUSION THERAPY

Infusion Nurses Society (INS). (2016a). *Policies and procedures for infusion therapy* (5th ed.). Norwood, MA: Author.

The Infusion Nurses Society is recognized as the global authority in infusion therapy. The *Infusion Nursing Standards of Practice* is an evidence-based document, providing policies and step-by-step procedures for nurses related to infusion therapy for use in all patient settings and addressing all patient populations.

Refer to thePoint° for additional research on related nursing topics.

Skill 15-2 ▶ **Changing an IV Solution Container and Administration Set**

Intravenous (IV) fluid administration frequently involves multiple bags or bottles of fluid infusion. Verify the amount and type of solution to be administered, as well as the prescribed infusion rate. Critically evaluating all patient orders prior to administration. Any concerns regarding the type or amount of therapy prescribed should be immediately and clearly communicated to the prescribing health care provider. Evaluate the patient's need for IV therapy, the type of solution being used, its desired effect, and potential adverse reactions and effects. Follow the facility's policies and guidelines to determine if the infusion should be administered by electronic infusion device or by gravity. Refer to Box 15-1 for guidelines to calculate the flow rate for gravity infusion. In addition, monitor these fluid infusions and replace the fluid containers, as needed. Focus on the following points:

• If more than one IV solution or medication is ordered, check facility policy and appropriate literature to make sure that the additional IV solution can be attached to the existing tubing.
• As one bag is infusing, prepare the next bag so it is ready for a change when less than 50 mL of fluid remains in the original container.
• Ongoing assessments related to the desired outcomes of the IV therapy, as well as assessing for both local and systemic IV infusion complications, are required. Refer to Fundamentals Review 15-3.
• Before switching the IV solution containers, check the date and time of the infusion administration set to ensure it does not also need to be replaced. Check facility policy for guidelines for changing IV administration sets. Refer to Box 15-2 for recommended administration set change guidelines.

Box 15-2 | Recommended Administration Set Change Schedule

Type of Infusion/Type of Device	Recommended Frequency
• Primary and secondary continuous administration sets used to administer fluids other than lipid, blood, or blood products	• Change no more frequently than every 96 hours.
• Anti-infective CVAD	• Change every 7 days.
• Primary intermittent administration sets	• Change every 24 hours.
• Secondary intermittent administration sets detached from the primary administration set	• Change every 24 hours.
• Administration sets used to administer parenteral nutrition	• Change at least every 24 hours; some guidelines recommend changing with each new PN container.
• Administration sets used to administer intravenous fat emulsions	• Change every 12 hours and/or with each new fat emulsion container.
• Administration sets used to administer blood and blood components	• Change after the completion of each unit or every 4 hours.

Source: Adapted from Infusion Nurses Society (INS). (2016b). Infusion therapy. Standards of practice. *Journal of Infusion Nursing, 39*(Suppl 1), S1–S159; O'Grady, N. P., Alexander, M., Burns, L. A., et al. (2011). Guidelines for the prevention of intravascular catheter-related infections. *American Journal of Infection Control, 39*(4 Supplement), S1–S34.

DELEGATION CONSIDERATIONS

The changing of an IV solution container and administration set is not delegated to nursing assistive personnel (NAP) or to unlicensed assistive personnel (UAP). Depending on the state's nurse practice act and the organization's policies and procedures, these procedures may be delegated to licensed practical/vocational nurses (LPN/LVNs). The decision to delegate must be based on careful analysis of the patient's needs and circumstances, as well as the qualifications of the person to whom the task is being delegated. Refer to the Delegation Guidelines in Appendix A.

EQUIPMENT

For solution container change:
- IV solution, as prescribed
- eMAR/MAR
- Time tape and/or label (for IV container)
- PPE, as indicated

For tubing change:
- Administration set
- Label for administration set (for next change date)

- Sterile gauze
- Nonallergenic tape
- IV securement/stabilization device, as appropriate
- Passive disinfection caps (based on facility policy)
- Clean gloves
- Additional PPE, as indicated
- Alcohol or other disinfectant wipes

ASSESSMENT

Review the patient's record for baseline data, such as vital signs, intake and output balance, and pertinent laboratory values, such as serum electrolytes. Assess the appropriateness of the solution for the patient. Review assessment and laboratory data that may influence solution administration.

Inspect the IV site. The dressing should be intact, adhering to the skin on all edges. Check for any leaks or fluid under or around the dressing. Inspect the tissue around the IV entry site for swelling, coolness, or pallor. These are signs of fluid infiltration into the tissue around the IV catheter. Also inspect the site for redness, swelling, and warmth. These signs might indicate the development of phlebitis or an inflammation of the blood vessel at the site. Ask the patient if he/she is experiencing any pain or discomfort related to the IV line. Pain or discomfort can be a sign of infiltration, extravasation, phlebitis, thrombophlebitis, and infection related to IV therapy. Refer to Fundamentals Review 15-3. Skill 15-3 provides additional detail related to monitoring an IV site.

NURSING DIAGNOSIS

Determine the related factors for the nursing diagnoses based on the patient's current status. Appropriate nursing diagnoses may include:

- Deficient fluid volume
- Risk for infection

- Impaired skin integrity

OUTCOME IDENTIFICATION AND PLANNING

The expected outcome to achieve when changing an IV solution container and tubing is that the prescribed IV infusion continues without interruption and no infusion complications are identified.

IMPLEMENTATION

ACTION	RATIONALE
1. Verify the IV solution order on the eMAR/MAR with the medical order. Consider the appropriateness of the prescribed therapy in relation to the patient. Clarify any inconsistencies. Check the patient's chart for allergies. Check solution for color, leaking, and expiration date. Know the purpose of the IV solution administration. Gather necessary supplies.	This ensures that the correct IV solution and rate of infusion, and/or medication will be administered. The nurse is responsible for critically evaluating all patient orders prior to administration. Any concerns regarding the type or amount of therapy prescribed should be immediately and clearly communicated to the prescribing health care provider. This knowledge and skill is essential for safe and accurate IV and medication administration. Preparation promotes efficient time management and an organized approach to the task.
2. Perform hand hygiene and put on PPE, if indicated.	Hand hygiene and PPE prevent the spread of microorganisms. PPE is required based on transmission precautions.
3. Identify the patient.	Identifying the patient ensures the right patient receives the intervention and helps prevent errors.

(continued)

Skill 15-2 ▶ Changing an IV Solution Container and Administration Set *(continued)*

ACTION	RATIONALE
4. Assemble equipment to the bedside stand or overbed table or other surface within reach.	Bringing everything to the bedside conserves time and energy. Arranging items nearby is convenient, saves time, and avoids unnecessary stretching and twisting of muscles on the part of the nurse.
5. Close the curtains around the bed and close the door to the room, if possible. Explain what you are going to do and why you are going to do it to the patient. Ask the patient about allergies to medications or tape, as appropriate.	This ensures the patient's privacy. Explanation relieves anxiety and facilitates cooperation. Possible allergies may exist related to the IV solution additive or tape.
6. Compare IV container label with the eMAR/MAR. Remove IV bag from the outer wrapper, if indicated. Check expiration dates. Scan bar code on container, if necessary (Figure 1). Compare patient identification band with the eMAR/MAR. Alternately, label the solution container with the patient's name, solution type, additives, date, and time. Complete a time strip for the infusion and apply to IV container.	Checking label with eMAR/MAR ensures the correct IV solution will be administered. Identifying the patient ensures the right patient receives the medications and helps prevent errors. Time strip allows for quick visual reference by the nurse to monitor infusion accuracy.

FIGURE 1. Scanning the bar code on container.

7. Maintain aseptic technique when opening sterile packages and IV solution. Remove administration set from the package. Apply label to the tubing reflecting the day/date for next set change, per facility guidelines.	Asepsis is essential for preventing the spread of microorganisms. Labeling the tubing ensures adherence to facility policy regarding administration set changes and reduces risk of spread of microorganisms. Refer to Box 15-2 for recommended administration set change guidelines.

To Change IV Solution Container

8. If using an electronic infusion device, pause the device or put on "hold." Close the slide clamp on the administration set closest to the drip chamber. If using gravity infusion, close the roller clamp on the administration set.	The action of the infusion device needs to be paused while the solution container is changed. Closing the clamp prevents the fluid in the drip chamber from emptying and air from entering the tubing during the procedure.
9. Carefully remove the cap on the entry site of the new IV solution container and expose the entry site, **taking care not to touch the exposed entry site.**	Touching the opened entry site on the IV container results in contamination and the container would have to be discarded.
10. Lift completed container off IV pole and invert it. Quickly remove the spike from the old IV container, **being careful not to contaminate it.** Discard old IV container.	Touching the spike on the administration set results in contamination and the tubing would have to be discarded.
11. Using a twisting and pushing motion, insert the administration set spike into the entry site of the IV container. Alternately, follow the manufacturer's directions for insertion. Hang the container on the IV pole.	Inserting the spike punctures the seal in the IV container and allows access to contents.

ACTION	RATIONALE

12. Alternately, hang the new IV fluid container on an open hook on the IV pole. Carefully remove the cap on the entry site of the new IV solution container and expose the entry site, **taking care not to touch the exposed entry site.** Lift completed container off the IV pole and invert it. Quickly remove the spike from the old IV container, **being careful not to contaminate it** (Figure 2). Discard old IV container. Using a twisting and pushing motion, insert the administration set spike into the entry port of the new IV container as it hangs on the IV pole (Figure 3).

Touching the opened entry site on the IV container or the administration set spike results in contamination and both would have to be discarded. Inserting the spike punctures the seal in the IV container and allows access to contents.

FIGURE 2. Removing administration spike from old IV fluid container.

FIGURE 3. Inserting administration set spike into entry port of new IV fluid container.

13. If using an electronic infusion device, open the slide clamp, check the drip chamber of the administration set, verify the flow rate programmed in the infusion device, and turn the device to "run" or "infuse."

Verifying the rate and device settings ensures the patient receives the correct volume of the solution.

14. If using gravity infusion, slowly open the roller clamp on the administration set and count the drops. Adjust until the correct drop rate is achieved (Figure 4).

Opening the clamp regulates the flow rate into the drip chamber. Verifying the rate ensures that the patient receives the correct volume of solution.

FIGURE 4. Reopening clamp and adjusting flow rate.

(continued)

Skill 15-2 ▶ Changing an IV Solution Container and Administration Set *(continued)*

ACTION	RATIONALE

To Change IV Solution Container and Administration Set

15. Prepare the IV solution and administration set. Refer to Skill 15-1, Steps 7–11.

16. Hang the new IV container on an open hook on the IV pole. Close the clamp on the existing IV administration set. Also, close the clamp on the short extension tubing connected to the IV catheter in the patient's arm.

Clamping the existing IV tubing prevents leakage of fluid from the administration set after it is disconnected. Clamping the tubing on the extension set prevents introduction of air into the extension tubing.

17. If using an electronic infusion device, remove the current administration set from the device. Following the manufacturer's directions, insert a new administration set into the infusion device.

Administration set has to be removed in order to insert a new tubing into the device.

18. Put on gloves. Remove the current infusion tubing from the needleless connector or end cap on the short extension IV tubing. Using an antimicrobial swab, vigorously scrub the needleless connector or end cap on the extension tubing and allow to dry. Remove the cap from the new administration set. Insert the end of the administration set into the needleless connector or end cap (Figure 5). Loop the administration set tubing near the entry site, and anchor with tape (nonallergenic) close to the site (Figure 6).

Venous access device entry points, end caps, and needleless connectors must be vigorously scrubbed and disinfected prior to each access to reduce the risk for introduction of microorganisms and prevent venous access device–related infection (Frimpong et al., 2015; Harper, 2014; INS, 2016b; The Joint Commission, 2018; Loveday et al., 2014). Friction is needed to physically remove microorganisms from the top, sides, and threads of the needleless connector or end cap. Allow the antiseptic to dry completely (15 to 30 seconds) to ensure complete effectiveness (Harper). Inserting the administration set allows initiation of the fluid infusion. The weight of the tubing is sufficient to pull it out of the vein if it is not well anchored. Nonallergenic tape is less likely to tear fragile skin.

FIGURE 5. Inserting the end of the administration set into the needleless connector or end cap.

FIGURE 6. Making sure clamp is open on new tubing, with short extension tubing taped in place.

19. Open the clamp on the extension tubing. Open the clamp on the administration set.

Opening clamps allows solution to flow to the patient.

20. If using an electronic infusion device, open the slide clamp, check the drip chamber of the administration set, verify the flow rate programmed in the infusion device, and turn the device to "run" or "infuse."

Verifying the rate and device settings ensures the patient receives the correct volume of solution.

21. If using gravity infusion, slowly open the roller clamp on the administration set and count the drops. Adjust until the correct drop rate is achieved.

Opening the clamp regulates the flow rate into the drip chamber. Verifying the rate ensures the patient receives the correct volume of solution.

ACTION	**RATIONALE**
22. Apply a passive disinfection cap to each access site on the administration set. Using an antimicrobial swab, vigorously scrub each access site cap on the administration set tubing and allow to dry. Attach a passive disinfection cap to each site.	Passive disinfection caps contain an antiseptic-impregnated sponge that dispenses the antiseptic over the connector's top and threads, and protect the hub from contamination by touch or airborne sources (Stango et al., 2014). Venous access device administration set entry points, end caps, and needleless connectors must be vigorously scrubbed and disinfected prior to each access to reduce the risk for introduction of microorganisms and prevent venous access device–related infection (Frimpong et al., 2015; Harper, 2014; INS, 2016b; The Joint Commission, 2018; Loveday et al., 2014). Friction is needed to physically remove microorganisms from the top, sides, and threads of the needleless connector or end cap. Allow the antiseptic to dry completely (15 to 30 seconds) to ensure complete effectiveness (Harper).
23. Remove equipment. Ensure the patient's comfort. Remove gloves. Lower the bed, if not in the lowest position.	Promotes patient comfort and safety. Removing gloves properly reduces the risk for infection transmission and contamination of other items.
24. Remove additional PPE, if used. Perform hand hygiene.	Proper removal of PPE reduces the risk for infection transmission and contamination of other items. Hand hygiene prevents transmission of microorganisms.
25. Return to check the flow rate and observe the IV site for infiltration and/or other complications 30 minutes after starting infusion, and at least hourly thereafter. Ask the patient if he/she is experiencing any pain or discomfort related to the IV infusion.	Continued monitoring is important to maintain the correct flow rate. Early detection of problems ensures prompt intervention.

EVALUATION

The expected outcome has been achieved when the IV solution container and administration set are changed; the IV infusion continues without interruption; and no infusion complications are identified.

DOCUMENTATION

Guidelines

Document the type of IV solution and the rate of infusion (often done in the eMAR/MAR); and the assessment of the access site. Record the patient's reaction to the procedure and pertinent patient teaching, such as alerting the nurse if the patient experiences any pain from the IV or notices any swelling at the site. Document the IV fluid solution on the intake and output record.

Sample Documentation

> <u>11/3/20</u> 1015 IV fluid changed from $D_5$1/2 NS with 20 mEq KCl/L at 125 mL/hr to D_5 0.9% NS with 20 mEq KCl/L at 80 mL/hr via infusion pump. IV site intact; no swelling, redness, or drainage noted.
>
> —S. Barnes, RN

UNEXPECTED SITUATIONS AND ASSOCIATED INTERVENTIONS

- *Infusion does not flow or flow rate changes after bag and tubing are changed:* Make sure that the flow clamp is open and the drip chamber is approximately half full. Check the electronic device for proper functioning. Check the IV site for possible problems with the catheter, such as bending of the catheter or the position of the patient's extremity, and inspect the IV site for signs and symptoms of complications. Readjust the flow rate.

(continued)

Skill 15-2 ▶ Changing an IV Solution Container and Administration Set *(continued)*

- *After attaching new IV tubing, you note air bubbles in the tubing:* If the bubbles are above the roller clamp, you can easily remove them by closing the roller clamp, stretching the tubing downward, and tapping the tubing with your finger so the bubbles rise to the drip chamber. If there is a larger amount of air in the tubing, swab the medication port on the tubing below the air with an antimicrobial solution and attach a syringe to the port below the air. Clamp the tubing below the access port. Aspirate the air from the tubing via the syringe. Remember that air bubbles in the tubing can be reduced if the tubing is primed slowly with fluid instead of allowing a wide-open flow of the solution.

EVIDENCE FOR PRACTICE ▶	**INFUSION NURSING STANDARDS OF PRACTICE** Infusion Nurses Society (INS). (2016b). Infusion therapy. Standards of practice. *Journal of Infusion Nursing, 39*(Suppl 1), S1–S159. Refer to details in Skill 15-1, Evidence for Practice, and refer to thePoint° for additional research on related nursing topics.

EVIDENCE FOR PRACTICE ▶	**INFUSION NURSING POLICIES AND PROCEDURES FOR INFUSION THERAPY** Infusion Nurses Society (INS). (2016a). *Policies and procedures for infusion therapy* (5th ed.). Norwood, MA: Author. Refer to details in Skill 15-1, Evidence for Practice, and refer to thePoint° for additional research on related nursing topics.

Skill 15-3 ▶ Monitoring an IV Site and Infusion

The nurse is responsible for monitoring the infusion rate and the IV site. This is routinely done as part of the initial patient assessment and at regular intervals, based on patient condition and facility policy. In addition, IV sites are checked at specific intervals and each time an IV medication is given, as dictated by the facility's policies. It is common to check the IV infusion and site every hour, but it is important to be familiar with the requirements of your facility. Monitoring the infusion rate is a very important part of the patient's overall management. If the patient does not receive the prescribed rate, he/she may experience a fluid volume deficit. In contrast, if the patient is administered too much fluid over a period of time, he/she may experience fluid volume overload. Other responsibilities involve checking the IV site for possible complications and assessing for both the desired effects of an IV infusion as well as potential adverse reactions to IV therapy.

DELEGATION CONSIDERATIONS	The monitoring of an IV site and infusion is not delegated to nursing assistive personnel (NAP) or to unlicensed assistive personnel (UAP). Depending on the state's nurse practice act and the organization's policies and procedures, these procedures may be delegated to licensed practical/vocational nurses (LPN/LVNs). The decision to delegate must be based on careful analysis of the patient's needs and circumstances, as well as the qualifications of the person to whom the task is being delegated. Refer to the Delegation Guidelines in Appendix A.
EQUIPMENT	• PPE, as indicated

ASSESSMENT	Inspect the IV infusion solution for any particulates and check the IV label. Confirm it is the solution prescribed. Assess the current rate of flow by verifying the settings on the electronic infusion device or timing the drops if it is a gravity infusion. Check the tubing for kinks or anything that might clamp or interfere with the flow of the solution. Inspect the IV site. The dressing should be intact, adhering to the skin on all edges. Check for any leaks or fluid under or around the dressing. Inspect the tissue around the IV entry site for swelling, coolness, or pallor. These are signs of fluid infiltration into the tissue around the IV catheter. Also inspect the site for redness, swelling, and warmth. These signs might indicate the development of phlebitis or an inflammation of the blood vessel at the site. Grade phlebitis, if present. Refer to Box 15-3. Ask the patient if he/she is experiencing any pain or discomfort related to the IV line. Pain or discomfort can be a sign of infiltration, extravasation, phlebitis, thrombophlebitis, and infection related to IV therapy. Refer to Fundamentals Review 15-3. Assess the patient's fluid intake and output. Assess the patient's knowledge of IV therapy.

Box 15-3 Phlebitis Scale

Grade and document phlebitis according to the most severe presenting indicator.

Grade	Clinical Criteria	Grade	Clinical Criteria
0	No symptoms	4	Pain at access site with erythema and/or edema
1	Erythema at access site with or without pain		Streak formation
2	Pain at access site with erythema and/or edema		Palpable venous cord >1 in in length
3	Pain at access site with erythema and/or edema Streak formation Palpable venous cord		Purulent drainage

Source: Adapted from Infusion Nurses Society (INS). (2016b). Infusion therapy. Standards of practice. *Journal of Infusion Nursing, 39*(Suppl 1), S96, http://www.ovid.com/site/catalog/books/8838.jsp, with permission.

NURSING DIAGNOSIS	Determine the related factors for the nursing diagnoses based on the patient's current status. Appropriate nursing diagnoses may include: • Excess fluid volume • Deficient fluid volume • Risk for infection
OUTCOME IDENTIFICATION AND PLANNING	The expected outcomes to be achieved when monitoring the IV infusion and site are the patient remains free of complications related to IV therapy, exhibits a patent IV site, and the IV solution infuses at the prescribed flow rate.

IMPLEMENTATION

ACTION	RATIONALE
1. Verify IV solution order on the eMAR/MAR with the medical order. Consider the appropriateness of the prescribed therapy in relation to the patient. Clarify any inconsistencies. Check the patient's medical record for allergies. Check for color, leaking, and expiration date. Know the purpose of the IV administration.	This ensures that the correct IV solution and rate of infusion, and/or medication will be administered. The nurse is responsible for critically evaluating all patient orders. Any concerns regarding the type or amount of therapy prescribed should be immediately and clearly communicated to the prescribing health care provider. This knowledge and skill is essential for safe and accurate IV and medication administration.

(*continued*)

Skill 15-3 ▶ Monitoring an IV Site and Infusion *(continued)*

ACTION	RATIONALE
2. Monitor IV infusion every hour or per facility policy. More frequent checks may be necessary if medication is being infused.	Promotes safe administration of IV fluids and medication.
3. Perform hand hygiene and put on PPE, if indicated.	Hand hygiene and PPE prevent the spread of microorganisms. PPE is required based on transmission precautions.
4. Identify the patient.	Identifying the patient ensures the right patient receives the intervention and helps prevent errors.
5. Close the curtains around the bed and close the door to the room, if possible. Explain what you are going to do and why you are doing it to the patient.	This ensures the patient's privacy. Explanation relieves anxiety and facilitates cooperation.
6. If an electronic infusion device is being used, check settings, alarm, and indicator lights. Check set infusion rate (Figure 1). Note position of fluid in IV container in relation to time tape. Teach the patient about the alarm features on the electronic infusion device.	Observation ensures that the infusion control device and the alarm are functioning. Lack of knowledge about "alarms" may create anxiety for the patient.
7. If IV is infusing via gravity, check the drip chamber and time the drops (Figure 2). Refer to Box 15-1 in Skill 15-1 to review calculation of IV flow rates for gravity infusion.	This ensures that the flow rate is correct. Use a watch with a second hand for counting the drops in regulating a gravity drip IV infusion.

FIGURE 1. Checking infusion device settings.

FIGURE 2. Checking drip chamber and timing drops.

8. Check the tubing for anything that might interfere with the flow (Figure 3). Be sure clamps are in the open position.	Any kink or pressure on the tubing may interfere with the flow.
9. Observe the dressing for leakage of IV solution.	Leakage may occur at the connection of the tubing with the hub of the needle or the catheter and allow for loss of IV solution.
10. Inspect the site for swelling, leakage at the site, coolness, or pallor, which may indicate infiltration (Figure 4). Ask if the patient is experiencing any pain or discomfort. If any of these symptoms are present, the IV will need to be removed and restarted at another site. Check facility policy for treating infiltration. See Fundamentals Review 15-3.	Catheter may become dislodged from the vein, and IV solution may flow into the subcutaneous tissue.

ACTION

RATIONALE

FIGURE 3. Checking tubing for anything that might interfere with flow rate.

FIGURE 4. Inspecting IV site.

11. Inspect the site for redness, swelling, and heat. Palpate for induration. Ask if the patient is experiencing pain. These findings may indicate phlebitis, making it necessary to discontinue and restart the IV at another site. Grade phlebitis (refer to Box 15-3 and Fundamentals Review 15-3). Check facility policy for treatment of phlebitis. Notify the primary health care provider for severe (Grade 3 or 4) phlebitis (INS, 2016a).

Chemical irritation, mechanical trauma, and bacteria cause injury to the vein and can lead to phlebitis.

12. Check for local manifestations (redness, pus, warmth, induration, and pain) that may indicate an infection is present at the site. Also check for systemic manifestations (chills, fever, tachycardia, hypotension) that may accompany local infection at the site. If signs of infection are present, discontinue the IV and notify the primary care provider. Be careful not to disconnect the IV tubing when putting on the patient's hospital gown or assisting the patient with movement.

Poor aseptic technique may allow bacteria to enter the needle, catheter insertion site, or the tubing connection and may occur with manipulation of equipment.

13. Be alert for additional complications of IV therapy, such as fluid overload or bleeding. Refer to Fundamentals Review 15-3.

Infusing too much IV solution results in an increased volume of circulating fluid volume.

   a. Fluid overload can result in signs of cardiac and/or respiratory failure. Monitor intake and output and vital signs. Assess for edema and auscultate lung sounds. Ask if the patient is experiencing any shortness of breath.

Older adults are most at risk for this complication due to possible decrease in cardiac and/or renal functions.

   b. Check for bleeding at the site.

Bleeding may be caused by anticoagulant medication. Bleeding at the site is most likely to occur when the IV is discontinued.

14. If appropriate, instruct the patient to call for assistance if any discomfort is noted at the site, solution container is nearly empty, flow has changed in any way, or if the electronic pump alarm sounds.

This facilitates patient cooperation and safe administration of IV solution.

 15. Remove PPE, if used. Perform hand hygiene.

Proper removal of PPE reduces the risk for infection transmission and contamination of other items. Hand hygiene prevents transmission of microorganisms.

(continued)

Skill 15-3 ▶ Monitoring an IV Site and Infusion *(continued)*

EVALUATION

The expected outcome has been achieved when the patient remains free of complications related to IV therapy, exhibits a patent IV site, and the IV solution infuses at the prescribed flow rate.

DOCUMENTATION

Guidelines

Document the type of IV solution as well as the infusion rate. Note the insertion site location and site assessment. Document the patient's reaction to the IV therapy as well as the absence of subjective reports that he/she is not experiencing any pain or other discomfort, such as coolness or heat associated with the infusion. In addition, record that the patient is not demonstrating any other IV complications, such as signs or symptoms of fluid overload. Document the IV fluid solution on the intake and output record.

Sample Documentation

> <u>11/6/20</u> 1020 IV site right forearm/cephalic vein intact without swelling, redness, or drainage. D_5 0.9% NS with 20 mEq KCl continues to infuse at 110 mL/hr. Patient instructed to call nurse with any swelling or pain.
>
> —S. Barnes, RN

UNEXPECTED SITUATIONS AND ASSOCIATED INTERVENTIONS

- *Patient's lung sounds were previously clear, but now some crackles in the bases are auscultated:* Notify the primary care provider immediately. The patient may be exhibiting signs of fluid overload. Be prepared to tell the health care provider what the past intake and output totals were, as well as the vital signs and pulse oximetry findings of the patient.
- *IV is not flowing as easily as it previously had been:* Check all clamps on the tubing and check the tubing for any kinking. Check that the patient is not lying on the tubing. If the IV is over a joint, reposition the extremity and see if this helps the flow. Attempt to flush the IV with 2 to 3 mL of normal saline. If the IV is painful or you meet resistance when attempting to flush, discontinue the IV and restart in another place.

EVIDENCE FOR PRACTICE ▶

INFUSION NURSING STANDARDS OF PRACTICE
Infusion Nurses Society (INS). (2016b). Infusion therapy. Standards of practice. *Journal of Infusion Nursing, 39*(Suppl 1), S1–S159.
   Refer to details in Skill 15-1, Evidence for Practice, and refer to thePoint® for additional research on related nursing topics.

EVIDENCE FOR PRACTICE ▶

INFUSION NURSING POLICIES AND PROCEDURES FOR INFUSION THERAPY
Infusion Nurses Society (INS). (2016a). *Policies and procedures for infusion therapy* (5th ed.). Norwood, MA: Author.
   Refer to details in Skill 15-1, Evidence for Practice, and refer to thePoint® for additional research on related nursing topics.

EVIDENCE FOR PRACTICE ▶

DECREASING INTRAVENOUS (IV) INFILTRATES
Infiltration is the inadvertent administration of nonvesicant (agent capable of causing tissue damage) solution or medication into the surrounding tissue (INS, 2016a). Infiltration of IV solution can cause local and systemic complications. Prevention and early recognition are critical nursing responsibilities. What can nurses do to decrease the risk of this potential complication of IV therapy?

Related Research
Major, T. W., & Huey, T. K. (2016). Decreasing IV infiltrates in the pediatric patient—System-based improvement project. *Pediatric Nursing, 42*(1), 14–49.

The goal of this quality improvement project was to achieve a 10% decrease in the baseline infiltrate rate over a 6-month period of time on two inpatient units and in the overall infiltrate rate across all of the pediatric units in a regional medical center. Improvement strategies focused on evidence-based education, IV catheter securement, and family engagement. Staff education was provided via 1-hour continuing education presentations. A knowledge assessment survey was administered to attendees immediately before and at completion of the educational sessions. Two IV dressing/catheter securement devices were put into use to replace traditional transparent dressings; in-service presentations were provided regarding use of the devices. Family engagement was addressed through provision of basic explanations of IV therapy, associated goals, and an explanation of what the IV site should look like. Nurses and family members assessed the IV site together and the family was encouraged to notify the nurse with any concerns. In addition, a daily question appeared on the institution's interactive television network; any negative response to the question "Does your child's IV look okay?" triggered an electronic signal informing the nurse of the negative response. The nurse was expected to immediately check the IV and discuss the concern with the family and/or child.

A comparative purposive sample was used to evaluate the pre- and postimplementation period to determine if desired project success measures were achieved. Data analysis determined positive results across all units, with the number of events and infiltration rates decreasing over a 3-month period. A decrease also occurred in the overall percent of IVs that infiltrated in the first 24 hours of implementation. A statistically significant increase was noted in nurses' education pre- and postassessment survey scores. The family engagement strategy revealed overall parental responses to be 88% positive. The authors concluded that by decreasing infiltrates, quality of care improved, resulting in the delivery of safe, effective, and patient-centered IV therapy and care.

Relevance for Nursing Practice

Nurses are responsible for identifying clinical practice concerns and possible solutions, working to improve patient care. Nurses should consider interventions to provide the best care for patients. This information can be used to assist in developing policies for nursing interventions and standards of practice related to management of peripheral IV access devices.

Refer to thePoint° for additional research on related nursing topics.

Skill 15-4 ▶ Changing a Peripheral Venous Access Site Dressing

The IV site is a potential entry point for microorganisms into the bloodstream. Maintenance of an intact and patent dressing at the insertion site is an important means of preventing infection and other complications. Transparent semipermeable membrane (TSM) dressings are commonly used to protect the insertion site. TSM dressings (e.g., Tegaderm or OpSite IV) allow easy inspection of the IV site and permit evaporation of moisture that accumulates under the dressing. Sterile gauze may also be used to cover the catheter site. A gauze dressing is recommended if the patient is diaphoretic or if the site is bleeding or oozing or has drainage from the exit site; replace it with a TSM once this is resolved (INS, 2016b; O'Grady et al., 2011).

Facility policy generally determines the type of dressing used and when these dressings are changed. Dressing changes for short peripheral catheters are performed every 5 to 7 days, or if the dressing becomes damp, loosened, and/or visibly soiled (INS, 2016b). However, dressing changes might be required more often, based on nursing assessment and judgment. Immediately change any dressing that is damp, loosened, or soiled. In the event of drainage, site tenderness, or other signs of infection, change the dressing. This allows for the opportunity to assess, cleanse, and disinfect the site (INS, 2016b, p. S82). Observe meticulous aseptic technique to minimize the possibility of contamination when changing these dressings.

(continued)

Skill 15-4 ▶ Changing a Peripheral Venous Access Site Dressing *(continued)*

DELEGATION CONSIDERATIONS	The changing of a peripheral venous access dressing is not delegated to nursing assistive personnel (NAP) or to unlicensed assistive personnel (UAP). Depending on the state's nurse practice act and the organization's policies and procedures, the changing of a peripheral venous access dressing may be delegated to licensed practical/vocational nurses (LPN/LVNs). The decision to delegate must be based on careful analysis of the patient's needs and circumstances, as well as the qualifications of the person to whom the task is being delegated. Refer to the Delegation Guidelines in Appendix A.

EQUIPMENT

- Transparent occlusive dressing
- Cleansing swabs (>0.5% chlorhexidine preferred; tincture of iodine, an iodophor [povidone-iodine], or 70% alcohol may also be used) (INS, 2016b; Mimoz et al., 2015; O'Grady et al., 2011)
- Adhesive remover (optional)
- Alcohol or other disinfectant wipes
- Skin protectant wipe (e.g., Skin-Prep)
- IV securement/stabilization device, as appropriate
- Tape
- Clean gloves
- Towel or disposable pad
- Additional PPE, as indicated

ASSESSMENT

Assess the IV site. The dressing should be intact, adhering to the skin on all edges. Check for any leaks or fluid under or around the dressing, or other indications that the dressing needs to be changed. Inspect the tissue around the IV entry site for swelling, coolness, or pallor. These are signs of fluid infiltration into the tissue around the IV catheter. Also inspect the site for redness, swelling, and warmth. These signs might indicate the development of phlebitis or an inflammation of the blood vessel at the site. Ask the patient if he/she is experiencing any pain or discomfort related to the IV line. Pain or discomfort can be a sign of infiltration, extravasation, phlebitis, thrombophlebitis, and infection related to IV therapy. Refer to Fundamentals Review 15-3. Note the insertion date and date of last dressing change, if different from insertion date. Assess the patient's need to maintain venous access. If the patient does not need the access, discuss the possibility of discontinuation with the primary health care provider. Ask the patient about any allergies.

NURSING DIAGNOSIS

Determine the related factors for the nursing diagnoses based on the patient's current status. Appropriate nursing diagnoses may include:

- Risk for infection
- Risk for injury
- Risk for impaired skin integrity

OUTCOME IDENTIFICATION AND PLANNING

The expected outcome to achieve when changing a peripheral venous access dressing is that the patient will exhibit an access site that is clean, dry, and without evidence of any signs and symptoms of infection, infiltration, or phlebitis. In addition, the dressing will be clean, dry, and intact and the patient will not experience injury.

IMPLEMENTATION

ACTION	**RATIONALE**
1. Determine the need for a dressing change. Check facility policy. Gather equipment.	The particular facility's policies determine the type of dressing used and when these dressings are changed. Dressing changes might be required more often, based on nursing assessment and judgment. Immediately change any access site dressing that is damp, loosened, or soiled. Preparation promotes efficient time management and an organized approach to the task.
2. Perform hand hygiene and put on PPE, if indicated.	Hand hygiene and PPE prevent the spread of microorganisms. PPE is required based on transmission precautions.

ACTION	RATIONALE

3. Identify the patient.

Identifying the patient ensures the right patient receives the intervention and helps prevent errors.

4. Assemble equipment to the bedside stand or overbed table or other surface within reach.

Bringing everything to the bedside conserves time and energy. Arranging items nearby is convenient, saves time, and avoids unnecessary stretching and twisting of muscles on the part of the nurse.

5. Close the curtains around the bed and close the door to the room, if possible. Explain what you are going to do and why you are going to do it to the patient. Ask the patient about allergies to tape and skin antiseptics.

This ensures the patient's privacy. Explanation relieves anxiety and facilitates cooperation. Possible allergies may exist related to tape or antiseptics.

6. Put on gloves. Place a towel or disposable pad under the arm with the venous access. If the solution is currently infusing, temporarily stop the infusion. Hold the catheter in place with your nondominant hand. Beginning at the device hub, **gently pull the dressing perpendicular to the skin toward the insertion site, carefully removing the old dressing and/or stabilization/securing device (Figure 1).** Avoid inadvertently dislodging the catheter, as it may be adhered to the dressing (INS, 2016a). Use adhesive remover as necessary. Discard the dressing.

Gloves prevent contact with blood and body fluids. The pad protects the underlying surface. Proper disposal of dressing prevents transmission of microorganisms.

7. **Inspect the IV site for the presence of phlebitis (inflammation), infection, or infiltration. If noted, discontinue and relocate IV. Refer to Fundamentals Review 15-3 and Box 15-3 (in Skill 15-3).**

Inflammation (phlebitis), infection, or infiltration causes trauma to tissues and necessitates removal of the venous access device.

8. **Cleanse the site with an antiseptic solution, such as chlorhexidine, or according to facility policy (Figure 2). Press the applicator against the skin and apply chlorhexidine using a gentle back and forth motion. Do not wipe or blot. Allow to dry completely for at least 30 seconds (INS, 2016a).**

Cleansing the skin is necessary because organisms on the skin can be introduced into the tissues or the bloodstream with the venous access. Use of >0.5% chlorhexidine in alcohol solution is preferred for skin antisepsis. If there is a contraindication to alcoholic chlorhexidine solution, tincture of iodine, an iodophor (povidone-iodine), or 70% alcohol may also be used (INS, 2016b; Mimoz et al., 2015; O'Grady et al., 2011). Povidone-iodine must remain on the skin for 1½ to 2 minutes or longer to completely dry for adequate antisepsis (INS, 2016a).

FIGURE 1. Carefully removing old dressing.

FIGURE 2. Cleansing the site with an antiseptic solution.

(continued)

Skill 15-4 ▶ Changing a Peripheral Venous Access Site Dressing *(continued)*

ACTION	RATIONALE
9. Open the skin protectant wipe. Apply it to the site, making sure to cover at minimum the area to be covered with the dressing (Figure 3). Allow to dry. Place the sterile transparent dressing and/or catheter securing/stabilization device over the venipuncture site (Figure 4).	Skin protectant aids in adhesion of the dressing and decreases the risk for skin trauma when the dressing is removed. Transparent dressing allows easy visualization and protects the site. Stabilization/securing devices preserve the integrity of the access device, minimize catheter movement at the hub, and prevent catheter dislodgement and loss of access (INS, 2016b). Some stabilization devices act as a site dressing also.

FIGURE 3. Applying skin protectant to site.

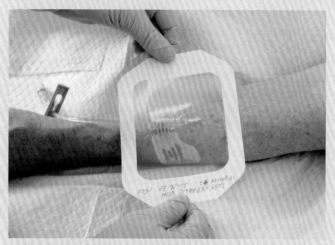

FIGURE 4. Applying transparent dressing to site.

ACTION	RATIONALE
10. Label the dressing with date, time of change, and initials. Loop the tubing near the entry site, and anchor with tape (nonallergenic) close to the site (Figure 5). Resume fluid infusion, if indicated. Check that IV flow is accurate and system is patent. Refer to Skill 15-3.	Other personnel working with the infusion will know what type of device is being used, the site, and when it was inserted.

FIGURE 5. Site dressing with label and anchored tubing.

ACTION	RATIONALE
11. Apply an IV securement/stabilization device if not already in place as part of the dressing, as indicated, based on facility policy. Explain to the patient the purpose of the device and the importance of safeguarding the site when using the extremity.	These systems are recommended for use on all venous access sites, and particularly central venous access sites, to preserve the integrity of the access device, minimize catheter movement at the hub, and prevent catheter dislodgement and loss of access (INS, 2016b). Some devices also act as a site dressing and may already have been applied.

ACTION	**RATIONALE**
12. Remove equipment. Ensure the patient's comfort. Remove gloves. Lower the bed, if not in the lowest position.	Promotes patient comfort and safety. Removing gloves properly reduces the risk for infection transmission and contamination of other items.
13. Remove additional PPE, if used. Perform hand hygiene.	Removing PPE properly reduces the risk for infection transmission and contamination of other items. Hand hygiene prevents transmission of microorganisms.

EVALUATION

The expected outcome has been met when the patient remains free of any signs and symptoms of infection, phlebitis, or infiltration at the venous access site. In addition, the access site dressing is clean, dry, and intact; and the patient has not experienced injury.

DOCUMENTATION

Guidelines

Document the location of the venous access as well as the condition of the site. Include the presence or absence of signs of erythema, redness, swelling, or drainage. Document the clinical criteria for site complications. Refer to Fundamentals Review 15-3 and Box 15-3 (in Skill 15-3). Record the subjective comments of the patient regarding the absence or presence of pain at the site. Record the patient's reaction to the procedure and pertinent patient teaching, such as alerting the nurse if the patient experiences any pain from the IV or notices any swelling at the site.

Sample Documentation

11/15/20 1120 Dressing change to IV site in L hand (dorsal metacarpal) complete. Transparent dressing and peripheral stabilization device applied. Site without erythema, redness, edema, or drainage. D_5 NS infusing at 75 mL/hr. Patient instructed to call nurse with any pain, discomfort, swelling, or questions.

—S. Barnes, RN

UNEXPECTED SITUATIONS AND ASSOCIATED INTERVENTIONS

- *Patient complains that IV site feels "funny" and hurts:* Observe the venous access site for redness, edema, and warmth and/or swelling, pallor, and coolness. If present, clamp the tubing to stop the IV solution flow, put on gloves and remove the catheter. Use a skin marker to outline the area with visible signs of infiltration to allow for assessment of changes. Secure gauze with tape over the insertion site without applying pressure. Assess the area distal to the venous access device for capillary refill, sensation, and motor function (INS, 2016a). Restart the IV in a new location. Estimate the volume of fluid that escaped into the tissue based on the rate of infusion and length of time since last assessment. Notify the primary health care provider and use an appropriate method for clinical management of the infiltrate site, based on infused solution and facility guidelines (INS, 2016b). Record site assessment and interventions, as well as the site for new venous access.
- *IV catheter is partially pulled out of insertion site (migrates externally):* Do not reinsert the catheter. Whether the IV is salvageable depends on how much of the catheter remains in the vein. Assess for proper placement in the vein before further use (INS, 2016b). If this catheter is not removed, monitor it closely for signs of infiltration and infection.

SPECIAL CONSIDERATIONS

General Considerations

- Use of >0.5% chlorhexidine is preferred for skin antisepsis for peripheral venous catheters; tincture of iodine, an iodophor (povidone-iodine), or 70% alcohol may also be used (INS, 2016b; Mimoz et al., 2015; O'Grady et al., 2011).
- Use of topical antibiotic ointments or creams on insertion sites is not recommended because of their potential to promote fungal infections and antimicrobial resistance (O'Grady et al., 2011).

(continued)

Skill 15-4 ▶ Changing a Peripheral Venous Access Site Dressing *(continued)*

- Chlorhexidine-impregnated dressings may be used over central venous access devices (CVADs) to reduce infection risk when the extraluminal route is the primary source of infection (INS, 2016b, p. S82).
- Do not submerge venous catheters and catheter sites in water; showering is permitted with use of impermeable coverings to protect the catheter and connecting device (O'Grady et al., 2011).

Infant and Child Considerations

- Use chlorhexidine with caution in infants under 2 months of age and premature infants due to the risk of skin irritation and chemical burns (INS, 2016b).
- For neonates with compromised skin integrity, remove dried povidone-iodine with normal saline wipes or sterile water (INS, 2016a).

Older Adult Considerations

- Avoid using vigorous friction at the insertion site, which can traumatize fragile skin and veins in older adults.

EVIDENCE FOR PRACTICE ▶

INFUSION NURSING STANDARDS OF PRACTICE

Infusion Nurses Society (INS). (2016b). Infusion therapy. Standards of practice. *Journal of Infusion Nursing, 39*(Suppl 1), S1–S159.

Refer to details in Skill 15-1, Evidence for Practice, and refer to thePoint® for additional research on related nursing topics.

EVIDENCE FOR PRACTICE ▶

INFUSION NURSING POLICIES AND PROCEDURES FOR INFUSION THERAPY

Infusion Nurses Society (INS). (2016a). *Policies and procedures for infusion therapy* (5th ed.). Norwood, MA: Author.

Refer to details in Skill 15-1, Evidence for Practice, and refer to thePoint® for additional research on related nursing topics.

Skill 15-5 ▶ Capping for Intermittent Use and Flushing a Peripheral Venous Access Device

When a continuous intravenous (IV) is no longer necessary, the primary IV line (short peripheral venous catheter or central venous access device [CVAD]) can be capped and converted to an intermittent infusion device. A capped line consists of the IV catheter connected to a short length of the extension tubing sealed with a needless connector or end cap. Capping of a short peripheral venous catheter is commonly referred to as a medication or saline lock. Capping of a vascular access device provides venous access for intermittent infusions or emergency medications. This can be accomplished in different ways. Refer to facility policy for the procedure to convert an access for intermittent use.

Vascular access devices used for intermittent infusions should be flushed with normal saline solution prior to each infusion as part of the assessment of catheter function. Flushing of the device is also required after each infusion to clear the infused medication or other solution from the catheter lumen. Vascular access devices should also be "locked" after completion of the flush solution at each use to decrease the risk of occlusion and catheter-related bloodstream infection (INS, 2016b). According to the guidelines from the INS (2016b), short peripheral catheters are locked with normal saline solution. If the device is not in use, periodic flushing according to facility policy is required to keep the catheter patent.

DELEGATION CONSIDERATIONS	Capping and flushing of a peripheral venous access device is not delegated to nursing assistive personnel (NAP) or to unlicensed assistive personnel (UAP). Depending on the state's nurse practice act and the organization's policies and procedures, these procedures may be delegated to licensed practical/vocational nurses (LPN/LVNs). The decision to delegate must be based on careful analysis of the patient's needs and circumstances, as well as the qualifications of the person to whom the task is being delegated. Refer to the Delegation Guidelines in Appendix A.
EQUIPMENT	<ul><li>End cap device</li><li>Clean gloves</li><li>Additional PPE, as indicated</li><li>4 × 4 gauze pad</li><li>Normal saline flush prepared in a syringe (1 to 3 mL) according to facility policy</li></ul> <ul><li>Passive disinfection caps (based on facility policy)</li><li>Alcohol or other disinfectant wipes</li><li>Tape</li></ul>
ASSESSMENT	Assess the insertion site for signs of any complications. Refer to Fundamentals Review 15-3 and Box 15-3 (in Skill 15-3). Verify the medical order for discontinuation of IV fluid infusion.
NURSING DIAGNOSIS	Determine the related factors for the nursing diagnoses based on the patient's current status. Appropriate nursing diagnoses may include: <ul><li>Risk for infection</li><li>Risk for injury</li></ul>
OUTCOME IDENTIFICATION AND PLANNING	The expected outcome to achieve when converting a primary peripheral IV line is that IV is converted for intermittent use; the patient remains free from injury and signs and symptoms of complications. In addition, the capped venous access device remains patent.

IMPLEMENTATION

ACTION	RATIONALE
1. Determine the need for conversion to an intermittent access. Verify medical order. Check facility policy. Gather equipment.	Ensures correct intervention for the correct patient. Preparation promotes efficient time management and an organized approach to the task.
2. Perform hand hygiene and put on PPE, if indicated.	Hand hygiene and PPE prevent the spread of microorganisms. PPE is required based on transmission precautions.
3. Identify the patient.	Identifying the patient ensures the right patient receives the intervention and helps prevent errors.
4. Assemble equipment to the bedside stand or overbed table or other surface within reach.	Bringing everything to the bedside conserves time and energy. Arranging items nearby is convenient, saves time, and avoids unnecessary stretching and twisting of muscles on the part of the nurse.
5. Close the curtains around the bed and close the door to the room, if possible. Explain what you are going to do and why you are going to do it to the patient. Ask the patient about allergies to tape and skin antiseptics.	This ensures the patient's privacy. Explanation relieves anxiety and facilitates cooperation. Possible allergies may exist related to tape or antiseptics.

(continued)

Skill 15-5 ▶ Capping for Intermittent Use and Flushing a Peripheral Venous Access Device *(continued)*

ACTION	**RATIONALE**
6. Assess the IV site. Refer to Skill 15-3.	Complications, such as infiltration, phlebitis, or infection, necessitate discontinuation of the IV infusion at that site.
7. If using an electronic infusion device, stop the device. Close the roller clamp on the administration set. If using gravity infusion, close the roller clamp on the administration set.	The action of the infusion device needs to be stopped and clamp closed to prevent leaking of fluid when the tubing is disconnected.
8. Put on gloves. Close the clamp on the short extension tubing connected to the IV catheter in the patient's arm.	Clamping the tubing on the extension set prevents introduction of air into the extension tubing.
9. Remove the administration set tubing from the needleless connector or end cap on the extension set. Using an antimicrobial swab, vigorously scrub the needleless connector or end cap on the extension tubing and allow to dry (Figure 1).	Removing the infusion tubing discontinues the infusion. Cleaning the cap reduces the risk for contamination. Venous access device entry points, end caps, and needleless connectors must be vigorously scrubbed and disinfected prior to each access to reduce the risk for introduction of microorganisms and prevent venous access device–related infection (Frimpong et al., 2015; Harper, 2014; INS, 2016b; The Joint Commission, 2018; Loveday et al., 2014). Friction is needed to physically remove microorganisms from the top, sides, and threads of the needleless connector or end cap. Allow the antiseptic to dry completely (15 to 30 seconds) to ensure complete effectiveness (Harper).
10. Insert the saline flush syringe into the needleless connector or end cap on the extension tubing. Pull back on the syringe to aspirate the catheter for positive blood return. If positive, instill the solution over 1 minute or flush the line according to facility policy (Figure 2). Remove the syringe and reclamp the extension tubing.	Positive blood return confirms patency before administration of medications and solutions (INS, 2016b). Flushing maintains patency of the IV line. Action of the positive pressure end cap is maintained with removal of the syringe before clamp is engaged. Clamping prevents air from entering the extension set.

FIGURE 1. Using an antimicrobial swab to vigorously scrub the needleless connector or end cap.

FIGURE 2. Flushing venous access device.

11. If necessary, loop the extension tubing near the entry site and anchor it with tape (nonallergenic) close to the site.	The weight of the tubing is sufficient to pull it out of the vein if it is not well anchored. Nonallergenic tape is less likely to tear fragile skin.

ACTION	**RATIONALE**
12. Using an antimicrobial swab, vigorously scrub the needle-less connector or end cap on the extension tubing and allow to dry. Attach a passive disinfection cap.	Passive disinfection caps contain an antiseptic-impregnated sponge that dispenses the antiseptic over the connector's top and threads, and protect the hub from contamination by touch or airborne sources (Stango et al., 2014). Venous access device entry points, end caps, and needleless connectors must be vigorously scrubbed and disinfected prior to each access to reduce the risk for introduction of microorganisms and prevent venous access device–related infection (Frimpong et al., 2015; Harper, 2014; INS, 2016b; The Joint Commission, 2018; Loveday et al., 2014). Friction is needed to physically remove microorganisms from the top, sides, and threads of the needleless connector or end cap. Allow the antiseptic to dry completely (15 to 30 seconds) to ensure complete effectiveness (Harper).
13. Remove equipment. Ensure the patient's comfort. Remove gloves. Lower the bed, if not in the lowest position.	Promotes patient comfort and safety. Removing gloves properly reduces the risk for infection transmission and contamination of other items.
14. Remove additional PPE, if used. Perform hand hygiene.	Proper removal of PPE reduces the risk for infection transmission and contamination of other items. Hand hygiene prevents transmission of microorganisms.

EVALUATION

The expected outcome has been met when the IV has been converted for intermittent use; and the patient is free from injury and signs and symptoms of complications. In addition, the capped venous access device is patent.

DOCUMENTATION

Guidelines

Document discontinuation of the IV fluid infusion. Record the condition of the venous access site. Document the flushing of the venous access device. This is often done in the eMAR/MAR. Record the patient's reaction to the procedure and any patient teaching that occurred.

Sample Documentation

> 12/13/20 1720 IV infusion capped per order. Peripheral site right forearm (cephalic) flushed without resistance using 3 mL of saline. Dressing remains intact. Site without redness, swelling, drainage, or heat. Patient denies discomfort. Patient verbalized an understanding of the need to maintain IV access.
>
> —A. Lynn, RN

UNEXPECTED SITUATIONS AND ASSOCIATED INTERVENTIONS

- *Peripheral venous access site leaks fluid when flushed:* To prevent infection and other complications, remove from site. Evaluate the need for continued access; if a clinical need is present, restart in another location.
- *IV does not flush easily:* Assess insertion site. Infiltration and/or phlebitis may be present. If present, remove the IV. Use a skin marker to outline the area with visible signs of infiltration to allow for assessment of changes. Secure gauze with tape over the insertion site without applying pressure. Assess the area distal to the venous access device for capillary refill, sensation, and motor function (INS, 2016a). Assess the need for continued venous access. If a clinical need is present, restart the IV in a new location. Estimate the volume of fluid that escaped into the tissue based on the rate of infusion and length of time since last assessment. Notify the primary health care provider and use an appropriate method for clinical management of the infiltrate site, based on infused solution and facility guidelines (INS, 2016b). Record site assessment and interventions, as well as the site for new venous access.

(continued)

Skill 15-5 ▶ Capping for Intermittent Use and Flushing a Peripheral Venous Access Device *(continued)*

- *IV does not flush easily:* The catheter may be blocked or clotted due to a kinked catheter at the insertion site. Aspirate and attempt to flush again. If resistance remains, do not force. Forceful flushing can dislodge a clot at the end of the catheter. Remove the IV. Assess the need for continued venous access. If a clinical need is present, restart the IV in a new location.
- *IV catheter is partially pulled out of insertion site (migrates externally):* Do not reinsert the catheter. Whether the IV is salvageable depends on how much of the catheter remains in the vein. Assess for proper placement in the vein before further use (INS, 2016b). If this catheter is not removed, monitor it closely for signs of infiltration and infection.

SPECIAL CONSIDERATIONS
- Some facilities may use end caps for venous access devices that are not positive pressure devices. In this case, flush with the recommended volume of saline, ending with 0.5 mL of solution remaining in the syringe. While maintaining pressure on the syringe, clamp the extension tubing. This provides positive pressure, preventing backflow of blood into the catheter, decreasing risk for occlusion.
- If the administration tubing was connected directly to the hub of the IV catheter when the access was initiated, short extension tubing should be added when the line is capped.

EVIDENCE FOR PRACTICE ▶
INFUSION NURSING STANDARDS OF PRACTICE
Infusion Nurses Society (INS). (2016b). Infusion therapy. Standards of practice. *Journal of Infusion Nursing, 39*(Suppl 1), S1–S159.
Refer to details in Skill 15-1, Evidence for Practice, and refer to thePoint° for additional research on related nursing topics.

EVIDENCE FOR PRACTICE ▶
INFUSION NURSING POLICIES AND PROCEDURES FOR INFUSION THERAPY
Infusion Nurses Society (INS). (2016a). *Policies and procedures for infusion therapy* (5th ed.). Norwood, MA: Author.
Refer to details in Skill 15-1, Evidence for Practice, and refer to thePoint° for additional research on related nursing topics.

Skill 15-6 ▶ Administering a Blood Transfusion

A blood transfusion is the infusion of whole blood or a blood component, such as plasma, red blood cells, cryoprecipitate, or platelets, into the patient's venous circulation (Table 15-1). A blood product transfusion is given when a patient's red blood cells, platelets, or coagulation factors decrease to levels that compromise a patient's health. Before a patient can receive a blood product, his/her blood must be typed to ensure that he/she receives compatible blood (**blood typing** and **crossmatching**). Otherwise, a serious and life-threatening transfusion reaction may occur involving clumping and hemolysis of the red blood cells and, possibly, death (Table 15-2). Alternately, a patient may receive an **autologous transfusion**, in which case, the potential for transfusion reaction is significantly decreased (Long et al., 2014). The nurse must also verify the infusion rate, based on facility policy or medical order. Follow the facility's policies and guidelines to determine if the transfusion should be administered by an electronic infusion device or by gravity. Refer to Box 15-1 in Skill 15-1 for guidelines to calculate the flow rate for gravity infusion. Patient monitoring during transfusion of blood products is essential because of continued risk for transfusion reaction (Menendez & Edwards, 2016).

DELEGATION CONSIDERATIONS
The administration of a blood transfusion is not delegated to nursing assistive personnel (NAP), to unlicensed assistive personnel (UAP), or to licensed practical/vocational nurses (LPN/LVNs).

Table 15-1	Blood Products

BLOOD PRODUCT	FILTER	RATE OF ADMINISTRATION	ABO COMPATIBILITY	DOUBLE-CHECKED BY TWO LICENSED PRACTITIONERS (e.g., registered nurse, physician)
Packed red blood cells	Yes	1 unit over 2–3 hours; no longer than 4 hours	Yes	Yes
Platelets	Yes	Over 30–60 minutes or as quickly as the patient can tolerate	No	Yes
Cryoprecipitate	Yes	As quickly as tolerated by the patient or over 30–60 minutes	Recommended	Yes
Fresh-frozen plasma	Yes	As quickly as tolerated by the patient or over 15–60 minutes	Yes	Yes
Albumin	Yes	1–10 mL/min (5%) 0.2–0.4 mL/min (25%)	No	No

Table 15-2	Transfusion Reactions

REACTION	SIGNS AND SYMPTOMS	NURSING ACTIVITY
Allergic reaction: allergy to transfused blood	Hives, itching Anaphylaxis	• Stop transfusion immediately and keep vein open with normal saline. • Notify primary care provider stat. • Administer antihistamine parenterally, as necessary.
Febrile reaction: fever develops during infusion	Fever and chills Headache Malaise	• Stop transfusion immediately and keep vein open with normal saline. • Notify primary care provider. • Treat symptoms.
Hemolytic transfusion reaction: incompatibility of blood product	Immediate onset Facial flushing Fever, chills Headache Low back pain Shock	• Stop infusion immediately and keep vein open with normal saline. • Notify primary care provider stat. • Obtain blood samples from site. • Obtain first voided urine. • Treat shock if present. • Send unit, tubing, and filter to laboratory. • Draw blood sample for serologic testing and send urine specimen to the laboratory.
Circulatory overload: too much blood administered	Dyspnea Dry cough Pulmonary edema	• Slow or stop infusion. • Monitor vital signs. • Notify primary care provider. • Place in upright position with feet dependent.
Bacterial reaction: bacteria present in blood	Fever Hypertension Dry, flushed skin Abdominal pain	• Stop infusion immediately. • Obtain culture of the patient's blood and return blood bag to laboratory. • Monitor vital signs. • Notify primary care provider. • Administer antibiotics as ordered.

(continued)

Skill 15-6 ▶ Administering a Blood Transfusion *(continued)*

EQUIPMENT

- Blood product
- Blood administration set (tubing with in-line filter, or add-on filter, and Y for saline administration)
- 0.9% normal saline for IV infusion
- IV pole
- Venous access; if peripheral site, initiated with a 20- to 24-gauge catheter (adults)
- Alcohol or other disinfectant wipes
- Clean gloves
- Additional PPE, as indicated
- Tape (hypoallergenic)
- Second registered nurse, other licensed practitioner (hospital/outpatient setting), or responsible adult (home setting) to verify blood product and patient information (INS, 2016b)

ASSESSMENT

Review the most recent laboratory values, in particular, the complete blood count (CBC). Ask the patient about any previous transfusions, including the number he/she has had and any reactions experienced during a transfusion. Inspect the IV insertion site, noting the gauge of the IV catheter. Blood or blood components may be transfused via a 20- to 24-gauge peripheral venous access device (adult). Central venous access devices (CVADs) may also be used to administer a transfusion. Baseline assessment prior to obtaining blood for transfusion should include measurement of vital signs, lung assessment, identification of conditions that may increase the risk of transfusion-related adverse reactions, the presence of an appropriate and patent vascular access device, and current laboratory values (INS, 2016b). Institution policies vary on the frequency of assessment. The Infusion Nurses Society Standards of Practice recommend checking the patient's vital signs prior to transfusion, within 5 to 15 minutes after initiating the transfusion, after the transfusion is completed, and as needed depending on patient condition (INS, 2016b, p. S136).

NURSING DIAGNOSIS

Determine the related factors for the nursing diagnoses based on the patient's current status. Appropriate nursing diagnoses may include:

- Risk for injury
- Excess fluid volume
- Decreased cardiac output

OUTCOME IDENTIFICATION AND PLANNING

The expected outcome to achieve when administering a blood transfusion is that the patient receives the blood transfusion without any evidence of a transfusion reaction or complications. In addition, the patient exhibits signs and symptoms of fluid balance, improved cardiac output, and enhanced peripheral tissue perfusion.

IMPLEMENTATION

ACTION	RATIONALE
1. Verify the medical order for transfusion of a blood product. Verify the completion of informed consent documentation in the medical record. Verify any medical order for pre-transfusion medication. If ordered, administer medication at least 30 minutes before initiating transfusion.	Verification of order ensures the right patient receives the correct intervention. Premedication is sometimes administered to decrease the risk for allergic and febrile reactions for patients who have received multiple previous transfusions.
2. Gather all equipment.	Preparation promotes efficient time management and an organized approach to the task.
3. Perform hand hygiene and put on PPE, if indicated.	Hand hygiene and PPE prevent the spread of microorganisms. PPE is required based on transmission precautions.

ACTION	RATIONALE
4. Identify the patient.	Identifying the patient ensures the right patient receives the intervention and helps prevent errors.
5. Assemble equipment to the bedside stand or overbed table or other surface within reach.	Bringing everything to the bedside conserves time and energy. Arranging items nearby is convenient, saves time, and avoids unnecessary stretching and twisting of muscles on the part of the nurse.
6. Close the curtains around the bed and close the door to the room, if possible. Explain what you are going to do and why you are going to do it to the patient. Ask the patient about previous experience with a transfusion and any reactions. Advise the patient to report any chills, itching, rash, or unusual symptoms.	This ensures the patient's privacy. Explanation relieves anxiety and facilitates cooperation. Previous reactions may increase the risk for reaction to this transfusion. Any reaction to the transfusion necessitates stopping the transfusion immediately and evaluating the situation.
7. Prime blood administration set with the normal saline IV fluid. Refer to Skill 15-2.	Normal saline is the solution of choice for blood product administration. Solutions with dextrose may lead to clumping of red blood cells and hemolysis.
8. Put on gloves. If the patient does not have a venous access device in place, initiate peripheral venous access. (Refer to Skill 15-1.) Connect the administration set to the venous access device via the extension tubing. (Refer to Skill 15-1.) Infuse the normal saline per facility policy.	Gloves prevent contact with blood and body fluids. Infusion of fluid via venous access maintains patency until the blood product is administered. Start an IV before obtaining the blood product in case the initiation takes longer than 30 minutes. Blood must be stored at a carefully controlled temperature (4°C) and transfusion must begin within 30 minutes of release from the blood bank.
9. Obtain blood product from blood bank according to facility policy. Scan the bar codes on blood products if required.	Bar codes on blood products are currently being implemented in some facilities to identify, track, and assign data to transfusions as an additional safety measure.
10. Two registered nurses (or other licensed practitioner [hospital/outpatient setting], or responsible adult [home setting]) compare and validate the following information in the presence of the patient with the medical record, patient identification band (hospital/outpatient setting), and the label of the blood product: • Medical order for transfusion of blood product • Informed consent • Patient identification number • Patient name • Blood group and type • Expiration date • Inspection of blood product for clots, clumping, gas bubbles	In the hospital or outpatient setting, this should be two practitioners trained in the identification of the recipient and blood components, such as registered nurses, advance practice nurses, or physicians. In home settings, it should be the registered nurse and a responsible adult (INS, 2016b). Most states/facilities require verification of the following information: unit numbers match; ABO group and Rh type are the same; expiration date (after 35 days, red blood cells begin to deteriorate); two patient identifiers. If clots or signs of contamination (clumping, gas bubbles) are present, return blood to the blood bank.
11. **Obtain baseline set of vital signs before beginning the transfusion.**	Any change in vital signs during the transfusion may indicate a reaction.
12. Put on gloves. If using an electronic infusion device, put the device on "hold." Close the roller clamp closest to the drip chamber on the saline side of the administration set. Close the roller clamp on the administration set below the infusion device. Alternately, if infusing via gravity, close the roller clamp on the administration set.	Gloves prevent contact with blood and body fluids. Stopping the infusion prevents blood from infusing to the patient before completion of preparations. Closing the clamp to saline allows blood product to be infused via electronic infusion device.

(continued)

Skill 15-6 ▶ Administering a Blood Transfusion *(continued)*

ACTION	RATIONALE
13. Close the roller clamp closest to the drip chamber on the blood product side of the administration set. Remove the protective cap from the access port on the blood container. Remove the cap from the access spike on the administration set. Using a pushing and twisting motion, insert the spike into the access port on the blood container, taking care not to contaminate the spike. Hang the blood container on the IV pole. Open the roller clamp on the blood side of the administration set. Squeeze drip chamber until the in-line filter is saturated (Figure 1). Remove gloves.	Filling the drip chamber prevents air from entering the administration set. The filter in the blood administration set removes particulate material formed during storage of blood. If the administration set becomes contaminated, the entire set would have to be discarded and replaced.
14. **Start administration slowly (approximately 2 mL per minute for the first 15 minutes) (INS, 2016b). Stay with the patient for the first 5 to 15 minutes of transfusion.** Open the roller clamp on the administration set below the infusion device. Set the flow rate and begin the transfusion. Alternately, start the flow of solution by releasing the clamp on the tubing and counting the drops. Adjust until the correct drop rate is achieved. Assess the flow of the blood and function of the infusion device. Inspect the insertion site for signs of infiltration.	Transfusion reactions typically occur during this period, and a slow rate will minimize the volume of red blood cells infused. Verifying the rate and device settings ensures the patient receives the correct volume of solution. If the catheter slips out of the vein, the blood will accumulate (infiltrate) into the surrounding tissue.
15. Observe the patient for flushing, dyspnea, itching, hives or rash, or any unusual comments.	These signs and symptoms may be an early indication of a transfusion reaction.
16. Reassess vital signs after 15 minutes (Figure 2). Obtain vital signs thereafter according to facility policy and nursing assessment.	Vital signs must be assessed as part of monitoring for possible adverse reaction. Facility policy and nursing judgment will dictate frequency.

FIGURE 1. Squeezing the drip chamber to saturate the filter.

FIGURE 2. Assessing vital signs after 15 minutes.

17. After the observation period (5 to 15 minutes) increase the infusion rate to the calculated rate to complete the infusion within the prescribed time frame, no more than 4 hours.	If no adverse effects occurred during this time, the infusion rate is increased. If complications occur, they can be observed and the transfusion can be stopped immediately. Verifying the rate and device settings ensures the patient receives the correct volume of solution. Transfusion must be completed within 4 hours due to potential for bacterial growth in blood product at room temperature.

CVADs provide access for a variety of IV fluids, medications, blood products, and TPN solutions and provide a means for hemodynamic monitoring and blood sampling. The patient's diagnosis, the type of care that is required, and other factors (e.g., limited venous access, irritating drugs, patient request, or the need for long-term intermittent infusions) determine the type of CVAD used.

Vascular access devices used for intermittent infusions should be flushed with normal saline solution (NSS) prior to each infusion as part of the assessment of catheter function. Flushing of the device is also required after each infusion to clear the infused medication or other solution from the catheter lumen. Vascular access devices should also be "locked" after completion of the flush solution at each use to decrease the risk of occlusion and catheter-related bloodstream infection (INS, 2016b). According to the guidelines from the INS (2016b), CVADs should be locked with either a heparin solution (10 units/mL) or normal saline solution after each intermittent use, according to the directions for use for the specific CVAD and needleless connector. If the device is not in use, periodic flushing according to facility policy is required to keep the catheter patent.

Dressings are placed at the insertion site to occlude the site and prevent the introduction of microorganisms into the bloodstream. Scrupulous care of the site is required to help control contamination and to help prevent the introduction of microorganisms into the bloodstream. Facility policy generally determines the type of dressing used and the intervals for dressing change.

Transparent semipermeable membrane (TSM) dressings are commonly used to protect the insertion site. TSM dressings (e.g., Tegaderm or OpSite IV) allow easy inspection of the IV site and permit evaporation of moisture that accumulates under the dressing. Sterile gauze may also be used to cover the catheter site. A gauze dressing is recommended if the patient is diaphoretic or if the site is bleeding or oozing, or has drainage from the exit site; replace it with a TSM once this is resolved (INS, 2016b; O'Grady et al., 2011). Chlorhexidine-impregnated dressings may be used over CVADs to reduce infection risk when the extraluminal route is the primary source of infection (INS, 2016b, p. S82).

Perform site care and replace TSM dressings on CVADs every 5 to 7 days and every 2 days for CVAD sites with gauze dressings (INS, 2016b; O'Grady et al., 2011). Immediately change any dressing that is damp, loosened, or soiled. In the event of drainage, site tenderness, or other signs of infection, change the dressing. This allows for the opportunity to assess, cleanse, and disinfect the site (INS, 2016b, p. S82). Do not submerge venous catheters and catheter sites in water; showering is permitted with use of impermeable coverings to protect the catheter and connecting device (O'Grady et al., 2011). Whenever these dressings need to be changed, it is important to observe meticulous aseptic technique to minimize the possibility of contamination.

DELEGATION CONSIDERATIONS	The changing of a CVAD dressing is not delegated to nursing assistive personnel (NAP) or to unlicensed assistive personnel (UAP). Depending on the state's nurse practice act and the organization's policies and procedures, the changing of a CVAD dressing may be delegated to licensed practical/vocational nurses (LPN/LVNs). The decision to delegate must be based on careful analysis of the patient's needs and circumstances, as well as the qualifications of the person to whom the task is being delegated. Refer to the Delegation Guidelines in Appendix A.

EQUIPMENT

- Sterile tape or Steri-Strips
- TSM dressing; antimicrobial dressing; or gauze pad for dressing, based on facility policy
- Several 2 × 2 gauzes
- Sterile towel or drape
- Cleansing swabs (>0.5% chlorhexidine preferred; tincture of iodine, an iodophor [povidone-iodine], or 70% alcohol may also be used) (INS, 2016b; Mimoz et al., 2015; O'Grady et al., 2011)
- NSS vial and 10-mL syringe or prefilled 10-mL NSS syringe; one for each lumen of the CVAD
- Heparin 10 units/mL in 10-mL syringe; one for each lumen of the CVAD (based on facility policy)
- Masks (2), depending on facility policy
- Clean gloves
- Sterile gloves
- Additional PPE, as indicated
- Skin protectant/barrier wipe (e.g., Skin-Prep)
- Alcohol or other disinfectant wipes
- Needleless connector or positive pressure end caps; one for each lumen of the CVAD
- IV securement/stabilization device, as appropriate
- Sterile measuring tape
- Bath blanket

(continued)

Skill 15-7 ▶ Changing the Dressing and Flushing Central Venous Access Devices *(continued)*

ASSESSMENT	Assess the CVAD site. The dressing should be intact, adhering to the skin on all edges. Check for any leaks or fluid under or around the dressing, or other indications that the dressing needs to be changed. Inspect the tissue around the entry site for redness, swelling, tenderness, and warmth. These signs might indicate the development of localized infection. Ask the patient if he/she is experiencing any pain or discomfort related to the venous access device, paresthesias, numbness or tingling. Pain or discomfort can be a sign of infiltration, extravasation, phlebitis, thrombophlebitis, deep vein thrombosis, and/or infection. Refer to Fundamentals Review 15-3. Note the insertion date/access date and the date of the last dressing change. Assess the catheter condition. Verify if the current locking solution dwelling in the CVAD needs to be aspirated and discarded or may be infused as part of the flushing procedure; all antimicrobial lock solutions, for example, must be aspirated and discarded (INS, 2016b).
NURSING DIAGNOSIS	Determine the related factors for the nursing diagnoses based on the patient's current status. Appropriate nursing diagnoses may include: • Risk for infection • Deficient knowledge • Risk for impaired skin integrity
OUTCOME IDENTIFICATION AND PLANNING	The expected outcome to achieve when changing a CVAD dressing is that site care will be provided and the dressing is replaced. In addition, the patient will remain free of any signs and symptoms of infection; the site will be clean and dry, with an intact dressing, and show no signs or symptoms of complications; and the CVAD will remain patent.

IMPLEMENTATION

ACTION	**RATIONALE**
1. Verify the medical order and/or facility policy and procedure. Determine the need for a dressing change. Often, the procedure for CVAD flushing and dressing changes will be a standing protocol. Gather equipment.	Ensures correct intervention for the correct patient. Preparation promotes efficient time management and an organized approach to the task.
2. Perform hand hygiene and put on PPE, if indicated.	Hand hygiene and PPE prevent the spread of microorganisms. Unclean hands and improper technique are potential sources for infecting a CVAD. PPE is required based on transmission precautions.
3. Identify the patient.	Identifying the patient ensures the right patient receives the intervention and helps prevent errors.
4. Assemble equipment to the bedside stand or overbed table or other surface within reach.	Bringing everything to the bedside conserves time and energy. Arranging items nearby is convenient, saves time, and avoids unnecessary stretching and twisting of muscles on the part of the nurse.
5. Close the curtains around the bed and close the door to the room, if possible. Explain what you are going to do and why you are going to do it to the patient. Ask the patient about allergies to tape and skin antiseptics.	This ensures the patient's privacy. Explanation relieves anxiety and facilitates cooperation. Possible allergies may exist related to tape or antiseptics.
6. Place a waste receptacle or bag at a convenient location for use during the procedure.	Having a waste container handy means the soiled dressing can be discarded easily, without the spread of microorganisms.
7. Adjust the bed to a comfortable working height, usually elbow height of the caregiver (VHACEOSH, 2016).	Having the bed at the proper height prevents back and muscle strain.

ACTION	**RATIONALE**
8. Assist the patient to a comfortable position that provides easy access to the CVAD insertion site and dressing. If the patient has a PICC, position the patient with the arm extended from the body below heart level. Use the bath blanket to cover any exposed area other than the site.	Patient positioning and use of a bath blanket provide for comfort and warmth. This position is recommended to reduce the risk of air embolism.
9. Apply a mask. Ask the patient to turn his/her head away from the access site. Alternately, have the patient put on a mask, depending on facility policy. Move the overbed table to a convenient location within easy reach. Set up a sterile field on the table. Open dressing supplies and add to sterile field. If IV solution is infusing via CVAD, interrupt and place on hold during dressing change. Apply slide clamp on each lumen of the CVAD.	Masks are recommended to help to deter the spread of microorganisms (INS, 2016b). The patient should wear a mask if unable to turn the head away from the site or if based on facility policy. Many facilities have all sterile dressing supplies gathered in a single package. Stopping infusion and clamping each lumen prevents air from entering CVAD.
10. Put on clean gloves. Assess the CVAD insertion site through the old dressing (Figure 4). (Refer to Assessment discussion above.) Palpate the site, noting pain, tenderness, or discomfort. Remove the old dressing, beginning at the device hub. Stabilize the catheter. Gently pull the dressing perpendicular to the skin toward the insertion site (INS, 2016b). Take care to avoid inadvertently dislodging the catheter/needle. Discard the dressing in a trash receptacle.	Gloves prevent contact with blood and body fluids. Pain, tenderness, or discomfort on palpation may be a sign of infection. The catheter/needle may be adhered to the dressing, increasing the risk of accidental dislodgment (INS, 2016b). Proper disposal of dressing prevents transmission of microorganisms.

FIGURE 4. Inspecting CVAD insertion site.

11. Based on the device in use, remove the stabilization device according to the manufacturer's directions. A subcutaneous external stabilization device is not removed with each dressing change (INS, 2016b). Note the status of any sutures or staples that may be present. Remove gloves and discard.	Stabilization device is changed with dressing change. Some CVADs may be sutured or stapled in place. Note how the CVAD is secured. If staples or sutures are loosened, other methods of stabilization may be necessary (INS, 2016b, p. 119). Removing gloves properly reduces the risk for infection transmission and contamination of other items.

(continued)

Skill 15-7 ▸ Changing the Dressing and Flushing Central Venous Access Devices *(continued)*

ACTION	RATIONALE

12. Perform hand hygiene. Put on sterile gloves. Starting at the insertion site and continuing in a circle, wipe off any old blood or drainage with a sterile antimicrobial wipe. Using the chlorhexidine swab, cleanse the site, covering at least a 2- to 3-in area. **Apply chlorhexidine using a gentle back and forth motion for at least 30 seconds (INS, 2016b). Do not wipe or blot. Allow to dry completely.**

Hand hygiene prevents transmission of microorganisms. Site care and replacement of the dressing are accomplished using sterile technique. Cleansing is necessary because organisms on the skin can be introduced into the tissues or the bloodstream with venous access. Use of >0.5% chlorhexidine in alcohol solution is preferred for skin antisepsis. If there is a contraindication to alcoholic chlorhexidine solution, tincture of iodine, an iodophor (povidone-iodine), or 70% alcohol may also be used (INS, 2016b; Mimoz et al., 2015; O'Grady et al., 2011). Povidone-iodine must remain on the skin for 1½ to 2 minutes or longer to completely dry for adequate antisepsis (INS, 2016a). The use of concentric circles or a back-and-forth motion has not been studied (INS, 2016b, p. 120).

13. Apply antimicrobial dressing, based on facility policy (Figure 5). Apply the skin protectant to the same 2- to 3-in area, avoiding direct application to the antimicrobial pad or gel component of the dressing or the insertion site, and allow to dry. Apply the securement/stabilization device, if used, and/or the TSM dressing, centering over the insertion site (Figure 6). Measure the length of the catheter that extends out from the insertion site.

An antimicrobial dressing may be used over CVADs to reduce infection risk when the extraluminal route is the primary source of infection (INS, 2016b, p. S82). Skin protectant under the antimicrobial dressing interferes with the action of the dressing. Skin protectant improves adhesion of the dressing and protects the skin from damage and irritation when the dressing is removed. The dressing prevents contamination of the IV catheter and protects the insertion site. Stabilization/securing devices preserve the integrity of the access device, minimize catheter movement at the hub, and prevent catheter dislodgement and loss of access (INS, 2016b). Some stabilization devices act as a site dressing also. Measurement of the extending catheter can be compared with the documented length at the time of insertion to assess if the catheter has migrated inward or moved outward.

![Applying antimicrobial dressing]

FIGURE 5. Applying antimicrobial dressing.

FIGURE 6. Applying site dressing.

14. Based on facility policy, replace end caps, as indicated. Working with one lumen at a time, remove the needleless connector or end cap. Using an antimicrobial swab, vigorously scrub the end of the lumen and apply a new needleless connector or end cap. Repeat for each lumen.

The catheter ends should be cleansed and injection caps changed to prevent infection.

ACTION

15. If required, flush each lumen of the CVAD. Amount of saline and heparin flushes varies depending on specific CVAD and facility policy.

16. Using an antimicrobial swab, vigorously scrub the needleless connector or end cap on one of the lumens and allow to dry. Insert the saline flush syringe into the needleless connector. Open the clamp on the lumen. Slowly inject the saline flush, noting any resistance or sluggishness, and slowly pull back on the syringe to aspirate for positive blood return. If positive, instill the solution over 1 minute or by using a pulsatile flushing technique of 10 short boluses of 1 mL interrupted by brief pauses; flush the line according to facility policy. Remove the syringe. Insert the locking solution syringe and instill the volume of solution designated by facility policy over 1 minute or according to facility policy. Remove the syringe and reclamp the lumen. Remove gloves.

17. Apply a passive disinfection cap to each needleless connector or end cap. Using an antimicrobial swab, vigorously scrub the needleless connector or end cap on the extension tubing and allow to dry. Attach a passive disinfection cap (Figure 7).

RATIONALE

Flushing maintains patency of CVAD.

Venous access device entry points, end caps, and needleless connectors must be vigorously scrubbed and disinfected prior to each access to reduce the risk for introduction of microorganisms and prevent venous access device–related infection (Frimpong et al., 2015; Harper, 2014; INS, 2016b; The Joint Commission, 2018; Loveday et al., 2014). Friction is needed to physically remove microorganisms from the top, sides, and threads of the needleless connector or end cap. Allow the antiseptic to dry completely (15 to 30 seconds) to ensure complete effectiveness (Harper). Positive blood return confirms patency before administration of medications and solutions (INS, 2011, p. S60). Flushing maintains patency of the IV line. A pulsatile flushing technique of 10 short boluses of 1 mL interrupted by brief pauses may be effective in removing solid deposits (INS, 2016b). Action of the positive pressure end cap is maintained with removal of the syringe before the clamp is engaged. Clamping prevents air from entering the CVAD. CVADs should be "locked" with either a heparin solution (10 units/mL) or normal saline solution after each intermittent use, according to the directions for use for the specific CVAD and needleless connector, to maintain patency (INS, 2016a). Removing gloves properly reduces the risk for infection transmission and contamination of other items.

Passive disinfection caps contain an antiseptic-impregnated sponge that dispenses the antiseptic over the connector's top and threads, and protect the hub from contamination by touch or airborne sources (Stango et al., 2014). Venous access device entry points, end caps, and needleless connectors must be vigorously scrubbed and disinfected prior to each access to reduce the risk for introduction of microorganisms and prevent venous access device–related infection (Frimpong et al., 2015; Harper, 2014; INS, 2016b; The Joint Commission, 2018; Loveday et al., 2014). Friction is needed to physically remove microorganisms from the top, sides, and threads of the needleless connector or end cap. Allow the antiseptic to dry completely (15 to 30 seconds) to ensure complete effectiveness (Harper).

FIGURE 7. Attaching a passive disinfection cap to each access site.

(continued)

Skill 15-7 ▶ Changing the Dressing and Flushing Central Venous Access Devices   *(continued)*

ACTION	RATIONALE
18. Label the dressing with the date, time of change, and initials. Resume fluid infusion, if indicated. Check that IV flow is accurate and system is patent. (Refer to Skill 15-3.)	Other personnel working with the infusion will know what type of device is being used, the site, and when the dressing was last changed.
19. Apply an IV securement/stabilization device if not already in place as part of the dressing, as indicated, based on facility policy. Explain to the patient the purpose of the device and the importance of safeguarding the site when using the extremity.	Weight of the tubing and/or tugging on the tubing could cause catheter dislodgement. Securing the catheter lumens and/or the tubing preserves the integrity of the access device, minimizes catheter movement at the hub, and prevents catheter dislodgement and loss of access (INS, 2016b). Some devices also act as a site dressing and may already have been applied.
20. Remove equipment. Ensure the patient's comfort. Lower the bed, if not in the lowest position.	Promotes patient comfort and safety.
21. Remove additional PPE, if used. Perform hand hygiene.	Proper removal of PPE reduces the risk for infection transmission and contamination of other items. Hand hygiene prevents transmission of microorganisms.

EVALUATION

The expected outcomes have been met when site care has been provided and the dressing has been replaced; the patient is free of any signs and symptoms of infection; the site is clean and dry, with an intact dressing, and shows no signs or symptoms of complications; and the CVAD remains patent.

DOCUMENTATION

Guidelines

Document the location, appearance, and condition of the CVAD site. Include the presence or absence of signs of erythema, redness, swelling, or drainage. Record if the patient is experiencing any pain or discomfort related to the CVAD. Document the clinical criteria for site complications. Refer to Fundamentals Review 15-3 and Box 15-3 (in Skill 15-3). Record the subjective comments of the patient regarding the absence or presence of pain at the site. Record the patient's reaction to the procedure and pertinent patient teaching, such as alerting the nurse if the patient experiences any pain from the site or notices any swelling at the site. The CVAD lumens should flush without difficulty. Report any abnormal findings, such as dislodgement of the CVAD, abnormal insertion assessment findings, or inability to flush the CVAD, to the primary health care provider.

Sample Documentation

> 11/12/20 0400 PICC line located in the right basilic vein. Old dressing removed, no drainage, redness, or swelling noted at site. Site care performed; transparent dressing applied and needleless connectors changed. Extending catheter length 5 cm. NSS flush per protocol without difficulty. Patient denies pain or discomfort. Patient instructed to inform nurse of any pain, swelling, or leakage related to PICC line.
>
> —S. Barnes, RN

UNEXPECTED SITUATIONS AND ASSOCIATED INTERVENTIONS

- *While dressing is being changed, PICC is inadvertently dislodged:* If PICC is not all the way out, notify the primary health care provider. The primary care provider will most likely want a chest x-ray to determine the location of the end of the PICC line. Before the chest x-ray, reapply a dressing so that the PICC is not further dislodged.
- *When the dressing is removed, purulent drainage is noted at the insertion site:* Obtain a culture of the site; clean the area; reapply a dressing; and then notify the primary care provider. This prevents the PICC line from being open to air and unprotected while you are notifying the primary care provider. In addition, the culture is obtained without having to remove the dressing a second time. If the primary care provider does not want the culture, discard it in the appropriate receptacle.
- *When flushing the catheter, you are unable to withdraw blood, there is a sluggish flow, and/or you are unable to flush or infuse through the CVAD:* These signs may indicate CVAD occlusion. Consult with the nurse IV team and the primary care provider for appropriate catheter clearance procedure to preserve the function of the CVAD.

SPECIAL CONSIDERATIONS	• Use a 10-mL syringe or a syringe specifically designed to generate lower injection pressure to assess CVAD patency (INS, 2016a). Syringes smaller than 10 mL may provide pressures great enough to damage the PICC.
	• Implanted ports require larger flush volumes due to volume required to fill the device.
	• Groshong devices do not require the use of heparin for flushing.
	• Some facilities call for a pulsatile flushing technique, which may be more effective in removing solid deposits from VAD lumens (INS, 2016a).
	• Heparin-induced thrombocytopenia (HIT) has been reported with the use of heparin flush solutions. Monitor all patients closely for signs and symptoms of HIT. If present or suspected, discontinue heparin (INS, 2016a).
	• Monitoring of platelet counts for HIT is not recommended in postoperative and medical patients receiving only heparin in the form of a catheter lock solution due to a very low incidence of HIT (INS, 2016a, p. S78).
	• Use of topical antibiotic ointments or creams on insertion sites is not recommended because of their potential to promote fungal infections and antimicrobial resistance (O'Grady et al., 2011).
	• Do not submerge access central venous devices in water; showering is permitted with the use of impermeable coverings to protect the catheter and connecting device (O'Grady et al., 2011).
Infant and Child Considerations	• Use chlorhexidine with caution in infants under 2 months of age and premature infants due to the risk of skin irritation and chemical burns (INS, 2016b).
	• For neonates with compromised skin integrity, remove dried povidone-iodine with normal saline wipes or sterile water (INS, 2016a).
Older Adult Considerations	• Avoid using vigorous friction at the insertion site, which can traumatize fragile skin and veins in older adults.
Home Care Considerations	• Instruct the patient or caregiver to check the CVAD site at least once a day for signs of complications. Signs and/or symptoms of complications or dressing dislodgement should be reported immediately (INS, 2016b, p. 117). Patient education plays a critical role in CVAD safety (Weingart, Hsieh, Lane, & Cleary, 2014).

EVIDENCE FOR PRACTICE ▶ **INFUSION NURSING STANDARDS OF PRACTICE**

Infusion Nurses Society (INS). (2016b). Infusion therapy. Standards of practice. *Journal of Infusion Nursing, 39*(Suppl 1), S1–S159.

Refer to details in Skill 15-1, Evidence for Practice, and refer to thePoint® for additional research on related nursing topics.

EVIDENCE FOR PRACTICE ▶ **INFUSION NURSING POLICIES AND PROCEDURES FOR INFUSION THERAPY**

Infusion Nurses Society (INS). (2016a). *Policies and procedures for infusion therapy* (5th ed.). Norwood, MA: Author.

Refer to details in Skill 15-1, Evidence for Practice, and refer to thePoint® for additional research on related nursing topics.

EVIDENCE FOR PRACTICE ▶ **DECREASING EXTERIOR CONTAMINATION OF IV ADMINISTRATION TUBING**

Continuous intravenous (IV) infusions into CVADs may involve administration tubing that is long in length. This extra length of tubing may drag on the floor, become entangled with other equipment, or even be run over by the IV pole used to administer the infusion, resulting in contamination of the exterior of the tubing, increasing the risk for central line–associated blood stream infection.

(continued)

Skill 15-7 ► **Changing the Dressing and Flushing Central Venous Access Devices** *(continued)*

Related Research

Herriage, T., Hooke, M. C., Streifel, A., & Slaker, B. (2016). Utilization of an intravenous line lifter within a pediatric oncology population. *Journal of Pediatric Oncology Nursing, 33*(2), 105–110.

The purpose of this clinical project was to evaluate the effectiveness of the IV Line Lifter in decreasing the contamination of exterior IV tubing in ambulatory pediatric oncology patients. The IV Line Lifter is a tubing management system which consists of a flexible device that is secured to the IV pole and keeps the IV tubing off the hospital floor. A nonrandomized comparative group of ambulatory pediatric oncology patients between the ages of 2 and 10 years were included in the study. Baseline bioluminescence tests were performed on the IV tubing of participants pre- and postimplementation.

Relevance for Nursing Practice

Nurses are responsible for identifying clinical practice concerns and possible solutions, working to improve patient care. Nurses should consider interventions to provide the best care for patients. This information can be used to assist in developing policies for nursing interventions and standards of practice related to management of peripheral IV access devices.

Refer to thePoint® for additional research on related nursing topics.

Skill 15-8 ► **Accessing an Implanted Port**

An implanted port consists of a subcutaneous injection port attached to a catheter. The distal catheter tip dwells in the lower segment of the superior vena cava at or near the cavoatrial junction (CAJ), the point at which the superior vena cava meets and melds into the superior wall of the right atrium (INS, 2016b), and the proximal end or port is usually implanted in a subcutaneous pocket of the upper chest wall (Figure 1). Implanted ports placed in the antecubital area of the arm are

Angled needle

Catheter entering subclavian vein

Implanted port in subcutaneous pocket

FIGURE 1. An implanted port with catheter inserted in subclavian vein and noncoring needle inserted into port.

referred to as peripheral access system ports. Confirmation of tip location either by postprocedure chest radiograph or by technology used during the placement procedure is required prior to use and should be documented in the patient's health record (INS, 2016b).

When not in use, no external parts of the system are visible. When venous access is desired, the location of the injection port must be palpated. A special angled, noncoring needle is inserted through the skin and septum and into the port reservoir to access the system. Once accessed, patency is maintained by periodic flushing. The length and gauge of the needle used to access the port should be selected based on the patient's anatomy, amount of subcutaneous tissue at the site, and anticipated infusion requirements. Access the port with the smallest-gauge noncoring needle to accommodate the prescribed therapy (INS, 2016a). The length of the noncoring needle should be such that it allows the needle to sit flushed to the skin and securely within the port, reducing the risk of needle dislodgement during access (INS, 2016a). Site dressings are maintained and changed as outlined in Skill 15-7.

Consider the use of methods to reduce pain and discomfort of catheter insertion, such as local anesthetic agents and adjunctive therapies (cognitive, behavioral, and complementary therapies) (INS, 2016a).

DELEGATION CONSIDERATIONS	Accessing an implanted port is not delegated to nursing assistive personnel (NAP), to unlicensed assistive personnel (UAP), or to licensed practical/vocational nurses (LPN/LVNs).
EQUIPMENT	• Sterile tape or Steri-Strips • TSM dressing; antimicrobial dressing; or gauze pad for dressing, based on facility policy • Several 2 × 2 gauzes • Sterile towel or drape • Cleansing swabs (>0.5% chlorhexidine preferred; tincture of iodine, an iodophor [povidone-iodine], or 70% alcohol may also be used) (INS, 2016b; Mimoz et al., 2015; O'Grady et al., 2011) • NSS vial and 10-mL syringe or prefilled 10-mL NSS syringe • Heparin 10 units/mL in 10-mL syringe • Noncoring safety needle of appropriate length and gauge • Local anesthetic (based on facility policy and/or if prescribed) • Masks (2), depending on facility policy • Clean gloves • Sterile gloves • Additional PPE, as indicated • Skin protectant/barrier wipe (e.g., Skin-Prep) • Alcohol or other disinfectant wipes • Needleless connector or positive pressure end caps; one for each lumen of the central venous access device (CVAD) • IV securement/stabilization device, as appropriate • Sterile measuring tape • Bath blanket
ASSESSMENT	Assess the port site. Inspect the skin over the port, looking for any swelling, redness, or drainage. Also assess the site over the port for any pain or tenderness. These signs might indicate the development of localized infection. Review the patient's history for the length of time the port has been in place. If the port has been placed recently, assess surgical incision. Note the presence of Steri-Strips, approximation, ecchymosis, redness, edema, and/or drainage. Verify if the current locking solution dwelling in the CVAD needs to be aspirated and discarded or may be infused as part of the flushing procedure; all antimicrobial lock solutions, for example, must be aspirated and discarded (INS, 2016b).
NURSING DIAGNOSIS	Determine the related factors for the nursing diagnoses based on the patient's current status. Appropriate nursing diagnoses may include: • Risk for infection • Deficient knowledge • Risk for impaired skin integrity

(continued)

Skill 15-8 ▶ Accessing an Implanted Port   *(continued)*

OUTCOME IDENTIFICATION AND PLANNING

The expected outcome to achieve when accessing an implanted port is that the port is accessed with minimal to no discomfort to the patient; the patient experiences no trauma to the site or infection; and the patient verbalized an understanding of care associated with the port.

IMPLEMENTATION

ACTION	RATIONALE
1. Verify medical order and/or facility policy and procedure. Often, the procedure for accessing an implanted port and dressing changes will be a standing protocol. Gather equipment.	Checking the order and/or policy ensures that the proper procedure is initiated. Preparation promotes efficient time management and an organized approach to the task.
2. Perform hand hygiene and put on PPE, if indicated.	Hand hygiene and PPE prevent the spread of microorganisms. Unclean hands and improper technique are potential sources for infecting a CVAD. PPE is required based on transmission precautions.
3. Identify the patient.	Identifying the patient ensures the right patient receives the intervention and helps prevent errors.
4. Assemble equipment to the bedside stand or overbed table or other surface within reach.	Bringing everything to the bedside conserves time and energy. Arranging items nearby is convenient, saves time, and avoids unnecessary stretching and twisting of muscles on the part of the nurse.
5. Close the curtains around the bed and close the door to the room, if possible. Explain what you are going to do, and why you are going to do it to the patient. Ask the patient about allergies to tape and skin antiseptics. If considering using a local anesthetic, inquire about allergies for these substances as well.	This ensures the patient's privacy. Explanation relieves anxiety and facilitates cooperation. Possible allergies may exist related to tape or antiseptics. Injectable anesthetic can result in allergic reactions and tissue damage.
6. If using a local anesthetic, explain the rationale and procedure to the patient. Apply the anesthetic as indicated to the port site. Allow sufficient time for the anesthetic to take effect.	Local anesthetic decreases the degree of pain felt at the insertion site. Some of the anesthetics take up to an hour to become effective. If using transdermal anesthetic cream, apply at least 1 hour prior to port access procedure (INS, 2016b).
7. Place a waste receptacle or bag at a convenient location for use during the procedure.	Having a waste container handy means the soiled dressing can be discarded easily, without the spread of microorganisms.
8. Adjust the bed to a comfortable working height, usually elbow height of the caregiver (VHACEOSH, 2016).	Having the bed at the proper height prevents back and muscle strain.
9. Assist the patient to a comfortable position that provides easy access to the port site. Use the bath blanket to cover any exposed area other than the site.	Patient positioning and use of a bath blanket provide for comfort and warmth.
10. Apply a mask. Ask the patient to turn his/her head away from the access site. Alternately, have the patient put on a mask, depending on facility policy. Move the overbed table to a convenient location within easy reach. Set up a sterile field on the table. Open dressing supplies and add to the sterile field.	Masks are recommended to help to deter the spread of microorganisms (INS, 2016b). The patient should wear a mask if unable to turn the head away from the site or if based on facility policy. Many facilities have all sterile dressing supplies gathered in a single package.
11. Put on clean gloves. Palpate the location of the port. Assess site. Note the status of any surgical incisions that may be present. Remove gloves and discard.	Knowledge of location and boundaries of port are necessary to access the site safely.

ACTION	RATIONALE
12. Put on sterile gloves. Connect the needleless connector or end cap to the extension tubing on the noncoring needle. Using an antimicrobial swab, vigorously scrub the needleless connector or end cap on the extension tubing and allow to dry. Insert a syringe with 10-mL normal saline into the needleless connector or end cap. Fill the extension tubing with normal saline and apply clamp. Remove the syringe. Place on sterile field.	Port access is accomplished using sterile technique. Organisms on the skin can be introduced into the tissues or the bloodstream with the needle. Priming the extension tubing removes air from tubing and prevents administration of air when connected to the port. Venous access device entry points, end caps, and needleless connectors must be vigorously scrubbed and disinfected prior to each access to reduce the risk for introduction of microorganisms and prevent venous access device–related infection (Frimpong et al., 2015; Harper, 2014; INS, 2016b; The Joint Commission, 2018; Loveday et al., 2014). Friction is needed to physically remove microorganisms from the top, sides, and threads of the needleless connector or end cap. Allow the antiseptic to dry completely (15 to 30 seconds) to ensure complete effectiveness (Harper).
13. Using the chlorhexidine swab, cleanse the port site, covering at least a 2- to 3-in area. **Apply chlorhexidine using a gentle back and forth motion for at least 30 seconds (INS, 2016b). Do not wipe or blot. Allow to dry completely.**	Use of >0.5% chlorhexidine in alcohol solution is preferred for skin antisepsis. If there is a contraindication to alcoholic chlorhexidine solution, tincture of iodine, an iodophor (povidone-iodine), or 70% alcohol may also be used (INS, 2016b; Mimoz et al., 2015; O'Grady et al., 2011). Povidone-iodine must remain on the skin for 1½ to 2 minutes or longer to completely dry for adequate antisepsis (INS, 2016a). The use of concentric circles or a back-and-forth motion has not been studied (INS, 2016b, p. 120).
14. Using the nondominant hand, locate the port by palpating the edges through the skin. Hold the port stable, keeping the skin taut (Figure 2).	The edges of the port must be palpated so that the needle can be inserted into the center of the port. Hold the port with your nondominant hand so that the needle is inserted into the port with the dominant hand.

FIGURE 2. Stabilizing port with nondominant hand.

(*continued*)

Skill 15-8 ▶ Accessing an Implanted Port *(continued)*

ACTION	RATIONALE

ACTION

15. Visualize the center of the port. Pick up the noncoring needle and extension tubing. Coil the extension tubing into the palm of your hand. Holding the needle at a 90-degree angle to the skin, insert **through the skin into the port septum (Figure 3) until the needle hits the back of the port (Figure 4).**

RATIONALE

To function properly, the needle must be located in the middle of the port and inserted to the back internal wall of the port.

FIGURE 3. Inserting needle through skin into port.

FIGURE 4. Noncoring (Huber) needle in place.

16. Using an antimicrobial swab, vigorously scrub the needleless connector or end cap on the extension tubing and allow to dry. Insert the syringe with normal saline. **Open the clamp on the extension tubing and flush with 3 to 5 mL of saline, while observing the site for fluid leak or infiltration. It should flush easily, without resistance.**

    Alert: if an antimicrobial locking solution was used when the port was last locked, withdraw the solution from the port prior to flushing and discard (INS, 2016a, p. 182).

Venous access device entry points, end caps, and needleless connectors must be vigorously scrubbed and disinfected prior to each access to reduce the risk for introduction of microorganisms and prevent venous access device–related infection (Frimpong et al., 2015; Harper, 2014; INS, 2016b; The Joint Commission, 2018; Loveday et al., 2014). Friction is needed to physically remove microorganisms from the top, sides, and threads of the needleless connector or end cap. Allow the antiseptic to dry completely (15 to 30 seconds) to ensure complete effectiveness (Harper). If the needle is not inserted correctly, fluid will leak into the tissue, causing the tissue to swell and producing signs of infiltration. Flushing without resistance is also a sign that the needle is inserted correctly.

Flushing an antibiotic solution into the patient's blood stream could increase development of antibiotic resistance and other adverse effects (INS, 2016a, p. 182).

17. Slowly pull back on the syringe plunger to aspirate for blood return (Figure 5). Do not allow blood to enter the syringe. If positive, instill the solution over 1 minute or by using a pulsatile flushing technique of 10 short boluses of 1 mL interrupted by brief pauses; flush the line according to facility policy. Remove the syringe. Insert the locking solution syringe and instill the volume of solution designated by facility policy over 1 minute or according to facility policy. Remove the syringe and reclamp the lumen. Alternately, if IV fluid infusion is to be initiated, do not flush with heparin.

Positive blood return confirms patency before administration of medications and solutions (INS, 2016b). Not allowing blood to enter the syringe ensures that the needle will be flushed with pure saline. A pulsatile flushing technique of 10 short boluses of 1 mL interrupted by brief pauses may be effective in removing solid deposits (INS, 2016b). Action of the positive pressure end cap is maintained with removal of the syringe before the clamp is engaged. Clamping prevents air from entering the CVAD. CVADs should be "locked" with either a heparin solution (10 units/mL) or normal saline solution after each intermittent use, according to the directions for use for the specific CVAD and needleless connector, to maintain patency (INS, 2016a).

ACTION	RATIONALE

FIGURE 5. Aspirating for blood return.

18. If using a "Gripper" needle, remove the gripper portion from the needle by squeezing the sides together and lifting off the needle while holding the needle securely to the port with the other hand (Figure 6).

Gripper facilitates needle insertion and needs to be removed before application of the dressing.

19. Apply the skin protectant to the site, avoiding direct application to the needle insertion site. Allow to dry.

Skin protectant improves adhesion of the dressing and protects the skin from damage and irritation when the dressing is removed.

20. Apply an antimicrobial dressing, a CVAD site dressing, and securement device, based on facility policy. Refer to Skill 15-7. Apply a passive disinfection cap to the needleless connector or end cap on the extension tubing (Figure 7).

An antimicrobial dressing may be used over CVADs to reduce infection risk when the extraluminal route is the primary source of infection (INS, 2016b, p. S82). A site dressing prevents contamination and protects the insertion site. Stabilization/securing devices preserve the integrity of the access device, minimize catheter movement at the hub, and prevent catheter dislodgement and loss of access (INS, 2016b). Some stabilization devices act as a site dressing also. Passive disinfection caps contain an antiseptic-impregnated sponge that dispenses the antiseptic over the connector's top and threads, and protect the hub from contamination by touch or airborne sources (Stango et al., 2014).

FIGURE 6. Removing gripper from needle.

FIGURE 7. Attaching a passive disinfection cap.

(*continued*)

Skill 15-8 ▶ Accessing an Implanted Port (continued)

ACTION	RATIONALE
21. Remove equipment. Ensure the patient's comfort. Lower the bed, if not in the lowest position.	Promotes patient comfort and safety.
22. Remove additional PPE, if used. Perform hand hygiene.	Proper removal of PPE reduces the risk for infection transmission and contamination of other items. Hand hygiene prevents transmission of microorganisms.

EVALUATION

The expected outcome has been met when the port was accessed without difficulty or pain; the patient is free of signs and symptoms of infection or trauma; and the patient verbalized an understanding of care related to the port.

DOCUMENTATION

Document the location of the port and the size of needle used to access the port. Document the presence of a blood return and the ease of ability to flush the port. Record the patient's reaction to the procedure and if the patient is experiencing any pain or discomfort related to the port. Document the assessment of the site. Record any appropriate patient teaching.

Sample Documentation

> 11/22/20 1245 Implanted port R chest wall. Site without drainage, swelling, or redness. 20-gauge 0.75-in Huber needle used to access port. Flushes easily with good blood return. Transparent dressing and external stabilization device applied. Patient denies pain or discomfort. Patient instructed to call nurse with any swelling, pain, or leaking.
>
> —S. Barnes, RN

UNEXPECTED SITUATIONS AND ASSOCIATED INTERVENTIONS

- *Port insertion site begins to swell when flushing with saline:* Stop flushing. Verify that the needle is in place and has not become dislodged. Attempt to flush. If swelling persists, stop flush. Remove the needle. Obtain additional supplies and reaccess port with a new needle. Check blood return and flush. If swelling persists, stop flush. Depending on facility policy, leave the access needle in place. Cover with transparent dressing. Notify the primary care provider. Anticipate diagnostic tests to determine patency of port.
- *Port does not flush:* Check clamp to make sure it is open. Gently push down on the needle and again try to flush. Ask the patient to perform a Valsalva maneuver. Try having the patient change position or place the affected arm over the head, or try raising or lowering the head of the bed. If the port still does not flush, remove the needle. Obtain additional supplies and reaccess with a new needle. Check blood return and flush. If still unable to flush, notify the primary care provider. Depending on facility policy, leave the access needle in place. Cover with transparent dressing. Anticipate diagnostic tests to determine patency of port.
- *Port flushes, but does not have a blood return:* Ask the patient to perform a Valsalva maneuver. Try having the patient change position or place the affected arm over the head, or try raising or lowering the head of the bed. If the port still does not have a blood return, remove the needle. Obtain additional supplies and reaccess with the new needle. Check blood return and flush. If it still does not have a blood return, notify the primary care provider. Depending on facility policy, leave the access needle in place. Cover with transparent dressing. Anticipate diagnostic tests to determine patency of the port and/or instillation of thrombolytic.

SPECIAL CONSIDERATIONS

General Considerations

- Consider orienting the bevel of the port access needle in the opposite direction from the outflow channel where the catheter is attached to the port body; a greater amount of protein is removed when flushing with this bevel orientation (INS, 2016b, p. S58).
- Lock accessed implanted vascular access ports daily (INS, 2016b).

- For vascular access ports that are not actively accessed for infusion therapy, there is insufficient evidence to recommend the optimal frequency for flushing and locking; refer to the manufacturers' directions for use and facility policy (INS, 2016a, p. 179).
- The most common practice is to replace the needle every 7 days when using a port for continuous infusions (INS, 2016a).
- Implanted ports require larger flush volumes due to volume required to fill the device.
- Groshong devices do not require the use of heparin for flushing.
- Some facilities call for a pulsatile flushing technique, which may be more effective in removing solid deposits from VAD lumens (INS, 2016a).
- Heparin-induced thrombocytopenia (HIT) has been reported with the use of heparin flush solutions. Monitor all patients closely for signs and symptoms of HIT. If present or suspected, discontinue heparin (INS, 2016a).
- Monitoring of platelet counts for HIT is not recommended in postoperative and medical patients receiving only heparin in the form of a catheter lock solution due to a very low incidence of HIT (INS, 2016a, p. S78).
- Use of topical antibiotic ointments or creams on insertion sites is not recommended because of their potential to promote fungal infections and antimicrobial resistance (O'Grady et al., 2011).
- Do not submerge accessed ports in water; showering is permitted with use of impermeable coverings to protect the catheter and connecting device (O'Grady et al., 2011).

Infant and Child Considerations

- Use chlorhexidine with caution in infants under 2 months of age and premature infants due to the risk of skin irritation and chemical burns (INS, 2016b).
- For neonates with compromised skin integrity, remove dried povidone-iodine with normal saline wipes or sterile water (INS, 2016a).

Older Adult Considerations

- Avoid using vigorous friction at the insertion site, which can traumatize fragile skin and veins in older adults.

Home Care Considerations

- Patients often are discharged with a CVAD. The patient and family or significant other require teaching to care for CVAD in the home.
- Instruct the patient or caregiver to check the port site at least once a day for signs of complications. Signs and/or symptoms of complications or dressing dislodgement should be reported immediately (INS, 2016b, p. 117).

EVIDENCE FOR PRACTICE ▶

INFUSION NURSING STANDARDS OF PRACTICE

Infusion Nurses Society (INS). (2016b). Infusion therapy. Standards of practice. *Journal of Infusion Nursing, 39*(Suppl 1), S1–S159.

Refer to details in Skill 15-1, Evidence for Practice, and refer to thePoint° for additional research on related nursing topics.

EVIDENCE FOR PRACTICE ▶

INFUSION NURSING POLICIES AND PROCEDURES FOR INFUSION THERAPY

Infusion Nurses Society (INS). (2016a). *Policies and procedures for infusion therapy* (5th ed.). Norwood, MA: Author.

Refer to details in Skill 15-1, Evidence for Practice, and refer to thePoint° for additional research on related nursing topics.

Skill 15-9 ▶ Deaccessing an Implanted Port

When an implanted port will not be used for a period of time, the port is deaccessed. Deaccessing a port involves flushing and locking the port and removing the needle.

DELEGATION CONSIDERATIONS	Deaccessing an implanted port is not delegated to nursing assistive personnel (NAP), to unlicensed assistive personnel (UAP), or to licensed practical/vocational nurses (LPN/LVNs).

EQUIPMENT

- Clean gloves
- Additional PPE, as indicated
- NSS vial and 10-mL syringe or prefilled 10-mL NSS syringe
- Heparin 10 U/mL in 10-mL syringe (based on facility policy)

- Sterile gauze sponge
- Alcohol or other disinfectant wipes
- Small adhesive bandage

ASSESSMENT	Assess the port site. Inspect the skin over the port, looking for any swelling, redness, or drainage. Also assess the site over the port for any pain or tenderness. These signs might indicate the development of localized infection. Review the patient's history for the length of time the port has been in place. If the port has been placed recently, assess surgical incision. Note presence of Steri-Strips, approximation, ecchymosis, redness, edema, and/or drainage.
NURSING DIAGNOSIS	Determine the related factors for the nursing diagnoses based on the patient's current status. Appropriate nursing diagnoses may include: • Risk for infection • Deficient knowledge • Risk for injury
OUTCOME IDENTIFICATION AND PLANNING	The expected outcome to achieve when deaccessing an implanted port is that the port is flushed and locked without adverse effect and the needle is removed with minimal to no discomfort to the patient; the patient experiences no trauma or infection; and the patient verbalizes an understanding of port care.

IMPLEMENTATION

ACTION	RATIONALE
1. Verify medical order and/or facility policy and procedure. Often, the procedure for deaccessing an implanted port will be a standing protocol. Gather equipment.	Checking the order and/or policy ensures that the proper procedure is initiated. Preparation promotes efficient time management and an organized approach to the task.
2. Perform hand hygiene and put on PPE, if indicated.	Hand hygiene and PPE prevent the spread of microorganisms. Unclean hands and improper technique are potential sources for infecting a CVAD. PPE is required based on transmission precautions.
3. Identify the patient.	Identifying the patient ensures the right patient receives the intervention and helps prevent errors.
4. Assemble equipment to the bedside stand or overbed table or other surface within reach.	Bringing everything to the bedside conserves time and energy. Arranging items nearby is convenient, saves time, and avoids unnecessary stretching and twisting of muscles on the part of the nurse.
5. Close the curtains around the bed and close the door to the room, if possible. Explain what you are going to do and why you are going to do it to the patient.	This ensures the patient's privacy. Explanation relieves anxiety and facilitates cooperation.

ACTION	**RATIONALE**
6. Adjust the bed to a comfortable working height, usually elbow height of the caregiver (VHACEOSH, 2016).	Having the bed at the proper height prevents back and muscle strain.
7. Assist the patient to a comfortable position that provides easy access to the port site. Use the bath blanket to cover any exposed area other than the site.	Patient positioning and use of a bath blanket provide for comfort and warmth.
8. Put on gloves. Using an antimicrobial swab, vigorously scrub the needleless connector or end cap on the extension tubing and allow to dry. Insert the syringe with normal saline. Unclamp the extension tubing and check for a blood return as indicated in Skill 15-8. If positive, instill the solution over 1 minute or by using a pulsatile flushing technique of 10 short boluses of 1 mL interrupted by brief pauses; flush the line according to facility policy (Figure 1).	Gloves prevent contact with blood and body fluids. Venous access device entry points, end caps, and needleless connectors must be vigorously scrubbed and disinfected prior to each access to reduce the risk for introduction of microorganisms and prevent venous access device–related infection (Frimpong et al., 2015; Harper, 2014; INS, 2016b; The Joint Commission, 2018; Loveday et al., 2014). Friction is needed to physically remove microorganisms from the top, sides, and threads of the needleless connector or end cap. Allow the antiseptic to dry completely (15 to 30 seconds) to ensure complete effectiveness (Harper). It is important to flush all substances out of the well of the implanted port, because it may be inactive for an extended period of time. Positive blood return confirms patency before administration of medications and solutions (INS, 2016b). Not allowing blood to enter the syringe ensures that the needle will be flushed with pure saline. A pulsatile flushing technique of 10 short boluses of 1 mL interrupted by brief pauses may be effective in removing solid deposits (INS, 2016b).

FIGURE 1. Flushing port with saline.

9. Remove the syringe. Using an antimicrobial swab, vigorously scrub the needleless connector or end cap on the extension tubing and allow to dry. Insert the locking solution syringe and instill the volume of solution designated by facility policy over 1 minute or according to facility policy. Remove the syringe and clamp the lumen.	Venous access device entry points, end caps, and needleless connectors must be vigorously scrubbed and disinfected prior to each access to reduce the risk for introduction of microorganisms and prevent venous access device–related infection (Frimpong et al., 2015; Harper, 2014; INS, 2016b; The Joint Commission, 2018; Loveday et al., 2014). Friction is needed to physically remove microorganisms from the top, sides, and threads of the needleless connector or end cap. Allow the antiseptic to dry completely (15 to 30 seconds) to ensure complete effectiveness (Harper). CVADs should be "locked" with either a heparin solution (10 units/mL) or normal saline solution after each intermittent use, according to the directions for use for the specific CVAD and needleless connector, to maintain patency (INS, 2016a).

(continued)

Skill 15-9 ▶ Deaccessing an Implanted Port *(continued)*

ACTION	RATIONALE
10. Remove the dressing and/or stabilization device, noting any drainage and discard (Refer to Skill 15-7).	Removal of the stabilization device and dressing is necessary to remove the access needle.
11. Stabilize the port on either side with the thumb and fore-finger of your nondominant hand. Grasp the needle/wings with the fingers of the dominant hand. Firmly and smoothly, pull the needle straight up at a 90-degree angle from the skin to remove it from the port septum (Figure 2). Engage needle guard, if not automatic on removal.	The port is held in place while the needle is removed.

FIGURE 2. Pulling needle from port with auto-engagement of needle guard.

ACTION	RATIONALE
12. Apply gentle pressure with the gauze to the insertion site. Apply a small adhesive bandage over the port if any oozing occurs. Otherwise, a dressing is not necessary. Remove gloves.	A small amount of blood may form from the needlestick. Intact skin provides a barrier to infection.
13. Ensure the patient's comfort. Lower the bed, if not in the lowest position. Put on one glove to handle the needle. Dispose of the needle with the extension tubing in the sharps container.	Promotes patient comfort and safety. Proper disposal of the needle prevents accidental injury.
14. Remove gloves and additional PPE, if used. Perform hand hygiene.	Removing PPE properly reduces the risk for infection transmission and contamination of other items. Hand hygiene prevents transmission of microorganisms.

EVALUATION

The expected outcome has been met when the port flushes easily; the needle is removed without difficulty; the site is clean, dry, without evidence of redness, irritation, or warmth; and the patient verbalizes an understanding of port care.

DOCUMENTATION

Guidelines

Document the location of the port, assessment of site, and the ease or difficulty of flushing the port. Record the locking of the port. This may be done on the eMAR/MAR. Document removal of the access needle. Record the appearance of the site, including if there is any drainage, swelling, or redness. Record any appropriate patient teaching.

Sample Documentation

> 11/13/20 1020 Implanted port L chest wall flushed without resistance using 10 mL of saline and 5 mL of heparin/10 U/mL. No hematoma noted. Access needle removed without difficulty. Site without redness, swelling, drainage, or heat. Patient denies discomfort. Patient verbalized an understanding of site care.
>
> —S. Barnes, RN

UNEXPECTED SITUATIONS AND ASSOCIATED INTERVENTIONS

- *Port does not flush:* Check clamp to make sure tubing is open. Gently push down on the needle and again try to flush. Ask the patient to perform a Valsalva maneuver. Have the patient change position or place the affected arm over the head and raise or lower the head of the bed. If the port still does not flush, notify the primary care provider.
- *Site does not stop bleeding:* Continue to hold pressure. If the patient has some clotting disturbances, pressure may need to be applied for a longer duration.

SPECIAL CONSIDERATIONS

General Considerations

- For vascular access ports that are not actively accessed for infusion therapy, there is insufficient evidence to recommend the optimal frequency for flushing and locking; refer to the manufacturers' directions for use and facility policy (INS, 2016a, p. 179).
- Implanted ports require larger flush volumes due to volume required to fill the device.
- Groshong devices do not require the use of heparin for flushing.
- Some facilities call for a pulsatile flushing technique, which may be more effective in removing solid deposits from VAD lumens (INS, 2016a).
- Heparin-induced thrombocytopenia (HIT) has been reported with the use of heparin flush solutions. Monitor all patients closely for signs and symptoms of HIT. If present or suspected, discontinue heparin (INS, 2016a).
- Monitoring of platelet counts for HIT is not recommended in postoperative and medical patients receiving only heparin in the form of a catheter lock solution due to a very low incidence of HIT (INS, 2016a, p. S78).

EVIDENCE FOR PRACTICE ▶

INFUSION NURSING STANDARDS OF PRACTICE

Infusion Nurses Society (INS). (2016b). Infusion therapy. Standards of practice. *Journal of Infusion Nursing, 39*(Suppl 1), S1–S159.

Refer to details in Skill 15-1, Evidence for Practice, and refer to thePoint' for additional research on related nursing topics.

EVIDENCE FOR PRACTICE ▶

INFUSION NURSING POLICIES AND PROCEDURES FOR INFUSION THERAPY

Infusion Nurses Society (INS). (2016a). *Policies and procedures for infusion therapy* (5th ed.). Norwood, MA: Author.

Refer to details in Skill 15-1, Evidence for Practice, and refer to thePoint' for additional research on related nursing topics.

Skill 15-10 ▶ Removing a Peripherally Inserted Central Catheter (PICC)

When PICC is no longer required or when the patient has developed complications, it will be discontinued. Nurses or specialized IV team nurses may be responsible for removing a PICC line. Specific protocols must be followed to prevent breakage or fracture of the catheter.

DELEGATION CONSIDERATIONS

The removal of a PICC is not delegated to nursing assistive personnel (NAP), to unlicensed assistive personnel (UAP), or to licensed practical/vocational nurses (LPN/LVNs).

(continued)

Skill 15-10 ▶ Removing a Peripherally Inserted Central Catheter (PICC) *(continued)*

EQUIPMENT	
• Clean gloves	• Sterile petroleum-based ointment
• Additional PPE, as indicated	• Transparent semipermeable membrane dressing
• Sterile gauze sponges	
• Suture removal set, as needed	• Disposable measuring tape

ASSESSMENT

Inspect the insertion site, looking for any swelling, redness, or drainage. Check pertinent laboratory values, particularly coagulation times and platelet counts. Patients with alterations in coagulation require that pressure be applied for a longer period of time after catheter removal. Measure the length of the PICC after removal.

NURSING DIAGNOSIS

Determine the related factors for the nursing diagnoses based on the patient's current status. Appropriate nursing diagnoses may include:

- Risk for infection
- Risk for injury
- Deficient knowledge

OUTCOME IDENTIFICATION AND PLANNING

The expected outcome to achieve when removing a PICC is that the PICC is removed with minimal to no discomfort to the patient and the patient experiences no adverse effect or infection.

IMPLEMENTATION

ACTION	RATIONALE
1. Verify medical order for PICC removal and facility policy and procedure. Gather equipment.	Checking the order and/or policy ensures that the proper procedure is initiated. Preparation promotes efficient time management and an organized approach to the task.
2. Perform hand hygiene and put on PPE, if indicated.	Hand hygiene and PPE prevent the spread of microorganisms. Unclean hands and improper technique are potential sources for infecting a CVAD. PPE is required based on transmission precautions.
3. Identify the patient.	Identifying the patient ensures the right patient receives the intervention and helps prevent errors.
4. Close the curtains around the bed and close the door to the room, if possible. Explain what you are going to do and why you are going to do it to the patient.	This ensures the patient's privacy. Explanation relieves anxiety and facilitates cooperation.
5. Adjust the bed to a comfortable working height, usually elbow height of the caregiver (VHACEOSH, 2016).	Having the bed at the proper height prevents back and muscle strain.
6. Assist the patient to a supine flat or Trendelenburg position with the arm straight and the catheter insertion site at or below heart level. Use the bath blanket to cover any exposed area other than the site.	This position is recommended to reduce the risk of air embolism. Use of a bath blanket provides for comfort and warmth.
7. Put on gloves. Stabilize catheter hub with your nondominant hand. Remove the dressing and/or stabilization device, noting any drainage and discard (Refer to Skill 15-7).	Gloves prevent contact with blood and body fluids. Removal of the stabilization device and dressing is necessary to remove PICC.
8. Instruct the patient to hold the breath, and perform a Valsalva maneuver as the last portion of the catheter is removed; if unable to do so, have the patient exhale (INS, 2016a).	Use of the Valsalva maneuver or other recommended intervention reduces the risk for air embolism (INS, 2016a; Feil, 2012).

ACTION	**RATIONALE**
9. Using the dominant hand, remove the catheter slowly. Grasp the catheter close to the insertion site and slowly ease it out, keeping it parallel to the skin. Continue removing in small increments, using a smooth and constant motion (Figure 1).	Gentle pressure reduces risk of breakage. Catheter should come out easily.

FIGURE 1. Removing PICC in small increments, using a smooth and constant motion. (*Photo by B. Proud.*)

10. After removal, apply pressure to the site with sterile gauze until hemostasis is achieved (minimum 1 minute). Apply petroleum-based ointment and a sterile occlusive dressing.	Adequate pressure prevents hematoma formation. Use of a petroleum-based ointment and a sterile dressing at the access site seals the skin-to-vein tract and decreases the risk of air embolus (INS, 2016b).
11. Measure the catheter and compare it with the length listed in the chart when it was inserted. Inspect the catheter for patency. Dispose of PICC according to facility policy.	Measurement and inspection ensures that the entire catheter was removed. Proper disposal reduces transmission of microorganisms and prevents contact with blood and body fluids.
12. Remove gloves. Ensure the patient's comfort. Lower the bed, if not in the lowest position.	Promotes patient comfort and safety.
13. Instruct the patient to remain in flat/supine position, if able, for 30 minutes postremoval.	Remaining in a flat or reclining position decreases the risk of air entering through an intact skin-to-vein tract (INS, 2016b).
14. Remove additional PPE, if used. Perform hand hygiene.	Proper removal of PPE reduces the risk for infection transmission and contamination of other items. Hand hygiene prevents transmission of microorganisms.
15. Leave the dressing in place for at least 24 hours (INS, 2016a). Change the dressing daily until the exit site has healed.	Maintenance of the dressing until the site heals prevents transmission and entry of microorganisms.

EVALUATION   The expected outcome has been met when the PICC is removed with minimal to no discomfort to the patient and without adverse event or infection.

DOCUMENTATION

Guidelines   Document the location of the PICC and its removal. Record the catheter length and patency. Record the appearance of the site, including if there is any drainage, swelling, or redness. Record any appropriate patient teaching.

(*continued*)

Skill 15-10 ▶ Removing a Peripherally Inserted Central Catheter (PICC) *(continued)*

Sample Documentation

4/1/15 1230 PICC removed from L brachial. Length of catheter 37.5 cm; entire length intact. Pressure applied to insertion site for 2 minutes; site without bleeding, ecchymosis, redness, drainage. Dry dressing applied. Patient instructed to notify nurse if pain or bleeding noted.

—S. Stone, RN

UNEXPECTED SITUATIONS AND ASSOCIATED INTERVENTIONS

- *You encounter resistance while attempting to remove the PICC:* If resistance is felt when removing a catheter, stop removal. Resistance typically may be caused by smooth muscle spasm inside the vein wall. Encourage the patient to relax and take deep breaths. Wait a few minutes and then try again (Hadaway, 2009). Do not forcibly remove the catheter (INS, 2016a). Replace the sterile dressing and notify the patient's primary health care provider.
- *You measure the catheter after removal and it is shorter than the documented length at insertion:* Notify the primary care provider. Monitor the patient for signs of distress. The piece of catheter could be lodged in the venous system or have migrated to the right atrium. Anticipate the need for radiology studies to locate the piece of catheter and possible surgery to retrieve the catheter.

SPECIAL CONSIDERATIONS

- When the Valsalva's maneuver is contraindicated, use a Trendelenburg or left lateral decubitus position (INS, 2016b).

EVIDENCE FOR PRACTICE ▶

INFUSION NURSING STANDARDS OF PRACTICE
Infusion Nurses Society (INS). (2016b). Infusion therapy. Standards of practice. *Journal of Infusion Nursing, 39*(Suppl 1), S1–S159.
  Refer to details in Skill 15-1, Evidence for Practice, and refer to thePoint® for additional research on related nursing topics.

EVIDENCE FOR PRACTICE ▶

INFUSION NURSING POLICIES AND PROCEDURES FOR INFUSION THERAPY
Infusion Nurses Society (INS). (2016a). *Policies and procedures for infusion therapy* (5th ed.). Norwood, MA: Author.
  Refer to details in Skill 15-1, Evidence for Practice, and refer to thePoint® for additional research on related nursing topics.

Enhance Your Understanding

Focusing on Patient Care: Developing Clinical Reasoning

Consider the case scenarios at the beginning of the chapter as you answer the following questions to enhance your understanding and apply what you have learned.

QUESTIONS

1. Simon Lawrence's mother is asking about the risks associated with IV placement. What would you tell her about the risks associated with IV placement and rehydration?

2. During the first 5 minutes of Melissa Cohen's transfusion of packed red blood cells, she reports a headache and low back pain. When you assess her, you find that she has a temperature of 101°F (up from 98.9°F earlier) and she is shivering. What actions would be most appropriate at this time?

3. Mr. Tracy asks about care of his recently implanted port. What are some topics you should discuss with him while he is at the outpatient chemotherapy center?

You can find suggested answers after the Bibliography at the end of this chapter.

Enhance Your Understanding (Continued)

Integrated Case Study Connection

The case studies in the back of the book focus on integrating concepts. Refer to the following case studies to enhance your understanding of the concepts and skills in this chapter.

- Intermediate Case Studies: Olivia Greenbaum, page 1113; Jason Brown, page 1119; Kent Clark, page 1121; Janice Romero, page 1124; Gwen Galloway, page 1125.
- Advanced Case Studies: Robert Espinoza, page 1132.

Taylor Suite Resources

Explore these additional resources to enhance learning for this chapter:

- NCLEX-Style Questions and other resources on thePoint®, http://thePoint.lww.com/Lynn5e
- *Skill Checklists for Taylor's Clinical Nursing Skills*, 5e
- *Taylor's Video Guide to Clinical Nursing Skills:* Intravenous Therapy and Central Venous Access Devices
- *Fundamentals of Nursing:* Chapter 40, Fluid, Electrolyte, and Acid–Base Balance
- *Lippincott DocuCare* Fundamentals cases

Bibliography

AABB. (n.d.) *Transfusion medicine. Clinical resources. Clinical guidelines and guidance.* Retrieved http://www.aabb.org/programs/clinical/Pages/default.aspx

Agency for Healthcare Research and Quality (AHRQ). (2011). *Blood transfusion: Indications, administration and adverse reactions.* Retrieved https://www.guideline.gov/summaries/summary/34955

American Red Cross. (n.d.a). *Blood testing.* Retrieved http://www.redcrossblood.org/learn-about-blood/what-happens-donated-blood/blood-testing

American Red Cross. (n.d.b). *Donating blood. Eligibility requirements.* Retrieved http://www.redcrossblood.org/donating-blood/eligibility-requirements

American Red Cross. (n.d.c). *Autologous and directed donations.* Retrieved http://www.redcrossblood.org/donating-blood/types-donations/autologous-and-directed

American Red Cross. (2013). *A compendium of transfusion practice guidelines* (2nd ed.). Retrieved http://www.redcrossblood.org/sites/arc/files/59802_compendium_brochure_v_6_10_9_13.pdf

Arbique, D., Boredelon, M., Dragoo, R., & Huckaby, S. (2014). Ultrasound-guided access for peripheral intravenous therapy. *Academy of Medical-Surgical Nurses, 23,* 9–15.

Bolton, D. (2015). Clinically indicated replacement of peripheral cannulas. *British Journal of Nursing, 24*(19), S4–S12.

Cameron-Watson, C. (2016). Port protectors in clinical practice: An audit. *British Journal of Nursing (IV Therapy Supplement), 25*(8), S25–S31.

Campbell, N., Cleaver, K., & Davies, N. (2014). Oral sucrose as an analgesia for neonates: How effective and safe is the sweet solution? A review of the literature. *Journal of Neonatal Nursing, 20*(6), 274–282.

Carson, J. L., Grossman, B. J., Kleinman, S., et al. (2012). Red blood cell transfusion: A clinical practice guideline from the AABB. *Annals of Internal Medicine, 157*(1), 49–58.

Centers for Disease Control and Prevention (CDC). (2013). *Blood safety.* Retrieved http://www.cdc.gov/bloodsafety/bbp/diseases_organisms.html

Cohen, B. J., & Hull, K. L. (2015). *Memmler's structure and function of the human body* (11th ed.). Philadelphia, PA: Wolters Kluwer.

Cook, L. S. (2013). Infusion-related air embolism. *Journal of Infusion Nursing, 36*(1), 26–36.

Dalton, M., Pheil, N., Lacy, J., & Dalton, J. (2014). Does sludge/debris exist in today's vascular access ports?. *Journal of the Association for Vascular Access, 19*(1), 23–26.

DeYoung Sullivan, K., Vu, T., Richardson, G., Castillo, E., & Martinez, F. (2015). Evaluating the frequency of vital sign monitoring during blood transfusion: An evidence-based practice initiative. *Clinical Journal of Oncology Nursing, 19*(5), 516–520.

Doenges, M. E., Moorhouse, M. F., & Murr, A. C. (2016). *Nursing diagnoses manual. Planning, individualizing, and documenting client care* (5th ed.). Philadelphia, PA: F.A. Davis.

Dougherty, L. (2013). Intravenous therapy in older patients. *Nursing Standard, 28*(6), 50–58.

Dudek, S. (2018). *Nutrition essentials for nursing practice* (8th ed.). Philadelphia, PA: Wolters Kluwer.

Dychter, S., Gold, D., Carson, D., & Haller, M. (2012). Intravenous therapy: A review of complications and economic considerations of peripheral access. *Journal of Infusion Nursing, 35*(2), 84–91.

Egan, G. M., Siskin, G. P., Weinmann IV, R., & Galloway, M. M. (2013). A prospective postmarket study to evaluate the safety and efficacy of a new peripherally inserted central catheter stabilization system. *Journal of Infusion Nursing, 36*(3), 181–188.

Eliopoulos, C. (2018). *Gerontological nursing* (9th ed.). Philadelphia, PA: Wolters Kluwer.

Feil, M.; Pennsylvania Patient Safety Authority. (2012). Pennsylvania patient safety advisory. Reducing risk if air embolism associated with central venous access devices. Retrieved http://patientsafetyauthority.org/ADVISORIES/AdvisoryLibrary/2012/Jun;9(2)/Pages/58.aspx

Fields, J. M., Piela, N. E., Au, A. K., & Ku, B. S. (2014). Risk factors associated with difficult venous access in adult ED patients. *American Journal of Emergency Medicine, 32*(10), 1179–1182.

Fischbach, F. T., & Dunning III, M. B. (2015). *A manual of laboratory and diagnostic tests* (9th ed.). Philadelphia, PA: Wolters Kluwer Health.

Freire, M. P., Pierrotti, L. C., Zerati, A. E., et al. (2013). Infection related to implantable central venous access devices in cancer patents: Epidemiology and risk factors. *Infection Control and Hospital Epidemiology, 34*(7), 671–677.

Frimpong, A., Caguioa, J., & Octavo, G. (2015). Promoting safe IV management in practice using H.A.N.D.S. *British Journal of Nursing (IV Therapy Supplement), 24*(2), S18–S23.

Grossman, S., & Porth, C. M. (2014). *Porth's pathophysiology: Concepts of altered health states* (9th ed.). Philadelphia, PA: Wolters Kluwer.

Hadaway, L. C. (2009). Central venous access devices. *Nursing 2009 Critical Care, 3*(5), 26–33.

Hale, A., & Hovey, M. J. (2014). *Fluid, electrolyte, and acid–base imbalances.* Philadelphia, PA: F.A. Davis Company.

Harper, D. (2014). I.V. Rounds. Infusion therapy: Much more than a simple task. *Nursing, 44*(7), 66–67.

Helton, J., Hines, A., & Best, J. (2016). Peripheral IV site rotation based on clinical assessment vs. length of time since insertion. *Medsurg Nursing, 25*(1), 44–49.

Herriage, T., Hooke, M. C., Streifel, A., & Slaker, B. (2016). Utilization of an intravenous line lifter within a pediatric oncology population. *Journal of Pediatric Oncology Nursing, 33*(2), 105–110.

Higginson, R. (2015). Intravenous therapy: Guidance and implications for practice. *British Journal of Healthcare Management, 21*(6), 264–268.

Hinkle, J. L., & Cheever, K. H. (2018). *Brunner & Suddarth's textbook of medical–surgical nursing* (14th ed.). Philadelphia, PA: Wolters Kluwer.

Houston, P. A. (2013). Obtaining vascular access in the obese patient population. *Journal of Infusion Nursing, 36*(1), 52–56.

Infusion Nurses Society (INS). (2016a). *Policies and procedures for infusion therapy* (5th ed.). Norwood, MA: Author.

Infusion Nurses Society (INS). (2016b). Infusion therapy. Standards of practice. *Journal of Infusion Nursing, 39*(Suppl 1), S1–S159.

Institute for Safe Medication Practices (ISMP). (2009a). *ISMP summit on the use of smart infusion pumps: Guidelines for safe implementation and use.* Retrieved http://www.ismp.org/tools/guidelines/smartpumps/default.asp

Jarvis, C. (2016). *Physical examination & health assessment* (7th ed.). St. Louis, MO: Elsevier.

Jensen, S. (2015). *Nursing health assessment: A best practice approach* (2nd ed.). Philadelphia, PA: Wolters Kluwer.

The Joint Commission. (2018). *National patient safety goals.* Retrieved https://www.jointcommission.org/standards_information/npsgs.aspx

Julian, M. K. (2013). Caring for your patient receiving TPN. *Nursing Made Incredibly Easy!, 11*(1), 8–11.

Karch, A. M. (2017). *Focus on nursing pharmacology* (7th ed.). Philadelphia, PA: Wolters Kluwer.

Kessler, C. (2013). Priming blood transfusion tubing: A critical review of the blood transfusion process. *Critical Care Nurse, 33*(3), 80–84.

Kyle, T., & Carman, S. (2017). *Essentials of pediatric nursing* (3rd ed.). Philadelphia, PA: Wolters Kluwer.

LeMone, P., Burke, K. M., Bauldoff, G., & Gubrud, P. (2015). *Medical-surgical nursing. Clinical reasoning in patient care* (6th ed.). New York: Pearson.

Long, M. -Y., Liu, Z. -H., & Zhu, J. -G. (2014). Comparative analysis of autologous blood transfusion and allogeneic blood transfusion in surgical patients. *International Journal of Clinical and Experimental Medicine, 7*(9), 2889–2894.

Loveday, H. P., Wilson, J. A., Pratt, R. J., et al. (2014). Epic3: National evidence-based guidelines for preventing healthcare-associated infections in NHS hospitals in England. *Journal of Hospital Infection, 86*(1), S1–S70.

Mace, S. E. (2016). Prospective, randomized, double-blind controlled trial comparing vapocoolant spray vs placebo spray in adults undergoing venipuncture. *American Journal of Emergency Medicine, 34*(5), 798–804.

Major, T. W., & Huey, T. K. (2016). Decreasing IV infiltrates in the pediatric patient-System-based improvement project. *Pediatric Nursing, 42*(1), 14–49.

Makic, M. B., Martin, S. A., Burns, S., Philbrick, D., & Rauen, C. (2013). Putting evidence into nursing practice: Four traditional practices not supported by the evidence. *Critical Care Nurse, 33*(2), 28–44.

Marsh, N., Webster, J., Mihala, G., & Rickard, C. M. (2015). Devices and dressings to secure peripheral venous catheters to prevent complications. *Cochrane Database of Systematic Reviews, (6)*, CD011070.

McClelland, M. (2014). IV therapies for patients with fluid and electrolyte imbalances. *Med-Surg Nursing, 23*(5), 4–8.

Menendez, B. J., & Edwards, B. (2016). Early identification of acute hemolytic transfusion reactions: Realistic implications for best practice in patient monitoring. *Medsurg Nursing, 25*(2), 88–109.

Mimoz, O., Lucet, J. C., Kerforne, T., et al. (2015). Skin antisepsis with chlorhexidine-alcohol versus povidone iodine-alcohol, with and without skin scrubbing, for prevention of intravascular-catheter-related infection (CLEAN): An open-label, multicenter, randomized, controlled, two-by-two factorial trial. *Lancet, 386*(10008), 2069–2077.

Moureau, N. (2013). Safe patient care when using vascular access devices. *British Journal of Nursing, 22*(2), S14–S21.

NANDA International, Inc.: *Nursing Diagnoses— Definitions and Classification 2018–2020* © 2017

NANDA International, ISBN 978-1-62623-929-6. Used by arrangement with the Thieme Group, Stuttgart/New York.

Nuttall, G. A., Stubbs, J. R., & Oliver, W. C. (2014). Transfusion errors: Causes, incidence, and strategies for prevention. *Current Opinion in Anaesthesiology, 27*(6), 657–659.

O'Grady, N. P., Alexander, M., Burns, L. A., et al; The Healthcare Infection Control Practices Advisory Committee (HICPAC). (2011). Guidelines for the prevention of intravascular catheter-related infections. *American Journal of Infection Control, 39*(4 Suppl), S1–S34.

Partovi-Deilami, K., Nielsen, J. K., Møller, A. M., Nesheim, S. S., & Jørgensen, V. L. (2016). Effect of ultrasound-guided placement of difficult-to-place peripheral venous catheters: A prospective study of a training program for nurse anesthetists. *AANA Journal, 84*(2), 86–92.

Perry, S. E., Hockenberry, M. J., Lowdermilk, D. L., & Wilson, D. (2014). *Maternal child nursing care* (5th ed.). St. Louis, MO: Elsevier Mosby.

Purnell, L. D. (2013). *Transcultural health care. A culturally competent approach* (4th ed.). Philadelphia, PA: F.A. Davis Company.

Stango, C., Runyan, D., Stern, J., Macri, I., & Vacca, M. (2014). A successful approach to reducing bloodstream infections based on a disinfection device for intravenous needleless connector hubs. *Journal of Infusion Nursing, 37*(6), 462–465.

Taylor, C., Lynn, P., & Bartlett, J. (2019). *Fundamentals of nursing: The art and science of person-centered care* (9th ed.). Philadelphia, PA: Wolters Kluwer.

Tuffaha, H. S., Rickard, C. M., Weber, J., et al. (2014). Cost-effectiveness analysis of clinically indicated versus routine replacement of peripheral intravenous catheters. *Applied Health Economics and Health Policy, 12*(1), 51–58.

Ullman, A. J., Cooke, M., & Rickard, C. M. (2015). Examining the role of securement and dressing products to prevent central venous access device failure: A narrative review. *Journal of the Association for Vascular Access, 20*(2), 99–110.

Van Leeuwen, A. M., & Bladh, M. L. (2015). *Davis's comprehensive handbook of laboratory & diagnostic tests with nursing implications* (5th ed.). Philadelphia, PA: F.A. Davis.

VHA Center for Engineering & Occupational Safety and Health (CEOSH). (2016). *Safe patient handling and mobility guidebook.* St. Louis, MO: Author. Retrieved http://www.tampavaref.org/safe-patient-handling.htm

Weingart, S. N., Hsieh, C., Lane, S., & Cleary, A. M. (2014). Standardizing central venous catheter care by using observations from patients with cancer. *Clinical Journal of Oncology Nursing, 18*(3), 321–326.

Willis, L. M. (2015). *Fluids & electrolytes made incredibly easy!* (6th ed.). Philadelphia, PA: Wolters Kluwer.

Woody, G., & Davis, B. A. (2013). Increasing nurse competence in peripheral intravenous therapy. *Journal of Infusion Nursing, 36*(1), 413–419.

SUGGESTED ANSWERS FOR FOCUSING ON PATIENT CARE: DEVELOPING CLINICAL REASONING

1. Explain the reason the IV access is necessary and the rationale for IV fluid replacement. Discuss the potential complications related to peripheral venous access and IV fluid infusion, including infiltration, phlebitis, and infection. Explain the steps the nurses will take to prevent these complications; discuss the steps Ms. Lawrence can take to help prevent complications, as well as the signs and symptoms of which she should be aware. Encourage her to continue to ask questions and report any signs or symptoms she feels her son exhibits. Discuss the advantages related to using a topical anesthetic before peripheral venous access insertion. Explain any securement/stabilization devices that will be used with Simon to prevent accidental dislodgement or removal of the venous access device.

2. Ms. Cohen is exhibiting signs and symptoms consistent with a hemolytic transfusion reaction. This type of reaction typically occurs immediately and is the result of incompatibility of the donor blood with the recipient's blood. Stop the blood immediately. Disconnect the blood and begin infusing normal saline via a different, new administration set. Notify the primary care provider immediately. Monitor vital signs and symptoms. Anticipate the administration of medications to treat the reaction, including hypotension. Prepare to obtain required blood samples for serologic testing and a urine specimen. Return blood product and administration tubing to laboratory.

3. Provide Mr. Tracy with information regarding skin care and assessment related to his port site. Inform him about how to care for his port if it is accessed. It is important that he is aware of signs and symptoms that he should report to his primary care provider. He also needs to be aware of the time interval for surgical follow-up and the interval for appointments to flush and lock the port, if not in use.

Cardiovascular Care

16

Focusing on Patient Care

This chapter will help you develop some of the skills related to cardiovascular care necessary to care for the following patients:

Coby Pruder, age 40, is to undergo an electrocardiogram as part of his physical examination. Although he considers himself healthy, he is nervous.

Harry Stebbings, age 67, is admitted to the emergency department for chest pain and cardiac monitoring.

Ann Kribell, age 54, is a patient in the cardiac care unit. She has been diagnosed with heart failure and is receiving cardiac monitoring. She needs to have arterial blood samples drawn from her arterial catheter.

Refer to Focusing on Patient Care: Developing Clinical Reasoning at the end of the chapter to apply what you learn.

Learning Objectives

After completing the chapter, you will be able to accomplish the following:

1. Perform cardiopulmonary resuscitation (CPR).
2. Perform emergency automated external defibrillation.
3. Perform emergency manual external defibrillation (asynchronous).
4. Obtain a 12-lead ECG.
5. Apply a cardiac monitor.
6. Apply and monitor an external pacemaker.
7. Obtain an arterial blood sample from an arterial catheter.
8. Remove a peripheral arterial catheter.

Key Terms

cardiac arrest: sudden cessation of functional circulation of the heart (pulse), such as asystole or defibrillation, typically caused by the occlusion of one or more of the coronary arteries or cardiomyopathy

cardiac monitoring: visualization and monitoring of the cardiac electrical activity stimulating the heartbeat

cardiopulmonary resuscitation (CPR): also known as basic life support: revival in the absence of spontaneous respirations and heartbeat to preserve heart and brain function while waiting for defibrillation and advanced cardiac life support care. Achieved by manually pumping the heart by compressing the sternum and forcing oxygen into the lungs using mouth-to-mouth or rescue breathing.

cardioversion: conversion of a pathologic cardiac rhythm to normal sinus rhythm through low doses of electricity, using a device that applies synchronized counter shocks to the heart

circulation: the continuous one-way circuit of blood through the heart and blood vessels, with the heart as the pump (Cohen & Hull, 2015)

defibrillation: the use of a large amount of electric current to the heart through the chest wall over a brief period of time to treat chaotic cardiac rhythms; temporarily depolarizes the myocardium, producing a momentary asystole (absence of ventricular activity), providing an opportunity for the heart's normal pacemaker to restore a normal rhythm

dysrhythmia: group of conditions in which the electrical activity of the heart is irregular or is faster or slower than normal

electrocardiogram (ECG): graphic record of the electrical activity of the heart

electrocardiography: the making and study of records of the electrical activity of the heart

fibrillation: small, local, involuntary contraction of muscle, resulting from spontaneous activation of a single muscle fiber or of an isolated bundle of nerve fibers (Grossman & Porth, 2014)

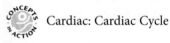

Cardiac: Cardiac Cycle

Cardiac: Myocardial Blood Flow

The cardiovascular system is composed of the heart and the blood vessels. The heart is the main organ of **circulation**, which is the continuous one-way circuit of blood through the blood vessels (Cohen & Hull, 2015). The heart is the circulatory pump, squeezing through the heart and out into the body. This is accomplished by contractions starting in the atria, followed by contraction of the ventricles, with a subsequent resting of the heart. Figure 16-1 provides an overview of cardiac anatomy. Deoxygenated blood (low in oxygen; high in carbon dioxide) is carried from the right side of the heart to the lungs, where oxygen is picked up and carbon dioxide is released, and then returned to the left side of the heart. This oxygenated blood (high in oxygen; low in carbon dioxide) is pumped out to all other parts of the body and back again (refer to Figure 14-2 in Chapter 14). The contraction of the muscles of the heart is controlled by electrical impulses produced in and carried over specialized tissue within the heart. These tissues make up the heart's conduction system. Figure 16-2 provides a review of the cardiac conduction system.

Assessment of cardiovascular function commonly involves noninvasive techniques such as inspection, auscultation, and palpation. Additional basic and important indicators of the heart's effectiveness are pulse rate, strength, and rhythm; blood pressure; skin color and temperature; and level of consciousness. Refer to Chapters 2 and 3 for additional information related to these assessments. Chapter 14 provides additional information related to oxygenation and cardiopulmonary function.

This chapter covers selected skills to assist the nurse in providing cardiovascular care. Should the heart stop pumping, it can be manually pumped via CPR until electrical **defibrillation** and additional medical support arrives. Noninvasive heart monitoring involves **electrocardiography** and **cardiac monitoring**. Figure 16-3 highlights cardiac landmark reference lines that are used in assessment and also for placing devices related to the application and use of an external pacemaker. Other electrical therapy devices are discussed in Fundamentals Review 16-1. The last two skills in the chapter focus on obtaining an arterial blood sample from an arterial catheter and removing a peripheral arterial catheter.

Invasive techniques, such as pulmonary artery pressure monitoring, Swan–Ganz catheterization, cardiac output determination, and cardiac support via an intra-aortic balloon pump (IABP) typically are used by trained critical care personnel to provide additional monitoring and support. These techniques are beyond the scope of this text.

Fundamentals Review 16-1

ELECTRICAL THERAPY DEVICES

In addition to defibrillation, electrical therapy may be delivered via the following devices:

- **Implantable cardioverter–defibrillator (ICD)** is a sophisticated device that automatically discharges an electric current to provide bradycardia and antitachycardia pacing, synchronized cardioversion, and defibrillation (convert abnormal cardiac rhythms to normal sinus rhythm) when it senses ventricular bradycardia and tachyarrhythmias. Patients with a history of ventricular fibrillation or ventricular tachycardia, with poor ejection fraction (<35%), or with nonischemic dilated cardiomyopathy (New York Heart Association [NYHA] functional class II or III), as well as patients with other conditions may be candidates for this type of device (Morton & Fontaine, 2018).
- **Synchronized cardioversion** is the treatment of choice for arrhythmias that do not respond to vagal maneuvers or to drug therapy, such as atrial tachycardia, atrial flutter, atrial fibrillation, and symptomatic ventricular tachycardia. Cardioversion is performed similarly to defibrillation but is synchronized with the heart rhythm and uses fewer joules. Cardioversion works by delivering an electrical charge to the myocardium at the peak of the R wave. This causes immediate depolarization, interrupting reentry circuits, and allowing the sinoatrial node to resume control. Synchronizing the electrical charge with the R wave ensures that the current will not be delivered on the vulnerable T wave and thus disrupting repolarization. It is usually performed in a critical care area, in the presence of a physician, an anesthesiologist, and emergency equipment. The patient is premedicated with pain medicine.

- **Pacemakers** are electronic devices that can be used to initiate the heartbeat when the heart's intrinsic electrical system cannot effectively generate a rate adequate to support cardiac output. Pacemakers help control abnormal heart rhythms (NHLBI, 2012). Pacemakers can be temporary: placed on the skin (transcutaneous); via temporary epicardial pacing wires inserted during surgery; or transvenous, via a pacing electrode wire passed through a vein (the brachial, internal, or external jugular, subclavian, or femoral) and into the right atrium or right ventricle. Pacemakers can also be permanent surgically implanted devices.
- **Biventricular pacemakers** (cardiac resynchronization therapy pacing device) use electrical current to improve synchronization of left ventricular contraction. Biventricular pacemakers are used in patients with heart failure (NYHA class III or IV), with an intraventricular conduction delay (QRS >120 ms), and in patients with left ventricular ejection fraction ≤35%. These devices improve right and left ventricle contraction, resulting in improved cardiac function, with improved ejection fraction (Cleveland Clinic, n.d.).

FIGURE 16-1. Cardiac anatomy.

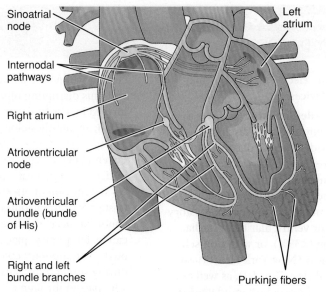

FIGURE 16-2. Cardiac conduction system.

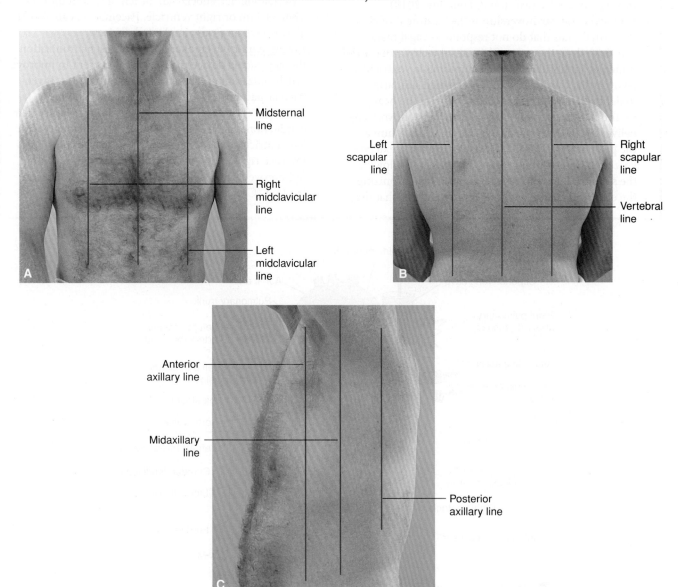

FIGURE 16-3. Cardiac landmarks: Reference lines. **A.** Anterior chest. **B.** Posterior chest. **C.** Lateral chest.

Skill 16-1 ▶ Performing Cardiopulmonary Resuscitation

Cardiopulmonary resuscitation (CPR), also known as basic life support, is used in any situation in which either breathing alone or breathing and a heartbeat are absent. It is a combination of chest compressions, which circulate blood, and mouth-to-mouth breathing, which supplies oxygen to the lungs. The brain is sensitive to hypoxia and will sustain irreversible damage after 4 to 6 minutes of no oxygen. The faster CPR is initiated, the greater the chance of survival.

The American Heart Association (AHA) identifies two "Chains of Survival" (AHA, 2015a). These pathways identify separate care for patients who experience a cardiac event in the hospital and those who experience an event in out-of-hospital settings. After checking the victim for a response, health care workers in the hospital activate the emergency response system, get an automated external defibrillator (AED) or defibrillator, and begin CPR.

In the health care setting, it is imperative that personnel be aware of the patient's stated instructions regarding any wish not to be resuscitated. This should be clearly expressed and documented in the patient's health record.

The AHA provides guidelines related to emergency interventions outside of health care facilities. Learning conventional CPR is still recommended, and trained lay rescuers should provide rescue breaths in addition to chest compressions (AHA, 2015b). However, the AHA guidelines recommend that when a teen or adult suddenly collapses, untrained lay rescuers should call 911 (activate the emergency response system) and push hard and fast in the center of the victim's chest. Studies of real emergencies that have occurred in homes, at work, or in public locations show that these two steps, called Hands-Only CPR, can be as effective as conventional CPR. Providing Hands-Only CPR to a teen or adult who has collapsed from a sudden **cardiac arrest** can more than double that person's chance of survival (AHA, 2016a).

DELEGATION CONSIDERATIONS	The initiation and provision of cardiopulmonary resuscitation is appropriate for all health care providers.
EQUIPMENT	• Personal protective equipment, such as a face shield or one-way valve mask and gloves, if available • Bag-valve-mask device and oxygen, if available
ASSESSMENT	Assess the patient's vital parameters and determine the patient's level of responsiveness. Check for partial or complete airway obstruction. Assess for the absence or ineffectiveness of respirations. Assess for the absence of signs of circulation and pulses.
NURSING DIAGNOSIS	Determine the related factors for the nursing diagnoses based on the patient's current status. Appropriate nursing diagnoses may include: • Decreased cardiac output • Impaired gas exchange • Impaired spontaneous ventilation
OUTCOME IDENTIFICATION AND PLANNING	The expected outcome to achieve when performing CPR is that CPR is performed effectively without adverse effect to the patient. Additional outcomes include the following: the patient regains a pulse and respirations; the patient's heart and lungs maintain adequate function to sustain life; advanced cardiac life support (ACLS) is initiated; and the patient does not experience serious injury.

IMPLEMENTATION

ACTION	RATIONALE
1. Verify scene safety. Assess responsiveness. Look for no breathing or only gasping. Call for help, pull call bell, and call the facility emergency response number. Call for emergency equipment and the AED or defibrillator, if available.	Assessing responsiveness prevents starting CPR on a conscious patient. Activating the emergency response system initiates a rapid response.

(continued)

Skill 16-1 ▶ Performing Cardiopulmonary Resuscitation *(continued)*

ACTION	RATIONALE
2. Put on gloves, if available. Position the patient supine on his or her back on a firm, flat surface, with arms alongside the body. If the patient is in bed, place a backboard or other rigid surface under the patient (often the footboard of the patient's bed). Position yourself at the patient's side.	Gloves prevent contact with blood and body fluids. The supine position is required for resuscitative efforts and evaluation to be effective. Backboard provides a firm surface on which to apply compressions.
3. **Provide defibrillation (if indicated) at the earliest possible moment, as soon as an AED becomes available.** Refer to Skills 16-2 and Skill 16-3.	The interval from collapse to defibrillation is one of the most important determinants of survival from sudden cardiac arrest with ventricular **fibrillation** or pulseless ventricular tachycardia (VT) (AHA, 2015b).
4. Simultaneously look for no breathing or only gasping and check for a pulse, palpating the carotid pulse. This assessment should take at least 5 seconds and no more than 10 seconds. If you do not definitely feel a pulse within 10 seconds, begin CPR using the compression:ventilation ratio of 30 compressions to 2 breaths, starting with chest compressions (CAB sequence). Alternately, if there is no normal breathing but the patient has a pulse, see Step 14.	Pulse assessment evaluates cardiac function. Delays in chest compressions should be minimized, so the health care provider should take no more than 10 seconds to check for a pulse. If it is not felt within that time period, chest compressions should be started (AHA, 2015b). Rescue breathing should be provided to maintain effective oxygenation and ventilation (AHA, 2015b).
5. Position the heel of one hand in the center of the chest between the nipples, directly over the lower half of the sternum. Place the heel of the other hand directly on top of the first hand. Extend or interlace fingers to keep fingers above the chest. Straighten arms and position shoulders directly over hands.	Proper hand positioning ensures that the force of compressions is on the sternum, thereby reducing the risk of rib fracture, lung puncture, or liver laceration.
6. Push hard and fast. Chest compressions should depress the sternum to a depth of at least 2 in (adult). Push straight down on the patient's sternum. Perform 30 chest compressions at a rate of 100/min, counting "1, 2, etc." up to 30, keeping elbows locked, arms straight, and shoulders directly over the hands. Allow full chest recoil (reexpand) after each compression (Figure 1). **Do not lean on chest wall between compressions.** Chest compression and chest recoil/relaxation times should be approximately equal.	Direct cardiac compression and manipulation of intrathoracic pressure supply blood flow during CPR. Compressing the chest at least 2 in ensures that compressions are not too shallow and provides adequate blood flow. Full chest recoil allows adequate venous return to the heart. Leaning on chest wall between compressions precludes full chest wall recoil (AHA, 2015a).

Upstroke
Downstroke
At least 2 in

FIGURE 1. Using correct body alignment for chest compressions. Depress the sternum 2 in.

ACTION

7. Ventilate using a barrier device (face mask or bag-valve-mask device, if available) (refer to Skill 14-14 in Chapter 14). Give 2 breaths (as described below) after each set of 30 compressions. Cycles of 30 compressions and 2 ventilations are recommended (AHA, 2015a).

8. Use the head tilt–chin lift maneuver to open the airway (Figure 2). Place one hand on the patient's forehead and apply firm, backward pressure with the palm to tilt the head back. Place the fingers of the other hand under the bony part of the lower jaw near the chin and lift the jaw upward to bring the chin forward and the teeth almost to occlusion.

9. If trauma to the head or neck is present or suspected, use the jaw-thrust maneuver to open the airway (Figure 3). Place one hand on each side of the patient's head. Rest elbows on the flat surface under the patient, grasp the angle of the patient's lower jaw, and lift with both hands.

RATIONALE

Breathing and compressions simulate lung and heart function, providing oxygen and circulation.

The head tilt–chin lift maneuver, recommended for use by health care providers, lifts the tongue, relieving airway obstruction by the tongue in an unresponsive person (AHA, 2015b).

The jaw-thrust maneuver may reduce neck and spine movement.

FIGURE 2. Using the head tilt–chin lift method to open the airway.

FIGURE 3. Using the jaw-thrust maneuver to open the airway.

10. Seal the patient's mouth and nose with the face shield, one-way valve mask (Figure 4A), or Ambu bag (handheld resuscitation bag), if available (refer to Skill 14-14 in Chapter 14) (Figure 4B). If not available, seal the patient's mouth with your mouth.

Sealing the patient's mouth and nose prevents air from escaping. Devices such as masks reduce the risk for transmission of infections.

A **B**

FIGURE 4. **A.** Using a one-way valve mask. **B.** Using a handheld resuscitation bag. (*Photo by B. Proud.*)

(*continued*)

Skill 16-1 ▶ Performing Cardiopulmonary Resuscitation *(continued)*

ACTION	**RATIONALE**
11. Instill 2 breaths, each lasting 1 second, making the chest rise.	Breathing into the patient provides oxygen to the patient's lungs. Hyperventilation results in increased positive chest pressure and decreased venous return. Blood flow to the lungs during CPR is only about 25% to 33% normal; patient requires less ventilation to provide oxygen and remove carbon dioxide. Longer breaths reduce the amount of blood that refills the heart, reducing blood flow generated by compressions. Delivery of large, forceful breaths may cause gastric inflation and distension (AHA, 2015b).
12. If you are unable to ventilate or the chest does not rise during ventilation, reposition the patient's head and reattempt to ventilate. If still unable to ventilate, resume CPR. Each subsequent time the airway is opened to administer breaths, look for an object. If an object is visible in the mouth, remove it. If no object is visible, continue with CPR.	Inability to ventilate indicates that the airway may be obstructed. Repositioning maneuvers may be sufficient to open the airway and promote spontaneous respirations. It is critical to minimize interruptions in chest compressions, to maintain circulatory perfusion.
13. After about 2 minutes (until prompted by AED or about 5 complete cycles of CPR), assess the patient's rhythm on the defibrillator. Defibrillate as indicated (see Skill 16-2 or Skill 16-3). If no pulse, continue CPR.	Evaluates cardiac function and the need for continuation of CPR.
14. Rescue breathing: If the patient has a pulse but remains without spontaneous breathing, continue with rescue breathing, without chest compressions. Administer rescue breathing at a rate of 1 breath every 5 to 6 seconds, for a rate of 10 to 12 breaths/min. If situation involves a possible opioid overdose, administer naloxone as per protocol. Check pulse about every 2 minutes. If no pulse, begin CPR (Step 5).	Rescue breathing maintains adequate oxygenation. For patients with suspected opioid overdose who are unresponsive with no normal breathing but have a pulse, administration of naloxone is indicated to reverse the opioid effects (AHA, 2015b).
15. If spontaneous breathing resumes, place the patient in the recovery position (Figure 5).	Prevents obstruction of airway.

FIGURE 5. Recovery position. (*Photo by B. Proud.*)

16. Otherwise, continue CPR until advanced care providers take over, the patient starts to move, you are too exhausted to continue, or an advanced health care provider discontinues CPR.	Once started, CPR must continue until one of these conditions is met. In an acute care setting, help should arrive within a few minutes.
17. Remove gloves, if used. Perform hand hygiene.	Proper removal of PPE reduces the risk for infection transmission and contamination of other items. Hand hygiene prevents transmission of microorganisms.

EVALUATION

The expected outcome has been achieved when CPR has been performed effectively without adverse effect to the patient; the patient regained a pulse and respirations; the patient's heart and lungs maintained adequate function to sustain life; ACLS was initiated; and the patient did not experience serious injury.

DOCUMENTATION

Guidelines

Document the time the patient was discovered unresponsive and CPR was initiated. Continued intervention, such as by the code team, is typically documented on a code form, which identifies the actions and drugs provided during the code. Provide a summary of these events in the patient's health record.

Sample Documentation

> <u>07/06/20</u> 2230 Called to patient's room by wife. Patient noted to be without evidence of respirations or circulation. Emergency response system activated, CPR initiated. See code sheet.
>
> —B. Clapp, RN

UNEXPECTED SITUATIONS AND ASSOCIATED INTERVENTIONS

- *When performing chest compression, there is an audible crack:* Be aware that this sound most commonly indicates cracking of the ribs. Recheck hand position. Then continue compressions.
- *You find a patient lying on the floor:* Determine the patient's level of responsiveness. If the patient is unresponsive, quickly clear an area, call for assistance and AED, and begin CPR as indicated.

SPECIAL CONSIDERATIONS

General Considerations

- **Every effort should be taken to minimize interruptions in chest compressions. Causes for not providing compressions may include prolonged pulse checks, taking too long to give breaths, moving the patient, and using the AED. Try to limit interruptions to less than 10 seconds (AHA, 2015b).**
- Perform CPR in the same manner if the patient is obese. Techniques may need to be adjusted in the presence of morbid obesity, due to the physical attributes of individual patients (AHA, 2015b).
- Perform CPR for pregnant patients using the same guidelines, with a few additional measures. Relief of aortocaval compression must be maintained continuously during resuscitative efforts (Jeejeebhoy et al., 2015, p. 5). If the fundus is at or above the level of the umbilicus, manual left uterine displacement (LUD) in the supine position should be performed to reduce aortic and vena cava compression and optimize the quality of compressions (AHA, 2015b). Manual LUD can be performed from the left of the patient, where the uterus is cupped and lifted up and leftward off the maternal vessels or from the right of the patient, where the uterus is pushed upward and leftward off the maternal vessels (Jeejeebhoy et al., 2015, p. 6). The same currently recommended protocol for chest compressions and defibrillation should be used in the pregnant patient as in the nonpregnant patient (Jeejeebhoy et al.). During cardiac arrest, if the pregnant woman with a fundus height at or above the umbilicus has not achieved "return to spontaneous circulation" with usual resuscitation measures, anticipate emergency cesarean delivery within 4 to 5 minutes (Jeejeebhoy et al., p. 6).
- If it is not possible to seal the patient's mouth completely for reasons such as oral trauma, perform mouth-to-nose breathing. If the patient has a tracheostomy, provide ventilation through the tracheostomy instead of the mouth.
- The AHA provides guidelines related to emergency interventions outside of health care facilities. Learning conventional CPR is recommended and trained lay rescuers should provide rescue breaths in addition to chest compressions (AHA, 2015b). However, when a teen or adult suddenly collapses, untrained lay rescuers should call 911 (to activate the emergency response system), and push hard and fast in the center of the victim's chest. Compression-only CPR should continue until the arrival of an AED or rescuers with additional training (AHA, 2015a). Studies of real emergencies that have occurred in homes, at work, or in public locations, show that these two steps, called Hands-Only CPR, can be as effective as conventional CPR. Providing Hands-Only CPR to a teen or adult who has collapsed from a sudden cardiac arrest can double or triple that person's chance of survival (AHA, 2016a).

(continued)

Skill 16-1 ▶ Performing Cardiopulmonary Resuscitation *(continued)*

- Be familiar with facility guidelines and/or standards of care related to family presence during resuscitation (FPDR), and advocate for the presence of a family facilitator and support for family needs. The presence of people who are relatives or significant others with whom the patient shares an established relationship during resuscitation or invasive procedures is controversial. Evidence in the literature suggests multiple benefits (American Association of Critical-Care Nurses [AACN], 2015; Emergency Nurses Association [ENA], 2009; McAlvin & Carew-Lyons, 2014; Pankop, Chang, Thorlton, & Spitzer, 2013). The AACN and the ENA recommend family members of all patients undergoing resuscitation and invasive procedures should be given the option of presence at the bedside, as well as recommending the development of related policies or standards of practice in all patient care areas (AACN, ENA). The AHA supports offering family members the opportunity to be present during resuscitation, assuming the patient has not indicated this is undesirable (AHA, 2015b). In addition, current guidelines from the AHA indicate resuscitation team members should be sensitive to the presence of family members, assign a team member to remain with the patient, answer questions, clarify information, and offer comfort (AHA, 2015b; Hassankhani, Zamanzadeh, Rahmani, Haririan, & Porter, 2017).

Infant and Child Considerations

- Once a child reaches puberty (breast development on the female; underarm hair on the male), use adult CPR guidelines for resuscitation (AHA, 2015b).
- As soon as it is determined that an infant or child is unresponsive and not breathing (or only gasping), shout for help to activate the emergency response system. Health care providers may take up to 10 seconds to attempt to feel for a pulse (brachial in an infant and carotid or femoral in a child). If within 10 seconds a pulse is not detected or not detected for certain, begin chest compressions. The only difference in chest compressions is for infants. A lone health care provider should use the two-finger compression technique for infants. The two-thumb–encircling hands technique is recommended when CPR is provided by two rescuers. If it is not possible to encircle the victim's chest, compress the chest with the two fingers (AHA, 2015b).
- Perform the head tilt–chin lift and give 2 breaths after 30 compressions (15 compressions if two rescuers) to deliver 8 to 10 breaths/min (AHA, 2015b).
- Children with sudden witnessed collapse are likely to have ventricular fibrillation or pulseless VT and need immediate CPR and rapid defibrillation.
- Children with unwitnessed collapse: Give 2 minutes of CPR, then leave the victim to activate the emergency response system and get the AED. Return and resume CPR; use the AED as soon as it is available (AHA, 2015a).
- Many AEDs are equipped to decrease (attenuate) the delivered energy to make them suitable for infants and children <8 years of age; an AED with a pediatric attenuator is preferred for infants and children (AHA, 2015b).

Older Adult Considerations

- Nurses can help promote informed decision making about CPR to older adults and their families. Educate, support, and advocate for patients as they face this critical choice. Provide evidence-based information, supportive listening, and a willingness to respect their choices (Anderson et al., 2016).

EVIDENCE FOR PRACTICE ▶

CARDIOPULMONARY RESUSCITATION AND EMERGENCY CARDIAC CARE

The AHA provides guidelines for cardiopulmonary resuscitation and emergency cardiac care and has incorporated these guidelines into the Basic Life Support and Advanced Life Support education for health care providers who respond to cardiovascular and respiratory emergencies.

- American Heart Association (AHA). (2015b). *2015 American Heart Association Guidelines for CPR & ECC.* Retrieved https://eccguidelines.heart.org/index.php/circulation/cpr-ecc-guidelines-2
- American Heart Association (AHA). (2015). *Basic life support (BLS) Provider manual.* Dallas, TX: Author.
- American Heart Association (AHA). (2015). *ACLS for experienced providers. Manual and resource text.* Dallas, TX: Author.

Refer to thePoint° for additional research on related nursing topics.

EVIDENCE FOR PRACTICE ▶

CARDIOPULMONARY RESUSCITATION AND FAMILY PRESENCE

The option for FPDR or invasive procedures is recommended by multiple professional organizations, but remains controversial among nurses (Powers, 2017). What educational interventions are available to improve nurses' support for FPDR?

Related Research

Powers, K. A. (2017). Educational interventions to improve support for family presence during resuscitation. A systematic review of the literature. *Dimensions of Critical Care Nursing, 36*(2), 125–138.

This systematic literature review examined research evidence regarding the use of education on nurses' and providers' support for FPDR. Quantitative studies included for review focused on the testing of the effect of education on nurses' and/or health care providers' support for FPDR and family presence during invasive procedures or trauma resuscitation. Articles involving FPDR education for nurses and health care providers from all settings and patient populations of care were included. A total of 16 articles met the identified eligibility criteria and included numerous educational approaches: classroom interventions, simulation interventions, mixed classroom and simulation interventions, and online interventions. Level of evidence was assigned using the Johns Hopkins Evidence Level and Quality Guide. All included studies provided level II evidence on FPDR educational interventions. Findings from 13 of the 16 studies demonstrated FPDR education had a positive effect on multiple factors related to FPDR: more favorable view of the risks and benefits of FPDR; increased comfort for working with families; improved self-confidence for implementing FPDR; improved support for giving family the choice for FPDR; increased support for FPDR; and increased intent to offer FPDR as an option. The authors concluded that these positive results suggest educational interventions are effective in improving support for FPDR.

Relevance for Nursing Practice

Nurses are important patient advocates. Evidence supports the development, implementation, and evaluation of family presence protocols to ensure that patient- and family-centered care is provided. Nurses should be active participants in the development of educational interventions to address options for FPDR. Nurse educators should consider implementing educational interventions to improve nurses' support for FPDR and prepare them to implement it in clinical practice.

Refer to thePoint® for additional research on related nursing topics.

Skill 16-2 ▶ Performing Emergency Automated External Defibrillation

Rapid defibrillation for shockable rhythms (ventricular fibrillation [VF] and pulseless ventricular tachycardia [VT]) is a critical part of Basic Life Support and administration of cardiopulmonary resuscitation (CPR) (see Skill 16-1) (AHA, 2015b). Early defibrillation is critical to increase patient survival (AHA, 2015b). Electrical therapy can be administered by defibrillation, **cardioversion**, or a pacemaker (see Fundamentals Review 16-1 at the beginning of the chapter).

Defibrillation delivers large amounts of electric current to a patient over brief periods of time. It is the standard treatment for VF and is also used to treat pulseless VT. The goal is to depolarize the irregularly beating heart temporarily and allow more coordinated contractile activity to resume. It does so by completely depolarizing the myocardium, producing a momentary asystole. This provides an opportunity for the natural pacemaker centers of the heart to resume normal activity.

(*continued*)

Skill 16-2 ▶ Performing Emergency Automated External Defibrillation *(continued)*

The automated external defibrillator (AED) is a portable external defibrillator that automatically detects and interprets the heart's rhythm and informs the operator if a shock is indicated (Figure 1). AEDs are appropriate for use in situations where the patient is unresponsive, not breathing, and has no pulse (AHA, 2015a). The defibrillator responds to the patient information by advising "shock" or "no shock." Fully automatic models automatically perform rhythm analysis and shock, if indicated. These are usually found in out-of-hospital settings. Semiautomatic models require the operator to press an "Analyze" button to initiate rhythm analysis and then press a "Shock" button to deliver the shock, if indicated. Semiautomatic models are usually found in acute care and other health care settings. An AED will not deliver a shock unless the electrode pads are correctly attached and a shockable rhythm is detected. Some AEDs have motion-detection devices that ensure the defibrillator will not discharge if there is motion, such as motion from personnel in contact with the patient. The strength of the charge is preset. Once the pads are in place and the device is turned on, follow the prompts given by the device. The following guidelines are based on the AHA (2015a) guidelines. AHA guidelines state that these recommendations may be modified for the in-hospital setting, where continuous electrocardiographic or hemodynamic monitoring may be in place. CPR should be immediately initiated (see Skill 16-1) and the AED/defibrillator should be used as soon as it is available.

Current recommendations call for the application of the AED as soon as it is available, allowing for analysis of cardiac status and delivery of an initial shock, if indicated, for adults and children. After an initial shock, resume CPR immediately for about 2 minutes (until prompted by AED to allow rhythm check). Provide sets of one shock alternating with 2 minutes of CPR until the AED indicates a "no shock indicated" message, the victim starts to move, or until advanced cardiac life support (ACLS) is available (AHA, 2015a).

In the health care setting, it is imperative that personnel be aware of the patient's stated instructions regarding a wish not to be resuscitated. This should be clearly expressed and documented in the patient's health record.

FIGURE 1. Automated external defibrillator (AED).

DELEGATION CONSIDERATIONS	The initiation and provision of CPR, including use of an AED, is appropriate for all health care providers.
EQUIPMENT	• AED (some models have the pads, cables, and AED preconnected) • Self-adhesive, pregelled electrode monitor-defibrillator pads (6) • Cables to connect the pads and AED • Razor • Towel
ASSESSMENT	Assess the patient for unresponsiveness, effective breathing, and signs of circulation. Assess the patient's vital parameters and determine the patient's level of responsiveness. Check for partial or complete airway obstruction. Assess for the absence or ineffectiveness of respirations. Assess

Box 16-1	Special Situations Related to Automated External Defibrillation (AED)

- **_The patient is in water._** Water is a good conductor of electricity. Do not use an AED in water. Defibrillation administered to a patient in water could result in shocking the AED operator and bystanders. Another possible effect is that water on the patient's skin will provide a direct path for the electrical current from one electrode to the other. The arcing of the electrical current between the electrodes bypasses the heart, resulting in the delivery of inadequate current to the heart. If the patient is in water, pull the patient out of the water. If water is covering the patient's chest, quickly dry the chest before attaching the AED pads. If the patient is lying on snow or in a small puddle, the AED may be used (AHA, 2015b).
- **_The patient has an implanted pacemaker or defibrillator._** If possible, avoid placing the AED pad directly over the implanted device, which will appear as a hard lump (half the size of a deck of cards) beneath the skin of the upper chest or abdomen with an overlying scar (AHA, 2016c, p. 39). If an AED electrode pad is placed directly over an implanted device, the device may block delivery of the shock to the heart.
- **_A transdermal medication patch or other object is located on the patient's skin where the electrode pads are to be placed._** Do not place AED pads directly on top of a medication patch. The patch may block the delivery of energy to the heart and cause small burns to the skin. If it will not delay shock delivery, remove the patch and wipe the area clean before attaching the electrode pads (AHA, 2016c, p. 39).

for the absence of signs of circulation and pulses. An AED should be used only when a patient is unresponsive, not breathing, or not breathing normally, and without signs of circulation (pulseless, lack of effective respirations, coughing, movement). Determine the age of the patient; some AED systems are designed to deliver both adult and child shock doses. Choose correct electrode pad for size/age of patient. If available, use child pads or a child system for children less than 8 years of age.

Determine whether special situations exist that require additional actions before the AED is used or that contraindicate its use (refer to Box 16-1 for details of these situations and appropriate actions).

NURSING DIAGNOSIS	Determine the related factors for the nursing diagnoses based on the patient's current status. Appropriate nursing diagnoses may include: • Decreased cardiac output • Impaired spontaneous ventilation • Risk for ineffective cerebral tissue perfusion
OUTCOME IDENTIFICATION AND PLANNING	The expected outcome to achieve when performing AED is that it is performed correctly without adverse effect to the patient, and the patient regains signs of circulation, with organized electrical rhythm and pulse. Additional outcomes include the following: the patient regains respirations; the patient's heart and lungs maintain adequate function to sustain life; the patient does not experience serious injury; and ACLS is initiated, as indicated.

IMPLEMENTATION

ACTION	RATIONALE
1. Verify scene safety. Assess responsiveness. Look for no breathing or only gasping. Call for help, pull call bell, and call the facility emergency response number. Call for emergency equipment and the AED or defibrillator, if available. Put on gloves, if available. Begin CPR (see Skill 16-1).	Assessing responsiveness prevents starting CPR on a conscious patient. Activating the emergency response system initiates a rapid response. Gloves prevent contact with blood and body fluids. Initiating CPR preserves heart and brain function while awaiting defibrillation.
2. **Provide defibrillation at the earliest possible moment, as soon as AED becomes available.**	The interval from collapse to defibrillation is one of the most important determinants of survival from sudden cardiac arrest with VF or pulseless VT (AHA, 2015b).

Skill 16-2

Performing Emergency Automated External Defibrillation *(continued)*

3. Prepare the AED. Power on the AED. Push the power button. Some devices will turn on automatically when the lid or case is opened.

4. Attach AED cables to the adhesive electrode pads (may be preconnected).

5. Stop chest compressions. Peel away the covering from the electrode pads to expose the adhesive surface. Attach the electrode pads to the patient's chest. Place one pad on the upper right sternal border, directly below the clavicle. Place the second pad lateral to the left nipple, with the top margin of the pad a few inches below the axilla (anterolateral positioning) (Figure 2). Alternately, if two or more rescuers are present, one rescuer should continue chest compressions while another rescuer attaches the AED pads. Attach the AED connecting cables to the AED box, if not preconnected.

6. Once the pads are in place and the device is turned on, follow the prompts given by the device. Clear the patient and analyze the rhythm. Ensure no one is touching the patient. Loudly state a "Clear the patient" message. Press "Analyze" button to initiate analysis, if necessary. Some devices automatically begin analysis when the pads are attached. Avoid all movement affecting the patient during analysis.

7. If a shockable rhythm is present, the device will announce that a shock is indicated and begin charging. Once the AED is charged, a message will be delivered to shock the patient.

8. **Before pressing the "Shock" button, loudly state a "Clear the patient" message. Visually check that no one is in contact with the patient or the bed (Figure 3). Press the "Shock" button. If the AED is fully automatic, a shock will be delivered automatically.**

Proper setup ensures proper functioning.

Proper setup ensures proper functioning.

Proper setup ensures proper functioning. The most common placement of the electrode pads is the anterior-lateral position (Morton & Fontaine, 2018). This placement puts the heart directly in the current pathway (Morton & Fontaine, 2018). Application by second rescuer minimizes interruptions in chest compressions.

Movement and electrical impulses cause artifact during analysis. Avoidance of artifact ensures accurate rhythm analysis. Avoidance of contact with the patient avoids accidental shock to personnel.

Shock message is delivered through a written or visual message on the AED screen, an auditory alarm, or a voice-synthesized statement.

Ensuring a clear patient avoids accidental shocking of personnel.

FIGURE 2. AED electrode pad placement.

FIGURE 3. Clearing the patient.

ACTION	RATIONALE
9. Immediately resume CPR, beginning with chest compressions. After about 2 minutes (until prompted by AED or about five complete cycles of CPR), allow the AED to analyze the heart rhythm. If a shock is not advised, resume CPR, beginning with chest compressions. Do not recheck to see if there is a pulse. Follow the AED voice prompts.	Resuming CPR provides optimal treatment. CPR preserves heart and neurologic function (based on AHA [2015a] recommended guidelines). Even when a shock eliminates the **dysrhythmia**, it may take several minutes for a heart rhythm to establish and even longer to achieve perfusion. Chest compressions can provide coronary and cerebral perfusion during this period. Some AEDs in the community for use by untrained lay rescuers are automatically programmed to cycle through three analysis/shock cycles in one set. This would necessitate turning off the AED after the first shock and turning it back on for future analysis and defibrillation. Be familiar with the type of AED available for use.
10. Continue CPR until advanced care providers take over, the patient starts to move, you are too exhausted to continue, or an advanced health care provider discontinues CPR.	Once started, CPR must continue until one of these conditions is met. In an acute care setting, help should arrive within a few minutes.
11. Remove gloves, if used. Perform hand hygiene.	Proper removal of PPE reduces the risk for infection transmission and contamination of other items. Hand hygiene prevents transmission of microorganisms.

EVALUATION

The expected outcomes have been achieved when defibrillation has been performed correctly without adverse effect to the patient; the patient regained signs of circulation, with organized electrical rhythm and pulse; the patient regained respirations; the patient's heart and lungs maintained adequate function to sustain life; the patient did not experience serious injury; and ACLS was initiated, as indicated.

DOCUMENTATION

Guidelines

Document the time you discovered the patient unresponsive and started CPR. Document the time(s) AED shocks are initiated. Continued intervention, such as by the code team, is typically documented on a code form, which identifies the actions and drugs provided during the code. Provide a summary of these events in the patient's health record.

Sample Documentation

07/06/20 2230 Called to patient's room by wife. Patient noted to be without evidence of respirations or circulation. Emergency response system activated, CPR initiated. AED applied at 2232. See code sheet.

—B. Clapp, RN

UNEXPECTED SITUATIONS AND ASSOCIATED INTERVENTIONS

- *You find a patient lying on the floor:* Determine the patient's level of responsiveness. If the patient is unresponsive, quickly clear an area, call for assistance and AED, and begin CPR.
- *A "Check pads" or "Check electrodes" message appears on the AED:* The electrode pads are not securely attached to the chest or the cables are not securely fastened. Check that the pads are firmly and evenly adhered to the patient's skin. Verify connections between the cables and the AED and the cables and electrode pads. Check that the patient is not wet or diaphoretic, or has excessive chest hair. See actions below for appropriate interventions in these situations.
- *The patient has a hairy chest:* The adhesive electrode pads may stick to the chest hair instead of to the skin, preventing adequate contact with the skin. Press firmly on the current pads to attempt to provide sufficient adhesion. If unsuccessful, briskly remove the current pads to remove a good portion of the chest hair. If a significant amount of hair remains, shave the area with the razor in the AED case. Apply a second set of electrode pads over the same sites. Continue with the procedure.
- *The patient is noticeably diaphoretic or the skin is wet:* The electrode pads will not attach firmly to wet or diaphoretic skin. Dry the chest with a cloth or towel before attaching the electrode pads.

Skill 16-2   Performing Emergency Automated External Defibrillation   *(continued)*

SPECIAL CONSIDERATIONS

General Considerations

- Every effort should be taken to minimize interruptions in chest compressions. Causes for not providing compressions may include prolonged pulse checks, taking too long to give breaths, moving the patient, and using the AED. Try to limit interruptions to less than 10 seconds to maximize effectiveness (AHA, 2015b).
- Most defibrillators use multifunctional electrode patches to both monitor and administer electrical therapy. Although paddles are still available, they are seldom used as positioning requires additional "hands off" time, which depletes myocardial oxygen and energy stores (Morton & Fontaine, 2018, p. 330).
- Nurses should know the distinction between automatic and automated AEDs. Automatic AECs charge and independently deliver a shock when indicated. Automated AEDs require action on the part of the user to deliver the shock. Familiarity with the device is important to its safe and effective use (Morton & Fontaine, 2018, p. 331).
- Appropriate maintenance of the AED is critical for proper operation. Check the AED for any visible signs of damage. Check the "ready for use" indicator on the AED daily. Perform maintenance according to the manufacturer's recommendations and facility policy.

Infant and Child Considerations

- Use the largest self-adhering electrodes that will fit on the infant's or child's chest without touching; when possible, leave about 3 cm between the electrodes (AHA, 2015b).
- "Adult size" self-adhering electrodes should be used for children >10 kg (> approximately 1 year of age) (AHA, 2015b).
- "Infant size" self-adhering electrodes should be used for infants <10 kg (AHA, 2015b).

Older Adult Considerations

- Nurses can help promote informed decision making about CPR to older adults and their families. Educate, support, and advocate for patients as they face this critical choice. Provide evidence-based information, supportive listening, and a willingness to respect their choices (Anderson et al., 2016).

EVIDENCE FOR PRACTICE ▶

CARDIOPULMONARY RESUSCITATION AND EMERGENCY CARDIAC CARE

The AHA provides guidelines for CPR and emergency cardiac care and has incorporated these guidelines into the Basic Life Support and Advanced Life Support education for health care providers who respond to cardiovascular and respiratory emergencies.

Refer to the Evidence for Practice in Skill 16-1 for details and refer to thePoint® for additional research on related nursing topics.

Skill 16-3   Performing Emergency Manual External Defibrillation (Asynchronous)

Rapid defibrillation for shockable rhythms (ventricular fibrillation [VF] and pulseless ventricular tachycardia [VT]) is a critical part of Basic Life Support and administration of cardiopulmonary resuscitation (CPR) (see Skill 16-1) (AHA, 2015b). Early defibrillation is critical to increase patient survival (AHA, 2015b). Electrical therapy can be administered by defibrillation, cardioversion, or a pacemaker (see Fundamentals Review 16-1 at the beginning of the chapter).

(continued)

Defibrillation delivers large amounts of electric current to a patient over brief periods of time. It is the standard treatment for VF and is also used to treat VT, in which the patient has no pulse. The goal is temporarily to depolarize the irregularly beating heart and allow more coordinated contractile activity to resume. It does so by completely depolarizing the myocardium, producing a momentary asystole. This provides an opportunity for the natural pacemaker centers of the heart to resume normal activity. The self-adhering electrode pads delivering the current are placed on the patient's chest; during cardiac surgery, electrode paddles are placed directly on the myocardium.

Manual defibrillation is accomplished with an external defibrillator (Figure 1) and depends on the operator for analysis of rhythm, charging, proper application of the self-adhering electrode pads to the patient's thorax, and delivery of the shock. It requires the user to have immediate and accurate dysrhythmia recognition skills. The following guidelines are based on the AHA (2015b) guidelines.

In the health care setting, it is imperative that personnel be aware of the patient's stated instructions regarding a wish not to be resuscitated. This should be clearly expressed and documented in the patient's health record.

FIGURE 1. External defibrillator. (Image from https://www.usa.philips.com/healthcare/product/HCM3535A/heartstart-mrx#galleryTab=PI Courtesy of Royal Philips ©.)

DELEGATION CONSIDERATIONS	The initiation and provision of manual external defibrillation should be performed by health care providers who are certified in advanced cardiac life support (ACLS) measures.
EQUIPMENT	• Defibrillator (monophasic or biphasic) • External self-adhering electrode pads (or internal paddles sterilized for cardiac surgery) • Electrocardiogram (ECG) monitor with recorder, depending on equipment available (usually part of the defibrillator) • Oxygen therapy equipment • Bag-valve-mask • Airway equipment • Emergency pacing equipment • Emergency cardiac medications
ASSESSMENT	Assess the patient for unresponsiveness, effective breathing, and signs of circulation. Assess the patient's vital parameters and determine the patient's level of responsiveness. Check for partial or complete airway obstruction. Assess for the absence or ineffectiveness of respirations. Assess for the absence of signs of circulation and pulses. Call for help and perform CPR until the defibrillator and other emergency equipment arrive.

Skill 16-3 ▶ Performing Emergency Manual External Defibrillation (Asynchronous) *(continued)*

NURSING DIAGNOSIS	Determine the related factors for the nursing diagnoses based on the patient's current status. Appropriate nursing diagnoses may include: • Decreased cardiac output • Impaired spontaneous ventilation • Risk for injury
OUTCOME IDENTIFICATION AND PLANNING	The expected outcome to achieve when performing manual external defibrillation is that it is performed correctly without adverse effect to the patient, and the patient regains signs of circulation with organized electrical rhythm and pulse. Additional outcomes may include the following: the patient regains respirations; the patient's heart and lungs maintain adequate function to sustain life; the patient does not experience serious injury; and ACLS is initiated, as indicated.

IMPLEMENTATION

ACTION	RATIONALE
1. Verify scene safety. Look for no breathing or only gasping. Call for help, pull call bell, and call the facility emergency response number. Call for emergency equipment and the automated external defibrillator (AED) or defibrillator, if available. Put on gloves, if available. Begin CPR, as indicated (see Skill 16-1).	Assessing responsiveness prevents starting CPR on a conscious victim. Activating the emergency response system initiates a rapid response. Gloves prevent contact with blood and body fluids. Initiating CPR preserves heart and brain function while awaiting defibrillation.
2. **Provide defibrillation at the earliest possible moment, as soon as AED becomes available.**	The interval from collapse to defibrillation is one of the most important determinants of survival from sudden cardiac arrest with VF or pulseless VT (AHA, 2015b).
3. Turn on the defibrillator.	Charging prepares for defibrillation.
4. Expose the patient's chest, and apply electrode pads to the chest. Place one pad on the upper right sternal border, directly below the clavicle. Place the second pad lateral to the left nipple, with the top margin of the pad a few inches below the axilla (anterolateral positioning) (Figure 2). Alternately, if two or more rescuers are present, one rescuer should continue chest compressions while another rescuer attaches the electrode pads. Assess the cardiac rhythm.	Proper setup ensures proper functioning. This placement puts the heart directly in the current pathway (Morton & Fontaine, 2018). Application by second rescuer minimizes interruptions in chest compressions. Connecting the monitor leads to the patient allows for assessment of the cardiac rhythm and determination of the need for defibrillation.

FIGURE 2. Anterolateral placement of self-adhering electrode pads.

ACTION	RATIONALE
5. Set the energy level for 360 J (joules) when using a mono-phasic defibrillator. Use clinically appropriate energy levels for biphasic defibrillators, beginning with 120 to 200 J, depending on device (Morton & Fontaine, 2018).	Proper setup ensures proper functioning and appropriate intervention.
6. If the patient remains in VF or pulseless VT, **loudly state a "Clear the patient" message. Visually check that no one is in contact with the patient or the bed.** Press the button to deliver the shock.	Standing clear of the bed and patient avoids accidental shock-ing of personnel. Pressing the shock button discharges the electric current for defibrillation.
7. After the shock, immediately resume CPR, beginning with chest compressions. After five cycles (about 2 minutes), reassess the cardiac rhythm. Continue until advanced care providers take over, the patient starts to move, you are too exhausted to continue, or an advanced health care provider discontinues CPR.	Even when a shock eliminates the dysrhythmia, it may take several minutes for a heart rhythm to establish and even lon-ger to achieve perfusion. Once started, CPR must continue until one of these conditions is met. In an acute care setting, help should arrive within a few minutes.
8. If necessary, prepare to defibrillate subsequent shocks per ACLS protocol.	Additional shocking may be needed to stimulate the heart.
9. Announce that you are preparing to defibrillate and follow the procedure described above.	Additional shocking may be needed to stimulate the heart.
10. If defibrillation restores a normal rhythm:	
a. Check for signs of circulation; check the central and peripheral pulses, and obtain a blood pressure reading, heart rate, and respiratory rate.	The patient will need continuous monitoring to prevent further problems. Continuous monitoring helps provide for early detection and prompt intervention should additional prob-lems arise.
b. If signs of circulation are present, check breathing. If breathing is inadequate, assist breathing. Administer rescue breathing at a rate of 1 breath every 5 to 6 seconds, for a rate of 10 to 12 breaths/min (refer to Skill 16-1).	Rescue breathing maintains adequate oxygenation.
c. If breathing is adequate, place the patient in the recovery position. Continue to assess the patient.	
d. Assess the patient's level of consciousness, cardiac rhythm, blood pressure, breath sounds, skin color, and temperature.	Reassessment determines the need for continued intervention. Provides optimal treatment.
e. Obtain baseline ABG levels (Skill 18-11) and a 12-lead ECG (Skill 16-4), if ordered.	These assessments provide data to help inform continued inter-vention and optimal treatment.
f. Provide supplemental oxygen, ventilation, and medica-tions, as needed.	Provides optimal treatment.
g. Anticipate the possible use of targeted temperature man-agement, including therapeutic hypothermia.	Lowering of a patient's core temperature after cardiac arrest may improve survival and functional recovery (Avery, O'Brien, Pierce, & Gazarian, 2015; Morton & Fontaine, 2018).
11. Keep electrode pads on in case of recurrent VT or VF.	Keeping pads in place provides preparation for future use.
12. Remove gloves, if used. Perform hand hygiene.	Proper removal of PPE reduces the risk for infection transmis-sion and contamination of other items. Hand hygiene pre-vents transmission of microorganisms.
13. Prepare the defibrillator for immediate reuse.	A patient may remain unstable and could require further intervention.

(continued)

Skill 16-3 ▶ Performing Emergency Manual External Defibrillation (Asynchronous)   *(continued)*

EVALUATION

The expected outcomes have been achieved when defibrillation has been performed correctly without adverse effect to the patient; the patient regained signs of circulation, with organized electrical rhythm and pulse; the patient regained respirations; the patient's heart and lungs maintained adequate function to sustain life; the patient did not experience serious injury; and ACLS was initiated, as indicated.

DOCUMENTATION

Guidelines

Document the time you discovered the patient unresponsive and started CPR. Document the procedure, including the patient's ECG rhythms both before and after defibrillation; the number of times defibrillation was performed; the voltage used during each attempt; whether a pulse returned; the dosage, route, and time of drug administration; whether CPR was used; how the airway was maintained; and the patient's outcome. Continued intervention, such as by the code team, is typically documented on a code form, which identifies the actions and drugs provided during the code. Provide a summary of these events in the patient's health record.

Sample Documentation

> <u>07/06/20</u> 2230 Called to patient's room by wife. Patient noted to be without evidence of respirations or circulation. Emergency response system activated, CPR initiated. Manual defibrillation initiated at 2232. See code sheet.
>
> —B. Clapp, RN

UNEXPECTED SITUATIONS AND ASSOCIATED INTERVENTIONS

- *The defibrillator fails to fire:* Check that the power is turned on. If the defibrillator is not plugged in, check if the battery is low. Check that it is fully charged.
- *The patient has a hairy chest:* The adhesive electrode pads may stick to the chest hair instead of to the skin, preventing adequate contact with the skin. Press firmly on the current pads to attempt to provide sufficient adhesion. If unsuccessful, briskly remove the current pads to remove a good portion of the chest hair. If a significant amount of hair remains, shave the area. Apply a second set of electrode pads over the same sites. Continue with the procedure.
- *The patient is noticeably diaphoretic or the skin is wet:* The electrode pads will not attach firmly to wet or diaphoretic skin. Dry the chest with a cloth or towel before attaching the electrode pads.

SPECIAL CONSIDERATIONS

General Considerations

- **Every effort should be taken to minimize interruptions in chest compressions. Causes for not providing compressions may include prolonged pulse checks, taking too long to give breaths, moving the patient, and using the defibrillator. Try to limit interruptions to less than 10 seconds to maximize effectiveness (AHA, 2015b).**
- Alternative placement of self-adhering electrode pads: Anterior–posterior placement. Place one pad anteriorly at the precordium to the left of the lower sternal border and the other pad posteriorly under the patient's body beneath the heart and immediately below the scapula (Figure 3).

FIGURE 3. Anteroposterior placement of self-adhering electrode pads.

- Most defibrillators use multifunctional electrode patches to both monitor and administer electrical therapy. Although paddles are still available, they are seldom used as positioning requires additional "hands off" time, which depletes myocardial oxygen and energy stores (Morton & Fontaine, 2018, p. 330).
- Defibrillation can cause accidental electric shock to those providing care.
- Defibrillators vary from one manufacturer to another, so familiarize yourself with your facility's equipment. Perform maintenance according to the manufacturer's recommendations and facility policy.

Infant and Child Considerations

- Use the largest self-adhering electrodes that will fit on the infant's or child's chest without touching; when possible, leave about 3 cm between the electrodes (AHA, 2015b).
- "Adult size" self-adhering electrodes should be used for children >10 kg (> approximately 1 year of age) (AHA, 2015b).
- "Infant size" self-adhering electrodes should be used for infants <10 kg (AHA, 2015b).

Older Adult Considerations

- Nurses can help promote informed decision making about CPR to older adults and their families. Educate, support, and advocate for patients as they face this critical choice. Provide evidence-based information, supportive listening, and a willingness to respect their choices (Anderson et al., 2016).

EVIDENCE FOR PRACTICE ▶

CARDIOPULMONARY RESUSCITATION AND EMERGENCY CARDIAC CARE
The AHA provides guidelines for CPR and emergency cardiac care and has incorporated these guidelines into the Basic Life Support and Advanced Life Support education for health care providers who respond to cardiovascular and respiratory emergencies.

Refer to the Evidence for Practice in Skill 16-1 for details, and refer to thePoint° for additional research on related nursing topics.

Skill 16-4 ▶ Obtaining an Electrocardiogram

Electrocardiography is one of the most valuable and frequently used diagnostic tools. Electrocardiography measures the heart's electrical activity. Impulses moving through the heart's conduction system create electric currents that can be monitored on the body's surface. Electrodes attached to the skin can detect these electric currents and transmit them to an instrument that produces a record, the **electrocardiogram (ECG)**, of cardiac activity. The data are graphed as waveforms (Figure 1). ECG can be used to identify myocardial ischemia and infarction, rhythm and conduction disturbances, chamber enlargement, electrolyte imbalances, and drug toxicity.

The standard 12-lead ECG uses a series of electrodes placed on the extremities and the chest wall to assess the heart from 12 different viewpoints (leads) by attaching 10 cables with electrodes to the patient's limbs and chest: 4 limb electrodes and 6 chest electrodes (Figure 2). Each lead provides an electrographic snapshot of electrochemical activity of the myocardial cell membrane. The ECG device measures and averages the differences between the electrical potential of the electrode sites for each lead and graphs them over time, creating the standard ECG complex,

FIGURE 1. Electrocardiogram (waveform) strip.   (*continued*)

Skill 16-4 ▶ Obtaining an Electrocardiogram *(continued)*

called PQRST (Box 16-2). These electrodes provide views of the heart from the frontal plane as well as the horizontal plane. It is essential that connection or placement of the ECG electrodes/leads is accurate to prevent misdiagnosis. The ECG tracing needs to be clear to enable accurate and reliable interpretation (Jevon, 2010).

An ECG is typically accomplished using a multichannel method. All electrodes are attached to the patient at once and the machine prints a simultaneous view of all leads. It is important to reassure the patient that the leads just sense and record and do not transmit any electricity. The patient must be able to lie still and refrain from speaking to prevent body movement from creating artifact in the ECG. Variations of standard ECG include exercise ECG (stress ECG) and ambulatory ECG (Holter monitoring).

Interpreting the ECG requires the following actions:

- Determine the rhythm.
- Determine the rate.
- Evaluate the P wave.
- Determine the duration of the PR interval.
- Determine the duration of the QRS complex.
- Evaluate the T wave.
- Determine the duration of the QT interval.
- Evaluate the ST segment.
- Evaluate any other components.

FIGURE 2. 12-lead ECG lead placement. (From Morton, P. G., & Fontaine, D. K. [2018]. *Essentials of critical care nursing. A holistic approach* [11th ed.]. Philadelphia, PA: Wolters Kluwer, with permission.)

Box 16.2 ECG Complex

The ECG complex consists of five waveforms labeled with the letters P, Q, R, S, and T. In addition, sometimes a U wave appears.

- **P wave:** Represents atrial depolarization (conduction of the electrical impulse through the atria); the first component of ECG waveform.
- **PR interval:** Tracks the atrial impulse from the atria through the AV node, from the SA node to the AV node. Measures from the beginning of the P wave to the beginning of the QRS complex. Normal PR is 0.12 to 0.2 seconds.
- **QRS complex:** Follows the PR interval and represents depolarization of the ventricles (the time it takes for the impulse to travel through the bundle branches to the Purkinje fibers) or impulse conduction and contraction of the myocardial cells (ventricular systole). The Q wave appears as the first negative deflection in the QRS complex, the R

wave as the first positive deflection. The S wave appears as the second negative deflection or the first negative deflection after the R wave. Normal QRS is 0.06 to 0.1 seconds.
- **ST segment:** Represents the end of ventricular conduction or depolarization and the beginning of ventricular recovery or repolarization; the J point marks the end of the QRS complex and the beginning of the ST segment.
- **T wave:** Represents ventricular recovery or repolarization.
- **QT interval:** Measures ventricular depolarization and repolarization; varies with the heart rate (i.e., the faster the heart rate, the shorter the QT interval); extends from the beginning of the QRS complex to the end of the T wave. Normal QT is <0.4 seconds, but can vary with heart rate.
- **U wave:** Represents the recovery period of the Purkinje fibers or ventricular conduction fibers; not present on every rhythm strip.

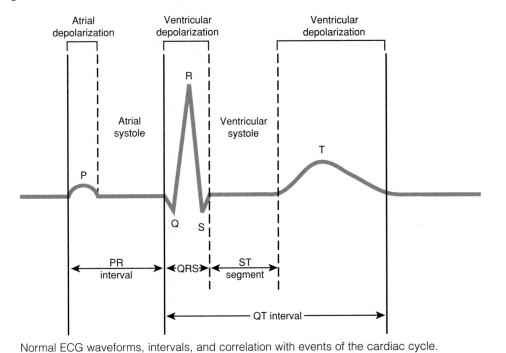

Normal ECG waveforms, intervals, and correlation with events of the cardiac cycle.

DELEGATION CONSIDERATIONS

Obtaining an ECG is not delegated to nursing assistive personnel (NAP) or to unlicensed assistive personnel (UAP); in some facilities, technicians are trained to obtain an ECG. Depending on the state's nurse practice act and the organization's policies and procedures, this procedure may be delegated to licensed practical/vocational nurses (LPN/LVNs). The decision to delegate must be based on careful analysis of the patient's needs and circumstances, as well as the qualifications of the person to whom the task is being delegated. Refer to the Delegation Guidelines in Appendix A.

EQUIPMENT

- ECG machine
- Recording paper
- Disposable pregelled electrodes
- Adhesive remover swabs
- 4 × 4 gauze pads
- Skin cleanser and water, if necessary
- Additional PPE, as indicated
- Bath blanket

(continued)

Skill 16-4 ▶ Obtaining an Electrocardiogram *(continued)*

ASSESSMENT	Review the patient's health record and care plan for information about the patient's need for an ECG. Assess the patient's cardiac status, including heart rate, blood pressure, and auscultation of heart sounds. If the patient is already connected to a cardiac monitor, remove the electrodes to accommodate the precordial leads and minimize electrical interference on the ECG tracing. Keep the patient away from objects that might cause electrical interference, such as equipment, fixtures, and power cords. Inspect the patient's chest for areas of irritation, breakdown, or excessive hair that might interfere with electrode placement.
NURSING DIAGNOSIS	Determine the related factors for the nursing diagnoses based on the patient's current status. Appropriate nursing diagnoses may include: • Decreased cardiac output • Activity intolerance • Acute pain
OUTCOME IDENTIFICATION AND PLANNING	The expected outcome to achieve is that an ECG is obtained without any complications and the patient demonstrates an understanding of the need for and about the ECG.

IMPLEMENTATION

ACTION	**RATIONALE**
1. Verify the order/prescription for an ECG in the patient's health record.	This ensures that the correct intervention is performed on the correct patient.
2. Gather all equipment.	Assembling equipment provides for an organized approach to the task.
3. Perform hand hygiene and put on PPE, if indicated.	Hand hygiene and PPE prevent the spread of microorganisms. PPE is required based on transmission precautions.
4. Identify the patient.	Identifying the patient ensures the right patient receives the intervention and helps prevent errors.
5. Close curtains around the bed and close the door to the room, if possible. As you set up the machine to record a 12-lead ECG, explain the procedure to the patient. Tell the patient that the test records the heart's electrical activity, and it may be repeated at certain intervals. Emphasize that no electrical current will enter his or her body. Tell the patient the test typically takes about 5 minutes. Ask the patient about allergies to adhesive, as appropriate.	This ensures the patient's privacy. Explanation relieves anxiety and facilitates cooperation. Possible allergies may exist related to adhesive on ECG leads.
6. Place the ECG machine close to the patient's bed, and plug the power cord into the wall outlet.	Having equipment available saves time and facilitates accomplishment of the task.
7. If the bed is adjustable, raise it to a comfortable working height, usually elbow height of the caregiver (VHACEOSH, 2016).	Having the bed at the proper height prevents back and muscle strain.
8. Ideally, position the patient supine in the center of the bed with the arms at the sides. Alternately, raise the head of the bed to a semi-Fowler's position, if necessary to promote comfort. Expose the patient's arms and legs, and drape appropriately. Encourage the patient to relax the arms and legs. Ensure the wrists do not touch the waist. Make sure the feet do not touch the bed's footboard.	Proper positioning helps promote patient comfort and will produce a better tracing. The standard and ideal patient positioning is in the supine position; however, if necessary for patient comfort, a recumbent (semi-Fowler's) position can be used. A change in patient position moves the heart, altering the ECG tracing (Garcia, 2015). Document the patient's position so that subsequent tracings are performed with the patient in the same position (Garcia, 2015; Morton & Fontaine, 2018). Proper positioning and relaxation of the arms and legs minimizes muscle tension and trembling and resulting electrical interference.

ACTION	RATIONALE

9. If necessary, prepare the skin for electrode placement. If an area is excessively hairy, clip the hair. **Do not shave hair.** Clean excess oil or other substances from the skin with skin cleanser and water. Use a gauze pad to vigorously rub and dry the skin.

Shaving causes microabrasions on the skin, possibly resulting in portals of entry for microorganisms. Oils and excess hair interfere with electrode contact and function. Rubbing with gauze abrades and dries the skin. Proper skin preparation is essential to reduce artifact in and increase quality of the ECG tracing (Garcia, 2015).

10. Apply the limb electrodes (Figure 3). Peel the contact paper off the self-sticking disposable electrode and apply directly to the prepared site, as recommended by the manufacturer. Connect the limb lead wires to the electrodes. The tip of each lead wire is lettered and color coded for easy identification. The white or RA lead goes to the right arm, just above the wrist bone; the green or RL lead to the right leg, just above the ankle bone; the red or LL lead to the left leg, just above the ankle bone; the black or LA lead to the left arm, just above the wrist bone. Refer to Figure 2 for electrode placement.

Use of recommended standard sites for limb electrodes is essential to obtain accurate recording (Garcia, 2015; Morton & Fontaine, 2018).

FIGURE 3. Applying limb electrode.

11. Expose the patient's chest. Apply the chest electrodes (Figure 4A). Peel the contact paper off the self-sticking, disposable electrode and apply directly to the prepared site, as recommended by the manufacturer. Connect the chest lead wires to the electrodes (Figure 4B). The tip of each

Proper lead placement is necessary for accurate test results (Garcia, 2015; Morton & Fontaine, 2018).

FIGURE 4. A. Applying chest electrode. **B.** Applying chest lead.

(continued)

Skill 16-4 ▸ Obtaining an Electrocardiogram *(continued)*

ACTION	**RATIONALE**

lead wire is lettered and color coded for easy identification. The V_1 to V_6 leads are applied to the chest. Position chest electrodes as follows (refer to Figure 2):

- V_1: (Red) Fourth intercostal space at right sternal border
- V_2: (Yellow) Fourth intercostal space at left sternal border
- V_3: (Green) Exactly midway between V_2 and V_4
- V_4: (Blue) Fifth intercostal space at the left midclavicular line
- V_5: (Orange) Left anterior axillary line, same horizontal plane as V_4 and V_6
- V_6: (Purple) Left midaxillary line, same horizontal plane as V_4 and V_5

12. After the application of all the leads (Figure 5), ensure that the cables are not pulling on the electrodes or lying over each other. Make sure the paper-speed selector is set to the standard 25 mm/sec and that the machine is set to full voltage.

Lack of pulling and tension minimizes electrical artifact and improves quality and accuracy of the ECG. Correct paper speed affects the timing of the ECG with respect to measurement of rate and duration of intervals (Garcia, 2015). The machine will record a normal standardization mark—a square that is the height of 2 large squares or 10 small squares on the recording paper.

13. Enter the appropriate patient identification data into the machine. Depending on facility policy, enter the patient's name, health record number, and age and sex.

This allows for proper identification of the ECG strip. The ECG device requires minimum data input of age and sex to correctly analyze the data (Garcia, 2015).

14. Ask the patient to relax and breathe normally. **Instruct the patient to lie still and not to talk while the ECG is being recorded.**

Lying still and not talking produce a better tracing.

15. Press the AUTO button. Observe the tracing quality (Figure 6). The machine will record all 12 leads automatically, recording 3 consecutive leads simultaneously. Some machines have a display screen so you can preview waveforms before the machine records them on paper. Adjust waveform, if necessary. If any part of the waveform extends beyond the paper when you record the ECG, adjust the normal standardization to half-standardization and repeat. Note this adjustment on the ECG strip, because this will need to be considered in interpreting the results.

Observation of tracing quality allows for adjustments to be made, if necessary. Notation of adjustments ensures accurate interpretation of results.

FIGURE 5. Completed application of 12-lead ECG.

FIGURE 6. Observing tracing quality.

ACTION	RATIONALE
16. When the machine finishes recording the 12-lead ECG (Figure 7), remove the electrodes and clean the patient's skin, if necessary, with adhesive remover for sticky residue.	Removal and cleaning promote patient comfort.

FIGURE 7. Normal 12-lead ECG configuration. (From Diepenbrock, N. [2011]. *Quick reference to critical care* [4th ed.]. Philadelphia, PA: Wolters Kluwer, with permission.)

ACTION	RATIONALE
17. After disconnecting the lead wires from the electrodes, dispose of the electrodes. Return the patient to a comfortable position. Lower bed height and adjust the head of bed to a comfortable position.	Proper disposal deters the spread of microorganisms. Positioning with head adjustment promotes patient comfort. Lowering the bed height promotes patient safety.
18. Clean the ECG machine per facility policy. If not done electronically from data entered into the machine, label the ECG with the patient's name, date of birth, location, date and time of recording, and other relevant information, such as symptoms that occurred during the recording. Note any deviations to the standard approach to the recording, such as alternative placement of leads (see Special Considerations below).	Cleaning equipment between each patient use decreases the risk for transmission of microorganisms. Accurate labeling ensures the ECG is recorded for the correct patient and accurate and reliable interpretation.
19. Remove additional PPE, if used. Perform hand hygiene.	Proper removal of PPE reduces the risk for infection transmission and contamination of other items. Hand hygiene prevents transmission of microorganisms.

EVALUATION

The expected outcomes have been achieved when an ECG is obtained without any complications and the patient demonstrated an understanding of the need for and about the ECG.

DOCUMENTATION

Guidelines

Document significant assessment findings, the date and time that the ECG was obtained, and the patient's response to the procedure. Label the ECG recording with the patient's name, room number, and facility identification number, if this was not done by the machine. Also record the date, time, and the patient's position, as well as any appropriate clinical information on the ECG, such as blood pressure measurement, if the patient was experiencing chest pain. Record any deviations to the standard approach to the recording, such as alternative placement of leads (see Special Considerations below).

Sample Documentation

<u>11/10/20</u> 1745 Patient admitted to room 663. Denies pain, nausea, and shortness of breath. Apical heart rate 82 and regular. Blood pressure 146/88. ECG obtained as per admission orders. Copy faxed to Dr. Martin.

—B. Clapp, RN

(continued)

Skill 16-4 ▶ Obtaining an Electrocardiogram *(continued)*

UNEXPECTED SITUATIONS AND ASSOCIATED INTERVENTIONS	• *An artifact appears on the tracing:* An artifact may be due to loose electrodes or patient movement. Reassess electrode connections. Ensure the ECG electrodes have not expired and are not dry; change electrodes, if necessary. Ask the patient to lie extremely still. Redo the ECG, if necessary. • *Minimal complexes are seen:* This may be due to extreme bradycardia. Run longer strips.
SPECIAL CONSIDERATIONS	• Nurses must be familiar with the particular equipment in use; accuracy of the information is dependent on following the specifications of the manufacturer (Garcia, 2015). • The standard limb electrode locations are slightly proximal (just above) to the wrist and ankle bones (Campbell et al., 2017). Limb electrodes may be placed on the inside or outside aspects of wrist and ankle. Allow patients to position themselves comfortably, and then use the most accessible aspect for electrode placement. Do not obtain recordings from any other limb position unless there is a clinical reason, such as an amputation, surgical wounds, or burns. In patients with amputations, it is important to place the electrodes in the same position bilaterally (Garcia, 2015). Upper arms and upper legs may be used as alternate sites in these situations. ECGs recorded using any other limb position or precordial positions must be labeled to account for changes that might affect the interpretation and clinical decisions made (Garcia, 2015). • To position the chest leads (V_1 to V_6) correctly, it is important to be able to accurately locate the relevant intercostal spaces (Garcia, 2015). • For female patients, place the V_4 electrode, as well as V_5 and V_6 as necessary, under the breast tissue as close to the chest wall as possible (Garcia, 2015). In a large-breasted woman, you may need to displace the breast tissue laterally and/or superiorly.

Skill 16-5 ▶ Applying a Cardiac Monitor

Bedside cardiac (electrocardiographic) monitoring provides continuous observation of the heart's electrical activity. It is used to monitor a patient's heart rate and rhythm or the effects of a therapy (Morton & Fontaine, 2018). Cardiac monitoring is used for patients with conduction disturbances and for those at risk for life-threatening arrhythmias, such as postoperative patients and patients who are sedated. As with other forms of electrocardiography, cardiac monitoring uses electrodes placed on the patient's chest to transmit electrical signals that are converted into a tracing of cardiac rhythm on an oscilloscope. Three- or five-lead systems may be used (Figure 1). The three-lead–wire monitoring system facilitates monitoring of the patient in leads I, II, and III limb leads (Morton & Fontaine, 2018). The five-lead–wire monitoring system facilitates monitoring of the patient in any one of the standard 12 leads.

Two types of monitoring may be performed: hardwire or telemetry. In hardwire monitoring, the patient is connected to a monitor at the bedside. The rhythm display appears at the bedside, but may also be transmitted to a console at a remote location. Telemetry uses a small transmitter connected to an ambulatory patient to send electrical signals to another location, where they are displayed on a monitor screen. Battery powered and portable, telemetry frees patients from cumbersome wires and cables and lets them be comfortably mobile. Telemetry is especially useful for monitoring arrhythmias that occur during sleep, rest, exercise, or stressful situations.

Regardless of the type, cardiac monitors can display the patient's heart rate and rhythm, produce a printed record of cardiac rhythm, and sound an alarm if the heart rate exceeds or falls below specified limits. Monitors also recognize and count abnormal heartbeats as well as changes. Cardiac monitoring systems may incorporate computer systems that store, analyze, and trend monitored data, automatic chart documentation, and wireless communication devices that provide data and alarms that can be carried by the nurse (Morton & Fontaine, 2018).

Gel foam electrodes are commonly used. Electrodes should be changed every 24 hours, or according to facility policy, to prevent skin irritation and maintain quality of data. Hypoallergenic electrodes are available for patients with hypersensitivity to tape or adhesive. Any loose or nonadhering electrode should be replaced immediately to prevent inaccurate or missing data.

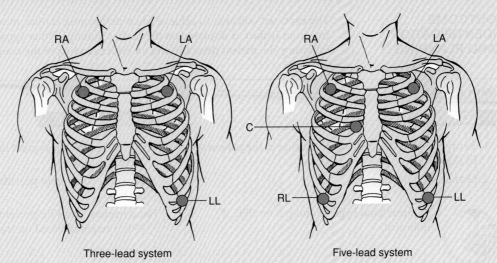

Three-lead system   Five-lead system

FIGURE 1. Electrode positions for three- (*left*) and five-lead (*right*) systems.

Positions for the three-lead system:
RA (white electrode) below right clavicle, second ICS, right midclavicular line
LA (black electrode) below left clavicle, second ICS, left midclavicular line
LL (red electrode) left lower rib cage, eighth ICS, left midclavicular line

Positions for the five-lead system:
RA (white electrode) below right clavicle, second ICS, right midclavicular line
RL (green electrode) right lower rib cage, eighth ICS, right midclavicular line
LA (black electrode) below left clavicle, second ICS, left midclavicular line
LL (red electrode) left lower rib cage, eighth ICS, left midclavicular line
Chest (brown electrode) any V lead position, usually V_1 (fourth ICS, right sternal border)

DELEGATION CONSIDERATIONS	The application of a cardiac monitor is not delegated to nursing assistive personnel (NAP) or to unlicensed assistive personnel (UAP); in some facilities, technicians are trained to apply the leads. Depending on the state's nurse practice act and the organization's policies and procedures, application of a cardiac monitor may be delegated to licensed practical/vocational nurses (LPN/LVNs). The decision to delegate must be based on careful analysis of the patient's needs and circumstances, as well as the qualifications of the person to whom the task is being delegated. Refer to the Delegation Guidelines in Appendix A.

EQUIPMENT

- Lead wires
- Pregelled (gel foam) electrodes (number varies from 3 to 5)
- Gauze pads
- Skin cleanser

- Patient cable for hardwire cardiac monitoring
- Transmitter, transmitter pouch, and telemetry battery pack for telemetry
- PPE, as indicated

ASSESSMENT	Review the patient's health record and care plan for information about the patient's need for cardiac monitoring. Assess the patient's cardiac status, including heart rate, blood pressure, and auscultation of heart sounds. Inspect the patient's chest for areas of irritation, breakdown, or excessive hair that might interfere with electrode placement. Electrode sites must be dry, with minimal hair. The patient may be sitting or supine, in a bed or chair.

NURSING DIAGNOSIS	Determine the related factors for the nursing diagnoses based on the patient's current status. Appropriate nursing diagnoses may include:

- Decreased cardiac output
- Excess fluid volume
- Deficient knowledge

(*continued*)

Skill 16-5 ▶ Applying a Cardiac Monitor *(continued)*

OUTCOME IDENTIFICATION AND PLANNING
The expected outcome to achieve when performing cardiac monitoring is that a clear waveform, free from artifact, is displayed on the cardiac monitor. Other appropriate outcomes may include the following: the patient demonstrates an understanding of the reason for monitoring.

IMPLEMENTATION

ACTION	RATIONALE
1. Verify the order for cardiac monitoring in the patient's health record.	This ensures that the correct intervention is performed on the correct patient.
2. Gather equipment.	Assembling equipment provides for an organized approach to the task.
3. Perform hand hygiene and put on PPE, if indicated.	Hand hygiene and PPE prevent the spread of microorganisms. PPE is required based on transmission precautions.
4. Identify the patient.	Identifying the patient ensures the right patient receives the intervention and helps prevent errors.
5. Close curtains around the bed and close the door to the room, if possible. Explain the procedure to the patient. Tell the patient that the monitoring records the heart's electrical activity. Emphasize that no electrical current will enter his or her body. Ask the patient about allergies to adhesive, as appropriate.	This ensures the patient's privacy. Explanation relieves anxiety and facilitates cooperation. Possible allergies may exist related to adhesive on ECG leads.
6. For hardwire monitoring, plug the cardiac monitor into an electrical outlet and turn it on to warm up the unit while preparing the equipment and the patient. For telemetry monitoring, insert a new battery into the transmitter. Match the poles on the battery with the polar markings on the transmitter case. Press the button at the top of the unit, test the battery's charge, and test the unit to ensure that the battery is operational.	Proper setup ensures proper functioning. Not all models have a test button. Test according to manufacturer's directions.
7. Insert the cable into the appropriate socket in the monitor.	Proper setup ensures proper functioning.
8. Connect the lead wires to the cable. In some systems, the lead wires are permanently secured to the cable. For telemetry, if the lead wires are not permanently affixed to the telemetry unit, attach them securely. If they must be attached individually, connect each one to the correct outlet.	Proper setup ensures proper functioning.
9. Connect an electrode to each of the lead wires, carefully checking that each lead wire is in its correct outlet.	Proper setup ensures proper functioning.
10. If the bed is adjustable, raise it to a comfortable working height, usually elbow height of the caregiver (VHACEOSH, 2016).	Having the bed at the proper height prevents back and muscle strain.
11. Expose the patient's chest and determine electrode positions, based on which system and leads are being used (refer to Figure 1). If necessary, clip the hair from an area about 10 cm in diameter around each electrode site. **Do not shave hair.** Clean excess oil or other substances from the skin with skin cleanser and water. Use a gauze pad to vigorously rub and dry the skin.	Shaving causes microabrasions on the skin, possibly resulting in portals of entry for microorganisms. Oils and excess hair interfere with electrode contact and function. Rubbing with gauze abrades and dries the skin. Proper skin preparation and application of electrodes are imperative for good ECG monitoring (Morton & Fontaine, 2018, p. 215).

ACTION	RATIONALE
12. Remove the backing from the pregelled electrode. Check the gel for moistness. If the gel is dry, discard it and replace it with a fresh electrode. **Apply the electrode to the site and press firmly to ensure a tight seal.** Repeat with the remaining electrodes to complete the three- or five-lead system (Figure 2).	Gel acts as a conduit and must be moist and secured tightly.

FIGURE 2. Applying the electrodes.

ACTION	RATIONALE
13. When all the electrodes are in place, connect the appropriate lead wire to each electrode. Check waveform for clarity, position, and size. **To verify that the monitor is detecting each beat, compare the digital heart rate display with an auscultated count of the patient's heart rate.** If necessary, use the gain control to adjust the size of the rhythm tracing, and use the position control to adjust the waveform position on the monitor.	This ensures accuracy of reading.
14. Set the upper and lower limits of the heart rate alarm, based on the patient's condition or unit policy.	Setting the alarm allows for audible notification if the heart rate is beyond limits. The default setting for the monitor automatically turns on all alarms; limits should be set for each patient.
15. For telemetry, place the transmitter in the pouch in the patient gown. If no pouch is available in the gown, use a portable pouch. Tie the pouch strings around the patient's neck and waist, making sure that the pouch fits snugly without causing discomfort. If no pouch is available, place the transmitter in the patient's bathrobe pocket.	Patient comfort leads to compliance.
16. Return the patient to a comfortable position. Lower the bed height and adjust the head of bed to a comfortable position.	Repositioning promotes patient comfort. Lowering the bed promotes patient safety.
17. To obtain a rhythm strip, press the RECORD key, either at the bedside for monitoring or at the central station for telemetry. Analyze the strip, as appropriate. If the rhythm strip is a printed copy, label the strip with the patient's name and room number, date, time, and rhythm identification. Place the rhythm strip in the appropriate location in the patient's health record, based on facility policy.	A rhythm strip provides a baseline for future comparison.

(continued)

Skill 16-5 ▶ Applying a Cardiac Monitor *(continued)*

ACTION	RATIONALE

 18. Remove additional PPE, if used. Perform hand hygiene.

Proper removal of PPE reduces the risk for infection transmission and contamination of other items. Hand hygiene prevents transmission of microorganisms.

EVALUATION

The expected outcomes have been achieved when a clear waveform, free from artifact, has been displayed on the cardiac monitor and the patient demonstrated an understanding of the reason for monitoring.

DOCUMENTATION

Guidelines

Record the date and time that monitoring begins and the monitoring lead used in the health record. Document a rhythm strip at least every 8 hours and with any changes in the patient's condition (or as stated by facility's policy). Label the rhythm strip with the patient's name and room number, date, and time.

Sample Documentation

> <u>12/16/20</u> 1615 Patient admitted to room. Cardiac telemetry monitor in place; monitoring in lead II. See EHR for assessment data and initial rhythm strip.
>
> —T. Shah, RN

UNEXPECTED SITUATIONS AND ASSOCIATED INTERVENTIONS

- *Low amplitude:* Assess if the size control is adjusted properly; poor contact between skin and electrodes; dried gel; broken or loose lead wires; poor connection between patient and monitor; or malfunctioning monitor. Check connections on all lead wires and monitoring cable. Replace electrodes, as necessary. Reapply electrodes, if required.
- *Wandering baseline:* Assess for poor position or contact between electrodes and skin, or thoracic movement with respirations. Reposition or replace electrodes.
- *Artifact (waveform interference):* Assess for patient movement, improperly applied electrodes, or static electricity. Check plugs to make sure prongs are not loose.
- *Skin excoriation under electrodes:* Assess for allergic reaction to electrode adhesive or electrodes being left on the skin too long. Remove electrodes and apply hypoallergenic electrodes and hypoallergenic tape, or remove electrode, clean site, and reapply electrode at new site.

SPECIAL CONSIDERATIONS

General Considerations

- Make sure all electrical equipment and outlets are grounded to avoid electric shock and interference (artifacts).
- Avoid opening the electrode package until just before using to prevent the gel from drying out.
- Avoid placing the electrodes on bony prominences, hairy locations, areas where defibrillator pads will be placed, or areas for chest compression.
- Assess skin integrity and examine the leads every 8 hours. Replace and reposition the electrodes, as necessary.
- If the patient is being monitored by telemetry, show him or her how the transmitter works. If applicable, identify the button that will produce a recording of the ECG at the central station. Instruct the patient to push the button whenever symptoms occur; this causes the central console to print a rhythm strip. Also, advise the patient to notify the nurse immediately if symptoms occur.
- If a medical order is in place, tell the patient to remove the transmitter during showering or bathing, if appropriate, but stress that he or she should let the nurse know the unit is being removed.

Infant and Child Considerations

- Having the infant or child wear a snug undershirt over the leads helps to keep the leads in place (Kyle & Carman, 2017).

EVIDENCE
FOR PRACTICE ▶

CARDIAC MONITORING

Many patients admitted to acute care settings with cardiac, respiratory, and other acute health problems are placed on electrocardiographic monitoring. This monitoring allows the health care providers, including nurses, to monitor the patient for the development of cardiac dysrhythmias. Frequent monitor alarms are distracting, interfere with the ability to perform critical tasks, and contribute to alarm fatigue (Walsh-Irwin & Jurgens, 2015). Does proper skin preparation and electrode placement impact the frequency of cardiac monitor alarms?

Related Research

Walsh-Irwin, C., & Jurgens, C. Y. (2015). Proper skin preparation and electrode placement decreases alarms on a telemetry unit. *Dimensions of Critical Care Nursing, 34*(3), 134–139.

Large numbers of technical alarms distract patient care providers and interfere with patient care. Frequent alarms may lead to errors of omission, inattention, and missed patient status alarms. This study examined the effects of proper skin preparation and electrode placement on the number of cardiac monitor alarms. Alarms were counted for 24 hours after patients were admitted to a telemetry hospital. Electrodes were replaced using proper skin preparation and application technique. Alarms were again counted for 24 hours after replacement. Electrocardiographic alarms decreased significantly ($p < 0.05$) after proper skin preparation and electrode placement. The authors concluded proper skin preparation and electrode placement reduces the number of cardiac monitor alarms.

Relevance for Nursing Practice

As primary care providers, nurses have the responsibility to include interventions to provide for the best patient care outcomes possible. Ensuring proper skin preparation before applying monitor electrodes and proper electrode placement are simple interventions that can be implemented by nurses. These interventions can lead to fewer cardiac monitor alarms, contributing to reduced alarm fatigue and increased patient safety.

Refer to thePoint* for additional research on related nursing topics.

Skill 16-6 ▶ Using a Transcutaneous (External) Pacemaker

Temporary cardiac pacing is used to correct life-threatening cardiac dysrhythmias and as an elective procedure, such as to evaluate the need for permanent pacing or after cardiac surgery. A temporary pacemaker consists of an external, battery-powered pulse generator and a lead or electrode system to electrically stimulate heartbeat. Transcutaneous pacing can temporarily supply an electrical current in the heart when electrical conduction is abnormal. This device works by sending an electrical impulse from the pulse generator to the patient's heart by way of two electrodes, which are placed on the front and back of the patient's chest. This stimulates the contraction of cardiac muscle fibers through electrical stimulation (depolarization) of the myocardium. Transcutaneous pacing is quick and effective, but is usually used as short-term therapy until the situation resolves or transvenous or permanent pacing can be initiated.

Transcutaneous pacing can cause significant discomfort. The patient should be informed and adequately sedated, whenever possible (Morton & Fontaine, 2018, p. 312). Provide analgesia as needed (Stout, 2017).

DELEGATION
CONSIDERATIONS

The use of a transcutaneous pacemaker is not delegated to nursing assistive personnel (NAP) or to unlicensed assistive personnel (UAP). Depending on the state's nurse practice act and the organization's policies and procedures, this procedure may be delegated to licensed practical/vocational nurses (LPN/LVNs). The decision to delegate must be based on careful analysis of the patient's needs and circumstances, as well as the qualifications of the person to whom the task is being delegated. Refer to the Delegation Guidelines in Appendix A.

(continued)

Skill 16-6 ▶ Using a Transcutaneous (External) Pacemaker *(continued)*

EQUIPMENT	• Transcutaneous noninvasive pacemaker • Transcutaneous pacing electrodes and cables • ECG electrodes and cables • Cardiac monitor • Medication for analgesia and/or sedation, as prescribed

ASSESSMENT

Review the patient's health record and care plan for information about the patient's need for pacing. Transcutaneous pacing is generally an emergency measure. Assess the patient's initial cardiac rhythm, including a rhythm strip and 12-lead ECG. Monitor heart rate, respiratory rate, level of consciousness, and skin color. If the patient is pulseless, initiate CPR.

NURSING DIAGNOSIS

Determine the related factors for the nursing diagnoses based on the patient's current status. Appropriate nursing diagnoses include:

• Decreased cardiac output
• Anxiety
• Risk for injury

OUTCOME IDENTIFICATION AND PLANNING

The expected outcome to achieve when using an external transcutaneous pacemaker is that it is applied correctly without adverse effect. Additional outcomes may include the following: the patient regains and/or maintains signs of adequate circulation, including the capture of at least the minimal set heart rate; and the patient does not experience injury.

IMPLEMENTATION

ACTION	**RATIONALE**
1. Verify the order for a transcutaneous pacemaker in the patient's health record.	This ensures that the correct intervention is performed on the correct patient.
2. Gather all equipment.	Assembling equipment provides for an organized approach to the task.
3. Perform hand hygiene and put on PPE, if indicated.	Hand hygiene and PPE prevent the transmission of microorganisms. PPE is required based on transmission precautions.
4. Identify the patient.	Verifying the patient's identity validates that the correct procedure is being done on the correct patient.
5. If the patient is responsive, explain the procedure to the patient. Explain that it involves some discomfort and that you will administer medication to keep him or her comfortable and help him or her to relax. **Administer analgesia and sedation, as ordered, if not an emergency situation.**	External pacemakers are typically used with unconscious patients because most alert patients cannot tolerate the uncomfortable sensations produced by the high energy levels needed to pace externally. If responsive, the patient will most likely be sedated (Morton & Fontaine, 2018).
6. Close curtains around the bed and close the door to the room, if possible. Obtain vital signs.	This provides for patient privacy. Vital signs provide baseline for assessing pacing effectiveness.
7. If necessary, clip the hair over the areas of electrode placement. **Do not shave the area.** Use a gauze pad to vigorously rub and dry the skin at the locations where the cardiac monitoring electrodes will be placed.	Shaving causes microabrasions on the skin, possibly resulting in portals of entry for microorganisms. Oils and excess hair interfere with electrode contact and function. Rubbing with gauze abrades and dries the skin. Proper skin preparation is essential to reduce artifact in and increase quality of the ECG tracing (Garcia, 2015).

ACTION

8. Attach cardiac monitoring electrodes to the patient in the lead I, II, and III positions. Do this even if the patient is already on telemetry monitoring. If you select the lead II position, adjust the left leg (LL) electrode placement to accommodate the anterior pacing electrode and the patient's anatomy.

9. Attach the patient monitoring electrodes to the ECG cable and into the ECG input connection on the front of the pacing generator. Set the selector switch to the "Monitor on" position.

10. Note the ECG waveform on the monitor. Adjust the R-wave beeper volume to a suitable level and activate the alarm by pressing the "Alarm on" button. Set the alarm for 10 to 20 beats lower and 20 to 30 beats higher than the patient's target pacing rate.

11. Press the "Start/Stop" button for a printout of the waveform.

12. Apply the two pacing electrodes. Make sure the patient's skin is clean and dry to ensure good skin contact. Pull the protective strip from the posterior electrode (marked "Back") and apply the electrode on the left side of the thoracic spinal column, just below the scapula (Figure 1).

RATIONALE

Cardiac monitoring electrodes must be placed in addition to the pacing electrodes in order for the pacemaker to read the patient's cardiac rhythm while the pacing electrodes deliver the energy needed to pace the heart (Stout, 2017). Connecting the telemetry electrodes to the pacemaker is required.

These actions ensure that the equipment is functioning properly.

These actions ensure that the equipment is functioning properly. Alarms alert the nurse to potential concerns regarding the patient's status.

A printout provides objective data.

This placement ensures that the electrical stimulus will travel only a short distance to the heart.

Anterior pacing electrode

Posterior pacing electrode

FIGURE 1. Transcutaneous pacemaker pads in place.

13. Apply the anterior pacing electrode (marked "Front"), which has two protective strips—one covering the gelled area and one covering the outer rim. Expose the gelled area and apply it to the skin in the anterior position, to the left of the precordium in the V_2 to the V_5 position (see Figure 1). Move this electrode around to get the best waveform. Then expose the electrode's outer rim and firmly press it to the skin.

14. Prepare to pace the heart. After making sure the energy output in milliamperes (mA) is on 0, connect the electrode cable to the monitor output cable.

15. Check the waveform, looking for a tall QRS complex in lead II.

This placement ensures that the electrical stimulus will travel only a short distance to the heart.

This sets the pacing threshold.

(continued)

Skill 16-6 ▶ Using a Transcutaneous (External) Pacemaker *(continued)*

ACTION	RATIONALE
16. Check the selector switch to "Pacer on." Select synchronous (demand) or asynchronous (fixed-rate or nondemand) mode, as prescribed. **Tell the patient he or she may feel a thumping or twitching sensation. Reassure the patient you will provide analgesic medication if the discomfort is intolerable.**	Asynchronous pacing delivers a stimulus at a set (fixed) rate regardless of the occurrence of spontaneous myocardial depolarizations (patient's own underlying heart rate). Synchronous pacing delivers a stimulus only when the heart's intrinsic pacemaker fails to function at a predetermined rate (if the patient's own heart rate drops below the demand rate set on the pacemaker). Analgesia and/or sedation may be administered, as prescribed and indicated, for discomfort associated with pacing (Morton & Fontaine, 2018; Stout, 2017).
17. Set the pacing rate dial to a target pacing rate of 60 to 70 beats/min. Look for pacer artifact or spikes, which will appear as you increase the rate.	Setting the pacing rate dial higher than the intrinsic rhythm ensures adequate cardiac output.
18. Set the pacing current output (in mA), if not automatically done by the pacemaker. For patients with bradycardia, start with the minimal setting and **slowly increase the amount of energy delivered to the heart by adjusting the "Output" mA dial. Do this until electrical capture is achieved: you will see a pacer spike followed by a widened QRS complex and a tall broad T wave that resembles a premature ventricular contraction.**	Setting the pacing current output ensures adequate cardiac output.
19. Increase output by 2 mA or 10% to ensure capture. **Do not go higher (unless prescribed or indicated) because of the increased risk of discomfort to the patient. Print a strip and place in the patient's health record.**	Increasing the output ensures consistent capture. With full capture, the patient's heart rate should be the same as the pacemaker rate shown on the machine. The usual pacing threshold is between 40 and 80 mA. Thresholds may vary due to recent cardiothoracic surgery, pericardial effusions, cardiac tamponade, acidosis, and hypoxia. These conditions may require higher thresholds. Printing a strip documents the patient's paced rhythm.
20. Assess for effectiveness of pacing and mechanical capture: observe for pacemaker spike with subsequent capture; assess heart rate and rhythm (using right carotid, brachial, or femoral artery); assess blood pressure; assess for signs of improved cardiac output (increased blood pressure, improved level of consciousness, improved body temperature).	Both electrical and mechanical capture must occur to benefit the patient (Stout, 2017). Use of patient's right side for pulse assessment avoids inaccuracy related to strong contractions from the pacemaker.
21. Secure the pacing leads and cable to the patient's body.	This prevents accidental displacement of the electrode, resulting in failure to pace or sense.
22. Remove PPE, if used. Perform hand hygiene.	Proper removal of PPE reduces the risk for infection transmission and contamination of other items. Hand hygiene and proper disposal of equipment reduce the transmission of microorganisms.
23. Continue to monitor the patient's heart rate and rhythm to assess ventricular response to pacing. Assess the patient's vital signs, skin color, level of consciousness, and peripheral pulses. Take blood pressure in both arms.	Assessment helps determine the effectiveness of the paced rhythm. If the blood pressure reading is significantly higher in one arm, use that arm for measurements.
24. Continue to assess the patient's pain and administer analgesia/sedation, as ordered, to ease the discomfort of chest wall muscle contractions (Morton & Fontaine, 2018).	Analgesia and sedation promote patient comfort.
25. Perform a 12-lead ECG and additional ECG daily or with clinical changes.	ECG monitoring provides a baseline for further evaluation.
26. Continually monitor the ECG readings, noting capture, sensing, rate, intrinsic beats, and competition of paced and intrinsic rhythms. If the pacemaker is sensing correctly, the sense indicator on the pulse generator should flash with each beat.	Continuous monitoring helps evaluate the patient's condition and determine the effectiveness of therapy.

EVALUATION

The expected outcomes have been achieved when the external transcutaneous pacemaker was applied correctly without adverse effect; the patient regained and/or maintained signs of adequate circulation, including the capture of at least the minimal set heart rate; and the patient did not experience injury.

DOCUMENTATION

Guidelines

Document the reason for pacemaker use, time that pacing began, electrode locations, pacemaker settings, patient's response to the procedure and to temporary pacing, complications, and nursing actions taken. Document the patient's pain intensity rating, analgesia or sedation administered, and the patient's response. If possible, obtain a rhythm strip before, during, and after pacemaker placement; anytime the pacemaker settings are changed; and whenever the patient receives treatment because of a complication due to the pacemaker.

Sample Documentation

> <u>1/2/20</u> 1218 Baseline rhythm strip obtained, sinus bradycardia at 43 beats/min; see flow sheet. External temporary pacemaker placed by Dr. Goodman. Cardiac monitoring electrodes placed in the lead I, II, and III positions. Pacer set in synchronous mode at rate of 80 beats/min; pacing current output 72 mA. Patient with strong femoral pulses; see flow sheet for vital signs. Patient reports chest discomfort of 4/10. Medicated with morphine 2 mg IV, per order. Pacer alarms set at 50 and 90 beats/min, per order.
> —*R. Robinson, RN*
>
> <u>1/2/20</u> 1250 Patient reports decreased pain, 1/10.
> —*R. Robinson, RN*

UNEXPECTED SITUATIONS AND ASSOCIATED INTERVENTIONS

- *Failure to pace:* This happens when the pacemaker either does not fire or fires too often. The pulse generator may not be working properly, or it may not be conducting the impulse to the patient. If the pacing or sensing indicator flashes, check the connections to the cable and the position/contact of the pacing electrodes on the patient. The cable may have come loose, or the electrode may not be making contact. If the pulse generator is turned on but the indicators still are not flashing, change the battery. If that does not help, use a different pulse generator. Check the settings if the pacemaker is firing too rapidly. If they are correct, or if altering them (according to your facility's policy or the prescribed order) does not help, change the pulse generator.
- *Failure to capture:* Pacemaker spikes are seen but the heart is not responding. The most common reason is failure to increase the current sufficiently. It may also be caused by changes in the pacing threshold from ischemia, an electrolyte imbalance (high or low potassium or magnesium levels), acidosis, an adverse reaction to a medication, or fibrosis. If the patient's condition has changed, notify the health care provider and ask for new settings. Carefully check all connections, making sure they are placed properly and securely. Increase the milliamperes slowly (according to your facility's policy or the prescribed order).
- *Failure to sense intrinsic beats:* This could cause ventricular tachycardia or ventricular fibrillation if the pacemaker fires on the vulnerable T wave. This could be caused by the pacemaker sensing an external stimulus as a QRS complex, which could lead to asystole, or by the pacemaker not being sufficiently sensitive, which means it could fire anywhere within the cardiac cycle. If the pacing is undersensing, turn sensitivity dial toward lower millivolt value. If it is oversensing, reduce sensitivity; value in millivolts should be larger to make pacer less sensitive (Morton & Fontaine, 2018). If the pacemaker is not functioning correctly, change the battery or the pulse generator.

SPECIAL CONSIDERATIONS

- Do not leave patients unattended during noninvasive pacing. It is safe to touch the patient and perform procedures during pacing (e.g., CPR). Gloves should be worn. Do not touch the conductive surface of the electrodes.
- Check the skin where the electrodes are placed for skin burns or tissue damage. Reposition, as needed.

(continued)

Skill 16-7   Obtaining an Arterial Blood Sample From an Arterial Catheter

Obtaining an arterial blood sample requires percutaneous puncture of the brachial, radial, or femoral artery (refer to Chapter 18). However, an arterial blood sample can also be obtained from an arterial catheter. Arterial catheters are used for hemodynamic monitoring, blood gas analysis, and obtaining blood samples. A pressure monitoring system (Figure 1) transmits pressures from the intravascular space or cardiac chambers through a catheter and fluid-filled tubing to a pressure transducer, which converts the physiologic signal from the patient to a pressure tracing and digital value. Patency of the system and prevention of backflow of blood through the catheter and tubing is maintained by using a continuous flush solution under pressure (Morton & Fontaine, 2018).

The procedure below describes obtaining a sample from an open, stopcock system. For information on obtaining an arterial blood sample from a closed reservoir system, please see the Skill Variation at the end of this skill.

Pressure infuser
Saline
Pressure gauge
Cable to monitor
Noncompliant tubing
Catheter
Stopcock
Transducer

FIGURE 1. Pressure monitoring system. (From Morton, P. G., & Fontaine, D. K. [2018]. *Essentials of critical care nursing. A holistic approach* [11th ed.]. Philadelphia, PA: Wolters Kluwer.)

DELEGATION CONSIDERATIONS	Obtaining an arterial blood sample from an arterial catheter is not delegated to nursing assistive personnel (NAP), unlicensed assistive personnel (UAP), or licensed practical/vocational nurses (LPN/LVNs).

EQUIPMENT

- Arterial blood gas (ABG) syringe with needleless cannula, rubber cap for ABG syringe hub, and ice-filled plastic bag or cup, if ABG is ordered
- Gloves
- Goggles

- Additional PPE, as indicated
- Vacutainer with needleless Luer adapter (or blunt cannula, for closed reservoir system) and appropriate blood collection tubes for ordered tests

- Two additional blood collection tubes, for discard blood volume
- Antimicrobial or chlorhexidine swabs, per facility policy
- Waterproof protective pad
- Passive disinfection caps (based on facility policy) or

- Sterile cap for arterial catheter stopcock (based on facility policy)
- Label with patient identification information
- Blank labels (2)
- Biohazard bag
- Bath blanket

ASSESSMENT	Review the patient's health record and care plan for information about the patient's need for an arterial blood sample. Assess the patient's cardiac status, including heart rate, blood pressure, and auscultation of heart sounds. Also assess the patient's respiratory status, including respiratory rate, excursion, lung sounds, and use of oxygen, if ordered. Check the patency and functioning of the arterial catheter. Assess the patient's understanding about the need for specimen collection.
NURSING DIAGNOSIS	Determine the related factors for the nursing diagnoses based on the patient's current status. Appropriate nursing diagnoses may include: • Impaired gas exchange • Decreased cardiac output • Excess fluid volume
OUTCOME IDENTIFICATION AND PLANNING	The expected outcome to achieve when obtaining an arterial blood sample is that a specimen is obtained without compromise to the patency of the arterial catheter. In addition, the patient experiences minimal discomfort, remains free from infection, and verbalizes an understanding of the rationale for and the steps of the procedure.

IMPLEMENTATION

ACTION	**RATIONALE**
1. Verify the order for laboratory testing in the patient's health record.	This ensures that the correct intervention is performed on the correct patient.
2. Gather all equipment.	Assembling equipment provides for an organized approach to the task.
3. Perform hand hygiene and put on PPE, if indicated.	Hand hygiene and PPE prevent the spread of microorganisms. PPE is required based on transmission precautions.
4. Identify the patient.	Identifying the patient ensures the right patient receives the intervention and helps prevent errors.
5. Close curtains around the bed and close the door to the room, if possible. Explain the procedure to the patient.	This ensures the patient's privacy. Explanation relieves anxiety and facilitates cooperation.
6. Assemble equipment on overbed table or other surface within reach.	Arranging items nearby is convenient, saves time, and avoids unnecessary stretching and twisting of muscles on the part of the nurse.
7. Adjust the bed to a comfortable working height, usually elbow height of the caregiver (VHACEOSH, 2016).	Having the bed at the proper height prevents back and muscle strain.
8. Compare specimen label with patient identification bracelet. Label should include patient's name and identification number, time specimen was collected, route of collection, identification of the person obtaining the sample, and any other information required by facility policy.	Verifying the patient's identity validates that the correct procedure is being done on the correct patient, and the specimen is accurately labeled.

(continued)

Skill 16-7 ▸ Obtaining an Arterial Blood Sample From an Arterial Catheter *(continued)*

ACTION	RATIONALE
9. Use blank labels to label the two blood sample collection tubes to be used for discard blood sample and discard flush.	Labeling of discard tubes prevents accidental confusion with blood specimen tubes.
10. Assist the patient to a comfortable position that provides easy access to the sampling site. Use the bath blanket to cover any exposed area other than the sampling site. Place a waterproof pad under the site.	Patient positioning and use of a bath blanket provide for comfort and warmth. Waterproof pad protects underlying surfaces.
11. Put on gloves and goggles or face shield.	Gloves and goggles (or face shield) prevent contact with blood and body fluids.
12. Temporarily silence the arterial pressure monitor alarms.	The integrity of the system is being altered, which will cause the system to sound an alarm. Facility policy may require the alarm be left on.
13. Locate the stopcock nearest the arterial line insertion site (see Figure 1). Remove the passive disinfection cap or nonvented cap from the stopcock. If a nonvented cap was removed, use an antimicrobial swab to vigorously scrub the sampling port on the stopcock. Allow to air dry.	Removal of stopcock cap allows access for blood sampling. Sampling port does not need to be scrubbed after passive disinfection cap is removed. Cleansing sampling port after removal of nonvented cap reduces the risk of contamination; entry points, end caps, and needleless connectors must be vigorously scrubbed and disinfected prior to each access to reduce the risk for introduction of microorganisms and prevent infection (Frimpong, Caguioa, & Octavo, 2015; Loveday et al., 2014). Friction is needed to physically remove microorganisms from the sampling port. Allow the antiseptic to dry completely (15 to 30 seconds) to ensure complete effectiveness (Harper, 2014).
14. Attach the needleless Luer adapter to the Vacutainer (Figure 2). Connect the needleless adapter of the Vacutainer to the sampling port of the stopcock. Turn off the stopcock to the flush solution. Insert the labeled blood sample tube for the discard sample into the Vacutainer (Figure 3). Follow facility policy for the volume of discard blood to collect (usually 5 to 10 mL).	A sufficient amount of discard volume needs to be withdrawn before obtaining the blood sample to be tested in the laboratory. This sample is discarded because it is diluted with flush solution, possibly leading to inaccurate test results. If an insufficient amount of discard volume is withdrawn, the specimen may be diluted and contaminated with flush solution. If an excessive amount of discard volume is withdrawn, the patient may experience an iatrogenic (treatment-induced) blood loss.

FIGURE 2. Blood sample tube holder with Monoject needleless Luer lock adapter. (© 2017 Cardinal Health. All rights reserved.)

FIGURE 3. Blood sample tube inserted in tube holder connected to the sampling port of stopcock.

ACTION	**RATIONALE**
15. Remove the discard syringe and dispose of appropriately, according to facility policy.	Proper disposal reduces the risk of accidental blood exposure and transmission of microorganisms.
16. Insert each blood sample collection tube into the Vacutainer, keeping the stopcock turned off to the flush solution. For each additional sample required, repeat this procedure. If coagulation tests are included in the required tests, obtain blood for this from the final sample. Apply the rubber cap to the ABG syringe hub, if necessary.	Turning the stopcock off to the flush solution allows for sampling and prevents dilution from the flush device. The Vacutainer is a nonvented system, preventing backflow of blood from the patient. Obtaining coagulation samples last prevents dilution from the flush device. The rubber cap on the ABG syringe hub prevents entry of air into the blood sample.
17. After obtaining the final blood sample, turn off the stopcock to the Vacutainer. Activate the in-line flushing device.	Turning the stopcock off and in-line flushing clears the tubing to maintain the integrity of the system and prevent clotting and infection.
18. Turn off the stopcock to the patient. Attach a labeled discard blood sample tube to the Vacutainer. Activate the in-line flushing device.	Turning the stopcock off and in-line flushing clears the stopcock sampling port to maintain the integrity of the system and prevent clotting and infection.
19. Turn off the stopcock to the sampling port. Remove the Vacutainer. Use an antimicrobial swab to vigorously scrub the sampling port on the stopcock. Allow to air dry. Place a new disinfection cap or sterile nonvented cap on the blood sampling port of the stopcock.	Entry points, end caps, and needleless connectors must be vigorously scrubbed and disinfected prior to each access to reduce the risk for introduction of microorganisms and prevent infection (Frimpong et al., 2015; Loveday et al., 2014). Friction is needed to physically remove microorganisms from the sampling port. Allow the antiseptic to dry completely (15 to 30 seconds) to ensure complete effectiveness (Harper, 2014). Capping the port maintains system integrity and reduces the risk for contamination and infection.
20. Remove gloves. Reactivate the monitor alarms. Record date and time the samples were obtained on the labels, as well as the required information to identify the person obtaining the samples. If ABG was collected, record oxygen flow rate (or room air) on label. Apply labels to the specimens, according to facility policy. Place in biohazard bags; place ABG sample in bag with ice.	Proper removal of PPE reduces the risk for infection transmission and contamination of other items. Reactivating the system ensures proper functioning. Proper labeling prevents error. Recording oxygen flow rate ensures accurate interpretation of results of ABG. Use of a biohazard bag prevents contact with blood and body fluids. Ice maintains integrity of the sample.
21. Check the monitor for return of the arterial waveform and pressure reading.	This ensures proper functioning and integrity of the system.
22. Return the patient to a comfortable position. Lower bed height, if necessary, and adjust head of bed to a comfortable position.	Repositioning promotes patient comfort. Lowering the bed promotes patient safety.
23. Remove goggles and additional PPE, if used. Perform hand hygiene. Send specimens to the laboratory immediately.	Proper removal of PPE reduces the risk for infection transmission and contamination of other items. Hand hygiene prevents transmission of microorganisms. Specimens must be processed in a timely manner to ensure accuracy.

EVALUATION   The expected outcomes have been achieved when an arterial specimen was obtained without compromise to the patency of the arterial catheter; the patient experienced minimal discomfort; the patient remained free from infection; and the patient verbalized an understanding of the rationale for and the steps of the procedure.

DOCUMENTATION

Guidelines   Document any pertinent assessments, the laboratory specimens obtained, date and time specimens were obtained, and disposition of specimens.

(continued)

Skill 16-7 ▸ Obtaining an Arterial Blood Sample From an Arterial Catheter *(continued)*

Sample Documentation

> 10/20/20 0230 Continuous heparin IV infusion at 900 units/hour via left subclavian central catheter. Blood specimens for repeat PT/PTT, CBC, and BMP obtained via right radial arterial catheter, per order. Catheter flushed, per policy; specimens sent to the laboratory.
>
> —R. Chin, RN

UNEXPECTED SITUATIONS AND ASSOCIATED INTERVENTIONS

- *The specimen obtained is dark:* Dark blood means a vein may have been accessed, or the blood may be poorly oxygenated. Ensure that the line from which you are obtaining the specimen is indeed an arterial catheter. Also, check the patient's oxygen saturation level to evaluate for possible hypoxemia.
- *When retracting the syringe for the discarded sample, you feel resistance:* Reposition the affected extremity and check the insertion site for obvious problems (e.g., catheter kinking). Then attempt to obtain the sample to be discarded. If resistance is still felt, notify the health care provider.
- *After obtaining the specimen and reactivating the arterial pressure monitoring system, no waveform is noted:* Check the stopcock to make sure that it is open to the patient and recheck all connections and components of the system to ensure proper setup. If necessary, rebalance the transducer or replace the system, as necessary. If problem persists, suspect a clotted catheter tip. Follow facility policy to troubleshoot a potentially clotted arterial catheter and notify the primary care provider.

SPECIAL CONSIDERATIONS

- If the patient is receiving oxygen, wait 30 minutes after a change in type or mode of oxygen delivery or rate for specimen collection for ABG analysis (Van Leeuwen & Bladh, 2017). Indicate on the laboratory request the amount and type of oxygen therapy the patient is receiving. Also note the patient's current temperature, most recent hemoglobin level, and current respiratory rate. If the patient is receiving mechanical ventilation, note the fraction of inspired oxygen and tidal volume.
- If the patient is not receiving oxygen, indicate that he or she is breathing room air on the laboratory request for an ABG analysis.
- If the patient has just received a nebulizer treatment, wait about 20 minutes before collecting the sample for ABG analysis.

Skill Variation ▸ Obtaining an Arterial Blood Sample From a Closed Reservoir System

1. Follow Steps 1 to 12 in Skill 16-7.
2. Locate the closed-system reservoir and blood-sampling site. Use an antimicrobial swab to vigorously scrub the sampling site. Allow to air dry.
3. Holding the reservoir upright, grasp the flexures and slowly fill the reservoir with blood over a 3- to 5-second period. If you feel resistance, reposition the extremity and check the catheter site for obvious problems (e.g., kinking of the tubing). Then continue with blood withdrawal.
4. Turn off the one-way valve to the reservoir by turning the handle perpendicular to the tubing.
5. Attach the blunt cannula to the Vacutainer or syringe, based on facility policy. Insert the blunt cannula into the sampling site. Insert the blood sample tubes into the Vacutainer. If coagulation tests have been ordered, collect those sample tubes last. After obtaining the final blood sample, grasp the cannula near the sampling site and remove the Vacutainer and blunt cannula as one unit.

6. Alternately, based on facility policy, attach the blunt cannula to the syringe. Insert the blunt cannula into the sampling site. Slowly fill the syringe. Then grasp the cannula near the sampling site and remove the syringe and cannula as one unit. Repeat the procedure, as needed, to fill the required number of syringes. If coagulation tests have been ordered, obtain blood for those tests from the final syringe.
7. After removal of blunt cannula and Vacutainer or syringe, turn the one-way valve to its original position, parallel to the tubing. Push down evenly on the plunger until the flexures lock in place in the fully closed position and all fluid has been reinfused. The fluid should be reinfused over a 3- to 5-second period. Activate the fast-flush release.

8. Use an antimicrobial swab to vigorously scrub the sampling site. Reactivate the monitor alarms. Transfer blood samples to the appropriate specimen tubes, if necessary. Record on the labels the date and time the samples were obtained, as well as the required information to identify the person obtaining the samples. Apply labels to the specimens according to facility policy. Place in biohazard bags; place ABG sample in bag with ice. Remove gloves.

9. Check the monitor for return of the arterial waveform and pressure reading.

10. Remove any remaining equipment. Remove goggles and additional PPE, if used. Perform hand hygiene. Send specimens to the laboratory immediately.

Skill 16-8 Removing Peripheral Arterial Catheters

Arterial catheters, which are used for intensive and continuous cardiac monitoring and intra-arterial access, are commonly placed in the radial or brachial arteries in adults to reduce the risk of infection (O'Grady et al., 2011), although the femoral site can be used as well. Alternative and less frequent sites include the axillary and dorsalis pedis arteries in adults and the temporal and umbilical arteries in neonates (Morton & Fontaine, 2018). As soon as the arterial catheter is no longer needed or has become ineffective, it should be removed (O'Grady et al.). Consult facility policy to determine whether nurses are permitted to perform this procedure. Two nurses should be at the bedside until bleeding is controlled, and to be available to give emergency medications or assistance, if necessary.

DELEGATION CONSIDERATIONS

Removal of an arterial catheter is not delegated to nursing assistive personnel (NAP), unlicensed assistive personnel (UAP), or licensed practical/vocational nurses (LPN/LVNs).

EQUIPMENT

- Sterile gloves
- Clean gloves
- Goggles or face shield
- Sterile gauze pads
- Waterproof protective pad
- Sterile suture removal set
- Transparent dressing
- Hypoallergenic tape

- For femoral catheter: small sandbag (5 to 10 lb), wrapped in a towel or pillowcase, based on facility policy
- Emergency medications (e.g., atropine, for a vasovagal response with femoral catheter removal) for emergency response, per facility policy and guidelines

ASSESSMENT

Review the patient's health record and care plan for information about discontinuation of the arterial catheter. Assess the patient's coagulation status, including laboratory studies, to reduce the risk of complications secondary to impaired clotting ability. Assess the patient's understanding of the procedure. Inspect the site for leakage, bleeding, or hematoma. Assess skin color and temperature and assess distal pulses for strength and quality. Mark distal pulses with an "X" for easy identification after the procedure. Assess the patient's blood pressure; systolic blood pressure should be less than 180 mm Hg before the catheter is removed.

NURSING DIAGNOSIS

Determine the related factors for the nursing diagnoses based on the patient's current status. Appropriate nursing diagnoses may include:

- Risk for injury
- Impaired skin integrity

- Risk for infection

(continued)

Skill 16-8 ▶ Removing Peripheral Arterial Catheters *(continued)*

OUTCOME IDENTIFICATION AND PLANNING

The expected outcome to achieve when removing an arterial catheter is that the catheter is removed intact and without injury to the patient. In addition, the patient maintains intact peripheral circulation and the site remains clean and dry, without evidence of infection, bleeding, or hematoma.

IMPLEMENTATION

ACTION	RATIONALE
1. Verify the order for removal of the arterial catheter in the patient's health record.	This ensures that the correct intervention is performed on the correct patient.
2. Gather all equipment.	Assembling equipment provides for an organized approach to the task.
3. Perform hand hygiene and put on PPE, if indicated.	Hand hygiene and PPE prevent the spread of microorganisms. PPE is required based on transmission precautions.
4. Identify the patient.	Identifying the patient ensures the right patient receives the intervention and helps prevent errors.
5. Close curtains around the bed and close the door to the room, if possible. Explain the procedure to the patient.	This ensures the patient's privacy. Explanation relieves anxiety and facilitates cooperation.
6. Maintain an IV infusion of normal saline via another venous access during the procedure, as ordered or per facility guidelines.	IV access may be needed in case of hypotension or bradycardia.
7. If the bed is adjustable, raise it to a comfortable working height, usually elbow height of the caregiver (VHACEOSH, 2016).	Having the bed at the proper height prevents back and muscle strain.
8. Put on clean gloves, goggles, and gown.	These prevent contact with blood and body fluids.
9. Turn off the monitor alarms and then turn off the flow clamp to the flush solution. Carefully remove the stabilization device and/or dressing over the insertion site. Remove any sutures using the suture removal kit; make sure all sutures have been removed.	These measures help prepare for withdrawal of the catheter.
10. **Withdraw the catheter using a gentle, steady motion. Keep the catheter parallel to the blood vessel during withdrawal. Watch for hematoma formation during catheter removal by gently palpating surrounding tissue. If hematoma starts to form, reposition your hands until optimal pressure is obtained to prevent further leakage of blood.**	Using a gentle, steady motion parallel to the blood vessel helps reduce the risk for traumatic injury.
11. **Immediately after withdrawing the catheter, apply pressure over and just above the cannula site with a sterile 4 × 4 gauze pad. Maintain pressure for at least 10 minutes, or per facility policy (longer if bleeding or oozing persists). Apply additional pressure to a femoral site or if the patient has a coagulation abnormality or is receiving anticoagulants (Infusion Nurses Society [INS], 2016).**	If sufficient pressure is not applied, a large, painful hematoma may form.
12. **Assess distal pulses every 3 to 5 minutes while pressure is being applied. Note: Dorsalis pedis and posterior tibial pulses should be markedly weaker from baseline if sufficient pressure is applied to the femoral artery.**	Assessment of distal pulses determines blood flow to the extremity. Pulses should return to baseline after pressure is released.
13. Cover the site with an appropriate dressing and secure the dressing with tape. If stipulated by facility policy, make a pressure dressing for a femoral site by folding four sterile 4 × 4 gauze pads in half, and then applying the dressing.	Sufficient pressure is needed to prevent continued bleeding and hematoma formation.

ACTION

14. Cover the dressing with a tight adhesive bandage, per facility policy. Remove goggles and gloves. *If the catheter was in a femoral site,* use these additional interventions: Cover the bandage with a sandbag, depending on facility policy; maintain the patient on bed rest, with the head of the bed elevated less than 30 degrees, for 6 hours with the sandbag in place; instruct the patient not to lift his or her head while on bed rest; and use logrolling to assist the patient in using the bedpan, if needed.

15. Lower the bed height. Remove additional PPE. Perform hand hygiene. Send specimens to the laboratory immediately.

16. Observe the site for bleeding. Assess circulation in the extremity distal to the site by evaluating color, pulse, and sensation. Repeat this assessment every 15 minutes for the first 1 hour, every 30 minutes for the next 2 hours, hourly for the next 2 hours, then every 4 hours, or according to facility policy.

RATIONALE

Sufficient pressure is needed to prevent continued bleeding and hematoma formation.
Proper removal of PPE reduces the risk for infection transmission and contamination of other items.
Raising the head increases intra-abdominal pressure, which could lead to bleeding from the site.

Lowering the bed promotes patient safety. Proper removal of PPE reduces the risk for infection transmission and contamination of other items. Hand hygiene prevents transmission of microorganisms. Specimens must be processed in a timely manner to ensure accuracy.

Continued assessment allows for early detection and prompt intervention, should problems arise.

EVALUATION

The expected outcomes have been met when the patient exhibited a clean and dry arterial catheter site without evidence of injury, infection, bleeding, or hematoma; and the patient demonstrated intact peripheral circulation.

DOCUMENTATION

Guidelines

Document the time the catheter was removed and how long pressure was applied. Document assessment of peripheral circulation, appearance of site, type of dressing applied, the timed assessments, patient's response, and any medications given.

Sample Documentation

> 12/20/20 1830 Right radial arterial catheter removed per order. Pressure applied to site for 10 minutes. Site intact without signs of hematoma; radial pulse present, +2 and regular. Hand warm and dry; hand skin tone consistent with left hand. Pressure dressing applied to site. Patient denies pain, nausea, shortness of breath. Vital signs stable before, during, and after procedure. See vital signs tab.
>
> —B. Clapp, RN

UNEXPECTED SITUATIONS AND ASSOCIATED INTERVENTIONS

- *Assessment reveals fresh blood on the site dressing:* Apply pressure. If bleeding continues, notify the health care provider.
- *The patient has a history of peripheral vascular disease:* Assess the peripheral circulation for changes; if necessary, apply slightly decreased pressure at the insertion site.
- *Affected extremity is cold and/or pulseless:* Immediately notify health care provider.
- *Patient complains of severe back pain or is noted to be hypotensive:* Symptoms may be due to retroperitoneal bleeding. Notify health care provider immediately.

SPECIAL CONSIDERATIONS

- Sometimes a culture of the catheter tip is ordered to aid in identifying the source of infection. If ordered, place the catheter tip on a 4 × 4 sterile gauze pad. After the bleeding is under control and the dressing is secure, hold the catheter over the sterile container. Cut the tip of the catheter with sterile scissors and allow it to fall into the sterile container. Label the specimen and send it to the laboratory.

(continued)

Enhance Your Understanding

Focusing on Patient Care: Developing Clinical Reasoning

Consider the case scenarios at the beginning of the chapter as you answer the following questions to enhance your understanding and apply what you have learned.

QUESTIONS

1. Coby Pruder becomes visibly anxious when you bring in the ECG machine and begin to open the supplies. What could you do to help alleviate his anxiety?

2. You go in to assess Harry Stebbings and find him unresponsive. How should you respond?

3. You meet resistance while attempting to draw the discard sample from Ann Kribell's arterial catheter. Should you use excessive pressure to try to obtain the discard sample? Discuss the appropriate actions to problem solve this unexpected situation.

You can find suggested answers after the Bibliography at the end of this chapter.

Integrated Case Study Connection

The case studies in the back of the book focus on integrating concepts. Refer to the following case studies to enhance your understanding of the concepts and skills in this chapter.

- Advanced Case Studies: Cole McKean, page 1128.

Taylor Suite Resources

Explore these additional resources to enhance your learning of this chapter:

- NCLEX-Style Questions and other resources on thePoint*, http://thePoint.lww.com/Lynn5e
- *Skill Checklists for Taylor's Clinical Nursing Skills,* 5e

Bibliography

American Association of Critical-Care Nurses (AACN). (2015). *AACN practice alert. Family presence during resuscitation and invasive procedures. Critical Care Nurse, 36*(1), e11–e14.

American Association of Critical-Care Nurses (AACN). (2017). In D. L. Wiegand (Ed.). *AACN procedure manual for high acuity, progressive, and critical care* (7th ed.). St. Louis, MO: Elsevier.

American Heart Association (AHA). (2015a). *Highlights of the 2015 American Heart Association Guidelines Update for CPR and ECC.* Dallas, TX: Author. Retrieved https://eccguidelines.heart.org/wp-content/uploads/2015/10/2015-AHA-Guidelines-Highlights-English.pdf

American Heart Association (AHA). (2015b). *2015 American Heart Association Guidelines for CPR & ECC.* Retrieved https://eccguidelines.heart.org/index.php/circulation/cpr-ecc-guidelines-2

American Heart Association (AHA). (2016a). *Hands-only CPR.* Retrieved http://cpr.heart.org/AHAECC/CPRAndECC/Programs/HandsOnlyCPR/UCM_473196_Hands-Only-CPR.jsp

American Heart Association (AHA). (2016b). *Implantable cardioverter defibrillator (ICD).* Retrieved http://www.heart.org/HEARTORG/Conditions/Arrhythmia/PreventionTreatmentofArrhythmia/Implantable-Cardioverter-Defibrillator-ICD_UCM_448478_Article.jsp#.WN6CIfnyuUk

American Heart Association (AHA). (2016c). *Basic life support (BLS). Provider manual.* USA: First American Heart Association Printing.

Anderson, P., Light, P., King, J. C., et al. (2016). Cardiopulmonary resuscitation knowledge and opinions on end of life decision making of older adults admitted to an acute medical service. *New Zealand Medical Journal, 129*(1428), 26–36.

Avery, K. R., O'Brien, M., Pierce, C. D., & Gazarian, P. K. (2015). Use of a nursing checklist to facilitate implementation of therapeutic hypothermia after cardiac arrest. *Critical Care Nurse, 35*(1), 29–37.

Bell, L. (2015). Family presence during invasive procedures. *American Journal of Critical Care, 24*(6), 539.

Campbell, B., Richley, D., Ross, C., & Eggett, C. J. (2017). *Clinical guidelines by consensus: Recording a standard 12-lead electrocardiogram. An approved method by the Society for Cardiological Science and Technology (SCST).* Retrieved http://www.scst.org.uk/resources/SCST_ECG_Recording_Guidelines_2017

Castro, M. C., Cruz, M., & Briones, R. (2014). Code blue: Overcoming the fear. *Nursing, 44*(6), 65–67.

Cleveland Clinic. (n.d.). *Biventricular pacemaker.* Retrieved http://my.clevelandclinic.org/heart/services/tests/procedures/biventricular_pm.aspx

Cohen, B. J., & Hull, K. (2015). *Memmler's structure and function of the human body* (11th ed.). Philadelphia, PA: Wolters Kluwer Health.

Delac, K., Blazier, D., Daniel, L., & N-Wilfong, D. (2013). Five alive: Using mock code simulation to improve responder performance during the first 5 minutes of a code. *Critical Care Nursing Quarterly, 36*(2), 244–250.

Diaz, M. C. G. (2013). Early use of AEDs can save kids' lives. *Contemporary Pediatrics, 30*(3), 12–20.

Doenges, M. E., Moorhouse, M. F., & Murr, A. C. (2016). *Nursing diagnoses manual: Planning, individualizing, and documenting client care* (5th ed.). Philadelphia, PA: F.A. Davis Company.

Dumas, F., Rea, T. D., Fahrenbruch, C., et al. (2013). Chest compression alone cardiopulmonary resuscitation is associated with better long-term survival compared with standard cardiopulmonary resuscitation. *Circulation, 127*(4), 435–441.

Emergency Nurses Association (ENA), ENA Emergency Nursing Resources Development Committee. (2009; Revised 2012, December). *Clinical practice guideline. Family presence during invasive procedures and resuscitation.* Retrieved https://www.ena.org/docs/default-source/resource-library/practice-resources/cpg/familypresencecpg3eaabb7cf0414584ac2291feba3be481.pdf?sfvrsn=9c167fc6_12

Frimpong, A., Caguioa, J., & Octavo, G. (2015). Promoting safe IV management in practice using H.A.N.D.S. *British Journal of Nursing (Mark Allen Publishing), 24*(2), S18, S20–S23.

Garcia, T. (2015). Acquiring the 12-lead electrocardiogram: Doing it right every time. *Journal of Emergency Nursing, 41*(6), 474–478.

Grossman, S., & Porth, C. M. (2014). *Porth's pathophysiology: Concepts of altered health states* (9th ed.). Philadelphia, PA: Wolters Kluwer Health.

Hanlon, P. (2016). Resuscitation: Access to AEDs a major challenge. *RT: The Journal for Respiratory Care Practitioners, 29*(10), 28–32.

Harper, D. (2014). Infusion therapy: Much more than a simple task. *Nursing, 44*(7), 66–67.

Hassankhani, H., Zamanzadeh, V., Rahmani, A., Haririan, H., & Porter, J. E. (2017). Family presence during resuscitation: A double-edged sword. *Journal of Nursing Scholarship, 49*(2), 127–134.

Hazinski, M. F., Nolan, J. P., Bhanji, F., et al. (2015). Part 1: Executive Summary: 2015 International consensus on cardiopulmonary resuscitation and emergency cardiovascular care science with treatment recommendations. *Circulation, 132*(16 Suppl 1), S2–S39.

Hinkle, J. L., & Cheever, K. H. (2018). *Brunner & Suddarth's textbook of medical-surgical nursing* (14th ed.). Philadelphia, PA: Wolters Kluwer.

Hogan-Quigley, B., Palm, M. L., & Bickley, L. (2017). *Bates' nursing guide to physical examination and history taking* (2nd ed.). Philadelphia, PA: Wolters Kluwer.

Infusion Nurses Society (INS). (2016). *Policies and procedures for infusion therapy* (5th ed.). Norwood, MA: Author.

Jarvis, C. (2016). *Physical examination and health assessment* (7th ed.). St. Louis, MO: Elsevier.

Jeejeebhoy, F. M., Zelop, C. M., Lipman, S., et al. (2015). Cardiac arrest in pregnancy. A scientific statement from the American Heart Association. *Circulation, 132*(18), 1747–1773.

Jensen, S. (2015). *Nursing health assessment: A best practice approach* (2nd ed.). Philadelphia, PA: Wolters Kluwer.

Jevon, P. (2010). Procedure for recording a standard 12-lead electrocardiogram. *British Journal of Nursing (Mark Allen Publishing), 19*(10), 649–651.

Knapp, R. (Ed.). (2016). *Hemodynamic monitoring made incredibly easy* (3rd ed.). Philadelphia, PA: Wolters Kluwer.

Kyle, T., & Carman, S. (2017). *Essentials of pediatric nursing* (3rd ed.). Philadelphia, PA: Wolters Kluwer.

LeMone, P., Burke, K. M., Bauldoff, G., & Gubrud, P. (2015). *Medical-surgical nursing: Clinical reasoning in patient care* (6th ed.). New York: Pearson.

Loveday, H. P., Wilson, J. A., Pratt, R. J., et al. (2014). Epic3: National evidence-based guidelines for preventing healthcare-associated infections in NHS hospitals in England. *The Journal of Hospital Infection, 86*(Suppl 1), S1–S70.

McAlvin, S. S., & Carew-Lyons, A. (2014). Family presence during resuscitation and invasive procedures in pediatric critical care: A systematic review. *American Journal of Critical Care, 23*(6), 477–484.

McLaughlin, M. A. (Ed.). (2014). *Cardiovascular care made incredibly easy* (3rd ed.). Philadelphia, PA: Wolters Kluwer.

Morton, P. G., & Fontaine, D. K. (2018). Essentials of *critical care nursing: A holistic approach* (11th ed.). Philadelphia, PA: Wolters Kluwer.

Mpotos, N., Decaluwe, K., Van Belleghem, V., et al. (2015). Automated testing combined with automated retraining to improve CPR skill level in emergency nurses. *Nurse Education in Practice, 15*(3), 212–217.

NANDA International, Inc.: *Nursing diagnoses–Definitions and classification 2018–2020* © 2017 NANDA International, ISBN 978-1-62623-929-6. Used by arrangement with the Thieme Group, Stuttgart/New York.

National Heart, Lung, and Blood Institute (NHLBI). (2012). *Pacemakers: What is a pacemaker?* Retrieved

https://www.nhlbi.nih.gov/health/health-topics/topics/pace

Oermann, M. H., Kardong-Edgren, S. E., & Odom-Maryon, T. (2012). Competence in CPR. *The American Journal of Nursing, 112*(5), 43–46.

O'Grady, N. P., Alexander, M., Burns, L. A., et al; Healthcare Infection Control Practices Advisory Committee (HICPAC). (2011). Guidelines for the prevention of intravascular catheter-related infections, 2011. *American Journal of Infection Control, 39*(4 Suppl), S1–S34. Retrieved http://www.cdc.gov/hicpac/BSI/BSI-guidelines-2011.html

Pankop, R., Chang, K., Thorlton, J., & Spitzer, T. (2013). Implemented family presence protocols: An integrative review. *Journal of Nursing Care Quality, 28*(3), 281–288.

Perkins, G. D., Travers, A. H., Berg, R. A., et al; Basic Life Support Chapter Collaborators. (2015). Part 3: Adult basic life support and automated external defibrillation: 2015 International Consensus on Cardiopulmonary Resuscitation and Emergency Cardiovascular Care Science with Treatment Recommendations. *Resuscitation, 95*, e43–e69.

Perry, S. E., Hockenberry, M. J., Lowdermilk, D. L., & Wilson, D. (2014). *Maternal child nursing care* (5th ed.). St. Louis, MO: Elsevier.

Powers, K. A. (2017). Educational interventions to improve support for family presence during resuscitation: A systematic review of the literature. *Dimensions of Critical Care Nursing, 36*(2), 125–138.

Richley, D. (2016). Understanding how to interpret ECGs in primary care. *Practice Nursing, 27*(3), 136–139.

Stout, K. (Ed.). (2017). *ACLS review made incredibly easy* (3rd ed.). Philadelphia, PA: Wolters Kluwer.

Taylor, C., Lynn, P., & Bartlett, J. (2019). *Fundamentals of nursing: The art and science of person-centered care* (9th ed.). Philadelphia, PA: Wolters Kluwer.

The Society for Cardiological Science & Technology (SCST). (2010). *Clinical guidelines by consensus: Recording a standard 12-lead electrocardiogram. An approved methodology.* Retrieved https://www.bcs.com/documents/consensus_guidelines.pdf

Twibell, R. S., Craig, S., Siela, D., Simmonds, S., & Thomas, C. (2015). Being there: Inpatients' perceptions of family presence during resuscitation and invasive cardiac procedures. *American Journal of Critical Care, 24*(6), e108–e115.

Van Leeuwen, A. M., & Bladh, M. L. (2017). *Davis's comprehensive handbook of laboratory & diagnostic tests with nursing implications* (7th ed.). Philadelphia, PA: F.A. Davis Company.

VHA Center for Engineering & Occupational Safety and Health (CEOSH). (2016). *Safe patient handling and mobility guidebook.* St. Louis, MO: Author. Retrieved http://www.tampavaref.org/safe-patient-handling.htm

Walsh-Irwin, C., & Jurgens, C. Y. (2015). Proper skin preparation and electrode placement decreases alarms on a telemetry unit. *Dimensions of Critical Care Nursing, 34*(3), 134–139.

SUGGESTED ANSWERS FOR FOCUSING ON PATIENT CARE: DEVELOPING CLINICAL REASONING

1. Explain the steps involved in obtaining an ECG. Tell Mr. Pruder that the test records the heart's electrical activity, and it may be repeated at certain intervals. Emphasize that no electrical current will enter his body and that the ECG will provide important information to help guide his health care. Tell him the test typically takes about 5 minutes.

2. Call for help, pull call bell, and call the facility emergency response number. Call for the automated external defibrillator (AED). Put on gloves, if available. Position Mr. Stebbings supine on his back on a firm, flat surface, with arms alongside the body. If he is in bed, place a backboard or other rigid surface under him (often the footboard of the patient's bed). Initiate CPR. Provide defibrillation as soon as an AED becomes available.

3. Do not use excessive pressure. Ask Ms. Kribell to reposition the affected extremity. Check the insertion site for obvious problems (e.g., catheter kinking). Attempt to obtain the sample to be discarded. If resistance is still felt, notify the primary care provider.

Neurologic Care

Focusing on Patient Care

This chapter will help you develop some of the skills related to neurologic care necessary for the following patients:

Aleta Jackson, age 68, was involved in a head-on collision. She has been prescribed and will be discharged with a cervical collar to stabilize her neck.

Yuka Chong, age 7, was recently diagnosed with epilepsy, and has arrived at the clinic for a follow-up visit. Her mothers have a lot of questions and concerns about how to react when Yuka has a seizure.

Nikki Gladstone, age 19, is in your intensive care unit following surgery related to a cranial malignancy. She has an external ventriculostomy device in place to monitor intracranial pressure.

Refer to Focusing on Patient Care: Developing Clinical Reasoning at the end of the chapter to apply what you learn.

Learning Objectives

After completing the chapter, you will be able to accomplish the following:

1. Apply a two-piece cervical collar.
2. Implement seizure precautions and seizure management.
3. Care for patient in halo traction.
4. Care for a patient with an external ventriculostomy device.
5. Care for a patient with a fiberoptic intracranial catheter.

Key Terms

aura: a premonitory or warning sensation of a seizure that can be visual, auditory, or olfactory

cerebral perfusion pressure (CPP): a way of calculating cerebral blood flow; the formula is mean arterial pressure (MAP) minus intracranial pressure (ICP) equals CPP; normal CPP for an adult is 50 to 70 mm Hg (Hickey, 2014)

coma: a pathologic state of unconsciousness characterized by an unarousable sleeplike state; eyes closed at all times; no speech or sound noted; no spontaneous movement of extremities (Hickey, 2014)

consciousness: the degree of wakefulness or ability to be aroused

decerebrate: abnormal body posture associated with severe brain injury; involves muscle tightening and rigidity; the arms and legs are held straight out, the toes are pointed downward, and the head and neck are arched backward

decorticate: abnormal body posture associated with severe brain injury; involves stiffness of the extremities; the arms are bent in toward the body, fists clenched, wrists are bent and held on the chest, and legs held out straight

intracranial compliance: the potential expandability of the brain; the ability of the brain to tolerate stimulation or an increase in intracranial volume without corresponding increase in pressure (Hickey, 2014; Morton & Fontaine, 2018)

intracranial pressure (ICP): pressure within the cranial vault; normal ICP is less than 15 mm Hg (Hickey, 2014)

seizure: temporary alteration in brain function due to abnormal electrical discharges of neurons in the brain that may result in uncontrolled body movements or a convulsion and alteration of consciousness (Hickey, 2014)

ventriculostomy: a catheter inserted through a hole made in the skull into the ventricular system of the brain; can be used to monitor ICP and/or drain cerebrospinal fluid

Many patients experience injury to the head, neck, or spinal column. In addition, numerous disorders, such as infections and tumors, can affect the brain and spinal cord, interfering with neurologic function. Specialized devices may be used to monitor and control ICP. Meticulous care is needed after injury or trauma to ensure that further injury does not occur. This chapter covers skills to assist the nurse in providing neurologic care. Behavioral scales are used to standardize observations for the objective and accurate assessment of level of **consciousness** (LOC) and monitor changes related to neurologic injury and **coma** (Hickey, 2014). The Glasgow Coma Scale (GCS) and the Full Outline of UnResponsiveness (FOUR) score are examples of two tools used to evaluate LOC. The FOUR score addresses many limitations that have been identified with the GCS, allowing more precise assessment of the extent of brainstem function, through eye response, motor response, brainstem reflexes, and respiratory pattern and drive (Hickey; Kocak, Ozturk, Ege, & Ekmekci, 2012). The FOUR score scale is very useful in evaluating patients who are endotracheally intubated (Czaikowski, Liang, & Stewart, 2014; Johnson & Whitcomb, 2013; Mink, 2012). Fundamentals Review 17-1 reviews a simple neurologic exam. Refer to Fundamentals Review 17-2 and Fundamentals Review 17-3 for the GCS and the FOUR Score assessment tools. Refer to Chapter 3 for a review of other components of a neurologic assessment.

Fundamentals Review 17-1

NEUROLOGIC EXAM

By assessing the patient's appearance and verbal and physical responses, you can obtain important information about the patient's neurologic status, including:

- Is it unchanged/changed from baseline?
- Has the patient developed changes that may indicate a problem with the nervous system?
- Are there symptoms that need further investigation?

This basic examination can be used during every patient encounter. Refer to Chapter 3 for details related to other components of a neurologic assessment.

What?	How?	Why?
<ul><li>Assess level of consciousness, cognition, position, posture, facial symmetry, respiratory pattern.</li><li>Assess ability to speak at normal conversational volume.</li><li>Identify external forces (e.g., medications, other injuries, or altered laboratory values) that may affect the patient's responses during the assessment.</li><li>Identify abnormalities that existed before the patient's current health problem (Mink, 2012).</li></ul>	Does the patient:<ul><li>Wake up easily?</li><li>Hear introduction and question?</li><li>Open both eyes and keep them open?</li><li>Pay attention to you and remain awake and alert?</li><li>Demonstrate behavior appropriate for situation?</li><li>Track you with head and eye movements as you move around room?</li><li>Speak clearly?</li><li>Provide appropriate responses?</li><li>Demonstrate symmetry of movement in extremities?</li></ul>	<ul><li>Alertness, attention, arousal: Assesses reticular activating system, hypothalamus, and thalamus</li><li>Interpretation of what is heard and responds appropriately: Assesses cerebral cortex</li><li>Motor function: Assesses corticospinal motor pathway and basal ganglia system</li><li>Clear, organized, and appropriate speech: Assesses motor speech and language centers in left cerebral hemisphere</li></ul>

Source: Adapted from Hickey, J. (2014). *The clinical practice of neurological and neurosurgical nursing* (7th ed.). Philadelphia, PA: Wolters Kluwer; McCallum, C., & Leonard, M. (2013). The connection between neurosciences and dialysis: A quick neurological assessment for hemodialysis nurses. *CANNT Journal, 23*(3), 20–26; and Mink, J. (2012). The neurologic assessment toolbox: Key assessments at critical times. *Nursing2012CriticalCare, 7*(3), 12–17.

Fundamentals Review 17-2

GLASGOW COMA SCALE

The Glasgow Coma Scale (GCS) evaluates three key categories of behavior that most closely reflect activity in the higher centers of the brain: eye opening, verbal response, and motor response. Within each category, each level of response is given a numerical value. The maximal score is 15, indicating a fully awake, alert, and oriented patient; the lowest score is 3, indicating deep coma (Hickey, 2014). The GCS is used in conjunction with other neurologic assessments, including pupillary reaction and vital sign measurement, to evaluate a patient's status.

Component	Score	Response
Eye opening	4	Opens eyes spontaneously when someone approaches
	3	Opens eyes in response to speech (normal tone or shouting)
	2	Opens eyes only to painful stimuli (apply pressure with a pen to the lateral outer aspect of the second or third finger, up to 10 seconds, then release)
	1	No response to painful stimuli
Best motor response	6	Accurately responds to instructions; obeys a simple command, such as "Lift your left hand off the bed"
	5	Localizes (moves hand to point of stimulation) to painful stimuli and attempts to remove source
	4	Flexion reflex action, but unable to locate the source of pain; purposeless movement in response to pain
	3	Flexes elbows and wrists while extending lower legs to pain; **decorticate** posturing
	2	Extends upper and lower extremities to pain; **decerebrate** posturing
	1	No motor response to pain on any limb
Best verbal response	5	Converses; oriented to time, place, and person
	4	Converses; disoriented to time, place, or person; any one or all indicators
	3	Converses only in words or phrases that make little sense in the context of the questions
	2	Responds with incomprehensible sounds; no understandable words and/or moaning, groaning, or crying in response to painful stimuli
	1	No response

Source: Adapted from Hickey, J. (2014). *The clinical practice of neurological and neurosurgical nursing* (7th ed.). Philadelphia, PA: Wolters Kluwer; Okamura, K. (2014). Glasgow Coma Scale flow chart: A beginner's guide. *British Journal of Nursing (Mark Allen Publishing)*, *23*(20), 1068–1073; and Teasdale, G., & Jennett, B. (1974). Assessment of coma and impaired consciousness. A practical scale. *Lancet*, *2*(7872), 81–84.

Fundamentals Review 17-3

THE FULL OUTLINE OF UNRESPONSIVENESS (FOUR)

Researchers at the Mayo Clinic designed the FOUR score coma scale, which has been proposed as an alternative to the Glasgow Coma Scale (GCS). The FOUR score assigns a value of 0 to 4 to each of four functional categories: eye response, motor response, brainstem reflexes, and respiration. In each of these categories, a score of 0 indicates nonfunctioning status, and a score of 4 represents normal functioning. The FOUR score may provide greater neurologic detail than the GCS due to its ability to evaluate brainstem reflexes and to recognize changes in breathing patterns and stages of brain herniation (Hickey, 2014; Kocak et al., 2012). The FOUR score is used in conjunction with other neurologic assessments and vital sign measurement to evaluate a patient's status.

Ec1316227-013-0

D.F. © MAYO 2008

Eye response (E):	E4 = eyelids open or opened, tracking or blinking to command
	E3 = eyelids open, but not tracking
	E2 = eyelids closed, but open to loud voice
	E1 = eyelids closed, but open to pain
Motor response (M):	M4 = demonstrated thumbs-up, fist, or peach sign to command
	M3 = localizing to pain
	M2 = flexion response to pain
	M1 = extensor posturing
	M0 = no response to pain or generalized myoclonus status epilepticus (prolonged repetitive epileptic myoclonic [involuntary twitching of a muscle] activity)
Brainstem reflexes (B):	B4 = pupil and corneal reflexes present
	B3 = one pupil wide and fixed
	B2 = pupil or corneal reflexes absent
	B1 = pupil and corneal reflexes absent
	B0 = absent pupil, corneal, and cough reflex
Respiration (R):	R4 = not intubated, regular breathing
	R3 = not intubated, Cheyne–Stokes breathing pattern
	R2 = not intubated, irregular breathing pattern
	R1 = breathes above ventilator rate
	R0 = breathes at ventilator rate or apnea

Skill 17-1 ▶ Applying a Two-Piece Cervical Collar

Patients suspected of having injuries to the cervical spine are often immobilized with a cervical collar to stabilize the neck and prevent further damage to the spinal cord. A cervical collar maintains the neck in a straight line, with the chin slightly elevated and tucked inward. The collar is removed as soon as is feasible after radiological clearance (Montgomery & Goode, 2014). Cervical collars may also be used to support the weight of the head and limit cervical motion as part of nonpharmacologic management of pain associated with degeneration in rheumatic disorders (Figure 1) (Hinkle & Cheever, 2018). Care must be taken, when applying the collar, not to hyperflex or hyperextend the patient's neck.

FIGURE 1. Cervical collar in place.

DELEGATION CONSIDERATIONS

Application of a cervical collar is not delegated to nursing assistive personnel (NAP) or to unlicensed assistive personnel (UAP). Depending on the state's nurse practice act and the organization's policies and procedures, application of a cervical collar may be delegated to licensed practical/vocational nurses (LPN/LVNs). The decision to delegate must be based on careful analysis of the patient's needs and circumstances, as well as the qualifications of the person to whom the task is being delegated. Refer to the Delegation Guidelines in Appendix A.

EQUIPMENT

- Nonsterile gloves
- Additional PPE, as indicated
- Tape measure
- Cervical collar of appropriate size
- Washcloth
- Disposable skin cleansing wipes or skin cleanser and water
- Towel

ASSESSMENT

Perform a neurologic assessment (see Fundamentals Review 17-1 and Chapter 3). Assess the patient's level of consciousness and ability to follow commands to determine any neurologic dysfunction.

If application of the cervical collar is in response to trauma or injury, assess for a patent airway. If airway is occluded, try repositioning using the jaw-thrust–chin lift method, which helps open the airway without moving the patient's neck. Inspect and palpate the cervical spine area for

(*continued*)

Skill 17-1 ▶ Applying a Two-Piece Cervical Collar *(continued)*

tenderness, swelling, deformities, or crepitus. Do not ask the patient to move the neck if a cervical spinal cord injury is suspected. If the patient is able to follow commands, instruct him or her not to move the head or neck. Have a second person stabilize the cervical spine by holding the patient's head firmly on either side directly above the ears.

NURSING DIAGNOSIS	Determine the related factors for the nursing diagnoses based on the patient's current status. Appropriate nursing diagnoses may include:

- Risk for injury
- Acute pain

OUTCOME IDENTIFICATION AND PLANNING	The expected outcome is that the patient's cervical spine is immobilized. Other outcomes that may be appropriate include the following: prevention of further injury to the spinal cord; the patient maintains head and neck without movement; the patient experiences minimal to no pain; and the patient demonstrates an understanding about the need for immobilization.

IMPLEMENTATION

ACTION	RATIONALE
1. Review the medical record and nursing care plan to determine the need for placement of a cervical collar. Identify any movement limitations. Gather the necessary supplies.	Reviewing the record and care plan validates the correct patient and correct procedure. Identification of limitations prevents injury. Assembling equipment provides for an organized approach to the task.
2. Perform hand hygiene and put on PPE, if indicated.	Hand hygiene and PPE prevent the spread of microorganisms. PPE is required based on transmission precautions.
3. Identify the patient.	Identifying the patient ensures the right patient receives the intervention and helps prevent errors.
4. Assemble equipment to the bedside stand or overbed table or other surface within reach.	Arranging items nearby is convenient, saves time, and avoids unnecessary stretching and twisting of muscles on the part of the nurse.
5. Close curtains around the bed and close the door to the room, if possible. Explain what you are going to do and why you are going to do it to the patient.	This ensures the patient's privacy. Explanation relieves anxiety and facilitates cooperation.
6. Assess the patient for any changes in neurologic status (see Fundamentals Review 17-1 and Chapter 3 for assessment details).	Patients with cervical spine injuries are at risk for problems with the neurologic system.
7. Place the bed at an appropriate and comfortable working height, usually elbow height of the caregiver (VHACEOSH, 2016). Lower the side rails as necessary.	Having the bed at the proper height and lowering the rails prevent back and muscle strain.
8. Gently clean the patient's face and neck with a skin cleanser and water. If the patient has experienced trauma, inspect the area for broken glass or other material that could cut the patient or the nurse. Pat the area dry.	Blood, glass, leaves, and twigs may be present on the patient's neck. The area should be clean before applying the cervical collar to prevent skin breakdown.
9. If the patient has experienced trauma or injury, have a second caregiver in position to hold the patient's head firmly on either side above the ears. Measure from the bottom of the chin to the top of the sternum, and measure around the neck. Match these height and circumference measurements to the manufacturer's recommended size chart.	This action stabilizes the cervical spine by holding the head firmly on either side above the ears. To immobilize the cervical spine and to prevent skin breakdown under the collar, the correct collar size must be used (Cooper, 2013).

ACTION	RATIONALE
10. Slide the flattened back portion of the collar under the patient's head (Figure 2). **The center of the collar should line up with the center of the patient's neck. Do not allow the patient's head to move when passing the collar under the head.**	Stabilizing the cervical spine is crucial to prevent the head from moving, which could cause further damage to the cervical spine. Placing the collar in the center ensures that the neck is aligned properly.
11. Place the front of the collar centered over the chin, while ensuring that the chin area fits snugly in the recess. Be sure that the front half of the collar overlaps the back half. Secure Velcro straps on both sides (Figure 3). Check to see that at least one finger can be inserted between collar and patient's neck.	The collar should fit snugly to prevent the patient from moving the neck and causing further damage to the cervical spine. Velcro will help hold the collar securely in place. Collar should not be too tight to cause discomfort.

FIGURE 2. Sliding the flattened back portion of the collar under the patient's head.

FIGURE 3. Securing the front and back halves of the cervical collar.

ACTION	RATIONALE
12. Raise the side rails. Place the bed in lowest position. Make sure the call bell is in reach.	Bed in lowest position and access to call bell contribute to patient safety.
13. Reassess the patient's neurologic status and comfort level.	Reassessment helps to evaluate the effects of movement on the patient.
14. Remove PPE, if used. Perform hand hygiene.	Proper removal of PPE reduces the risk for infection transmission and contamination of other items. Hand hygiene prevents transmission of microorganisms.
15. **Assess the skin under the cervical collar and at contact points on the chin, shoulder, and ear at least every 4 hours for any signs of skin breakdown. Remove the collar every 8 to 12 hours and inspect and cleanse the skin under the collar, drying well before replacement. When the collar is removed, if the patient has experienced trauma or injury, have a second person immobilize the cervical spine.**	Skin breakdown may occur under the cervical collar and at contact points. The neck is particularly prone to sweating, necessitating cleansing of the skin and thorough drying, to prevent increased risk of skin breakdown (Cooper, 2013).

EVALUATION

The expected outcomes have been met when the cervical collar has been placed without adverse effect and the patient's cervical spine has been immobilized without further injury; the patient maintained head and neck without movement; and the patient demonstrated an understanding of the rationale for cervical spine immobilization.

(continued)

Skill 17-1 ▶ Applying a Two-Piece Cervical Collar (continued)

DOCUMENTATION

Guidelines

Document the application of the collar, including size and any skin care necessary before the application, condition of skin under the cervical collar and at pressure points, patient's pain level, and neurologic and any other assessment findings.

Sample Documentation

> <u>11/22/20</u> 0900 Patient arrived on unit; cervical spine immobilized; medium cervical collar applied. Patient awake, alert, and oriented. Admits to right neck pain; denies other pain. See flow sheet for neurologic assessment. Skin pink, warm, and dry. A 3-cm laceration noted on R anterior side of neck. Wound cleansed and antibiotic ointment applied. Patient instructed to refrain from moving without assistance; call bell placed in right hand.
>
> —B. Clapp, RN

UNEXPECTED SITUATIONS AND ASSOCIATED INTERVENTIONS

- *The height and neck circumference measurements are between two sizes:* Start with the smaller size. If the collar is too large, the neck may not be immobilized.
- *Skin breakdown is noted on the shoulder, neck, or ear:* Apply a protective dressing over the area and continue to assess for further skin breakdown. Assess for continued need for the application of the collar (Cooper, 2013).
- *Patient complains that the collar is "choking" him:* If not contraindicated, place the patient in the reverse Trendelenburg position to see if this helps. Elevation of the upper body lessens pressure on the head and neck from the collar. Assess the tightness of the cervical collar; at least one finger should slide under the collar.
- *Patient is able to move head from side to side with cervical collar on:* Tighten the cervical collar, if possible. If the collar is as tight as possible, apply a collar one size smaller and evaluate for a better fit.

SPECIAL CONSIDERATIONS

- Cervical collar-related pressure injuries may develop on the occiput, chin, ears, mandible, suprascapular area, and over the larynx. Padded collars may prevent pressure injury development if used appropriately (Ackland et al., 2007, as cited in Cooper, 2013).
- If collar has removable inner pads, obtain an extra set of pads to remove and replace pads to allow for cleansing and complete drying of soiled pads (Cooper, 2013). Change and wash the pads every 24 hours and as needed (Cooper, 2013).

EVIDENCE FOR PRACTICE ▶

EVIDENCE-BASED PRACTICE GUIDELINE: PREVENTING PRESSURE INJURIES

Cooper, K. L. (2013). Evidence-based prevention of pressure ulcers in the intensive care unit. *CriticalCareNurse, 33*(6), 57–66.

Patients with critical health problems in intensive care units have multiple factors that increase the risk of the development of pressure injuries. The use of devices such as cervical collars increases the risk for development of pressure injuries at various contact points. The development of stage III or IV ulcers is considered a never event (Patient Safety Network, n.d.). This evidence-based practice review discusses the multiple risk factors present in critical care for the development of pressure injuries, current practices, and evidence for interventions aimed at preventing pressure injuries, including those related to the use of cervical collars.

Patient Safety Network. (n.d.). *Never events.* Retrieved https://psnet.ahrq.gov/primers/primer/3/never-events.

Refer to thePoint® for additional research on related nursing topics.

Skill 17-2 ▶ Employing Seizure Precautions and Seizure Management

Seizures occur when the electrical system of the brain malfunctions. Sudden abnormal and excessive discharge from cerebral neurons results in episodes of abnormal motor, sensory, autonomic, or psychic activity, or a combination of these (Hickey, 2014). A **seizure** manifests as an alteration in sensation, behavior, movement, perception, or consciousness that may be barely noticeable to abnormal, involuntary contractions and rapid shaking (convulsion) with loss of consciousness (Centers for Disease Control and Prevention [CDC], 2014; Hinkle & Cheever, 2018).

During a seizure, patients are at risk for hypoxia, vomiting, and pulmonary aspiration. Patients who are at risk for seizures and those who have had a seizure(s) are often placed under seizure precautions to minimize the risk of physical injury. Causes of seizures include cerebrovascular disease, hypoxemia, head injury, hypertension, central nervous system infections, metabolic and toxic conditions, brain tumor, drug and alcohol withdrawal, allergies, and a history of epilepsy (seizure disorder) (Hinkle & Cheever, 2018). Seizure management includes interventions by the nurse to prevent aspiration, protect the patient from injury, provide care after the seizure, and observe and document the details of the event (Hickey, 2014; Hinkle & Cheever, 2018). Figure 1 illustrates nursing measures to protect the patient from injury.

FIGURE 1. Protecting patient from injury. (Hinkle, J. L., & Cheever, K. H. (2018). *Brunner & Suddarth's textbook of medical-surgical nursing* (14th ed.). Philadelphia, PA: Wolters Kluwer; and adapted from American Association of Neuroscience Nurses [AANN]. [2016]. *Care of adults and children with seizures and epilepsy: AANN clinical practice guideline series.* Chicago, IL: Author.)

DELEGATION CONSIDERATIONS	The implementation of seizure precautions may be delegated to nursing assistive personnel (NAP) or to unlicensed assistive personnel (UAP). The implementation of seizure management may not be delegated to nursing assistive personnel (NAP) or to unlicensed assistive personnel (UAP). Implementation of seizure precautions as well as seizure management may be delegated to licensed practical/vocational nurses (LPN/LVNs). The decision to delegate must be based on careful analysis of the patient's needs and circumstances, as well as the qualifications of the person to whom the task is being delegated. Refer to the Delegation Guidelines in Appendix A.

(continued)

Skill 17-2 ▶ Employing Seizure Precautions and Seizure Management *(continued)*

EQUIPMENT	• PPE, as indicated
	• Portable or wall suction unit with tubing
	• A commercially prepared suction kit with an appropriate size catheter or:
	  • Sterile suction catheter with Y-port of the appropriate size (adult: 10 to 16 Fr)
	  • Sterile disposable container
	  • Sterile gloves
	• Oral airway
	• Bed rail padding
	• Oxygen apparatus
	• Nasal cannula or mask to deliver oxygen
	• Handheld bag valve/resuscitation bag

ASSESSMENT	Assess for pre-existing conditions that increase the patient's risk for seizure activity. For example, assess for a history of seizure disorder or epilepsy, cerebrovascular disease, hypoxemia, head injury, hypertension, central nervous system infections, metabolic conditions (e.g., renal failure, hypocalcemia, hypoglycemia), brain tumor, drug/alcohol withdrawal, or allergies. Assess circumstances before the seizure, such as visual, auditory, or olfactory stimuli, tactile stimuli, emotional or psychological disturbances, sleep, or hyperventilation. Assess for the occurrence of an **aura**. Note where the movements or stiffness begin; and the gaze position and position of the head when the seizure begins. Assess the body part(s) and the type of movement(s) involved in the seizure. Assess pupil sizes; if eyes remained open during seizure; and whether eyes or head turned to one side. Assess for the presence or absence of repeated involuntary motor activity (e.g., repeated swallowing); incontinence of urine or stool; duration of seizure; presence of unconsciousness and duration; obvious paralysis or weakness of arms or legs after seizure; and inability to speak, movements, sleeping, and/or confusion after seizure. Assess the patient's neurologic status (refer to Fundamentals Review 17-1 and Chapter 3) and for injury after the seizure is over.
NURSING DIAGNOSIS	Determine the related factors for the nursing diagnoses based on the patient's current health status. Appropriate nursing diagnoses may include: • Risk for injury • Deficient knowledge • Risk for aspiration
OUTCOME IDENTIFICATION AND PLANNING	The expected outcome to achieve when implementing seizure precautions and seizure management is that the patient remains free from injury and that the sequence of signs and symptoms is observed and recorded. Other specific outcomes will be formulated depending on the identified nursing diagnosis.

IMPLEMENTATION

ACTION	**RATIONALE**
1. Review the health record and nursing care plan for conditions that would place the patient at risk for seizures. Review the medical orders and the nursing care plan for orders for seizure precautions.	Reviewing the order and care plan validates the correct patient and correct procedure.
Seizure Precautions	
2. Gather the necessary supplies.	Preparation promotes efficient time management and an organized approach to the task.
3. Perform hand hygiene and put on PPE, if indicated.	Hand hygiene and PPE prevent the spread of microorganisms. PPE is required based on transmission precautions.
4. Identify the patient.	Identifying the patient ensures the right patient receives the intervention and helps prevent errors.

ACTION	**RATIONALE**
5. Assemble equipment to the bedside stand or overbed table or other surface within reach.	Arranging items nearby is convenient, saves time, and avoids unnecessary stretching and twisting of muscles on the part of the nurse.
6. Close curtains around the bed and close the door to the room, if possible. Explain what you are going to do and why you are going to do it to the patient.	This ensures the patient's privacy. Explanation relieves anxiety and facilitates cooperation.
7. Place the bed in the lowest position with two to three side rails elevated. Apply padding to the side rails.	Bed in lowest position promotes safety and decreases risk of injury. Rail padding decreases the risk of injury.
8. Attach oxygen apparatus to oxygen access in the wall at the head of the bed. Place nasal cannula or mask equipment in a location where it can be easily reached, if needed.	During a seizure, patients are at risk for hypoxia, vomiting, and pulmonary aspiration. Ready access ensures availability of oxygen in the event of a seizure.
9. Attach suction apparatus to vacuum access in the wall at the head of the bed. Place suction catheter, oral airway, and resuscitation bag in a location where they are easily reached, if needed.	During a seizure, patients are at risk for hypoxia, vomiting, and pulmonary aspiration. Ready access ensures availability of suction in the event of a seizure. Oral airway and resuscitation bag ensure availability of emergency ventilation in the event of respiratory arrest.
10. Remove PPE, if used. Perform hand hygiene.	Proper removal of PPE reduces the risk for infection transmission and contamination of other items. Hand hygiene prevents the spread of microorganisms.

Seizure Management

11. For patients with known seizures, be alert for the occurrence of an aura, if known. If the patient reports experiencing an aura, have the patient lie down.	Some patients report a warning or premonition before seizures occur; an aura can be a visual, auditory, or olfactory sensation that indicates a seizure is going to occur. Lying down prevents injury that might occur if the patient falls to the floor.
12. Once a seizure begins, close the curtains around the bed and close the door to the room, if possible.	Closing the door or curtain provides for patient privacy.
13. If the patient is seated, ease the patient to the floor.	Getting the patient to the floor prevents injury that might occur if the patient falls to the floor.
14. Remove patient's eyeglasses. Loosen any constricting clothing. Place something flat and soft, such as a folded blanket, under the head. Push aside furniture or other objects in area.	Removing objects and loosening clothing prevent possible injury. Blanket prevents injury from striking a hard surface (floor).
15. If the patient is in bed, remove the pillow, place bed in lowest position, and raise side rails.	Prevents injury.
16. Do not restrain patient. Guide movements, if necessary. Do not try to insert anything in the patient's mouth or open jaws.	Guiding movements prevents injury. Restraint can injure the patient. Attempting to open the mouth and/or insert anything into the mouth can result in broken teeth, and injury to mouth, lips, or tongue.
17. If possible, place patient on the side with the head flexed forward, head of bed elevated 30 degrees. Begin administration of oxygen, based on facility policy. Clear airway using suction, as appropriate (refer to Skill 14-5 in Chapter 14).	During a seizure, patients are at risk for hypoxia, vomiting, and pulmonary aspiration. This position allows the tongue to fall forward, and facilitates drainage of saliva and mucus and minimizes risk for aspiration. Oxygen supports the increased metabolism associated with neurologic and muscular hyperactivity. Patent airway is necessary to support ventilation.
18. Provide supervision throughout the seizure and time the length of the seizure.	Supervision of the patient ensures safety. Timing of event contributes to accurate information and documentation.
19. Establish/maintain intravenous access, as necessary. Administer medications, as appropriate, based on medical order and facility policy.	Pharmacologic therapy may be appropriate, based on patient history and medical diagnoses. Intravenous access is necessary to administer emergency medications.

(continued)

Skill 17-2 ▶ Employing Seizure Precautions and Seizure Management *(continued)*

ACTION	RATIONALE
20. After the seizure, place the patient in a side-lying position. Clear airway using suction, as appropriate.	Side-lying position facilitates drainage of secretions. Patent airway is necessary to support ventilation.
21. Monitor vital signs, oxygen saturation, response to medications administered, and capillary glucose, as appropriate.	Monitoring of parameters provides information for accurate assessment of patient status.
22. Place the bed in the lowest position. Make sure the call bell is in reach.	Bed in lowest position and access to call bell contribute to patient safety.
23. Reassess the patient's neurologic status and comfort level.	Reassessment helps to evaluate the effects of the event on the patient.
24. Allow the patient to sleep after the seizure. On awakening, orient and reassure the patient. Reassess, as indicated.	The patient will probably experience an inability to recall the seizure; patients may also experience confusion, anxiety, embarrassment, and/or fatigue after a seizure. Reassessment helps to evaluate the effects of the event on the patient.
25. Remove PPE, if used. Perform hand hygiene.	Proper removal of PPE reduces the risk for infection transmission and contamination of other items. Hand hygiene prevents the spread of microorganisms.

EVALUATION

The expected outcomes have been met when the patient remains free from injury and the sequence of signs and symptoms was observed and recorded.

DOCUMENTATION

Guidelines

Document initiation of seizure precautions, including specific interventions put in place. Document if the beginning of the seizure was witnessed. If so, record noted circumstances before the seizure, such as visual, auditory, or olfactory stimuli, tactile stimuli, emotional or psychological disturbances, sleep, or hyperventilation. Note the occurrence of an aura; where the movements or stiffness began; gaze position and position of the head when the seizure began. Record the body part(s) and the type of movement(s) involved in the seizure. Document pupil sizes; if eyes remained open during seizure; whether eyes or head turned to one side; presence or absence of repeated involuntary motor activity (e.g., repeated swallowing); incontinence of urine or stool; duration of seizure; presence of unconsciousness and duration; obvious paralysis or weakness of arms or legs after seizure; and inability to speak, movements, sleeping, and/or confusion after seizure. Document oxygen administration, airway suction, safety measures, and medication administration, if used. If the patient was injured during the seizure, document assessment of injury.

Sample Documentation

> 1/22/20 0745 Patient bathing with assistance. Stated "I don't feel right." Patient suddenly verbally unresponsive, stiff contractions of legs and arms, with arms extended, lasting approximately 15 seconds; 5-second period of apnea; and bladder incontinence. Continued with approximately 30 seconds of muscle contraction of extremities; eyes closed, facial grimacing. Patient then appeared to sleep; BP 102/68; P 88; R 16; oxygen saturation 94%. Patient awakened after 20 minutes, complaining of headache and fatigue and returned to sleep. Dr. Mason notified of events and assessment. Seizure precautions implemented.
>
> —D. Tyne, RN

UNEXPECTED SITUATIONS AND ASSOCIATED INTERVENTIONS

• *You enter room and find patient in the midst of a seizure:* Initiate seizure management interventions outlined above. Note in documentation that the seizure onset was not initially witnessed.

SPECIAL CONSIDERATIONS

Infant and Child Considerations

- Most seizures in children are caused by disorders that originate outside of the brain, such as high fever, infection, head trauma, toxins, or cardiac arrhythmias. Febrile seizures are the most common type during childhood and are usually benign (Kyle & Carman, 2017).
- Seizures in newborns are associated with underlying conditions, such as hypoxic ischemic encephalopathy, hypoglycemia, hypocalcemia, meningitis, encephalitis, and intracranial hemorrhage. The prognosis depends on the underlying cause and severity of the seizure (Kyle & Carman, 2017).
- Children with recurrent seizures should wear a medical alert bracelet.
- Provide education regarding prescribed medications, including administration, potential side effects, and the importance of not running out of medication (El-Radhi, 2015).
- Encourage patients and their families to keep a seizure diary (El-Radhi, 2015).
- Encourage the use of showers instead of baths, to reduce the risk of drowning (El-Radhi, 2015).
- Encourage regular sleep and avoidance of fatigue (El-Radhi, 2015; Smith, Wagner, & Edwards, 2015).
- Explain that swimming should be supervised (El-Radhi, 2015).
- Emergency assistance should be obtained for multiple or prolonged (>5 minutes in duration) seizures.
- Provide information about support groups for children, parents, and families adjusting to a diagnosis of epilepsy.
- Suggest that families have periodic "seizure drills" to practice what every family member should do if the child has a seizure (Smith et al., 2015).

Home Care Considerations

- Include patient and family/significant other teaching for patients with documented seizures, as well as those at risk for seizures. Teaching should include basic first aid management and the following tips:
  - Help person to lie down.
  - Remove eyeglasses and loosen constrictive clothing.
  - Clear the area around the person of anything hard or sharp.
  - Place something flat and soft (e.g., a folded jacket) under the head. Turn the person gently on the side, if possible.
  - Do not try to force anything into the patient's mouth.
  - Stay with the person during the seizure.
  - Remain calm.
  - Time the seizure.
  - After the seizure, place the person on his or her side and stay with the patient until consciousness is regained; reorient as necessary.
- Patients with recurrent seizures should wear a medical alert bracelet.
- Teach the patient and family/significant other guidelines about when to seek emergency medical assistance. Instruct patients' families and significant others to call for emergency assistance if the person has never had a seizure before; the seizure lasts more than 5 minutes; occurs in water; if the person has trouble breathing or waking afterward; the person has one seizure soon after the first one; if the patient is injured during the seizure; or if the person has a health condition such as diabetes or heart disease or is pregnant (CDC, 2015).

Skill 17-3 ▶ Caring for a Patient in Halo Traction

Halo traction provides stabilization of the cervical spine for patients with spinal cord injury. Halo traction consists of a metal ring that fits over the patient's head, connected with skull pins into the skull, and metal bars that connect the ring to a vest that distributes the weight of the device around the chest. This type of traction immobilizes the head and neck after traumatic injury to the cervical vertebrae and allows early mobility (Hinkle & Cheever, 2018). It is also used to apply spinal traction.

Nursing responsibilities include reassuring the patient, maintaining the device, monitoring neurovascular status, monitoring respiratory status, promoting exercise, preventing complications from the therapy, preventing infection by providing pin-site care, and providing teaching to ensure compliance and self-care. A growing evidence base supports effective management of pin sites, but there

(continued)

Skill 17-3 ▶ Caring for a Patient in Halo Traction *(continued)*

is no clear consensus (Cam & Korkmaz, 2013; Ktistakis, Guerado, & Giannoudis, 2015; Lagerquist, Dabrowski, & Dock, 2012; Lethaby, Temple, & Santy-Tomlinson, 2013). Pin-site care often varies based on primary care provider and facility policy. Dressings are often applied for the first 48 to 72 hours, and then sites may be left open to air. Pin-site care may be performed frequently in the first 48 to 72 hours after application, when drainage may be heavy; other evidence suggests pin care should begin after the first 48 to 72 hours. Routine pin-site care may then be done on a daily or weekly basis (Lagerquist et al., 2012; Timms & Pugh, 2012). Pin-site care is completed using aseptic technique in the immediate postoperative period. Refer to specific patient medical orders and facility guidelines.

DELEGATION CONSIDERATIONS	The care of a patient with halo traction may not be delegated to nursing assistive personnel (NAP) or to unlicensed assistive personnel (UAP). Depending on the state's nurse practice act and the organization's policies and procedures, care for these patients may be delegated to licensed practical/vocational nurses (LPN/LVNs). The decision to delegate must be based on careful analysis of the patient's needs and circumstances, as well as the qualifications of the person to whom the task is being delegated. Refer to the Delegation Guidelines in Appendix A.
EQUIPMENT	• Basin of warm water, bath towels and skin cleanser, based on facility policy • Antimicrobial ointment, per primary care provider order or facility policy • Sterile applicators • Sterile container • Cleansing agent for pin care, usually sterile normal saline, but may be an antimicrobial such as chlorhexidine, per primary care provider order or facility policy • Sterile gauze or dressing per primary care provider order or facility policy • Analgesic, as ordered • Clean gloves, if appropriate, for bathing under the vest • Sterile gloves for performing pin care, depending on facility policy • Additional PPE, as indicated
ASSESSMENT	Review the patient's health record, medical orders, and nursing care plan to determine the type of device being used and the prescribed care. Assess the halo traction device to ensure proper function and position. Perform respiratory, neurologic, and skin assessments. Inspect the pin-insertion sites for inflammation and infection, including swelling, cloudy or offensive drainage, pain, or redness. Assess the patient's knowledge regarding the device and self-care activities and responsibilities, and his or her feelings related to treatment.
NURSING DIAGNOSIS	Determine the related factors for the nursing diagnoses based on the patient's current status. Appropriate nursing diagnoses may include: • Disturbed body image • (Bathing-; Dressing-; Feeding-; Toileting-) Self-care deficit • Risk for infection
OUTCOME IDENTIFICATION AND PLANNING	The expected outcome to achieve when caring for a patient with halo traction is that the patient maintains cervical alignment. Additional outcomes that may be appropriate include that the patient shows no evidence of infection; and the patient is free from injury.

IMPLEMENTATION

ACTION	RATIONALE
1. Review the health record and the nursing care plan to determine the type of device being used and prescribed care.	Reviewing the health record and care plan validates the correct patient and correct procedure.
2. Gather the necessary equipment.	Preparation promotes efficient time management and an organized approach to the task.
3. Perform hand hygiene and put on PPE, if indicated.	Hand hygiene and PPE prevent the spread of microorganisms. PPE is required based on transmission precautions.

ACTION	RATIONALE

4. Identify the patient.

Identifying the patient ensures the right patient receives the intervention and helps prevent errors.

5. Assemble equipment to the bedside stand or overbed table or other surface within reach.

Arranging items nearby is convenient, saves time, and avoids unnecessary stretching and twisting of muscles on the part of the nurse.

6. Close curtains around the bed and close the door to the room, if possible. Explain what you are going to do and why you are going to do it to the patient.

This ensures the patient's privacy. Explanation relieves anxiety and facilitates cooperation.

7. Assess the patient for possible need for nonpharmacologic, pain-reducing interventions or analgesic medication before beginning. Administer appropriate prescribed analgesic. Allow sufficient time for analgesic to achieve its effectiveness before beginning the procedure.

Pain is a subjective experience influenced by past experience. Pin care may cause pain for some patients.

8. Place a waste receptacle at a convenient location for use during the procedure.

Having a waste container handy means that the soiled dressing may be discarded easily, without the spread of microorganisms.

9. Adjust bed to comfortable working height, usually elbow height of the caregiver, if the patient will remain in bed (VHACEOSH, 2016). Alternatively, have the patient sit up, if appropriate.

Having the bed at the proper height prevents back and muscle strain.

10. Assist the patient to a comfortable position that provides easy access to the head. Place a waterproof pad under the head if the patient is lying down.

Patient positioning provides for comfort. Waterproof pad protects underlying surfaces.

11. Monitor vital signs and perform a neurologic assessment, including level of consciousness, motor function, and sensation, per facility policy (see Fundamentals Review 17-1 and Chapter 3). This is usually at least every 2 hours for 24 hours, or possibly every hour for 48 hours.

Changes in the neurologic assessment could indicate spinal cord trauma, which would require immediate intervention.

12. Examine the halo vest unit every 8 hours for stability, secure connections, and positioning (Figure 1). Make sure the patient's head is centered in the halo without neck flexion or extension. Check each bolt for loosening.

Assessment ensures correct function of the device and patient safety. Loose bolts require attention from an appropriate advanced practice professional to maintain correct positioning, proper alignment, and unit stability.

FIGURE 1. Examining halo vest for stability, secure connections, and positioning.

(*continued*)

Skill 17-3 ▶ Caring for a Patient in Halo Traction *(continued)*

ACTION	RATIONALE
13. Check the fit of the vest. With the patient in a supine position, you should be able to insert one or two fingers under the jacket at the shoulder and chest.	Checking the fit prevents compression on the chest, which could interfere with respiratory status.
14. Put on nonsterile gloves, if appropriate. Remove patient's shirt or gown. Wash the patient's chest and back daily. Loosen the bottom Velcro straps. Protect the vest liner with a waterproof pad.	Gloves prevent contact with blood and body fluids. Removal of clothing from torso allows visualization of, and access to, appropriate areas. Daily cleaning prevents skin breakdown and allows assessment. Loosening the straps allows access to the chest and back. Waterproof pad keeps the vest liner dry and prevents skin irritation and breakdown.
15. Wring out a bath towel soaked in warm water (and skin cleanser, depending on facility policy). Pull the towel back and forth in a drying motion beneath the front.	Using an overly wet towel could lead to skin maceration and breakdown.
16. Thoroughly dry the skin in the same manner with a dry towel. Inspect the skin for tender, reddened areas or pressure spots. Do not use powder or lotion under the vest.	Drying prevents skin irritation and breakdown. Powders and lotions can cause skin irritation.
17. Turn the patient on his or her side, less than 45 degrees if lying supine, and repeat the process on the back. Remove waterproof pad from the vest liner. Close the Velcro straps. Assist the patient with putting on a new shirt, if desired.	Doing so prevents skin breakdown. Cleansers and lotions can cause skin irritation.
18. Perform a respiratory assessment. Check for respiratory impairment, such as absence of breath sounds, the presence of adventitious sounds, reduced inspiratory effort, or shortness of breath.	The halo vest limits chest expansion, which could lead to alterations in respiratory function. Pulmonary embolus is a common complication associated with spinal cord injury.
19. Assess the pin sites for redness, tenting of the skin; prolonged or purulent drainage; swelling; and bowing, bending, or loosening of the pins. Monitor body temperature.	Pin sites provide an entry for microorganisms. Assessment allows for early detection and prompt intervention should problems arise.
20. Perform pin-site care (Figure 2) (see Skills 9-19 and 9-20 in Chapter 9).	Pin-site care reduces the risk of infection and subsequent osteomyelitis.

FIGURE 2. Cleansing pin sites.

21. Depending on medical order and facility policy, apply antimicrobial ointment to pin sites and a dressing.	Antimicrobial ointment helps prevent infection. Dressing provides protection and helps contain any drainage.
22. Remove gloves and dispose of them appropriately. Raise rails, as appropriate, and place the bed in the lowest position. Assist the patient to a comfortable position.	Disposing of gloves reduces the risk of microorganism transmission. Rails assist with patient positioning. Proper bed height ensures patient safety.

ACTION	RATIONALE
23. Remove additional PPE, if used. Perform hand hygiene.	Proper removal of PPE reduces the risk for infection transmission and contamination of other items. Hand hygiene prevents the spread of microorganisms.

EVALUATION

The expected outcomes have been met when the patient maintained cervical alignment; has no evidence of infection; and the patient is free from injury.

DOCUMENTATION

Guidelines

Document the time, date, and type of device in place. Include the skin assessment, pin-site assessment, personal hygiene, and pin-site care. Document the patient's response to the device and the neurologic assessment and respiratory assessment.

Sample Documentation

> <u>11/10/20</u> 2030 Halo traction in place. Skin care provided under jacket; two fingers fit at shoulders and chest. Skin intact without redness or irritation. Pin-site care performed. Pin sites cleaned with normal saline and open to the air. Sites without redness, swelling, and drainage. Neurovascular status intact. Patient reports pain at pin sites 4/10. Medicated with ibuprofen 600 mg per order. Will reevaluate pain in 1 hour.
>
> —*M. Leroux, RN*

UNEXPECTED SITUATIONS AND ASSOCIATED INTERVENTIONS

- *A patient being treated with halo traction complains of a headache after the physician or advanced practice professional has tightened the skull pins:* This is a common complaint; obtain an order for and administer an analgesic. However, if the pain is associated with jaw movement, notify the primary health care provider immediately, because the pins may have slipped onto the temporal plate.

SPECIAL CONSIDERATIONS

General Considerations

- Always keep wrenches specific for the vest at the bedside for emergency removal of the anterior portion of the vest should it be necessary to perform CPR.
- Patient teaching to prevent injury is very important. Patients need to learn to turn slowly and refrain from bending forward to avoid falls.
- Stress to the frame could cause misalignment of the spine and straining or tearing of the skin. Do not use the frame as handles to transfer or position the patient.
- If a pin site becomes unusually painful or tender, or if you notice any fluid discharge, it may be a signal that the pin has loosened or become infected. In the event of unusual pain or irritation, notify the primary care provider (American Association of Critical-Care Nurses [AACN], 2017). Pin loosening may also be indicated by a "tight" feeling or a "clicking" sound (Lagerquist et al., 2012).

Older Adult Considerations

- Restrictions imposed by a halo vest can be detrimental to older adults, who may be at greater risk for complications, including death (Sharpe, Magnotti, Weinberg, Schroeppel, Fabian, & Croce, 2016).

Home Care Considerations

- Patients and families require information and guidance about the care of their halo in the community. Written information, as well as specific discharge teaching, is important in helping to prevent complications. Teaching should include the importance of vigilant skin care and signs and symptoms of pin-site infection.
- Encourage exercise by walking; teach patient to avoid other exercise activities.
- Keeping hair clean is important. Hair should be shampooed regularly. This can be accomplished by having the patient lie supine in bed, with the head out over foot of the mattress so it is suspended beyond the mattress; shoulders should remain on the mattress with a towel or plastic bag along the back and shoulders of the vest to keep it from getting wet. A garbage can under the patient's head can be used to catch the water. Alternately, the patient could rest on the edge of a bathtub, with a towel on the edge of the tub for padding, resting elbows on edge for support. Use a spray attachment or pitcher of water to wash hair.

(*continued*)

Skill 17-3 ▶ Caring for a Patient in Halo Traction *(continued)*

EVIDENCE FOR PRACTICE ▶

EXTERNAL FIXATOR PIN SITES-CLINICAL EVIDENCE REVIEW

Lethaby, A., Temple, J., & Santy-Tomlinson, J. (2013). Pin site care for preventing infections associated with external bone fixators and pins (Review). (2013). *Cochrane Database of Systematic Reviews, (12)*, CD004551. DOI: 10.1002/14651858.CD004551.pub3.

This clinical evidence review was conducted the Cochrane Wounds Group Specialised Register; The Cochrane Central Register of Controlled Trials (CENTRAL) (*The Cochrane Library*); Ovid MEDLINE; Ovid MEDLINE (In-Process & Other Nonindexed Citations); Ovid EMBASE; and EBSCO CINAHL. The authors evaluated all randomized controlled trials that compared the effect on infection and other complication rates of different methods of cleansing or dressing orthopedic percutaneous pin sites. Eleven trials with 572 participants but not all participants contributed data to each comparison. Three trials examined cleansing regimen with no cleansing; three trials compared alternative sterile cleansing solutions; three trials compared methods of cleansing; one trial compared daily site care with no care; and six trials compared different dressings. The authors concluded the evidence was not extensive, was very heterogeneous, and generally of poor quality, so there was no strong evidence that one pin care technique was any better than any other and there was insufficient evidence to identify a strategy of pin-site care that minimizes infection rates.

Refer to thePoint* for additional research on related nursing topics.

Skill 17-4 ▶ Caring for a Patient With an External Ventriculostomy (Intraventricular Catheter–Closed Fluid-Filled System)

Intracranial pressure (ICP) is the pressure inside the cranium. The components that occupy the intracranial space, blood, tissue, and cerebrospinal fluid (CSF) circulating in the ventricles and subarachnoid space, contribute to the ICP (Hickey, 2014). ICP monitoring is used to assess cerebral perfusion. When ICP increases, as a result of conditions such as a mass (e.g., a tumor), bleeding into the brain or fluid around the brain, or swelling within the brain matter itself, neurologic consequences may range from minor to severe, including death. Normal ICP is less than 15 mm Hg. Elevated ICP, intracranial hypertension, is a sustained ICP of 20 to 25 mm Hg or higher for greater than 5 minutes (Hickey, 2014). Box 17-1 identifies signs and symptoms of increased ICP in adults.

An external **ventriculostomy** is one method used to monitor ICP. It is part of a system that includes an external drainage system and an external transducer. This device is inserted into a ventricle of the brain, most commonly the nondominant lateral ventricle, through a hole drilled into the skull. The catheter is connected by a fluid-filled system to a transducer, which records the

Box 17-1   Signs and Symptoms of Increased Intracranial Pressure in Adults

- Decreased level of consciousness
- Changes in mental status
- Lethargy
- Coma
- Headache
- Confusion
- Restlessness, agitation
- Irritability
- Hypoactive reflexes
- Slowed response time
- Ataxia

- Aphasia
- Slowed speech
- Progressively severe headache
- Nausea and vomiting (usually projectile vomiting)
- Seizures
- Changes in pupil size; unequal pupils
- Slowed or lack of pupillary response to light
- Widening of pulse pressure
- Respiratory pattern changes
- Leakage of clear yellow or pinkish fluid from ear or nose

pressure in the form of an electrical impulse (Hinkle & Cheever, 2018). The ventriculostomy can be used to measure the ICP, to drain CSF, such as removing excess fluid associated with hydrocephalus, or to decrease the volume in the cranial vault, thereby decreasing the ICP, and to instill medications. ICP and blood pressure measurements are used to calculate **cerebral perfusion pressure (CPP)**, the blood pressure gradient across the brain and the pressure necessary to maintain an adequate force for blood throughout the brain, to prevent cerebral ischemia (Hickey, 2014). ICP monitoring also provides information about **intracranial compliance**, the ability of the brain to change volume related to a change in pressure; to tolerate stimulation or increase in intracranial volume without an increase in pressure through waveform assessment (Box 17-2) (Hickey, 2014; Morton & Fontaine, 2018).

Ventricular drainage is associated with an increased risk of infection. Strict sterile technique should be observed when manipulating the ventricular drain (AACN, 2017; Hickey, 2014).

Box 17-2 | Interpreting ICP Waveforms

Sustained periods (>5 minutes) of ICPs greater than 20 mm Hg are considered significant and can be extremely dangerous. Sustained periods of ICPs greater than 60 mm Hg are usually fatal (Morton & Fontaine, 2018, p. 667). A normal waveform correlates with hemodynamic changes. Plotting extended periods of increased ICP measurements over time provides patterns known as A, B, and C waves (waveform trends).

Normal Intracranial Waveform

A normal ICP waveform typically shows a steep upward slope followed by a downward slope with three descending peaks that correlate with hemodynamic changes (forces related to the circulation of blood). P1 correlates with systole; P2 most directly reflects the state of intracranial compliance, so as ICP rises, P2 elevates; P3 tapers down to correlate with diastole (Morton & Fontaine, 2018). In normal circumstances, this waveform occurs continuously and indicates an ICP between 0 and 15 mm Hg—normal pressure. The amplitude of P2 may exceed P1 with increased ICP or decreased intracranial compliance (Morton & Fontaine).

A Waves

A waves are produced by spontaneous, transient, rapid increases of pressure over a period of time (ICP values of 50 to 200 mm Hg, lasting 5 to 20 minutes) and are associated with compromised cerebral perfusion and deteriorating neurologic status.

B Waves

B waves, which appear sharp and rhythmic with a sawtooth pattern, are shorter (30 seconds to 2 minutes) with ICP values of 20 to 50 mm Hg. They are seen in patients with intracranial hypertension and decreased intracranial compliance. B waves are an early indication of deteriorating neurologic status and may precede A waves.

C Waves

C waves are rapid and rhythmic, but they are not as sharp as B waves. C waves are associated with ICPs as high as 20 mm Hg that persist for less than 5 minutes. They may fluctuate with respirations or systemic blood pressure changes and are without clinical significance (AACN, 2017).

Source: Adapted from Morton, P. G., & Fontaine, D. K. (2018). *Critical care nursing. A holistic approach* (11th ed.). Philadelphia, PA: Wolters Kluwer; Hinkle, J. L., & Cheever, K. H. (2018). *Brunner & Suddarth's textbook of medical-surgical nursing* (14th ed.). Philadelphia, PA: Wolters Kluwer; and American Association of Critical-Care Nurses (AACN). (2017). In D. L. Wiegand (Ed.). *AACN procedure manual for high acuity, progressive, and critical care* (7th ed.). St. Louis, MO: Elsevier.

(continued)

Skill 17-4 ▶ Caring for a Patient With an External Ventriculostomy (Intraventricular Catheter–Closed Fluid-Filled System) *(continued)*

DELEGATION CONSIDERATIONS	The care of a patient with an external ventriculostomy may not be delegated to nursing assistive personnel (NAP) or to unlicensed assistive personnel (UAP). Depending on the state's nurse practice act and the organization's policies and procedures, care for these patients may be delegated to licensed practical/vocational nurses (LPN/LVNs). The decision to delegate must be based on careful analysis of the patient's needs and circumstances, as well as the qualifications of the person to whom the task is being delegated. Refer to the Delegation Guidelines in Appendix A.
EQUIPMENT	• Ventriculostomy setup • Carpenter level, bubble-line level, or laser level, according to facility policy • PPE, as indicated
ASSESSMENT	Assess the color of the fluid draining from the ventriculostomy. Normal CSF is clear or straw colored. Cloudy CSF may suggest an infection. Red or pink CSF may indicate bleeding. Assess vital signs, because changes in vital signs can reflect a neurologic problem. Assess the patient's pain level. The patient may be experiencing pain at the ventriculostomy insertion site. Perform a neurologic assessment (see Fundamentals Review 17-1 and Chapter 3). Assess the patient's level of consciousness (LOC). If the patient is awake, assess for his or her orientation to person, place, and time. If the patient's LOC is decreased, note the patient's ability to respond and to be aroused. Inspect pupil size and response to light. Pupils should be equal and round and should react to light bilaterally. Any changes in LOC or pupillary response may suggest a neurologic problem. If the patient can move the extremities, assess strength of hands and feet (see Chapter 3 for detailed instructions on assessing muscle strength). A change in strength or a difference in strength on one side compared with the other may indicate a neurologic problem.
NURSING DIAGNOSIS	Determine the related factors for the nursing diagnoses based on the patient's current status. Appropriate nursing diagnoses may include: • Risk for injury • Risk for ineffective cerebral tissue perfusion • Risk for infection
OUTCOME IDENTIFICATION AND PLANNING	The expected outcome to achieve is that the patient maintains ICP at less than 15 mm Hg and CPP at 50 to 70 mm Hg (Hickey, 2014, pp. 266, 270–271). Other outcomes that may be appropriate include the following: patient is free from infection and the patient/significant others understand the need for the ventriculostomy.

IMPLEMENTATION

ACTION	**RATIONALE**
1. Review the medical orders and patient health record for specific information about ventriculostomy parameters.	The nurse needs to know the most recent order for the height of the ventriculostomy. For example, if the health care practitioner has ordered that the ventriculostomy is to be at 10 cm, this means the patient's ICP must rise above 10 cm before the ventriculostomy will drain CSF.
2. Gather the necessary supplies.	Preparation promotes efficient time management and an organized approach to the task.
3. Perform hand hygiene and put on PPE, if indicated.	Hand hygiene and PPE prevent the spread of microorganisms. PPE is required based on transmission precautions.
4. Identify the patient.	Identifying the patient ensures the right patient receives the intervention and helps prevent errors.

ACTION	RATIONALE
5. Assemble equipment to the bedside stand or overbed table or other surface within reach.	Arranging items nearby is convenient, saves time, and avoids unnecessary stretching and twisting of muscles on the part of the nurse.
6. Close curtains around the bed and close the door to the room, if possible. Explain what you are going to do and why you are going to do it to the patient.	This ensures the patient's privacy. Explanation relieves anxiety and facilitates cooperation.
7. Assess patient for any changes in neurologic status (see Fundamentals Review 17-1 and Chapter 3 for details of assessment).	Patients with ventriculostomies are at risk for problems with the neurologic system.
8. Set the zero reference level. **Assess the height of the ventriculostomy system to ensure that the stopcock is at the appropriate reference point: the tragus of the ear (Figure 1), the outer canthus of the patient's eye, or the patient's external auditory canal** (American Association of Neuroscience Nurses [AANN], 2011) using carpenter level, bubble-line level, or laser level, according to facility policy. Adjust the height of the system, if needed.	For measurements to be accurate, the stopcock must be at a reference point to approximate the catheter tip at the level of the foramen of Monro. Use of the same reference point for all readings is critical to ensure accuracy. Use of a carpenter level, bubble-line level, or laser level, ensures accuracy (Hickey, 2014). If the ventriculostomy is used just to measure the ICP and not to drain the CSF, the stopcock will be turned off to the drip chamber.

FIGURE 1. Transducer leveled with tragus. (© Copyright 2011 by AANN. All rights reserved.)

ACTION	RATIONALE
9. Set the pressure level based on prescribed pressure. Move the drip chamber to the ordered height. Assess the amount of CSF in the drip chamber if the ventriculostomy is draining.	When the ICP is higher than the prescribed pressure level, CSF will drain into the drip chamber. If the ventriculostomy is to drain CSF, the nurse must turn the stopcock off to the drip chamber to obtain a measurement of ICP. After the ICP value is obtained, remember to turn the stopcock back off to the transducer so that CSF is allowed to drain.
10. **Zero the transducer.** Turn the stopcock off to the patient. Remove the cap from the transducer, being careful not to touch the end of the cap. Press and hold the calibration button on the monitor until the monitor beeps. Return the cap to the transducer. **Turn the stopcock off to the drip chamber to obtain an ICP reading and waveform tracing. After obtaining a reading, turn the stopcock off to the transducer.**	The readings would not be considered accurate if the transducer had not been recently zeroed. If the stopcock is not turned off to the patient, when opened to room air, CSF will flow out of the stopcock. The end of the cap must remain sterile to prevent an infection. The stopcock must be off to the drip chamber (open to the transducer) to obtain an ICP. If the ventriculostomy is to drain CSF, the nurse must turn the stopcock off to the drip chamber. After the ICP value is obtained, remember to turn the stopcock back off to the transducer so that CSF is allowed to drain into the drip chamber.

(continued)

Skill 17-4   Caring for a Patient With an External Ventriculostomy (Intraventricular Catheter–Closed Fluid-Filled System) *(continued)*

ACTION	RATIONALE
11. Adjust the ventriculostomy height to prevent too much drainage, too little drainage, or inaccurate ICP readings.	If the patient's head is lower than the ventriculostomy, the drainage of CSF will slow or stop. If the patient's head is higher than the ventriculostomy, the drainage of CSF will increase. Any ICP readings taken when the ventriculostomy is not level with the outer canthus of the eye would be inaccurate.
12. Care for the insertion site according to the facility's policy. Maintain the system using strict sterile technique. Assess the site for any signs of infection, such as purulent drainage, redness, or warmth. Ensure the catheter is secured at site per facility policy. If the catheter is sutured to the scalp, assess integrity of the sutures (Figure 2).	Site care varies, possibly ranging from leaving the site open to air to applying antibiotic ointment and gauze. Sterile technique helps to prevent infection (AACN, 2017; Hickey, 2014). Securing the catheters after insertion prevents dislodgement and breakage of the device.

FIGURE 2. Sutured external ventriculostomy catheter.

ACTION	RATIONALE
13. Calculate the CPP, if necessary. Calculate the difference between the systemic MAP and the ICP.	CPP is an estimate of the adequacy of the blood supply to the brain.
14. Remove PPE, if used. Perform hand hygiene.	Proper removal of PPE reduces the risk for infection transmission and contamination of other items. Hand hygiene prevents the spread of microorganisms.
15. Assess ICP, MAP, and CPP continuously or intermittently as prescribed (AACN, 2017). Note drainage amount, color, clarity. If there is an increase in the ICP, the value should be obtained more often, as often as every 15 minutes (AANN, 2011).	Frequent assessment provides valuable indicators for identifying subtle trends that may suggest developing problems.

ACTION	RATIONALE
16. Assess ICP drainage system at least every 4 hours, checking the insertion site, all drainage system tubing and parts, for cracks in the system, or leakage from insertion site or system. Label external ventriculostomy tubing and access ports clearly.	Frequent monitoring allows for early identification of problems and prompt intervention. Clear labeling prevents accidental use as an intravenous access.

EVALUATION

The expected outcomes have been achieved when the patient maintains ICP at less than 15 mm Hg and CPP at 50 to 70 mm Hg (Hickey, 2014, pp. 266, 270–271); the patient is free from infection; and the patient/significant others verbalized an understanding of the need for the ventriculostomy.

DOCUMENTATION

Guidelines

Document the following information: amount and color of CSF, ICP, and CPP; pupil status; motor strength bilaterally; orientation to time, person, and place; LOC; vital signs; pain; assessment of insertion site; and height of ventriculostomy.

Sample Documentation

> 11/2/20 1410 External ventriculostomy zeroed; transducer level with outer canthus of eye, drip chamber 10 cm; draining cloudy, straw-colored CSF (12 mL), Dr. Hill notified of clarity. ICP 10 mm Hg; CPP 83 mm Hg, see attached wave tracing. Ventriculostomy insertion site with small amount of serosanguineous drainage; open to air. Strong equal grip bilaterally. Patient awake, alert, and oriented to person, place, and time. Pupils equal, round, and reactive to light 6/4 bilaterally. See graphics for vital signs. Patient denies pain.
>
> —B. Traudes, RN

UNEXPECTED SITUATIONS AND ASSOCIATED INTERVENTIONS

- *ICP exceeds established parameters:* Notify primary care provider immediately. If no parameter is specified, notify primary care provider if ICP is >20 to 25 mm Hg (AANN, 2011; Hickey, 2014).
- *CSF stops draining:* Assess for any kinks or narrowing of tubing. Assess that all connections on the tubing are well connected and that CSF is not leaking anywhere from the tubing. Assess the height of the system and the height of the drip chamber. If the system is too high, the CSF drainage will taper off. Assess for any liquid on the sheets around the patient's head. If the ventriculostomy has become clogged, the CSF may begin to leak around the insertion site. Assess the patency of the ventriculostomy catheter. Raise and lower the system. If the ventriculostomy catheter is patent, the fluid in the tube will tidal, or rise and fall with the position change. If CSF still is not draining or if you believe that the tube is clogged, notify the primary care provider. The tube may need to be flushed using sterile technique to ensure patency.
- *The amount of CSF drainage increases:* Assess the height of the system and the height of the drip chamber. If the system is too low, the amount of CSF drainage will increase. If CSF continues to drain at an increased amount, notify the primary care provider. The height of the drip chamber may need to be increased.
- *CSF has changed from clear to cloudy:* Notify the primary care provider immediately. This can signify an infection, and antibiotics may need to be started.
- *CSF has changed from straw-colored to pink tinged or serosanguineous:* Notify the primary care provider immediately. This can signify bleeding in the ventricles of the brain.
- *Catheter is accidentally dislodged:* Notify the primary care provider immediately. Put on sterile gloves and cover the insertion site with sterile gauze. Monitor for color and amount of CSF if draining from site.

SPECIAL CONSIDERATIONS

- Secure and label the catheters according to facility policy after insertion, and use care when moving patients to prevent dislodgement and breakage of these devices.
- Repositioning is important to prevent skin alterations and to decrease the risks associated with immobility. During position changes, clamp the ventriculostomy; after repositioning, maintain

(*continued*)

Skill 17-4 ▶ Caring for a Patient With an External Ventriculostomy (Intraventricular Catheter–Closed Fluid-Filled System) *(continued)*

the reference level and ensure the system is patent (AACN, 2017). Modest, initial increases in ICP experienced with repositioning quickly return to baseline after repositioning is complete (McNett & Olson, 2013). Turn and position the patient in proper body alignment, avoiding angulation of body parts. Extreme hip flexion or flexion of upper legs can increase intra-abdominal pressure, leading to increased ICP. Maintain the neck in neutral position at all times to avoid neck vein compression, which can interfere with venous return (Hickey, 2014).

- Maintain the head of the bed elevated 30 degrees to promote venous return from the brain, depending on medical orders and facility procedure (AACN, 2017; Hickey, 2014).
- Endotracheal suctioning episodes should be limited to one to two passes of the catheter (Hickey, 2014). The ICP increases associated with suctioning, tracheal stimulation, and coughing are modest and transient (McNett & Olson, 2013).
- Oral care is a safe intervention; ICP increases experienced with oral care are modest, transient, and resolve quickly when oral care is complete (McNett & Olson, 2013).
- Auditory stimulation for critically ill neurologically impaired patients does not increase ICP and is considered a safe intervention (McNett & Olson, 2013).
- Plan care to avoid grouping activities and procedures known to increase ICP. Bathing, turning, and other routine care often have a cumulative effect to increase ICP when performed in succession. Allow rest periods between procedures and carefully assess the patient's response to interventions (Hickey, 2014).

EVIDENCE FOR PRACTICE ▶

CLINICAL PRACTICE GUIDELINE: UNIVERSAL STANDARD FOR EXTERNAL VENTRICULAR DRAIN CARE

Hepburn-Smith, M., Dynkevich, I., Spektor, M., Lord, A., Czeisler, B., & Lewis, A. (2016). Establishment of an external ventricular drain best practice guideline: The quest for a comprehensive, universal standard for external ventricular drain care. *Journal of Neuroscience Nursing*, 48(1), 54–65.

An interdisciplinary team of nurses, advanced practice nurses, and neurointensivists reviewed medical and nursing literature as well as research-based institutional protocols on external ventricular drain (EVD) insertion and maintenance to determine global best practices. The resulting guideline addresses preinsertion hair removal and skin preparation, aseptic technique, catheter selection, monitoring of EVD insertion technique using a bundle approach, postinsertion dressing type and frequency of dressing changes, techniques for maintenance and CSF sampling, duration of catheter placement, and staff education/competence, and surveillance.

Refer to thePoint® for additional research on related nursing topics.

EVIDENCE FOR PRACTICE ▶

CLINICAL PRACTICE GUIDELINE: INTRACRANIAL PRESSURE MONITORING/ EXTERNAL VENTRICULAR DRAINAGE OR LUMBAR DRAINAGE

American Association of Neuroscience Nurses (AANN). (2011). *Care of the patient undergoing intracranial pressure monitoring/external ventricular drainage or lumbar drainage.* Glenview, IL: Author.

The AANN is a professional nursing organization committed to the advancement of neuroscience nursing as a specialty through the development and support of nurses to promote excellence in patient care. The AANN provides continuing education, information dissemination, standard setting, and advocacy on behalf of neuroscience patients, families, and nurses. This evidence-based practice guideline is a resource for registered nurses (RNs), patient care units, and facilities in providing safe and effective care to patients undergoing ICP monitoring via an external ventricular drainage device (EVD) or those undergoing subarachnoid drainage of CSF with a lumbar drainage device (LDD).

Refer to thePoint® for additional research on related nursing topics.

See additional Evidence for Practice related to caring for patients with ICP monitoring at the end of Skill 17-5, and refer to thePoint® for additional research on related nursing topics.

Skill 17-5 ▶ Caring for a Patient With a Fiber Optic Intracranial Catheter

Intracranial pressure (ICP) is the pressure inside the cranium. The components that occupy the intracranial space, blood, tissue, and cerebrospinal fluid circulating in the ventricles and subarachnoid space, contribute to the ICP (Hickey, 2014). ICP monitoring is used to assess cerebral perfusion. When ICP increases, as a result of conditions such as a mass (e.g., a tumor), bleeding into the brain or fluid around the brain, or swelling within the brain matter itself, neurologic consequences may range from minor to severe, including death. Normal ICP is less than 15 mm Hg. Elevated ICP, intracranial hypertension, is a sustained ICP of 20 to 25 mm Hg or higher for greater than 5 minutes (Hickey, 2014). Refer to Box 17-1 in Skill 17-4 for signs and symptoms of increased ICP in adults.

Fiber optic catheters are one method used to monitor ICP. Fiber optic catheters directly monitor ICP using an intracranial transducer located in the tip of the catheter. A miniature transducer in the catheter tip is coupled by a long, continuous wire or fiber optic cable to an external electronic module. This device can be inserted into the lateral ventricle, subarachnoid space, subdural space, brain parenchyma, or under a bone flap (Figure 1). These devices are not fluid-filled systems, eliminating the problems associated with an external transducer and pressure tubing, such as an external ventriculostomy (Skill 17-4). Fiber optic catheters can be used to monitor the ICP and cerebral perfusion pressure (CPP). These devices are calibrated by the manufacturer and zero-balanced only once at the time of insertion.

ICP and blood pressure measurements are used to calculate CPP, the blood pressure gradient across the brain and the pressure necessary to maintain an adequate force for blood throughout the brain, to prevent cerebral ischemia (Hickey, 2014). ICP monitoring also provides information about intracranial compliance, the ability of the brain to tolerate stimulation or increase in intracranial volume without an increase in pressure through waveform assessment (Hickey, 2014; Hinkle & Cheever, 2018). Box 17-2 in Skill 17-4 reviews ICP waveforms.

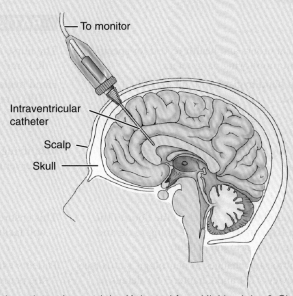

FIGURE 1. Fiber optic catheter in ventricle. (Adapted from Hinkle, J. L., & Cheever, K. H. [2018]. *Brunner & Suddarth's textbook of medical-surgical nursing* [14th ed.]. Philadelphia, PA: Wolters Kluwer, p. 1981.)

DELEGATION CONSIDERATIONS

The care of a patient with a fiber optic intracranial catheter may not be delegated to nursing assistive personnel (NAP) or to unlicensed assistive personnel (UAP). Depending on the state's nurse practice act and the organization's policies and procedures, care for these patients may be delegated to licensed practical/vocational nurses (LPN/LVNs). The decision to delegate must be based on careful analysis of the patient's needs and circumstances, as well as the qualifications of the person to whom the task is being delegated. Refer to the Delegation Guidelines in Appendix A.

EQUIPMENT

• PPE, as indicated

(continued)

Skill 17-5 ▶ Caring for a Patient With a Fiber Optic Intracranial Catheter *(continued)*

ASSESSMENT

Perform a neurologic assessment (see Fundamentals Review 17-1 and Chapter 3). Assess the patient's level of consciousness (LOC). If the patient is awake, assess the patient's orientation to person, place, and time. If the patient's LOC is decreased, note the patient's ability to respond and to be aroused. Inspect pupil size and response to light. Pupils should be equal and round and should react to light bilaterally. Any changes in LOC or pupillary response may suggest a neurologic problem. If the patient can move the extremities, assess strength of hands and feet (see Chapter 3 for detailed instructions on assessing muscle strength). A change in strength or a difference in strength on one side compared with the other may indicate a neurologic problem. Assess vital signs, because changes in vital signs can reflect a neurologic problem. Assess the patient's pain level. The patient may be experiencing pain at the fiber optic catheter insertion site.

NURSING DIAGNOSIS

Determine the related factors for the nursing diagnoses based on the patient's current status. Appropriate nursing diagnoses may include:

- Risk for infection
- Risk for injury
- Risk for ineffective cerebral tissue perfusion

OUTCOME IDENTIFICATION AND PLANNING

The expected outcome to achieve is that the patient maintains ICP at less than 15 mm Hg and CPP at 50 to 70 mm Hg (Hickey, 2014, pp. 266, 270–271). Other outcomes that may be appropriate include the following: patient is free from infection and the patient/significant others understand the need for the ventriculostomy.

IMPLEMENTATION

ACTION	RATIONALE
1. Review the medical orders and health record for specific information about monitoring parameters.	The nurse needs to know the most recent order for acceptable ICP and CPP values.
2. Perform hand hygiene and put on PPE, if indicated.	Hand hygiene and PPE prevent the spread of microorganisms. PPE is required based on transmission precautions.
3. Identify the patient.	Identifying the patient ensures the right patient receives the intervention and helps prevent errors.
4. Close curtains around the bed and close the door to the room, if possible. Explain what you are going to do and why you are going to do it to the patient.	This ensures the patient's privacy. Explanation relieves anxiety and facilitates cooperation.
5. Assess the patient for any changes in neurologic status (see Fundamentals Review 17-1 and Chapter 3 for details of assessment).	Patients with ventriculostomies are at risk for problems with the neurologic system.
6. Assess ICP, MAP, and CPP continuously or intermittently as prescribed (AACN, 2017). Note ICP value and waveforms as shown on the monitor. If there is an increase in the ICP, the value should be obtained more often, as often as every 15 minutes (AANN, 2011).	Frequent assessment provides valuable indicators for identifying subtle trends that may suggest developing problems.
7. Care for the insertion site according to the facility's policy. Maintain the system using strict sterile technique. Assess the site for any signs of infection, such as drainage, redness, or warmth. Ensure the catheter is secured at site per facility policy.	Site care varies, possibly ranging from leaving the site open to air to applying antibiotic ointment and gauze. Site care aids in reducing the risk for infection. Sterile technique helps to prevent infection (AACN, 2017; Hickey, 2014). Securing the catheters after insertion prevents dislodgement and breakage of the device.

ACTION	**RATIONALE**
8. Calculate the CPP, if necessary. Calculate the difference between the systemic MAP and the ICP.	CPP is an estimate of the adequacy of the blood supply to the brain.
9. Remove PPE, if used. Perform hand hygiene.	Proper removal of PPE reduces the risk for infection transmission and contamination of other items. Hand hygiene prevents the spread of microorganisms.

EVALUATION

The expected outcomes have been achieved when the patient maintains ICP at less than 15 mm Hg and CPP at 50 to 70 mm Hg (Hickey, 2014, pp. 266, 270–271); the patient is free from infection; and the patient/significant others verbalized an understanding of the need for the ventriculostomy.

DOCUMENTATION

General Guidelines

Document the following information: neurologic assessment; ICP and CPP; vital signs; pain; assessment of insertion site.

Sample Documentation

> <u>11/2/20</u> 1710 Patient sedated; disoriented and combative when awake. Pupils equal round and reactive to light 6/4 bilaterally. See graphics for vital signs. ICP 22 mm Hg; CPP 61 mm Hg; primary care provider notified. Dopamine drip increased to 8 μg/kg/min. Insertion site with small amount of serosanguineous drainage.
>
> —*B. Traudes, RN*

UNEXPECTED SITUATIONS AND ASSOCIATED INTERVENTIONS

- *ICP exceeds established parameters:* Notify primary care provider immediately. If no parameter is specified, notify primary care provider if ICP is >20 to 25 mm Hg (AANN, 2011; Hickey, 2014).
- *Fiber optic catheter is accidentally dislodged:* Notify the primary care provider immediately. Put on sterile gloves and cover the site with sterile gauze. Observe for any CSF leakage from the site.
- *Waveforms are not changing with procedures known to cause an increase in the ICP (e.g., suctioning):* Fiber optic catheter may be damaged. Check the manufacturer's instructions for troubleshooting. Notify the primary care provider.
- *CSF is leaking from insertion site:* Notify the primary care provider. CSF is a prime medium for bacteria, and leakage can lead to an infection. Follow the facility's policy. Some facilities may have the nurse apply a sterile dressing around the insertion site; others may require more frequent cleansing of the area.

SPECIAL CONSIDERATIONS

- Label and secure the catheters according to facility policy after insertion and use care when moving patients to prevent dislodgement and breakage.
- Repositioning is important to prevent skin alterations and to decrease the risks associated with immobility. Modest, initial increases in ICP experienced with repositioning quickly return to baseline after repositioning is complete (McNett & Olson, 2013). Turn and position the patient in proper body alignment, avoiding angulation of body parts. Extreme hip flexion or flexion of upper legs can increase intra-abdominal pressure, leading to increased ICP. Maintain the neck in neutral position at all times to avoid neck vein compression, which can interfere with venous return (Hickey, 2014).
- Maintain the head of the bed elevated 15 to 30 degrees to promote venous return from the brain, depending on medical orders and facility procedure (AACN, 2017; Hickey, 2014).
- Limit endotracheal suctioning episodes to one to two passes of the catheter (Hickey, 2014). The ICP increases associated with suctioning, tracheal stimulation, and coughing are modest and transient (McNett & Olson, 2013).
- Oral care is a safe intervention; ICP increases experienced with oral care are modest, transient, and resolve quickly when oral care is complete (McNett & Olson, 2013).

(continued)

Skill 17-5 ▶ Caring for a Patient With a Fiber Optic Intracranial Catheter *(continued)*

- Auditory stimulation for critically ill neurologically impaired patients does not increase ICP and is considered a safe intervention (McNett & Olson, 2013).
- Plan care to avoid grouping activities and procedures known to increase ICP. Bathing, turning, and other routine care often have a cumulative effect to increase ICP when performed in succession. Allow rest periods between procedures and carefully assess the patient's response to interventions (Hickey, 2014).

EVIDENCE FOR PRACTICE ▶

NURSING INTERVENTIONS FOR PATIENTS WITH INTRACRANIAL PRESSURE MONITORING

McNett, M. M., & Olson, D. M. (2013). Evidence to guide nursing interventions for critically ill neurologically impaired patients with ICP monitoring. *Journal of Neuroscience Nursing, 45*(3), 120–123.

This Executive Summary addresses the research evidence for common nursing interventions for critically ill neurologically impaired patients with ICP monitoring. The interventions addressed include oral care, endotracheal suctioning, patient repositioning, chest physiotherapy, and auditory stimulation.

See additional Evidence for Practice related to caring for patients with ICP monitoring at the end of Skill 17-4, and refer to thePoint® for additional research on related nursing topics.

Enhance Your Understanding

Focusing on Patient Care: Developing Clinical Reasoning

Consider the case scenarios at the beginning of the chapter as you answer the following questions to enhance your understanding and apply what you have learned.

QUESTIONS

1. Aleta Jackson, age 68, was involved in a head-on collision. She has begun to complain that the cervical collar is hurting her neck. How should you address this issue?

2. Yuka Chong has not had a seizure since being diagnosed with epilepsy. Her mothers seem anxious and fearful and have a lot of questions and concerns about what to do if Yuka has a seizure. What information should be included in teaching for Yuka's mothers?

What safety interventions are appropriate to prevent potential injury during a seizure? How will the mothers know when it is necessary to call for emergency assistance related to a seizure?

3. Mr. and Mrs. Gladstone ask about "the tube coming out of Nikki's head," referring to her ventriculostomy. What should you tell them regarding the ventriculostomy? What should be included in the teaching for her parents? What guidelines regarding positioning and turning Nikki should you keep in mind when caring for her?

You can find suggested answers after the Bibliography at the end of this chapter.

Integrated Case Study Connection

The case studies in the back of the book focus on integrating concepts. Refer to the following case studies to enhance your understanding of the concepts and skills in this chapter.

- Intermediate Case Studies: Kent Clark, page 1121.

Taylor Suite Resources

Explore these additional resources to enhance learning for this chapter:

- NCLEX-Style Questions and other resources on thePoint®, http://thePoint.lww.com/Lynn5e
- *Skill Checklists for Taylor's Clinical Nursing Skills, 5e*

Bibliography

American Association of Critical-Care Nurses (AANN). (2017). In D. L. Wiegand (Ed.). *AACN procedure manual for high acuity, progressive, and critical care* (7th ed.). St. Louis, MO: Elsevier.

American Association of Neuroscience Nurses (AANN). (2011). *Care of the patient undergoing intracranial pressure monitoring/external ventricular drainage or lumbar drainage.* Glenview, IL: Author.

American Association of Neuroscience Nurses (AANN). (2014). *Cervical spine surgery: A guide to preoperative and postoperative patient care.* Glenview, IL: Author.

American Association of Neuroscience Nurses (AANN). (2016). *Care of adults and children with seizures and epilepsy: AANN clinical practice guideline series.* Chicago, IL: Author.

Buelow, J. M. (2013). Kathleen Mears Memorial Lecture: An update on patient safety issues in the epilepsy monitoring unit. *Neurodiagnostic Journal, 53*(2), 104–113.

Cam, R., & Korkmaz, F. D. (2013). The effect of long-term care and follow-up on complications in patients with external fixators. *International Journal of Nursing Practice, 20*(1), 89–96.

Centers for Disease Control and Prevention (CDC). (2014). *Epilepsy. Types of seizures.* Retrieved https://www.cdc.gov/epilepsy/basics/types-of-seizures.htm

Centers for Disease Control and Prevention (CDC). (2015). *Epilepsy. Seizure first aid.* Retrieved https://www.cdc.gov/epilepsy/basics/first-aid.htm

Cohen, B. J., & Hull, K. L. (2016). *Memmler's structure and function of the human body* (11th ed.). Philadelphia: Wolters Kluwer.

Conrad, B. P., Del Rossi, G., Horodyski, M. B., Prasarn, M. L., Alemi, Y., & Rechtine, G. R. (2012). Eliminating log rolling as a spine trauma order. *Surgical Neurology International, 3*(Suppl 3), S188–S197.

Cooper, K. L. (2013). Evidence-based prevention of pressure ulcers in the intensive care unit. *CriticalCareNurse, 33*(6), 57–66.

Czaikowski, B. L., Liang, H., & Stewart, C. T. (2014). A pediatric FOUR Score Coma Scale: Interrater reliability and predictive validity. *Journal of Neuroscience Nursing, 46*(2), 79–87.

Doenges, M. E., Moorhouse, M. F., & Murr, A. C. (2016). *Nursing diagnoses manual: Planning, individualizing, and documenting client care* (5th ed.). Philadelphia, PA: F.A. Davis Company.

El-Radhi, A. S. (2015). Management of seizures in children. *British Journal of Nursing (Mark Allen Publishing), 24*(3), 152–155.

Epilepsy Foundation. (2013). *Seizure first aid.* Retrieved http://www.epilepsy.com/learn/treating-seizures-and-epilepsy/seizure-first-aid

Epilepsy Foundation. (2014). *What happens during a seizure.* Retrieved http://www.epilepsy.com/learn/epilepsy-101/what-happens-during-seizure

Fritz, D., & Musial, M. K. (2016). Neurological assessment. *Home Healthcare Now, 34*(1), 16–22.

Geyer, K., Meller, K., Kulpan, C., & Mowery, B. D. (2013). Traumatic brain injury in children: Acute care management. *Pediatric Nursing, 39*(6), 283–289.

Grossman, S., & Porth, C. M. (2014). *Porth's pathophysiology: Concepts of altered health states* (9th ed.). Philadelphia, PA: Wolters Kluwer Health

Ham, H. W., Schoonhoven, L., Galer, A. A., & Shortridge-Baggett, L. L. (2014). Cervical collar-related pressure ulcers in trauma patients in intensive care unit. *Journal of Trauma Nursing, 21*(3), 94–102.

Hepburn-Smith, M., Dynkevich, I., Spektor, M., Lord, A., Czeisler, B., & Lewis, A. (2016). Establishment of an external ventricular drain best practice guideline: The quest for a comprehensive, universal standard for external ventricular drain care. *Journal of Neuroscience Nursing, 48*(1), 54–65.

Hickey, J. (2014). *The clinical practice of neurological and neurosurgical nursing* (7th ed.). Philadelphia, PA: Wolters Kluwer.

Hinkle, J. L., & Cheever, K. H. (2018). *Brunner & Suddarth's textbook of medical-surgical nursing* (14th ed.). Philadelphia, PA: Wolters Kluwer.

Hogan-Quigley, B., Palm, M. L., & Bickley, L. (2017). *Bates' nursing guide to physical examination and history taking* (2nd ed.). Philadelphia, PA: Wolters Kluwer.

Iacono, L. A., Wells, C., & Mann-Finnerty, K. (2014). Standardizing neurological assessments. *Journal of Neuroscience Nursing, 46*(2), 125–132.

Jarvis, C. (2016). *Physical examination and health assessment.* (7th ed.). St. Louis, MO: Elsevier.

Jensen, S. (2015). *Nursing health assessment: A best practice approach* (2nd ed.). Philadelphia, PA: Wolters Kluwer.

Johnson, V. D., & Whitcomb, J. (2013). Neuro/trauma intensive care unit nurses' perception of the use of the full outline of unresponsiveness score versus the Glasgow Coma Scale when assessing the neurological status of intensive care unit patients. *Dimensions of Critical Care Nursing, 32*(4), 180–183.

Kocak, Y., Ozturk, S., Ege, F., & Ekmekci, H. (2012). A useful new coma scale in acute stroke patients: FOUR score. *Anaesthesia and Intensive Care, 40*(1), 131–136.

Ktistakis, I., Guerado, E., & Giannoudis, P. V. (2015). Pin-site care: Can we reduce the incidence of infections? *Injury, 46*(Suppl 3), S35–S39.

Kyle, T., & Carman, S. (2017). *Essentials of pediatric nursing* (3rd ed.). Philadelphia, PA: Wolters Kluwer.

Lagerquist, D., Dabrowski, M., Dock, C., et al. (2012). Care of external fixator pin sites. *American Journal of Critical Care, 21*(4), 288–292.

LeMone, P., Burke, K. M., Bauldoff, G., & Gubrud, P. (2015). *Medical-surgical nursing: Clinical reasoning in patient care* (6th ed.). New York: Pearson.

Lethaby, A., Temple, J., & Santy-Tomlinson, J. (2013). Pin site care for preventing infections associated with external bone fixators and pins (Review). *Cochrane Database of Systematic Reviews*, (12), CD004551. DOI: 10.1002/14651858.CD004551.pub3.

Mayo Foundation for Medical Education and Research (MFMER). (2012). *Spinal injury: First aid.* Retrieved http://www.mayoclinic.org/first-aid/first-aid-spinal-injury/basics/art-20056677

McCallum, C., & Leonard, M. (2013). The connection between neurosciences and dialysis: A quick neurological assessment for hemodialysis nurses. *CANNT Journal, 23*(3), 20–26

McNett, M. M., & Olson, D. M. (2013). Evidence to guide nursing interventions for critically ill neurologically impaired patients with ICP monitoring. *Journal of Neuroscience Nursing, 45*(3), 120–123.

Mink, J. (2012). The neurologic assessment toolbox: Key assessments at critical times. *Nursing2012 CriticalCare, 7*(3), 12–17.

Montgomery, N., & Goode, D. (2014). Managing patients with cervical spine injury. *Emergency Nurse, 22*(2), 18–22.

Morton, P. G., & Fontaine, D. K. (2018). *Critical care nursing: A holistic approach* (11th ed.). Philadelphia, PA: Wolters Kluwer.

NANDA International, Inc.: *Nursing diagnoses – Definitions and classification 2018–2020* © 2017 NANDA International, ISBN 978-1-62623-929-6. Used by arrangement with the Thieme Group, Stuttgart/New York.

National Institute of Neurological Disorders and Stroke. (n.d.). *The epilepsies and seizures: Hope through research.* Retrieved https://www.ninds.nih.gov/Disorders/Patient-Caregiver-Education/Hope-Through-Research/Epilepsies-and-Seizures-Hope-Through#230383109

Okamura, K. (2014). Glasgow Coma Scale flow chart: A beginner's guide. *British Journal of Nursing (Mark Allen Publishing), 23*(20), 1068–1073

Olson, D. M., McNett, M. M., Lewis, L. S., Riemen, K. E., & Bautista, C. (2013). Effects of nursing interventions on intracranial pressure. *American Journal of Critical Care, 22*(5), 431–438.

Patchen, S. J., Timyam, L., & Atherton, S. (2010). *Patient information manual: Your life in a halo made easier.* Miami, FL: University of Miami School of Medicine/ Össur. Retrieved https://assets.ossur.com/library/18099/ReSolve-Halo-Patient-Information-Manual.pdf

Patient Safety Network. (n.d.). *Never events.* Retrieved https://psnet.ahrq.gov/primers/primer/3/never-events

Perry, S. E., Hockenberry, M. J., Lowdermilk, D. L., & Wilson, D. (2014). *Maternal child nursing care* (5th ed.). St. Louis, MO: Elsevier.

Rank, W. (2013). Performing a focused neurologic assessment. *Nursing, 43*(12), 37–40.

Sharpe, J. P., Magnotti, L. J., Weinberg, J. A., Schroeppel, T. J., Fabian, T. C., & Croce, M. A. (2016). The old man and the C-spine fracture: Impact of halo vest stabilization in patients with blunt cervical spine fractures. *Journal of Trauma and Acute Care Surgery, 80*(1), 76–80.

Smith, G., Wagner, J. L., & Edwards, J. C. (2015). Epilepsy update, part 2: Nursing care and evidence-based treatment. *American Journal of Nursing, 115*(6), 34–44.

Spray, J. (2015). Seizures: Awareness and observation in the ward environment. *British Journal of Nursing (Mark Allen Publishing), 24*(19), 946–955.

Szabo, C. M., Grap, M. J., Munro, C. L., Starkweather, A., & Merchant, R. E. (2014). The effect of oral care on intracranial pressure in critically ill adults. *Journal of Neuroscience Nursing, 46*(6), 321–329.

Taylor, C., Lynn, P., & Bartlett, J. (2019). *Fundamentals of nursing: The art and science of person-centered care* (9th ed.). Philadelphia, PA: Wolters Kluwer.

Timms, A., & Pugh, H. (2012). Pin site care: Guidance and key recommendations. *Nursing Standard, 27*(1), 50–55.

VHA Center for Engineering & Occupational Safety and Health (CEOSH). (2016). *Safe patient handling and mobility guidebook.* St. Louis, MO: Author. Retrieved http://www.tampavaref.org/safe-patient-handling.htm

Warren, E. (2016). Epilepsy: What general practice nurses need to know. *Practice Nurse, 46*(6), 26–30.

Wijdicks, E. F., Bamlet, W. R., Maramattom, B. V., Manno, E. M., & McClelland, R. L. (2005) Validation of a new coma scale: The FOUR score. *Annals of Neurology, 58*(4), 585–593.

SUGGESTED ANSWERS FOR FOCUSING ON PATIENT CARE: DEVELOPING CLINICAL REASONING

1. Check the fit and placement of the collar. The center of the collar should line up with the center of the patient's neck. Center the front of the collar over the patient's chin, ensuring that the chin area fits snugly in the recess of the collar. Be sure that the front half of the collar overlaps the back half. Check to see that at least one finger can be inserted between collar and patient's neck. Check the skin under the cervical collar for any signs of skin breakdown. Have a second person immobilize the cervical spine. Remove the top half of the collar and cleanse the skin under the collar. Assess the skin for signs of irritation and/or breakdown. If not contraindicated, place the patient in the reverse Trendelenburg position to see if this helps. After replacing the collar, assess the tightness of the cervical collar; at least one finger should slide under the collar.

2. Patient and family education should include not only important information related to epilepsy and patient care, but

encouragement and support for the patient and family as well. Provide the following in discussions with Yuka and her mothers: Provide education regarding prescribed medications, including administration, potential side effects, and the importance of not running out of medication (El-Radhi, 2015). Yuka and her mothers should be encouraged to keep a seizure diary (El-Radhi, 2015). Suggest that Yuka and her mothers have periodic "seizure drills" to practice what every family member should do if Yuka has a seizure (Smith, 2015). Provide information regarding the actions to take if Yuka has a seizure. Encourage the use of showers instead of baths, to reduce the risk of drowning (El-Radhi, 2015). Encourage regular sleep and avoidance of fatigue (El-Radhi, 2015; Smith, 2015). Explain that swimming should be supervised. Emergency assistance should be obtained for prolonged seizures (>5 minutes in duration); if Yuka has trouble breathing or waking after a seizure; if Yuka has one seizure soon after the first one; or if Yuka is injured during the seizure (CDC, 2015). Provide information about support groups for Yuka, her mothers and families dealing with a diagnosis of epilepsy. Inform Yuka and her mothers that Yuka should wear a medical alert bracelet.

3. Include the following in discussions with the patient and her family: Explain what a ventriculostomy is, the rationale for placing it, and how it helps with the patient's care. Answer any questions they may have regarding the equipment. When positioning and turning the patient, be aware of the location of the ventriculostomy and attached tubing. Ensure that the tubing is not kinked or obstructed by the activity. After positioning the patient, reassess the height of the system to ensure that the location of the stopcock remains at the appropriate reference point: the tragus of the ear, the outer canthus of the patient's eye, or the patient's external auditory canal (AACN, 2017). Turn and position the patient in proper body alignment, avoiding angulation of body parts. Avoid extreme hip flexion or flexion of upper legs, which can increase intra-abdominal pressure, leading to increased ICP. Maintain the neck in a neutral position at all times to avoid neck vein compression, which can interfere with venous return (Hickey, 2014). Keep the head of the bed elevated at 30 degrees to promote venous return from the brain, depending on medical orders and facility procedure (AACN, 2017; Hickey, 2014). Bathing, turning, and other routine care often have a cumulative effect to increase ICP when performed in succession. Allow rest periods between procedures and carefully assess the patient's response to interventions (Hickey, 2014).

Laboratory Specimen Collection

Learning Objectives

After completing the chapter, you will be able to accomplish the following:

1. Obtain a nasal swab.
2. Obtain a nasopharyngeal swab.
3. Collect a sputum specimen (expectorated) for culture.
4. Obtain a urine specimen (clean catch, midstream).
5. Obtain a urine specimen from an indwelling urinary catheter.
6. Test a stool specimen for occult blood.
7. Collect a stool specimen.
8. Obtain a capillary blood sample for glucose testing.
9. Collect a venous blood specimen by venipuncture for routine laboratory testing.
10. Obtain a venous blood specimen for culture and sensitivity.
11. Obtain an arterial blood specimen for blood gas analysis.

Key Terms

arterial blood gas (ABG): a laboratory test that evaluates the adequacy of oxygenation, ventilation, and acid–base status

expectorate: expel from the mouth; spit

indole: produced by decomposition of tryptophan in the intestine; contributes to the peculiar odor of feces

lancet: a small, sharp device for piercing the skin

nares: plural for naris

naris: oval openings at the base of the nose

nasopharynx: upper portion of the throat (pharynx) located behind the nasal cavity

occult blood: blood that is hidden in a stool specimen or cannot be seen on gross examination

protocol: written plan that details the nursing activities to be executed in specific situations

skatole: produced by protein decomposition in the intestine; contributes to the peculiar odor of feces

standard: acceptable, expected level of performance established by authority, custom, or consent

Standard Precautions: precautions used in the care of all hospitalized people, regardless of their diagnosis or possible infection status; these precautions apply to blood, all body fluids, secretions, and excretions (except sweat), nonintact skin, and mucous membranes

sterile technique: involves practices used to render and keep objects and areas free from microorganisms

venipuncture: piercing a vein with a needle to obtain a venous blood sample

Laboratory specimens are collected to aid in the screening and diagnosing of patient health problems, in directing treatment, and in monitoring the treatment effectiveness. Blood, urine, and stool samples are commonly collected types of specimens. Follow facility **protocol** to collect, handle, and transport specimens. Always observe **Standard Precautions** and use **sterile technique** where appropriate. It is very important to adhere to protocols and **standards**, collect the appropriate amount, use appropriate containers and media, and store and transfer the specimen within specified timelines. It is also extremely important to ensure accurate labeling of any specimen collected, according to facility policy. These measures prevent invalid and inaccurate test results.

Patient teaching is an important part of specimen collection. Explain the rationale for the sample collection and the process for obtaining the specimen. Evaluate the patient's ability to follow the specific procedure for collecting the specimen.

When collecting a specimen, take care to prevent the outside of the container from becoming contaminated with any secretions or body fluids. Place all laboratory specimens in plastic bags marked "Biohazard" and seal the bags to prevent leakage during transportation.

This chapter reviews methods to obtain specimens for common laboratory tests. Nurses must also be knowledgeable about normal and abnormal findings associated with these laboratory tests. Fundamentals Review 18-1 and 18-2 highlight the normal findings associated with urine and stool specimens.

Fundamentals Review 18-1

CHARACTERISTICS OF URINE

Characteristic	Normal Findings	Special Considerations
Color	A freshly voided specimen is pale yellow, straw-colored, or amber, depending on its concentration.	Urine is darker than normal when it is scanty and concentrated. Urine is lighter than normal when it is excessive and diluted. Certain drugs, such as cascara, L-dopa, and sulfonamides, alter the color of urine. Some foods can alter the color; for example, beets can cause urine to appear red in color.
Odor	Normal urine smell is aromatic. As urine stands, it often develops an ammonia odor because of bacterial action.	Some foods cause urine to have a characteristic odor; for example, asparagus causes urine to have a strong, musty odor. Urine high in glucose content has a sweet odor. Urine that is heavily infected has a fetid odor.
Turbidity	Fresh urine should be clear or translucent; as urine stands and cools, it becomes cloudy.	Cloudiness observed in freshly voided urine is abnormal and may be due to the presence of red blood cells, white blood cells, bacteria, vaginal discharge, sperm, or prostatic fluid.
pH	The normal pH is about 6.0, with a range of 4.6 to 8. (Urine alkalinity or acidity may be promoted through diet to inhibit bacterial growth or urinary stone development or to facilitate the therapeutic activity of certain medications.) Urine becomes alkaline on standing when carbon dioxide diffuses into the air.	A high-protein diet causes urine to become excessively acidic. Certain foods tend to produce alkaline urine, such as citrus fruits, dairy products, and vegetables, especially legumes. Certain foods, such as meats, tend to produce acidic urine. Certain drugs influence the acidity or alkalinity of urine; for example, ammonium chloride produces acidic urine, and potassium citrate and sodium bicarbonate produce alkaline urine.
Specific gravity	This is a measure of the concentration of dissolved solids in the urine. The normal range is 1.015 to 1.025.	Concentrated urine will have a higher-than-normal specific gravity, and diluted urine will have a lower-than-normal specific gravity. In the absence of kidney disease, a high specific gravity usually indicates dehydration and a low specific gravity indicates overhydration.
Constituents	*Organic* constituents of urine include urea, uric acid, creatinine, hippuric acid, indican, urine pigments, and undetermined nitrogen. *Inorganic* constituents are ammonia, sodium, chloride, traces of iron, phosphorus, sulfur, potassium, and calcium.	*Abnormal constituents* of urine include blood, pus, albumin, glucose, ketone bodies, casts, gross bacteria, and bile.

Fundamentals Review 18-2

CHARACTERISTICS OF STOOL

Characteristic	Normal Findings	Special Considerations for Observation
Volume	Variable	Volume of the stool depends on the amount the person eats and the nature of the diet. For example, a diet high in roughage produces more feces than a soft, bland diet. Consistently large diarrheal stools suggest a disorder in the small bowel or proximal colon; small, frequent stools with urgency to pass them suggest a disorder of the left colon or rectum.
Color	Infant: Yellow to brown Adult: Brown	The brown color of the stool is due to stercobilin, a bile pigment derivative. The rapid rate of peristalsis in the breastfed infant causes the stool to be yellow. Stool color is influenced by diet. For example, the stool will be almost black if the person eats red meat and dark green vegetables, such as spinach. The stool will be light brown if the diet is high in milk and milk products and low in meat. The absence of bile may cause the stool to appear white or clay colored. Certain drugs influence the color of the stool. For example, iron salts cause the stool to be black. Antacids cause it to be whitish. Bleeding high in the intestinal tract causes a stool to be black due to the digestion of the blood. Bleeding low in the intestinal tract results in fresh blood in the stool. The stool darkens with standing.
Odor	Pungent; may be affected by foods ingested.	The characteristic odor of the stool is due to **indole** and **skatole**, caused by putrefaction and fermentation in the lower intestinal tract. Stool odor is influenced by its pH value, which normally is neutral or slightly alkaline. Excessive putrefaction causes a strong odor. The presence of blood in the stool causes a unique odor.
Consistency	Soft, semisolid, and formed	Stool consistency is influenced by fluid and food intake and gastric motility. The less time stool spends in the intestine (or the shorter the intestine), the more liquid the stool. Many pathologic conditions influence consistency.
Shape	Formed stool is usually about 1 in (2.5 cm) in diameter and has the tubular shape of the colon, but may be larger or smaller, depending on the condition of the colon.	A gastrointestinal obstruction may result in a narrow, pencil-shaped stool. Rapid peristalsis thins the stool. Increased time spent in the large intestine may result in a hard, marble-like fecal mass.
Constituents	Waste residues of digestion: bile, intestinal secretions, shed epithelial cells, bacteria, and inorganic material (chiefly calcium and phosphates); seeds, meat fibers, and fat may be present in small amounts.	Internal bleeding, infection, inflammation, and other pathologic conditions may result in abnormal constituents. These include blood, pus, excessive fat, parasites, ova, and mucus. Foreign bodies also may be found in the stool.

Skill 18-1 ▶ Obtaining a Nasal Swab

A nasal swab provides a sample that can be cultured, which will aid in the diagnosis of infection and detect the carrier state for certain organisms. A nasal swab may be used to diagnose infectious respiratory tract diseases, such as influenza. It is commonly used to detect the presence of organisms, such as *Staphylococcus aureus*, which may colonize on the skin in the nose, skin folds, hairline, perineum, and navel. These organisms often survive in these areas without causing infection, unless the organism invades the skin or deeper tissues (Centers for Disease Control and Prevention [CDC], 2011). Some strains of *S. aureus* have developed resistance to antibiotics. A nasal swab can be part of the screening process to detect infection with drug-resistant microorganisms, such as methicillin-resistant *S. aureus* (CDC, 2016).

DELEGATION CONSIDERATIONS	Obtaining a nasal swab is not delegated to nursing assistive personnel (NAP) or to unlicensed assistive personnel (UAP). Depending on the state's nurse practice act and the organization's policies and procedures, this procedure may be delegated to licensed practical/vocational nurses (LPN/LVNs). The decision to delegate must be based on careful analysis of the patient's needs and circumstances, as well as the qualifications of the person to whom the task is being delegated. Refer to the Delegation Guidelines in Appendix A.

EQUIPMENT

- Nasal swab
- Sterile water (optional)
- Nonsterile gloves
- Goggles and face mask, or face shield
- Additional PPE, as indicated
- Biohazard bag
- Appropriate label for specimen, based on facility policy and procedure

ASSESSMENT	Assess the patient's understanding of the collection procedure, reason for testing, and ability to cooperate. Inspect the patient's **nares** and for the presence of nasal symptoms, such as discharge, erythema, or congestion. Assess for conditions that would contraindicate obtaining a nasal swab, such as injury to the nares or nose, and surgery of nose.

NURSING DIAGNOSIS

Determine the related factors for the nursing diagnoses based on the patient's current status. Appropriate nursing diagnoses may include:

- Risk for infection
- Acute pain
- Deficient knowledge

OUTCOME IDENTIFICATION AND PLANNING	The expected outcome to achieve is that an uncontaminated specimen is obtained without injury to the patient and sent to the laboratory promptly. Additional outcomes that may be appropriate include the following: the patient verbalizes an understanding of the rationale for and the steps of the procedure.

IMPLEMENTATION

ACTION	RATIONALE
1. Verify the order for a nasal swab in the patient's health record. Gather equipment. Check the expiration date on the swab package.	Verifying the prescribed intervention is crucial to ensuring that the proper procedure is administered to the right patient. Assembling equipment provides for an organized approach to the task. Swab package is sterile and should not be used past the expiration date.
2. Perform hand hygiene and put on PPE, if indicated.	Hand hygiene and PPE prevent the transmission of microorganisms. PPE is required based on transmission precautions.
3. Identify the patient.	Identifying the patient ensures the right patient receives the intervention and helps prevent errors.

(continued)

Skill 18-1 ▶ Obtaining a Nasal Swab *(continued)*

ACTION	RATIONALE
4. Explain the procedure to the patient. Discuss with the patient the need for a nasal swab. Explain to the patient the process by which the specimen will be collected.	Discussion and explanation help to allay some of the patient's anxiety and prepare the patient for what to expect.
5. Check the specimen label with the patient identification bracelet. Label should include the patient's name and identification number, time specimen was collected, route of collection, identification of the person obtaining the sample, and any other information required by facility policy.	Confirmation of patient identification information ensures the specimen is labeled correctly for the right patient.
6. Assemble equipment on overbed table or other surface within reach.	Arranging items nearby is convenient, saves time, and avoids unnecessary stretching and twisting of muscles on the part of the nurse.
7. Close curtains around the bed or close the door to the room, if possible.	Closing the door or curtain provides for patient privacy.
8. Put on goggles and face mask, or face shield and nonsterile gloves.	Goggles, face mask, face shield, and gloves protect the nurse from exposure to blood or body fluids and prevent the transmission of microorganisms. Irritation to nose during collection of the nasal swab may cause the patient to sneeze or cough.
9. Place the bed at an appropriate and comfortable working height, usually elbow height of the caregiver (VHACEOSH, 2016). Ask the patient to tip his or her head back slightly. Assist, as necessary.	Having the bed at the proper height prevents back and muscle strain. Tilting the head allows optimal access to the nares, which is where the swab will be inserted.
10. Peel open the swab kit packaging to expose the swab and collection tube. Remove the white plug from the collection tube and discard. Remove the swab from packaging by grasping the exposed end. Take care not to contaminate the swab by touching it to any other surface. Moisten with sterile water, depending on facility policy.	Swab must remain sterile to ensure the specimen is not contaminated. Moistening the end of the swab minimizes discomfort to the patient.
11. Insert swab 2 cm into one **naris** and rotate against the anterior nasal mucosa for 3 seconds or five rotations, depending on facility policy, and then keep it in place for 15 seconds (Figure 1).	Contact with the mucosa is necessary to obtain potential pathogens.

FIGURE 1. Inserting nasal swab into naris.

| 12. Remove the swab and repeat in the second naris, using the same swab. | Repeating in the second naris ensures accurate specimen. |

ACTION	RATIONALE
13. Insert the swab fully into the collection tube, taking care not to touch any other surface. The handle end of the swab should fit snugly into the collection tube and the end of swab should be in the culture medium at the distal end of the collection tube. Lightly squeeze the bottom of the collection tube as necessary, depending on type of tube in use in facility, to break the seal on the culture medium.	Swab must remain uncontaminated to ensure accurate results. Full insertion of the swab ensures it will remain in the collection tube. Placement of swab end in culture medium and releasing the liquid transport medium are necessary to ensure accurate specimen processing.
14. Dispose of used equipment per facility policy. Remove gloves. Perform hand hygiene.	Proper disposal of equipment reduces the transmission of microorganisms. Removing gloves properly reduces the risk for infection transmission and contamination of other items. Hand hygiene reduces the transmission of microorganisms.
15. Place label on the collection tube per facility policy. Place container in plastic, sealable biohazard bag.	Ensures specimen is labeled correctly for the right patient and ensures proper processing of the specimen. Packaging the specimen in a biohazard bag prevents the person transporting the container from coming in contact with the specimen.
16. Remove face shield and other PPE, if used. Perform hand hygiene.	Proper removal of PPE reduces the risk for infection transmission and contamination of other items. Hand hygiene reduces the transmission of microorganisms.
17. Transport specimen to the laboratory immediately. If immediate transport is not possible, check with laboratory personnel or policy manual whether refrigeration is contraindicated.	Timely transport ensures accurate results.

EVALUATION

The expected outcomes have been achieved when an uncontaminated specimen has been obtained without injury to the patient and sent to the laboratory promptly; and the patient verbalized an understanding of the rationale for and the steps of the procedure.

DOCUMENTATION

Guidelines

Record the time the specimen was collected and sent to the laboratory. Document any pertinent assessments of the patient's nares and the presence of nasal symptoms, such as discharge, erythema, or congestion.

Sample Documentation

> 8/21/20 1545 Nasal swab collected and sent to the laboratory. Patient's nares noted to be patent without drainage, congestion, and erythema.
>
> —S. Turner, RN

UNEXPECTED SITUATIONS AND ASSOCIATED INTERVENTIONS

- *Swab touches surface other than inner aspect of nares on entry or exit:* Discard the swab, obtain a new culture swab, and recollect the specimen.

SPECIAL CONSIDERATIONS

- If the patient has injury to the nares or nose or has had nose surgery, the nurse should contact the health care provider to discuss collection of the specimen. These conditions may prohibit collection.
- If possible, ensure the specimen is obtained before antibiotics are started (Fischbach & Dunning, 2015).

(continued)

Skill 18-2 ▶ Obtaining a Nasopharyngeal Swab

A nasopharyngeal swab provides a sample that can be cultured to aid in the diagnosis of infection and to detect the carrier state for certain organisms. A swab on a flexible wire collects a specimen from the posterior **nasopharynx**. It can be used to detect viral and bacterial infections, including *Bordetella pertussis*, respiratory syncytial virus, *Neisseria meningitidis*, methicillin-resistant *Staphylococcus aureus*, and influenza (U.S. National Library of Medicine, National Institutes of Health, MedlinePlus, 2017).

DELEGATION CONSIDERATIONS	Obtaining a nasopharyngeal swab is not delegated to nursing assistive personnel (NAP) or to unlicensed assistive personnel (UAP). Depending on the state's nurse practice act and the organization's policies and procedures, this procedure may be delegated to licensed practical/vocational nurses (LPN/LVNs). The decision to delegate must be based on careful analysis of the patient's needs and circumstances, as well as the qualifications of the person to whom the task is being delegated. Refer to the Delegation Guidelines in Appendix A.

EQUIPMENT

- Nasopharyngeal swab (flexible wire)
- Penlight
- Tongue depressor
- Facial tissue
- Nonsterile gloves
- Additional PPE, as indicated
- Biohazard bag
- Appropriate label for specimen, based on facility policy and procedure

ASSESSMENT

Assess the patient's understanding of the collection procedure, reason for testing, and ability to cooperate. Assess the patient's nares and for the presence of nasal symptoms, such as discharge, erythema, or congestion. Inspect the patient's nasopharynx. Assess for conditions that would contraindicate obtaining a nasopharyngeal swab, such as injury to the nares or nose, and surgery of the nose or throat.

NURSING DIAGNOSIS

Determine the related factors for the nursing diagnoses based on the patient's current status. Appropriate nursing diagnoses may include:

- Risk for infection
- Acute pain
- Deficient knowledge

OUTCOME IDENTIFICATION AND PLANNING

The expected outcome to achieve is that an uncontaminated specimen is obtained without injury to the patient and sent to the laboratory promptly. Additional outcomes that may be appropriate include the following: the patient verbalizes an understanding of the rationale for and the steps of the procedure.

IMPLEMENTATION

ACTION	**RATIONALE**
1. Verify the order for a nasopharyngeal swab in the patient's health record. Gather equipment. Check the expiration date on the swab package.	Verifying the medical order is crucial to ensuring that the proper procedure is administered to the right patient. Assembling equipment provides for an organized approach to task. Swab package is sterile and should not be used past the expiration date.
2. Perform hand hygiene and put on PPE, if indicated.	Hand hygiene and PPE prevent the transmission of microorganisms. PPE is required based on transmission precautions.
3. Identify the patient.	Identifying the patient ensures the right patient receives the intervention and helps prevent errors.
4. Discuss with patient the need for a nasopharyngeal swab. Explain to patient the process by which the specimen will be collected. Inform the patient that he or she may experience slight discomfort and may gag.	Discussion and explanation help to allay some of the patient's anxiety and prepare the patient for what to expect.

ACTION	RATIONALE
5. Check the specimen label with the patient's identification bracelet. Label should include the patient's name and identification number, time specimen was collected, route of collection, identification of person obtaining the sample, and any other information required by facility policy.	Confirmation of patient identification information ensures the specimen is labeled correctly for the right patient.
6. Assemble equipment on overbed table or other surface within reach.	Arranging items nearby is convenient, saves time, and avoids unnecessary stretching and twisting of muscles on the part of the nurse.
7. Close curtains around the bed or close the door to the room, if possible.	Closing the door or curtain provides for patient privacy.
8. Put on goggles and face mask, or face shield and nonsterile gloves.	Goggles, face mask, face shield, and gloves protect the nurse from exposure to blood or body fluids and prevent the transmission of microorganisms. Irritation to nose and pharynx during collection of the nasal swab may cause the patient to sneeze or cough.
9. Place the bed at an appropriate and comfortable working height, usually elbow height of the caregiver (VHACEOSH, 2016). Ask the patient to blow his or her nose into facial tissue. Ask the patient to cough into facial tissue, and then to tip back his or her head. Assist, as necessary.	Having the bed at the proper height prevents back and muscle strain. Blowing of nose clears nasal passages and coughing clears the nasopharynx of material that may interfere with accurate sampling. Tilting the head allows optimal access to the nares, where the swab will be inserted.
10. Peel open the swab packaging to expose the swab and collection tube. Remove the cap from the collection tube and discard. Remove the swab from packaging by grasping the exposed end. Take care not to contaminate the swab by touching it to any other surface.	Swab must remain sterile to ensure specimen is not contaminated.
11. Ask the patient to open the mouth. Inspect the back of the patient's throat using the tongue depressor.	The swab must make contact with mucosa to ensure collection of potential pathogens.
12. Continue to observe the nasopharynx and gently insert the swab straight back into the nostril, aiming posteriorly along the floor of the nasal cavity (Figure 1A). Insert approximately 6 in (adult) (approximately the distance from the nose to the ear) to the posterior wall of the nasopharynx (Figure 1B). **Do not insert the swab upward. Do not force the swab.** Rotate the swab. Leave the swab in the nasopharynx for 15 to 30 seconds and remove. Take care not to touch the swab to the patient's tongue or sides of the nostrils.	Observation of the nasopharynx during collection ensures an accurate specimen is collected. Swab must remain uncontaminated to ensure accurate results.

A

B

FIGURE 1. A. Observing the nasopharynx and inserting swab. **B.** Nasopharyngeal swab inserted to the posterior wall of the nasopharynx.

(*continued*)

Skill 18-2 ▶ Obtaining a Nasopharyngeal Swab *(continued)*

ACTION	RATIONALE
13. Insert the swab fully into the collection tube, taking care not to touch any other surface. The handle end of the swab should fit snugly into the collection tube and the end of swab should be in the culture medium at the distal end of the collection tube. Lightly squeeze the bottom of the collection tube as necessary, depending on type of tube in use in facility, to break the seal on the culture medium.	Swab must remain uncontaminated to ensure accurate results. Full insertion of the swab ensures it will remain in the collection tube. Placement of the swab end in culture medium and releasing of liquid transport medium is necessary to ensure accurate specimen processing.
14. Dispose of used equipment per facility policy. Remove gloves. Perform hand hygiene.	Proper disposal of equipment reduces the transmission of microorganisms. Removing gloves properly reduces the risk for infection transmission and contamination of other items. Hand hygiene reduces the transmission of microorganisms.
15. Place label on the collection tube per facility policy. Place container in plastic, sealable biohazard bag.	Ensures specimen is labeled correctly for the right patient and also ensures proper processing of specimen. Packaging the specimen in a biohazard bag prevents the person transporting the container from coming in contact with the specimen.
16. Remove other PPE, if used. Perform hand hygiene.	Proper removal of PPE reduces the risk for infection transmission and contamination of other items. Hand hygiene reduces the transmission of microorganisms.
17. Transport the specimen to the laboratory immediately. If immediate transport is not possible, check with laboratory personnel or policy manual whether refrigeration is contraindicated.	Timely transport ensures accurate results.

EVALUATION

The expected outcome is met when an uncontaminated specimen has been obtained without injury to the patient and sent to the laboratory promptly; and the patient verbalized an understanding of the rationale for and the steps of the procedure.

DOCUMENTATION

Guidelines

Record the time the specimen was collected and sent to the laboratory. Document any pertinent assessments of the patient's nares and the presence of nasal symptoms, such as discharge, erythema, or congestion. Record significant assessments of the patient's oral cavity and throat.

Sample Documentation

8/21/20 1545 Nasopharyngeal swab specimen collected and sent to laboratory. Patient's nares noted to be patent without drainage, congestion, and erythema; nasopharynx bright red with tan discharge.

—S. Turner, RN

UNEXPECTED SITUATIONS AND ASSOCIATED INTERVENTIONS

- *The patient gags as soon as the tongue depressor is placed in the mouth:* Depress the tongue with the tongue depressor by pushing down halfway back on the tongue. Press slightly off center to avoid eliciting the gag reflex (Jarvis, 2016).

SPECIAL CONSIDERATIONS

General Considerations

- Warn the patient that the procedure may cause slight discomfort.
- Caution the patient that the procedure may cause gagging.

• If possible, ensure the specimen is obtained before antibiotics are started (Fischbach & Dunning, 2015).
• Do not force the swab. Forcing could cause injury. If an obstruction is encountered, try the other nostril (CDC, 2015).

Infant and Child Considerations

• A young child will require restraint so the nurse can depress the tongue and visualize the back of the mouth without injuring the child (Kyle & Carman, 2017).

Skill 18-3 ▶ Collecting a Sputum Specimen for Culture

Sputum production is the result of the reaction of the lungs to any constant recurring irritant (Hinkle & Cheever, 2018). A sputum specimen comes from deep within the bronchi, not from the postnasal region. Sputum analysis is used to diagnose disease, test for drug sensitivity, and guide patient treatment. Sputum may be obtained to identify pathogenic organisms, determine if malignant cells are present, and assess for hypersensitivity states. A sputum specimen may be ordered if a bacterial, viral, or fungal infection of the pulmonary system is suspected.

A sputum specimen can be collected by having the patient cough into a sterile container, by endotracheal suctioning, during bronchoscopy, and via transtracheal aspiration. Because secretions have accumulated during the night, it is desirable to collect an expectorated sputum specimen first thing in the morning when the patient rises, which aids in the collection process (Hess, MacIntyre, Galvin, & Mishoe, 2016). Characteristics of sputum and potential causes are outlined in Box 18-1. The following procedure describes collecting an expectorated sample. Collecting a sputum specimen by suctioning via an endotracheal tube is discussed in the Skill Variation at the end of this skill.

Box 18-1   Characteristics of Sputum and Potential Causes

Sputum Characteristic	Potential Cause
• Thick and yellow or green (purulent)	Bacterial infection
• Thin, white, or clear, mucoid (mucous)	Colds, viral infections, bronchitis
• Rust colored	Tuberculosis, pneumococcal pneumonia
• Gradual increase of sputum over time	Chronic bronchitis
• Pink-tinged, mucoid (mucous) sputum	Lung tumor, tuberculosis
• Profuse, frothy, pink sputum	Pulmonary edema
• Foul-smelling sputum and bad breath	Lung abscess, bronchiectasis, anaerobic infection

Source: Adapted from Hinkle, J. L., & Cheever, K. H. (2018). *Brunner & Suddarth's textbook of medical-surgical nursing* (14th ed.). Philadelphia, PA: Wolters Kluwer; Jarvis, C. (2016). *Physical examination and health assessment* (7th ed.). St. Louis, MO: Elsevier; and Jensen, S. (2015). *Nursing health assessment: A best practice approach* (2nd ed.). Philadelphia, PA: Wolters Kluwer.

DELEGATION CONSIDERATIONS

Obtaining a sputum specimen is not delegated to nursing assistive personnel (NAP) or to unlicensed assistive personnel (UAP). Obtaining a sputum specimen may be delegated to licensed practical/vocational nurses (LPN/LVNs). The decision to delegate must be based on careful analysis of the patient's needs and circumstances, as well as the qualifications of the person to whom the task is being delegated. Refer to the Delegation Guidelines in Appendix A.

EQUIPMENT

• Sterile sputum specimen container
• Nonsterile gloves
• Goggles or safety glasses or face shield
• Additional PPE, as indicated
• Biohazard bag
• Appropriate label for specimen, based on facility policy and procedure

(continued)

Skill 18-3 ▶ Collecting a Sputum Specimen for Culture *(continued)*

ASSESSMENT	Assess the patient's lung sounds. Patients with a productive cough may have crackles, rhonchi, wheezing, or diminished lung sounds. Monitor oxygen saturation levels, as patients with excessive pulmonary secretions may have decreased oxygen saturation. Assess the patient's level of pain. Consider administering pain medication before obtaining the sample, because the patient will have to cough. Assess the characteristics of the sputum: color, quantity, presence of blood, and viscosity.
NURSING DIAGNOSIS	Determine the related factors for the nursing diagnoses based on the patient's current status. Appropriate nursing diagnoses may include: • Acute pain • Ineffective airway clearance • Impaired gas exchange
OUTCOME IDENTIFICATION AND PLANNING	The expected outcome to achieve when collecting a sputum specimen is that the patient produces an adequate sample (based on facility policy) from the lower respiratory tract. Other outcomes that may be appropriate include the following: airway patency is maintained; and the patient demonstrates an understanding about the need and process for specimen collection.

IMPLEMENTATION

ACTION	RATIONALE
1. Verify the order for a sputum specimen collection in the patient's health record. Gather equipment.	Verifying the medical order is crucial to ensuring that the proper procedure is administered to the right patient. Assembling equipment provides for an organized approach to the task.
2. Perform hand hygiene and put on PPE, if indicated.	Hand hygiene and PPE prevent the transmission of microorganisms. PPE is required based on transmission precautions.
3. Identify the patient.	Identifying the patient ensures the right patient receives the intervention and helps prevent errors.
4. Explain the procedure to the patient. Administer pain medication (if ordered) if the patient might have pain with coughing. If the patient can perform the task without assistance after instruction, leave the container at bedside with instructions to call the nurse as soon as a specimen is produced.	Explanation provides reassurance and promotes cooperation. Pain relief facilitates compliance.
5. Check specimen label with the patient's identification bracelet. Label should include the patient's name and identification number, time specimen was collected, route of collection, identification of the person obtaining the sample, and any other information required by facility policy.	Confirmation of patient identification information ensures the specimen is labeled correctly for the right patient.
6. Assemble equipment on overbed table or other surface within reach.	Arranging items nearby is convenient, saves time, and avoids unnecessary stretching and twisting of muscles on the part of the nurse.
7. Close curtains around the bed and close the door to the room, if possible.	Closing the curtain or door provides for patient privacy.
8. Put on disposable gloves and goggles, safety glasses or face shield, as indicated.	Gloves and eye protection prevent contact with blood and body fluids. Eye protection may be indicated based on the patient's underlying health concerns and risk for contact with body fluids.

ACTION

9. Place the bed at an appropriate and comfortable working height, usually elbow height of the caregiver (VHACEOSH, 2016). Lower side rail closest to you. Place patient in semi-Fowler's position. **Have patient clear nose and throat and rinse mouth with water before beginning procedure.**

10. Caution the patient to avoid spitting saliva secretion into the sterile container. Explain the importance of obtaining sputum from lower respiratory tract. **Instruct the patient to inhale deeply two or three times and cough with exhalation.** If the patient has had abdominal surgery, assist the patient to splint the abdomen.

11. If the patient produces sputum, open the lid to the container and have the patient **expectorate** the specimen into the container (Figure 1). Caution the patient to avoid touching the edge or the inside of the collection container.

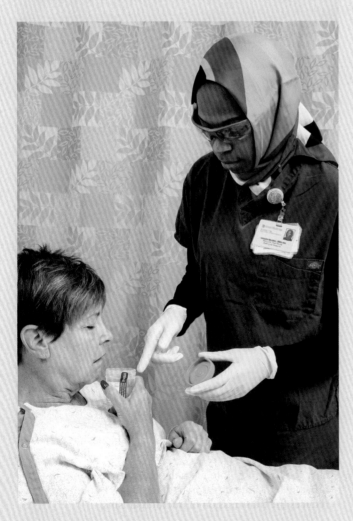

12. If patient believes he or she can produce more sputum for the specimen, have the patient repeat the procedure. Collect a volume of sputum based on facility policy.

RATIONALE

Having the bed at the proper height prevents back and muscle strain. The semi-Fowler's position will help the patient to cough and expectorate the sputum specimen. Water will rinse the oral cavity of saliva and any food particles.

Saliva can contaminate the sputum specimen. The specimen will need to come from the lungs; saliva is not acceptable. Splinting helps to reduce the pain in the abdominal incision.

The specimen needs to come from the lungs; saliva is not acceptable. Touching the edge or inside of the sterile collection container contaminates the specimen.

FIGURE 1. Instructing patient to expectorate into the collection container.

This ensures an adequate amount of sputum specimen is obtained for analysis.

(continued)

Skill 18-3 ▶ Collecting a Sputum Specimen for Culture *(continued)*

ACTION	RATIONALE
13. Close the container lid. Offer oral hygiene to the patient.	Closing the container prevents contamination of the specimen and possible infection transmission. Oral hygiene helps to remove pathogens from the oral cavity.
14. Remove equipment and return the patient to a position of comfort. Raise side rails and lower bed.	Repositioning promotes patient comfort. Raising rails promotes safety.
15. Remove gloves and goggles. Perform hand hygiene.	Removing gloves and goggles properly reduces the risk for infection transmission and contamination of other items. Hand hygiene reduces the transmission of microorganisms.
16. Place label on the container per facility policy (Figure 2). Place container in plastic, sealable biohazard bag (Figure 3).	Proper labeling of the specimen ensures the specimen is for the right patient. Packaging the specimen in a biohazard bag prevents the person transporting the container from coming in contact with the specimen.

FIGURE 2. Labeling specimen container.

FIGURE 3. Placing specimen container in biohazard bag.

ACTION	RATIONALE
17. Remove other PPE, if used. Perform hand hygiene.	Proper removal of PPE reduces the risk for infection transmission and contamination of other items. Hand hygiene reduces the transmission of microorganisms.
18. Transport the specimen to the laboratory immediately. If immediate transport is not possible, do not refrigerate specimens (Fischbach & Dunning, 2015).	Timely transport ensures accurate results.

EVALUATION

The expected outcomes have been met when the patient has produced an adequate sample (based on facility policy) from the lower respiratory tract; airway patency has been maintained; and the patient demonstrated an understanding about the need and process for specimen collection.

DOCUMENTATION

Guidelines

Record the time the sputum specimen was collected and sent to the laboratory, and the characteristics and amount of secretions. Document the tests for which the specimen was collected. Note the respiratory assessment pre- and postcollection. Note antibiotics administered in the past 24 hours on the laboratory request form, if required by the facility.

Sample Documentation

> 9/13/20 0615 Respirations unlabored; lungs with decreased breath sounds at posterior bases. Sputum specimen obtained; patient has moderate amount of thick, yellow sputum; specimen sent to laboratory for culture and sensitivity.
>
> —C. Bausler, RN

UNEXPECTED SITUATIONS AND ASSOCIATED INTERVENTIONS

- *Patient produced a specimen but did not tell you, so you do not know how long the specimen has been sitting at the bedside:* Unless the patient is able to tell you when the specimen was produced, discard the sample and recollect. Specimens should be sent to the laboratory as soon as possible to ensure valid results.
- *Patient spits saliva into container, without specimen from lungs:* Instruct the patient that the specimen needs to come from the lungs. Review the procedure for collection. Discard the contaminated container, obtain a new container and recollect a sample.

SPECIAL CONSIDERATIONS

General Considerations

- If possible, collect sputum sample when patient arises in the morning, to improve chances of obtaining an adequate amount of sputum. Specimens from deep in the lungs are obtained in the early morning after secretions have accumulated overnight (Hess et al., 2016; Hinkle & Cheever, 2018).
- If possible, ensure the specimen is obtained before antibiotics are started (Fischbach & Dunning, 2015).
- Instruct the patient to not use mouthwash before collecting a sputum sample because it may contain antibacterial agents (Hess et al., 2016).
- At least three consecutive sputum specimens are needed for diagnostic purposes for patients suspected of having tuberculosis (CDC, 2013b). Sputum specimens for acid-fast bacilli (AFB; to test for tuberculosis) should be collected at least 8 to 24 hours apart, with at least one specimen produced in the early morning (CDC, 2013b).
- If the patient understands directions and is able to cooperate, the specimen collection container may be left at bedside for the patient to collect sputum when available. Container lid should remain in place until the patient is ready to expectorate sputum. Instruct the patient to call to inform staff as soon as sputum is produced, so it can be transported to laboratory in a timely manner.

Home Care Considerations

- If the patient is to collect specimen at home, ensure that he or she has a clear understanding of the collection procedure and that the specimen needs to be transported immediately to the laboratory. Reinforce to the patient that it is important not to touch the inside of the collection container.

(continued)

Skill 18-3 ▶ Collecting a Sputum Specimen for Culture *(continued)*

Skill Variation ▶ Collecting Sputum Specimen via Endotracheal Suctioning

1. Sputum specimens can be collected by suctioning an endotracheal tube or tracheostomy tube. A sterile collection receptacle is attached between the suction catheter and the suction tubing to trap sputum as it is removed from the patient's airway, before reaching the suction collection canister.
2. Refer to Skills 14-7, 14-8, and 14-10 for the procedure for endotracheal suctioning.
3. After checking suction pressure (Step 10, Skill 14-7; Step 9, Skill 14-8; Step 10, Skill 14-10), attach a sterile specimen trap to the suction tubing, taking care to avoid contaminating the open ends (Figure A).

FIGURE A. Suction trap for sputum collection.

4. Continue with Step 11, Skill 14-7; Step 10, Skill 14-8; Step 11, Skill 14-10, taking care to handle the suction tubing and sputum trap with your nondominant hand. Proceed with suction procedure.
5. After first suction pass, if 2 to 3 mL of sputum has been obtained, disconnect the specimen container, and set aside (Fischbach & Dunning, 2015). If less than this amount has been collected, resuction the patient after waiting the appropriate amount of time for the patient to recover.
6. If secretions are extremely thick or tenacious, flush the catheter with a small amount (1 to 2 mL) of sterile normal saline to aid in moving the secretions into the trap.
7. Once the sputum trap is removed, connect suction tubing to the suction catheter. The catheter may then be flushed with normal saline before suctioning again. Continue with the suctioning procedure, if necessary, based on remaining steps in Skill 14-7, Skill 14-8, or Skill 14-10.
8. When suctioning is completed, check the specimen label with the patient's identification bracelet. Label should include the patient's name and identification number, time specimen was collected, route of collection, identification of person obtaining the sample, and any other information required by facility policy. Place label on the container per facility policy. Place container in plastic, sealable biohazard bag and send to the laboratory immediately.

Skill 18-4 ▶ Collecting a Urine Specimen (Clean Catch, Midstream)

Obtaining a urine specimen for random collection, urinalysis, and culture is an assessment measure to determine the characteristics of a patient's urine. A voided urine specimen for culture is collected midstream to provide a specimen that most closely reflects the characteristics of the urine being produced by the body. If the patient is able to understand and follow the procedure, the patient may collect the sample on his or her own, after explanation and instruction.

DELEGATION CONSIDERATIONS   Obtaining a urine specimen by midstream collection may be delegated to nursing assistive personnel (NAP) or to unlicensed assistive personnel (UAP), as well as to licensed practical/vocational nurses (LPN/LVNs). The decision to delegate must be based on careful analysis of the patient's needs and circumstances, as well as the qualifications of the person to whom the task is being delegated. Refer to the Delegation Guidelines in Appendix A.

EQUIPMENT	<ul><li>Moist cleansing towelettes or skin cleanser, water, and washcloth</li><li>Nonsterile gloves</li><li>Additional PPE, as indicated</li><li>Sterile specimen container; urine collection tubes, based on facility policy</li></ul>	<ul><li>Biohazard bag</li><li>Appropriate label for specimen, based on facility policy and procedure</li></ul>

ASSESSMENT

Ask the patient about any medications that he or she is taking, because medications may affect the results of the test. Assess for any signs and symptoms of a urinary tract infection, such as burning, pain (dysuria), or frequency. Assess the patient's ability to cooperate with the collection process. Determine the patient's need for assistance to obtain specimen correctly.

NURSING DIAGNOSIS

Determine the related factors for the nursing diagnoses based on the patient's current status. Possible nursing diagnoses may include:

- Impaired urinary elimination
- Deficient knowledge

OUTCOME IDENTIFICATION AND PLANNING

The expected outcome to achieve is that an adequate amount of urine is obtained from the patient without contamination. Other outcomes include the following: the patient demonstrates an understanding of the need and process for specimen collection.

IMPLEMENTATION

ACTION	RATIONALE
1. Verify the order for a urine specimen collection in the patient's health record. Gather equipment.	Verifying the medical order is crucial to ensuring that the proper procedure is administered to the right patient. Assembling equipment provides for an organized approach to the task.
2. Perform hand hygiene and put on PPE, if indicated.	Hand hygiene and PPE prevent the transmission of microorganisms. PPE is required based on transmission precautions.
3. Identify the patient.	Identifying the patient ensures the right patient receives the intervention and helps prevent errors.
4. Explain the procedure to the patient. If the patient can perform the task without assistance after instruction, leave the container at bedside with instructions to call the nurse as soon as a specimen is produced.	Explanation provides reassurance and promotes cooperation. Timely transport of the specimen ensures accurate results.
5. Check the specimen label with the patient's identification bracelet. Label should include the patient's name and identification number, time specimen was collected, route of collection, identification of the person obtaining the sample, and any other information required by facility policy.	Confirmation of patient identification information ensures the specimen is labeled correctly for the right patient.
6. Assemble equipment on overbed table or other surface within reach.	Arranging items nearby is convenient, saves time, and avoids unnecessary stretching and twisting of muscles on the part of the nurse.
7. Have the patient perform hand hygiene, if performing self-collection.	Hand hygiene prevents the transmission of microorganisms.
8. Close curtains around the bed and close the door to the room, if possible.	Closing the door or curtain provides for patient privacy.

(continued)

Skill 18-4 ▸ Collecting a Urine Specimen (Clean Catch, Midstream) *(continued)*

ACTION	RATIONALE
9. Put on nonsterile gloves. Assist the patient to the bathroom, or onto the bedside commode or bedpan. Instruct the patient not to defecate or discard toilet paper into the urine (Figure 1).	Gloves reduce the transmission of microorganisms. Stool and/or toilet paper may contaminate the specimen.

FIGURE 1. Instructing patient about urine collection procedure.

| 10. Instruct the female patient to separate the labia for cleaning of the area and during collection of urine. Female patients should use the towelettes or wet washcloth to clean each side of the urinary meatus, then the center over the meatus, from front to back, using a new wipe or a clean area of the washcloth for each stroke. Instruct the female patient to **keep the labia separated after cleaning and during collection (Figure 2)**. Male patients should use a towelette to clean the area around the meatus of the penis, wiping in a circular motion away from the urethral meatus. Instruct the uncircumcised male patient to retract the foreskin before cleaning and during collection (Figure 3). | Cleaning the perineal area or penis reduces the risk for contamination of the specimen. Separation of labia avoids contamination by perineal skin and hair. Retraction of foreskin avoids contamination by skin. |

FIGURE 2. Cleaning female perineum. Separating labia and cleansing from front to back.

FIGURE 3. Cleaning male perineum. Wiping in a circular motion away from urethra.

ACTION	**RATIONALE**
11. Do not let the container touch the perineal skin or hair during collection. Do not touch the inside of the container or the lid. Have patient void a small amount (approximately 25 to 30 mL/1 oz) of urine into the toilet, bedpan, or commode. The patient should then stop urinating briefly, and then continue voiding into the collection container. Collect the urine specimen (3 to 5 mL is sufficient), and then instruct the patient to finish voiding in the toilet, bedpan, or commode. Instruct the uncircumcised male patient to replace the foreskin after collection.	Collecting a midstream specimen ensures that fresh urine is analyzed. Some urine may have collected in the urethra from the last void. By voiding a little before collecting the specimen, the specimen will contain only fresh urine.
12. Place lid on container. If necessary, transfer the specimen to appropriate containers/tubes for specific test ordered, according to facility policy.	Placing the lid on the container helps to keep the specimen clean and prevents spills.
13. Assist the patient from the bathroom, off the commode, or off the bedpan. Provide perineal care, if necessary.	Perineal care promotes patient comfort and hygiene.
14. Remove gloves and perform hand hygiene.	Removing gloves properly reduces the risk for infection transmission and contamination of other items. Hand hygiene reduces the transmission of microorganisms.
15. Place label on the container per facility policy. Note specimen collection method, according to facility policy. Place container in plastic, sealable biohazard bag.	Proper labeling ensures accurate reporting of results. Packaging the specimen in a biohazard bag prevents the person transporting the container from coming in contact with urine.
16. Remove other PPE, if used. Perform hand hygiene.	Proper removal of PPE reduces the risk for infection transmission and contamination of other items. Hand hygiene reduces the transmission of microorganisms.
17. Transport the specimen to the laboratory as soon as possible. If unable to take the specimen to the laboratory immediately, refrigerate it (Fischbach & Dunning, 2015).	If not refrigerated immediately, urine may act as a culture medium, allowing bacteria to multiply and skewing the results of testing. Refrigeration prevents the bacteria from multiplying.

EVALUATION   The expected outcomes have been met when an adequate amount of urine has been obtained from the patient without contamination; and the patient demonstrated an understanding of the need and process for specimen collection.

DOCUMENTATION

Guidelines   Document that the specimen was collected and sent to the laboratory. Note the specimen collection method. Note the characteristics of the urine, including odor, amount (if known), color, and clarity. Include any significant patient assessments, such as patient complaints of burning or pain on urination.

Sample Documentation

> 7/10/20 2200 Patient instructed to collect midstream urine sample. Verbalized understanding of directions; 70 mL of cloudy, odorless, yellow urine sent to the laboratory. Patient denies pain or discomfort on urination.
>
> —A. Blitz, RN

UNEXPECTED SITUATIONS AND ASSOCIATED INTERVENTIONS

- *Patient cannot provide a sufficient urine sample:* Offer the patient fluids to drink, although drinking too much fluid may dilute the urine, invalidating the test. Patient may return later in day to supply sample. Offer patient assistance with the next void.

(continued)

Skill 18-4 > Collecting a Urine Specimen (Clean Catch, Midstream) *(continued)*

- *Patient missed voiding into the specimen container but did void into the collection receptacle in the toilet:* Do not use this urine as a sample for a culture; it could be heavily contaminated with bacteria and give a misleading result. Attempt to collect urine with next void. Offer patient assistance when trying to collect sample.

SPECIAL CONSIDERATIONS

General Considerations

- For many urine tests, such as a urinalysis, drug testing, or diabetes testing, the specimen does not need to be sterile and does not need to be collected as a midstream specimen. However, in the case of urinalysis, if the specimen shows nitrates and white blood cells, a culture of a urine specimen may be ordered as well.
- Because the first voiding of the day contains the highest bacterial counts, collect this sample whenever possible (Fischbach & Dunning, 2015).
- If possible, ensure the specimen is obtained before antibiotics are started (Fischbach & Dunning, 2015).
- Urine specimens may also be obtained by direct urethral catheterization. Refer to Skills 12-6 and 12-7 for catheterization procedure.
- Urine specimens may also be obtained from urinary diversions. See the accompanying Skill Variation below.

Infant and Child Considerations

- The most reliable method to obtain a urine specimen for culture (associated with lower contamination rates) in neonates and young infants is to perform a suprapubic aspiration or transurethral catheterization (Cheek, Craig, Seith, & West, 2015). Discuss sampling options with the health care provider and the patient's parents. Suprapubic aspiration is painful; pain management during the procedure is important—topical anesthetic cream should be used when time permits, as well as age-appropriate distraction techniques (Cheek et al., 2015).
- Midstream collection can be accomplished with children older than 2 years of age, provided the child is able to follow direction and will cooperate with the nurse. Try having the child sit facing the back of the toilet, straddling the toilet seat. The nurse or parent can position themselves behind the child, holding the sterile container for urine collection.
- Infants and toddlers who are not toilet trained may require a urine bag for urine collection. A sterile urine bag is required for a urine culture; a clean bag for routine urinalysis (Kyle & Carman, 2017, p. 764). Refer to the accompanying Skill Variation for the steps used to obtain a bagged urine specimen from an infant or young child.
- Familiar terms, such as "pee-pee," "potty" or "tinkle," may be used with young children to ensure they understand what is being explained and gain cooperation (Kyle & Carman, 2017, p. 767). Enlist the assistance of the patient's parents or significant others to identify appropriate terms.

Home Care Considerations

- If the patient is to collect a specimen at home, ensure that the patient has a clear understanding of collection procedure, understands the need to transport the specimen immediately to the laboratory, and has obtained the necessary equipment from his or her health care provider or laboratory. Reinforce that the patient cannot touch the inside of the collection container. Urine specimens must be refrigerated until they can be brought to the laboratory.

Skill Variation > Obtaining a Bagged Urine Specimen for Urinalysis From an Infant or Young Child

1. Follow Steps 1 to 3 in Skill 18-4.
2. Identify the patient. Explain the steps to a young child, if old enough, and to the parents. Talk to the child at the child's level, stressing that no pain will be involved.
3. Check specimen label with the patient's identification bracelet. Label should include the patient's name and

identification number, time specimen was collected, route of collection, identification of the person obtaining sample, and any other information required by facility policy.

4. Remove the diaper or underwear. Perform thorough perineal care with skin cleanser and water: for girls, spread labia and cleanse area; for boys, retract foreskin

Skill Variation Obtaining a Bagged Urine Specimen for Urinalysis From an Infant or Young Child *(continued)*

if intact and cleanse glans of penis. Pat skin dry. Consider application of a skin barrier, such as Skin-Prep, to the skin around the scrotum or vulvar area to aid with urine bag adhesion and reduce the risk of skin irritation.

5. Remove paper backing from adhesive faceplate. Apply faceplate over labia or over penis. Gently push faceplate so that seal forms on skin (Figure A). For boys, ensure the penis is fully inside the bag; a portion of the scrotum may or may not be inside the bag, depending on scrotal size (Kyle & Carman, 2017, p. 767). For girls, apply the narrow portion of the bag on the perineal space between

FIGURE A. Applying infant urine collection bag.

the anal and vulvar areas first, then spread the remaining adhesive section (Kyle & Carman, 2017).

6. Apply clean diaper or underwear over bag to help prevent dislodgement. Remove gloves and perform hand hygiene. **Check bag every 15 minutes to see whether the child has voided.**

 7. As soon as the patient has voided, perform hand hygiene and put on nonsterile gloves. Gently remove bag by pushing skin away from bag. Transfer urine to appropriate containers/tubes for specific test ordered, according to facility policy.

8. Perform perineal care and reapply diaper or clothing.

9. Remove gloves. Perform hand hygiene.

10. Place label on the container per facility policy. Place container in plastic, sealable biohazard bag.

 11. Remove other PPE, if used. Perform hand hygiene.

12. Transport the specimen to the laboratory as soon as possible. If unable to take the specimen to the laboratory immediately, refrigerate it.

13. If the collection bag falls off or does not adhere completely, remove the bag, perform perineal care, and apply a new collection bag.

Skill Variation   Obtaining a Urine Specimen From a Urinary Diversion

Equipment: Cleansing solution, based on facility policy; sterile gauze; sterile water or saline, or other cleansing solution for stoma site (povidone-iodine, chlorhexidine, soap and water), based on facility policy; double-lumen or straight catheter (16 Fr); sterile water-based lubricant if catheter not self-lubricated; sterile specimen container and urine collection tubes, based on facility policy; sterile and nonsterile gloves; new ostomy appliance; skin cleanser; disposable washcloth or washcloth and towel

1. Follow Steps 1 to 6 in Skill 18-4.
2. Put on nonsterile gloves. Remove ostomy appliance. If one-piece system is in place, remove entire appliance. If

two-piece system is in place, remove collection pouch only, leaving appliance pouch only, leaving faceplate wafer intact on skin.

3. Using a circular motion from stoma opening outward, clean the stoma site with the sterile water, sterile saline, or other cleansing solution, based on facility policy.
4. Remove gloves and put on sterile gloves. Blot stoma with sterile gauze.
5. Place open end of urinary catheter into specimen container. Lubricate the catheter with water-soluble lubricant. If using straight catheter, gently insert the urinary catheter into the stoma site and advance no more than

(continued)

Skill 18-4 ▶ Collecting a Urine Specimen (Clean Catch, Midstream) *(continued)*

Skill Variation ▶ Obtaining a Urine Specimen From a Urinary Diversion *(continued)*

2 to 3 in (5 to 7.5 cm). If using a double-lumen catheter, gently insert catheter tip into stoma and advance the inner catheter approximately 1 to 2 in (2.5 to 5 cm) (Mahoney et al., 2013).

6. Hold the catheter in position until urine begins to drip. **If you meet resistance, rotate the catheter gently until it slides forward. Do not force the catheter. If you continue to meet resistance, do not force it any further.** If urine does not flow into the catheter, ask the patient to shift position and/or cough to mobilize urine (Williams, 2012).

7. Collect approximately 5 to 10 mL of urine before removing catheter. This may take 5 to 15 minutes (Mahoney et al., 2013). Once catheter is removed, cap the specimen container. Clean and dry the stoma and peristomal skin. Replace ostomy appliance; refer to Skill 12-11. If necessary, transfer the specimen to appropriate containers/tubes for specific test ordered, according to facility policy.

8. Remove gloves and perform hand hygiene.

9. Continue with Steps 15 to 17 in Skill 18-4.

10. Alternately, once appliance is removed and stoma cleansed, hold the sterile specimen cup under the stoma to collect urine (Mahoney et al., 2013; Williams, 2012).

EVIDENCE FOR PRACTICE ▶

PRACTICE GUIDELINES: URINE SAMPLES AND URINARY DIVERSIONS

Mahoney, M., Baxter, K., Burgess, J., et al. (2013). Procedure for obtaining a urine sample from a urostomy, ileal conduit, and colon conduit. A best practice guideline for clinicians. *Journal of Wound, Ostomy and Continence Nursing, 40*(3), 277–279.

This best practice guideline was developed by a panel of certified ostomy nurses serving on the Wound, Ostomy and Continence Nurses (WOCN) Society's Clinical Practice Ostomy Committee. This guideline has been validated by the WOCN Society.

Refer to thePoint® for additional research on related nursing topics.

Skill 18-5 ▶ Obtaining a Urine Specimen From an Indwelling Urinary Catheter

Indwelling catheter drainage tubes have special sampling ports in the tubing for removal of urine for testing. Most sampling ports are needleless systems. However, some ports require the use of a needle or blunt cannula to access the sampling port. The drainage tubing below the access port may be bent back on itself or clamped so that urine collects near the port, unless contraindicated, based on the patient's condition. **Do not open the drainage system to obtain urine specimens, to avoid contamination of the system and bladder infection. Never take urine specimens from the catheter drainage bag because the urine is not fresh and bacteria may be present in the bag** (Fischbach & Dunning, 2015).

DELEGATION CONSIDERATIONS

Obtaining a urine specimen from an indwelling catheter may be delegated to nursing assistive personnel (NAP) or to unlicensed assistive personnel (UAP), as well as licensed practical/vocational nurses (LPN/LVNs). The decision to delegate must be based on careful analysis of the patient's needs and circumstances, as well as the qualifications of the person to whom the task is being delegated. Refer to the Delegation Guidelines in Appendix A.

EQUIPMENT	• 10-mL sterile syringe • Blunt cannula or 18-gauge needle, if needed, based on specific catheter in use • Alcohol or other antimicrobial wipe • Nonsterile gloves • Additional PPE, as indicated • Sterile specimen container; urine collection tubes, based on facility policy • Biohazard bag • Appropriate label for specimen, based on facility policy and procedure

ASSESSMENT

After verifying the order for specimen collection, review the patient's health record for, or question the patient about, information about any medications that the patient is taking, because medications may affect the results of the test. Assess the characteristics of the urine draining from the catheter. Inspect the catheter tubing to identify the type of sampling port.

NURSING DIAGNOSIS

Determine the related factors for the nursing diagnoses based on the patient's current status. Possible nursing diagnoses may include:

• Impaired urinary elimination
• Risk for infection

• Deficient knowledge

OUTCOME IDENTIFICATION AND PLANNING

The expected outcome to achieve is that an adequate amount of urine is obtained without contamination or adverse effect. Other outcomes that may be appropriate include the following: the patient demonstrates an understanding of the need and process for specimen collection.

IMPLEMENTATION

ACTION	**RATIONALE**
1. Verify the order for a urine specimen collection in the patient's health record. Gather equipment.	Verifying the medical order is crucial to ensuring that the proper procedure is administered to the right patient. Assembling equipment provides for an organized approach to the task.
2. Perform hand hygiene and put on PPE, if indicated.	Hand hygiene and PPE prevent the transmission of microorganisms. PPE is required based on transmission precautions.
3. Identify the patient.	Identifying the patient ensures the right patient receives the intervention and helps prevent errors.
4. Explain the procedure to the patient.	Explanation provides reassurance and promotes cooperation.
5. Check the specimen label with the patient's identification bracelet. Label should include the patient's name and identification number, time specimen was collected, route of collection, identification of person obtaining the sample, and any other information required by facility policy.	Confirmation of patient identification information ensures the specimen is labeled correctly for the right patient.
6. Assemble equipment on overbed table or other surface within reach.	Arranging items nearby is convenient, saves time, and avoids unnecessary stretching and twisting of muscles on the part of the nurse.
7. Close curtains around the bed and close the door to the room, if possible.	Closing curtain or door provides for patient privacy.
8. Put on nonsterile gloves.	Gloves reduce the transmission of microorganisms.

(continued)

Skill 18-5 ▶ Obtaining a Urine Specimen From an Indwelling Urinary Catheter *(continued)*

ACTION	RATIONALE
9. Clamp the catheter drainage tubing or bend it back on itself distal to the port. If an insufficient amount of urine is present in the tubing, allow the tubing to remain clamped up to 30 minutes, to collect a sufficient amount of urine, unless contraindicated. Remove lid from specimen container, keeping the inside of the container and lid free from contamination.	Clamping the tubing ensures the collection of an adequate amount of fresh urine. Clamping for an extended period of time leads to overdistention of the bladder. Clamping may be contraindicated based on the patient's condition (e.g., after bladder surgery). The container needs to remain sterile so as not to contaminate the urine.
10. **Scrub aspiration port vigorously with alcohol or other disinfectant wipe and allow port to air dry.**	Cleaning with alcohol or other antimicrobial deters entry of microorganisms when the needle punctures the port.
11. Attach the syringe to the needleless port. Alternately, insert the blunt-tipped cannula into the port. Slowly aspirate enough urine for specimen (usually 3 to 5 mL is adequate; check facility requirements) (Figure 1). Remove the syringe from the port. Engage the needle guard, if needle was used. **Unclamp the drainage tubing.**	Using a leur-lock syringe or blunt-tipped needle prevents a needlestick. Collecting urine from the port ensures that the specimen will contain fresh urine. Unclamping catheter drainage tubing prevents overdistention of and injury to the patient's bladder.

FIGURE 1. Attaching the syringe to the needleless aspiration port and slowly withdrawing urine specimen.

ACTION	RATIONALE
12. If a needle or blunt-tipped cannula was used on the syringe, remove from the syringe before emptying the urine from the syringe into the specimen cup. Place the needle into a sharps collection container. **Slowly inject urine into the specimen container. Take care to avoid touching the syringe tip to any surface. Do not touch the edge or inside of the collection container.**	Forcing urine through the needle breaks up cells and impedes accurate results of microscopic urinalysis. If the urine is injected quickly into the container, it may splash out of the container or into the nurse's eyes. Avoid touching edge or inside of container to avoid contamination.
13. Replace lid on container. If necessary, transfer the specimen to appropriate containers/tubes for specific test ordered, according to facility policy. Dispose of syringe in a sharps collection container.	Proper disposal of equipment prevents injury and transmission of microorganisms. Safe disposal of sharps prevents accidental injury.
14. Remove gloves and perform hand hygiene.	Removing gloves properly reduces the risk for infection transmission and contamination of other items. Hand hygiene reduces the transmission of microorganisms.
15. Place label on the container per facility policy. Note specimen collection method, according to facility policy. Place container in plastic sealable biohazard bag.	Proper labeling ensures accurate reporting of results. Packaging the specimen in a biohazard bag prevents the person transporting the container from coming in contact with the specimen.
16. Remove other PPE, if used. Perform hand hygiene.	Proper removal of PPE reduces the risk for infection transmission and contamination of other items. Hand hygiene reduces the transmission of microorganisms.

ACTION	RATIONALE
17. Transport the specimen to the laboratory as soon as possible. If unable to take the specimen to the laboratory immediately, refrigerate it (Fischbach & Dunning, 2015).	If not refrigerated immediately, urine may act as a culture medium, allowing bacteria to multiply and skewing the results of testing. Refrigeration prevents the bacteria from multiplying.

EVALUATION

The expected outcomes have been met when an adequate amount of urine has been obtained without contamination or adverse effect; and the patient demonstrated an understanding of the need and process for specimen collection.

DOCUMENTATION

Guidelines

Document the method used to obtain the specimen, type of specimen sent, and characteristics of urine. Note any significant patient assessments. Record urine volume on intake and output record, if appropriate.

Sample Documentation

> <u>10/20/20</u> 1515 Patient with indwelling urinary catheter in place. Urine noted to be dark yellow and cloudy. Patient's temperature 103°F, pulse 96, respirations 18, BP 118/64. Dr. Burning notified. Specimen for urine culture obtained from indwelling catheter and catheter removed per order. Patient due to void by 2115.
>
> —B. Clapp, RN

UNEXPECTED SITUATIONS AND ASSOCIATED INTERVENTIONS

- *No urine or insufficient amount noted in catheter tubing:* Clamp tubing below access port for up to 30 minutes, according to facility policy, unless contraindicated by patient condition.

SPECIAL CONSIDERATIONS

- Never obtain a urine specimen for culture from the urine collection bag that is part of an indwelling urinary catheter drainage system (Fischbach & Dunning, 2015).
- The routine collection of urine cultures is not recommended for patients with indwelling urinary catheters. If a patient has a catheter-associated urinary tract infection (CAUTI), the old catheter should be removed and the specimen should be collected using sterile technique when the new catheter is placed (Society of Urologic Nurses and Associates [SUNA], 2015).
- It is very important to remove the clamp from the drainage tubing as soon as the specimen is collected, unless there is a specific order to leave the tubing clamped, to prevent overdistention of the patient's bladder and injury.
- If possible, ensure the specimen is obtained before antibiotics are started (Fischbach & Dunning, 2015).

EVIDENCE FOR PRACTICE ▶

Centers for Disease Control and Prevention (CDC). (2015). *Healthcare-associated infections (HAI). Catheter-associated urinary tract infections (CAUTI).* Retrieved https://www.cdc.gov/HAI/ca_uti/uti.html.

This site provides resources for health care providers and patients, including the CDC guidelines for prevention of catheter-associated infections. These guidelines recommend considering use of alternatives to indwelling urethral catheterization in selected patients, when appropriate, such as the use of external urinary sheaths in cooperative male patients without urinary retention or bladder outlet obstruction.

Refer to thePoint® for additional research on related nursing topics.

Skill 18-6 ▶ Testing Stool for Occult Blood

Fecal occult blood testing (FOBT) is used to detect **occult blood** in the stool. It is used for initial screening for disorders such as cancer and for gastrointestinal bleeding in conditions such as ulcer disease, inflammatory bowel disorders, and intestinal polyps. Three consecutive stool samples should be collected over several days to provide the most effective screening for colon cancer (American Association for Clinical Chemistry [AACC], 2015; Fischbach & Dunning, 2015). FOBT may be performed within an institution, collected at the bedside, and sent to the laboratory for analysis. It may also be collected by the patient at home and delivered or mailed to the health care provider's office or to the laboratory for analysis.

The *guaiac fecal occult blood test* (gFOBT) is a chemical test that detects the enzyme peroxidase in hemoglobin molecules when blood is present in the stool sample. A positive gFOBT result indicates that abnormal bleeding is occurring somewhere in the digestive tract. Certain medications, such as a salicylate intake of more than 325 mg daily, other nonsteroidal anti-inflammatory drugs, steroids, iron preparations, and anticoagulants, may also lead to *false-positive* readings (AACC, 2015; Fischbach & Dunning, 2015). Previously, ingestion of certain foods and medications before specimen collection were thought to possibly cause *false-positive* test results. This is no longer believed to be true and the patient does not need to restrict their diet before testing (Bechtold, Ashraf, & Nguyen, 2016; Doubeni, 2015). The ingestion of vitamin C can produce *false-negative* results even if bleeding is present.

The *fecal immunochemical test* (FIT) uses antibodies directed against human hemoglobin to detect blood in the stool. A positive FIT is more specific for bleeding in the lower gastrointestinal tract (Fischbach & Dunning, 2015). No drug restrictions are required for the FIT.

The following are recommendations for the patient preparing for a fecal occult blood test:

- Do not use laxatives, enemas, or suppositories for 3 days before testing.
- Postpone the test until 3 days after her period has ended if a woman is menstruating.
- Postpone the test if hematuria or bleeding hemorrhoids are present.
- Postpone the test if the patient has had a recent nose or throat bleed.

In clinical settings, these restrictions are usually not practical. Be sure to note the presence of any of the previously mentioned conditions in the clinical setting.

A positive result from either the gFOBT or the FIT requires follow-up testing, such as a sigmoidoscopy or colonoscopy (AACC, 2015; U.S. Preventive Services Task Force, 2016).

DELEGATION CONSIDERATIONS

Obtaining a stool specimen for FOBT may be delegated to nursing assistive personnel (NAP) or to unlicensed assistive personnel (UAP), as well as to licensed practical/vocational nurses (LPN/LVNs). Developing the FOBT at the point of care is not delegated to nursing assistive personnel (NAP) or to unlicensed assistive personnel (UAP). Developing the FOBT at the point of care may be delegated to LPN/LVNs. The decision to delegate must be based on careful analysis of the patient's needs and circumstances, as well as the qualifications of the person to whom the task is being delegated. Refer to the Delegation Guidelines in Appendix A.

EQUIPMENT

- Nonsterile gloves; other PPE as indicated
- Wooden applicator
- gFOBT: Wooden applicator, testing card, and developer (if processing is being done at point of care)
- FIT: Applicator stick or brush, depending on collection kit in use
- Bedpan, or plastic collection receptacle for commode or toilet
- Biohazard bag
- Appropriate label for specimen, based on facility policy and procedure

ASSESSMENT

Assess the patient's understanding of the collection procedure and ability to cooperate. Assess the patient for a history of gastrointestinal bleeding. Review prescribed restrictions for medications and evaluate patient compliance with required restrictions. Assess patient for any blood in the perineal area, including hemorrhoids, menstruation, urinary tract infection, or vaginal or rectal tears. Blood may be from a source other than the gastrointestinal tract.

NURSING DIAGNOSIS	Determine the related factors for the nursing diagnoses based on the patient's current status. Appropriate nursing diagnoses may include: • Deficient knowledge • Anxiety

OUTCOME IDENTIFICATION AND PLANNING	The expected outcome to achieve is that an uncontaminated stool sample is obtained, following collection guidelines, and then transported to the laboratory within the recommended time frame. Other outcomes may include the following: the patient demonstrates accurate understanding of testing instructions and rationale for use.

IMPLEMENTATION

ACTION	RATIONALE
1. Verify the order for a stool specimen collection in the patient's health record. Gather equipment.	Verifying the medical order is crucial to ensuring that the proper procedure is administered to the right patient. Assembling equipment provides for an organized approach to the task.
2. Perform hand hygiene and put on PPE, if indicated.	Hand hygiene and PPE prevent the transmission of microorganisms. PPE is required based on transmission precautions.
3. Identify the patient.	Identifying the patient ensures the right patient receives the intervention and helps prevent errors.
4. Discuss with the patient the need for a stool sample. Explain to the patient the process by which the stool will be collected, either from a bedpan, commode, or plastic receptacle in the toilet.	Discussion and explanation help to allay some of the patient's anxiety and prepare the patient for what to expect.
5. If sending the specimen to the laboratory, check specimen label with patient identification bracelet. Label should include the patient's name and identification number, time specimen was collected, route of collection, identification of the person obtaining the sample, and any other information required by facility policy.	Facilities may allow point-of-service testing (at bedside or on unit) or the specimen may have to be sent to the laboratory for testing. Confirmation of patient identification information ensures the specimen is labeled correctly for the right patient.
6. Assemble equipment on overbed table or other surface within reach.	Arranging items nearby is convenient, saves time, and avoids unnecessary stretching and twisting of muscles on the part of the nurse.
7. Close curtains around the bed or close the door to the room, if possible.	Closing the door or curtain provides for patient privacy.
8. Place the plastic collection receptacle in the toilet, if applicable. Assist the patient to the bathroom or onto the bedside commode, or onto the bedpan. Instruct the patient not to urinate or discard toilet paper with the stool.	Proper collection into an appropriate receptacle for stool prevents inaccurate results. Urine or toilet paper can contaminate the specimen, interfering with accurate results.
9. After the patient defecates, assist the patient out of the bathroom, off the commode, or remove the bedpan. Perform hand hygiene and put on disposable gloves.	Hand hygiene deters the spread of microorganisms. Gloves protect the nurse from microorganisms in feces.

(*continued*)

Skill 18-6 ▶ Testing Stool for Occult Blood *(continued)*

ACTION	RATIONALE

If using gFOBT:

10. Open flap on sample side of card. With wooden applicator, apply a small amount of stool from the center of the bowel movement onto one window of the testing card. With the opposite end of the wooden applicator, obtain another sample of stool from another area and apply a small amount of stool onto second window of testing card (Figure 1).

Two separate areas of the same stool sample are tested to ensure accuracy. By using opposite ends of the wooden applicator, cross-contamination is avoided.

FIGURE 1. Using a wooden applicator to transfer stool specimen to window of testing card.

11. Close flap over stool samples.

Closing the flap prevents contamination of the samples.

12. If sending stool to the laboratory, label the specimen card per facility policy. Place in a sealable plastic biohazard bag and send to the laboratory immediately.

Facilities may allow point-of-service testing (at bedside or on unit) or the specimen may have to be sent to the laboratory for testing. Correct labeling is necessary to ensure accurate results. Packaging the specimen in a biohazard bag prevents the person transporting the container from coming in contact with the specimen.

13. If testing at the point of care, wait 3 to 5 minutes before developing. Open flap on opposite side of card and place two drops of developer over each window and **wait the time stated in the manufacturer's instructions (Figure 2).**

If immediate testing is required, waiting 3 to 5 minutes before developing allows adequate time for the sample to penetrate the test paper and dry (Fischbach & Dunning, 2015). The developer will react with any blood in the stool. Following the manufacturer's instructions promotes accuracy of results.

14. Observe card for any blue areas (Figure 3).

Any blue coloring on the card indicates a positive test result for blood.

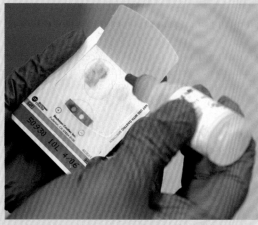

FIGURE 2. Applying developer to card windows.

FIGURE 3. Observing windows on card for blue areas.

ACTION	RATIONALE
If using FIT:	
15. Open flap on sample side of card. With applicator, brush, or sampling probe, apply a small amount of stool from the center of the bowel movement onto the top half of window of the testing card. With the opposite end of the device, obtain another sample of stool from another area and apply a small amount of stool onto the bottom half of window of testing card.	Two separate areas of the same stool sample are tested to ensure accuracy. By using opposite ends of the wooden applicator, cross-contamination is avoided.
16. Use the applicator to mix the samples and spread samples over entire window. Close flap over sample. Allow card to dry.	Drying of sample stabilizes hemoglobin, if present.
17. If sending to the laboratory, label the specimen card per facility policy. Place in a sealable plastic biohazard bag and send to the laboratory immediately.	Facilities may allow point-of-service testing (at bedside or on unit) or the specimen may have to be sent to the laboratory for testing. Correct labeling is necessary to ensure accurate results. Packaging the specimen in a biohazard bag prevents the person transporting the container from coming in contact with the specimen.
18. If testing at the point of care, open collection card according to manufacturer's instructions. Add three drops of developer to center of sample on Sample Pad. Developer should flow through the test (T) line and through the control (C) line. Snap Test Device closed.	The developer will react with any blood in the stool. Following the manufacturer's instructions promotes accuracy of results.
19. Wait 5 minutes, or time specified by manufacturer. Observe card for pink color on the test (T) line. The control (C) line must also turn pink within 5 minutes (Figure 4). If the control (C) line turns pink, read and report the result.	The developer will react with any blood in the stool. Following the manufacturer's instructions promotes accuracy of results. Any pink color on the test (T) line indicates a positive result.

FIGURE 4. Observing for pink color on test (T) line and the control (C) line. (Image courtesy of Beckman Coulter, Inc.)

(continued)

Skill 18-6 ▸ Testing Stool for Occult Blood *(continued)*

ACTION	RATIONALE

 20. After reading results, discard testing slide appropriately, according to facility policy. Remove gloves and any other PPE, if used. Perform hand hygiene.

Proper removal of PPE reduces the risk for infection transmission and contamination of other items. Hand hygiene and proper disposal of equipment reduces the transmission of microorganisms.

EVALUATION

The expected outcomes have been met when an uncontaminated stool sample has been obtained, following collection guidelines, and transported to the laboratory within the recommended time frame; the patient demonstrated accurate understanding of testing instructions and rationale for use.

DOCUMENTATION

Guidelines

Document the method used to obtain the specimen and transport it to the laboratory. If testing is done by the nurse, document results and communication of results to the health care provider. Document significant assessment findings and stool characteristics.

Sample Documentation

> 07/12/20 1040 Stool sample obtained from bowel movement. Labeled and sent to laboratory for occult blood testing. Stool noted to be semi-formed, dark brown, without evidence of gross blood.
>
> —K. Sanders, RN

UNEXPECTED SITUATIONS AND ASSOCIATED INTERVENTIONS

- *When developing a gFOBT, one window tests positive, whereas the second window tests negative:* This could indicate that the blood is from a source other than the gastrointestinal tract. Document these results and notify the primary care provider.
- *When developing an FIT test, the control (C) line does not turn pink:* This is an invalid test; do not report result. Repeat the test with a new collection card and test device (Beckman Coulter, 2013a).

SPECIAL CONSIDERATIONS

General Considerations

- *gFOBT* testing can be developed and used as a point-of-care test, but interpretation is considered subjective (Kessenich & Cronin, 2013).
- *gFOBT* testing must be repeated with three different samples of stool (Kessenich & Cronin, 2013).
- *FIT* sample collection is simpler, requiring only one to two different samples of stool (Bechtold et al., 2016; Kessenich & Cronin, 2013).
- Positive *FIT* test results may appear before 5 minutes. To verify a negative result, wait the full 5 minutes after closing the Test Device. Do not interpret *FIT* results after 5 minutes (Beckman Coulter, 2013a).
- Specimen can be collected from an ostomy appliance. Apply a clean ostomy appliance and obtain a sample as soon as patient passes stool into the appliance.

Infant and Child Considerations

- Stool can be collected from the diaper of an infant or child, as long as the specimen is not contaminated with urine.

Home Care Considerations

- Patients are often instructed on how to collect stool specimens for occult blood at home and bring the samples to the office, clinic, or laboratory. Patients should understand that it is important to follow instructions carefully to ensure validity of results. Any clean, dry container can be used to collect stool before contact with toilet bowl water. Patients are responsible only for obtaining a sample of stool and applying it to the collection card. Testing is done at the clinic, office, or laboratory.
- Some FIT collection kits use a sampling probe; the patient inserts the probe in the stool sample and inserts the probe in the collection device before returning for testing.
- Once the samples are collected, the collection devices can remain at room temperature until they are mailed or delivered to the testing location.

Skill 18-7 ▶ Collecting a Stool Specimen

A stool specimen may be ordered to screen for pathogenic organisms, such as bacteria associated with enteric infection or ova and parasites; the presence of toxins indicating *Clostridium difficile* infection; or for electrolytes, fat, and leukocytes. The nurse is responsible for obtaining the specimen according to facility procedure, labeling the specimen, and ensuring that the specimen is transported to the laboratory in a timely manner. The facility's policy and procedure manual or laboratory manual identifies specific information about the amount of stool needed, the time frame during which stool is to be collected, and the type of specimen container to use.

Usually, 1 in (2.5 cm) of formed stool or 15 to 30 mL of liquid stool is sufficient. If portions of the stool include visible blood, mucus, or pus, include these with the specimen. Also be sure that the specimen is free of any barium or enema solution. Because a fresh specimen produces the most accurate results, send the specimen to the laboratory immediately. If this is not possible, refrigerate it, unless contraindicated, such as when testing for ova and parasites. Refrigeration will affect parasites. Ova and parasites are best detected in warm stool. Some institutions require ova and parasite specimens to be placed in a container filled with preservatives; consult facility policy.

DELEGATION CONSIDERATIONS	Obtaining a stool specimen may be delegated to nursing assistive personnel (NAP) or to unlicensed assistive personnel (UAP), as well as to licensed practical/vocational nurses (LPN/LVNs). The decision to delegate must be based on careful analysis of the patient's needs and circumstances, as well as the qualifications of the person to whom the task is being delegated. Refer to the Delegation Guidelines in Appendix A.
EQUIPMENT	• Tongue blade (2) • Clean specimen container (or container with preservatives for ova and parasites) • Biohazard bag • Nonsterile gloves • Additional PPE, as indicated • Appropriate label for specimen, based on facility policy and procedure
ASSESSMENT	Assess the patient's understanding of the need for the test and the requirements of the test. Assess the patient's understanding of the collection procedure and ability to cooperate. Ask the patient when his or her last bowel movement was, and check the patient's health record for this information.
NURSING DIAGNOSIS	Determine the related factors for the nursing diagnoses based on the patient's current status. Appropriate nursing diagnoses include: • Deficient knowledge • Diarrhea
OUTCOME IDENTIFICATION AND PLANNING	The expected outcome to achieve is that an uncontaminated specimen is obtained and sent to the laboratory promptly. Additional outcomes that may be appropriate include the following: the patient demonstrates an understanding of the need and process for specimen collection.

IMPLEMENTATION

ACTION	RATIONALE
1. Verify the order for a stool specimen collection in the patient's health record. Gather equipment.	Verifying the medical order is crucial to ensuring that the proper procedure is administered to the right patient. Assembling equipment provides for an organized approach to the task.
2. Perform hand hygiene and put on PPE, if indicated.	Hand hygiene and PPE prevent the transmission of microorganisms. PPE is required based on transmission precautions.
3. Identify the patient.	Identifying the patient ensures the right patient receives the intervention and helps prevent errors.

(continued)

Skill 18-7 ▶ Collecting a Stool Specimen *(continued)*

ACTION	RATIONALE
4. Discuss with the patient the need for a stool sample. Explain to the patient the process by which the stool will be collected, either from a bedpan, commode, or plastic receptacle in the toilet (Figure 1) to catch stool without urine. Instruct the patient to void first and not to discard toilet paper with stool. Tell the patient to call you as soon as a bowel movement is completed.	Discussion and explanation help to allay some of the patient's anxiety and prepare the patient for what to expect. The patient should void first because the laboratory study may be inaccurate if the stool contains urine. Placing a container in the toilet or bedside commode aids in obtaining a clean stool specimen uncontaminated by urine.
5. Check specimen label with the patient's identification bracelet. Label should include the patient's name and identification number, time specimen was collected, route of collection, identification of the person obtaining the sample, and any other information required by facility policy.	Confirmation of patient identification information ensures the specimen is labeled correctly for the right patient.
6. Assemble equipment on overbed table or other surface within reach.	Arranging items nearby is convenient, saves time, and avoids unnecessary stretching and twisting of muscles on the part of the nurse.
7. After the patient has passed a stool, put on gloves. Use the tongue blades to obtain a sample, free of blood or urine, and place it in the designated clean specimen container (Figure 2).	The container does not have to be sterile, because stool is not sterile. To ensure accurate results, the stool should be free of urine or menstrual blood.

FIGURE 1. Plastic specimen collection receptacle in toilet to catch stool.

FIGURE 2. Transferring stool to specimen container.

8. Collect as much of the stool as possible to send to the laboratory.	Different tests and laboratories require different amounts of stool. Collecting as much as possible helps to ensure that the laboratory has an adequate amount of specimen for testing.
9. Place lid on container. Dispose of used equipment per facility policy. Remove gloves and perform hand hygiene.	Proper disposal of equipment reduces the transmission of microorganisms. Removing gloves properly reduces the risk for infection transmission and contamination of other items. Hand hygiene deters the spread of microorganisms.

ACTION

10. Place label on the container per facility policy. Place container in plastic, sealable biohazard bag (Figure 3).

RATIONALE

Correct labeling is necessary to ensure accurate results. Packaging the specimen in a biohazard bag prevents the person transporting the container from coming in contact with stool.

FIGURE 3. Placing specimen container in biohazard bag.

 11. Remove other PPE, if used. Perform hand hygiene.

Proper removal of PPE reduces the risk for infection transmission and contamination of other items. Hand hygiene reduces the transmission of microorganisms.

12. Transport the specimen to the laboratory while stool is still warm. If immediate transport is impossible, check with laboratory personnel or policy manual whether refrigeration is contraindicated.

Most tests have better results with fresh stool. Different tests may require different preparation if the test is not immediately completed. Some tests will be compromised if the stool is refrigerated.

EVALUATION

The expected outcomes have been met when an uncontaminated specimen has been obtained and sent to the laboratory promptly; and the patient demonstrated an understanding of the need and process for specimen collection.

DOCUMENTATION

Guidelines

Document amount, color, and consistency of stool obtained, time of collection, specific test for which the specimen was collected, and transport to laboratory.

Sample Documentation

7/12/20 2045 Large amount of pasty, green stool sent to laboratory for ova and parasite testing.

—K. Sanders, RN

UNEXPECTED SITUATIONS AND ASSOCIATED INTERVENTIONS

• *Patient is menstruating or has discarded toilet paper into commode with stool:* Call laboratory to discuss possible effects on test results. Not all tests will be affected by contaminants. The laboratory may accept the specimen even with the contaminant. Make notation in the information submitted with specimen.

(*continued*)

Skill 18-7 ▶ Collecting a Stool Specimen *(continued)*

- *Specimen is inadvertently left on counter instead of being sent to laboratory:* Call laboratory to discuss possible effects on test results. Not all tests will be affected by leaving the specimen on the counter for a period of time. The laboratory may accept the specimen even though it has been sitting out. Make sure that the time documented in the information submitted with the specimen accurately reflects the actual time the specimen was obtained.

SPECIAL CONSIDERATIONS

General Considerations

- Do not retrieve stool from the toilet for specimen use (Fischbach & Dunning, 2015).
- At least three stool specimens collected on separate days are recommended for stool cultures related to potential bacterial infection (Fischbach & Dunning, 2015).
- If possible, ensure specimens for culture are obtained before antibiotics are started, as therapy with antibiotics before specimen collection may decrease the type and the amount of bacteria (Fischbach & Dunning, 2015; Van Leeuwen & Bladh, 2017).
- If patient is wearing an adult incontinence brief, the stool may be collected from the brief as long as it is not contaminated with urine.
- Barium procedures and laxatives should be avoided for 1 week before specimen collection (Fischbach & Dunning, 2015).
- Specimen can be collected from ostomy appliance. Apply a clean ostomy appliance and obtain sample as soon as patient passes stool into the appliance.
- If a timed stool test is ordered, such as fecal fat, the entire amount of stool produced for 24 to 72 hours is sent to the laboratory. Be sure to follow instructions for storage while collection is ongoing.

Infant and Child Considerations

- Stool can be collected from the diaper of an infant or child, as long as the specimen is uncontaminated with urine.

Home Care Considerations

- Patients are often instructed on how to collect stool specimens at home and bring the samples to the office, clinic, or laboratory. Patients should understand that it is important to follow instructions carefully to ensure validity of results. Ensure the patient understands the proper procedure for sample storage before bringing it to the laboratory or office.

Skill 18-8 ▶ Obtaining a Capillary Blood Sample for Glucose Testing

Blood glucose monitoring provides information about how the body is controlling glucose metabolism. Controlling the patient's blood glucose levels is an important part of care for patients with many conditions, including diabetes, seizures, enteral and parenteral feeding, liver disease, pancreatitis, head injury, stroke, alcohol and drug intoxication, sepsis, and in patients prescribed corticosteroids. Point-of-care testing (testing done at the bedside, where samples are not sent to the laboratory) provides a convenient, rapid measurement of blood glucose. Patients with diabetes use this type of testing as an important part of disease management to monitor blood glucose and adjust lifestyle interventions and treatment (U.S. Food and Drug Administration [FDA], 2016). Blood samples are commonly obtained from the edges of the fingers for adults, but samples can be obtained from the palm of the hand, forearm, upper arm, calf, and anterior thigh, depending on the time of testing and monitor used (U.S. FDA, 2016). Avoid fingertips, because they are more sensitive. Rotate sites to prevent skin damage. It is important to be familiar with and follow the manufacturer's guidelines and facility policy and procedure to ensure accurate results. Blood glucose target levels are individualized for patients with diabetes, based on such things as duration of diabetes, comorbid conditions, and individual patient considerations (American Diabetes Association [ADA], 2016). Normal fasting glucose for adults without diabetes is less than 99 mg/dL (National Institute of Diabetes and Digestive and Kidney Diseases [NIDDK], 2016).

| DELEGATION CONSIDERATIONS | Obtaining a capillary blood sample for glucose testing may be delegated to nursing assistive personnel (NAP) or to unlicensed assistive personnel (UAP), as well as to licensed practical/vocational nurses (LPN/LVNs). The decision to delegate must be based on careful analysis of the patient's needs and circumstances, as well as the qualifications of the person to whom the task is being delegated. Refer to the Delegation Guidelines in Appendix A. |

EQUIPMENT

- Blood glucose meter
- Sterile lancet
- Cotton balls or gauze squares
- Testing strips for meter
- Nonsterile gloves
- Additional PPE, as indicated
- Skin cleanser and water or alcohol swab

ASSESSMENT

Assess the patient's history for indications necessitating the monitoring of blood glucose levels, such as high-carbohydrate feedings, history of diabetes mellitus, or corticosteroid therapy. Assess for signs and symptoms of hypoglycemia and hyperglycemia. In addition, assess the patient's knowledge about monitoring blood glucose. Inspect the area of the skin to be used for testing. Avoid bruised and open areas.

NURSING DIAGNOSIS

Determine the related factors for the nursing diagnoses based on the patient's current status. Possible nursing diagnoses may include:

- Risk for unstable blood glucose level
- Deficient knowledge
- Anxiety

OUTCOME IDENTIFICATION AND PLANNING

The expected outcome to achieve is that the blood glucose level is measured accurately without adverse effect. In addition, the patient demonstrates an understanding of the need and process for specimen collection.

IMPLEMENTATION

ACTION	RATIONALE
1. Check the patient's health record or nursing care plan for monitoring schedule. You may decide that additional testing is indicated based on nursing judgment and the patient's condition.	This confirms scheduled times for checking blood glucose. Independent nursing judgment may lead to the decision to test more frequently, based on the patient's condition.
2. Gather equipment. Check expiration date on blood test strips.	This provides an organized approach to the task. Blood test strips that are past expiration date could cause inaccurate results and should not be used.
3. Perform hand hygiene and put on PPE, if indicated.	Hand hygiene and PPE prevent the transmission of microorganisms. PPE is required based on transmission precautions.
4. Identify the patient. Explain the procedure to the patient and instruct the patient about the need for monitoring blood glucose.	Identifying the patient ensures the right patient receives the intervention and helps prevent errors. Explanation helps to alleviate anxiety and facilitate cooperation.
5. Close curtains around the bed and close the door to the room, if possible.	Closing the curtain or door provides for patient privacy.
6. Turn on the monitor.	The monitor must be on for use.

(continued)

Skill 18-8 ▷ Obtaining a Capillary Blood Sample for Glucose Testing *(continued)*

ACTION	RATIONALE
7. Enter the patient's identification number or scan his or her identification bracelet, if required, according to facility policy.	Use of identification number allows for electronic storage and accurate identification of patient data.
8. Put on nonsterile gloves.	Gloves protect the nurse from exposure to blood or body fluids.
9. Prepare **lancet** using aseptic technique.	Aseptic technique maintains sterility.
10. Remove test strip from the vial. **Recap container immediately. Test strips also come individually wrapped. Check that the code number for the strip matches the code number on the monitor screen.**	Immediate recapping protects strips from exposure to humidity, light, and discoloration. Matching code numbers on the strip and glucose monitor ensures that the machine is calibrated correctly.
11. Insert the strip into the meter according to directions for that specific device. Alternately, strip may be placed in meter after collection of sample on test strip, depending on meter in use.	Correctly inserted strip allows meter to read blood glucose level accurately.
12. **Have the patient wash hands with skin cleanser and warm water and dry thoroughly. Alternately, cleanse the skin with an alcohol swab. Allow skin to dry completely.**	Washing with skin cleanser and water or alcohol cleanses the puncture site. Warm water also helps to cause vasodilation. Alcohol can interfere with accuracy of results if not completely dried.
13. Choose a skin site that is intact, warm, and free of calluses and edema (Van Leeuwen & Bladh, 2017).	Areas with lesions are not suitable for capillary sampling. Calluses, edema, and vasoconstriction (cool to palpation) interfere with the ability to obtain a blood sample.
14. Hold lancet perpendicular to skin and pierce skin with lancet (Figure 1).	Holding lancet in proper position facilitates proper skin penetration.
15. Encourage bleeding by lowering the hand, making use of gravity. Lightly stroke the finger, if necessary, until a sufficient amount of blood has formed to cover the sample area on the strip, based on monitor requirements (check instructions for monitor). Take care not to squeeze the finger, not to squeeze at puncture site, or not to touch puncture site or blood.	An appropriate-sized droplet facilitates accurate test results. Squeezing can cause injury to the patient and alter the test result (WHO, 2010).
16. Gently touch a drop of blood to the test strip without smearing it (Figure 2). Depending on meter in use, insert strip into meter after collection of sample on test strip.	Smearing blood on the strip may result in inaccurate test results.

FIGURE 1. Piercing patient's finger with lancet.

FIGURE 2. Applying blood to test strip.

ACTION	**RATIONALE**
17. Apply pressure to puncture site with a cotton ball or dry gauze. **Do not use alcohol wipe.**	Pressure causes hemostasis. Alcohol stings and may prolong bleeding.
18. Read blood glucose results and document the results in EHR or other designated location, based on facility policy. Inform patient of test result.	Timing depends on type of meter.
19. Turn off meter, remove test strip, and dispose of supplies appropriately. Place lancet in sharps container.	Proper disposal prevents exposure to blood and accidental needlestick.
20. Remove gloves and any other PPE, if used. Perform hand hygiene.	Proper removal of PPE reduces the risk for infection transmission and contamination of other items. Hand hygiene reduces the transmission of microorganisms.

EVALUATION

The expected outcomes have been achieved when the patient's blood glucose level has been measured accurately without adverse effect; and the patient demonstrated an understanding of the need and process for testing.

DOCUMENTATION

Guidelines

Document blood glucose level in the patient's health record, according to facility policy. Document pertinent patient assessments, any intervention related to glucose level, and any patient teaching. Report abnormal results and/or significant assessments to the health care provider.

Sample Documentation

DocuCare Practice documenting blood glucose testing in *Lippincott DocuCare.*

> <u>11/1/20</u> 0800 Patient performed own fingerstick blood glucose test with minimal guidance. Verbalized rationale for fasting measurement and able to state symptoms of hypoglycemia. Patient's fingerstick blood glucose level 168. Four units regular Humulin insulin given per sliding scale, in addition to 10 units NPH Humulin insulin scheduled for 0800. Patient encouraged to review written guidelines for subcutaneous insulin administration; will review procedure and plan to have patient administer insulin at dinnertime. Patient verbalized an understanding.
>
> —B. Clapp, RN

UNEXPECTED SITUATIONS AND ASSOCIATED INTERVENTIONS

- *Extremity is pale and cool to the touch:* Begin by warming the extremity. Have adult patients warm their hands by rubbing them together. Warm, moist compresses may also be used.
- *Blood glucose level results are above or below normal parameters:* Assess the patient for signs of hyperglycemia or hypoglycemia, respectively. Check patient's health record for ordered interventions, such as insulin dosage or glucose-containing carbohydrate administration (ADA, 2017). Notify health care provider of results and assessment.

SPECIAL CONSIDERATIONS

General Considerations

- If the selected site feels cool or appears pale, warm compresses can be applied for 3 to 5 minutes to dilate the capillaries
- Sampling of blood from an alternative site other than fingertips may have limitations. Blood in the fingertips shows changes in glucose levels more quickly than blood in other parts of the body. This means that alternative site test results may differ from fingertip test results when glucose

(continued)

Skill 18-8 ▶ Obtaining a Capillary Blood Sample for Glucose Testing *(continued)*

levels are changing rapidly (e.g., after a meal, taking insulin, or during or after exercise) because the results may be inaccurate. Caution patients to use a fingertip sample if it is less than 2 hours after eating, less than 2 hours after injecting rapid-acting insulin, during exercise or within 2 hours of exercise, when sick or under stress, when having symptoms of hypoglycemia, if unable to recognize symptoms of hypoglycemia, or if site results do not agree with the way the patient feels (U.S. FDA, 2016).

- Meters require calibration at least monthly or according to the manufacturer's recommendation, and when a new bottle of test strips is opened. Manufacturer's directions for calibration should be followed. After calibration, the meter is checked for accuracy by testing a control solution containing a known amount of glucose.

- Inadequate sampling can cause errors in the results. It is very important to be aware of requirements for the specific monitor used.

- Continuous glucose monitoring systems use sensors placed just below the skin to check glucose levels in tissue fluid. A transmitter sends information about glucose levels from the sensor to a wireless monitor. These devices provide real-time measurements of glucose levels every few minutes (NIDDK, 2017). These systems supplement standard fingerstick meters and provide a way to see glucose trends, and track patterns (NIDDK, n.d.).

Infant and Child Considerations

- Heel sticks, using the outer aspect of the heel, may be used for infants. Warming the heel for 5 to 10 minutes before the sample is taken dilates the blood vessels in the area and aids in sampling (Perry, Hockenberry, Lowdermilk, & Wilson, 2014). This technique is not without controversy, as it is painful and can lead to fibrosis, scarring, and necrotizing osteochondritis (from puncture of the heel bone) (Perry et al., 2014). Venipuncture by a skilled phlebotomist is suggested instead of heel lance methods due to the increased pain from heel lance (Infusion Nurses Society [INS], 2016b).

Older Adult Considerations

- Meters are available with large digital readouts or audio components for patients with visual impairments.

Home Care Considerations

- Patients monitor blood glucose levels routinely at home. Provide education focusing on important elements of diabetes education to assist patients in managing their diabetes, including the signs, symptoms, and management of hypoglycemia and hyperglycemia; correct administration of oral hypoglycemic agents and/or insulin; fingerstick blood glucose monitoring; and the accurate use of fingerstick blood glucose monitoring equipment.

- Many different types of monitors are available. Assist patients to identify desirable features for individual use.

EVIDENCE FOR PRACTICE ▶

STANDARDS OF MEDICAL CARE IN DIABETES—2017

American Diabetes Association (ADA). (2017). Standards of medical care in diabetes—2017. *Diabetes Care, 40*(Suppl 1): S11–S66. Retrieved http://professional.diabetes.org/sites/professional.diabetes.org/files/media/dc_40_s1_final.pdf.

These standards of care provide clinicians, patients, researchers, payers, and other interested people with the components of diabetes care, general treatment goals, and tools to evaluate the quality of care. The recommendations included are screening, diagnostic, and therapeutic actions that are known or believed to favorably affect health outcomes of patients with diabetes.

Refer to thePoint® for additional research on related nursing topics.

Skill 18-9 ▶ Using Venipuncture to Collect a Venous Blood Sample

Venipuncture involves piercing a vein with a needle to obtain a venous blood sample, which is collected in a syringe or tube. The superficial veins of the arm in the antecubital fossa, which include the basilic, median cubital, and cephalic veins, are typically used for venipuncture (Figure 1) (Van Leeuwen & Bladh, 2017). However, venipuncture can be performed on a vein in the dorsal forearm, the dorsum of the hand, or another accessible location. When performing a venipuncture, remember the following:

- Do not use the inner wrist because of the high risk for damage to underlying structures.
- Avoid areas that are edematous, paralyzed, burned, scarred, have a tattoo, or are on the same side as a mastectomy, arteriovenous shunt, or graft.
- Avoid an extremity affected by a cerebrovascular accident, areas of infection, or areas with abnormal skin conditions.
- Do not draw blood from the same extremity being used for administration of intravenous medications, fluids, or blood transfusions. Some facilities will allow use of such sites as a "last resort," after the infusion has been held for a period of time. If necessary, choose a site distal to the intravenous access site. Check facility policy and procedure (INS, 2016b; Van Leeuwen & Bladh, 2017).

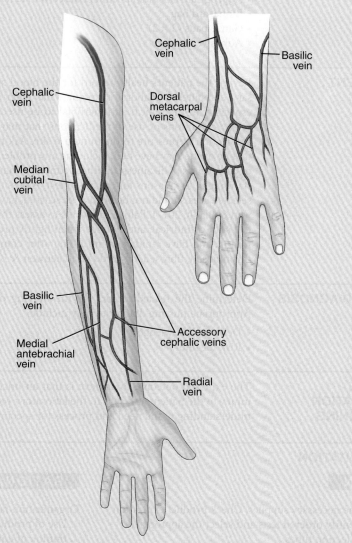

FIGURE 1. Blood vessels in the arm typically used for venipuncture.

(*continued*)

Skill 18-9 ▶ Using Venipuncture to Collect a Venous Blood Sample *(continued)*

Explanation and communication with patients about the need for venipuncture can reduce anxiety. It is important to explain carefully the information about the need for blood tests to ensure patient understanding.

DELEGATION GUIDELINES

The use of venipuncture to obtain a blood sample may be delegated to nursing assistive personnel (NAP) or to unlicensed assistive personnel (UAP) in some settings, as well as to licensed practical/vocational nurses (LPN/LVNs). The decision to delegate must be based on careful analysis of the patient's needs and circumstances, as well as the qualifications of the person to whom the task is being delegated. Refer to the Delegation Guidelines in Appendix A.

EQUIPMENT

- Tourniquet
- Nonsterile gloves
- Additional PPE, as indicated
- Antimicrobial swab, such as chlorhexidine or alcohol
- Sterile needle, gauge appropriate to the vein and sampling needs, using the smallest possible
- Vacutainer needle adaptor
- Blood collection tubes appropriate for ordered tests
- Appropriate label for specimen, based on facility policy and procedure
- Biohazard bag
- Gauze pads (2 × 2)
- Adhesive bandage

ASSESSMENT

Review the patient's health record for the blood specimens to be obtained. Ensure that the necessary computerized laboratory request has been completed. Assess the patient for any allergies, especially to the topical antimicrobial to be used for skin cleansing. Investigate for the presence of any conditions or use of medications that may prolong bleeding time, necessitating additional application of pressure to the puncture site. Ask the patient about any previous laboratory testing that he or she may have had, including any problems, such as difficulty with venipuncture, fainting, or complaints of dizziness, lightheadedness, or nausea. Assess the patient's anxiety level and understanding of the reasons for the blood test. Assess the patency of the veins in both upper limbs. The selected area should not be burned or scarred, have a tattoo, or have hematoma present (Van Leeuwen & Bladh, 2017). Palpate the veins to assess the condition of the vessel; vein should be straight, feel soft, cylindrical, and bounce when lightly pressed. Appropriate vessels will compress without rolling, and have rapid rebound filling after compression. Avoid veins that are tender, sclerosed, thrombosed, fibrosed, or hard (Van Leeuwen & Bladh, 2017).

NURSING DIAGNOSIS

Determine the related factors for the nursing diagnoses based on the patient's current status. Appropriate nursing diagnoses may include:

- Deficient knowledge
- Risk for injury
- Risk for infection

OUTCOME IDENTIFICATION AND PLANNING

The expected outcome to achieve is that an uncontaminated specimen will be obtained without injury to the patient and sent to the laboratory promptly. In addition, the patient demonstrates an understanding of the need and process for specimen collection.

IMPLEMENTATION

ACTION	RATIONALE
1. Gather the necessary supplies. Check product expiration dates. Identify ordered tests and select the appropriate blood collection tubes.	Organization facilitates efficient performance of the procedure. Use of products that have not expired ensures proper functioning of equipment. Using correct bottles ensures accurate blood sampling.

ACTION	**RATIONALE**
2. Perform hand hygiene and put on PPE, if indicated.	Hand hygiene and PPE prevent the transmission of microorganisms. PPE is required based on transmission precautions.
3. Identify the patient.	Identifying the patient ensures the right patient receives the intervention and helps prevent errors.
4. Explain the procedure to the patient. Allow the patient time to ask questions and verbalize concerns about the venipuncture procedure.	Explanation provides reassurance and promotes cooperation.
5. Check the specimen label with the patient's identification bracelet. Label should include the patient's name and identification number, time specimen was collected, route of collection, identification of the person obtaining the sample, and any other information required by facility policy.	Confirmation of patient identification information ensures the specimen is labeled correctly for the right patient.
6. Assemble equipment on overbed table or other surface within reach.	Arranging items nearby is convenient, saves time, and avoids unnecessary stretching and twisting of muscles on the part of the nurse.
7. Close curtains around the bed and close the door to the room, if possible.	Closing the door or curtain provides for patient privacy.
8. Provide for good light. Artificial light is recommended. Place a trash receptacle within easy reach.	Good lighting is necessary to perform the procedure properly. Having the trash receptacle within easy reach allows for safe disposal of contaminated materials.
9. Assist the patient to a comfortable position, either sitting or lying. If the patient is lying in bed, raise the bed to a comfortable working height, usually elbow height of the caregiver (VHACEOSH, 2016).	Proper positioning allows easy access to the site and promotes patient comfort and safety. Proper bed height helps reduce back strain while performing the procedure.
10. Determine the patient's preferred site for the procedure based on his or her previous experience. Expose the arm, supporting it in an extended position on a firm surface, such as a tabletop. Position self on the same side of the patient as the site selected. Apply a tourniquet to the upper arm on the chosen side approximately 3 to 4 in above the potential puncture site. Apply sufficient pressure to impede venous circulation but not arterial blood flow.	Patient preference promotes patient participation in treatment and gives the nurse information that may aid in site selection. Positioning close to the chosen site reduces back strain. Use of a tourniquet increases venous pressure to aid in vein identification. Tourniquet should remain in place no more than 60 seconds to prevent stasis and hemoconcentration (Fischbach & Dunning, 2015).
11. Put on gloves. Assess the veins using inspection and palpation to determine the best puncture site. Refer to the Assessment section above.	Gloves reduce transmission of microorganisms. Using the best site reduces the risk of injury to the patient. Observation and palpation allow for making distinction between other structures, such as tendons and arteries, in the area to avoid injury.
12. **Release the tourniquet. Check that the vein has decompressed.**	Releasing the tourniquet reduces the length of time the tourniquet is applied. Tourniquet should remain in place no more than 60 seconds to prevent injury, stasis, and hemoconcentration, which may alter results (Fischbach & Dunning, 2015). Thrombosed veins will remain firm and palpable and should not be used for venipuncture.
13. Attach the needle to the Vacutainer device. Place first blood collection tube into the Vacutainer, but not engaged in the puncture device in the Vacutainer.	Device is prepared for use to ensure efficiency with the task.

(continued)

Skill 18-9 ▶ Using Venipuncture to Collect a Venous Blood Sample *(continued)*

ACTION	RATIONALE
14. Clean the patient's skin at the selected puncture site with the antimicrobial swab (Figure 2). If using chlorhexidine, use a gentle back and forth motion for at least 30 seconds or use the procedure recommended by the manufacturer (INS, 2016a). If using alcohol, wipe in a circular motion spiraling outward. Allow the skin to dry before performing the venipuncture. Do not wipe or blot. Allow to dry completely.	Cleaning the patient's skin reduces the risk for transmission of microorganisms. Allowing the skin to dry maximizes antimicrobial action and prevents contact of the substance with the needle on insertion, thereby reducing the sting associated with insertion.
15. Reapply the tourniquet approximately 3 to 4 in above the identified puncture site (Figure 3). Apply sufficient pressure to impede venous circulation but not arterial blood flow. After disinfection, do not palpate the venipuncture site unless sterile gloves are worn.	Use of a tourniquet increases venous pressure to aid in vein identification. Tourniquet should remain in place no more than 60 seconds to prevent injury, stasis, and hemoconcentration, which may alter results (Fischbach & Dunning, 2015).

FIGURE 2. Cleaning the patient's skin at the venipuncture site.

FIGURE 3. Reapplying the tourniquet.

ACTION	RATIONALE
16. Hold the patient's arm in a downward position with your nondominant hand. Align the needle and Vacutainer device with the chosen vein, holding the Vacutainer and needle in your dominant hand. Use the thumb or first finger of your nondominant hand to apply pressure and traction to the skin about 1 to 2 in below the identified puncture site (Van Leeuwen & Bladh, 2017).	Applying pressure helps immobilize and anchor the vein. Taut skin at entry site aids smooth needle entry.
17. Inform the patient that he or she is going to feel a pinch. With the bevel of the needle up, insert the needle into the vein at a 15 to 30 degree angle to the skin (Van Leeuwen & Bladh, 2017) (Figure 4).	Warning the patient prevents reaction related to surprise. Positioning the needle at the proper angle reduces the risk of puncturing through the vein.

FIGURE 4. Inserting the needle at a 15-degree angle, with the bevel up.

ACTION	RATIONALE
18. Grasp the Vacutainer securely to stabilize it in the vein with your nondominant hand, and push the first collection tube into the puncture device in the Vacutainer, until the rubber stopper on the collection tube is punctured. You will feel the tube push into place on the puncture device. Blood will flow into the tube automatically (Figure 5).	The collection tube is a vacuum; negative pressure within the tube pulls blood into the tube.

FIGURE 5. Observing blood flowing into the collection tube.

ACTION	RATIONALE
19. **Remove the tourniquet as soon as blood flows adequately into the tube.**	Tourniquet removal reduces venous pressure and restores venous return to help prevent bleeding and bruising (Van Leeuwen & Bladh, 2017).
20. Continue to hold the Vacutainer in place in the vein and continue to fill the required tubes, removing one and inserting another. Gently rotate each tube as you remove it.	Filling the required tubes ensures that the sample is accurate. Gentle rotation helps to mix any additive in the tube with the blood sample.
21. After you have drawn all required blood samples, remove the last collection tube from the Vacutainer. **Place a gauze pad over the puncture site and slowly and gently remove the needle from the vein. Engage needle guard. Do not apply pressure to the site until the needle has been fully removed.**	Slow, gentle needle removal prevents injury to the vein. Releasing the vacuum before withdrawing the needle prevents injury to the vein and hematoma formation. Use of a needle guard prevents accidental needlestick injuries.
22. Apply gentle pressure to the puncture site for 2 to 3 minutes or until bleeding stops.	Applying pressure to the site after needle removal prevents injury, bleeding, and extravasation into the surrounding tissue, which can cause a hematoma.
23. After bleeding stops, apply an adhesive bandage.	The bandage protects the site and aids in applying pressure.
24. Remove equipment and return the patient to a position of comfort. Raise side rail and lower bed.	Repositioning promotes patient comfort. Raising rails promotes safety.
25. Discard Vacutainer and needle in sharps container.	Proper disposal of equipment reduces transmission of microorganisms.
26. Remove gloves and perform hand hygiene.	Removing gloves properly reduces the risk for infection transmission and contamination of other items.
27. Place label on the container per facility policy. Place container in plastic, sealable biohazard bag.	Proper labeling ensures accurate reporting of results. Packaging the specimen in a biohazard bag prevents the person transporting the container from coming in contact with blood and body fluids.
28. Check the venipuncture site to see if a hematoma has developed.	Development of a hematoma requires further intervention.

(continued)

Skill 18-9 ▶ Using Venipuncture to Collect a Venous Blood Sample *(continued)*

ACTION	RATIONALE

 29. Remove other PPE, if used. Perform hand hygiene.

Proper removal of PPE reduces the risk for infection transmission and contamination of other items. Hand hygiene reduces the transmission of microorganisms.

30. Transport the specimen to the laboratory immediately. If immediate transport is not possible, check with laboratory personnel or policy manual whether refrigeration is contraindicated.

Timely transport ensures accurate results.

EVALUATION

The expected outcomes have been achieved when an uncontaminated specimen has been obtained without injury to the patient and has been sent to the laboratory promptly; and the patient demonstrated an understanding of the need and process for specimen collection.

DOCUMENTATION

Guidelines

Record the date, time, and site of the venipuncture; the name of the test(s); the time the sample was sent to the laboratory; the amount of blood collected, if required; and any significant assessments or patient reactions.

Sample Documentation

> 6/10/20 0945 Blood specimen for CBC with differential obtained from right antecubital space. Approximately 8 mL of blood collected and sent to laboratory. No evidence of bleeding or hematoma at venipuncture site. Patient denied any complaints of pain or feelings of lightheadedness.
>
> —C. Lewis, RN

UNEXPECTED SITUATIONS AND ASSOCIATED INTERVENTIONS

- *After applying the tourniquet, you have trouble finding a distended vein:* Have the patient make a fist, or try tapping the skin over the vein lightly several times. **Do not have the patient pump the fist as this may increase plasma potassium levels** (Fischbach & Dunning, 2015; INS, 2016b). If unsuccessful, remove the tourniquet and try lowering the patient's arm to allow blood to pool in the veins. If necessary, apply warm compresses for about 10 minutes before reapplying the tourniquet.
- *Patient has large, distended, highly visible veins:* Perform venipuncture without a tourniquet to minimize the risk for hematoma (Fischbach & Dunning, 2015).
- *Patient has a clotting disorder or is receiving anticoagulant therapy:* Maintain firm pressure on the venipuncture site for at least 5 minutes after withdrawing the needle to prevent hematoma formation.
- *Oozing or bleeding continues from the puncture site for more than a few minutes:* Elevate the area and apply a pressure dressing. If bleeding is excessive or persists for longer than 10 minutes, notify the health care provider.
- *A hematoma develops at the venipuncture site:* Apply pressure until you are sure bleeding has stopped (about 5 minutes). Notify the health care provider. Document size and appearance of hematoma, notification of primary health care provider, and any ordered interventions.
- *Patient reports feeling lightheaded and says she is going to faint:* Stop the venipuncture. If the patient is in bed, have the patient lie flat and elevate the feet. If the patient is in a chair, have the patient put her head between her knees. Encourage the patient to take slow, deep breaths. Call for assistance and stay with the patient. Obtain vital signs, if possible.

SPECIAL CONSIDERATIONS

General Considerations

- **Obtain only the volume of blood needed for accurate testing.** Phlebotomy (drawing blood) contributes to iron deficiency and blood loss in newborns and critically ill patients. Consider interventions to conserve blood, including the use of low-volume blood collection tubes, recording the volume of blood obtained for laboratory testing, avoidance of routine testing, and consolidation of all daily tests with one blood draw (INS, 2016b, p. S86).

- Be aware of the facility's policy regarding order of collection of multiple tubes of blood to ensure accurate results.
- If the flow of blood into the collection tube or syringe is sluggish, leave the tourniquet in place longer, but always remove it before withdrawing the needle. Do not leave the tourniquet on for more than 60 seconds.
- If necessary, use a blood pressure cuff inflated to a point between systolic and diastolic pressure values as an alternative to a tourniquet (Fischbach & Dunning, 2015).
- Avoid collecting blood from edematous areas, arteriovenous shunts, an upper extremity on the same side as a previous lymph node dissection or mastectomy, infected sites, same extremity as an intravenous infusion, and sites of previous hematomas or vascular injury.
- Avoid previous sites of venipuncture to reduce the potential for infection (Van Leeuwen & Bladh, 2017).
- Do not use veins in the lower extremities for venipuncture, because of an increased risk of thrombophlebitis. Some facilities allow collection from lower extremities with a health care provider's order to collect blood from a leg or foot vein. Check your facility's policies.
- Apply warm compresses to the selected site 15 to 20 minutes before venipuncture to aid in distending veins that are difficult to locate.
- Consider the use of topical anesthetic creams to minimize discomfort and pain for the patient, based on facility policy. Allow 60 seconds after application for patients with light skin tones and 120 seconds for patients with dark skin tones before performing the venipuncture (Fischbach & Dunning, 2015). Be familiar with requirements and specifications for a particular product available for use. Application needs to occur sufficiently in advance to allow enough time to become effective.
- Use distraction, if appropriate. Distraction has been shown to be of benefit in reducing anxiety related to venipuncture, especially with children (da Silva et al., 2016; Mutlu & Balcı, 2015bib19). Asking the patient to concentrate on relaxing; performing deep breathing may help the patient relax.

Infant and Child Considerations

- Use smaller-gauge needles with infants and children because their veins are smaller and more fragile.
- Consider automatically applying warm compresses to distend the small veins of infants and young children before attempting any venipuncture.
- Use butterfly needles, as appropriate, for obtaining blood from infants and small children.
- Venipuncture by a skilled phlebotomist is suggested instead of heel lance methods due to the increased pain from heel lance (INS, 2016b).
- Administer oral sucrose/glucose beginning 1 to 2 minutes before the venipuncture procedure for young infants, to decrease the incidence of procedure-related pain (Sethi & Nayak, 2015; Uzelli & Güneş, 2015).
- Consider using topical anesthetic creams or gels, refrigerant spray, or iontophoresis (application of electric current to carry ionized lidocaine through the skin) with infants and children, to decrease the incidence of procedure-related pain (Baxter, Ewing, Young, Ware, Evans, & Manworren, 2013; Kearl, Yanger, Montero, Morelos-Howard, & Claudius, 2015). Apply the product for sufficient time to reach maximal effectiveness.
- Consider the use of distraction to decrease the incidence of procedure-related pain (da Silva et al., 2016; Mutlu & Balcı, 2015bib19).
- Consider the use of self-adhesive wrap instead of tape to avoid damage to delicate skin. A section of self-adhesive wrap is placed over the gauze at the venipuncture site and wrapped several times around the gauze. The wrap sticks to itself instead of the skin to hold the gauze in place. Self-adhesive wrap is available in numerous colors; this, combined with elimination of adhesion to the skin, makes it an attractive alternative to tape for infants and children (Van Leeuwen & Bladh, 2017).

(continued)

Skill 18-9 ▶ Using Venipuncture to Collect a Venous Blood Sample *(continued)*

Older Adult Considerations

- Keep in mind that the veins of an older adult are fragile and may collapse easily. In addition, the skin is less elastic and may be more difficult to pull taut.
- The superficial veins of the hands of older adults are fragile and venipuncture can cause a hematoma to form. Additionally, these veins move due to the age-related loss of supportive muscle and connective tissue, making it difficult to enter the lumen of the vein (Malarkey & McMorrow, 2012).
- Consider performing venipuncture without a tourniquet for older adults to prevent rupture of capillaries. Instruct the patient to make a tight fist before needle insertion. Do not have the patient pump the fist, because this may increase plasma potassium levels (Fischbach & Dunning, 2015; INS, 2016b).
- Consider the use of self-adhesive wrap instead of tape to avoid damage to delicate skin. A section of self-adhesive wrap is placed over the gauze at the venipuncture site and wrapped several times around the gauze. The wrap sticks to itself instead of the skin to hold the gauze in place, eliminating adhesion to the skin and resulting skin damage (Van Leeuwen & Bladh, 2017).

EVIDENCE FOR PRACTICE ▶

RELIEF OF PAIN DURING BLOOD SPECIMEN COLLECTION IN PEDIATRIC PATIENTS

Needle insertion for venipuncture is painful, frightening, and distressful for children. What interventions can assist nurses to reduce the emotional and physical effects of painful procedures, such as venipuncture, in children?

Related Research

Mutlu, B., & Balcı, S. (2015). Effects of balloon inflation and cough trick methods on easing pain in children during the drawing of venous blood samples: A randomized controlled trial. *Journal for Specialists in Pediatric Nursing, 20*(3), 178–186.

The purpose of this prospective randomized, controlled study was to investigate the effects of balloon inflation and cough trick methods on easing pain in children during blood specimen collection. Children aged 9 to 12 years who required blood tests and met the inclusion criteria were randomly assigned to a control group (no intervention) or an experimental group that utilized balloon inflation or a cough trick. Participants in the experimental groups were asked to inflate balloons (balloon group) or cough (cough trick group) during the venipuncture procedure. The Facial Pain Scale-Revised (FPS-R) was used to evaluate expected pain before and perceived pain during the venipuncture procedure. All groups of children expected similar, moderate pain levels before the procedure. Children in the control group reported experiencing the pain they had expected to feel during the procedure. The pain reported by the children in the balloon and cough trick groups was noticeably and significantly lower than they had expected ($p < 0.001$). There was no statistically significant within-group difference in the mean pain scores of the children in the balloon and cough trick groups. The authors concluded the use of distraction, specifically through balloon inflation and coughing during venipuncture, decreased perceived pain during blood specimen collection.

Relevance for Nursing Practice

Nurses are often responsible for obtaining blood samples from their patients, including children. Using the most efficient techniques can result in decreased pain and anxiety for both the children and their parents. This study suggests a method of reducing pain associated with venipuncture and should be taken into consideration when caring for these young patients.

Refer to the Evidence for Practice in Skill 18-10 and to thePoint® for additional research on related nursing topics.

Skill 18-10

Obtaining a Venous Blood Specimen for Culture and Sensitivity

Normally bacteria-free blood is susceptible to infection through infusion lines as well as from thrombophlebitis, surgical drains, infected shunts, and bacterial endocarditis due to prosthetic heart-valve replacements. Bacteria may also move into the bloodstream through the lymphatic system from an infection of a specific body site when the person's immune system cannot contain the infection at its source, such as the bladder or kidneys, from a urinary tract infection. Patients with a compromised immune system are at higher risk for septicemia.

Blood cultures are performed to detect bacterial invasion (bacteremia) or fungi (fungemia) and the systemic spread of such an infection (septicemia) through the bloodstream. In this procedure, a venous blood sample is collected by venipuncture into two bottles (one set), one containing an anaerobic medium and the other an aerobic medium. The bottles are incubated, encouraging any organisms present in the sample to grow in the media. Two or three sets of cultures from different venipuncture sites, each collected 30 to 60 minutes apart, should be obtained (Van Leeuwen & Bladh, 2017). In general, no more than three sets of blood specimens over a 24-hour period should be collected; more than three sets of cultures per day do not significantly add to the likelihood of pathogen capture (Van Leeuwen & Bladh, 2017).

The main problem encountered with blood culture testing is that the specimen is easily contaminated with bacteria from the environment. Care must be taken to clean the skin at the venipuncture site properly to prevent contamination with skin flora, and aseptic technique must be used during the procedure. In addition, the access ports on the blood culture bottles must be properly cleaned before use.

Refer to Skill 18-9 for additional considerations related to venipuncture and blood sample collection.

DELEGATION GUIDELINES	The use of venipuncture to obtain a blood sample for blood culture may be delegated to nursing assistive personnel (NAP) or to unlicensed assistive personnel (UAP) in some settings, as well as to licensed practical/vocational nurses (LPN/LVNs). The decision to delegate must be based on careful analysis of the patient's needs and circumstances, as well as the qualifications of the person to whom the task is being delegated. Refer to the Delegation Guidelines in Appendix A.

EQUIPMENT

- Tourniquet
- Nonsterile gloves
- Additional PPE, as indicated
- Antimicrobial swabs, such as chlorhexidine, per facility policy, for cleaning skin and culture bottle tops
- Vacutainer needle adaptor
- Sterile butterfly needle, gauge appropriate to the vein and sampling needs, using the smallest possible, with extension tubing
- Two blood culture collection bottles for each set being obtained: one anaerobic bottle and one aerobic bottle
- Appropriate label for specimen, based on facility policy and procedure
- Biohazard bag
- Nonsterile gauze pads (2 × 2)
- Sterile gauze pads (2 × 2)
- Adhesive bandage

ASSESSMENT

Review the patient's health record for the number and type of blood cultures to be obtained. Ensure that the appropriate computer laboratory request has been completed. Assess the patient for signs and symptoms of infection, including vital signs, and note any antibiotic therapy being administered. Inspect any invasive monitoring insertion sites or incisions for indications of infection. Assess the patient for any allergies, especially related to the topical antimicrobial used for skin cleansing. Assess for presence of any conditions or use of medications that may prolong bleeding time, necessitating additional application of pressure to the puncture site. Ask the patient about any previous laboratory testing that he or she may have had, including any problems, such as difficulty with venipuncture, fainting, or complaints of dizziness, lightheadedness, or nausea. Assess the

(continued)

Skill 18-10 ▶ Obtaining a Venous Blood Specimen for Culture and Sensitivity *(continued)*

patient's anxiety level and understanding about the reasons for the blood test. Assess the patency of the veins in both upper limbs. The selected area should not be burned or scarred, have a tattoo, or have hematoma present (Van Leeuwen & Bladh, 2017). Palpate the veins to assess the condition of the vessel; vein should be straight, feel soft, cylindrical, and bounce when lightly pressed. Appropriate vessels will compress without rolling, and have rapid rebound filling after compression. Avoid veins that are tender, sclerosed, thrombosed, fibrosed, or hard (Van Leeuwen & Bladh, 2017).

NURSING DIAGNOSIS	Determine the related factors for the nursing diagnoses based on the patient's current status. Appropriate nursing diagnoses may include: • Deficient knowledge • Risk for infection • Risk for injury
OUTCOME IDENTIFICATION AND PLANNING	The expected outcome to achieve is that an uncontaminated specimen will be obtained without injury to the patient and sent to the laboratory promptly. In addition, the patient demonstrates an understanding of the need and process for specimen collection.

IMPLEMENTATION

ACTION	RATIONALE
1. Gather the necessary supplies. Check product expiration dates. Identify ordered number of blood culture sets and select the appropriate blood collection bottles (at least one anaerobic and one aerobic bottle). **If tests are ordered in addition to the blood cultures, collect the blood culture specimens before other specimens.**	Organization facilitates efficient performance of the procedure. Use of products that have not expired ensures proper functioning of equipment. Using correct tubes ensures accurate blood sampling.
2. Perform hand hygiene and put on PPE, if indicated.	Hand hygiene and PPE prevent the transmission of microorganisms. PPE is required based on transmission precautions.
3. Identify the patient.	Identifying the patient ensures the right patient receives the intervention and helps prevent errors.
4. Explain the procedure. Allow the patient time to ask questions and verbalize concerns about the venipuncture procedure.	Explanation provides reassurance and promotes cooperation.
5. Check specimen label with the patient's identification bracelet. Label should include the patient's name and identification number, time specimen was collected, route of collection, identification of person obtaining the sample, and any other information required by facility policy.	Confirmation of patient identification information ensures the specimen is labeled correctly for the right patient.
6. Assemble equipment on overbed table or other surface within reach.	Arranging items nearby is convenient, saves time, and avoids unnecessary stretching and twisting of muscles on the part of the nurse.
7. Close curtains around the bed and close the door to the room, if possible.	Closing the door or curtain provides for patient privacy.
8. Provide for good light. Artificial light is recommended. Place a trash receptacle within easy reach.	Good lighting is necessary to perform the procedure properly. Having the trash receptacle within easy reach allows for safe disposal of contaminated materials.

ACTION

9. Assist the patient to a comfortable position, either sitting or lying. If the patient is lying in bed, raise the bed to a comfortable working height, usually elbow height of the caregiver (VHACEOSH, 2016).

10. Determine the patient's preferred site for the procedure based on his or her previous experience. Expose the arm, supporting it in an extended position on a firm surface, such as a tabletop. Position self on the same side of the patient as the site selected. Apply a tourniquet to the upper arm on the chosen side approximately 3 to 4 in above the potential puncture site (Figure 1). Apply sufficient pressure to impede venous circulation, but not arterial blood flow.

RATIONALE

Proper positioning allows easy access to the site and promotes patient comfort and safety. Proper bed height helps reduce back strain while performing the procedure.

Patient preference allows the patient to be involved in treatment and gives the nurse information that may aid in site selection. Positioning close to the chosen site reduces back strain. Use of a tourniquet increases venous pressure and distention to aid in vein identification. Tourniquet should remain in place no more than 60 seconds to prevent stasis and hemoconcentration (Fischbach & Dunning, 2015).

FIGURE 1. Applying the tourniquet.

11. Put on nonsterile gloves. Assess the veins using inspection and palpation to determine the best puncture site. Refer to the Assessment section above.

12. **Release the tourniquet. Check that the vein has decompressed.**

Gloves reduce transmission of microorganisms. Using the best site reduces the risk of injury to the patient. Palpation allows for making a distinction between other structures, such as tendons and arteries, in the area to avoid injury.

Tourniquet should remain in place no more than 60 seconds to prevent injury, stasis, and hemoconcentration, which may alter results (Fischbach & Dunning, 2015). Thrombosed veins will remain firm and palpable and should not be used for venipuncture.

13. Attach the butterfly needle extension tubing to the Vacutainer device.

14. Move collection bottles to a location close to the arm.

15. **Clean the patient's skin at the selected puncture site with the antimicrobial swab, according to facility policy. If using chlorhexidine, use a gentle back and forth motion for at least 30 seconds or use the procedure recommended by the manufacturer (INS, 2016a). Allow the skin to dry before performing the venipuncture. Do not wipe or blot. Allow to dry completely.**

Connection prepares device for use.

Bottles must be close enough to reach easily once venipuncture is successful.

Cleaning the patient's skin reduces the risk for transmission of microorganisms. Allowing the skin to dry maximizes antimicrobial action and prevents contact of the substance with the needle on insertion, thereby reducing the sting associated with insertion.

(continued)

Skill 18-10 ▶ Obtaining a Venous Blood Specimen for Culture and Sensitivity *(continued)*

ACTION	RATIONALE
16. Using a new antimicrobial swab, clean the stoppers of the culture bottles with the appropriate antimicrobial, per facility policy. Cover bottle top with sterile gauze square, based on facility policy.	Cleaning the bottle top reduces the risk for transmission of microorganisms into the bottle. Covering the top reduces risk of contamination.
17. Reapply the tourniquet approximately 3 to 4 in above the identified puncture site. Apply sufficient pressure to impede venous circulation, but not arterial blood flow. **After disinfection, do not palpate the venipuncture site unless sterile gloves are worn.**	Use of tourniquet increases venous pressure to aid in vein identification. Tourniquet should remain in place no more than 60 seconds to prevent injury, stasis, and hemoconcentration, which may alter results (Fischbach & Dunning, 2015). Palpation is a potential cause of blood culture contamination (Denno & Gannon, 2013; Fischbach & Dunning; Marini & Truog, 2013).
18. Hold the patient's arm in a downward position with your nondominant hand. Align the butterfly needle with the chosen vein, holding the needle in your dominant hand. Use the thumb or first finger of your nondominant hand to apply pressure and traction to the skin about 1 to 2 in below the identified puncture site (Van Leeuwen & Bladh, 2017) (Figure 2). **Do not touch the insertion site.**	Applying pressure helps immobilize and anchor the vein. Taut skin at the entry site aids smooth needle entry. Not touching the insertion site helps to prevent contamination. Palpation is a potential cause of blood culture contamination (Denno & Gannon, 2013; Fischbach & Dunning; Marini & Truog, 2013).
19. **Inform the patient that he or she is going to feel a pinch.** With the bevel of the needle up, insert the needle into the vein at a 15 to 30 degree angle to the skin (Malarkey & McMorrow, 2012; Van Leeuwen & Bladh, 2017). You should see a flash of blood in the extension tubing close to the needle when the vein is entered (Figure 3).	Warning the patient prevents reaction related to surprise. Positioning the needle at the proper angle reduces the risk of puncturing through the vein. Flash of blood indicates entrance into the vein.

FIGURE 2. Aligning the butterfly needle with the chosen vein.

FIGURE 3. Inserting the needle with the bevel up at a 15- to 30-degree angle.

20. **Keeping the specimen bottle upright,** fill the aerobic bottle first (Fischbach & Dunning, 2015; Laboratory Alliance of Central New York, LLC, 2017; Van Leeuwen & Bladh, 2017). Grasp the butterfly needle securely to stabilize it in the vein with your nondominant hand, and push the Vacutainer onto the first collection bottle (aerobic bottle), until the rubber stopper on the collection bottle is punctured (Figure 4). You will feel the bottle push into place on the puncture device. Blood will flow into the bottle automatically. Fill to the level indicated on the bottle; do not overfill (Fischbach & Dunning, 2015).	Specimen bottles should remain upright to prevent backflow of contents to patient. The collection bottle is a vacuum; negative pressure within the bottle pulls blood into the bottle.

ACTION

RATIONALE

FIGURE 4. Stabilizing the butterfly needle and pushing the Vacutainer onto the aerobic collection bottle, keeping the bottle upright while filling.

21. **Remove the tourniquet as soon as blood flows adequately into the bottle.**

Tourniquet removal reduces venous pressure and restores venous return to help prevent bleeding and bruising (Van Leeuwen & Bladh, 2017).

22. Continue to hold the butterfly needle in place in the vein. Once the first bottle is filled, remove it from the Vacutainer and insert the second bottle. After the blood culture specimens are obtained, continue to fill any additional required tubes, removing one and inserting another. Gently rotate each bottle and tube as you remove it.

Filling the required bottles ensures that the sample is accurate. Gentle rotation helps to mix any additive in the tube with the blood sample.

23. After you have drawn all required blood samples, remove the last collection tube from the Vacutainer. **Place a gauze pad over the puncture site and slowly and gently remove the needle from the vein. Engage needle guard. Do not apply pressure to the site until the needle has been fully removed.**

Slow, gentle needle removal prevents injury to the vein. Releasing the vacuum before withdrawing the needle prevents injury to the vein and hematoma formation. Use of a needle guard prevents accidental needlestick injuries.

24. Apply gentle pressure to the puncture site for 2 to 3 minutes or until bleeding stops.

Applying pressure to the site after needle removal prevents injury, bleeding, and extravasation into the surrounding tissue, which can cause a hematoma.

25. After bleeding stops, apply an adhesive bandage.

The bandage protects the site and aids in applying pressure.

26. Remove equipment and return patient to a position of comfort. Raise side rails and lower bed.

Repositioning promotes patient comfort. Raising rails promotes safety.

27. Discard Vacutainer and butterfly needle in sharps container.

Proper disposal of equipment reduces transmission of microorganisms.

28. Remove gloves and perform hand hygiene.

Removing gloves properly reduces the risk for infection transmission and contamination of other items. Hand hygiene reduces the transmission of microorganisms.

(continued)

Skill 18-10 ▶ Obtaining a Venous Blood Specimen for Culture and Sensitivity *(continued)*

ACTION	RATIONALE
29. Place label on the container, per facility policy (Figure 5). Place containers in plastic, sealable biohazard bag (Figure 6). Refer to facility policy regarding the need for separate biohazard bags for blood culture specimens and other blood specimens.	Proper labeling ensures accurate reporting of results. Packaging the specimen in a biohazard bag prevents the person transporting the container from coming in contact with blood or body fluids. Some facility policies call for individual bagging.

FIGURE 5. Placing a label on specimen container.

FIGURE 6. Placing specimen containers in biohazard bag.

ACTION	RATIONALE
30. Check the venipuncture sites to see if a hematoma has developed.	Development of a hematoma requires further intervention.
31. Remove other PPE, if used. Perform hand hygiene.	Proper removal of PPE reduces the risk for infection transmission and contamination of other items. Hand hygiene reduces the transmission of microorganisms.
32. Transport the specimen to the laboratory immediately. If immediate transport is not possible, check with laboratory personnel or policy manual as to appropriate handling.	Timely transport ensures accurate results.

EVALUATION

The expected outcomes have been achieved when an uncontaminated specimen has been obtained without injury to the patient and has been sent to the laboratory promptly; and the patient demonstrated an understanding of the need and process for specimen collection.

DOCUMENTATION

Guidelines

Record the date, time, and site of the venipunctures; the name of the test(s); the time the sample was sent to the laboratory; the amount of blood collected, if required; and any significant assessments or patient reactions.

Sample Documentation

> 6/6/20 1710 Patient's temperature increased to 104.2°F. Patient very lethargic, pale, diaphoretic; with cool, clammy skin. Bradycardic with pulse rate of 56 beats/min and hypotensive with blood pressure of 90/50 mm Hg. Dr. Barrie notified. Blood cultures ×2 ordered; first set obtained from right antecubital vein. No evidence of bleeding or hematoma at venipuncture site.
>
> —B. Pearson, RN

UNEXPECTED SITUATIONS AND ASSOCIATED INTERVENTIONS

- *After applying the tourniquet, you have trouble finding a distended vein:* Have the patient make a fist, or try tapping the skin over the vein lightly several times. **Do not have the patient pump the fist as this may increase plasma potassium levels** (Fischbach & Dunning, 2015; INS, 2016b). If unsuccessful, remove the tourniquet and try lowering the patient's arm to allow blood to pool in the veins. If necessary, apply warm compresses for about 10 minutes before reapplying the tourniquet.
- *Patient has large, distended, highly visible veins:* Perform venipuncture without a tourniquet to minimize the risk for hematoma (Fischbach & Dunning, 2015).
- *Patient has a clotting disorder or is receiving anticoagulant therapy:* Maintain firm pressure on the venipuncture site for at least 5 minutes after withdrawing the needle to prevent hematoma formation.
- *Oozing or bleeding continues from the puncture site for more than a few minutes:* Elevate the area and apply a pressure dressing. If bleeding is excessive or persists for longer than 10 minutes, notify the health care provider.
- *A hematoma develops at the venipuncture site:* Apply pressure until you are sure bleeding has stopped (about 5 minutes). Notify the patient's health care provider. Document size and appearance of hematoma, notification of primary health care provider, and any ordered interventions.
- *Patient reports feeling lightheaded and says she is going to faint:* Stop the venipuncture. If the patient is in bed, have the patient lie flat and elevate the feet. If the patient is in a chair, have the patient put her head between her knees. Encourage the patient to take slow, deep breaths. Call for assistance and stay with the patient. Obtain vital signs, if possible.

SPECIAL CONSIDERATIONS

General Considerations

- Be aware that the size of the culture bottles may vary according to facility policy, but the sample dilution should always be 1:10.
- If possible, ensure the specimen is obtained before antibiotics are started (Fischbach & Dunning, 2015; Van Leeuwen & Bladh, 2017). The use of antimicrobial removal devices (ARDs) may be ordered if antibiotic therapy is initiated prior to specimen collection (Van Leeuwen & Bladh, 2017). This involves transferring some of the blood sample into a special vial containing absorbent resins that remove antibiotics from the sample before the culture is performed (Van Leeuwen & Bladh, 2017, p. 659). The use of ARDs is costly and controversial with respect to their effectiveness versus standard culture techniques (Van Leeuwen & Bladh, 2017).
- Draw blood from different peripheral venipuncture sites and document each site. This increases the likelihood of detecting a bloodstream infection and helps differentiate true bacteremia from a false-positive finding due to skin contamination. Peripheral sites are preferred (Denno & Gannon, 2013; Kyle & Carman, 2017; Septimus, 2015; Van Leeuwen & Bladh, 2017).
- In the case of suspected catheter-related bloodstream infection, one set of blood cultures should be drawn through the device and one set from a separate venipuncture (Septimus, 2015). Clearly document site of collection.
- Avoid collecting blood from edematous areas, arteriovenous shunts, an upper extremity on the same side as a previous lymph node dissection or mastectomy, infected sites, same extremity as an intravenous infusion, and sites of previous hematomas or vascular injury.
- Avoid previous sites of venipuncture to reduce the potential for infection (Van Leeuwen & Bladh, 2017).
- Do not use veins in the lower extremities for venipuncture, because of an increased risk of thrombophlebitis. However, some facilities do allow collection from lower extremities with a health care provider's order to collect blood from a leg or foot vein. Check your facility's policies.
- Apply warm compresses to the selected site 15 to 20 minutes before venipuncture to aid in distending veins that are difficult to locate.
- Consider the use of topical anesthetic creams to minimize discomfort and pain for the patient, based on facility policy. Allow 60 seconds after application for patients with light skin tones and 120 seconds for patients with dark skin tones before performing the venipuncture (Fischbach & Dunning, 2015). Be familiar with requirements and specifications for a particular product available for use. Application needs to occur sufficiently in advance to allow enough time to become effective.

(continued)

Skill 18-10 ▶ Obtaining a Venous Blood Specimen for Culture and Sensitivity *(continued)*

- Use distraction, if appropriate. Distraction has been shown to be of benefit in reducing anxiety related to venipuncture, especially with children (da Silva et al., 2016; Mutlu & Balcı, 2015bib19). Asking the patient to concentrate on relaxing; performing deep breathing may help the patient relax.
- The application of molecular diagnostics techniques using identification of specific sequences of DNA and the development of automated instruments that can identify pathogens from a small amount of blood has made faster diagnosis of bloodstream infections and detection of antibiotic resistance possible (Liesenfeld, Lehman, Hunfeld, & Kost, 2014; Van Leeuwen & Bladh, 2017).

Infant and Child Considerations

- Consider automatically applying warm compresses to distend the small veins of infants and young children before attempting any venipuncture.
- Venipuncture by a skilled phlebotomist is suggested instead of heel lance methods due to the increased pain from heel lance (INS, 2016b).
- Administer oral sucrose/glucose beginning 1 to 2 minutes before the venipuncture procedure for young infants, to decrease the incidence of procedure-related pain (Sethi & Nayak, 2015; Uzelli & Güneş, 2015).
- Consider using topical anesthetic creams or gels, refrigerant spray, or iontophoresis (application of electric current to carry ionized lidocaine through the skin) with infants and children, to decrease the incidence of procedure-related pain (Baxter et al., 2013; Kearl et al., 2015). Apply the product for sufficient time to reach maximal effectiveness.
- Consider the use of distraction to decrease the incidence of procedure-related pain (da Silva et al., 2016; Mutlu & Balcı, 2015bib19).
- Consider the use of self-adhesive wrap instead of tape to avoid damage to delicate skin. A section of self-adhesive wrap is placed over the gauze at the venipuncture site and wrapped several times around the gauze. The wrap sticks to itself instead of the skin to hold the gauze in place. Self-adhesive wrap is available in numerous colors; this, combined with elimination of adhesion to the skin, makes it an attractive alternative to tape for infants and children (Van Leeuwen & Bladh, 2017).

Older Adult Considerations

- Keep in mind that the veins of an older adult are fragile and may collapse easily. In addition, the skin is less elastic and may be more difficult to pull taut.
- The superficial veins of the hands of older adults are fragile and venipuncture can cause a hematoma to form. Additionally, these veins move due to the age-related loss of supportive muscle and connective tissue, making it difficult to enter the lumen of the vein (Malarkey & McMorrow, 2012).
- Consider performing venipuncture without a tourniquet, for older adults, to prevent rupture of capillaries.
- Consider the use of self-adhesive wrap instead of tape to avoid damage to delicate skin. A section of self-adhesive wrap is placed over the gauze at the venipuncture site and wrapped several times around the gauze. The wrap sticks to itself instead of the skin to hold the gauze in place, eliminating adhesion to the skin and resulting skin damage (Van Leeuwen & Bladh, 2017).

EVIDENCE FOR PRACTICE ▶

RELIEF OF PAIN DURING BLOOD SPECIMEN COLLECTION IN ADULT PATIENTS
Needle insertion for venipuncture is painful. What interventions can assist nurses to reduce the pain associated with venipuncture in adults?

Related Research
Mace, S. E. (2016). Prospective, randomized, double-blind controlled trial comparing vapocoolant spray vs placebo spray in adults undergoing venipuncture. *American Journal of Emergency Medicine, 34*(5), 798–804.

 This prospective randomized, double-blind controlled trial examined the use of vapocoolant versus placebo spray in 100 adults, ages 18 to 80, requiring venipuncture in a hospital emergency department or observation unit. Participants were randomly assigned to a control group (placebo spray) or experimental group (vapocoolant spray). Procedure-related pain was scored immediately after venipuncture, measured on a 10-point numerical scale. Local adverse effects (edema, erythema, blanching) and changes in vital signs postapplication were also recorded. Participants in the control group reported a median pain score related to venipuncture of 3. Participants in the intervention group reported a median pain score related to venipuncture of 1. The pain reported by the intervention group was significantly lower than the control group ($p < 0.001$). Minor adverse effects were observed, related to use of the vapocoolant and resolved quickly; minimal blanching (4% of participants) and minimal erythema which resolved within 5 minutes (18% of participants). No visible skin changes were noted in the placebo group. Photographs at 5 and 10 minutes revealed no visible skin changes in any patient. No significant changes in vital signs were noted pre- and postintervention in either group. The authors concluded the vapocoolant significantly decreased venipuncture pain in adults compared with the placebo and was well tolerated with minor adverse effects that resolved quickly.

Relevance for Nursing Practice

Nurses are often responsible for obtaining blood samples from their patients. Using the most efficient techniques can result in decreased pain and anxiety related to venipuncture. The use of a vapocoolant spray is an easy and effective method to reduce venipuncture-associated pain and should be considered as part of providing patient care related to venipuncture to obtain laboratory specimens and venous access.

Refer to the Evidence for Practice in Skill 18-9 and to thePoint° for additional research on related nursing topics.

Skill 18-11 ▶ Obtaining an Arterial Blood Specimen for Blood Gas Analysis

Arterial blood gases (ABGs) are obtained to determine the adequacy of oxygenation and ventilation, to assess acid–base status, and to monitor the effectiveness of treatment. The most common site for sampling arterial blood is the radial artery. Other arteries may be used, but an advanced health care provider's order may be required to obtain the sample from another artery.

Analysis of ABGs evaluates ventilation by measuring blood pH and the partial pressure of arterial oxygen (Pao_2) and partial pressure of arterial carbon dioxide ($Paco_2$). Blood pH measurement reveals the blood's acid–base balance. Pao_2 indicates the amount of oxygen that the lungs deliver to the blood, and $Paco_2$ indicates the lungs' capacity to eliminate carbon dioxide. ABG samples can also be analyzed for oxygen content and saturation, and for bicarbonate values. Table 18-1

Table 18-1 Arterial Blood Gas: Normal Values

PARAMETER	NORMAL VALUE
pH	7.35–7.45
$PaCO_2$	35–45 mm Hg
HCO_3	22–26 mEq/L
SaO_2	Oxygen saturation >95%
PaO_2	>80–100 mm Hg
Base excess or deficit	±2 mEq/L

(continued)

Skill 18-11 ▶ Obtaining an Arterial Blood Specimen for Blood Gas Analysis *(continued)*

highlights the normal values for ABG. A respiratory technician or specially trained nurse can collect most ABG samples, but an advanced practice professional usually performs collection from the femoral artery, depending on facility policy. An Allen's test should always be performed before using the radial artery to determine whether the ulnar artery delivers sufficient blood to the hand and fingers, in case there is damage to the radial artery during the blood sampling. Refer to the guidelines in this skill for performing an Allen's test.

DELEGATION CONSIDERATIONS	Obtaining an arterial blood specimen for blood gas analysis is not delegated to nursing assistive personnel (NAP) or to unlicensed assistive personnel (UAP). Depending on the state's nurse practice act and the organization's policies and procedures, obtaining an arterial blood specimen for blood gas analysis may be delegated to licensed practical/vocational nurses (LPN/LVNs). The decision to delegate must be based on careful analysis of the patient's needs and circumstances, as well as the qualifications of the person to whom the task is being delegated. Refer to the Delegation Guidelines in Appendix A.
EQUIPMENT	• ABG kit, *or* heparinized self-filling 10-mL syringe with 22-gauge, 1-in needle attached • Airtight cap for hub of syringe • 2 × 2 gauze pad • Band-Aid • Antimicrobial swab, such as chlorhexidine, per facility policy • Biohazard bag • Appropriate label for specimen, based on facility policy and procedure • Cup or bag of ice and water • Nonsterile gloves • Goggles • Additional PPE, as indicated • Rolled towel
ASSESSMENT	Review the patient's health record and nursing care plan for information about the need for an ABG specimen. Assess the patient's cardiac status, including heart rate, blood pressure, and auscultation of heart sounds. Also assess the patient's respiratory status, including respiratory rate, excursion, lung sounds, and use of oxygen, including the amount being used, if ordered. Determine the adequacy of peripheral blood flow to the extremity to be used by performing the Allen's test (detailed below). If Allen's test reveals little or no collateral circulation to the hand, do not perform an arterial stick to that artery. Assess the patient's radial pulse. If unable to palpate the radial pulse, consider using the other wrist. Assess the patient's understanding about the need for specimen collection. Ask the patient if he or she has ever felt faint, sweaty, or nauseated when having blood drawn.
NURSING DIAGNOSIS	Determine the related factors for the nursing diagnoses based on the patient's current status. Appropriate nursing diagnoses may include: • Impaired gas exchange • Risk for injury • Acute pain
OUTCOME IDENTIFICATION AND PLANNING	The expected outcome to achieve is that an uncontaminated specimen will be obtained without injury to the patient or damage to the artery and sent to the laboratory promptly. In addition, the patient demonstrates an understanding of the need and process for specimen collection.

IMPLEMENTATION

ACTION	RATIONALE

1. Gather the necessary supplies. Check product expiration dates. Identify ordered arterial blood gas analysis. Check the chart to make sure the patient has not been suctioned within the past 20 to 30 minutes. Check facility policy and/or procedure for guidelines on administering local anesthesia for arterial punctures. Administer anesthetic and allow sufficient time for full effect before beginning procedure.

Organization facilitates efficient performance of the procedure. Use of products that have not expired ensures proper functioning of equipment. Suctioning may change the oxygen saturation and is a temporary change not to be confused with baseline for the patient. Arterial puncture is a source of pain and discomfort. Intradermal injection of lidocaine around the puncture site has been shown to decrease the incidence and severity of localized pain when used before arterial puncture (American Association of Critical-Care Nurses [AACN], 2017).

2. Perform hand hygiene and put on PPE, if indicated.

Hand hygiene and PPE prevent the transmission of microorganisms. PPE is required based on transmission precautions.

3. Identify the patient.

Identifying the patient ensures the right patient receives the intervention and helps prevent errors.

4. Explain the procedure to the patient. Tell the patient you need to collect an arterial blood sample and the needlestick will cause some discomfort but that he or she must remain still during the procedure.

Explanation facilitates cooperation and provides reassurance for the patient.

5. Check specimen label with the patient's identification bracelet. Label should include patient's name and identification number, time specimen was collected, route of collection, identification of person obtaining the sample, amount of oxygen the patient is receiving, type of oxygen administration device, patient's body temperature, and any other information required by facility policy.

Confirmation of patient identification information ensures the specimen is labeled correctly for the right patient. Oxygen information and patient's body temperature are required for accurate analysis.

6. Assemble equipment on overbed table or other surface within reach.

Arranging items nearby is convenient, saves time, and avoids unnecessary stretching and twisting of muscles on the part of the nurse.

7. Close curtains around the bed and close the door to the room, if possible.

Closing the door or curtain provides for patient privacy.

8. Provide for good light. Artificial light is recommended. Place a trash receptacle within easy reach.

Good lighting is necessary to perform the procedure properly. Having the trash receptacle in easy reach allows for safe disposal of contaminated materials.

9. If the patient is on bed rest, ask him or her to lie in a supine position, with the head slightly elevated and the arms at the sides. Ask an ambulatory patient to sit in a chair and support the arm securely on an armrest or a table. Place a waterproof pad under the site and a rolled towel under the wrist.

Positioning the patient comfortably helps minimize anxiety. Using a rolled towel under the wrist provides for easy access to the insertion site.

10. **Perform Allen's test (Figure 1) before obtaining a specimen from the radial artery.**

Allen's testing assesses patency of the ulnar and radial arteries.

a. Have the patient clench the fist to minimize blood flow into the hand.

b. Using your index and middle fingers, press on the radial and ulnar arteries (Figure 1A). Hold this position for a few seconds.

(continued)

Skill 18-11 ▶ Obtaining an Arterial Blood Specimen for Blood Gas Analysis *(continued)*

ACTION	RATIONALE

c. Without removing your fingers from the arteries, ask the patient to unclench the fist and hold the hand in a relaxed position (Figure 1B). The palm will be blanched because pressure from your fingers has impaired the normal blood flow.

d. Release pressure on the ulnar artery (Figure 1C). If the hand becomes flushed, which indicates that blood is filling the vessels, it is safe to proceed with the radial artery puncture. This is considered a positive test. If the hand does not flush, perform the test on the other arm.

A

B

C

FIGURE 1. Performing Allen's test. **A.** Compressing the arteries with the patient's fist closed. **B.** Maintaining compression as patient unclenches fist. **C.** Compressing only the radial artery.

11. Put on nonsterile gloves. Locate the radial artery and lightly palpate it for a strong pulse.

Gloves reduce transmission of microorganisms. If you push too hard during palpation, the radial artery will be obliterated and hard to palpate.

12. **Clean the patient's skin at the puncture site with the antimicrobial swab, according to facility policy. If using chlorhexidine, use a gentle back and forth motion for at least 30 seconds or use the procedure recommended by the manufacturer (INS, 2016a). Do not wipe or blot. Allow to dry completely. After disinfection, do not palpate the site unless sterile gloves are worn.**

Site cleansing prevents potentially infectious skin flora from being introduced into the vessel during the procedure. Palpation after cleansing contaminates the area.

ACTION	**RATIONALE**

13. Stabilize the hand with the wrist extended over the rolled towel, palm up. Palpate the artery above the puncture site with the index and middle fingers of your nondominant hand while holding the syringe over the puncture site with your dominant hand. **Do not directly touch the area to be punctured.**

Stabilizing the hand and palpating the artery with one hand while holding the syringe in the other provides better access to the artery. Palpating the area to be punctured would contaminate the clean area.

14. Hold the needle bevel up at a 45- to 60-degree angle at the site of maximal pulse impulse, with the shaft parallel to the path of the artery.

The proper angle of insertion ensures correct access to the artery. The artery is shallow and does not require a deeper angle to penetrate.

15. **Inform the patient that he or she is going to feel a pinch.** Puncture the skin and arterial wall in one motion. Watch for blood backflow in the syringe (Figure 2). Pulsating blood will flow into the syringe. Do not pull back on the plunger. Collect 2 to 3 mL (Hess et al., 2016).

Warning the patient prevents reaction related to surprise. Positioning the needle at the proper angle reduces the risk of puncturing through the artery. The blood should enter the syringe automatically due to arterial pressure.

FIGURE 2. Observing blood backflow into syringe. (*Photo by B. Proud.*)

16. After collecting the sample, withdraw the syringe while your nondominant hand is beginning to place pressure proximal to the insertion site with the 2 × 2 gauze. **Press a gauze pad firmly over the puncture site until the bleeding stops—at least 5 minutes. If the patient is receiving anticoagulant therapy or has a blood dyscrasia, apply pressure for 10 to 15 minutes; if necessary, ask a coworker to hold the gauze pad in place while you prepare the sample for transport to the laboratory, but do not ask the patient to hold the pad.**

If insufficient pressure is applied, a large, painful hematoma may form, hindering future arterial puncture at the site.

17. When the bleeding stops and the appropriate time has lapsed, apply a small adhesive bandage or small pressure dressing (fold a 2 × 2 gauze into fourths and firmly apply tape, stretching the skin tight).

Applying a dressing also prevents arterial hemorrhage and extravasation into the surrounding tissue, which can cause a hematoma.

(*continued*)

Skill 18-11 ▶ Obtaining an Arterial Blood Specimen for Blood Gas Analysis *(continued)*

ACTION	RATIONALE
18. Once the sample is obtained, check the syringe for air bubbles. If any appear, remove them by holding the syringe upright and slowly ejecting some of the blood onto a 2 × 2 gauze pad.	Air bubbles can affect the laboratory values.
19. Engage the needle guard and remove the needle. Place the airtight cap on the syringe. Gently rotate the syringe. Do not shake.	Engaging the needle guard prevents accidental needlestick injury. Using an airtight cap prevents the sample from leaking and keeps air out of the syringe, because blood will continue to absorb oxygen and will give a false reading if allowed to have contact with air. Rotating the syringe ensures proper mixing of heparin in syringe with the sample; heparin prevents blood from clotting. Vigorous shaking may cause hemolysis.
20. Place label on the syringe per facility policy. Place syringe in plastic, sealable biohazard bag. Insert the syringe into a cup or bag of ice water.	Labeling ensures the specimen is the correct one for the right patient. Packaging the specimen in a biohazard bag prevents the person transporting the samples from coming in contact with blood. Ice prevents the blood from degrading.
21. Remove equipment and return the patient to a position of comfort. Raise side rail and lower bed.	Repositioning promotes patient comfort. Raising rails promotes safety.
22. Discard the needle in sharps container. Remove gloves and perform hand hygiene.	Proper disposal of equipment prevents accidental injury and reduces transmission of microorganisms. Removing gloves properly reduces the risk for infection transmission and contamination of other items. Hand hygiene reduces transmission of microorganisms.
23. Check the puncture site for bleeding and to see if a hematoma has developed.	Continued bleeding or development of a hematoma requires further intervention.
24. Remove other PPE, if used. Perform hand hygiene.	Proper removal of PPE reduces the risk for infection transmission and contamination of other items. Hand hygiene reduces the transmission of microorganisms.
25. Transport the specimen to the laboratory immediately.	Timely transport ensures accurate results.

EVALUATION

The expected outcomes have been achieved when an uncontaminated specimen has been obtained without injury to the patient and has been sent to the laboratory promptly; and the patient demonstrated an understanding of the need and process for specimen collection.

DOCUMENTATION

Guidelines

Document results of Allen's test, time the sample was drawn, arterial puncture site, amount of time pressure was applied to the site to control bleeding, type and amount of oxygen therapy that the patient was receiving, pulse oximetry values, respiratory rate, respiratory effort, patient's other vital signs, and any other significant assessments.

Sample Documentation

> 9/22/20 1245 Allen's test positive at R radial artery. ABG obtained using R radial artery. Pressure applied to site for 5 minutes. Patient receiving 3 L/NC oxygen, pulse oximetry 94%, respirations even/unlabored, respiratory rate 18 breaths/min, oral temperature 98.9°F, patient denies dyspnea.
>
> —C. Bausler, RN

UNEXPECTED SITUATIONS AND ASSOCIATED INTERVENTIONS

- *While you are attempting to puncture the artery, the patient complains of severe pain:* Using too much force may cause the needle to touch bone, causing the patient pain. Too much force may also result in advancing the needle through the opposite wall of the artery. If this happens, slowly pull the needle back a short distance and check to see if blood returns. If blood still fails to enter the syringe, withdraw the needle completely and restart the procedure.
- *You cannot obtain a specimen from the same site after two attempts:* Stop. Do not make more than two attempts from the same site. Probing the artery may injure it and the radial nerve.
- *Blood will not flow into the syringe:* Typically, this occurs as a result of arterial spasm. Replace the needle with a smaller one and try the puncture again. A smaller-bore needle is less likely to cause arterial spasm.
- *After inserting the needle, you note that the syringe is filling sluggishly with dark red/purple blood:* If the patient is in critical condition, this may be arterial blood. But if the patient is awake and alert with a pulse oximeter reading within normal parameters, you have most likely obtained a venous sample. Discard the sample and redraw.
- *Patient is on anticoagulant therapy:* Expect to hold pressure on the puncture site for at least 10 minutes. If pressure is not held sufficiently long, a hematoma may form, place pressure on the artery, and decrease the flow of blood.
- *Blood was drawn without incident, but now, 2 hours later, the patient is complaining of tingling in the fingers and the hand is cool and pale:* Notify the health care provider. An arterial thrombosis may have formed. If not treated, the thrombosis can lead to tissue necrosis on the extremity.
- *Puncture site continues to ooze:* If the site is not actively bleeding, consider placing a small pressure bandage on the insertion site. This will prevent the artery from continuing to ooze. Continually check the site for bleeding and assess the extremity to ensure that blood flow is adequate.
- *The Allen's test is negative:* Try the other extremity. If the other extremity has a positive result (collateral circulation), use that extremity. If the Allen's test is negative in both extremities, notify the health care provider.

SPECIAL CONSIDERATIONS

General Considerations

- Be aware that use of a particular arterial site is contraindicated for the following reasons: absence of a palpable radial artery pulse; Allen's test showing only one artery supplying blood to the hand; Allen's test showing obstruction in the ulnar artery; cellulitis or infection at the site; presence of arteriovenous fistula or shunt; severe thrombocytopenia (platelet count 20,000/mm³ or less, or based on facility policy); a prolonged prothrombin time or partial thromboplastin time, or elevated INR; or significant or uncontrolled bleeding disorder (Fischbach & Dunning, 2015; Van Leeuwen & Bladh, 2017).
- If the patient is receiving oxygen, wait 30 minutes after a change in type or mode of oxygen delivery or rate for specimen collection for arterial blood gas analysis (Van Leeuwen & Bladh, 2017). Indicate on the laboratory request, the amount and type of oxygen therapy the patient is receiving. Also note the patient's current temperature, most recent hemoglobin level, and current respiratory rate. If the patient is receiving mechanical ventilation, note the fraction of inspired oxygen and tidal volume.
- If the patient is not receiving oxygen, indicate that he or she is breathing room air on the laboratory request for an arterial blood gas analysis.
- If the patient has just received a nebulizer treatment, wait about 20 minutes before collecting the sample for arterial blood gas analysis.
- Specimens collected within 20 to 30 minutes of respiratory passage suctioning or other respiratory therapy will not be accurate (Van Leeuwen & Bladh, 2017).
- Consider obtaining an order for the use of a local anesthetic solution (1% lidocaine solution), gel, or cream to minimize discomfort and pain for the patient, based on facility policy (AACN, 2017). The use of 1% lidocaine without epinephrine injected intradermally around the artery puncture site has been shown to decrease the incidence of localized pain (AACN). Be familiar with requirements and specifications for particular products available for use. Application needs

(continued)

| **Skill 18-11** | **Obtaining an Arterial Blood Specimen for Blood Gas Analysis** *(continued)* |

to occur sufficiently far in advance to allow enough time to become effective, which may be contraindicated by the patient's condition. Consider such use of lidocaine carefully because it can delay the procedure. The patient may be allergic to the drug, or the resulting vasoconstriction may prevent successful puncture.

- Consider the use of topical anesthetic creams to minimize discomfort and pain for the patient, based on facility policy. Allow 60 seconds after application for patients with light skin tones and 120 seconds for patients with dark skin tones before performing the venipuncture (Fischbach & Dunning, 2015). Be familiar with requirements and specifications for a particular product available for use. Application needs to occur sufficiently in advance to allow enough time to become effective.
- If the femoral site is used for the procedure, apply pressure for a minimum of 10 minutes.
- Arterial lines may be used to obtain blood samples (refer to Skill 16-7 in Chapter 16). When sampling from arterial lines, record the amount of blood drawn for each sampling. Frequent sampling can result in significant amount of blood being removed.
- Capillary blood gas samples may be used to estimate pH and PCO_2 in infants or other people when arterial blood gas analysis is indicated but arterial access is difficult (Hess et al., 2016).

Infant and Child Considerations

- Administer oral sucrose/glucose beginning 1 to 2 minutes before the venipuncture procedure for young infants, to decrease the incidence of procedure-related pain (Sethi & Nayak, 2015; Uzelli & Güneş, 2015).
- Consider using topical anesthetic creams or gels, refrigerant spray, or iontophoresis (application of electric current to carry ionized lidocaine through the skin) with infants and children, to decrease the incidence of procedure-related pain (Baxter et al., 2013; Kearl et al., 2015). Apply the product for sufficient time to reach maximal effectiveness.
- Consider the use of distraction to decrease the incidence of procedure-related pain (da Silva et al., 2016; Mutlu & Balcı, 2015).
- Consider the use of self-adhesive wrap instead of tape to avoid damage to delicate skin. A section of self-adhesive wrap is placed over the gauze at the venipuncture site and wrapped several times around the gauze. The wrap sticks to itself instead of the skin to hold the gauze in place. Self-adhesive wrap is available in numerous colors; this, combined with elimination of adhesion to the skin, makes it an attractive alternative to tape for infants and children (Van Leeuwen & Bladh, 2017).

Older Adult Considerations

- Consider the use of self-adhesive wrap instead of tape to avoid damage to delicate skin. A section of self-adhesive wrap is placed over the gauze at the venipuncture site and wrapped several times around the gauze. The wrap sticks to itself instead of the skin to hold the gauze in place, eliminating adhesion to the skin and resulting skin damage (Van Leeuwen & Bladh, 2017).

EVIDENCE FOR PRACTICE ▶

RELIEF OF PAIN DURING BLOOD SPECIMEN COLLECTION
Needle insertion for venipuncture is painful. What interventions can assist nurses to reduce the pain associated with venipuncture and arterial puncture?

Related Research
Mace, S. E. (2016). Prospective, randomized, double-blind controlled trial comparing vapocoolant spray vs placebo spray in adults undergoing venipuncture. *American Journal of Emergency Medicine, 34*(5), 798–804.

Mutlu, B., & Balcı, S. (2015). Effects of balloon inflation and cough trick methods on easing pain in children during the drawing of venous blood samples: A randomized controlled trial. *Journal for Specialists in Pediatric Nursing, 20*(3), 178–186.

Refer to the details in the Evidence for Practice in Skills 18-9 and 18-10 and to thePoint® for additional research on related nursing topics.

Enhance Your Understanding

Focusing on Patient Care: Developing Clinical Reasoning

Consider the case scenarios at the beginning of the chapter as you answer the following questions to enhance your understanding and apply what you have learned.

QUESTIONS

1. The nurse explained to Mr. Conklin the procedure for obtaining the required urine specimens. Unfortunately, it becomes clear that the patient is too confused at this time to follow the directions and obtain the specimen by himself. How would you handle this situation? How would you successfully obtain an uncontaminated specimen from a patient who is unable to cooperate?

2. Huana Yon's health care provider provides pre- and postappointment education and information for the patients in the practice. Part of the nurse's responsibilities when contacting patients before their scheduled visit is to provide information related to anticipated laboratory tests and any necessary patient preparation.

What information would you include if you were calling this patient before her visit in relation to collecting a stool specimen for occult blood? What medications or other habits would you question her about? What information would you give her to prepare for the test?

3. The nurse assigned to Mrs. Yeletsky questions her about her blood glucose testing at home. Mrs. Yeletsky states, "I never really figured out how to work the machine they gave me the last time I saw the doctor. The buttons are too small, and I can't see the writing on the screen very well. Besides, I'm only a little diabetic." What additional information would you want to obtain from this patient? How would you address her possible lack of understanding regarding diabetes? What interventions could you attempt to aid her in managing her blood glucose levels? What other aspects of her health habits would you want to assess?

You can find suggested answers after the Bibliography at the end of this chapter.

Integrated Case Study Connection

The case studies in the back of the book focus on integrating concepts. Refer to the following case studies to enhance your understanding of the concepts and skills in this chapter.

- Basic Case Studies: Joe LeRoy, page 1108; Tula Stillwater, page 1111.
- Intermediate Case Studies: Victoria Holly, page 1115.
- Advanced Case Studies: Cole McKean, page 1128.

Taylor Suite Resources

Explore these additional resources to enhance learning for this chapter:

- NCLEX-Style Questions and other resources on thePoint*, http://thePoint.lww.com/Lynn5e
- *Skill Checklists for Taylor's Clinical Nursing Skills*, 5e
- *Lippincott DocuCare* Fundamentals cases

Bibliography

American Association for Clinical Chemistry (AACC). (2015). *Lab Tests Online*: Fecal occult blood test and fecal immunochemical test. Retrieved https://labtestsonline.org/understanding/analytes/fecal-occult-blood/tab/glance

American Association of Critical-Care Nurses (AACN). (2012). *AACN practice alert: Catheter-associated urinary tract infections. Critical Care Nurse (CCN), 32*(2), 75.

American Association of Critical-Care Nurses (AACN). (2017). In D. L. Wiegand (Ed.). *AACN procedure manual for high acuity, progressive, and critical care* (7th ed.). St. Louis, MO: Elsevier.

American Diabetes Association (ADA). (2016). *Checking your blood glucose.* Retrieved http://www.diabetes.org/living-with-diabetes/treatment-and-care/blood-glucose-control/checking-your-blood-glucose.html?referrer=https://www.google.com

American Diabetes Association (ADA). (2017). Standards of medical care in diabetes—2017. *Diabetes Care, 40*(Suppl 1), S11–S66. Retrieved http://professional.diabetes.org/sites/professional.diabetes.org/files/media/dc_40_s1_final.pdf

Austin, M. M. (2013). The two skill sets of self-monitoring of blood glucose education: The operational and the interpretive. *Diabetes Spectrum, 26*(2), 83–90.

Baxter, A. L., Ewing, P. H., Young, G. B., Ware, A., Evans, N., & Manworren, R. C. (2013). EMLA application exceeding two hours improves pediatric emergency department venipuncture success. *Advanced Emergency Nursing Journal, 35*(1), 67–75.

Bechtold, M. L., Ashraf, I., & Nguyen, D. L. (2016). A clinician's guide to fecal occult blood testing for colorectal cancer. *Southern Medical Journal, 109*(4), 248–255.

Beckman Coulter. (n.d.). *Patient education and sample collection videos.* Retrieved https://www.beckmancoulter.com/wsrportal/wsr/support/training-education/patient-education-and-sample-collection-videos/index.htm

Beckman Coulter. (2013a). *Hemoccult^{BRAND}ICT: Fecal immunochemical test (FIT).* Retrieved https://www.beckmancoulter.com/wsrportal/bibliography?docname=IB-17781A+Laminated+Hemoccult+ICT+Test+Procedure.pdf

Beckman Coulter. (2013b). *Hemoccult^{BRAND}: Fecal occult blood tests. Interpreting the Hemoccult and Hemoccult SENSA tests.* Retrieved https://www.beckmancoulter.com/wsrportal/bibliography?docname=FL-16681B%20Interpreting%20the%20Hemoccult%20and%20Hemoccult%20SENSA%20Tests.pdf

Centers for Disease Control and Prevention (CDC). (n.d.). *Influenza specimen collection.* Retrieved https://www.cdc.gov/flu/pdf/freeresources/healthcare/flu-specimen-collection-guide.pdf

Centers for Disease Control and Prevention (CDC). (2011). *Healthcare-associated infections (HAIs). Staphylococcus aureus in healthcare settings.* Retrieved https://www.cdc.gov/HAI/organisms/staph.html

Centers for Disease Control and Prevention (CDC). (2013a). *Colorectal (colon) cancer. Colorectal cancer screening tests.* Retrieved http://www.cdc.gov/cancer/colorectal/basic_info/screening/guidelines.htm

Centers for Disease Control and Prevention (CDC). (2013b). *Chapter 4: Diagnosis of tuberculosis disease.* Retrieved https://www.cdc.gov/tb/education/corecurr/pdf/chapter4.pdf

Centers for Disease Control and Prevention (CDC). (2015). *Pertussis (whooping cough). Specimen collection. Pertussis testing video: Collecting a nasopharyngeal swab clinical specimen.* Retrieved https://www.cdc.gov/pertussis/clinical/diagnostic-testing/specimen-collection.html

Centers for Disease Control and Prevention (CDC). (2016). *Methicillin-resistant Staphylococcus aureus (MRSA): Precautions to prevent spread of MRSA.* Retrieved https://www.cdc.gov/mrsa/healthcare/clinicians/precautions.html

Cheek, J. A., Craig, S. S., Seith, R. W., & West, A. (2015). Urine collection in young children. *Emergency Medicine Australasia, 27*(4), 348–350.

Cohen, B. J., & Hull, K. L. (2015). *Memmler's structure and function of the human body* (11th ed.). Philadelphia: Wolters Kluwer.

da Silva, J. R., Pizzoli, L. M., Amorim, A. R., et al. (2016). Using therapeutic toys to facilitate venipuncture procedure in preschool children. *Pediatric Nursing, 42*(2), 61–68.

Denno, J., & Gannon, M. (2013). Practical steps to lower blood culture contamination rates in the emergency department. *Journal of Emergency Nursing, 39*(5), 459–464.

Doenges, M. E., Moorhouse, M. F., & Murr, A. C. (2016). *Nursing diagnoses manual: Planning, individualizing, and documenting client care* (5th ed.). Philadelphia, PA: F.A. Davis Company.

Dolan, V. J., & Cornish, N. E. (2013). Urine specimen collection: How a multidisciplinary team improved patient outcomes using best practice. *Urologic Nursing, 33*(5), 249–256.

Doubeni, C. (2015). UpToDate®. *Tests for screening for colorectal cancer: Stool tests, radiologic imaging and endoscopy.* Wolters Kluwer. Retrieved http://www.uptodate.com/contents/tests-for-screening-for-colorectal-cancer-stool-tests-radiologic-imaging-and-endoscopy?source=machineLearning&search=barium±enema&selectedTitle=1~79&sectionRank=1&anchor=H9#H9

Downie, P. (2013). Practical aspects of capillary blood glucose monitoring: A simple guide for primary care. *Diabetes & Primary Care, 15*(3), 149–153.

Eliopoulos, C. (2018). *Gerontological nursing* (9th ed.). Philadelphia, PA: Wolters Kluwer.

Fischbach, F. T., & Dunning III, M. B. (2015). *A manual of laboratory and diagnostic tests* (9th ed.). Philadelphia, PA: Wolters Kluwer Health.

Grossman, S., & Porth, C. M. (2014). *Porth's pathophysiology: Concepts of altered health states* (9th ed.). Philadelphia, PA: Wolters Kluwer Health.

Hess, D. R., MacIntyre, N. R., Galvin, W. F., & Mishoe, S. C. (2016). *Respiratory care. Principles and practice* (3rd ed.). Sudbury, MA: Jones & Bartlett Learning.

Hinkle, J. L., & Cheever, K. H. (2018). *Brunner & Suddarth's textbook of medical-surgical nursing* (14th ed.). Philadelphia, PA: Wolters Kluwer.

Hogan-Quigley, B., Palm, M. L., & Bickley, L. (2017). *Bates' nursing guide to physical examination and history taking* (2nd ed.). Philadelphia, PA: Wolters Kluwer.

Holt, P. (2014). Blood glucose monitoring in diabetes. *Nursing Standard, 28*(27), 52–58.

Infusion Nurses Society (INS). (2016a). *Policies and procedures for infusion therapy* (5th ed.). Norwood, MA: Author.

Infusion Nurses Society (INS). (2016b). Infusion therapy. Standards of practice. *Journal of Infusion Nursing, 39*(Suppl 1), S1–S159.

Jarvis, C. (2016). *Physical examination and health assessment* (7th ed.). St. Louis, MO: Elsevier.

Jensen, S. (2015). *Nursing health assessment: A best practice approach* (2nd ed.). Philadelphia, PA: Wolters Kluwer.

The Joint Commission. (2017). *National patient safety goals®.* Retrieved https://www.jointcommission.org/standards_information/npsgs.aspx

Jones, K., Sibai, J., Battjes, R., & Fakih, M. G. (2016). How and when nurses collect urine cultures on catheterized patients: A survey of 5 hospitals. *American Journal of Infection Control, 44*(2), 173–176.

Kearl, Y. L., Yanger, S., Montero, S., Morelos-Howard, E., & Claudius, I. (2015). Does combined use of the J-tip® and Buzzy® device decrease the pain of venipuncture in a pediatric population? *Journal of Pediatric Nursing, 30*(6), 829–833.

Kessenich, C. R., & Cronin, K. (2013). Fecal occult blood testing in older adult patients with anemia. *The Nurse Practitioner, 38*(1), 6–8.

Knapp, R. (Clinical Editor). (2016). *Hemodynamic monitoring made incredibly visual* (3rd ed.). Philadelphia, PA: Wolters Kluwer.

Kyle, T., & Carman, S. (2017). *Essentials of pediatric nursing* (3rd ed.). Philadelphia, PA: Wolters Kluwer.

Laboratory Alliance of Central New York, LLC. (2017). *Collection and inoculation of blood specimens for routine culture (Bacterial, T.B. or fungus).* Retrieved http://laboratoryalliance.com/healthcare-providers/laboratory-services/specimen-collection-documents/collection-and-inoculation-of-blood-specimens-for-routine-culture-bacterial-t-b-or-fungus

LeFever Kee, J. (2017). *Pearson handbook of laboratory and diagnostic tests with nursing implications* (8th ed.). Boston, MA: Pearson.

LeMone, P., Burke, K. M., Bauldoff, G., & Gubrud, P. (2015). *Medical-surgical nursing: Clinical reasoning in patient care* (6th ed.). New York: Pearson.

Liesenfeld, O., Lehman, L., Hunfeld, K. P., & Kost, G. (2014). Molecular diagnosis of sepsis: New aspects and recent developments. *European Journal of Microbiology & Immunology, 4*(1), 1–25. Retrieved https://www.ncbi.nlm.nih.gov/pmc/articles/PMC3955828

Lopez, O., Subramanian, P., Rahmat, N., Theam, L. C., Chinna, K., & Rosli, R. (2015). The effect of facilitated tucking on procedural pain control among premature babies. *Journal of Clinical Nursing, 24*(1–2), 183–191.

Mace, S. E. (2016). Prospective, randomized, double-blind controlled trial comparing vapocoolant spray vs placebo spray in adults undergoing venipuncture. *American Journal of Emergency Medicine, 34*(5), 798–804.

Mahoney, M., Baxter, K., Burgess, J., et al. (2013). Procedure for obtaining a urine sample from a urostomy, ileal conduit, and colon conduit. A best practice guideline for clinicians. *Journal of Wound, Ostomy and Continence Nursing, 40*(3), 277–279.

Malarkey, L. M., & McMorrow, M. E. (2012). *Saunders nursing guide to laboratory and diagnostic tests* (2nd ed.). St. Louis, MO: Elsevier Saunders.

Mariani, H. S., Layden, B. T., & Aleppo, G. (2017). Continuous glucose monitoring: A perspective on its past, present, and future applications for diabetes management. *Clinical Diabetes, 35*(1), 60–65.

Marini, M. A., & Truog, A. W. (2013). Reducing false-positive peripheral blood cultures in a pediatric emergency department. *Journal of Emergency Nursing, 39*(5), 440–446.

McGoldrick, M. (2015). Urine specimen collection and transport. *Home Healthcare Now, 33*(5), 284–285.

Moore, N. (2016). Rapid point-of-care assays for influenza testing. *MLO: Medical Laboratory Observer, 48*(11), 18–20.

Morton, P. G., & Fontaine, D. K. (2018). *Critical care nursing: A holistic approach* (11th ed.). Philadelphia, PA: Wolters Kluwer.

Mutlu, B., & Balcı, S. (2015). Effects of balloon inflation and cough trick methods on easing pain in children during the drawing of venous blood samples: A randomized controlled trial. *Journal for Specialists in Pediatric Nursing, 20*(3), 178–186.

NANDA International, Inc.: *Nursing diagnoses—Definitions and classification 2018–2020* © 2017 NANDA International, ISBN 978-1-62623-929-6. Used by arrangement with the Thieme Group, Stuttgart/New York.

National Institute of Diabetes and Digestive and Kidney Diseases (NIDDK). (n.d.). *Continuous glucose monitoring.* Retrieved https://www.niddk.nih.gov/health-information/diabetes/overview/managing-diabetes/continuous-glucose-monitoring

National Institute of Diabetes and Digestive and Kidney Diseases (NIDDK). (2016). *Diabetes tests & diagnosis.* Retrieved https://www.niddk.nih.gov/health-information/diabetes/overview/tests-diagnosis

Novotne, T. A., & Kaseb, H. O. (2013). The changing face of *Clostridium difficile* in critical care. *Nursing2013 Critical Care, 8*(3), 26–34.

Perry, S. E., Hockenberry, M. J., Lowdermilk, D. L., & Wilson, D. (2014). *Maternal child nursing care* (5th ed.). St. Louis, MO: Elsevier.

Reyhani, T., Aemmi, S. Z., Mohebbi, T., & Boskabadi, H. (2014). The effect of facilitated tucking (FT) during venipuncture on duration of crying in preterm infants. *International Journal of Pediatrics, 2*(4-3), 431–435.

Septimus, E. (2015). *Clinician guide for collecting cultures.* Centers for Disease Control and Prevention (CDC). Retrieved https://www.cdc.gov/getsmart/healthcare/implementation/clinicianguide.html

Sethi, R., & Nayak, G. (2015). Effect of 24% oral sucrose in pain reduction during venipuncture in neonates. *Asian Journal of Nursing Education and Research, 5*(4), 457–460.

Society of Urologic Nurses and Associates (SUNA). (2010). *Clinical practice guidelines: Prevention & control of catheter-associated urinary tract infection (CAUTI). [Brochure].* Pitman, NJ: Author.

Society of Urologic Nurses and Associates (SUNA). (2015). *Clinical practice guidelines: Care of the patient with an indwelling catheter. [Brochure].* Pitman, NJ: Author.

Taylor, C., Lynn, P., & Bartlett, J. (2019). *Fundamentals of nursing: The art and science of person-centered care* (9th ed.). Philadelphia, PA: Wolters Kluwer.

U.S. Food & Drug Administration (FDA). (2016). *Blood glucose monitoring devices.* Retrieved https://www.fda.gov/%20medicaldevices/productsandmedicalprocedures/invitrodiagnostics/glucosetestingdevices/default.htm

U.S. National Library of Medicine, National Institutes of Health, MedlinePlus. (2017). *Nasopharyngeal culture.* Retrieved https://medlineplus.gov/ency/article/003747.htm

U.S. Preventive Services Task Force. (2016). *Final recommendation statement. Colorectal cancer: Screening.* Retrieved https://www.uspreventiveservicestaskforce.org/Page/Document/RecommendationStatementFinal/colorectal-cancer-screening2#tab

Uzelli, D., & Güneş, Ü. Y. (2015). Oral glucose solution to alleviate pain induced by intramuscular injections in preterm infants. *Journal for Specialists in Pediatric Nursing, 20*(1), 29–35.

Van Leeuwen, A. M., & Bladh, M. L. (2017). *Davis's comprehensive handbook of laboratory & diagnostic tests with nursing implications* (7th ed.). Philadelphia, PA: F.A. Davis Company.

VHA Center for Engineering & Occupational Safety and Health (CEOSH). (2016). *Safe patient handling and mobility guidebook.* St. Louis, MO: Author. Retrieved http://www.tampavaref.org/safe-patient-handling.htm

Wallymahmed, M. (2013). Encouraging people with diabetes to get the most from blood glucose monitoring: Observing and acting upon blood glucose patterns. *Journal of Diabetes Nursing, 17*(1), 6–13.

Washer, L. L., Chenoweth, C., Kim, H. W., et al. (2013). Blood culture contamination: A randomized trial evaluating the comparative effectiveness of 3 skin antiseptic interventions. *Infection Control and Hospital Epidemiology, 34*(1), 15–21.

Williams, J. (2012). Stoma care: Obtaining a urine specimen from a urostomy. *Gastrointestinal Nursing, 10*(5), 11–12.

World Health Organization (WHO). (2010). *WHO guidelines on drawing blood: Best practices in phlebotomy.* Geneva, Switzerland: Author. Retrieved http://www.euro.who.int/__data/assets/pdf_file/0005/268790/WHO-guidelines-on-drawing-blood-best-practices-in-phlebotomy-Eng.pdf?ua-1

SUGGESTED ANSWERS FOR FOCUSING ON PATIENT CARE: DEVELOPING CLINICAL REASONING

1. Obtaining a urine specimen is a priority in Mr. Conklin's care. Results will help determine the underlying cause of his symptoms and direct treatment. As a result, you will have to take a more involved role in the collection. You will have to obtain the specimen. Continue to reinforce the need for the urine specimen. Gather the necessary supplies and place them in the patient's room or bathroom. Plan to obtain the specimen the next time Mr. Conklin has to void. Share the plan with other caregivers. When the patient communicates his need to void, put on nonsterile gloves. Assist him to the bathroom. Explain again the need and rationale for the urine specimen. Explain that you are going to clean his penis to get the specimen. Clean his penis according to the guidelines in the procedure. Ask Mr. Conklin to void into the toilet; be ready to place the specimen cup in the stream of urine to obtain a sample. Put the lid on the specimen container. After assisting the patient with the rest of his toileting needs, clean the outside of the container, if urine contacted the outside during sampling. Label the sample and transport it to the laboratory.

2. Explain the reason for the test and the procedure for stool collection. Ask about any hematuria, bleeding hemorrhoids, or recent nose or throat bleeding. These situations would require the test to be postponed. Question Ms. Yon regarding medications she uses, including certain medications, such as a salicylate intake of more than 325 mg daily, steroids, iron preparations, and anticoagulants, that may lead to false-positive readings, and use of vitamin C, as this may lead to false-negative results. Ask about the use of laxatives, enemas, or suppositories for 3 days before testing. Ms. Yon should understand that she should collect the specimen the morning of her appointment and know how to handle the specimen once she has obtained it.

3. Assess Mrs. Yeletsky's knowledge regarding her understanding of what diabetes is, its effects on the body, possible complications, dietary guidelines, medications she is prescribed to treat her diabetes, activity level/habits, and personal hygiene, particularly foot care. You should incorporate education regarding diabetes, including simple explanations of the definition of diabetes, normal blood glucose ranges, effect of insulin and exercise, effect of food and stress, and basic treatment approaches. A referral to the diabetic clinical specialist, if available, would be appropriate, as well as a referral for outpatient follow-up. Review her understanding of blood glucose monitoring and the use of the blood glucose monitor. Investigate alternate blood glucose monitors; models are available to aid people with impaired vision. Explore the support she has available and the possibility of a significant other assisting with her diabetes management, if appropriate.

Integrated Case Studies

UNIT III

These case studies are designed to focus on integrating concepts. They are not meant to be all-inclusive. The critical thinking questions should guide your discussions of related issues. The discussion within the integrated nursing care section represents possible nursing care solutions to problems; you may find other solutions that are equally acceptable.

Basic Case Studies

Case Study

Abigail Cantonelli

Abigail Cantonelli, age 80, injured her left knee and wrist when she fell on an icy sidewalk. She has been on your orthopedic and neurologic unit for several days. She has a history of cardiomyopathy, for which she receives furosemide. Her vital signs are stable and she rates her pain as aching, intermittent, and a 2 on a scale of 1 to 10 (10 = worst pain). Because Mrs. Cantonelli has an increased risk of falling, her health care provider has ordered physical therapy and cane-walking instructions before discharge. Although the physical therapy staff has already initiated the cane-walking instructions, you will need to ambulate Mrs. Cantonelli with her cane during your shift. While you are ambulating down the hall, she says, "Oh, dear! I feel dizzy." She begins to lose her balance and begins to fall toward you.

Prescribed Interventions

Physical therapy for cane-walking instruction
Ambulate every shift with cane assistance
Furosemide 20 mg PO every morning

Potassium chloride 10 mEq PO every day
Naprosyn 275 mg PO q6–8h prn pain

Developing Clinical Reasoning

- Identify Mrs. Cantonelli's risk factors for falling.

- Considering these risk factors, what special assessments and precautions should you implement before assisting her to ambulate or while assisting her with ambulation?

- Describe the actions you would implement when Mrs. Cantonelli begins to fall.

continued

Abigail Cantonelli (continued)

Suggested Responses for Integrated Nursing Care

- Falls are the leading cause of unintentional injury death in people aged 65 and over (National Center for Health Statistics, 2015). Because of Mrs. Cantonelli's age, history of falls, and impaired mobility, she continues to be at risk for falls. Her weakness and pain from her injuries also contribute to this risk. In addition, she is taking furosemide, which is a diuretic. This medication contributes to an increased risk for falling and subsequent injury (Taylor et al., 2019). Implement fall prevention interventions (Refer to Chapter 4).

- Before ambulating Mrs. Cantonelli, it is a good idea to implement several assessments and precautions to prevent orthostatic hypotension. Have her sit on the side of the bed for a few minutes and make sure she does not feel dizzy, weak, or lightheaded (refer to Chapter 9). Because she has a history of cardiomyopathy, assess for shortness of breath and chest pain. If she cannot tolerate sitting up on the side of the bed without having these symptoms, then she will not tolerate standing up or ambulating. Assess her pain level immediately before ambulation. If you have to medicate her for pain, then wait until the pain medicine has had time to take effect before ambulating. Because she is weaker on her left side, assess strength on her right side to ensure she will be able to support her weight with the cane (refer to Chapter 9).

- If she has difficulty maintaining her balance, apply a safety belt (gait belt) before she begins to ambulate with the cane (some institutions require the use of a safety belt).

- While Mrs. Cantonelli is ambulating with her cane, observe her closely. Assess her technique with the cane. Observe for symptoms such as dizziness, chest pain, and shortness of breath. As she continues ambulating, evaluate how she tolerates this activity. Before she is discharged from the hospital, assess her self-confidence as well as her overall ability to use the cane.

- If Mrs. Cantonelli begins to fall, it is important to protect her while also protecting yourself. If you feel her start to fall, maintain a wide base of support, grasp the safety belt firmly, and place her weight against your body. You can then gently and slowly guide her down toward the floor (refer to Chapter 9). Assess her orientation and stay with her while waiting for help from another health care provider. Take her vital signs to determine if there is a change from baseline. Thoroughly explore other factors that may have contributed to her fall, and plan interventions that will prevent future falls. If Mrs. Cantonelli continues to have problems with falling or difficulty using the cane, consider having her use a walker.

Case Study

Tiffany Jones

Tiffany Jones, age 17, is scheduled to undergo an ovarian cyst biopsy under local anesthesia. She has been NPO since midnight. Her ID bracelet is on and her consent form is signed. Her mother is in the waiting room. You are to provide Tiffany's immediate preoperative care. You place an IV in her left hand without difficulty. The next procedure is to insert an indwelling urinary (Foley) catheter. You set up the sterile field between her legs. As you clean the urinary meatus, Tiffany keeps drawing her legs closer together. When you remind her, she opens her legs and says, "Sorry, I didn't mean to move." As you insert the catheter into the urethra, Tiffany is startled and slams her knees together. When she opens her knees, the catheter appears to be inserted, but no urine is flowing.

Prescribed Interventions

Intravenous fluids: D5 ½ NSS at 50 mL/hr

Foley catheter to straight drainage

continued

Developing Clinical Reasoning

- Where might the urinary catheter be positioned, and should you advance the catheter further?

- Identify issues of concern to patients before surgery.

- How do you determine whether the catheter and the sterile field are still sterile?

- Describe methods of responding to Tiffany's nervousness.

- How could you have set up a more stable sterile field?

Suggested Responses for Integrated Nursing Care

- The female urethra is short, only about 1.5 to 2.5 in long. If the catheter is advanced that far and no urine is flowing, the catheter may be in the vagina. Do not remove the catheter; it will serve as a guide to locate the urethral opening, which is just above the vagina (refer to Chapter 12). You would not advance the catheter further even if it were in the urethra, because when Tiffany closed her legs, the catheter probably came into contact with her skin and is no longer sterile. Advancing a nonsterile catheter into the urethra would increase her risk for developing a urinary tract infection. Because you are not certain whether her legs touched the sterile field, the sterile field is also no longer considered sterile (refer to Chapters 1 and 12).

- You will need to obtain another complete catheter insertion kit. Cover Tiffany and verify that she understands your plans. As you set up the new kit, place it on the bedside table, not between her legs, to prevent accidental contamination (refer to Chapter 12).

- Teenagers are generally uncomfortable with urinary catheterization because in this procedure, the nurse must look at and touch a very private area. Such an invasion of privacy is traumatic at an age when girls are easily embarrassed. Teenage girls may have "nervous legs": As you touch their inner thighs or labia, the knees slam shut almost involuntarily. Have a second nurse or a relative attend to the teenager. The nurse or relative can distract and soothe the teen, minimizing the unpleasantness of the experience, and can also keep a "reminder" hand on Tiffany's open knee to help you maintain sterility.

- As with most preoperative patients, Tiffany has several reasons to feel nervous. She is facing surgery, an unknown and anxiety-producing experience. The preoperative procedures, such as IV insertion and urinary catheterization, are unpleasant and uncomfortable. You can implement several strategies to reduce preoperative patients' anxiety. Have a familiar person stay with the patient. Tell the patient your name. Clearly explain procedures and provide instructions to the patient before you begin. Instructions should include the rationale and the length of time the procedure will take. For urinary catheterization, the patient may also want to know how long he or she will have the catheter in place. Emphasize to the patient that it is all right to ask questions. Describe how the procedure will feel to the patient—for example, "when I clean you, it will feel cold and wet." Keep your voice calm and very matter-of-fact throughout the procedure (refer to Chapters 6 and 12).

Case Study

James White

James White, a patient with an exacerbation of chronic obstructive pulmonary disease (COPD), is on your medical-surgical unit. You need to obtain his vital signs and give him a bath. His vital signs at 0800 were as follows: temperature, 98.4°F; pulse, 86 beats/min and regular; respirations, 18 breaths/min; blood pressure, 130/68 mm Hg. The physical therapist who is working with this patient on conditioning therapy has just brought him back from his exercises. You notice that his breathing is labored, with audible expiratory wheezes. While you are obtaining his oral temperature and vital signs, you continue to hear audible expiratory wheezing. His vital signs now are as follows: temperature, 96.8°F; pulse, 106 beats/min and irregular; respirations, 26 breaths/min; blood pressure, 140/74 mm Hg.

Prescribed Interventions

Daily physical therapy for conditioning

Oxygen at 2 L via nasal prongs prn for pulse oximetry <90%

Vital signs q4h

Oxygen saturation levels via pulse oximeter every shift and prn

Developing Clinical Reasoning

- Did you take the second set of vital signs at the most appropriate time? Why or why not?

- Describe the timing and type of bath you think Mr. White requires and the degree of assistance he will need. Explain your rationale.

- How has Mr. White's physical activity affected the accuracy of his vital signs?

- What would be your course of action in response to his labored breathing?

Suggested Responses for Integrated Nursing Care

- Always compare vital signs with the baseline before making further clinical decisions (refer to Chapter 2). As you compare the previous vital signs with the ones you just obtained, you notice that Mr. White's pulse rate, respiratory rate, and blood pressure are elevated. Your assessment of his pulse also indicates that his pulse is now irregular. Mr. White has just experienced a significant increase in activity; waiting until he has recovered from the exertion would be more appropriate in order to obtain a resting set of vital signs.

- What does the very low temperature indicate? Remember, you continued to hear Mr. White's heavy breathing while obtaining the remainder of the vital signs. Mr. White could not keep his lips pursed in a seal around the thermometer, and this often gives an inaccurate temperature. Mouth breathing and respiratory distress are contra-indications for obtaining an oral temperature. As a nurse, you are responsible for determining the most appropriate site to obtain the temperature (refer to Skill 2-1).

continued

- Does Mr. White's elevated respiratory rate and noisy breathing indicate respiratory distress or a need for oxygen? Obtain an oxygen saturation level via pulse oximetry. If the oxygen saturation level is satisfactory for Mr. White, then you can be confident his body is compensating for the increased oxygen demand. Allow him to rest, with the head of his bed elevated, and retake his vital signs in 15 to 30 minutes. Take vital signs as often as the patient's condition warrants. If Mr. White's oxygen saturation and vital signs continue to deviate from baseline after a rest period, notify the health care provider (refer to Chapter 2).

- A bath represents another increase in activity. Mr. White needs time to recover from the physical therapy exercises before attempting the bath. He should be able to sit in a chair and, in fact, will breathe more comfortably sitting up than lying down. Having him lie flat could make him decompensate (deterioration in respiratory function), so you should not perform occupied bed-making. If encouraged to sit up, he will probably be able to complete much of his bath by himself.

Case Study

Naomi Bell

Naomi Bell, age 90, was admitted to the hospital yesterday after experiencing chest pain. She wears a hearing aid in her left ear. In the report you were told that she is "confused" and "doesn't answer questions appropriately." Her vital signs overnight were as follows: temperature, 98.0°F; pulse, 62 beats/min; respirations, 18 breaths/min; blood pressure, 132/86 mm Hg. She is due for her morning medications. As you give Mrs. Bell her medications and state their purpose, she points to the digoxin and says, "Honey, I don't take that pill."

Prescribed Interventions

Digoxin 0.125 mg PO every morning
Enteric-coated aspirin 81 mg PO every day
Furosemide 20 mg PO every morning

Famotidine 20 mg PO BID
Potassium chloride 10 mEq PO every morning
Captopril 50 mg PO TID

Developing Clinical Reasoning

- How would you respond to Mrs. Bell's statement, "Honey, I don't take that pill"?

- Describe factors that can contribute to inappropriate answers, and identify nursing actions to diminish these factors.

- Suggest ways in which you can confirm you are giving Mrs. Bell the correct medications.

- How would you determine Mrs. Bell's level of confusion, if any?

- Identify the medications that require assessment before administration.

continued

Naomi Bell (continued)

Suggested Responses for Integrated Nursing Care

- When patients question you regarding their medications, listen to them. Questions like this should send a "red flag" to the nurse. Often, patients are familiar with what they normally take and can alert you that this may not be the right medication. Do not insist that Mrs. Bell take the digoxin until you confirm the accuracy of the order. In this case, it could be that Mrs. Bell just did not hear what you said. Always confirm what patients say to you by restating it back to them. It could also be that she is more familiar with the trade name for this drug or the medication may look different from the medication she uses at home.

- You should use multiple safety checks to give medications safely. Some measures include researching the drug before administration and double-checking all of the "rights." Compare the Medication Administration Record with the original order in the medical record. If the order still remains unclear to you, call the prescriber to clarify it (refer to Chapter 5).

- Some medications require assessment before you administer them to the patient. In this case, Mrs. Bell takes four medications that will require assessment before administration. Digoxin, furosemide, and captopril will affect pulse and blood pressure. In addition, laboratory test results should be available on potassium and digoxin levels. If Mrs. Bell has a low pulse rate, low blood pressure, or a toxic laboratory value, you will not administer these medications and will notify the health care provider (refer to Chapter 5).

- Sometimes, older patients become confused in unfamiliar settings—in this case—the hospital. However, do not assume this is always the case. The nurse who gave you the report may have assumed that Mrs. Bell's inappropriate answers were due to confusion, when in fact they may be related to Mrs. Bell's hearing problem. When patients with a hearing impairment are in an unfamiliar setting, such as a hospital admission, encourage them to wear their hearing aids and help them check their batteries to ensure they are working. If you are still unclear whether Mrs. Bell is confused, perform a standard mental status examination used by your institution (refer to Chapter 3). This will establish a baseline assessment of her mental status that you can use to individualize her nursing care plan.

- If you determine Mrs. Bell is confused, assess the source of confusion. Given Mrs. Bell's cardiac condition, assess her respiratory status and oxygen saturation level via pulse oximetry to determine whether she is experiencing hypoxia or ischemia. If the cause is physiologic, notify the health care provider immediately. Another source contributing to confusion could be isolation caused by hearing loss. One way to reduce possible confusion for Mrs. Bell is to improve communication. Ensure that her hearing aid battery is operating and that the unit is placed correctly. Other ways to improve communication include talking to her at eye level, facing her directly when speaking, or even speaking into her unaffected ear. If Mrs. Bell's vision is better than her hearing, you can also give her pertinent information in writing.

Case Study

John Willis

You are a nursing student in your first semester of nursing school. Your assigned patient has been discharged before your arrival. Your instructor provides you with the name of another patient to care for, based on the recommendation of the staff. Before you can review the information about the patient with your instructor, she is called to consult with another student and a physician about an emergent patient situation. You read the clinical pathway for John Willis and find that he has methicillin-resistant *Staphylococcus aureus* (MRSA) in his sputum and suspected pulmonary tuberculosis (TB). You remember reviewing these topics in class

continued

and in the learning resource center. Because your instructor is still occupied with the patient emergency, you decide to begin caring for your new patient, instead of wasting time waiting to review the information with her. When you go to your patient's room, you see the isolation cart containing the transmission-based precaution supplies outside the room, with the hospital's policy and procedure posted for precautions to use for TB and MRSA. You see there are individual masks in plastic bags with different people's names on them, as well as masks with protective eye shields. You recall something from class about wearing a specially fitted mask when implementing these precautions, but realize you do not remember as much as you thought you did. You are unsure of exactly what you need to do. You find the staff nurse assigned to the patient in another patient's room, interrupt his conversation, and say, "I don't have a mask to care for my patient." The nurse sharply responds, "Just go get started. I'm in the middle of something." You consider just going in and introducing yourself and checking on the patient's status. Should you "borrow" a mask from one of the bags? You think it is your duty to care for this patient, but think you may need more information to be safe.

Prescribed Interventions

Airborne precautions

Contact precautions

Sputum specimen for culture and sensitivity and acid-fast bacillus (AFB)

Vital signs every shift

Developing Clinical Reasoning

- Compare the mode of transmission for TB and MRSA.

- Describe another way in which you could have approached this situation.

- What may have led to the nurse's abrupt and sharp response?

- What are potential consequences of a lack of use of appropriate transmission-based precautions?

- Identify the appropriate protective equipment needed to care for a patient with TB and a patient with MRSA.

continued

John Willis (continued)

Suggested Responses for Integrated Nursing Care

- Pulmonary TB transmission occurs through the air from one person to another. MRSA transmission can occur through direct contact with contaminated blood or body fluids. MRSA can be spread by direct or indirect contact. In this case, MRSA could be transmitted indirectly by coming into contact with items used to care for the patient, such as blood pressure cuffs or linen, or contact with contaminated surfaces in the room.

- Facilities require the use of appropriate personal protective equipment (PPE), including gowns, gloves, and masks, when caring for patients with TB and MRSA. Unique to the Airborne Precautions needed for TB is the use of specially fitted masks, either a high-efficiency particulate air (HEPA) filter respirator or N95 respirator mask certified by NIOSH to prevent the inspiration of airborne microorganisms (refer to Chapter 1). N95 respirators require fit-testing to ensure the mask is on correctly and adjusted to fit properly. If a fit-tested mask is required by your facility, you would either need to be fit-tested for a mask (often done by Employee Health) or reassigned to another patient. In addition, to protect yourself whenever there is the potential for contamination to your eyes, such as coughing, you should wear goggles or a mask with a face shield. Institutions vary greatly in their supplies. If you do not take the appropriate transmission-based precautions, you put yourself at risk for exposure to disease; in this case, TB and MRSA. In addition, entering other patients' rooms results in the potential for transmission of microorganisms and infection. It is always your responsibility, even as a student, to follow the policies and procedures of the facility where you are placed for clinical experiences.

- Hospitals are stressful places. Understanding when and how to communicate with others is an invaluable set of skills. Waiting for the nurse to complete a conversation and task before asking for guidance would have been the ideal situation. Nurses have to prioritize the care they provide. Asking, "Do you have a moment to review something with me?" is a good way to ensure getting the time and attention you need. Because there was no emergency to obtain the vital signs and sputum specimen, they can wait until you are sure you can provide safe care.

- You were right to question the appropriateness of caring for this patient and in thinking you may need more information to be safe. In this situation, waiting to review the patient information with your instructor is the ideal solution. Your instructor did not have all the information about the patient before being called away to an emergency. She would not have assigned this patient to you after reviewing his diagnosis, realizing that you would need a specially fitted mask to care for the patient. While waiting for your instructor, you should obtain as much information as possible. Background research and knowledge are powerful tools. Examples of resources you can access include the hospital policies and procedure files, the infection control manual, the infection control nurse, and experienced staff members, provided they are able to take time out from their patient care responsibilities. Then, when your instructor is available, you can share this information with him or her to plan your care for that day.

Case Study

Claudia Tran

Claudia Tran, age 84, has been on your skilled nursing unit following a cerebral vascular accident (CVA). Her neurologic checks and vital signs are unchanged from her baseline admission. Her CVA has impaired her ability to chew and swallow and she is receiving weekly vitamin B_{12} injections for pernicious anemia. She has left-sided weakness, with flaccidity of her left hand. Ms. Tran is emaciated and her skin is very fragile. She has reddened areas on her coccyx, heels, left hip, and elbows. Over the past week, Ms. Tran has become increasingly confused and incontinent. She has a gastric tube for

continued

feedings, which she receives every 8 hours. Ms. Tran constantly pulls at her feeding tube and has had to have it reinserted today after pulling it out. Because of this, a soft wrist restraint has been ordered for the next four hours. You check the gastric residual prior to administering the gastric tube feeding and it is 380 mL.

Prescribed Interventions

Soft wrist restraint for safety for the next 4 hours (end 1330), then reevaluate

Vitamin B_{12} injection 1,000 mcg IM weekly

Gastric tube feedings—FiberSOURCE HN 320 mL q8h

Hold feeding for gastric residual ≥200 mL and notify health care provider

Physical therapy daily, passive and active range of motion (ROM) as tolerated

Developing Clinical Reasoning

- Considering Ms. Tran's condition, what special safety measures should be implemented related to the use of the wrist restraint?

- What are the risks of falling for this patient?

- Identify the risks associated with gastric tube feeding for this patient.

- Identify risk factors and preventive measures to maintain the integrity of Ms. Tran's skin.

- Identify appropriate sites and administration considerations related to the vitamin B_{12} injections prescribed for Ms. Tran.

Suggested Responses for Integrated Nursing Care

- Restraints are used only as a last resort after all other measures have failed. Implement alternatives to the use of restraints (refer to Chapter 4). Other measures could include placing her bed in a low position, having a family member sit with her, and placing her in a room near the nurses' station. Only use restraints with an order from the health care provider, and follow facility guidelines to protect the patient. Because Ms. Tran already has skin breakdown, pad the restraints and make sure they are the correct size. An additional safety measure would be performing frequent neurovascular checks to the extremity, including checking warmth, sensation, and capillary refill. Restraints are released at specified frequencies. This will improve the circulation to her extremities, reduce the chance of skin breakdown, and give you an opportunity to assess the site. Ms. Tran has left-sided weakness; therefore, applying a restraint on her flaccid arm could cause harm and is not needed (refer to Chapter 4).

- Ms. Tran has many factors that increase her risk for alterations in skin integrity, including decreased mobility, malnutrition, altered mental status, advanced age, incontinence, and positioning for tube feedings. A multifaceted approach is necessary to reduce

her risk and prevent further alterations in her skin integrity (refer to Chapter 8). It is essential to develop a schedule for repositioning (refer to Chapter 9). Ms. Tran could benefit from a special type of mattress, such as one with a pressure-reducing surface. Implementing a physical therapy program of active and passive ROM exercises would be helpful. Arrange for a nutritional consult to ensure she will receive adequate protein, as well as other vitamins and minerals essential to maintain skin integrity.

- What complications could result from the combination of decreased mobility and incontinence? A noninvasive way to reduce the chance of recurrent incontinence is to offer Ms. Tran a bedpan at regular intervals. Frequent skin care and use of a skin protectant/barrier to prevent damage from excessive moisture is an important part of her nursing care (refer to Chapter 7).

- Because Ms. Tran is older, confused, and in a restraint, her risk for falling is high. Keep her bed in a low position at all times and make sure her call light is within reach. Frequently check on patients such as Ms. Tran to decrease isolation, provide reorientation, and assess for patient needs.

continued

Claudia Tran (continued)

- Ms. Tran is receiving tube feedings and has an excessive gastric residual. She is at increased risk for aspiration of tube feedings into her lungs if positioned supine. To decrease the risk for aspiration, check the residual amount before every feeding. Additional assessments should include auscultating for the presence of bowel sounds, abdominal distension, and abdominal tenderness. In this situation, Ms. Tran's gastric residual was greater than 200 mL. Therefore, keep her head elevated, hold her tube feeding (based on the prescribed orders), and contact her health care provider as soon as possible to confer about the appropriate course of action (refer to Chapter 11).

- When giving Ms. Tran vitamin B_{12} injections, use larger muscles and rotate sites. Implement the rotation schedule for this injection in her care plan. This is particularly important because Ms. Tran is emaciated and does not have good muscle mass. Avoid areas that are reddened or have palpable nodules and scars. Because vitamin B_{12} injections can be irritating, inject the medication using the Z-track method to minimize pain, trauma, and discomfort (refer to Chapter 5) (Taylor et al., 2019).

Case Study

Joe LeRoy

Joe LeRoy, age 60, was brought in by his daughter and admitted to your small rural hospital. He has had the stomach flu at home for several days and is suffering from dehydration. He has right-sided hemiplegia due to a cerebral vascular accident (CVA) 3 years ago. Mr. LeRoy has remained in bed during his hospital stay due to extreme weakness and fatigue.

You received the report from the previous nurses related to your five patients. From the report, you note that Mr. LeRoy continues to have frequent liquid stools (averaging about three or four times per shift). The doctor has ordered a stool sample for culture and sensitivity. When entering your patient's room, you notice his sheets are very dirty and he has a strong body odor.

Prescribed Interventions

Intravenous fluids: D5 ½ NSS at 125 mL/hr
Stool sample for culture and sensitivity

Vital signs every shift

Developing Clinical Reasoning

- Develop your priorities and rationales for the following nursing care for Mr. LeRoy:
  - Considerations when collecting the stool sample
  - Changing his sheets
  - Completing the initial nursing assessment

- Are there any assessments that you would want to pay particular attention to during your nursing care?
  - Obtaining vital signs
  - Collecting the sample
  - Giving a bath

continued

- Describe how your attitude and nonverbal behavior could affect Mr. LeRoy's hospital experience.

Suggested Responses for Integrated Nursing Care

- Prioritizing care is sometimes a difficult, but important skill for all nurses. Determine whether Mr. LeRoy can provide his own personal care, although this is unlikely due to his hemiplegia and weakness. If you need to assist him with his personal care, determine the needs of your other patients before beginning this task. Before leaving Mr. LeRoy, let him know your plan and the time he can expect to have assistance with his bath. Another alternative is to delegate the bath and changing of bed linens to nursing assistive personnel (NAP) or unlicensed assistive personnel (UAP). During your initial assessment of Mr. LeRoy, cover any very obviously dirty areas of his sheets with a blue waterproof pad or a clean sheet. You could also offer him a wet, warm washcloth and a dry towel for initial cleaning while you are completing the nursing assessment. You should also inform Mr. LeRoy of the need for a stool specimen.

- If an NAP or UAP is not available, return to his room after completing your other patient assessments. First, obtain the warm stool sample, give the bath, and then change his linens. This sequence saves time and energy for both the nurse and the patient, because the linens may become soiled when providing a bed bath or assisting a patient on a bedpan.

- While wearing gloves, collect and send the stool specimen promptly to the laboratory. Specimens should be sent while still warm, because the microorganisms present at body temperature may die when the specimen temperature changes, and this would produce a false-negative result (refer to Chapter 18).

- During your assessment, pay particular attention to Mr. LeRoy's skin. Mr. LeRoy is at risk for alterations in skin integrity and pressure injury due to his age, diarrhea, altered nutrition, and immobility. Assist Mr. LeRoy to turn over so that you can inspect his back and bony prominences, the most likely areas for alterations in skin integrity. Institute nursing interventions to prevent pressure injury. If you notice any skin breakdown, institute appropriate nursing interventions, based on facility policy, and notify the health care provider.

- A nurse's nonverbal behavior can have a dramatic impact on a patient's health care experience. Projecting a positive attitude and providing nonjudgmental care help a patient cope with hospitalization. You may be offended by Mr. LeRoy's body odor and the smell of his stool, but as a nurse you need to learn strategies to manage strong odors and make sure that your facial expressions or body language do not convey discomfort or disgust.

Case Study

Kate Townsend

Kate Townsend, a 70-year-old patient with chronic obstructive pulmonary disease (COPD), has just returned to your medical-surgical unit from surgery for repair of a bowel obstruction and lysis of intestinal adhesions. She has a midline abdominal transverse incision secured with sutures and covered with a dry sterile dressing. She has a right peripheral IV with D5 ½ NSS at 75 mL/hr. She has a history of long-term steroid use for her COPD. She has a nasogastric (NG) tube in her right naris, which is clamped at this time. The health care provider orders oxygen 2 L/min via nasal cannula. The patient's primary nurse asks you to place the patient on oxygen. When you attempt to place the cannula in the patient's naris with the NG

continued

tube, you think it is uncomfortable and a little odd. For comfort, you consider placing a simple oxygen mask on Mrs. Townsend instead. Her vital signs are as follows: temperature, 99.6°F; pulse, 76 beats/min; respirations, 24 breaths/min; blood pressure, 110/70 mm Hg; oxygen saturation (O_2 2 L/min), 92%.

Prescribed Interventions

NG tube to low intermittent suction

Cough and deep breathe/Incentive spirometry every hour while awake

Morphine sulfate 1 to 2 mg IV q4h prn pain

Oxygen 2 L/min via nasal cannula

Intravenous fluid: D5 ½ NSS at 75 mL/hr

Developing Clinical Reasoning

- What is the difference between oxygen given by nasal cannula and that given via a simple oxygen mask?

- What comfort measures would you want to provide for Mrs. Townsend?

- What do you need to consider in changing to a simple oxygen mask for delivery of the oxygen?

- Develop a discharge plan for Mrs. Townsend.

- Considering Mrs. Townsend's chronic lung disease, what complications can occur postoperatively, and what nursing interventions could decrease these complications?

Suggested Responses for Integrated Nursing Care

- Several delivery systems exist to provide oxygen to patients, and they deliver varying amounts of oxygen. Oxygen delivered via a nasal cannula set at 2 L/min would deliver about 28% oxygen, whereas oxygen delivered in a simple mask could deliver 40% to 60% oxygen, depending on the flow meter setting (refer to Chapter 14). Oxygen is considered a medicine, so it is not a nursing order but a health care provider order. The oxygen concentration and delivery system are adjusted according to orders or parameters from a physician or other advanced practice professional.

- When changing Mrs. Townsend for comfort reasons from the nasal cannula to the mask, you could increase the delivery of oxygen anywhere from 12% to 32%; a change in delivery method may have significant implications. Although it is not entirely comfortable to have an NG tube, much less another tube

in the naris, it is not unusual for this to occur. Both will fit with some manipulation by the nurse. Oxygen is considered a medicine, so it is not a nursing order but a health care provider order. The oxygen concentration and delivery systems are adjusted according to orders or parameters from a physician or other advanced practice professional.

- Patients with chronic lung disease are at increased risk after surgery for pulmonary complications, including atelectasis and pneumonia. General anesthesia alters all of the muscles involved in breathing and clearing the airway. COPD is a restrictive lung disease, meaning that the patient's lungs lose their elasticity and become less compliant. For Mrs. Townsend, this combination of underlying disease and the effects of surgery results in a decreased ability to mobilize secretions, which could lead to

continued

atelectasis and possibly pneumonia. Mrs. Townsend may be experiencing atelectasis, indicated by her temperature of 99.6°F. Other signs of atelectasis would be decreased breath sounds and/or crackles in the lung bases, shortness of breath, increased respiratory rate, and decreased oxygen saturation of pulse oximetry. Without nursing intervention, atelectasis could lead to pneumonia. Measures to facilitate lung expansion and mobilization of secretions will minimize atelectasis. These nursing measures include elevation of the head of her bed, deep-breathing and coughing exercises, incentive spirometry, adequate pain control, and early ambulation.

- Long-term steroid use can make the skin very fragile, increase the potential for alterations in skin integrity, and delay wound healing. To prevent this, observe the skin under her NG tube and oxygen cannula tubing. The pressure of the tubes on her face and behind her ears could cause a break in skin integrity. Repositioning the tape that is holding the NG tube

may make it more comfortable. You may need to protect the skin under the cannula tubing with a hydrocolloid dressing (refer to Chapter 8), especially if the skin becomes reddened. There are many commercial products to hold oxygen nasal cannulas, as well as NG tubes, which may also increase her comfort.

- Discharge plans for Mrs. Townsend would need to address both her underlying lung disease as well as her recent intestinal surgery. Patient education should focus on measures that enable Mrs. Townsend to improve her lung compliance and increase her oxygenation. Deep breathing, coughing, and a daily activity schedule are imperative. Due to her prolonged use of steroids, she may also experience delayed wound healing at her incision site. Patient education should address optimal nutrition and prevention of infection. Before discharge, validate Mrs. Townsend's knowledge of measures to prevent pulmonary and wound complications.

Case Study

Tula Stillwater

Tula Stillwater is a 36-year-old woman who has had diabetes since age 26. Ms. Stillwater weighs 218 lb, is gravida 1 para 1, and delivered a 9 lb, 6 oz boy via cesarean section 3 days ago, resulting in a transverse abdominal incision with staples. She reports tenderness on the right side of the incision, but acute pain on the left side of the incision. Her 0800 vital signs are as follows: temperature, 101.6°F; pulse, 76 beats/min; respirations, 18 breaths/min; blood pressure, 134/78 mm Hg. Her blood glucose before breakfast is 185 mg/dL; her blood glucose on previous days had ranged from 90 to 124 mg/dL.

On initial assessment, you note the dressing is intact on her incision. The staples are intact in the incision; the incision is well approximated and without erythema on the right side. However, the left side of the incision is pulling apart and is edematous and warm to the touch, with a scant amount of purulent drainage.

Prescribed Interventions

Vital signs q4h
Fingerstick blood glucose before meals and at bedtime
Regular insulin per sliding scale

Standing orders:
- Remove staples before discharge.
- Discharge on third day, if stable.

continued

Developing Clinical Reasoning

- What is your interpretation of her vital signs? Who should be notified and when?

- How would you determine whether Ms. Stillwater meets the criteria for discharge?

- What is the relationship between Ms. Stillwater's diabetes and her postsurgical condition?

- What factors affect her staple removal?

- How should you respond to her fingerstick blood glucose level?

- What nursing interventions do you foresee performing?

- Describe the timing and the technique for administering her insulin.

Suggested Responses for Integrated Nursing Care

- Ms. Stillwater's vital signs and other symptoms should alert you to a potential complication. She may have an infection related to her incision, as evidenced by her increased temperature and her subjective report of acute pain at the incision. Her blood pressure could be a result of her pain, but you should compare it with her baseline and continue to monitor it. You inspected the incision carefully for signs of infection. Notify her health care provider immediately of this potential complication.

- Wound healing may be impaired in people with diabetes, so any patient with diabetes requires vigilant wound assessment. Additionally, the stress of surgery usually results in increased blood glucose levels. Ms. Stillwater's fingerstick blood sugar is elevated from her baseline, another symptom of a possible infection. When you see a dramatic increase in blood sugar in a patient with diabetes, consider the possible causes.

- Despite the urgency of this new complication of wound infection, Ms. Stillwater should receive her insulin and breakfast as she usually would. Administer her insulin in a subcutaneous site; she can help you identify the site where she should receive her insulin. Patients who are accustomed to managing their diabetes at home will have preferences when in the hospital, and you should honor these preferences when possible (refer to Chapter 5).

- Many women who have had cesarean sections are discharged on the third day. One of the expected outcomes for discharge would include being free of infection. Ms. Stillwater is not free of infection; she has pain at her incision site, a fever, incision assessment findings indicating alterations in healing, and an elevated fingerstick blood sugar. When you notify the health care provider of these symptoms, a complete blood count, a wound culture, incision site care, and cancellation of the discharge are ordered.

- Given the delayed discharge and impaired wound healing, you would not want to remove the staples from this incision because removing the staples at this time could place Ms. Stillwater at risk for dehiscence. Another factor affecting the risk for dehiscence and impaired wound healing is Ms. Stillwater's increased subcutaneous fat.

- Did you foresee obtaining a complete blood count and a wound culture and performing incision site care? Did you also anticipate that this patient should not be discharged nor have her staples removed? In addition, although her physiologic care is very important, you will also need to relieve anxiety related to this infection and acknowledge her disappointment and potential concerns regarding the care of her son, since she cannot go home today.

Intermediate Case Studies

Case Study

Olivia Greenbaum

Olivia Greenbaum is a 9-month-old infant admitted to the hospital with respiratory syncytial virus (RSV). She was born prematurely at 30 weeks' gestation. Her complications at birth included respiratory distress syndrome (RDS), suspected sepsis, and formula intolerance. She was discharged home after 8 weeks on soy-based formula. This is her first hospitalization since her birth. Olivia is Mr. and Mrs. Greenbaum's only child, and they are very anxious. Mrs. Greenbaum is her primary caregiver.

Olivia is receiving supplemental humidified oxygen administered via oxygen tent at 40%. She is very fussy and is not tolerating separation from her mother well. She has a peripheral IV inserted in her right hand with D5 ¼ NSS with 10 mEq of potassium chloride infusing at 20 mL/hr. It is covered with a sock puppet. She is wearing a T-shirt and a disposable diaper. She is quite active within the crib. Her previous vital signs were as follows: temperature, 36.4°C (97.5°F); pulse, 84 beats/min; respirations, 38 breaths/min; blood pressure, 94/58 mm Hg.

Mrs. Greenbaum spent the night and is currently sleeping in the recliner in Olivia's room. You enter the room and observe Olivia sleeping. She is pale with circumoral cyanosis. Her respiratory rate is 40 breaths/min with an audible expiratory wheeze. Her heart rate on the monitor is 86 beats/min; her pulse rate on the pulse oximeter is 62 beats/min. The pulse oximeter is currently showing an oxygen saturation level of 68%.

Prescribed Interventions

Vital signs q4h

Encourage coughing

Oxygen via tent at 40%

Continuous pulse oximetry when quiet; may obtain qh intermittent pulse oximeter readings when active

Maintain O₂ saturation 93%–97%. Adjust O₂ in increments of 2% up to a max of 50%.

Isomil 6–8 oz q4h when awake

Intravenous fluids: D5 ¼ NSS with 10 mEq potassium chloride at 20 mL/hr

Heart rate/resp. monitor

continued

Developing Clinical Reasoning

- What is your first priority after observing Olivia sleeping?

- Should you increase the oxygen being administered?

- What is your interpretation of her vital signs and oxygen saturation?

- Give examples of how to manage thermoregulation within an oxygen tent.

- Identify factors that affect the accuracy of the oxygen saturation reading.

- How frequently should Olivia's IV site be assessed? What is the function of the sock puppet?

- How do you encourage coughing in a 9-month-old baby?

Suggested Responses for Integrated Nursing Care

- Your first priority is to establish whether Olivia is hypoxic. You noted a rapid respiratory rate and circumoral cyanosis, both potential symptoms of hypoxia. The pulse oximeter heart rate does not match the cardiac monitor heart rate. Gently, without disturbing Olivia, you remove and replace the pulse oximeter.

- Your preliminary assessment is that the pulse oximeter is not accurately assessing her oxygenation. You are able to hold the probe to her toe and get a reading of 95%. Olivia begins to wake up. Take her apical heart rate, which is the most reliable site for infants and small children (see Chapter 2).

Compare her apical pulse rate with the heart rate on the pulse oximeter as well as the heart rate on the cardiac monitor. Nurses must always verify that the equipment is accurately reflecting the patient's status. Next, you take her temperature, which is 36.2°C (97.1°F). The humidified oxygen is also cooling Olivia, making her hands, feet, and lips appear cold, blue, and dusky (see Chapter 14).

- Once Olivia is awake, she will not tolerate having the pulse oximeter probe on her toe and will keep pulling it off. You will need to check the oxygen saturation intermittently. Your next priority is to warm her up. When children become chilled, they have increased

continued

energy expenditure. When infants are stressed beyond aerobic metabolism, they use anaerobic metabolism. This produces lactic acid, which increases the acidity of the blood, exacerbating respiratory distress. Urge her mother to bring in more clothes and to layer her clothes to keep Olivia thermoregulated within the humidified tent. You do not need to increase the oxygen level; what at first looked like hypoxia is in fact hypothermia!

- The accuracy of a pulse oximetry reading is affected by several factors, including patient perfusion and peripheral vasoconstriction. Other factors that prevent the detection of oxygen saturation may be as simple as nail polish or artificial nails (see Chapter 14).
- Encouraging coughing in an infant is accomplished either through crying or laughing. Crying and laugh-ing require deep breaths and will cause a patient to cough, thus promoting airway clearance. If the infant is periodically crying vigorously, that is sufficient. You can try tickling or playing peekaboo to get a 9 month old to laugh.

- Check this patient's IV site every hour to ensure there are no signs of infiltration. The sock puppet is one way to disguise the IV site dressing while leaving it accessible for examination. If a young child can see the IV site dressing, he or she will often persist in try-ing to remove the tape and dressing despite all your efforts. If you cover the site, the child will not remem-ber it is there. Piaget's theory of cognitive develop-ment includes the concept of object permanence. At 9 months old, a child cannot imagine what he or she cannot see—in other words, what is out of sight is out of mind.

Case Study

Victoria Holly

Victoria Holly, age 68, is newly admitted to the hospital due to anemia and severe dehydration. She has been prescribed an IV of D5 ½ NSS infusing into the right hand to address the dehydration. Mrs. Holly has a second IV access in her left arm to be used for blood administration only. She recently received 2 units of packed red blood cells, in response to the anemia. You have prescribed orders to draw a complete blood count (CBC) and a complete metabolic profile (CMP). Mrs. Holly also has an ileostomy, which she has managed for several years on her own. Upon your initial nursing assessment of Mrs. Holly, you find her vital signs are as follows: temperature, 97.2°F; pulse, 96 beats/min; respirations, 18 breaths/min; blood pressure, 88/50 mm Hg. Her skin is "tenting" and you are having difficulty palpating her peripheral pulses. Her lips are dry and cracked. The skin around her stoma site is bright red and open in areas. You notice that her ostomy pouch was cut much larger than the stoma site. She reports she is very tired and "lacks energy." Her family informs you that she has always been a very independent person but in the last couple of months she just "hasn't been herself."

Prescribed Interventions

Intravenous fluids: D5 ½ NSS IV at 125 mL/hr
Strict I&O

Daily weights
CBC and CMP stat.

continued

Developing Clinical Reasoning

- Identify the equipment needed and appropriate sites to consider to obtain the blood samples.

- Describe how you would assess Mrs. Holly's peripheral circulation.

- What concerns you about Mrs. Holly's present condition in relationship to performing her activities of daily living (ADLs) independently?

- What is alarming about the assessment of her ileostomy? Identify possible explanations for the stoma's condition.

- What are measurable physical parameters you can use to determine whether the fluid replacement therapy and blood administration have had a therapeutic effect?

- Develop a discharge teaching plan for Mrs. Holly related to ostomy care.

Suggested Responses for Integrated Nursing Care

- You cannot obtain the specimen from above the IV in her right hand because the specimen will be diluted with the D5 ½ NSS solution and, thus, will be inaccurate. It is not considered best practice to draw laboratory specimens from an IV site unless absolutely necessary, according to facility policy. Also, you cannot draw blood specimens from a dedicated IV access such as the one Mrs. Holly has for blood administration. Collect Mrs. Holly's laboratory work from her left arm via venipuncture, avoiding the right arm due to the IV infusion.

- When a patient has no peripheral pulses, you must investigate further. Never ignore the absence of pulses, as this could signal a life-threatening condition. Have another nurse check the pulses, or use a Doppler. Upon checking Mrs. Holly's pulses with a Doppler device, you were able to hear them and marked them with an "x" to facilitate future assessments. In your initial assessment, you were not surprised that Mrs. Holly's pulses were nonpalpable, as she has a very low circulating volume (see Chapter 2).

- Mrs. Holly's vital signs are disconcerting because her blood pressure is low. Because of her hypotension, ADLs may unduly tax her. Until you see a positive change in her vital signs, provide assistance with her ADLs (see Chapter 7). In addition, Mrs. Holly has an IV in each arm. It may be difficult for her to care for the ostomy and perform personal care when one or both of the access sites are used for infusions.

- Mrs. Holly's ileostomy site is very red and excoriated. You are alarmed, as this could place her at risk for infection. Do not assume that a health care provider has seen the excoriation around the ostomy site. If the patient came into the hospital with more pressing matters, such as decreased blood pressure, the health care provider may not have observed the ileostomy. Notify the health care provider. Mrs. Holly may lack knowledge about the appropriate method for sizing and cutting her ostomy appliance. You suspect that she may be cutting the faceplate in such a way as to leave her skin exposed to the liquid stool, which is then causing the excoriation (see Chapter 13).

continued

- One therapeutic outcome to anticipate with Mrs. Holly would be an increase in blood pressure. Other outcomes include palpable peripheral pulses and normal skin turgor. Subjectively, Mrs. Holly should report that her energy has increased. Her family may also comment that she is becoming more "like herself." Sometimes health care workers make judgments about older adults, thinking that they are always tired. Since health care workers are often unfamiliar with their patients' normal conditions, comments made by family members can often be very helpful in determining progress. This is especially true if your patient cannot communicate. Objectively, one outcome would be that Mrs. Holly becomes more active in her own care.

- One area you should investigate is Mrs. Holly's ability to care for the ostomy before she came to the hospital. It is possible that her skin around the stoma site has looked like this for some time. Before her hospital discharge, evaluate her knowledge through return demonstration to ensure that she can care for the stoma and can identify possible family resources. She may benefit from a home health referral to ensure she is caring for her stoma properly.

Case Study

Tula Stillwater

It is now day 5 in the hospital for Ms. Stillwater (Refer to Case Study in the Basic Case Studies section on p. 1111). She has developed a staphylococcal infection in her cesarean section incision. This is the second time you have cared for this patient. You are familiar with her diabetic status, baseline vital signs, and routine postpartum care. She is currently receiving an IV antibiotic. Her vital signs are as follows: temperature, 99.2°F; pulse, 74 beats/min; respirations, 18 breaths/min; blood pressure, 130/80 mm Hg. Her fingerstick blood glucose before breakfast is 120 mg/dL.

You learned in report that her incision is intact and healing on the right side, but the far left side of her incision is being treated with a calcium alginate wound dressing. The open part of the incision is approximately 1″ long, 0.5″ wide, and 1″ deep. This part of her incision is draining copious amounts of foul-smelling, yellow to green purulent drainage. The incision is very painful. Ms. Stillwater reports her pain as a constant, stabbing, and burning pain at a 6 on a scale of 1 to 10 (10 = worst) before her pain medication is administered.

Ms. Stillwater's 5-day-old boy is now bottle-feeding regularly. He is taking 3 oz of Similac with Iron every 4 hours. Ms. Stillwater is eager to assume the majority of his care.

Prescribed Interventions

Medication or saline lock; flush every shift and prn

Vancomycin 1.0 g IV q12h

Sterile dressing change with calcium alginate wound dressing; pack loosely, change when outer dressing is saturated with drainage. Irrigate wound with normal saline before removing dressing.

Irrigate wound with NSS with dressing change

Fingerstick blood glucose before meals and at bedtime

Humalog insulin per sliding scale

Vital signs q4h

ibuprofen 600 mg po q4–6h prn pain

hydrocodone 5 mg and acetaminophen 325 mg po q4–6h prn pain unrelieved by ibuprofen

continued

Developing Clinical Reasoning

- How will you plan the dressing change for Ms. Stillwater and what equipment will you need?

- What techniques can you show Ms. Stillwater to improve her mobility and ability to hold and care for her infant?

- Describe your assessment and interventions for this wound.

- Identify factors that will promote wound healing in Ms. Stillwater.

- How will you organize your nursing care to provide uninterrupted time for Ms. Stillwater to care for her 5-day-old son?

- Describe the procedure you will use to administer the IV antibiotic.

Suggested Responses for Integrated Nursing Care

- Ms. Stillwater's dressing change will be stressful and uncomfortable. To manage the pain, perform the dressing change after she has taken her pain medication and you have allowed enough time for it to be effective. Given her diabetic status, allow her to eat her breakfast and receive her insulin before you begin her dressing change. Ms. Stillwater's focus is probably on her son. Encourage her to give him his morning bottle and to be satisfied that he is comfortable before you begin the dressing change.

- Review Chapter 8 to develop the list of equipment you will need for the dressing change. You will need to set up a sterile field and maintain the sterility during the dressing change. Ms. Stillwater can be positioned supine and rotated slightly to her left to promote drainage of the wound during irrigation.

- Make sure your assessment of the wound includes the size, the presence of granulation tissue, a description of the drainage, wound color, the

presence of edema and erythema, and temperature (see Chapter 8). Note the condition of the skin at the wound edges as well as the surrounding skin, including the location of the dressing tape. Look for changes in the condition of the wound and note how Mrs. Stillwater is tolerating the dressing change. If she will be taught to care for this wound and perform the dressing changes at home, instruction and return demonstration would become part of her discharge planning.

- For Ms. Stillwater's wound to heal, the infection must be resolved and the wound edges will need to become approximated. To optimize wound healing, Ms. Stillwater will need a diet high in protein, calories, and minerals. Obtain a nutritional consultation.

- The care of her infant son is a priority for Ms. Stillwater. Cluster your nursing care, such as wound dressing changes, vital signs, and medication administration, to allow her sufficient time to provide care for her son.

continued

- Make sure Ms. Stillwater knows how to use a splint, such as a pillow or folded blanket, across her abdomen to give support to her abdominal musculature when moving or coughing (see Chapter 6). Spending time in a comfortable chair may be preferable to getting in and out of bed. Assess that Ms. Stillwater is using the "football hold" to feed and comfort her son. The advantage of this position is that the infant does not rest on the mother's abdomen. Ms. Stillwater should have several pillows available to provide support for her arms when holding her infant.

- To give the IV antibiotic, assess the IV site for patency, flush the IV per facility policy prior to administration, administer the antibiotics according to the facility and/or manufacturer's guidelines, and then flush the medication or saline lock after the antibiotic is infused (see Chapter 5).

Case Study

Jason Brown

Jason Brown is a 21-year-old college football player. It is the second post-op day following surgical repair of a fracture of his right tibia and fibula. He has sutures over the anterior knee and lateral malleolus and a posterior splint on the right leg. He continues to report considerable pain. His vital signs at midnight were as follows: temperature, 98.3°F; pulse, 58 beats/min; respirations, 12 breaths/min; blood pressure 118/70 mm Hg. He reported his incisional pain as sharp, stabbing, and a 3 on a scale of 1 of 10 (10 = worst) at about 10 PM. He has a peripheral IV in his left forearm infusing D5 ½ NSS at a rate of 20 mL/hr. He is using a PCA pump for pain relief. The nursing care for the morning includes routine AM care, cast care, and a trip to physical therapy (PT). Shortly after morning report, the unit secretary catches you and says, "Jason says he needs a nurse. He is in terrible pain."

You enter the room. Jason is pale and diaphoretic. His sheets are damp with some wet spots. He says, "My leg hurts. It really hurts." You ask him to rate his pain, and he answers, "At least an 8. I've been pushing my pain pump but I'm still in pain." His IV site looks okay. You say, "I'm going to find out why it is hurting. I need to get your vital signs first." His vital signs now are as follows: temperature, 98.9°F; pulse, 72 beats/min; respirations, 20 breaths/min; blood pressure, 124/78 mm Hg.

Prescribed Interventions

Vital signs q4h

Intravenous fluids: D5 ½ NSS at 20 mL/hr

PCA—Morphine sulfate 1 mg/mL, 1 mg q6min; lockout max 10 mg in 1 hr

Zolpidem 5 mg prn at bedtime for sleep

PT for weight bearing, as tolerated

continued

Developing Clinical Reasoning

- What is the significance of the changes in Jason's vital signs?

- What interventions for Jason's pain must occur immediately before administering nursing care and PT?

- How do you assess the following:
  - Infection versus inflammation?
  - Neurovascular compromise?
  - IV patency?

Suggested Responses for Integrated Nursing Care

- Always compare vital signs with a baseline and the previous vital signs (see Chapter 2). While Jason's temperature is elevated slightly, it has not increased dramatically, as it would be with an infection. His respiratory rate and pulse rate were quite low at midnight. Since he is a young, healthy athlete, his resting pulse rate may be lower than what is often considered as the norm. You notice that his resting pulse rates on the night shift have been running from 56 to 60 beats/min. Another factor contributing to his decreased pulse rate may be the effect of the zolpidem that he took at 2200 to help him sleep. Therefore, while his morning respiratory rate and pulse rate are still within normal range, they represent a significant increase from his resting baseline. These are objective assessments supporting his assertion of increased pain.

- One reason for an increase in pain with any post-surgical patient is the possibility of infection. Quickly assess all surgical incision sites and observe for redness, swelling, or a foul odor (Chapter 8). Due to short hospital stays, signs and symptoms of infection do not usually appear until after the patient is discharged. The assessment of the surgical site should also include checking for bleeding. Hemorrhage in the postoperative period is always a potential complication (see Chapter 6).

- In addition to infection, Jason is at risk for neurovascular compromise because of the trauma to his right leg as well as from the splint and dressing. Assess for neurovascular compromise and perform cast care (see Chapter 9). Jason's fracture has been placed in a splint rather than a cast, which is a more current surgical practice, but nurses still refer to the care of the affected extremity as "cast care." Determine whether there are any signs of compartment

syndrome (see Chapter 9). You need no additional equipment for this assessment, and it should take very little time; do this immediately.

- Upon assessment, you find that Jason's foot and leg are pink and warm with 2+ pulses, no edema, full sensation, motion, and capillary refill measuring less than 3 seconds. The incision sites show no redness, swelling, drainage, or foul odor, and no bleeding is evident.

- Another possible reason for his pain is that his IV may no longer be patent and, therefore, he would not be receiving any pain medication. You remember the wet spots on the bed as you begin systematically checking each of the IV administration-set connections. Your assessment of the IV site shows no swelling, and he reports no pain at the site. Your next check should be from the IV site to the IV tubing. You find that the connection of the IV tubing to the IV insertion catheter is loose and leaking. Determine whether the IV site is still patent (see Chapter 15). If the IV is still patent, replace the IV tubing (see Chapter 15). Check the medication in the PCA pump to ensure it is the correct medication. You will be required to check the PCA history to determine the amount of medication used as well as the amount remaining every 4 hours or according to facility policy (see Chapter 10).

- Contact the health care provider to explain that the PCA pain medication was infusing onto the bed linens, and obtain an order for an appropriate bolus dose so that Jason can obtain immediate pain relief. After 30 minutes, obtain another set of vital signs and perform a pain assessment. Document the evaluation of your interventions. Jason's pain will need to be controlled before initiating additional nursing care. Coordinating with PT to reschedule his therapy until his pain is controlled is a nursing responsibility.

Case Study

Kent Clark

Kent Clark, age 29, was admitted 24 hours ago for observation related to a suspected closed head injury following a motor vehicle accident (MVA). Mr. Clark's baseline vital signs are stable. He has a cervical collar and is scheduled to undergo an MRI to determine if he has a cervical spine injury. The health care provider has asked you to reduce his activity until cervical spinal injuries are ruled out.

Currently, Mr. Clark is awake, alert, and oriented (to person, place, and time); his pupils are equally round and reactive to light and accommodation (PERRLA). He moves all four extremities bilaterally. His head is elevated 30 degrees to minimize increased intracranial pressure (ICP) and edema. A peripheral IV in his right arm is infusing D5 ½ NSS at 40 mL/hr.

Just before you are scheduled to take him to Special Procedures for the MRI, Mr. Clark becomes restless and anxious. During the neuro check, you notice that his right pupil is sluggish. Although he denies pain, he says, "I don't care what the doctors say. I am not going to stay in this bed any longer!" When you call the health care provider, she orders lorazepam 0.5 mg IV push. However, as you give the IV push medication to Mr. Clark, you notice a cloudy substance forming in the IV line and the patient reports a slight burning at his IV insertion site.

Prescribed Interventions

Bed rest
Intravenous fluids: D5 ½ NSS at 40 mL/hr
HOB elevated 30 degrees

Neurologic checks q2h
Lorazepam 0.5 mg IV push now x one dose
Cervical collar

Developing Clinical Reasoning

- What clinical symptoms alert you that Mr. Clark's condition is changing? What additional assessments will you do?

- Identify the source of the pain at the IV insertion site and the cloudy substance in the IV tubing.

- Describe special positioning and transfer techniques to be followed for Mr. Clark.

- What could you have done to prevent these complications, and how will you intervene now?

- How will you handle Mr. Clark's anger and maintain reduced activity?

continued

Suggested Responses for Integrated Nursing Care

- In a patient with a closed head injury, bleeding or swelling may occur within the confines of the skull, leading to increased ICP. This increased ICP could cause extensive brain damage. Mr. Clark became increasingly restless and anxious, which could be a subtle sign of increased ICP. Even slow bleeding inside the cranium can cause changes. When you observe a change, immediately perform a neurologic assessment to determine if there are further neurologic alterations. When Mr. Clark became restless, you noticed that his right pupil was more sluggish to light than the left, which is another sign of increased ICP. Complete neurologic checks as often as his condition warrants, and immediately report subtle changes in neurologic checks to the health care provider. Meticulous documentation of baseline neurologic checks and subsequent assessments is important to detect subtle neurologic changes (see Chapter 17).

- Cervical spinal injuries can vary in severity, and even hairline fractures can become unstable if the patient is not positioned and transferred correctly. Mr. Clark has a cervical collar and the health care provider has asked you to minimize his movement. If you need to turn Mr. Clark, keep his head lowered and then logroll him as a unit without flexing or turning his neck. Obtain help from additional staff so that you can stabilize his head, neck, and torso in straight alignment while he is being turned. When Mr. Clark is transferred from the bed to a stretcher, use a friction-reducing sheet or lateral transfer device to move him gently and carefully as a unit. Even though he has a cervical collar, do not assume that it is safe for him to sit up further in the bed or get up and move around.

- Mr. Clark is angry and wants to get out of bed. For Mr. Clark, careful pharmacologic sedation may be a good option. The health care provider has ordered lorazepam to reduce his agitation and anxiety. Another possible intervention is to help Mr. Clark feel more in control of his environment. This could be as simple as having a family member stay with him, and frequently checking his needs. Restraints would be the least desirable option for him. At this time, placing restraints on him could increase his agitation and make him feel more trapped, and this could increase his ICP (see Chapter 4).

- Pain at the IV site could mean that the IV is not patent. Carefully observe the IV site for any signs of phlebitis or infiltration before and while giving the IV push. If you determine that Mr. Clark's IV has a good blood return and is not infiltrated, the burning sensation at his IV site may be related to the administration of the lorazepam IV. Medications given by intravenous (IV) bolus can be irritating. Give the medication and the flush that follows at a slower rate. If not contraindicated, some medications can also be diluted, based on facility policy and/or as prescribed.

- The most probable cause for the cloudy appearance in Mr. Clark's IV line is precipitation of the drug due to chemical incompatibility of the lorazepam and the IV fluid of D5 ½ NSS. When giving any medication through an IV line, you must know whether the drug and IV solution are chemically compatible (see Chapter 5). When IV drugs are not compatible, a reaction immediately occurs that may or may not be visible to the eye, but nevertheless can be dangerous. To prevent this, flush the IV line before and after medication administration per facility policy. Since a precipitate has already formed, clamp the tubing off using the clamp closest to Mr. Clark and make sure that the cloudy substance does not reach him (see Chapter 5). Some facilities require discontinuing the IV and restarting another IV with new IV tubing; other hospitals require changing only the IV tubing. If signs of incompatibility occur, notify the health care provider and continue to assess Mr. Clark's need for further medication.

Case Study

Lucille Howard

Lucille Howard, age 78, is in the hospital for a severe urinary tract infection (UTI). She has a history of urinary retention and UTIs. She is overweight, has a history of heart failure, and is allergic to many medications, including several antibiotics. Twenty-four hours ago she had severe nausea and vomiting and was ordered nothing by mouth (NPO). She has an IV catheter inserted in her left arm, infusing D5 ½ NSS at 75 mL/hr. While caring for Ms. Howard, you notice that she begins to have some coarse audible breath sounds and difficulty breathing. She reports pain in her abdomen.

Medical Orders

Intravenous fluids: D5 ½ NSS at 75 mL/hr

ciprofloxacin 200 mg IV q12h

NPO

Strict I&O

Developing Clinical Reasoning

- What are possible causes of Ms. Howard's current symptoms?

- How would you identify the source of her current symptoms?

- What actions will you take?

Suggested Responses for Integrated Nursing Care

- There are several potential causes for Ms. Howard's symptoms. In light of her drug sensitivities, she may be allergic to the amphotericin B. Allergic responses can include difficulty breathing as well as itching and a rash. Another source of her symptoms could be related to her heart problems. People with heart problems can easily become overloaded with fluid. Symptoms of fluid overload, a common problem for patients with heart failure, include crackles in the lungs, abnormal heart sounds, and possibly edema.

- To determine the cause of Ms. Howard's symptoms, you need to perform several assessments. First, auscultate her heart and lung sounds and palpate her abdomen. Assess for edema. Also assess for a rash on her skin, and ask her if she has any itching. Review her voiding history and volume of urine per episode of voiding.

- If her heart and lung sounds are normal, but her abdominal discomfort persists, she may have to

urinate. Review the method she has been using to void. Ms. Howard is overweight and positioning on a bedpan may be difficult and is not conducive to emptying of her bladder. Arrange for and encourage her to get out of bed to void; use of a bedside commode is probably the best intervention, as she is experiencing some difficulty breathing and probably has decreased energy related to her acute illness. Consider checking postvoid residual to confirm she is emptying her bladder (see Chapter 12). Consult a safe patient handling algorithm to help you make decisions about safe patient handling and movement (see Chapter 9). Utilize appropriate transfer devices and the assistance of others when assisting Ms. Howard out of bed.

- If Ms. Howard seems to be emptying her bladder and the postvoid bladder scans reveal minimal retention, her discomfort could be related to the UTI. Collaborate with the health care provider regarding appropriate analgesia.

continued

- You should also review the patient's intake and output, for the most recent hours and for the last 24 hours. Currently, Ms. Howard is getting 75 mL/hr of IV fluid. She should be voiding an average of at least 30 mL/hr, the least amount of urine you would expect to see in an hour (30 mL). You could weigh the patient and compare today's weight with her admission weight. The record of a patient's daily weight may more accurately depict fluid balance status, due to possible numerous sources of inaccuracies in fluid intake and output measurement. Weigh the patient at the same time every day. If Ms. Howard's input is higher than her output, she is at risk for overload. New or worsening edema or significantly increased body weight in 24 hours indicates an accumulation of fluid related to fluid overload or worsening heart failure.

- If Ms. Howard is having an allergic reaction, hold any dose of the ciprofloxacin that may be due, follow anaphylaxis protocol, and notify the health care provider. If she is beginning to have problems with fluid overload due to her heart problems, reduce the IV rate to a keep open rate (20 to 40 mL/hr), and contact the health care provider for further orders. Continue to monitor Ms. Howard until you are certain she is stabilized and her symptoms have resolved.

Case Study

Janice Romero

Janice Romero, age 24, has recently been diagnosed with acute lymphocytic leukemia (ALL). To provide long-term venous access, she is having an implanted port placed. She had a 21-gauge peripheral IV inserted in her right arm prior to surgery. After her port was placed, Mrs. Romero's health care provider ordered 2 units of packed red blood cells (PRBCs). You note an order for the use of a blood warmer for the transfusions. When you talk to Mrs. Romero about the blood transfusion, she tells you that the last time she received blood she had chills and fever during the transfusion.

Prescribed Interventions

2 units packed RBCs via blood warmer stat.

Intravenous fluids: D5 ½ NSS at 50 mL/hr

Developing Clinical Reasoning

- Identify the site you will use to administer blood to Mrs. Romero. Why did you choose this site?

- Describe the technique you will use to administer blood to Mrs. Romero.

- Identify the purposes for warming blood, and describe the safest way to warm blood.

- Considering Mrs. Romero's history and diagnosis, describe the precautions you will implement before giving her blood.

continued

Suggested Responses for Integrated Nursing Care

- Before Mrs. Romero can receive blood, you must select an appropriate site (see Chapter 15). Site selection depends on the gauge of the IV and the fluid infusing in the IV. Blood must be given through a large-bore catheter to prevent red blood cell damage. Since dextrose will cause hemolysis, blood can be administered only with normal saline. For these two reasons, the optimal site for blood administration is her implanted port. Before you give her blood through the port, be certain that the port is not dedicated for other infusions, such as chemo.

- Since the implanted port is new, check the patient's health record for indications that the port has been approved for use; confirmation of location of the tip of the port catheter either by postprocedure chest radiograph or by technology used during the placement procedure is required prior to use and should be documented in the patient's health record. Maintain sterile technique when accessing the port and wear a mask (see Chapter 15). Ensure that the port is patent prior to use. Check the port for patency and blood return per facility policy. Infuse the normal saline slowly while you observe the implanted port site for signs of swelling and pain. If the port shows any sign of infiltration, notify the health care provider and choose another site to give her blood.

- Some patients may need to have their blood warmed before it is administered. This includes patients who are at risk for cardiac arrhythmias, patients with unusual immune responses, as well as neonatal and pediatric patients. A health care provider must prescribe warming of blood products during transfusion. Various devices exist to warm blood. Do not use the microwave to warm any blood product: It coagulates the proteins of the blood and causes severe hemolysis in the patient, which could be fatal. Whenever you need to warm blood, always use a blood warmer approved by your facility.

- Mrs. Romero's history of chills and fever are signs of a possible transfusion reaction; thus, she is at increased risk for a transfusion reaction. Ensure that she has a signed consent form and that she fully understands her need for the blood. The health care provider should be aware of this history of a transfusion reaction. The health care provider may order premedication with diphenhydramine, acetaminophen, or steroids prior to blood administration to reduce the risk for developing another reaction. Stay with the patient for at least 15 minutes at the beginning of the transfusion. Continue to monitor her vital signs frequently per hospital policy. When you leave her room, make sure her call light is available, and instruct her to contact you if she has any symptoms.

Case Study

Gwen Galloway

Mrs. Galloway, age 64, had a left-sided mastectomy and is now receiving follow-up chemotherapy for recurrent breast cancer with axillary node involvement at the outpatient oncology center. She reports intermittent pain and soreness on her left side and under her left arm. She has a CVAD (double-lumen Hickman catheter) inserted in the right side of her chest. Recent laboratory work shows a low white blood cell count of $1,800/mm^3$ and a low platelet count of $39,000/mm^3$. She also bleeds and bruises very easily. You have to obtain vital signs and draw a complete blood count (CBC). The dressing on her CVAD must be changed.

Prescribed Interventions

Vital signs on arrival

CBC on arrival

Acetaminophen 650 mg po q6h prn pain

Change central line dressing q week

continued

Gwen Galloway (continued)

Developing Clinical Reasoning

- What special precautions should you take while obtaining Mrs. Galloway's vital signs?

- Explain why some sites would be contraindicated when taking Mrs. Galloway's temperature.

- Identify your interventions when changing Mrs. Galloway's central line dressing and the rationale for these interventions.

- Describe the special precautions you would take when drawing blood from Mrs. Galloway. Identify the site where you would draw the blood.

Suggested Responses for Integrated Nursing Care

- To individualize care, always assess your patient's condition and special needs. When a patient undergoes a mastectomy, she will often have lymph nodes removed from the affected side. Taking a blood pressure reading in the affected arm could interfere with circulation and harm the extremity (see Chapter 2). In Mrs. Galloway's case, her affected side is on the left, so take her blood pressure on the right side.

- Mrs. Galloway has a low platelet count, which places her at risk for bleeding. In addition, her low white blood cell count places her at risk for infection and other complications. Therefore, taking a rectal temperature would be contraindicated for Mrs. Galloway. It would also be contraindicated to take a left-sided axillary temperature on Mrs. Galloway because she is still having some discomfort due to her recent mastectomy (see Chapter 2).

- Given Mrs. Galloway's risk for bleeding, would a peripheral venipuncture be the best choice to

obtain her CBC? Due to the risk for prolonged bleeding, her central line may provide the best access for a blood specimen. Determine whether her health care provider has restricted her central line for chemotherapy. If her central line is dedicated to chemotherapy only, obtain a blood specimen via venipuncture. If you needed to do a venipuncture, using Mrs. Galloway's left side would be contraindicated due to the mastectomy. You will need to apply pressure to the site for a longer period of time because of her increased risk for bleeding.

- When changing Mrs. Galloway's central line dressing, use sterile technique due to her increased risk for infection. Maintain sterile technique when changing the CVAD dressing and wear a mask (see Chapter 15). Ensure that the CVAD is patent prior to use. Check the CVAD for patency and blood return per facility policy. To prevent bleeding and bruising at the central line site, do not move or pull on the catheter as you are manipulating the central line dressing.

Case Study

George Patel

George Patel, age 64, was admitted to your floor 3 days ago following surgical insertion of a tracheostomy tube. His diagnosis prior to surgery was acute upper airway obstruction. He has a medication (saline) lock. Currently, he is receiving oxygen via his tracheostomy at 40%. His pulse oximetry readings have been consistently running in the low 90s. He quickly becomes short of breath when his oxygen is interrupted during suctioning. During

continued

your shift, you will have to suction Mr. Patel as needed and provide routine tracheostomy care. You will also need to transport him with portable oxygen to radiology for his chest x-ray (AP and lateral).

Prescribed Interventions

Morphine sulfate 1 to 4 mg IV q3h prn for pain
AP and lateral chest x-ray
Pulse oximetry every shift and prn
Oxygen via trach Venturi mask at 40%

Tracheostomy care every shift and prn
Medication or saline lock, flush every shift
Tracheal suctioning prn

Developing Clinical Reasoning

- How would you determine when Mr. Patel needs to be suctioned?

- How would you determine when Mr. Patel needs to have tracheostomy care?

- Describe expected outcomes when suctioning and providing tracheostomy care.

- When transporting Mr. Patel to the radiology department, what interventions should you implement to ensure his safety?

Suggested Responses for Integrated Nursing Care

- To evaluate the need for suctioning, first assess Mr. Patel's respiratory status. Examine his oxygen saturation and compare it with his baseline. If his oxygen saturation is decreased from his baseline, this may be an indication that he needs to be suctioned. Observe his respirations to determine if they are more labored than usual. Listen to his lung sounds for crackles or wheezes. Also, listen around his tracheostomy for gurgling. Does he have a productive cough? All of these signs and symptoms are indications that he needs to be suctioned.

- To assess the need for tracheostomy care (see Chapter 14), closely examine his tracheostomy as well as the tracheostomy holder/ties and precut gauze dressing. If it appears wet or moist, tracheostomy care would be indicated. If his tracheostomy dressing appears dry and intact, you may want to wait until later in your shift to do tracheostomy care. Suctioning and subsequent coughing will often soil the tracheostomy dressings, so wait until after suctioning to change the tracheostomy dressing.

- Your expected outcomes when suctioning a tracheostomy include minimizing hypoxia, discomfort, and fatigue. Hypoxia may be reduced by hyperoxygenating the patient before suctioning

according to facility policy. When you suction Mr. Patel, limit the length of suction time to 10 to 15 seconds and allow him to rest before suctioning him again (see Chapter 14). During tracheostomy care or repeat suctioning, quickly replace his oxygen source and limit the time his oxygen is interrupted. Since Mr. Patel has a new tracheostomy, it is very likely he will need to be premedicated with morphine for pain. Morphine may depress respirations, so continually assess Mr. Patel's respiratory status after administering the pain medication. In addition, adequate rest periods are needed to minimize fatigue from suctioning. Mr. Patel may require a rest period between suctioning the tracheostomy and his tracheostomy care.

- Important interventions when transporting Mr. Patel focus on providing adequate oxygenation. First, assess Mr. Patel's oxygen saturation and respiratory status prior to transport. If indicated, suction Mr. Patel before he leaves his room. You must also check that the portable oxygen tank is full and the label says "oxygen." Before turning off his wall oxygen, make sure the portable oxygen tank is working properly and that the equipment is ready. This avoids interruption of the oxygen supply while placing him on the portable oxygen.

Advanced Case Studies

Case Study

Cole McKean

Cole McKean is a 4-year-old boy in the pediatric intensive care unit (PICU). He weighs 22 kg. He was admitted 3 days ago after nearly drowning in a neighbor's pool. He was submerged for 5 to 10 minutes. The neighbor initiated CPR and the rescue team had a heart rate established within 10 minutes of their arrival. The aspirated pool water caused a severe inflammatory response resulting in pulmonary edema. Cole is intubated with an endotracheal tube (ETT) and is on a mechanical ventilator. Throughout the past 2 days, he has been producing copious bronchial secretions and has required suctioning about every 2 hours. Today, his breath sounds are clearer and he requires less frequent suctioning. He is being weaned off oxygen. The care plan for today includes possible extubation. An arterial line is in place in his left radial artery, infusing NSS at 2 to 3 mL/hr. A peripherally inserted central catheter (PICC) line with an infusion of D5 ½ NSS at 75 mL/hr is inserted into his right arm. His heart rate, respiratory rate, and arterial waveform are being monitored. The pulse oximeter sensor is applied to his right toe. He has an indwelling urinary catheter to gravity drainage and a nasogastric tube in place and set to low intermittent suction. Cole is receiving sedation but is opening his eyes at times and moving his extremities. He is becoming more active.

Suddenly, the alarm goes off on the ventilator. You look at Cole. His eyes are open and he is making crying sounds. You know when a child is properly intubated he or she cannot make sounds. You notice that his oxygen saturation level has dropped to 81% and his color is dusky. He is breathing on his own around the tube and his abdomen is rounded. You and the pediatric intensivist assess Cole's respiratory status and oxygenation and decide to remove the ETT and begin oxygen at 40% via face mask. When you place Cole on the face mask, his oxygen saturation returns to the mid-90s. The health care provider says, "This little fellow was ready to get rid of his tube." She orders a follow-up arterial blood gas (ABG) to be drawn in 15 minutes.

continued

Prescribed Interventions

Continuous pulse oximetry

Foley to gravity

Maintain O_2 saturation 92% to 98%

I&O

Oxygen 40% via face mask

Nasogastric tube to low intermittent suction

Vital signs q1h

Neurologic checks q1h

Intravenous fluids: D5 ½ NS at 75 mL/hr

Endotracheal suctioning prn

Arterial line: NSS 2 to 3 mL/hr

Developing Clinical Reasoning

- Describe your initial actions in response to a possible extubation.

- How can the technique of drawing ABGs be adapted for a pediatric patient?

- How will Cole's response be evaluated now that he is on an oxygen mask?

- Develop a care plan that will allow Cole rest and sleep periods, but also allow hourly assessments.

- Identify the nursing skills involved in monitoring Cole's respiratory status.

Suggested Responses for Integrated Nursing Care

- When a patient is intubated, the patency of this airway is a critical priority. When you hear Cole cry, you must determine if his ETT is in the proper place. Listen with your stethoscope over the lung fields and abdomen. If you do not hear ventilator-induced breath sounds over the lung fields, then the ETT is not in place. Because a child's neck is so short, it is not difficult to displace a tracheal tube into the esophagus. If this occurs, you may hear ventilator-cycled sounds in the abdomen. Signs that an ETT is not in the correct position include unstable oxygen saturation levels, cyanosis, and abdominal distention. In Cole's situation, you determine that the ETT is no longer in the lungs. All patients on mechanical ventilation must have an Ambu bag and a mask of the correct size at the bedside. Cole did not require mask-bag respirations at this time, but he has the potential for this need.

- When you are evaluating Cole's response, the ABG results will guide clinical decision making regarding oxygen delivery. In Cole's case, 10 to 15 minutes after changing to the 40% oxygen mask, you draw an ABG (see Chapter 18). The results come back as follows: Pao_2, 82 mm Hg; $Paco_2$, 46 mm Hg; pH, 7.34; Hco_3, 20 mEq/L. This ABG shows that Cole's oxygen level is acceptable and there is no indication to support immediate reintubation. Continue to assess Cole's respiratory status and oxygenation and obtain ABGs periodically, as ordered, to evaluate Cole's response to treatment.

- Monitor and assess Cole's respiratory status: observe his work of breathing, count his respiratory rate,

observe his color, and auscultate breath sounds. If he shows no significant respiratory distress and has a stable respiratory rate and clear breath sounds, he is responding well to the change in his oxygen source. In addition, continuously monitor the oxygen saturation level via pulse oximetry. Immediately report any increases or decreases in oxygen saturation to the health care provider.

- Because children have a small total blood volume, the blood drawn back in the arterial line is usually not discarded but returned to the patient after the laboratory sample is drawn. Smaller volumes of blood are sent to the laboratory in pediatric specimen tubes. The setup for a pediatric arterial line delivers a smaller volume of fluid when the in-line flushing device is activated (see Chapter 16).

- When a patient, especially a child, is critically ill, cluster your hands-on care so that the patient will have a significant amount of time to sleep and rest between interventions. One of the initial assessments a nurse makes in an intensive care setting is to determine that each of the monitoring devices is accurately displaying the patient's status (see Chapters 14 and 16). After you determine that the monitors accurately reflect the patient's vital signs, obtaining alternating sets of vital signs from the patient and from the monitor may be permitted, according to hospital policy. Maintain a quiet environment. Because of the noise and activity of the intensive care unit, many infant and child intensive care units dim the lights at night to create day/night cycles for the children.

Case Study

Damian Wallace

Damian Wallace, age 19, was admitted to the emergency department approximately 4 hours ago with a stab wound to the chest that he received in a knife fight while intoxicated. You are asked to care for Damian while his nurse attends to a new emergency. She gives you the following report: He was admitted in respiratory distress and bleeding from the stab wound. His wound is on the right side at the sixth intercostal space and is approximately 1 in in length, sutured and intact. The chest x-ray confirmed a right hemothorax and, as a result, the ED physician inserted a chest tube. The chest tube is connected to a disposable drainage system and placed to suction at –20 cm H_2O. The chest tube is draining a small amount of dark-red blood. There has not been any new drainage for the past 2 hours.

Damian's most recent vital signs were as follows: temperature, 98.4°F; pulse, 88 beats/min; respirations, 24 breaths/min; blood pressure, 112/74 mm Hg. He is receiving oxygen via face mask at 30% and is on continuous pulse oximetry. The oxygen saturation level is currently 96%. He says he feels short of breath. He does not have labored breathing and is not using accessory muscles. He reports pain at the chest tube insertion site and stab wound site. He has a patent IV infusing in his left forearm. His laboratory work reported a blood alcohol level of 0.12. The nurse giving report says, "Good luck—He says he's in pain, but I think he already drank his pain medication from a bottle."

Damian turns on his call light. When you approach him, you notice his breathing is labored with subclavicular retractions. The pulse oximeter reads 95%. Damian says, "This thing in my side really hurts."

You take another set of vital signs: temperature, 98.6°F; pulse, 90 beats/min; respirations, 37 breaths/min; blood pressure, 118/78 mm Hg. You find the breath sounds are diminished on the right. The chest drainage tubing is in the bed without a dependent loop, and Damian has been lying on a segment of the tubing. You ask him to describe his pain and rate it on a scale of 1 to 10 (10 = worst), and he says, "Really bad, sharp, about a 5, like I'm being stabbed again!" You ask if the medicine he got earlier helped with the pain, and he replies, "it didn't help one bit!" When you review the eMAR, you find that Damian has been prescribed ketorolac 30 mg IV, which was given 3 hours ago, and hydrocodone 5 mg and acetaminophen 325 mg po for pain unrelieved by ketorolac, which has not been administered. You find his nurse and ask if pain medication was administered. The nurse responds, "Are you kidding? If he's tough enough to drink and fight, he's tough enough for a little chest tube. If the anti-inflammatory doesn't help, he doesn't deserve anything stronger."

continued

Prescribed Interventions

Chest tube with drainage system to suction at −20 cm H_2O

Intravenous fluids: NSS at 100 mL/hr

Oxygen at 30% via face mask

Ketorolac 30 mg IV q6h prn pain

Hydrocodone 5 mg and acetaminophen 325 mg po q4–6h prn pain unrelieved by ketorolac

Continuous pulse oximetry

Developing Clinical Reasoning

- Which of Damian's needs is your first priority? Describe your assessments related to your first priority.

- How would you troubleshoot his chest tube drainage system? What could be the source of his respiratory distress?

- Describe the purpose of a chest tube drainage system for a hemothorax.

- Discuss valid reasons a nurse might not give a pain medication when there is a prn order.

- Discuss prejudices nurses may have that may prohibit adequate pain management.

Suggested Responses for Integrated Nursing Care

- Your first priority is Damian's increased respiratory distress. Although the change in oxygen saturation levels is very small, this is only because Damian's body is compensating for it now. Damian's work of breathing has dramatically changed, signaling a change in his respiratory status. Your preliminary assessment showed a respiratory rate of 37 breaths/ min, up significantly from his earlier respiratory rate of 24. When you inspected the chest, you found sub-clavicular retractions; this indicates that Damian is using his intercostal muscles to breathe. When you auscultated breath sounds, you found decreased air movement on the right, indicating a hemothorax.

- In a hemothorax, blood collects in the pleural space and compresses a lung. The purpose of the chest tube is to evacuate the blood and allow the lung to expand fully. In Damian's case, the stab wound created a puncture in the pleura, allowing blood to accumulate within the pleural space. It is impor-tant to evaluate the right lung on a routine basis to make sure the blood in the pleural space has been removed so that the lung can reexpand. Any change in respiratory status may indicate a problem with the chest tube drainage system.

- As you noted in this case, Damian has had a change in his respiratory status. Since you have completed his assessment, now begin inspecting the equipment. As with any equipment check, begin inspection at the patient and move to the equipment. Start your inspection at the insertion site of the chest tube. Observe the dressing to ensure it is occlusive and inspect the tubing for leaks, kinks, and

dependent loops. Compare the amount of recent drainage in the drainage system, with the volume of old drainage, and check the amount of suction (see Chapter 14). In this case, Damian has been lying on his tubing, which would prevent it from draining properly. When you reposition Damian's tubing, approximately 60 mL of dark old blood flows into the drainage set. His respiratory status improves quickly. Thus, this accumulated blood in the pleural space was the source of his respiratory distress.

- There are several situations in which giving an opioid analgesic may be contraindicated. During a life-saving procedure, pain is not always a priority. In this case, Damian did not receive pain medication before the insertion of his chest tube, because he was at risk for respiratory arrest. Opioids may also be contraindicated when it is critical to assess mental status, because the opioid might mask neurologic changes. Opioid analgesics also are associated with the adverse effects of respiratory depression and vital sign changes. Patients sometimes do not receive the pain medication ordered because the nurse is worried about these adverse effects. Because of this, controversy exists as to whether the benefit of pain control outweighs the risk of adverse drug reactions. Many hospitals have committees that can assist with these ethical decisions. Collaboration among nurses, doctors, and pharmacists can result in optimal pain control with minimal adverse effects. Speak with the health care provider before indepen-dently deciding to withhold pain medication, to pre-vent adverse drug reactions.

continued

Damian Wallace (continued)

- Another reason nurses may withhold medication is their own preconception of the patient's pain and their own prejudices. Some nurses are not even aware that they have these feelings. As a nursing student, you need to understand how you will respond to patients, and you need to explore your own beliefs and prejudices. The accepted standard in nursing is that a patient defines his or her own pain and that it is the nurse's responsibility to manage it properly. Guidelines for pain management have been written by state Boards of Nursing, the U.S. Department of Health and Human Services, the World Health Organization, as well as other professional organizations.

Case Study

Robert Espinoza

Robert Espinoza, age 44, has just had exploratory abdominal surgery. The postanesthesia recovery room (PACU) nurse calls at 1410 to provide report for Mr. Espinoza and tells you he has a peripheral IV inserted in his right arm, infusing NSS at 50 mL/hr. He has a midline abdominal dressing that is dry and intact with two Jackson–Pratt (JP) drains in place. He also has a nasogastric (NG) tube and an indwelling urinary catheter to gravity drainage. The nurse reports that his NG tube has been checked for placement and has been draining moderate amounts of yellow-green contents. His vital signs in the PACU are as follows: temperature, 98.0°F; pulse, 86 beats/min; respirations, 16 breaths/min; blood pressure, 134/80 mm Hg. At 1400, he received 4 mg morphine sulfate IV for sharp incisional pain reported as 8 on a scale of 1 to 10 (10 = worst).

At 1500, you receive Mr. Espinoza on your medical-surgical unit via stretcher by a hospital transporter. The NG tube tape that secured the NG to his nose is no longer in place. You also notice that the urinary drainage bag lying on top of his legs has a small amount of amber urine in the reservoir. While you are in his room, Mr. Espinoza says, "Hey, it feels like there's something wet under my back." His vital signs on arrival are as follows: temperature, 98.0°F; pulse, 130 beats/min; respirations, 18 breaths/min; and blood pressure, 100/68 mm Hg. His respirations are regular and unlabored and his skin color is pink. He now rates his pain as dull and 2 on a scale of 1 to 10 (10 = worst). Mr. Espinoza's family is anxiously waiting in the waiting room on your unit.

Prescribed Interventions

Indwelling urinary catheter to gravity × 24 hours; discontinue at 0800 on 8/24

Routine JP drain care

Strict I&O

Routine postoperative vital signs

NG tube to intermittent suction; 30 mL NSS flush q4h

Intravenous fluids: NSS at 50 mL/hr

Morphine sulfate 3 mg IV q4h prn for pain

continued

Developing Clinical Reasoning

- Considering Mr. Espinoza's immediate postoperative status, describe how you would transfer him from the stretcher to his bed.

- Prioritize, with rationales, your assessments and nursing care for Mr. Espinoza in the following areas:
  - Immediate assessments and interventions
  - Assessment and management of tubes
  - Pain management and comfort level
  - Care of his family

Suggested Responses for Integrated Nursing Care

- When transferring Mr. Espinoza to his bed, consider the following factors: minimizing his pain level, protecting his incision, and protecting the patency of his tubes. Excessive strain from moving can cause disruption and bleeding to his abdominal incision. Per facility policy, carefully transfer him, utilizing appropriate transfer devices and the assistance of others. Consult a safe patient handling algorithm to help you make decisions about safe patient handling and movement (see Chapter 9). During transfer, be careful not to disrupt his tubes or dressings. Once Mr. Espinoza is in his bed, place his urinary drainage bag on the bed frame so that it hangs below the level of his bladder. This position will allow the urine to drain by gravity and decrease the possibility of a urinary tract infection (see Chapter 12).

- Because Mr. Espinoza is a new postoperative patient, your first priority is to perform an assessment based on the airway, breathing, and circulation (ABC) criteria. Compare his vital signs on arrival with his baseline vital signs. Mr. Espinoza's respiratory rate has not changed significantly from his baseline. If not contraindicated, elevate his head to facilitate deep breathing and continue to assess his airway and respiratory status (see Chapter 6).

- Circulation is the next immediate priority. In Mr. Espinoza's case, his blood pressure has decreased and his heart rate has increased from his baseline in the PACU. Both of these changes could indicate decreased blood volume related to bleeding. Therefore, assess Mr. Espinoza's abdominal dressing to evaluate if it is dry and intact. Never assume that an incision is dry just because you cannot see any blood on top of the dressing. If the abdominal dressing is covered by foam tape, blood underneath the tape may not be easily visualized. Look under the patient to see if blood has trickled underneath the dressing. Mr. Espinoza said that he felt something "wet" under his back, and when turning him, you discover that there is a large puddle of bright-red blood underneath him that is caused by acute bleeding from his abdominal incision. Do not remove the abdominal dressing. You may, however, reinforce the dressing if you have an order.

- Identify all other possible sources of bleeding. When you assess the JP drains, note the color, amount, and consistency of blood. Assess his abdomen for signs of internal bleeding, such as abdominal distention. Also check for decreased urine output, another sign indicating a possible decrease in blood volume. A urine output of less than 30 mL/hr may be a sign of hypovolemic shock. Although Mr. Espinoza is bleeding and has signs of decreased blood volume, he is not yet in hypovolemic shock. If Mr. Espinoza's blood pressure continues to drop, elevate his feet to increase venous return. Report all indications of internal and/or external bleeding and other assessment findings to the health care provider. Acute postoperative bleeding may require surgical repair.

- Your next priority is to ensure that all of his tubes are intact and working properly. One of the first tubes you want to assess for patency is his IV, particularly because he may be returning to surgery. The next tubes you want to examine are the JP drains. To maintain suction, a JP drain must be less than half full. Assess the color and other characteristics of the JP drainage (see Chapter 8). Next, assess his NG tube. Mr. Espinoza's NG tube tape is not secure, so you cannot assume that the tube is still in his stomach. Check the NG for placement; assess the color, pH, and amount of the return; measure the length of the exposed tube and compare it with the length documented at the time of insertion; and then, once correct placement is verified, place the NG to intermittent suction (see Chapter 13). Next, evaluate his urinary catheter to determine if it is draining properly (see Chapter 12).

- The next priority is to monitor Mr. Espinoza's pain level. If he is in acute pain, immediately consider incisional disruption. Because Mr. Espinoza is bleeding, you may need to give small increments as opposed to large amounts of morphine to prevent a further drop in his blood pressure; consult with the health care provider in light of the assessment findings and changes from baseline. In addition to his physical comfort, attend to potential anxiety about returning to the operating room. Maintain a calm voice and demeanor when caring for Mr. Espinoza.

continued

- Notify the health care provider of all assessment findings.
- Do not forget Mr. Espinoza's family, who are anxious to see him. It is helpful to send another staff nurse to keep them updated while you are busy in his room.

When his condition stabilizes and before the family visits him, tell them about the tubes that they will see, including the reason for and function of each of the tubes. Be flexible when allowing the family to come in and visit Mr. Espinoza.

Case Study

George Patel, Gwen Galloway, Claudia Tran, and James White

This is your first week as an RN in a small rural hospital. You work the night shift on a medical-surgical unit. Tonight your only unlicensed assistive personnel (UAP) and a staff nurse have called in sick, which makes the unit short-staffed. You have notified the night supervisor that you need help, and she sends a USP from another floor to assist you. She tells you she can send another nurse in about an hour, and instructs you to take care of the priority cases until that time.

You have six relatively uncomplicated patients; caring for them involves checking their vital signs and giving medications. You instruct the aide to obtain vital signs for these patients and report the results back to you. A quick review of the medications reveals nothing that is urgent; you can wait and have the second nurse administer the medications when he or she arrives. You have four other patients with more complicated issues, who require additional assessments and urgent care:

- *George Patel, a 64-year-old patient with a tracheostomy, has gurgling sounds coming from his tracheostomy and a frequent, nonproductive cough. His oxygen saturation level via pulse oximetry is 88%. You have orders to suction his tracheostomy prn.*

- *Gwen Galloway had been receiving chemotherapy and has now come back to the hospital with gastroenteritis. When you arrive on your shift, she is experiencing bouts of nausea and vomiting.*

- *Claudia Tran, an 84-year-old patient from a skilled nursing unit, is post-CVA. She has a stage III pressure injury on her coccyx and a stage I pressure injury on her left hip. She needs to be turned every 30 minutes because of rapidly developing erythema on bony prominences. She is confused and has fallen the past two nights when left unattended, even with implementation of fall precautions. Her family is visiting her now but plans to leave in 30 minutes.*

- *James White has COPD. The UAP reports that the blood pressure from the automatic cuff is 168/100 mm Hg; his baseline is usually 130/70 mm Hg. The UAP also reports that he is complaining of a severe headache, but has no other complaints.*

continued

Developing Clinical Reasoning

- Identify the order in which you would provide care to these patients. Explain your rationales as well as your interventions.

Suggested Responses for Integrated Nursing Care

- Mr. Patel is having difficulty with airway clearance and oxygenation, so he will be your first priority. Nursing priorities follow the ABCs: airway, breathing, and circulation. He will require prompt tracheal suctioning and further evaluation of his respiratory status (see Chapter 14).

- Next, address the dramatic change in vital signs that Mr. White is experiencing. Mr. White is at risk for adverse effects and possible stroke if his blood pressure continues to stay elevated and is not controlled. Before planning any other interventions, verify the blood pressure by taking it yourself with a manual cuff (see Chapter 2). Initial nursing assessment includes assessing the accuracy of the equipment as well as the accuracy of the information reported to you by assistive personnel. The blood pressure you obtain is 190/110 mm Hg. Check for the health care provider's orders regarding possible prn blood pressure medication to administer. Call the health care provider right away and notify him or her of the change in Mr. White's status.

- You know that Ms. Tran is at high risk for falls if left unattended, and she may injure herself seriously if this occurs. Reducing her risk for injury is your next priority (see Chapter 4). In Ms. Tran's case, you could ask a family member to stay the night, or at least until you get more help on the unit. Many families are willing to help if you make them aware of such situations. If the family leaves, ask the UAP to make sure the bed is in a low position, and stay with Ms. Tran until you get further help. You can delegate Ms. Tran's positioning schedule to the aide.

- Despite the obvious distress of vomiting, this is not a life-threatening situation for Mrs. Galloway. Therefore, her condition is a lower priority than that of the other three patients. Mrs. Galloway requires comfort. Check

if an antiemetic medication has been ordered; if not, call the health care provider and obtain an order. Other interventions you can perform until her medication takes effect are lowering the lights, applying a cool cloth to the neck, decreasing noises, removing substances that may have a strong odor (e.g., food and vomitus), and keeping her head elevated.

- When prioritizing and delegating care, here are some questions that might help guide your decision-making process:
  - Is the situation life threatening?
  - How rapidly could this patient's condition deteriorate?
  - How quickly can you remedy the problem?
  - Who can provide assistance?

- Whenever a patient's airway, breathing, or circulation is jeopardized, this is a life-threatening emergency. Base your priorities on the ABC criteria. Mr. Patel is your first priority because his airway and oxygenation are a problem. When a patient's condition has the potential to deteriorate rapidly, this is also a priority. In Mr. White's case, because of the spike in his blood pressure, he has the potential for a stroke. Preventing this life-threatening event requires immediate action. When two patients have problems of similar urgency, such as oxygenation, respond to the problem that you can remedy the quickest. Sometimes when you have many activities to accomplish in a short period of time, it is difficult to take time to seek additional help. Many hospitals will have night supervisors to assist you with problem solving. Additionally, health care providers are available by phone or in the hospital. UAP are sometimes available to assist with noncritical tasks. A nursing skill to develop is prioritization of nursing care and delegation of appropriate tasks and care.

Case Study References

Centers for Disease Control and Prevention (CDC). (2007a; updated 2012). *Airborne infection isolation precautions. Excerpted from guideline for isolation precautions: Preventing transmission of infectious agents in healthcare settings.* Retrieved https://www.cdc.gov/infectioncontrol/guidelines/isolation/index.html

Centers for Disease Control and Prevention (CDC). (2007b; updated 2012). *Standard precautions. Excerpted from guideline for isolation precautions: Preventing transmission of infectious agents in healthcare settings.* Retrieved https://www.cdc.gov/infectioncontrol/guidelines/isolation/index.html

Centers for Disease Control and Prevention (CDC). (2014a). *Sequence for putting on personal protective*

equipment (PPE). [Poster]. Retrieved http://www.cdc.gov/hai/pdfs/ppe/PPE-Sequence.pdf

Centers for Disease Control and Prevention (CDC). (2014b). *Guidance for the selection and use of personal protective equipment (PPE) in healthcare settings.* Retrieved http://www.cdc.gov/HAI/pdfs/ppe/PPEslides6-29-04.pdf

Centers for Disease Control and Prevention (CDC). (2016). *Methicillin-resistant Staphylococcus aureus (MRSA).* Retrieved https://www.cdc.gov/mrsa/index.html

U.S. Department of Health and Human Services, Centers for Disease Control and Prevention, National Center for Health Statistics. (2015, May). *Deaths from unintentional injury among adults aged 65 and over:*

United States, 2000–2013. NCHS Data Brief. No. 199. Retrieved https://www.cdc.gov/nchs/data/databriefs/db199.pdf

Institute for Safe Medication Practices (ISMP). (n.d.). *ISMP and FDA campaign to eliminate use of error-prone abbreviations.* Retrieved www.ismp.org/tools/abbreviations

The Joint Commission. (2017). *National patient safety goals.* Retrieved https://www.jointcommission.org/hap_2017_npsgs

Taylor, C., Lynn, P., & Bartlett, J. (2019). *Fundamentals of nursing: The art and science of person-centered care* (9th ed.). Philadelphia, PA: Wolters Kluwer.

GUIDELINES FOR DELEGATION DECISION MAKING

INTRODUCTION

Delegation involves the transfer of responsibility for the performance of an activity to another person while retaining accountability for the outcome. Used appropriately, delegation can result in safe and effective nursing care. Delegation can free the registered nurse (RN) to focus on assessment and development or revision of the nursing care plan (Trossman, 2012). Delegation allows the RN to attend to more complex patient care needs, develops the skills of nursing assistive personnel, and promotes cost containment for the health care organization. The RN determines appropriate nursing practice by using nursing knowledge, professional judgment, and the legal authority to practice nursing (American Nurses Association [ANA], 2007).

In delegating, the RN must ensure appropriate assessment, planning, implementation, and evaluation. Decision making about delegation is a continuous process. These guidelines provide a quick reference for the delegation decision-making information found in each skill.

DELEGATION CRITERIA

Three criteria to be considered by the RN when deciding to delegate care activities (National Council of State Boards of Nursing [NCSBN], 2005) are:

1. The State Nursing Practice Act must permit delegation and outline the authorized task(s) to be delegated or authorize the RN to decide delegation.
2. The person delegating has the appropriate qualifications: appropriate education, skills and experience, as well as current competency.
3. The person receiving the delegation must have the appropriate qualifications: appropriate education, training, skills and experience, as well as evidence of current competency.

In addition, according to the ANA and NCSBN (2006), the delegated task(s) must not require critical thinking or professional judgment.

DELEGATION PROCESS

Delegation is a multi-step, continuous process.

1. The RN must be fully aware of the parameters for delegation as outlined in their state's Nurse Practice Act as well as the employing organization's policies and procedures regarding delegation (Daley, 2013).
2. The RN must assess the situation, identifying the needs of the patient, considering the circumstances and setting, as well as the competence of the person to whom the task is being delegated. The RN may proceed with delegation if patient needs, circumstances, and available resources indicate patient safety will be maintained with delegated care.
3. The RN plans for and communicates clearly the specific task(s) to be delegated. The RN may proceed with delegation if the nature of the task, competence of the person receiving the delegation, and patient implications indicate patient safety will be maintained with delegated care.
4. The RN assures appropriate accountability. The RN may proceed with delegation if the RN and person receiving the delegation accept the accountability for their respective roles in the delegated patient care.
5. The RN supervises performance of the delegated task(s), providing directions and clear expectations of how the task(s) is to be performed. The RN monitors performance, intervenes if necessary, and ensures the appropriate documentation.
6. The RN must evaluate the entire delegation process, evaluating the patient, the performance of the task(s), and obtain and provide feedback.
7. The RN must reassess and adjust the overall plan of care, as needed.

FIVE RIGHTS OF DELEGATION

The Five Rights of Delegation provide a resource to facilitate decisions about delegation. The NCSBN (2016) identifies the Five Rights of Delegation as follows:

- **Right Task:** One that is delegable for a specific patient.
- **Right Circumstances:** Appropriate patient setting, available resources, and other relevant factors considered.
- **Right Person:** Right person is delegating the right task to the right person to be performed on the right person.
- **Right Direction/Communication:** Clear, concise description of the task, including its objective, limits, and expectations.
- **Right Supervision/Evaluation:** Appropriate monitoring, evaluation, intervention, as needed, and feedback.

"DO-NOT-DELEGATE" CARE

Nursing care or tasks that should never be delegated except to another RN include:

- Initial and ongoing nursing assessment of the patient and his or her nursing care needs

- Determination of the nursing diagnosis, nursing care plan, evaluation of the patient's progress in relation to the care plan, and evaluation of the nursing care delivered to the patient
- Supervision and education of nursing personnel; patient teaching that requires an assessment of the patient and his or her education needs
- Any other nursing interventions that requires professional nursing knowledge, judgment, and/or skill

DELEGATION DECISION TREE

Using skills, knowledge, and professional judgment, the RN determines appropriate nursing practice based on the state practice act and professional scope of practice, the standards and code of ethics, and the organization's policies and procedures related to delegation (ANA & NCSBN, 2006).

The Decision Tree for Delegation by Registered Nurses distributed by the American Nurses Association and the National Council of State Boards of Nursing can assist nurses with delegation decisions. The Decision Tree for Delegation can be found at https://www.ncsbn.org/Delegation_joint_statement_NCSBN-ANA.pdf.

Taylor Suite Resources

Explore these additional resources for more information on delegation:

- Online resource, http://thepoint.lww.com/Lynn5E
- *Fundamentals of Nursing*: Chapter 17, *Implementing*; Chapter 10, *Nurse Leader, Manager, and Care Coordinator*

References and Resources

American Nurses Association (ANA). (2007). Registered nurses utilization of nursing assistive personnel in all settings. Position statement. Retrieved https://www.nursingworld.org/practice-policy/nursing-excellence/official-position-statements/id/RN-utilization-of-nursing-assistive-personnel-in-all-settings

American Nurses Association (ANA). (2012). *Principles for delegation by registered nurses to unlicensed assistive personnel*. Silver Spring, MD: Author.

American Nurses Association (ANA) and National Council of State Boards of Nursing (NCSBN). (2006). *Joint statement on delegation*. Retrieved https://www.ncsbn.org/Delegation_joint_statement_NCSBN-ANA.pdf

Daley, K. (2013). Helping nurses strengthen their delegation skills. *American Nurse Today, 8*(3), 18.

National Council of State Boards of Nursing (NCSBN). (n.d.). *Delegation*. Retrieved https://www.ncsbn.org/1625.htm

National Council of State Boards of Nursing (NCSBN). (2005). *Working with others: A position paper*. Retrieved https://www.ncsbn.org/Working_with_Others.pdf

National Council of State Boards of Nursing (NCSBN). (2016). National guidelines for nursing delegation. *Journal of Nursing Regulation, 7*(1), 5–12.

Trossman, S. (2012). Is it OK to delegate?: Revised principles, resources aim to help RNs answer the question. *The American Nurse, 44*(6), 1, 6.

Note: Page number followed by b, f, and t indicates text in box, figure, and table respectively.